Burger's Medicinal
Chemistry and Drug Discovery

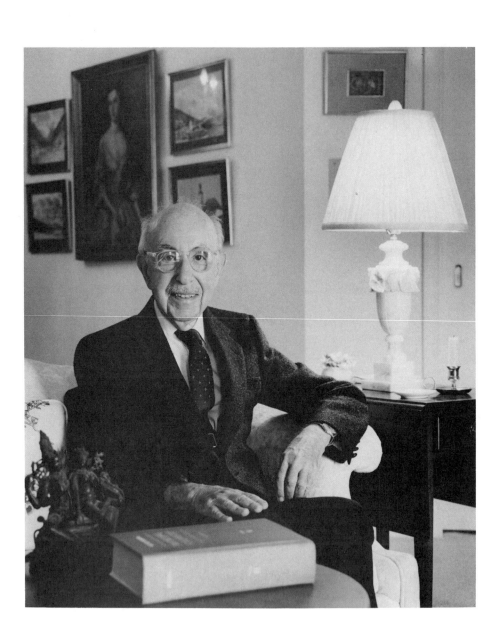

BURGER'S MEDICINAL CHEMISTRY AND DRUG DISCOVERY

Fifth Edition
Volume I: Principles and Practice

Edited by

Manfred E. Wolff

ImmunoPharmaceutics, Inc.
San Diego, California

A WILEY-INTERSCIENCE PUBLICATION

JOHN WILEY & SONS, Inc., New York · Chichester · Brisbane · Toronto · Singapore

Notice Concerning Trademark or Patent Rights.
The listing or discussion in this book of any drug in
respect to which patent or trademark rights may exist
shall not be deemed, and is not intended as
a grant of, or authority to exercise, or an
infringement of, any right or privilege protected by
such patent or trademark.

This text is printed on acid-free paper.

Copyright © 1995 by John Wiley & Sons, Inc.

All rights reserved. Published simultaneously in Canada.

Reproduction or translation of any part of this work beyond
that permitted by Section 107 or 108 of the 1976 United
States Copyright Act without the permission of the copyright
owner is unlawful. Requests for permission or further
information should be addressed to the Permissions Department,
John Wiley & Sons, 605 Third Avenue, New York, NY
10158-0012.

Library of Congress Cataloging in Publication Data:
Burger, Alfred, 1905–
    [Medicinal chemistry]
    Burger's medicinal chemistry and drug discovery. -- 5th ed. /
edited by Manfred E. Wolff.
        p.   cm.
    "A Wiley-Interscience publication."
    Contents: v. 1. Principles and practice
    Includes bibliographical references and index.
    ISBN 0-471-57556-9
    1. Pharmaceutical chemistry.   I. Wolff, Manfred E.   II. Title.
    III. Title: Medicinal chemistry and drug discovery.
    RS403.B8   1994
    615'. 19--dc20   94-12687

Printed in the United States of America

10 9 8 7 6 5 4 3 2

Preface

Did we know the mechanical affectations of the particles of rhubarb, opium, and a man, as a watchmaker does those of a watch, whereby it performs its operations, and of a file which by rubbing on them will alter the figure of any of the wheels; we should be able to tell beforehand that rhubarb will purge, hemlock kill and opium make a man sleep.

John Locke, Essay on the Human Understanding, 1690

Drug discovery has its roots in the beginnings of mankind. Even our phylogenetic cousins, the chimpanzees, have been observed to chew certain leaves to alleviate gastrointestinal distress. Likewise, in the evolution of the early hunter–gatherer communities it was only a short step from gathering vegetation to be eaten to assuage the pangs of hunger, to gathering material to be ingested to diminish the pain and discomfort of illness or injury. Thus, drug discovery has been important in every society, whether in the primitive tribes of North America or Africa, in the advanced classical Egyptian, Greek, and Roman civilizations, or in the more recent cultures of Europe, Asia, India, and elsewhere.

Today we are in the midst of an explosive expansion in the organized, purposeful discovery of drugs—an expansion that has occurred in the fifteen years that have elapsed since the previous edition of this series. Three forces are responsible for this growth. The first is the dawn of the golden age of biology, the stunning progress that has been made in structural biology and molecular biology, and its impact on the drug discovery process. The second is the information processing and transfer revolution that has made it possible to utilize all of the older and contemporary knowledge effectively in our new information society. And the third is the dramatic increase in the size of the world pharmaceutical market.

Science has never been confined by geographic boundaries. But in the past fifteen years, globalization, not only of technology itself, but of an appetite for the fruits of technology, has proceeded at an ever faster rate—the revolution of rising expectations. Nowhere is this more evident than in the desire of individuals everywhere to have the benefit of the best drugs available anywhere. The result has been to triple the world pharmaceutical market in ten years to $145 billion in 1989, compared to about $50 billion in 1979. Only six countries, the United States, Japan, Germany, Italy, France and the United Kingdom, are responsible for $113 billion (78%) of this sum. These countries represent only a fraction of the world population, and it is obvious that even greater growth is probable. In the past, a substantial part of such increases has resulted from simple price elevation. But the drive for cost containment in healthcare will ensure that most future growth will come from innovative new products and from market expansion.

The widening of the world pharmaceutical market has resulted in two collateral expansions. The first is in drug discovery research and development, both in absolute magnitude as well as in proportion to

v

product sales. For example, global R&D spending of PMA member companies as a percentage of sales changed from about 9% in 1980 to more than 15% in 1990. In addition, the absolute magnitude of U.S. R&D spending by PMA companies rose from about $2 billion in 1980 to about $7 billion in 1989. These increases have resulted in a dramatic expansion in the growth rate of pharmaceutical R&D spending in the U.S., as well as in the EC and Japan. Adjusted for inflation, the real growth in U.S. pharmaceutical R&D spending during 1975–1980 was only 3.5% per year. By contrast, during 1980–1990, the period since the publication of the preceding edition of this series, it was nearly 11% per year.

A second collateral expansion driven by the rapidly widening world pharmaceutical market has been in the number of pharmaceutical companies in operation, and being newly formed. It is a remarkable fact that there are hundreds of these, principally in the U.S., but also in the EC and elsewhere.

That these companies are attractive to the sources of financial capital necessary for their existence and operation is due to their potential for new drug discovery, and to the expectation of substantial profits from the sale of these new drugs. For this reason, such companies collectively employ thousands of scientists in the drug discovery area—scientists in laboratories and research programs that did not exist only a few years ago.

Not only has the scope and magnitude of drug discovery efforts expanded greatly, but the complexity, management challenges, and human resource requirements of the task have been correspondingly magnified. The new technologies, molecular biology, computational chemistry, the new analytical methods, and others, have combined to produce a more intellectually satisfying and effective, albeit more complex process. At the same time, increasingly stringent regulatory requirements with respect to novelty, efficacy and safety have made the development phase following drug discovery a more difficult undertaking. It is important that these later hurdles be fully appreciated by those workers active in the earlier aspects of drug discovery.

During the past decade, these drastically changed circumstances surrounding drug discovery created a much enlarged group of individuals involved in the search for new drugs. That group comprises not only academic and industrial scientists in the disciplines of biology, biotechnology, chemistry, physics, pharmaceutics and mathematics, but also clinicians, regulatory experts, financial analysts, lawyers, managers, and of course students and postdoctorals in all of these areas.

For success in the search for new drugs, full and complete communication is necessary between these many different individuals and disciplines. Drug discovery is above all an interdisciplinary effort—a team effort. As such, a contract lawyer may need to be aware of issues involved in the receptor specificity of ligands. A chemist may need to be conversant with aspects of patent law. A financial analyst may need to understand the potential of 3D database searches. A senior manager may need to appreciate the timing requirements of clinical trials. In this volume we attempt to inform such individuals in all of these areas.

Because numerous new factors must be considered in drug discovery, and a variety of individuals with widely divergent backgrounds now take part in it, the prophetic words of John Locke, which appeared in past editions and are given again at the beginning of this preface, address only a part of the task. Indeed, there are cases now where an x-ray crystallographic image of an enzyme inhibitor complex satisfies Locke's requirement for knowledge of the "mechanical affectations" of the drug and the patient. But we know now that this is not enough—that we must also have knowl-

One Hundred Newer Pharmaceutical Companies

Advanced Tissue Sciences	Creative Biomolecules	Magainin
Affinity Biotechnology	Curative Technologies	Matrix
Affymax	Cytel Corp.	Medarex
Agouron	Cytogen	MedImmune
Alkermes	Cyto Therapeutics	NeoRx
Alpha-Beta	DNX Corporation	Oculon
Alteon	Emisphere	Oncogene Science
Amgen	Enzon	Ogranogenesis
Amylin	Genelabs Technologies	Osteotech
Anergen	Genentech	PerSeptive Biosystems
Applied Immune Sciences	Genetic Therapy	Procyte
Arris	Genetics Institute	Protein Design Labs
Athena Neurosciences	Gensia	Regeneron
Autoimmune	Genta	Repligen
Biocryst	Genzyme	Ribi ImmunoChem
Biogen	Gilead Sciences	Scios Nova
Biomatrix	Glycomed	Sergen
Biomira	ICOS	Shaman Pharmaceuticals
BioSurface	IDEC	Somatogen
Bio-Technology General	IGI, Inc.	Sphinx
British Bio-Technology	ImClone	Synergen
Cambridge Biotechnology	ImmuLogic	SyStemix
Cambridge Neurosciences	Immune Response	T Cell Sciences
Cellcor	Immunex	Telios
Cell Genesys	ImmunoGen	Texas Biotechnology
CellPro	Immunomedics	TSI Corp.
Celtrix	ImmunoPharmaceutics	Univax Biologics
Centocor	Isis Pharmaceuticals	US Bioscience
Cephalon	LifeCell	Vertex
Chiron	Ligand	Vestar
CoCensys	Liposome Company	Xenova
COR Therapeutics	Liposome Technology	Xoma
Cortech		Zynaxis
Corvas		

edge of drug metabolism, toxicity, a means to demonstrate decisive clinical efficacy, and a host of other matters, in order to be able to discover new drugs. An attempt has been made to provide an overview of all of these areas in this volume, entitled "Principles and Practices".

In preparing this new edition of these volumes founded through the vision of Alfred Burger, an effort has been made to incorporate the new developments into the discussion in every place where it has been possible. In this first volume, particular attention has been paid to product development questions which should be considered early in the discovery phase. We begin with a consideration of the conceptual background of medicinal chemistry by Alfred Burger, and continue with the management of drug discovery and the accessing and protection of information and intellectual property. In the second section, product development issues that are important to the discovery process are reviewed—questions of ADME, toxicity and drug allergy, and clinical trial issues. In part III, the extensive advances that have been made in the structural biology of drug action are considered. And in the final section, the technologies for drug discovery, largely developed in the years since the preceding edition, are examined.

As indicated above, we hope that this volume will prove useful to all practitioners of drug discovery as well as graduate students and postdoctorals with these interests. We hope also that it will inform those interested in other types of biological actions of chemicals and biotechnology products, such as the environmental toxicity of herbicides and pesticides, or the effects of food additives. And, finally, we hope that it will serve as a suitable introduction and companion volume for the specialized chapters in the other volumes of this series.

I wish to express my sincere gratitude to the many persons who have made this new edition possible. Most of all, I thank the dedicated, knowledgeable authors, who have given so generously of their time in order to pass their expertise on to others, and many of whom have shared with me the benefit of their own views on the general topic of drug discovery. They and others have helped me enormously in defining the scope of this first volume, but ultimately the responsiblity for any deficiencies in this regard is mine alone. I am grateful to the editorial staff of John Wiley & Sons for their longstanding interest in this series. I wish especially to express my sincere appreciation to Lisa Trout, who organized and kept track of the voluminous correspondence resulting from so many interactions, and who tactfully managed finally to get all the manuscripts out of the hands of the authors. And finally I thank my wife, Gloria, for her enduring support and sustenance for all of my efforts.

MANFRED E. WOLFF

San Diego, California
January, 1995

Contents

Part I   The Drug Discovery Process, 1

1. THE CONCEPTUAL BACK-
   GROUND AND DEVELOPMENT
   OF MEDICINAL CHEMISTRY, 3

   Alfred Burger
   Charlottesville, Virginia, USA

2. THE MANAGEMENT OF DRUG
   DISCOVERY, 9

   Ralph E. Christofferson and J. Joseph
   Marr
   Ribozyme Pharmaceuticals, Inc.
   Boulder, Colorado, USA

3. INTELLECTUAL PROPERTY IN
   DRUG DISCOVERY AND BIO-
   TECHNOLOGY, 37

   Richard A. Kaba, David A. Crossman
   and Julius Tabin
   Fitch, Even, Tabin Flannery
   Chicago, Illinois, USA

4. INFORMATION SCIENCE IN
   DRUG DISCOVERY, 103

   Y. Lin Chang and Linda M. Klug
   Marion Merrell Dow, Inc.
   Kansas City, Missouri, USA

Part II   Product Development Issues, 111

5. DRUG ABSORPTION, DISTRI-
   BUTION AND ELIMINATION, 113

   Leslie Z. Benet and Beatrice Y. T.
   Perotti
   Department of Pharmacy
   University of California
   San Francisco, California, USA

6. DRUG METABOLISM, 129

   Bernard Testa
   Institut de Chimie Thérapeutique
   Ecole de Pharmacie
   Université de Lausanne
   Lausanne, Switzerland

7. DRUG ALLERGY, 181

   Charles W. Parker
   Department of Medicine
   Washington University School of
   Medicine
   St. Louis, Missouri, USA

8. THE APPLICATION OF STRUC-
   TURAL CONCEPTS TO THE
   PREDICTION OF THE CAR-
   CINOGENICITY OF THERA-
   PEUTIC AGENTS, 223

   Herbert S. Rosenkrantz
   Department of Environmental and
   Occupational Health

Graduate School of Public Health
University of Pittsburgh
Pittsburgh, Pennsylvania, USA

Gilles Klopman
Department of Chemistry
Case Western Reserve University
Cleveland, Ohio, USA

9. FROM DISCOVERY TO MARKET:
   THE DEVELOPMENT OF
   PHARMACEUTICALS, 251

Jan I. Drayer and James P. Burns
G.H. Besselaar Associates
Princeton, New Jersey, USA

Part III   Structural Medicinal Chemistry, 301

10. THREE DIMENSIONAL
    STRUCTURE-AIDED DRUG
    DESIGN, 303

B. Veerapandian
La Jolla Cancer Research
Foundation
La Jolla, California, USA

11. DRUG RECEPTORS, 349

Michael Williams, Darlene C. Deecher
and James P. Sullivan
Pharmaceutical Products Division
Abbott Laboratories
Abbott Park, Illinois, USA

12. DRUG-TARGET BINDING
    FORCES, 399

Peter A. Kollman
Department of Pharmaceutical
Chemistry
School of Pharmacy
University of California
San Francisco, California, USA

Part IV   Drug Discovery Technologies, 413

13. CHEMICAL INFORMATION
    COMPUTING SYSTEMS IN DRUG
    DISCOVERY, 415

Stephen W. Dietrich
Molecular Computing Systems, Inc.
Bothell, Washington, USA

14. THE QUANTITATIVE ANALYSIS
    OF STRUCTURE-ACTIVITY
    RELATIONSHIPS, 497

Dr. Hugo Kubinyi
Wirkstoffdesign
BASF Aktiengesellschaft
Ludwigshafen, Germany

15. MOLECULAR MODELING IN
    DRUG DESIGN, 573

Garland R. Marshall
Center for Molecular Design
Washington University
St. Louis, Missouri, USA

16. APPLICATION OF RECOMBI-
    NANT DNA TECHNOLOGY IN
    MEDICINAL CHEMISTRY AND
    DRUG DISCOVERY, 661

Michael C. Venuti
Parnassus Pharmaceuticals, Inc.
Alameda, California, USA

17. MASS LIGAND SCREENING AS A TOOL FOR DRUG AND DEVELOPMENT DISCOVERY, 697

Paul M. Sweetnam
Pfizer Central Research
Groton, Connecticut, USA

Christopher H. Price
Medical Innovation Partners
Minneapolis, Minnesota, USA

John W. Ferkany
Nova Screen and Oceanix Biosciences Corp.
Baltimore, Maryland, USA

18. APPROACHES TO THE RATIONAL DESIGN OF ENZYME INHIBITORS, 733

Angelika Muscate and George L. Kenyon
School of Pharmacy
University of California
San Francisco, California, USA

19. ANALOG DESIGN, 783

Joseph G. Cannon
College of Pharmacy
University of Iowa
Iowa City, Iowa, USA

20. PEPTIDOMIMETICS FOR DRUG DESIGN, 803

Murray Goodman
Department of Chemistry
University of California, San Diego
San Diego, California, USA

Seonggu Ro
Research and Development Park of LUCKY Ltd.
Biotechnology Science Town
Daejon, Korea

21. OLIGONUCLEOTIDE THERAPEUTICS, 863

Stanley T. Crooke
Isis Pharmaceuticals
Carlsbad, California, USA

22. CARBOHYDRATE-BASED THERAPEUTICS, 901

John H. Musser, Péter Fügedi and Mark Brian Anderson
Glycomed Inc.
Alameda, California, USA

23. METABOLIC CONSIDERATIONS IN PRODRUG DESIGN, 949

L. P. Balant and E. Doelker
Institutions Universitaires de Psychiatrie de Genève
Unité de Recherche Clinique
Genève, Switzerland

24. NATURAL PRODUCTS AS LEADS FOR NEW PHARMACEUTICALS, 983

Dr. A. D. Buss
Department of Natural Products Discovery
Glaxo Research and Development Ltd.
Middlesex, England

R. D. Waigh
Department of Pharmaceutical Sciences
Royal College
University of Strathclyde
Glasgow, Scotland

INDEX, 1035

Burger's Medicinal
Chemistry and Drug Discovery

PART I
THE DRUG DISCOVERY PROCESS

CHAPTER ONE

The Conceptual Background and Development of Medicinal Chemistry

ALFRED BURGER

CONTENTS

1 Introduction, 3
2 Natural Products, 3
3 Molecular Modification, 4
4 "Lead" Compounds, 5
5 Receptors, 6

1 INTRODUCTION

Medicinal chemistry had its beginning when chemists, pharmacists, and physicians isolated and purified active principles of plant and animal tissues and later from microorganisms and their fermentation products. Some of these chemicals had been associated with therapeutic properties in often ill-defined disease conditions. During the latter decades of the 20th century, the traditional dividing lines between biological, chemical, and physical sciences were erased, and new borderline investigations such as molecular biology, molecular pharmacology, biomedicine, and others began to capture the interest of medicinal scientists. Medicinal chemistry which had leaned on the classical fields of chemistry, especially organic chemistry, biology and some areas of physics extended new roots into these emerging topics. Problems in hitherto unapproachable chemical studies with therapeutic implications became accessible and revised the choice of researches to the benefit of all the scientific doctrines involved.

2 NATURAL PRODUCTS

The elucidation of the structure and function of natural products, especially those with a history of biological properties, has been an important incentive for organic

Burger's Medicinal Chemistry and Drug Discovery,
Fifth Edition, Volume 1: Principles and Practice,
Edited by Manfred E. Wolff.
ISBN 0-471-57556-9 © 1995 John Wiley & Sons, Inc.

chemistry. Learning how Nature handles the synthesis and degradation of such substances is a deeply fulfilling and exciting goal of organic and medicinal chemists and of biochemists. One can never stop marvelling at the ingenuity of Nature which creates unexpected and often amazingly novel structures by biosynthetic and degradative reactions. The apparent purpose of these metabolic chemical reactions is to rid the parent organism of unwanted or toxic substances. In some cases, toxic metabolites may be useful in protecting the organism against predators or environmental hazards. There is no support for the belief that natural metabolites of plants and animals are produced for therapeutic uses by humans, even though humans have learned to harvest and process some of them for the maintenance of their homeostasis.

Over the last 200 years, natural products have been screened by experimental biologists who devised increasingly meaningful animal models of clinical pathologies. More recently, *in vitro* inhibition data of enzyme systems have simplified some of these tests and deepened our understanding of the mode of action of drugs.

A limited number of natural products can serve directly as therapeutic agents although lack of specificity frequently limits their application in human and veterinary medicine and in analogous pesticidal and other uses in agriculture. However, their never-ending variety and novelty serves as a source of prototype compounds for molecular modification. By dissecting the structure of a natural product chemically, one arrives at its therapeutically significant molecular sections, the pharmacophores. The portions that can be deleted are of no interest as components of drug action; they are regarded as the result of the biosynthetic efforts of the parent organism to construct materials for its own metabolic or defensive purposes.

Some structurally relatively uncomplicated biocatalysts such as several hormones and vitamins were originally regarded as uniquely designed for their biological mission and chemists were reluctant to interfere. It is now hard to imagine what impact their first molecular modifications had on contemporary thinking (1–5).

3 MOLECULAR MODIFICATION

When synthetic organic chemicals overtook the number of natural products, synthetic compounds offered an opportunity to medicinal screening. Some kind of selection of candidate compounds had to be made because dipping blindly into the supply of millions of synthetic compounds would have put the lottery to shame. Therefore, synthetic derivatives and structural analogues of biologically interesting substances were tested first for activities associated with the "lead" compound. Such programs included the branching, lengthening or shortening of chain structures, the variation of the kinds and positions of substituents, the replacement of rings by similar cyclic structures, and other empirical molecular modifications within the framework of reasonably close analogy. Functional groups were replaced by similar reactive radicals and occasionally an unorthodox change was tried. Many of the alterations were dictated by synthetic accessibility in a given structural series, without regard to biochemical reasoning.

As could be expected, close structural analogues of a biologically active material had a better chance of being similarly active than more remote analogues. The batting average among random variations was and still is low, ranging from 1:5,000 to even 1:10,000 for elaborating a drug that can survive screening and preclinical evaluation. Such systematic molecular modifications are not profitable; nevertheless, they remain the principal approach to new drug structures. It is a monument to human patience that so many valuable drugs have been developed by this method.

We can now think of Paul Ehrlich's syntheses of organic arsenical chemotherapeutics as a transition to planned molecular modification. Inorganic arsenicals had proved toxic to several pathogens, and it was hoped that organic derivatives of arsenic would be more acceptable pharmacologically to the infected host. These experiments may be regarded as the first work in modern medicinal chemistry (6,7).

Early experiments to rationalize general thinking in drug design occurred in the 1930s with the application of isosteric replacements in biologically active "lead" compounds (8,9). This method requires correlations of chemical and physical properties. Among these is hydrophobicity, determined from the partition of a compound between aqueous and lipid environments. Hydrophobicity is a measure of a substance's ability to cross the essentially lipid membranes of cells. In practice it is modeled by the distribution of a compound between water and a solvent of low water solubility such as 1-octanol (10). The solution of problems of structure–activity relationships in drug design is contingent on factoring in as many properties as feasible. The general use of computers facilitates these calculations.

The increasingly routine determination of spectra of ligating conditions, molecular weights, and other properties by instrumental means has deepened our understanding of many research results including those in medicinal chemistry. Accuracy of analytical data and interpretation of atomic and molecular properties of a compound as well as the ability to picture steric changes in flexible structures have become a prerequisite for the progress of the field.

4 "LEAD" COMPOUNDS

The most vexing problem of medicinal chemistry is the discovery of prototype ("lead") compounds for a given biochemical or biological activity. With natural products, we have become accustomed to take potluck as such substances become available. Exploratory searches of exotic poisonous plants, of marine flora and fauna in tropical waters, and of random soil samples, fungi, microbes, and other sources of potential antibiotics are still conducted based on hope, and on hearsay of useful biological significance. The various products isolated from living organisms can then serve as "leads" for improvement of their therapeutic potential by molecular modification. Hundreds of alkaloids, nucleosides, and animal and plant hormones have served as metabolite prototypes for analogues with modified activity. The same procedure can serve to choose synthetic chemicals as "leads" but here one does not enjoy the luxury of biological or medicinal folklore that sometimes narrows the choice of biologically attractive natural products. This is balanced by the increasing demand of toxicity determinations for industrial chemicals which provides some insight into their biological behavior.

Some organic chemists who had not been steeped in the biological sciences confessed openly that they chose candidate test compounds solely on the basis of their interest in a given reaction, synthetic sequence, or structural series. As one may expect, the success rate of such programs was low but there were notable exceptions. The most surprising example may have been the benzodiazepine CNS depressants (11); their biological activities became known before the structure of their ring system had been elucidated. Persistent synthetic studies then added an increasing number of derivatives perceived on purely chemical grounds, which responded positively to some biological screening procedure.

The emergence of medicinal chemistry as a combination of chemical and biological sciences no longer permits such approaches to therapeutic planning. Biological considerations are now universally involved in drug design. Efforts to combine chemical and biological factors are seen in the pro-drug concept which unmasks functional groups of an inactive compound to yield an active drug by metabolic transformation within the host, e.g. by enzymatic hydrolysis, oxidation, or reduction (12).

Biotransformation of drugs and other xenobiotics usually leads to more polar metabolites that favor excretion, thereby ridding the organism of the foreign agent (13). In quite a few instances, however, biologically active metabolites more toxic than the administered drug are formed, increasing side effects or presenting new activities that may be unrelated to the originally observed and even planned action of the drug under study (14–16). Such active metabolites also often have a longer biological half life and are more difficult to detoxify.

5 RECEPTORS

Drug receptors had been conceived one hundred years ago and had been interpreted rather naively as bifunctional chemicals ready to ligate a suitable therapeutic agent (17). These ideas remained almost unchanged for seventy years. Their vagueness led to the claim that drugs might be at best "magic bullets" that hit a biological target whose very outlines remained unknown. The reason for this ignorance was the slow recognition that drug receptors must have macromolecular structures and that chemistry was not ready to define details of such macromolecules. Nor was it possible to study such receptors because their minute amounts did not permit an accumulation of sufficient material for a multifaceted investigation. This situation changed only when cloning of proteins became possible.

The complete chemical structures of an increasing number of enzymes has become known through a combination of X-ray diffraction and NMR measurements. Not only has the amino acid composition been sequenced but in many cases the secondary and tertiary peptide structure has been determined. This permits a description of the active site(s) of these enzymes and the participation of side chains of non-neighboring amino acids in the steric structures of those sites. The same type of information is now accumulating for transmembrane receptors and other receptor types. In the case of a few enzymes that contain coenzyme molecules (riboflavin in monoamine oxidases) or essential metal ions, the covalent ligating of small-molecular inhibitors is now understood. Ligating through hydrogen bonding can also be determined. Thus, the mechanism of action of several known drugs has become a detailed matter of record.

The active sites of polypeptide enzymes and protein receptors are not the only drug receptors. Nucleic acids also recognize drug molecules and ligate them by intercalation between helical turns.

For several decades it was assumed that a drug is carried by the circulating fluids to its receptor where it is recognized as a complementary molecule that could fit sterically to the active site of the receptor, bind to it, and initiate a reaction. The binding of a drug to a preexisting receptor is but the first step in the expression of biological activity. It sets into motion a cascade of biochemical events which culminate in an observable biological or therapeutic effect. This means that the medicinal chemist must consider the design of agents that will interfere with *any* of the enzymes participating in the pertinent sequence of biochemical reactions.

Virtually all drugs have multiple effects. In 1948, a study of adrenergic agents led to the conclusion that more than one receptor may be involved in the action of a drug

(18). In this case, inotropic action was attributed to a receptor subtype designated α, while the increase in heart rate was thought to be due to action on β receptors. As pharmacological observations were refined, both of these receptor subtypes had to be subdivided further, and α_1, α_2 etc., receptors were postulated. Similar classification of receptors for other drugs with multiple activities followed soon.

Enzymes which can be solubilized can be purified more readily than receptor proteins. The active sites of many enzymes are now well defined. In some cases they are cavities or clefts whose shape and size can be measured accurately (19). But inhibitors of such enzymes which fit into these cavities are still being discovered by conventional empirical methods. Why can they not yet be designed to fit the active sites? The answer seems to lie in our yet incomplete knowledge of ligating conditions, and more likely of the steric adaptations that both the "walls" of active sites and the drug or substrate molecules can undergo. These steric changes will determine which covalent, ionic and hydrogen-bridged linkages between the peptide chains surrounding the active sites and the ligands can be established. Thus, an important research problem for drug designers will be studies of these steric approaches. Isosteric comparisons carefully coupled with estimates of conformational adaptations especially of proposed enzyme inhibitors should lead us slowly to the design of as yet unknown drugs based on the increasing understanding of active sites of enzymes and inhibitors. This method now appears as a possibility on the horizon.

A number of computer-aided techniques for predicting pharmacophoric features of ligands at active sites have been described. Hydrogen bonding, negatively charged groups, and hydrophobic areas have been integrated into computer programs for this purpose. Three-dimensional software programs hold out hope of improving the design of flexible active-site ligands. Other programs concentrate on inspecting one molecular component placed there by damaged genes and correcting it by "vaccination" with the proper complete genes. Thus, tumor necrosis factor has been introduced into the genes of certain cancer patients, and interleukin-2 has been increased in cells modified with genes for this protein (17).

These advances in gene and tissue therapy, including human gene therapy (18,19), and the increased emphasis on discovering "lead" compounds based on three-dimensional relationships to the structures of active sites of enzymes and other receptors have raised some doubts (20) whether medicinal chemistry, as we have known it for a century, will survive the emerging biotechnology-oriented approach to new drugs. In addition, techniques such as chemically generated molecular diversity (21) and new synthetic routing to chiral drugs (22) have been recommended for the development of new therapeutic agents, and have suggested that classical drug discovery should be relegated to a less prominent place.

However, systematic screening of chemical libraries and other collections of thousands of compounds, aided by computer-assisted selection of related structures (23), is still one of the acknowledged ways of medicinal chemistry, especially if the biochemical cause of a disease has not yet been pinpointed. Medicinal research scientists will therefore have to acquire experience both in classical and the most innovative methodologies of drug discovery. This will mean a reorientation of their education, and dedication to learning every novel technique and line of thought, and an adaptation to emphasize such changes in their work. The future medicinal chemist will be more biochemically oriented than heretofore, but will derive a much greater intellectual satisfaction from this widening interest and causal understanding.

REFERENCES

1. G. Barger and H. H. Dale, *J. Physiol.* (London), **41**, 19 (1910).

2. H. Konzett, *Arch. Exp. Pathol. Pharmakol.*, **197**, 27 (1940).

3. R. Hunt and R. DeM. Taveau, *U.S. Hyg. Lab. Bull.*, No. 73, Washington, D.C., 1911.

4. J. Fried and E. Sabo, *J. Am. Chem. Soc.*, **76**, 1455 (1954).

5. H. L. Herzog, A. Nobile, S. Tolksdorf, W. Cherney, E. B. Hershberg, and P. L. Perlman, *Science*, **121**, 176 (1955).

6. P. Ehrlich and K. Shiga, *Klin. Wochenschr.*, **41**, 329, 362 (1904).

7. U.S. Pat. 986,148 (1911), P. Ehrlich and A. Bertheim (to Hoechst A.G.).

8. H. Erlenmeyer and M. Leo, *Helv. Chim. Acta*, **15**, 117 (1932).

9. A. Burger, in E. Jucker, ed., *Progress Drug Research*, Birkhäuser Basel, Vol. 37, 1991, p. 287.

10. C. Hansch, *J. Med. Chem.*, **19**, 1 (1976).

11. L. Sternbach, *J. Med. Chem.*, **22**, 1 (1979).

12. P. Ehrlich, *Chem. Ber.*, **42**, 17 (1909); *Z. Angew. Chem.*, **23**, 2 (1910); *Lancet*, **2**, 445 (1913).

13. R. P. Ahlquist, *Am. J. Physiol.*, **153**, 586 (1948).

14. W. Bode and R. Huber, *Eur. J. Biochem.*, **204**, 433 (1992).

15. S. Borman, *C & E. News*, 18 (Aug. 10, 1992).

16. L. H. Pinto, L. J. Holsinger, and R. A. Lamb, *Cell*, **69**, 517 (1992).

17. W. F. Anderson, *Science*, **256**, 808 (1992).

18. L. Thompson, *Science*, **258**, 744 (1992).

19. G. J. McGarrity and Y. Chiang, *Annu. Repts. Med. Chem.*, **28**, 267 (1993).

20. D. J. Triggle, *Annu. Repts. Med. Chem.*, **28**, 341 (1993).

21. W. H. Moos, G. D. Green, and M. R. Pavia, *Annu. Repts. Med. Chem.*, **28**, 315 (1993).

22. S. C. Stinson, *C & E. News*, 38–65 (Sept. 27, 1993).

23. J. C. Barrish and R. Zahler, *Annu. Repts. Med. Chem.*, **28**, 131–137 (1993).

CHAPTER TWO

The Management of Drug Discovery

RALPH E. CHRISTOFFERSEN
J. JOSEPH MARR

Ribozyme Pharmaceuticals, Inc.,
Boulder, Colorado, USA

CONTENTS

1 Introduction, 10
2 The Discovery Process, 10
  2.1 Definition of *drug discovery*, 10
  2.2 Stages of drug discovery, 12
    2.2.1 Basic research, 13
    2.2.2 Feasibility studies, 13
    2.2.3 Programs, 15
    2.2.4 Nonclinical development, 16
    2.2.5 Initial clinical development, 18
  2.3 Role of drug discovery in development, 20
3 Strategic Issues in Drug Discovery, 20
  3.1 Drug discovery criteria, 20
    3.1.1 Basic research, 21
    3.1.2 Feasibility studies, 21
    3.1.3 Programs, 22
    3.1.4 Nonclinical development, 23
    3.1.5 Early clinical development, 24
  3.2 Portfolio management issues, 25
  3.3 External issues, 26
4 Organizational Issues in Drug Discovery, 27
  4.1 Discipline versus therapeutic organizational structure, 27
  4.2 Matrix versus line organizational issues, 28
  4.3 Geographic issues, 29
  4.4 Rewards, 30
  4.5 Scientific versus management career paths, 31
  4.6 Rose of committees, 32
  4.7 Industrial and academic collaborations, 32
  4.8 Biotech companies versus large pharmaceutical companies, 33
5 Management Strategies for the Future, 34

Burger's Medicinal Chemistry and Drug Discovery,
Fifth Edition, Volume 1: Principles and Practice,
Edited by Manfred E. Wolff.
ISBN 0-471-57556-9   © 1995 John Wiley & Sons, Inc.

1 INTRODUCTION

The current environment for discovery and development of new pharamaceutical agents could hardly be more challenging. Public policies and attitudes are requiring reduction in health care expenditures and increased efficiencies, resulting in major health care reform in the United States. At the same time, major diseases remain untreated and, paradoxically, scientific progress continues with ever-increasing acceleration.

These economic and other pressures have already resulted in a number of mergers and acquisitions among pharmaceutical companies in an attempt to create more effective worldwide organizations (e.g., Ciba-Geigy, Bristol-Myers Squibb, SmithKine-Beecham, Rhone-Poulenc Rorer, and Kodak-Sterling). Among the results of that process has been the creation of large research and development (R&D) organizations, and one of the important associated questions is how such organizations should be managed.

In considering management options of large, new R&D organizations, one of the first questions typically asked is whether "synergies" can be found in the combination of the two organizations. This usually translates in practice into a question of whether R&D staffing levels can be decreased instead of allowing a larger critical mass of personnel to be constructed. At the very least, such corporate formations usually impose serious cost constraints on existing pharmaceutical R&D activities.

At the other end of the spectrum, many small biotechnology companies have been formed over the last several decades. These companies have been based on a variety of research portfolios, from broad, enabling technologies to narrow, single-product portfolios. In virtually all of them, however, there is a belief that both the internal organizations and processes used for drug discovery and development have significant advantages over large organizations. Thus precisely the opposite view from that of large R&D organizations is espoused, i.e., smaller is better.

At the same time, the drug discovery–development process has become both longer and more complex. Partly this is due to increased understanding of biological processes at a molecular level and a desire to characterize new drugs fully. It is also due to increased complexity and length of regulatory review processes. The not surprising result of such effects has been to increase, not decrease, R&D costs. These and other financial pressures have also led senior management to focus on finding breakthrough drugs, because of both the medical implications and economic consequences.

All of these factors have led to significant efforts to examine alternative approaches to drug discovery and development. In this chapter, the drug discovery component of the overall process will be reviewed to consider alternative structures and approaches. While neither the most expensive nor longest portion of the overall process of bringing new drugs to the market, drug discovery is the most complex and difficult to manage portion of the overall process. Furthermore, it has the highest potential impact on the resulting product and is, therefore worth examining in detail.

2 THE DISCOVERY PROCESS

2.1 Definition of *Drug Discovery*

It is important at the outset to note that *drug discovery* is not an unambiguous term in the pharmaceutical R&D world. For example, it can be defined using either programmatic or organizational approaches (or both), with several options in each category. Hence, it is important first to understand this variability and to adopt a specific definition for the purpose of this discussion.

From a programmatic perspective, perhaps the broadest definition of *drug discovery* is one defined as a process that starts with the identification of a disease and therapeutic target of interest and includes methodology and assay development, lead identification and characterization *in vitro*, formulation, animal pharmacology studies, pharmacokinetic and safety studies in animals, followed by Phase I and Phase II clinical studies in humans. The rationale for such a broad definition is that, in general, the studies just listed cannot be carried out sequentially. Instead, each step in the process can require, and frequently does require, iteration with previous studies, as the results of one investigation may provide insights that require rethinking of the results of the previous step(s) and a redesign–repeat of the experiments.

For example, animal pharmacokinetic data frequently are unpredictable, and corresponding studies in humans either rule out or enhance the viability of a drug candidate in surprising ways, thus requiring rethinking of the animal data and their interpretation. Thus, drug discovery in this definition includes both laboratory and clinical studies in practice and does not end until the essential elements of the safety and efficacy profile of the drug are established in humans.

At the other extreme, drug discovery can be thought of as consisting only of the process by which the lead is found. In such a case, development of the core technology or new assays needed may be thought of as "basic research support," and any studies beyond animal pharmacology research would be considered part of "drug development."

Clearly, there are many intermediate concepts of drug discovery that fall between these two extremes, and none of these can be shown to be "correct" in the sense that others have fatal flaws. Instead, they are all correct in the sense that each can be included in a self-consistent description of the drug discovery and development process. Hence, the definition of *drug discovery* is a matter of taste and organizational convenience, not the logical conclusion of a reasoned argument.

Among the other terms that are sometimes used to characterize certain drug discovery processes is *rational drug design*. This is intended to indicate that the rationale for identifying a lead compound has been based on a molecular understanding of the drug and its receptor. This is frequently accomplished by the use of three-dimensional data to model the drug itself or the drug–receptor complex.

While such approaches are clearly desirable, they often lead to misunderstanding. For example, if these approaches are "rational," does it not imply that other approaches are "irrational"? More seriously, while the geometric and electronic structural features of drugs and their receptors are indeed important components of a drug's behavior, creation of a safe and efficacious drug requires much more information than the interaction of the drug with its receptor, regardless of the level of detail known about the latter. Such additional information includes pathology, toxicology, formulation, pharmacokinetics, and metabolism data, which should also be obtained in a rational manner if the overall process is to be referred to as rational drug design. Semantics aside, however, the use of quantitative physical and chemical information, techniques, and concepts to help understand the complex biological events taking place in the diagnosis and treatment of human disease is an important trend and will almost certainly become more pervasive and important in the years ahead.

In addition, molecular modeling need not be restricted only to the design of totally new structures. For instance, by considering examples from a database of existing compounds, it is frequently possible to extract information concerning components from different classes of molecules that should be included (or excluded) in new leads, which can lead to a substantial improvement in an existing drug or class of drugs.

Sometimes thought of as the opposite of rational drug design, screening approaches also are important components of the drug discovery process. One form of this approach uses a biological endpoint to identify leads, without concern for the structure or mechanism by which the agent is acting to achieve the end point. Using such screens to identify new types of antibiotics from fermentation "beers" is an example of an approach that has been successful historically (1), and many of the different structural classes of antibiotics now on the market came from such screens.

Screening approaches can and are also used in approaches that are quite detailed in their use of molecular aspects of the drug–receptor process. For example, screens using cloned receptors to test large numbers of diverse chemical structures are now being used to discover new structural leads that act specifically at a chosen receptor (2). Clearly, rational drug design and screening approaches are not mutually exclusive.

Turning to different organizational approaches, drug discovery is typically defined in one of two basic ways. The first is based on a discipline approach, and the extent of the drug discovery organization depends on the number of disciplines included. For example, in the definition of drug discovery that limits activities only to those leading up to and including animal pharmacology, the disciplines typically included are medicinal chemistry, structural chemistry, biochemistry, cell biology, pharmacology (both *in vitro* and *in vivo*), molecular biology (including both cloning and expression), and immunology. To focus efforts on drug design for specific diseases, members of the various discipline-based

groups are assembled, using a "matrix" approach to interdisciplinary discovery teams. These teams typically remain in existence until a lead compound has been advanced into development or the approach has been deemed to be unsuccessful.

If a broader definition of drug discovery is used, more disciplines are included in the interdisciplinary discovery team. For example, clinicians and personnel having pathology, toxicology, drug metabolism, formulation and chemical scale-up expertise may be added.

The opposite organizational approach to drug discovery uses units that are more or less permanently organized into areas of medical or therapeutic interest, e.g., central nervous system (CNS) discovery, antibiotics discovery, and cardiovascular discovery. Within these units, persons having expertise in each of the disciplines necessary to carry out the research are included, and the interdisciplinary unit is maintained indefinitely to maximize the continued focus on the disease or therapeutic category of interest while encouraging interdisciplinary interaction.

For our purposes, it is appropriate to define drug discovery from a programmatic point of view and to discuss organizational options within such a definition. Furthermore, we shall define drug discovery in the most encompassing manner discussed above, to allow the full complexities and nuances of the process to be revealed. Hence, *drug discovery* encompasses all studies necessary to find and characterize a drug *in vivo*, including technology development and all activities from disease and target identification through Phase II clinical studies.

2.2 Stages of Drug Discovery

To structure the discussion of the drug discovery process, five stages will be identified; basic research, feasibility studies, programs, preclinical development, and initial clinical development. They are roughly sequential through time but, as noted above, are frequently interactive and iterative.

2.2.1 BASIC RESEARCH. Basic research that is relevant to the drug discovery process is nearly impossible to define or limit, primarily because the number of disciplines and the speed of discoveries within disciplines that are important to drug discovery continue to increase in apparent exponential fashion. Examples of disciplines now actively employed in the drug discovery process that would have been considered esoteric intellectual activities a few decades ago include quantum mechanics, drug and drug–receptor computer modeling, x-ray crystallography, multidimensional nuclear magnetic resonance (NMR) imaging, cloning ("traditional" and expression), polymerase chain reaction analysis (PCR), repertoire creation and screening, creation of human monoclonal antibodies, receptor isolation and characterization, molecular characterization of biological processes, artificial intelligence, macromolecular folding predictions, and a variety of noninvasive technologies to measure biological and/or clinical endpoints.

In a typical pharmaceutical research environment, both scientists and managers must be alert to new basic research concepts and technology developments and identify those having the potential for applicability in the discovery of new therapeutics, especially in areas where the medical need and market opportunities are significant. This latter point is nontrivial, because there is little to be gained in using a new and typically more expensive technology for drug discovery if there is no significant benefit to its use later in the process.

Progress in basic research that results in techniques relevant to drug discovery continues apace, and continued monitoring of activities is essential. Within a pharmaceutical or biotechnology R&D organization, however, there is typically little or no control on the type of basic research that is pursued or attempts to identify its relevance to existing R&D priorities, except to account for the time spent on such activities. Sources for ideas in this area are equally diverse, although the current literature, scientific meetings, and personal contact among scientists from academia, national laboratories, and the private sector represent typical mechanisms by which such activities are identified and initiated.

A wide range of estimates can be obtained as to how much time is typically spent on such activities, depending on the type of organization and accuracy of reporting. In large pharmaceutical research organizations, an average range of 5% to 10% of a scientist's activities would typically be found in this category. In smaller biotechnology companies, the percentage can easily be 50% or greater, especially in early start-up companies.

2.2.2 FEASIBILITY STUDIES. One of the most difficult steps in a typical drug discovery effort is identification of a lead compound. There can be several reasons for this situation, involving either the lack of information about the physiological mechanism of action of the disease or lack of a chemical/biological structural lead that is known to interfere with the disease process.

CNS diseases provide good examples of the former case, for which the details of physiological and/or biochemical mechanisms that give rise to diseases such as Alzheimer's, anxiety, sleeplessness, and most other CNS malfunctions are poorly if at all understood. In such cases, identification of leads is typically accomplished via "functional" screens (3), by which diverse chemical structures are tested to see if the biochemical or physiological behaviors of cells or animals that are believed to be correlated with disease characteristics are modified by a particular chemical. Clearly, the success of such drug discovery processes depends on having access to a diverse chemical database, and recent developments of importance in this area include technologies that can create large, diverse repertoires of structures that can be searched conveniently (4).

Inability to define a structural lead can be encountered in several different ways. For example, if the natural agonist against a particular receptor is not known and the receptor structure is unavailable, design of an antagonist to the receptor is difficult. In practice, differing chemical structures that have different biological effects at the receptor can provide inferential data about structural features of importance, which may lead to a new structural lead. However, such occurrences are rare, and discovery of a truly new structural lead in this circumstance is difficult and seldom accomplished.

Even if the receptor has been characterized, design of a structural lead can be difficult. For example, the interleukin-1 (IL-1) cytokine and its receptor have each been characterized in some detail (5), but identification of a small molecule antagonist for the IL-1 receptor has not occurred. In such cases, it may be that future studies will reveal features of the receptor that will allow a small molecular antagonist to be designed. Perhaps more likely is the conclusion that multiple epitopes are required for activation (or antagonism) of the IL-1 receptor and are relatively widely separated in space. In such a case, only macromolecules (e.g., proteins) may have sufficiently structured and spatially separated epitopes to be effective. In addition, search for a small molecule antagonist in such a situation would be continually ineffective.

Another circumstance in which a new structural lead is hard to find is when therapeutic approaches to treatment of a disease are relatively mature. In such cases, e.g., in the treatment of hypertension (6), several classes of chemical structures already exist that are used in treatment of the disease, and finding a new structural class is typically as difficult as the case in which little data are known about the receptor.

These examples illustrate that determination of the particular biochemical pathway or receptor of importance to the pathology of the disease, coupled with identification of a unique structural lead that will modulate the receptor's activity or biochemical pathway, is a key part of the overall drug discovery process. At the same time it is also the part of the overall process that typically requires the most creativity, as knowledge of the particular receptor or biochemical process of importance is most often not obvious, or other researchers would have focused on them much earlier. In addition, it is the part of the process in which the risk of failure is usually the highest, because even if the receptor or biochemical process that has been identified is characterized and a chemical lead that affects it has been found, there is no way to predict if the resulting effect will have any relevance to treatment of the disease.

Hence, the design and execution of studies that identify receptors or biochemical pathways that are relevant to disease pathology, plus identification of ways in which their action can be modulated, are important parts of the drug discovery process. In many organizations, such studies are referred to as *feasibility studies*, and it will be convenient to use such a definition in this discussion.

The appearance of a recent article, a paper presented at a scientific meeting, or the extrapolated "hunch" of a scientist may be the source of a new feasibility study. In any case, formalization of the idea typically takes place via preparation of a proposal whose goal is to demonstrate that interference with a particular biochemical pathway or receptor will have an effect that can be used for therapeutic purposes. A small interdisciplinary group (typically six or fewer persons) is then assembled to work on the feasibility study. The team members represent disciplines such as cell biology, biochemistry, molecular genetics, and sometimes medicinal chemistry. The time frame for such studies is usually kept short (6–9 months), in part because of the high likelihood of failure and the associated difficulty that the project may take on a scientific life of its own, unrelated to the therapeutic goals of the organization, if allowed to go on longer. If successful, however, the result of such efforts will be identification of a new biochemical process or receptor of relevance to the disease pathology, along with identification of a new structural class of chemicals that can modulate the effect of the receptor or biochemical pathway.

2.2.3 PROGRAMS. If a feasibility study has been successful, the process of drug discovery continues, typically in a significantly expanded scale, by formation of a *program* and associated *program team*. Such a team will typically be larger than the feasibility study's and may consist of 15 to 25 persons. Membership usually includes individuals from medicinal chemistry, pharmacology, drug delivery, cell biology, biochemistry, molecular genetics, and protein chemistry and perhaps others from patent law, toxicology, drug metabolism, project management, and scale-up chemistry. Leadership of program teams is frequently, but not always, appointed from the pharmacology area, as the animal studies that will be crucial to the success of the candidate are typically carried out by pharmacologists. However, if the program is highly chemically driven or if the agents of interest are macromolecules, then the program team leader may be a medicinal chemist or a molecular geneticist. In any case, it is important that, regardless of his or her

discipline, the leader serve not only as team leader but also as "champion" for the program both to R&D management and within the team itself.

The goals of the program team include preparation of a critical path of activities that will result in a *drug candidate*, i.e., a compound that will enter formal development and human clinical studies. Activities in such studies include preparation of sufficient amounts of the target (e.g., the receptor of interest) and, especially if the new structural lead is a small molecule (molecular weight <500), synthesis of a variety of chemical structures that allow characterization of the structure–activity relationships of the structural class. As many as several hundred structures may be synthesized and characterized during program activities, and 1 to 2 yr are frequently needed to complete program team activities.

Included in the characteristics of potential drug candidates to be determined in such studies are the feasibility of chemical synthesis at the gram level (and preferably at the kilogram level), demonstrated potency as measured in *in vitro* cell culture assays, acceptable relative and absolute bioavailability of the drug in animals when delivered via the route to be used in human clinical studies, demonstrated efficacy in one or more animal models (including determination of the dose-response behavior of the candidate drug) believed to be predictive of the human clinical situation, and if indicated by the structural features of the class of drugs under consideration, initial toxicity and drug metabolism studies.

If the candidate drug is a macromolecule, the process may differ substantially in both the approach and the nature of activities that are desired and required from a regulatory point of view. For example, if the candidate is an endogenous protein, issues of safety are quite different (7) from that for small molecules (i.e., are much reduced in general), and much greater emphasis is placed on methods and cost of synthesis.

If successful, the result will be a compound (or sometimes a few similar compounds) that is believed to be sufficiently efficacious and safe in animal studies for recommendation to enter into formal development, i.e., a *drug candidate proposal* is prepared. The content of such proposals vary from company to company, but they typically contain the current status of information regarding *in vitro* biochemical and pharmacological assays, animal pharmacology, method of synthesis and cost, pharmaceutical information (e.g., stability, salt form, etc), patent opinion, general plan for nonclinical and clinical development, available safety data, possible regulatory issues, the status of competition, and perhaps comments about the commercial potential of the drug.

2.2.4 NONCLINICAL DEVELOPMENT. *General Comments.* Assuming acceptance of the drug candidate proposal, the drug(s) will enter formal development (sometimes referred to as *safety assessment*, and a *development team* will replace the earlier program team. Ideally, the development team will be a continuation of the program ("early discovery") team, but the composition of the individuals whose main focus was the earlier aspects of drug discovery are replaced by persons with expertise in toxicology, formulation, metabolism, clinical pharmacology, regulatory affairs, scale-up of manufacturing processes, and sometimes marketing.

As indicated, formation of the development team not only assembles a relatively large number of persons but allows for integration of activities both with earlier discovery efforts and with future clinical studies. In addition, it is the first time that a formal plan for the development of the drug candidate is prepared. It will include estimates of the likely clinical indications,

mode of delivery, method of synthesis, and the timeline and critical questions to be answered before filing the investigational new drug (IND) application.

The importance of integrating disciplines in these latter stages of drug discovery cannot be overemphasized. For example, clinical expertise can provide valuable comparisons of clinical experience with modes of therapy costs, indications, etc., that are proposed for the candidate. In addition, such expertise can be helpful in distinguishing improvements in therapy or simply an improvement in science. Conversely, early discovery efforts may identify potential toxicological problems, formulation and/or bioavailability issues, or manufacturing scale-up issues that must be considered in IND application preparation. Such examples illustrate again how drug discovery is a process that extends well into the clinic and can be quite iterative.

The benefits of such an integrated approach are also seen in financial terms. For example, it will allow critical questions (e.g., about potential toxicities) to be asked at an early point in the process. Because approximately 80% of drug candidates fail to reach this point, elimination of candidates at an early stage has significant resource-saving implications. Furthermore, if there are multiple similar candidates under consideration, early nonclinical studies can frequently be used to choose the best from among the group. This type of integration of nonclinical studies into early discovery efforts is quite desirable and will be discussed in greater detail below.

However, in contrast to the diversity of approaches to early drug discovery, the safety and other nonclinical studies on a drug candidate(s) are usually quite similar, regardless of company or type of drug candidate. In particular, while the details may differ, the process applies in general to small molecules as well as to proteins or oligonucleotides.

Within the context of this discussion,

however, the goal of early nonclinical studies is clear: to determine whether the candidate is considered to be sufficiently safe to submit an investigational new drug application to the U.S. Food and Drug Administration (FDA) (or analogous regulatory agency in other countries) for approval to administer the drug to humans.

Toxicology, Mutagenicity, and Carcinogenicity Studies. While detailed discussion of nonclinical studies needed for IND filing and later is provided elsewhere in this volume, it is useful to outline the kinds of studies needed, so that they can be related to other aspects of the drug discovery process. What will not be outlined here are chronic, long-term studies, such as carcinogenicity testing and chronic toxicology for certain kinds of drugs, which are not usually relevant to the discovery process. While important to the overall drug development process, they may require 2 yr of study and typically will run in parallel with Phase II and Phase III clinical trials. At that point, the discovery process is largely complete, unless an unexpected, untoward event occurs as larger numbers of patients are included in trials. Of more importance to the discovery process are short-term toxicology, pathogenicity, metabolism, and formulation studies.

In vitro mutagenicity studies are an important part of discovery activities and are frequently critical in determining the future of a drug candidate. A drug candidate that is active in a mutagenicity test (e.g., the Ames test (8)) or that produces mutagenic metabolites by activation in a microsomal enzyme system generally will be discarded in favor of a backup candidate. However, available mutagenicity tests are not necessarily predictive of activity or pathology in humans. In many cases, the observance of activity in mutagenicity assays serves more as a guide to needed metabolism or other pharmacology studies than as a fatal flaw.

The nature and duration of toxicology studies depend on the route of delivery chosen for the drug candidate, the proposed duration of therapy, and the structural or metabolic relationship of the drug candidate to molecules related to it. Formal toxicology studies to be used in IND filing are done under good laboratory practice (GLP) conditions, which are used across the drug industry and provide assurance that stringent laboratory and toxicological standards have been met.

However, GLP studies needed for IND applications are frequently augmented by less formal, more probing studies that are of particular interest to the drug discovery process. For example, if a drug candidate is administered to a small group of animals, generally rodents at blood concentrations approximately 10-fold higher than the estimated effective blood concentration for 1 week without untoward effects, then the drug candidate generally will move forward quickly, and formal toxicology studies can be more easily designed. On the other hand, if toxic effects are seen (including metabolites, clinical pathology observation, and histological observation), then the candidate is typically either discarded or modified as part of the discovery process to eliminate the portion of the molecule thought to be responsible for the adverse toxicological profile. In either case, considerable resource savings occur, due to avoidance of nonclinical and/or clinical activities that would have taken place only to have the candidate fail later because of its toxicology profile.

Metabolism studies are sometimes done in conjunction with drug discovery efforts, but are more commonly carried out only in formal GLP studies due to their cost and complexity. In the former case, tissue culture derived from human cells, especially primary human tissue culture, will be used to predict human metabolism. While such studies are not necessarily predictive, they can frequently be used to eliminate candidates that show adverse metabolic properties that are characteristic of the class of molecules represented by the candidate or, conversely, identify candidates that may be exceptions to the rule. In any case, such studies can be quite useful in the drug discovery process.

Formulation and Bioavailability. Historically, formulation has typically been considered to be an issue considered only when formal development has been initiated. This was particularly the case when the molecules involved had low molecular weight and high bioavailability. In such cases, clinical convenience and cost were the driving factors, thus allowing formulation issues to wait until the development process had formally started. However, given the trend toward design of agents against specific molecular targets and the emergence of protein as well as peptide and peptidomimetic agents as important new classes of therapeutic agents, the situation has changed substantially.

For example, establishment of acceptable bioavailability may be absolutely essential if a peptidomimetic is to be carried forward into formal development. In such cases, development of a suitable formulation is not simply an issue of cost, but the process becomes integrally linked to the rest of the discovery process. It may entail chemical modification of the drug candidate to improve bioavailability, use of controlled-release vehicles, use of alternative delivery sites (e.g., nasal and transdermal), or even the development of a new type of delivery system (e.g., retroviral delivery) for the drug candidate to be successful. To complicate the situation, it is frequently the case that animal bioavailability models are not consistent or reliable indicators of human bioavailability, thus coupling the discovery process in yet another way from early chemical design and synthesis through early clinical evaluation.

Synthesis and Scale-up. When animal safety and human clinical studies are to begin, the amount of material needed increases dramatically. Instead of using milligrams of material in a given experiment, tens of grams may be needed. In addition, as this is the point at which data will be generated for regulatory use, it is necessary that the synthetic procedures comply with good manufacturing practices (GMP). Finally, the cost of goods is considered seriously, to ensure that if successfully developed the drug can be manufactured profitably.

The result of these new considerations is typically that the synthetic procedures are reviewed in great detail, and new procedures are developed for at least the most expensive and/or time-consuming parts of the synthetic process. Such development and optimization of synthetic procedures are needed regardless of the nature of the molecule under development, i.e., they are necessary whether the candidate is a small organic molecule or a macromolecule.

To be successful, e.g., to be able to produce approximately 100 g of GMP material for animal safety and other early nonclinical studies, it is typically necessary for process development personnel to interact closely with the chemists and biologists who have created the drug to understand the rate-determining steps and options available. Hence, the early discovery process and later steps are seen to be linked yet again.

2.2.5 INITIAL CLINICAL DEVELOPMENT. *Phase I Clinical Studies.* Following drug safety studies in animals, an IND application is filed with the FDA, and if objections are not received within 30 days of filing, initiation of the first studies of the drug in human subjects may begin. These clinical studies (known as Phase I studies) are designed to demonstrate the safety of the drug candidate in human subjects.

Because evaluation of safety is the primary goal of these studies, normal male volunteers have generally been used as the clinical population, although normal female volunteers are increasingly sought. These studies are an important part of the discovery process, as it is only at this point that obvious toxic effects in humans may be found and questions of bioavailability, blood levels, tissue distribution, metabolism, and routes of excretion can be addressed and correlated with previous *in vitro* and animal studies.

In Phase I studies, a relatively small number of subjects is employed from as few as 10 or 20 to as high as 100. Questions of clinical end points or modulation of disease progression are generally not asked in Phase I studies, although monitoring of enzymatic alterations and other biochemical endpoints frequently provides clues regarding likely efficacy of the drug in diseased patients. Instead, the primary end points of interest are those regarding safety and acceptability of pharmaceutical and other properties, e.g., is the drug orally bioavailable, is the half-life sufficiently long enough to provide dosing that is appropriate, are toxic metabolites formed, is the route of excretion the same as that shown in animals, does the drug distribute into the appropriate tissue compartments, are any of the standard clinical chemistry tests affected by the drug, and are other normal clinical parameters affected by the drug (electrocardiograms, heart rate, blood pressure, mental function)? If any of the results are not what is desired or expected, the Development Team must reconsider the drug candidate, either to terminate its development or to modify its characteristics chemically, via alternative formulations, or in other ways.

At this point, questions may not only be scientific, but may involve clinical judgment or marketing strategy. For example, in the absence of a safety issue the judgments are much more subjective. If a half-life is not as long as desired, then a judgement re-garding market risk must be made; if a drug causes an elevation of liver enzymes in the clinical chemistry panel that are not consistent with significant hepatic damage, then the question of whether this represents a potential market, regulatory, or other risk needs to be answered.

Answers to these questions often are not simple yes-or-no decisions but involve a risk–benefit judgment based on the severity of the disease to be treated versus the potential risk of the drug itself. Furthermore, these judgments are fluid in that the criteria change with time. As other drugs come into the marketplace that address the same disease, subsequent drug candidates must be of sufficient improvement to existing therapy that the risk of use is acceptable relative to the disease process and other existing therapies. A good example of this is isoniazid (9), which was used in the treatment of tuberculosis 30 yr ago. It causes the elevation of certain liver enzymes in 20% of patients. However, at the time it was an excellent drug, and there was nothing equal to it for therapy; therefore, this complication was accepted as a risk of therapy. A similar antituberculosis drug that caused this complication today, would not be accepted. In any case, one of the challenges in the design of these and later clinical studies is to create definite go–no go decision criteria prospectively and to use them to eliminate candidates as soon as possible.

Phase II Clinical Studies. The final phase of drug discovery as defined here is associated with the earliest studies of the drug in patients having the disease of interest. At this time, clinical measures of efficacy become the primary end points, to be correlated with previous *in vitro* and animal efficacy studies. In addition, if multiple drug candidates having similar profiles have been entered into clinical studies, their relative efficacy will allow the choice of a single lead candidate. Not only will these studies define whether a candidate can be taken forward for further development, but they will frequently result in a number of additional animal or *in vitro* studies to clarify unexpected clinical observations and to provide a better characterization of the drug candidate.

2.3 Role of Drug Discovery in Development

As the previous discussion has illustrated, the discovery process continues through early Phase II studies, and should be a continuous and iterative process if it is to be maximally effective. Interdisciplinary interactions are needed, and minimization of disciplinary barriers through appropriate organizational structures is essential to accomplish such interactions. In the following sections, the various factors and approaches that can be used to ensure a continuous, interactive, and interdisciplinary process will be discussed along with recommendations for choice of strategies that will optimize the discovery process.

3 STRATEGIC ISSUES IN DRUG DISCOVERY

While the previous discussion has pointed out the many options and complexities of the drug discovery process, it is also important to note that the overall cost of product innovation in the pharmaceutical industry is high. In particular, data from 93 new chemical entities (NCE) have been used to estimate that the average out-of-pocket cost of an NCE is $114 million (1987 dollars), and total costs of $231 million are incurred to the point of marketing approval (10).

One of the reasons for such high costs is the fact that the failure rate for drug candidates is quite high, e.g., in a survey of 49 companies covering 1972 to 1992, the mean number of compounds synthesized for every NCE marketed was 3,645 (11). Similar estimates (5,000–10,000 compounds/NCE) have been made by others (12). It is of interest in this regard to note that, while formal surveys have not been carried out, it is likely that the number of compounds/NCE when dealing with protein agents or other macromolecules as therapeutic agents is likely to be lower. This is partly because many of these agents occur naturally, thus mitigating many safety issues and increasing the probability of success.

Thus it is seen that drug discovery management includes a highly complex and iterative scientific and managerial process, with many options for organizational and programmatic approaches, along with high costs and relatively high failure rates. Given that situation, it is essential that managers of this process have a clear vision of what goals are to be accomplished and equally clear criteria (established in advance) to measure progress and to allow resource reallocation, including termination of efforts, when appropriate.

3.1 Drug Discovery Criteria

Among the most important criteria to be established in advance of initiating activities are the criteria to be used for starting and stopping activities. Not surprisingly, it is much easier to start than to stop, thus making the criteria for stopping the more difficult and important criteria to define prospectively. Also, from the description of the various stages of drug discovery described earlier, it is expected that the start and stop criteria will vary from one stage to another.

Regardless of the choice of criteria, one of the ways in which they can be applied uniformly is to have a single person or group make all discovery start and stop decisions. In most large organizations, a small group is typically used, which includes the senior managers of the disciplines involved in the drug discovery process. However, it is important that the group be kept small (e.g., less than six persons) if it is to be effective.

Another general point that should be obvious in the design of criteria is that these drug candidates are designed for human use, thus making human clinical data the only data on which definitive conclusions can be reached in general. This also implies that the studies carried out before human clinical studies should be the minimum necessary to ensure safety for human clinical studies. In other words, the goal should be to obtain data in the species of interest as soon as possible, consistent with safety, and early entry into human clinical studies is more important than full *in vitro* and animal characterization. As obvious as such a criterion is, frequently multiple *in vitro* or animal studies are proposed (which represent good science and will add to the overall portfolio of knowledge on the drug candidate) that are not essential to the information needed to initiate clinical trials. Such studies should be eliminated without hesitation.

A current example that illustrates this point is in the design of agents for the treatment of AIDS. Although there is a simian model of AIDS and there are transgenic animals whose immunological characteristics have been modified to mimic the human immune system, it is unfortunately true that a satisfactory predictive animal model of AIDS does not currently exist. This implies that, in the development of possible new treatments for HIV infection and replication, *in vitro* measures of efficacy and animal safety studies are the measures that are relevant before human clinical studies.

To understand this idea more generally, it is instructive to ask the following question of a proposed animal model efficacy or safety study: "If the results of the study are inconclusive or negative, will it cause a recommendation to discontinue the development of the drug?" If the answer is no, then the study is not essential and should be eliminated from the critical path of activities. As to specific criteria that can be used for start and stop decisions, there are few absolutes, but a few examples will illustrate how such criteria can be constructed.

3.1.1 BASIC RESEARCH.   As implied above, basic research is an essential activity, but the nature and amount will vary greatly, depending on the organization, and will be essentially driven completely by individual scientists. As a result, usual start and stop criteria are not appropriate here. Instead, only the relative amount of time to be spent on basic research activities at various scientific levels in the organization must be identified in advance (e.g., 5% of overall scientific activity) and monitored over time to ensure that such levels of effort are maintained.

Perhaps surprisingly, it is frequently the case in large organizations that the amount of basic research is far below the limit set, and encouragement needs to be given to increase basic research efforts. This is typically because scientists want to be involved in later discovery and development efforts of drug candidates that have arisen from their efforts, and they find it difficult to let go. Thus it is important to encourage researchers to attend external scientific meetings, monitor recent research reports, attend seminars, and otherwise find new techniques of possible interest.

3.1.2 FEASIBILITY STUDIES.   Because the feasibility study is the point at which new approaches to therapy will typically be verified or discarded, design of start and stop criteria are particularly important. If a new biochemical pathway or mediator is involved, then important criteria to be established in advance are how to determine if the pathway or mediator exists and how to determine if its modulation has the desired physiological effect. Because negative results in such experiments typically lead to new experiments, it is equally important to place time limits for achievement of such criteria and to terminate the activity if time limits are exceeded. However, it must be recognized that using deadlines as a means of terminating activities will almost always be viewed negatively by those doing the work, as scientists typically are optimistic and are "certain" that the next set of experiments will be successful.

When the biochemical pathway or target is established in advance, the criterion of importance is the successful identification of a new class of lead. Since the definition of a *new class* is open to interpretation, both scientifically and from a patent perspective, it is important to determine the definition in advance and, as in the previous case, couple the activity with a time limit. Although it may not be satisfying to have carried out a screening activity for months unsuccessfully and have the activity terminated because a new class of lead has not been found, it is essential to the long-term success of discovery activities. Furthermore, it may be that such screening activities have previously been quite successful, making it even more difficult to accept termination of efforts (e.g., in screening fermentation beers for new classes of antibiotic leads).

A general issue that sometimes arises during feasibility study design is whether screening or rational drug design should be used to identify a new lead. At the current time, it is apparent that neither is appropriate separately but that both are appropriate if used together. Hence, the issue is really a nonissue.

More specifically, given the rapid increase in identification of specific receptors and biochemical and physiological pathways relevant to disease pathology, it is

clearly desirable to use such receptors and/ or pathways in the design of feasibility studies, including structural data and modeling as appropriate. In that sense, rational drug design is essential in contemporary drug design. On the other hand, knowledge of a specific receptor or biochemical pathway can frequently allow design of a high throughput screen that is capable of screening large libraries of chemicals to identify new classes of agents that are effective only at specific receptors or within unique biochemical pathways. Hence, the best of both worlds is frequently possible.

3.1.3 PROGRAMS. Once a lead has been found and a formal *program* has been established, start and stop criteria become somewhat easier to identify (but not necessarily to achieve). However, these criteria will still be specific to the target and lead under consideration, and an absolute set of criteria cannot be given. In fact, the *critical path* of activities will typically contain several start and stop criteria, and failure to achieve any one will result in termination of the program. Among the kinds of criteria used are

1. Demonstration of *in vitro* potency (e.g., inhibition of a target enzyme with nanomolar concentrations of the drug in cell culture).
2. Demonstration of *in vivo* efficacy in one or more animal model (usually a rodent and nonrodent) of the human disease of interest.
3. Demonstration of suitable dose-response curves both *in vitro* and *in vivo*.
4. Determination of patentability (in the opinion of patent counsel).
5. Demonstration of acceptable formulation, stability, and bioavailability in one or more animal models
6. Demonstration that methods appropriate for synthesis of sufficient material

for subsequent animal and human clinical studies are available.

7. Verification that gross toxicologic effects are absent (including the lack of specific toxicological effects known for molecules having similar structural features).

The quantitative form of these criteria will vary from case to case and may be affected by data available for alternative therapeutic approaches and drugs currently available for treatment of the disease in question. In any case, it is important that quantitative criteria be agreed in advance, and not reinterpreted in the light of data that are generated.

Furthermore, it should be recognized that, if the program effort is successful, the recommendation to proceed with subsequent studies leading to human clinical evaluation of the drug candidate is a very important one. This is partially because it begins the commitment of significant amounts of human and financial resources over a long period of time. In addition, the drug candidate will take its place in the overall portfolio of drug candidates under consideration, will use scarce resources that are almost always maximally committed, and hence will receive considerable upper-management attention. As a result, determination as to whether criteria have been successfully met or not is particularly important at this stage.

Among the "surprises" that sometimes accompany a successful candidate into the next stage of drug discovery, which can be avoided if considered appropriately at the program stage, is the question of production of sufficient material for subsequent animal and human clinical studies. If the candidate is a small molecule, it has typically been produced for studies thus far by synthetic procedures designed to produce large numbers of compounds in small amounts, so that screening can be relatively comprehensive. At the point at which animal safety and human clinical studies are contemplated, multiple gram amounts of high quality material are needed, which frequently cannot be produced by the procedures used in previous studies.

Thus, to improve the efficiency of the overall process, reduce the time needed to prepare necessary materials, and in general, to make the drug discovery process into more of a parallel series of interactive activities, it is usually appropriate to engage the efforts of process development chemists during program activities. These efforts should be designed to produce large amounts of material (e.g., at least 100 g), using GMP procedures. As a result, the activities may require development of entirely new synthetic procedures as well as optimizing individual steps in reactions. The cost of such syntheses also becomes an issue to consider but is typically not a go–no go issue at this time.

3.1.4 NONCLINICAL DEVELOPMENT. At this stage, the start and stop criteria begin to be driven by multiple agenda, not the least of which are regulatory criteria that must be met for the type of drug under consideration. Clearly, there must be demonstration of sufficient safety (typically in more than one species) and lack of target organ toxicity at anticipated doses in human clinical studies to allow both corporate and regulatory approval to proceed in human clinical studies.

Such studies also typically include estimates of mutagenicity, although the reliability of current methods of estimating mutagenic potential have been questioned (13). Today, use of multiple mutagenicity tests is typically advisable to mitigate the relative uncertainty of an individual test. Unfortunately, the unavailability of truly predictive mutagenicity tests makes it difficult to devise prospective go–no go decision criteria, and the relevance of the results of such tests is frequently the source of considerable discussion both internally and with regulatory agencies.

Studies of the relative and absolute bioavailability of the drug in animal models represent another example of studies at this stage for which the relevance of results must be considered carefully. For animal models of diseases that have been well characterized and correlated with subsequent human clinical studies and when the drug under consideration has structural features mostly similar to other drugs, the results of bioavailability studies can be expected to be quite predictive. However, for diseases with few or no animal models (e.g., HIV), or when new forms of administration (e.g., inhalation and retroviral vectors) or a new class of drug (e.g., peptides and peptide mimetics) are being used, it is difficult to devise prospective criteria that need to be satisfied in animal studies to proceed into human clinical studies. In such cases, the severity of the disease and availability of alternative treatments may result in alteration of the criteria and risk to be taken.

Finally, it is at this stage that GMP manufacturing criteria must be satisfied. Both facilities and processes for production of material must be approved by the relevant regulatory agency, and all materials to be used in clinical studies must be produced in these facilities, using these processes. In the case of small molecules, GMP facilities usually exist already, and no significant capital expenditure is required to produce the materials.

However, such facilities may not exist internally for the production of biologicals (e.g., proteins), and so it may be necessary to gain access to GMP manufacturing capabilities. To do so at this early stage of development frequently presents a difficult business decision. In particular, access to such capabilities requires either a contract for manufacturing of GMP material from another supplier (which is not typically desirable) or the construction of a GMP facility. The latter situation can be expensive and represents a major capital expenditure at a stage when there may not be much information on the drug candidate; hence the decision is one of high risk.

3.1.5 EARLY CLINICAL DEVELOPMENT. Once internal and external regulatory approvals have been obtained to initiate human clinical studies, the kinds of strategic issues that arise change substantially from those encountered earlier. In particular, issues related to clinical observations dominate, and commercial implications become increasingly important. Hence, it is important to identify prospective quantitative criteria for success and failure.

Examples of such success and failure criteria for use in early clinical studies are overall clinical safety, bioavailability, metabolism, distribution and route(s) of excretion, dosing schedule and dose response, target organ toxicity, cost of goods, and clinical measures of efficacy (including target patient population). While the particular quantification of these criteria will vary from one case to another, it should be emphasized that these criteria must be defined prospectively and rigorously adhered to. In part, this will allow a much higher probability of success in subsequent (more expensive) studies. In addition, it will allow for much better commercial estimates of the market potential for the drug candidate to be made.

Note that the commercial potential of a drug candidate cannot be reliably determined until the clinical safety and efficacy profile is understood in some detail. In practice, such a determination ought to be possible by the end of Phase II clinical trials, i.e., by the end of the discovery studies discussed here. In addition, it is typically helpful to have representation from the commercial organization on development teams so that the characteristics of the drug candidate can be better understood. However, attempts to determine likely market potential, sales estimates, net present value, etc. before the end of Phase

II studies will not produce reliable data for decision making. Hence among the issues to be resolved early in the characterization of a drug are the point at which commercial considerations will be a part of the go–no go decision process and what kinds of data will be included.

3.2 Portfolio Management Issues

In addition to issues specific to the particular discovery activity under consideration, there are a number of overall portfolio management issues that need to be considered.

Among the most important of these is management of the overall composition of the portfolio. In large companies with diverse portfolios, this issue consumes a significant portion of senior research management's time and effort. Typical approaches to the overall management of the portfolio emphasize inclusion of a mixture of high risk and low risk candidates, acute and chronic treatment approaches, and limitation of the number of therapeutic areas under consideration. Although it may appear that achievement of a "balanced" portfolio is easily accomplished, it is frequently difficult to accomplish in practice. For example, the timing of various activities and their production of drug candidates may not allow portfolio balancing to occur, and even if an appropriate balance is created in early activities, the success and failure rates of various steps are essentially unpredictable. Hence prioritization of the portfolio to provide an appropriate balance is an issue that must be addressed continuously and should be carried out by the senior manager in drug discovery.

In small companies, this issue is generally handled more easily, as the number of drug discovery activities is frequently the maximum that can be handled, and the company is betting that the current choices will be successful. Of course, the risks associated with such a situation are considerably higher than if a larger portfolio is present.

Within the overall portfolio balancing process, there are several other issues that frequently arise. For example, creating a balance of high and low risk projects is sometimes translated into a different set of issues that are driven from a commercial perspective. In particular, high and low risk are sometimes translated into "breakthrough" and "me-too" classifications. This is a particularly undesirable result, for several reasons.

First, it implies that "me-too" projects are of marginal innovative value from a scientific or medical perspective, which is frequently not the case at all. For example, formulation changes that increase patient compliance substantially or the creation of second or third generations of a given class of drugs that use the same mechanism of action but improve the side effect profile (and thus the safety of the drug) are often important both medically and commercially, but they are labeled "me-too" and thus receive lower priority. Second, "breakthrough" activities are interpreted in some commercial organizations as activities that produce billion-dollar products, and thus they received a high priority, sometimes without the consideration of the concomitant risk of such projects.

Another issue that has significant resource as well as programmatic implications in drug discovery relates to the role that is envisioned for biologicals. In particular, as the biotechnologies have provided significant new tools for the discovery of new therapeutic agents, a general issue has arisen within many large research organizations as to whether the focus should be toward creating biologicals as agents (i.e., drugs) or targets (i.e., entities to be used to create other drugs). In a sense this ought to be a nonissue, because both uses are entirely appropriate and important. However, the identification of new targets (e.g., receptors) is now occurring at a rate at which (even if only a fraction of potentially interesting targets was cloned and expressed for use internally in screening programs) the demands will far exceed any likely available resources and will preclude any other activity by professionals in molecular genetics.

On the other hand, many important biological agents (e.g., proteins such as tissue plasminogen activator, human growth hormone, and erythropoietin) have been discovered that have significant commercial and scientific potential. To find, characterize, and develop these agents, it is necessary first to devote sufficient personnel and expertise (perhaps at the expense of target generation). In addition, production of significant quantities of biologicals requires substantial capital investment. However, the technologies available for production (e.g., prokaryotic expression and eukaryotic expression systems) continue to evolve rapidly and are frequently product dependent, thus the capital investment is more difficult and risky. As a result, an issue of importance to drug discovery efforts that needs continual consideration is what the balance should be between seeking biologicals as agents or targets.

3.3 External Issues

There are also several issues that relate to external influences on drug discovery that must be considered. From an historical perspective, one is the perceived difference between academic research and industrial drug discovery research. For the most part, this issue no longer exists, due to the creation of state-of-the-art facilities and programs in industrial settings on the one hand, and the direct applicability of basic research programs in universities to contemporary drug discovery research on the other. Indeed, it is possible to cite indus-

trial efforts that represent major contributions to basic research (e.g., the discovery of PCR technology (14)) and university efforts that have provided key technologies used in contemporary drug discovery research (e.g., the discovery of ribozymes (15)).

As a result, contemporary drug discovery research is found in both university and commercial laboratories, and exchange of personnel from one setting to the other is becoming much more common. In addition, many university administrations are creating policies that encourage entrepreneurship by their faculty within appropriate constraints as faculty members, and commercial organizations are increasingly recognizing the importance of supporting general university research (as opposed to "contract" research) and other activities. It is anticipated that such interactions will increase in the future, further blurring traditional roles, integrating research in universities and industrial organizations, and making this issue one of historical importance only.

On the other hand, technology transfer efforts between the private sector and government organizations are at an early stage, and many problems remain to be solved before such interactions can be as productive as the university–industry interactions just described. Both bureaucracy and public policy issues exist that have significantly hindered progress. In the United States, for example, cooperative research and development agreements (CRADAs) are frequently not only difficult to negotiate but contain provisions that are potentially onerous to the industrial organization. In addition, the constraints placed on government employees in consulting, participation in equity, and other relationships with private sector organizations are so serious that effective interactions are often not possible. Hence a significant nonresolved issue is a public policy issue: How can an expeditious and effective transfer of technology from the government to the private sector take place?

4 ORGANIZATIONAL ISSUES IN DRUG DISCOVERY

4.1 Discipline Versus Therapeutic Organizational Structure

In Section 2.1 of this chapter, two extremes of organizational approaches to drug discovery were outlined. The "discipline" approach places all personnel in discipline-based organizations and uses a matrix approach to drug discovery against a particular therapeutic target by forming (temporary) interdisciplinary teams for drug discovery. The "therapeutic" approach places individuals representing all scientific disciplines needed for drug discovery in a particular therapeutic area (e.g., cardiovascular diseases or inflammatory diseases) into individual therapeutic organizational units on a permanent basis. The question of which of these (or other) organizational structures to use is debated endlessly, because there is no single correct answer.

In part, the structure may be simply a reflection of the evolution of the company. Small companies tend to be organized around disciplines, since a new technology often is their reason for existence. Larger companies, which have built a broader technology base, will typically have several major emphases in therapeutic areas of interest, and drug discovery is often organized around these. As smaller companies emerge from the technology development into product development, a formal emphasis on therapeutic areas of interest, or at least a specific disease process, will emerge. During this evolution, a balance develops that is appropriate for the company at a particular stage. Any successful company must evolve, to some degree, into an organization that emphasizes therapeutic areas. Without this, there is not likely to

be a champion for a compound, and an efficient mechanism to move a compound from the early discovery stages through the development process will not be present. However, this does not imply that a pure therapeutic organizational structure as described above should be adopted.

To understand the issue further, it is instructive to examine the strengths and weaknesses of the two organizational extremes. A discipline organizational structure, for example, is especially useful if the discipline is rapidly evolving (e.g., as in many of the biotechnologies). In such a case it is important to keep sufficient personnel in a separate group to ensure that the state of the art can be maintained internally. Such an organization also enhances the probability that advances in the discipline can be made internally, through synergistic interactions among scientists within the unit.

On the other hand, a discipline structure is frequently difficult to organize into a focused effort on particular therapeutic areas. Interdisciplinary project teams are the usual mechanism used, but the heads of such teams (project managers) frequently do not have line authority. This usually results in the project managers acting only as facilitators, and the resource allocations needed to achieve progress are only obtained if the line managers of the discipline organizations agree to the request. This also makes prioritization among various therapeutic target activities difficult.

A therapeutic organization is, in many ways, the inverse of the discipline organization, in that the strengths of the discipline organization are usually the weaknesses of the therapeutic organization and vice versa. In a therapeutic organization, there is a clear focus on the therapeutic targets of interest. Prioritization of targets within the therapeutic area is easily accomplished, and because the unit is dealing with targets only within their therapeutic area, the question of prioritization across therapeutic areas does not generally arise. This ease of administration and resource allocation can result in increased speed in drug discovery, if managed appropriately. In addition, having all appropriate disciplines in the same therapeutic unit enhances the interdisciplinary interactions that are essential to effective drug design.

On the other hand, there are a number of disadvantages to such a structure. For example, there are generally only a few members of any particular discipline within a therapeutic unit, resulting in a lack of critical mass to ensure maintenance of state of the art and a lack of career development or upward mobility in the discipline. Furthermore, if all disciplines needed to carry drug discovery activities through initial human efficacy studies are included in the therapeutic unit, the size of the unit may become too large to be effectively managed. In addition, and probably most significant, a therapeutic organization will have a vested interest in continuing its current activities, which frequently leads to a "not-invented-here" syndrome and a lack of receptivity to new approaches. It also makes it difficult to impose change on such a group, as significant change may require dissolution of a large administrative unit.

In either organizational structure, individuals charged with the management of particular disciplines are, of necessity, preoccupied with the refinement of that discipline to reflect the state of the scientific art. However, enhancement of a particular technique within a discipline must sometimes be set aside to develop a drug candidate more expeditiously. In such cases, those in charge of disciplines must respond by recognizing that the goals of the company supersede those of a particular discipline.

In the case of therapeutic organizations, the individual in charge of a therapeutic area must cross a number of disciplines to ensure the rapid and efficient development of a drug candidate. This requires not only scientific knowledge and organizational skills but the diplomacy to persuade those engaged in a particular discipline to devote the appropriate time and effort to the furthering of the drug candidate.

In practice, most companies that are older than 1 or 2 yr will have some core disciplines that are integral to the development of their product lines and some therapeutic areas relevant to the company's goals. As the company matures, or as market forces supervene, the areas of therapeutic interest will receive increasing emphasis and particular disciplines will be restricted to the appropriate size consistent with the furthering of the therapeutic goals of the company.

It should be clear that one of the most difficult management issues in drug discovery is the balance of effort and resources between discipline-related groups and groups concerned with the movement of a drug candidate toward a therapeutic goal. Members of both types of groups have scientific and emotional involvement in their work. Frequently, they are reluctant to allow anything to impede what they view as the most important function within the company, i.e., whatever they happen to be working on at a particular time. Hence keeping the corporate perspective as the driving force in balancing this resource allocation is essential for success.

4.2 Matrix Versus Line Organizational Issues

Except for a large "pure" therapeutic organization that includes all disciplines needed through Phase II clinical studies, matrix organizational constructs cannot be avoided. As soon as therapeutic activities are organized (e.g., feasibility studies, program, and project teams), they require activities that cut across the line organizations of various disciplines, and a matrix organization is needed.

For example, after chemists synthesize potential drug candidates and begin to establish structure–activity relationships, they draw largely on members of similar disciplines, such as computational chemists. However, they also require the expertise of biologists doing tissue culture and animal pharmacologists to do preliminary efficacy studies. Thus different disciplines are needed at different times during the discovery process, and this requires coordination through some form of matrix organizational structure to be effective. The types of structures that are used are illustrated in Table 2.1, where persons from appropriate disciplinary units are assembled into project teams.

It should also be noted that because the nature of activities changes throughout the drug discovery process the membership of matrix organizations must change accordingly. Hence it is to be expected that only a few persons will be part of the project team from inception to conclusion, and that many others will come and go as the activities dictate.

Finally, as noted earlier, these matrix organizations also require project managers with special talents. In particular, these individuals should be credible scientists in their own disciplines, but must also possess the interpersonal skills to convince others to join in the pursuit of a particular goal, even though they may lack the managerial authority to force the cooperation. This is a delicate and difficult management exercise, but it is fundamental to the success of the R&D efforts of the company.

4.3 Geographic Issues

If other factors are equivalent, a single R&D site is obviously always better. It enhances communication and organizational cohesiveness, provides one home with which all employees can identify, and fosters a communal atmosphere. It also minimizes costs to run the infrastructure of the company, reduces travel, and allows for maximum synergies to occur.

However, as companies and R&D efforts grow (e.g., through acquisitions or to gain access to specialized expertise), the option to use other sites may arise. In the case of an acquisition, it is typically argued that it will be more efficient in the short term to use the additional site than to close it, considering personnel relocation costs, building closing costs, and time that would be lost in the process of closing the site. However, there are other significant issues that may substantially affect the potential advantages. For example, if the drug dis-

Table 2.1 Examples of Project Team Formation Using a Discipline Organizational Structure

Discipline	Therapeutic Project #1	Therapeutic Project #2	Therapeutic Project #3	
Chemistry	X		X	
Molecular biology		X	X	
Drug delivery	X	X	X	
Pharmacology	X	X	X	
Computational chemistry	X		X	
Toxicology			X	
.				
.				
.				

covery effort is to be divided among sites, it requires a leader at each site and a determination of who is in charge of the function overall. The resulting personnel and communication challenges may be great, and duplication of efforts may be costly.

When the alternate site is in another country, the management problems increase exponentially. Time differences alone may prove a significant challenge to effective operation and communication. Variations in customs, labor laws, and traditions all render the maintenance of a common corporate culture virtually impossible. In effect, the result is usually several different companies under the rubric of a single name. To be managed, these large organizations require considerable travel by upper management and scientists, which typically leads to inefficiencies due to the difficulty of scheduling and the amount of time needed for travel.

If it is necessary to have a multinational organization, it is generally best to locate complete functions in a single location (e.g., locate all CNS therapeutic activities in one location). However, it must be recognized that duplication of efforts is inevitable, e.g., when basic discipline support cannot be provided by mail or electronically in a time frame appropriate for discovery efforts. Video teleconferencing should be used as much as possible, but it should be remembered that such communication devices work well for some agendas (e.g., information transfer) but not for others (e.g., negotiation).

4.4 Rewards

It is somewhat surprising that the issue of how to motivate and reward scientific efforts arises frequently. This can be illus-trated by the tale of the Sun and the Wind, who were challenged to persuade a man to remove his coat. The Wind blew harder and harder, but this caused the man to wrap his coat more tightly around him. The Wind finally acknowledged failure, and the Sun took over. The Sun began to shine, and within a few minutes, the man removed his coat. You can catch more flies with honey than with vinegar! While it is true that a few individuals will respond only to coercion, most respond readily to reward and react negatively to threats.

These rewards should obviously include rewards for projects successfully completed but should also include rewards for definitive results that may lead to the elimination of a project from the portfolio. Both results are valuable to the company. Indeed, because drug discovery and development is so costly and time-consuming, establishing clear reasons for eliminating an approach or particular compound at an early stage can save significant resources and time. In addition, it should be remembered that many times the work that is to be rewarded has been carried out by a team and not one individual. In such cases, the entire team should receive the reward.

The nature of the reward may be less important than the fact that it is given. Monetary rewards are important, but scientists, perhaps more than others, tend to be motivated by other tangible recognitions of their efforts. For example, ceremonies that acknowledge patents, the acceptance of papers in particularly prestigious journals, and invitations to speak at important international conferences can provide nonmonetary ways to recognize research accomplishments. Other ceremonial occasions at which team efforts are recognized by management and peers are also valuable, not only for the morale of those receiving the awards but also for others who will recognize that teamwork does not go unnoticed.

4.5 Scientific Versus Management Career Paths

Virtually every company beyond its initial organizational stage has titles that are recognized as being associated with either scientific or management career paths. Historically, most individuals enter a company as either scientists or managers and tend to stay in those roles throughout their careers. For those who do change career paths, the switch is almost always from scientist to manager. Because of the extensive knowledge base required to be a scientist, the shift from manager to scientist almost never occurs.

Generally, the compensation provided for managers is higher than that for scientists, even though the knowledge, experience, and talents of the individuals may be comparable. The reason usually cited for this is that the decisions required by managers typically have more overall impact on the corporation and, therefore, carry more responsibility and should be compensated appropriately higher. However, while historically true, these compensation differentials usually provide a significant additional hurdle to change from a manager to scientist. They also give rise to animosity by scientists, who perceive that their contributions are not being recognized appropriately.

Furthermore, R&D managers often quickly become scientifically out of touch and focus only on the administrative aspects of their positions (e.g., budget and personnel). This causes rapid loss of credibility within the scientific community and decreased effectiveness of such managers. It also means that their decisions on scientific strategy and tactics will be much less effective.

On the scientific side, there is reduced motivation for continued development and expansion of responsibilities, because it is perceived that appropriate compensation and career development is not possible without becoming a manager.

Providing alternatives to such scenarios is not easy, but several possibilities, exist. Perhaps the most effective is to provide dual career paths, with titles and responsibilities in both the scientific and managerial ranks that provide comparable compensation until very high in the compensation scale. In particular, the highest ranking scientists should have responsibilities and compensation comparable to the highest R&D managers. To justify such compensation for scientists, it is also appropriate to bring them into high level scientific decision-making processes. For example, participation in the review of feasibility studies, program or project proposals, persons proposed for promotion to high scientific rank, and the scientific aspects of potential corporate acquisitions or collaborations represent activities in which the experience of senior scientists would be of considerable value to the corporation. In addition, such scientists should be expected to act as mentors to younger scientists.

On the managerial side, it is important that scientific activities be continued in some form throughout the managerial ranks. For lower management, continuation of laboratory work is important, although probably at a lower level than when such personnel were full-time scientists. At higher ranks, it is important that scientific activities also be continued, but they will obviously not involve laboratory work. Examples of ways in which scientific activities can be continued in such positions include writing review articles, participation in external review panels (e.g., for granting agencies or journals), and general "management by walking around" in the laboratories.

If such actions are taken, movement back and forth from the scientific to managerial career paths becomes possible, at least at the lower levels. Such a situation is highly desirable because, e.g., not all persons who enter into the managerial ranks will be effective, and alternatives that allow movement back into the scientific ranks with sufficient expertise and knowledge to be effective is important. In addition, the mutual respect and job satisfaction of persons in each career path will be increased.

4.6 Role of Committees

Committees are necessary to the function of larger organizations, because they provide working groups to deal with tasks that must be parceled out if management is to avoid paralysis. However, while the necessary interdisciplinary interactions in the discovery process require that committee structures be used, explicit and on-going efforts to minimize the number of committees should take place. The reasons for such efforts are intuitively obvious but cannot be overemphasized.

Committees tend to produce decisions that are the lowest common denominator, i.e., they offend the fewest number of people. Committees are useful when multiple input is required or when consensus is important, but they may significantly impede progress when a' rapid decision is essential or when risks are associated with the decision. In addition, most scientific questions are better addressed by small teams whose members are familiar with the scientific and technical issues. These small groups will focus more quickly on the issue at hand, will have less difficulty scheduling meetings, and thus will make decisions more efficiently.

More generally, the function of committees can be improved by defining their task and time of existence very tightly. For example, timelines for completion of goals should be agreed on in advance, and the committee should disband on completion of the goal. The chairperson of the committee should be responsible for minutes that have specific conclusions and an action plan that emerges from each meeting. While such steps seem obvious, they are frequently not easily accomplished, e.g., when the chairperson does not have line authority over the members of the committee. In such cases, consensus building and leadership by the chairperson are essential, and the committee members must be willing to act in the best interests of the team and not their own. It also emphasizes why committees should be kept small, so that the consensus process does not become unwieldy.

4.7 Industrial and Academic Collaborations

Because scientific progress in fields of direct interest to drug discovery continues to accelerate and because the number of disciplines and persons working in these fields is correspondingly increasing, it is not possible to create a drug discovery organization that is scientifically self-sufficient. Hence devising mechanisms for effective collaborations with external investigators, whether in the public sector or in other companies, is an important component of a drug discovery organization. For such collaborations to be useful to a drug discovery organization, they should be well defined. It is rare that unfocused scientific collaborations result in products for the company. Thus, the time frame for collaborations should be relatively short and the expected contributions of each of the collaborators should be well understood.

Collaborations are best undertaken when the company lacks a particular technology, type of assay, or particular knowledge. This is often the case when the technology is in early stages of development. In such cases, provision of resources (both financial and personnel) to accelerate the development of the technology can be a wise investment that can benefit the investigator, the company, and science in general. Of course, the success of such studies cannot be predicted, and it should be expected that many such investments will not produce a technology or entity that is directly useful to drug discovery.

In addition to the inherent uncertainty of such activities, there are other issues that frequently arise. For example, the time line and agenda of an external investigator may not be easily adapted to the focused goals of drug discovery programs, resulting in missed schedules and disappointment on the part of both scientists and managers of the funding agency. Issues of focus and time lines are particularly important to the success of small companies. Larger companies with a broad product base may have more flexibility. In general, however, time lines for achievement of scientific milestones should be short, usually not more than 1 yr, so that appropriate review and approval of future milestones can be accomplished.

Another set of issues that needs resolution before initiating external collaborations relates to intellectual property and long-term compensation to collaborators and their institutions. Fortunately, the importance of reaching an equitable resolution of these issues is now widely recognized, and processes and guidelines exist in many cases to help the discussions. However, the implications of such issues can be quite broad, making the process of their resolution difficult.

Public institutions (e.g., colleges, universities, and national laboratories) need to protect the academic freedom of their faculty, staff, and students involved in such collaborations. Publication of the results in peer-reviewed journals must be ensured in general, and particular care is needed if the thesis work of graduate students is involved. More generally, the agency must ensure that the results inure to the benefit of the public in as efficient a manner as possible. Companies, on the other hand, cannot be assured of the ability to commer-

cialize products without appropriate intellectual property coverage. This usually means exclusivity, which requires careful consideration relative to the need for general public benefit.

An agreement is usually reached to license patents resulting from the collaboration to the company, with appropriate compensation to the public agency and investigator in the form of continued research payments, royalties, etc. However, while both public agencies and private corporations have made significant strides in creating appropriate policies for collaborations that protect and benefit both parties, the negotiation of each specific arrangement continues to be done on a case-by-case basis.

4.8 Biotech Companies Versus Large Pharmaceutical Companies

There are many differences between biotech companies and large pharmaceutical companies, both conceptually and in scale. As a result, the management of discovery research in biotech firms raises several issues that are not usually found in larger companies.

First, there is the general approach to risk management. A typical biotech company is limited to a particular technology, product, or area of science and is focused very narrowly. In addition, limited resources are available to bring products to the marketplace. As a result, there is a high risk of failure, because of both the inherent uncertainty of science and the difficulty in maintaining the necessary focus on product development while simultaneously developing the technology.

Large pharmaceutical companies, on the other hand, usually have many areas of internal scientific interest, actively license compounds and technologies from external sources, and have a number of products that provide a stable commercial base. This reduces the risk associated with the overall discovery and development programs, because of a broad portfolio and a relatively secure source of financing.

Curiously, an interested but uninformed observer might conclude that the risk strategies just described for each type of organization are exactly opposite to what might be expected to be most appropriate. Large stable organizations can afford significant risk but typically are risk averse, and vice versa for biotech companies. In any case, the risks in either type of organization present issues that should not be ignored, either in the internal management or in the discussion of possible relationships between a biotechnology firm and pharmaceutical company.

Within a large organization, other issues arise relating to size. For example, increasing the number of personnel increases the infrastructure and cost of doing business. Substantial energy is devoted simply to maintaining the organization, and few companies have escaped this trap.

Within a biotech company different but equally difficult issues arise. The evolutionary process from startup to public company is compressed and intense. There are usually few if any committees, as decisions are made by a small management group or small team of scientists. This means that problems are raised, discussed, and addressed in a short time. The luxury of protracted discussion is not available, because financial pressures are ever present. Scientists usually must work with greater intensity to provide drug candidates that will serve as credible potential products to the investment community. Because there is no broad portfolio to rely on, drug candidates must be studied intensively and scrutinized carefully for potential flaws. A product failure in a company that has only one or two potential products can be disastrous.

Correspondingly, the management of a biotech firm must be continually alert to any issue that slows scientific progress, must balance the development of technology against the need to develop products, and must be aware of external forces that may compromise its position in the market. Pressure from the investment community on management of biotech companies is constant. However, too early a focus in science can be as bad as not focusing at all, and thus management must live with the science almost as intensively as the scientists themselves.

5 MANAGEMENT STRATEGIES FOR THE FUTURE

Given the scientific and managerial complexities of the drug discovery process, it is not surprising that a single set of principles and organizational structures for the management of drug discovery does not exist. However, regardless of the nature of the company and organizational structure chosen, there are several principles that appear to be broadly valid and, therefore, can be suggested for adoption in general.

The most important of these is remarkably obvious: periodic, frequent review of progress and justification of a project. This includes creation of prospective go–no go criteria, insistence on milestone judgments, time limits, repeated scientific and commercial justification of the activity, and elimination of unsuccessful projects as early as possible. Successful implementation of these principles is rarely accomplished.

Another general principle relates to scientific renewal, by which some fraction of an individual scientist's time is spent on basic research or another form of "skunkworks" project. This is sometimes difficult to justify to management, but it is essential if maintenance of state-of-the-art technologies and approaches are to be achieved and individual creativity is to be preserved. Good scientists can be as temperamental and fragile as any other creative person, and the self-renewal provided by this process should not be underestimated. The difficulty in achieving this is generally not a matter of accepting the idea in principle. Instead, as product development accelerates, the temptation to allocate most if not all resources to that end is often irresistible. At times this reallocation is necessary, especially in small companies, to preserve the organization or to bring a product to market in a timely manner. But the return to a milieu that encourages the creative process should occur as rapidly as possible.

Given the interactive nature of the discovery process, it is also recommended that organizational structures reflect the broad definition of drug discovery used above. This will ensure the interdisciplinary interactions necessary for success, yet retain the flexibility to change therapeutic goals and directions as needed. An organizational structure that includes both core technologies and therapeutic groups appears to come closest to achieving these goals. Core technologies include disciplines such as chemistry, molecular genetics, enzymology, computational chemistry, toxicology, metabolism, etc; therapeutic (or product-oriented) groups include individuals with specialized expertise in animal and clinical pharmacology. When specific projects are formed, members from both core technologies and therapeutic groups should be included as appropriate, and the composition of these groups should change as a project evolves. The formation of such project teams is illustrated in Table 2.2, where the members of specific project teams (e.g., PT1 and PT2) from a given therapeutic unit (e.g., central nervous system diseases) may not be the same.

As noted, geographic considerations often become important as companies grow, acquire other companies, or expand their research efforts by collaboration. As such expansions occur, maintaining a single site for R&D is far more desirable than multiple sites, as the difficulty of managing research and development in multiple sites increases exponentially with the number of sites. When multiple sites are required, the organization must consciously strive to maintain efficiency and avoid redundancy.

At the same time, therapeutic areas should be separated into self-contained units as soon as the size begins to create problems of communication and management. Of course, splitting a therapeutic area geographically into two or more units complicates its management significantly and virtually mandates redundancy. On a given site, organizational structures should

Table 2.2 Example of Project Team (PT) Formation, Using a Combination of Core Technology and Therapeutic Area Organizational Structures

Discipline	Central Nervous System Diseases	Cardiovascular Diseases	Infectious Diseases	· · ·
Chemistry	PT1, PT2	PT3	PT5	
Molecular biology		PT4	PT5	
Drug delivery	PT1, PT2	PT3, PT4	PT5	
Computational chemistry	PT1		PT5	
Toxicology		PT4		
.				
.				
.				

be kept as small as possible while maintaining critical mass. The benefits of more effective management, team building, and speed of decision making of such smaller organizations will, in general, outweigh the cost of duplication.

Finally, ensuring appropriate career development in the scientific ranks and creating mechanisms for transfer between scientific and managerial ranks should be encouraged. Only if both of these are accomplished can it be ensured that appropriate scientific career development and continued motivation will be possible and that scientists can become managers (and vice versa) without creating the impression that either move is necessarily a promotion or demotion.

Drug discovery remains a challenging, rewarding, and frequently frustrating activity. It requires a management that is conversant enough with the science to enjoy the respect of its scientific staff, is sensitive to the needs and aspirations of the scientists, but that can still focus on the objectives of the company. Moreover, as science and the scientific staff become increasingly sophisticated and complicated, management challenges will increase.

REFERENCES

1. H. C. Neu and K. P. Fu, *Antimicrob. Agents Chemother.*, **14**, 650–655 (1978).

2. J. Hodgson, *BioTechnology*, **11**, 683 (1993).

3. T. Gordh, I. Jansson, P. Hartvig, P. G. Gillberg, and C. Post, *Acta Anaesthesiol. Scand.*, **33**, 39–47 (1989).

4. S. Brenner and R. A. Lerner, *Proc. Nat. Acad. Sci. U. S. A.*, **89**, 5381–5383 (1992).

5. C. A. Dinarello, *Blood*, **77**, 1627 (1991).

6. M. H. Weinberger, "Systemic Hypertension," in *Textbook of Internal Medicine*, W. N. Kelley, Ed., J. B. Lippincott, New York, 1992, pp. 236–247.

7. "Pre-Clinical Safety of Biotechnology Products Intended for Human Use," in *Progress in Clinical and Biological Research*, **235**, C. E. Graham, Ed., A. Liss, Inc., New York, 1987.

8. B. N. Ames, J. McCann, and E. Yamasaki, *Mutat. Res.*, **31**, 347–364 (1975).

9. Public Health Service, U. S. Dept. of Health, Education and Welfare, Centers for Disease Control, *MMWR*, **23**, 97–98 (1974).

10. J. A. DiMasi, R. W. Hansen, H. G. Grabowski, and L. Lasagna, *J. Health Econ.*, **10**, 107 (1991).

11. R. G. Halliday, S. R. Walker, and C. E. Lumley, *J. Pharm. Med.*, **2**, 139–154 (1992).

12. J. S. G. Cox and A. E. J. Styles, *R&D Manage.*, **9**, 125 (1979).

13. B. N. Ames and L. S. Gold, *Monog. Natl. Cancer Inst.*, **12**(32), 125–132 (1992).

14. N. Arnheim and H. Erlich, *Ann. Rev. Biochem.*, **61**, 131–156 (1992).

15. T. R. Cech and B. L. Bass, *Ann. Rev. Biochem.*, **55**, 599–629 (1986).

CHAPTER THREE

Intellectual Property in Drug Discovery and Biotechnology

RICHARD A. KABA,
DAVID A. CROSSMAN and
JULIUS TABIN

Fitch, Even, Tabin & Flannery
Chicago, Illinois, USA

CONTENTS

1 Overview, 38

2 Patent Protection and Strategy, 43
2.1 Patent strategy, 44
2.2 First to invent versus first to file, 46
2.3 Absolute novelty, 47

3 Requirements for Patents, 48
3.1 Patentable subject matter in the United States, 48
3.2 Patentable subject matter outside the United States, 50
3.3 Patent specification, 51
3.3.1 Written description, 52
3.3.2 Enablement, 52
3.3.3 Best mode, 54
3.3.4 Claims, 55
3.4 Invention must be new and unobvious, 55
3.4.1 Novelty under 35 U.S.C. § 102, 56
3.4.2 Obviousness under 35 U.S.C. § 103, 57
3.5 Procedure for obtaining patents in the U.S. PTO, 60
3.6 Interference proceedings, 63
3.7 Correction of patents, 66

4 Enforcement of Patents, 67
4.1 Patent infringement, 67
4.2 Defenses to infringement, 69
4.3 Remedies for infringement, 71

5 Worldwide Patent Protection, 72
5.1 International agreements, 73
5.2 PCT patent practice, 75

Burger's Medicinal Chemistry and Drug Discovery,
Fifth Edition, Volume 1: Principles and Practice,
Edited by Manfred E. Wolff.
ISBN 0-471-57556-9 © 1995 John Wiley & Sons, Inc.

5.3 Other aspects of patent laws in other
    countries, 76
6 Trademarks,   78
    6.1 Trademarks as marketing tools, 79
    6.2 Selection of trademarks, 80
    6.3 Registration process, 82
    6.4 Oppositions and cancellations, 84
    6.5 Preserving trademark rights through proper
        use, 85
    6.6 Worldwide trademark rights, 85
    6.7 Other rights under the Lanham Act, 86
7 Trade Secrets,   87
    7.1 Trade secret definition, 88
    7.2 Requirements for trade secret protection, 88
    7.3 Enforcement of trade secrets, 89
    7.4 Relationship of trade secrets and patents, 90
    7.5 Freedom of Information Act, 91
    7.6 Trade secret protection outside the United
        States, 92
8 Other Forms of Protection,   94
9 Conclusion,   95

1 OVERVIEW

Intellectual property is the branch of law that protects and, indeed, encourages the creation of certain products of the human mind or intellect. This chapter is intended to provide a basic understanding and appreciation of intellectual property law, especially as it relates to patents, trademarks, and trade secrets, in the United States and, to a lesser extent, in the remainder of the world (1). Issues and concerns particularly related to the drug discovery and development process are emphasized.

This chapter cannot, of course, provide the reader with sufficient detail to allow him or her to protect drug-related technology effectively and comprehensively. It is imperative to obtain competent legal counsel specializing in the area of intellectual property and technology transfer, preferably counsel with the appropriate drug research and biotechnology experience, as early in the research and development process as possible. This chapter should enable the reader to communicate and interact more effectively with counsel as

they jointly fashion, within the ongoing research and development process, the appropriate legal protection for the particular technology under development.

By making effective use of the legal protection afforded by the intellectual property laws in the United States and elsewhere, the drug discovery or biotechnology organization can protect its investment, enhance the value of the technology being developed, and earn a profit sufficient to allow and encourage further research into improving existing drugs and therapies as well as developing new drugs and therapies. By better understanding these intellectual property laws, the drug developer, together with experienced intellectual property counsel, can develop an effective intellectual property strategy. In this way, new and emerging technologies as well as new drug discoveries can be identified, managed, and protected as an integral part of an organization's research and development activities to create a strong intellectual property portfolio.

The rewards flowing from the development of a strong intellectual property portfolio can be significant. A patent allows the patent holder to exclude others from making, using, or selling the patented invention during the term of the patent. A carefully crafted intellectual property portfolio (including pending patent applications, issued patents, trademarks, and trade secrets) can serve many other purposes. It can be used defensively to prevent others from patenting the invention. It can present legitimate barriers to competitors attempting to enter a new field. It can allow time for recouping investments and establishing market position and identity. It can be used to generate revenues through licensing arrangements or outright sales of patent applications, issued patents, trademarks and associated goodwill, or trade secrets. It can be useful in obtaining outside financing or entering into shared research arrangements, joint ventures, or cross-licensing arrangements. In many instances, a startup biotechnology company's only marketable asset is its intellectual property. A carefully crafted and maintained patent portfolio can be an especially beneficial asset when seeking outside funding or negotiating an agreement with a large, well-established, and well-funded partner.

The application of intellectual property law to the field of drug discovery and biotechnology presents unique and challenging issues for the individual researcher, the research organization or company, and the intellectual property counsel. These issues arise mainly because of the fast-developing nature of the drug discovery and biotechnology field, the enormous investment in time and money required in the current regulatory climate to develop a new drug or treatment process and bring it to the marketplace, and the opportunity derived from the "biotechnology revolution" to achieve rapid breakthroughs in the health care area with the potential for substantial economic rewards. How the industry meets these challenges and how the legal system evolves and adapts to this rapidly changing field will significantly affect the development of the burgeoning biotechnology–pharmaceutical industry and the health care system in general. How well individual companies or research organizations protect their intellectual property will determine, to a significant degree, who will survive and prosper.

The development of a drug or treatment process from its conception to its introduction in the marketplace generally requires 6 to 10 yr, sometimes even more. This delay is generally the result of the time required for research and development, pilot plant studies, scale-up studies, animal studies, clinical studies, the necessary regulatory approvals (e.g., from the U.S. Food and Drug Administration (FDA)), marketing studies, and the like. A successful drug development program can cost hundreds of millions of dollars. The ability to protect that human and economic investment has become an increasingly important factor in the drug discovery and development process. A business organization, whether a startup company or an established pharmaceutical giant, often cannot justify the necessary investment if its intellectual property cannot be reasonably protected. Without such protection, a so-called free rider could offer the same or very similar drug or treatment process based on the developer's own research data at a significantly lower cost. Without the ability to protect and recover one's investment and earn a profit, drug discovery and development, for all practical purposes, could only be carried out or sponsored by governments or large nonprofit organizations. This would severely limit the number of persons generating new ideas, decrease the number of new drugs entering the marketplace, and increase the time required for the development of new drugs or treatment processes.

Intellectual property law—the body of law that includes patents, trademarks, trade secrets, and copyrights—provides the framework and mechanism by which investment in intellectual property can be protected. The drug discovery process, especially as it has developed in response to federal regulation and the recent biotechnology revolution, faces new and difficult challenges and issues within the field of intellectual property law. The biotechnology–pharmaceutical industry must recognize and understand these challenges and issues to take advantage of the protection now offered and to be prepared to adapt to modifications that may be made in intellectual property law in the future.

Patents are generally considered the strongest form of protection available for intellectual property and, therefore, should be the cornerstone of the intellectual property protection strategy. An effective patent strategy or program must first identify new and emerging technologies and inventions. A significant part of this program is educating researchers and other employees about the importance of protecting intellectual property and providing mechanisms and incentives to encourage them to bring forward their ideas and innovations for appropriate evaluation. Next, the patent strategy should provide a mechanism to evaluate the inventions and determine whether to file a patent application on a given invention and, if so, when and where to file throughout the world. It must also determine whether and when to update pending patent applications when new information and data become available. This will generally require a careful case-by-case evaluation of each invention, including determination of the likelihood of patentability and success in the ongoing research and FDA approval process. Unfortunately, such decisions must almost always be made without complete data or information and long before concrete assessments and estimates can be made concerning the ultimate technological and economic success of the invention.

Drug discovery has accelerated over the past several decades due to the continuous and phenomenally rapid advance of the underlying technology. The amount of information and data in the literature is enormous and is growing at an increasing rate. What is unobvious today to one of "ordinary skill in the art" may well be obvious tomorrow, next week, or next month. This rapidly expanding body of technical information dramatically increases the pressure to seek patent protection as early as possible—oftentimes before the invention is fully developed and its ramifications and significance are fully known.

Drug discovery technology has become increasingly complex and multidisciplinary. It is increasingly difficult for meaningful research to be carried out by individuals or even small research teams. Rather, large multidisciplinary teams bringing wide-ranging expertise to bear on a given problem are generally needed to stay ahead of the competition. The existence and requirements of such teams may have a significant effect on the patentability of drugs and treatment processes.

In addition to being new or novel, a product or process to be patentable must not have been obvious at the time the invention was made to "a person having ordinary skill in the art to which said subject matter pertains" (2). Just who is a person of ordinary skill in the drug discovery area? Clearly a person of ordinary skill in the art of drug discovery is at least a highly skilled individual, probably with an advanced degree. Does that person have a master's or Ph.D. degree in the field to which the invention is most closely related? Or does that person have advanced-level knowledge in more than one field associated with the invention? If so, in how many fields? Is the person of ordinary skill a single individual or a mythical person having the combined knowledge and skill of a multidisciplinary team in which each member possesses ordinary skill in a specific art? These questions remain for the

U.S. Patent and Trademark Office (PTO), and ultimately the courts, to decide. (The chapters of this book, each written by experts in their fields, illustrate the multidisciplinary nature of the technology and the difficulty in defining a person of "ordinary skill in the art.") Whatever the resolution, this determination will dramatically affect the patentability of drug-related inventions.

The complexity of this technology has already had a significant effect on the patent system. The level of expertise required of patent examiners in the PTO and the patent bar has significantly increased in the last 15 yr. The PTO has attempted to upgrade the educational level and background of the examiners assigned to drug discovery and biotechnology arts. The typical PTO examiner assigned to handle the first biotechnology patent applications was likely a bachelor-degree chemist with, perhaps, some biology background. Now, many examiners in this art have graduate-level degrees in biotechnology-related disciplines. In mid-1993, more than 65% of these examiners had advanced degrees, including over 45% with doctoral-level degrees (3). Similarly, the technological skills required by the patent bar preparing and prosecuting such patent applications has increased dramatically. Although there have been enormous gains, there still remains a significant shortage of examiners in the PTO and members of the patent bar who can readily handle this technology. This shortage is likely to become even more severe as the number of biotechnology patent applications increases over the next several years. For example, in 1988, the PTO's Biotechnology Art Unit received 9,790 patent applications. In 1992, the number of applications increased to 11,711 (3).

Another unique aspect of the drug discovery industry is that the majority of research is directed toward a relatively limited number of well-known target diseases or disorders (e.g., AIDS and cancer) and enabling technologies (e.g., receptors) that are useful in drug discovery. Due to the importance of these diseases and enabling technologies, and the potentially huge economic rewards, many research groups and organizations have turned their resources toward these relatively few targets (4). While one hopes that this intense competition will lead to near-term breakthroughs in new drugs, methods of treatment, and cures, the intense competition makes it more difficult to protect inventions made along the way. Also, because of the large number of groups working and filing patent applications in the same or closely related biotechnology research areas, the number of potential invention priority contests between rival inventors (i.e., patent interferences; see section 3.6 below) within the PTO is likely to be significantly higher than in other technologies. The increased possibility of interferences in the areas of drug discovery and treatment processes contributes to the pressure to file as quickly as possible.

Throughout most of the world outside the United States, patents are granted to the first to file rather than the first to invent. In such countries, the failure to file quickly can result in loss of valuable patent rights. And, if others independently make the same invention and obtain a patent, the inventor who files late may be prevented from using the very technology on which vast sums and significant human resources were spent.

The changing pathway for drug discovery also influences the way in which inventors or their assignees interact with the patent system (5). Historically, drug discovery and development was carried out by large pharmaceutical companies. More and more, the basic discovery and initial stages of drug development are being carried out by university research teams and startup or relatively small biotechnology companies. These groups generally do not have the internal economic resources to seek worldwide patent protection or to carry a new drug or therapy through the clinical stages. Outside funding, strategic alliances, or licensing arrangements are usually necessary as the research and development progresses. In seeking funding or other business arrangements, researchers are generally required to disclose at least basic business and/or technical information. On the other hand, extreme care should be taken to prevent public disclosure of inventions before the appropriate patent applications are filed. The United States has a 1-yr grace period in which a patent application can be filed after the first public disclosure, public use, or offer for sale of the subject matter of the invention. In most other countries, however, there is an "absolute novelty" requirement—public disclosure of the subject matter of the invention anywhere in the world before filing the patent application will likely preclude patent protection (see section 2.3 below). It is critical, therefore, that secrecy be maintained until the initial patent application is filed covering the invention. Once the initial patent application is filed (usually in the country where the invention is made or developed), corresponding applications can be filed within 1 year in most countries under prevailing international agreements (i.e., the Paris Convention; see section 5.1 below), claiming the benefit of the filing date of the initial application.

Secrecy may be difficult to maintain if one is seeking outside funding. Most potential investors demand significant business and technical details before making the desired investment. To the extent possible, however, the amount of technical information provided should be strictly limited and its use and dissemination carefully controlled. Confidentiality agreements are helpful in maintaining secrecy and are highly recommended when seeking private funding or joint research arrangements. Public funding and offerings, which trigger

the disclosure requirements of the Securities Act, the Securities Exchange Commission (SEC), and state Blue Sky laws, present even more difficult problems. Delaying public offerings until patent applications are filed is, when possible, generally recommended. A public disclosure, even if accidental or in violation of a confidentiality agreement, can preclude patent protection in most countries of the world. Once again, there is great pressure for filing patent applications as quickly as possible.

The requirements set forth in the patent law and as dictated by procedures for obtaining research funding—both in the United States and the rest of the world—also strongly encourage filing a patent application covering a new drug or treatment process as soon as possible. In many cases, it may be desirable or even necessary to file the patent application before complete data are available. For example, a patent application covering a protein for which only a partial DNA coding sequence has been determined may be filed in the United States to establish an early priority date for the invention. This would permit such preliminary information to be disclosed with reduced risk of losing valuable patent rights. Once the sequence is complete, a continuation-in-part (CIP) application, including the additional data, may be filed in the United States (and, if appropriate, the original application abandoned). The new material added in the CIP application receives the priority date of the actual CIP filing date. In some cases, it may be desirable to file several CIP applications as new data and/or discoveries are made. Using such an approach, however, has risks. In the United States, a patent application must be "enabling," i.e., it must provide a "written description of the invention, and of the manner and process of making and using it, in such full, clear, concise, and exact terms as to enable any person skilled in the art to which it pertains, or with which it is most nearly connected, to make and use the same" (6). If a patent application is filed too early, before sufficient data are available to allow an enabling disclosure, the application may be rejected or any resulting patent may be invalid. In the protein example, if it is determined that a complete DNA sequence is required for enablement, the first filed patent application would not be legally sufficient; the CIP application containing the full sequence, however, would be enabling.

One must take into account that the United States generally has a more stringent enablement requirement than many other countries. Thus, in the DNA sequencing example above, a partial sequence may be sufficient in other parts of the world. In such countries, a patent application having only a partial sequence and an earlier filing date may have priority over a second patent application filed by another party where the second application is based on a U.S. application, the filing of which was delayed because the full sequence was not yet complete (7).

This chapter presents a discussion of utility patents, trademarks, and trade secrets and emphasizes their use in protecting intellectual property in the drug discovery and biotechnology areas. Other forms of protection will be mentioned briefly.

2 PATENT PROTECTION AND STRATEGY

The U.S. Constitution provides that "Congress shall have [the] power . . . [t]o promote the progress of science and useful arts by securing for limited times to authors and inventors the exclusive right to their respective writings and discoveries" (8). In exercising that power, Congress has established a system for granting utility patents, design patents, and plant patents. Utility patents protect the functional aspects of products or processes and are granted for a term of 17 yr. Design patents protect the

ornamental design or aspect of a useful product and are granted for a term of 14 yr. Plant patents grant the right to exclude others from reproducing, selling, or using an asexually reproduced plant variety for a term of 17 yr. Certain sexually reproduced plant varieties can be protected under the Plant Variety Protection Act of 1970 for a term of 18 yr; plant variety "certificates" under this program are issued by the U.S. Department of Agriculture. Although design and plant patents can, in some cases, be an important part of a company's portfolio, this chapter concentrates on utility patents.

Utility patents (hereinafter *patents*) are generally considered the strongest form of legal protection for intellectual property. They grant the patent holder a "legal monopoly" on the invention for 17 yr in the United States. During the term of the patent, the patent holder can prevent others from making, using, or selling the patented invention in the United States (9). In exchange for this limited right to exclude, the patentee must fully disclose the invention to the public; at the end of the patent term, the invention is dedicated to the public.

Patent protection is limited geographically. For the most part, a U.S. patent does not provide legal protection from, or prevent, an act occurring outside the United States (and its territories and possessions) although that same act would fall within the scope of patent protection if carried out in the United States (the one exception is discussed in section 4). The same is generally true for other countries. Thus a comprehensive patent strategy should take into account the possibility of obtaining patent protection in all countries where an invention will be exploited (i.e., sold, manufactured, or used).

The U.S. patent system is designed to protect new and nonobvious products and processes. It protects the application of ideas and laws of nature; it does not protect the ideas or laws of nature themselves. Thus Einstein's $E = mc^2$ equation would not have been patentable, even though Einstein or others might have obtained patent protection for a nuclear power plant, a nuclear engine, or the myriad other products and processes derived from this basic principle. The idea or basic principle itself is available for all to use and develop.

In the United States, the 17-yr term of a patent is measured from its actual issue date. Largely because of the time involved in the FDA approval process and associated clinical trials, a considerable portion of the patent term can elapse before a patented drug can be sold in the marketplace. Thus the period effectively available for the drug developer to recoup its investment and earn a profit can be considerably shorter than the 17-yr patent term.

Beginning in the early 1980s, Congress has taken steps to significantly strengthen and improve the patent system. These steps include adding a reexamination process, authorizing the formation of the U.S. Court of Appeals for the Federal Circuit to hear appeals from the PTO and in patent infringement cases, and providing for the extension of the patent term for certain drug-related inventions. The patent system now provides substantially better and more consistent protection to technology in general than in the past and is now an even more attractive mechanism for the drug discovery and biotechnology industry to protect its intellectual property. As part of this revitalization, Congress provided a legal mechanism for extending the patent term up to 5 yr for qualifying drugs, medical devices, food additives, and methods "primarily us[ing] recombinant DNA technology in the manufacture of the product" to compensate for certain, but not all, delays in the regulatory and approval process (10). The patent term may be extended only if the approval of the first commercial use of the patented product occurs during the original patent term and the extension is applied for within 60 days of the approval. Due to the limited time in which to apply for the extension, it is important that patent counsel be informed when approval of a drug, medical device, or process is granted, so that the application for term extension can be filed within the required time period. The patent term extension process is jointly administered by the PTO and the FDA. The PTO determines whether a patent qualifies for the extension, and the FDA determines the allowable extension term.

2.1 Patent Strategy

Pharmaceutical and other high-technology industries are increasingly global in nature. More and more, competition in global markets requires effective global protection for intellectual property. As barriers to trade decrease and the legal mechanisms for protecting intellectual property are strengthened around the world, such protection will become even more important. It is an important part of any drug discovery organization's intellectual property strategy to determine how best to protect its intellectual property throughout its global market.

The simplest strategy would be to file patent applications for each invention in each and every country having a patent system. Such a strategy could, of course, be prohibitively expensive and in most cases less than cost-effective. A cost-benefit strategy should be applied to each particular invention and its uses. It is essential to evaluate the market potential of the invention around the world and the ability to control that market based on patent protection in key countries. For countries with interrelated markets, it may be possible to protect technology effectively in one country with a patent in another country.

Appropriate technical, business, marketing, and legal personnel should be involved in the decision-making process so that all relevant factors can be considered in determining whether to file a patent application on a given invention, and if so, when and where to file. The relevant factors will, of course, vary from case to case, as will their relative importance. For example, a startup company interested in developing a single drug or family of drugs may have a strong interest in obtaining as comprehensive patent coverage as possible. Unfortunately, a startup company may not have the resources necessary to seek such comprehensive patent coverage. A pioneer invention (i.e., one that breaks new ground or provides an important technical breakthrough and will likely dominate a particular industry segment) generally warrants wider patent protection than an invention that provides only an incremental improvement in an existing technology. Patent protection around the world is further discussed in section 5.

Improvements of previously patented inventions deserve special consideration in developing a patent strategy. Patents covering even relatively minor improvements can be important elements in expanding and extending protection of a basic technology. If the inventor or assignee of the improved invention is also the holder of the patent on the basic invention, there are generally two options. The improvement can either be kept as a trade secret or patented. Although a trade secret potentially has an unlimited lifetime (i.e., until secrecy is lost), the actual lifetime is likely to be much shorter, especially in the drug industry where detailed FDA disclosures are required. However, if the improvement is only an obvious variation of a basic invention, reliance on trade secret law may be the only option.

Generally, however, patent protection of the improvement is the preferred option. A patent for an improved drug or process may allow for additional patent protection for commercially significant embodiments past the term of the basic patent on the original invention. Obtaining such improvement patents will also make it more difficult for competitors to penetrate or expand into a market. "Driving stakes in the ground" in the form of improvement patents all around the basic or core invention makes it more difficult for any potential competitor to carve out a niche in the market.

In most cases where the developer of the improvement does not hold the patent on the basic or core invention, keeping the improvement as a trade secret is not a realistic option unless the patent covering the basic invention is due to expire in a relatively short time. Therefore, seeking patent protection is generally the best option. Assume the basic drug X is protected by a patent held by Company A and that Competitor B develops and patents a significantly improved drug formulation Y containing drug X. Company A can continue to market drug X but cannot offer drug formulation Y. Competitor B cannot offer either drug X alone or in the form of formulation Y. Competitor B may wish simply to license the improvement to Company A and collect revenues through a license. Or Competitor B can use its patent position on formulation Y as leverage in seeking access to the market. In many cases, Company A and Competitor B will agree to cross-license each other so that each can offer the improved formulation Y. Thus, for a competitor seeking to enter a market otherwise closed by another's patent position, improvement patents can provide valuable leverage.

Several differences between U.S. patent law and the patent law of almost every other country also significantly affect patent strategy, especially the determination of when to file a patent application in the United States. Some of the most important of these differences include the rules for determining priority and the requirement of "absolute novelty," which exists essentially everywhere except the United States. These differences are discussed directly below.

2.2 First to Invent Versus First to File

In our world of rapidly advancing technology, and particularly for active research areas such as drug discovery and biotechnology, investigators at different locations are often working in the same general area, often on the same specific research topic, and frequently discover essentially the same invention within a very short time of each other. Thus the issue often arises as to which of two (or more) inventors is entitled to a patent on a contemporaneously discovered invention.

U.S. patent law establishing entitlement to a patent in the case of essentially simultaneous invention is different from the law of substantially all other countries throughout the world. Nearly all countries award the patent to the first party who files a patent application (i.e., the first-to-file rule) (11). The United States, however, follows the first-to-invent rule whereby, at least in theory, the first to invent is generally entitled to the patent even though he or she was not the first to file a patent application. Thus it is possible that one party (i.e., the first to invent) who loses the race to the PTO may be entitled to patent protection in the United States while another party (i.e., the first to file) may be entitled to patent protection for the same invention in most other countries. This possibility increases the incentive for a party to file a patent application covering the invention as quickly as possible.

The U.S. PTO, on discovering that two or more parties have copending patent applications or a patent application and a recently issued patent claiming the same invention, may set up an interference

proceeding to determine which party is the first inventor of the subject matter. Such a determination is not straightforward. In an attempt to make the procedure as predictable as possible, a great number of rules—both substantive and procedural—have been adopted by the PTO to govern the proceedings and the gathering of the evidence necessary to establish the facts surrounding the making of the invention by each party. These rules give the party who was the first to file (the senior party) significant substantive and procedural advantages that significantly increase the senior party's chances of prevailing in the interference proceeding.

Generally, in the United States, the party who is first to "reduce an invention to practice" is given priority and awarded the patent, unless another party who reduced the invention to practice at a later date can prove that he or she was the first to conceive the invention and worked diligently to reduce it to practice from a time before the other party's date of conception (12). Reduction to practice may be an "actual reduction to practice" (physically making or carrying out the invention) or a "constructive reduction to practice" (filing a patent application). Therefore, in the United States, at least in theory, the filing date of a U.S. patent application may not control the outcome of the priority contest between parties who each actually reduced the invention to practice. As just noted, however, the party who files first has certain practical advantages in the interference proceeding.

Currently there is considerable interest in the world community for the United States to harmonize its laws with the rest of the industrialized world and adopt the first-to-file system. There is at least some likelihood that, within the next decade, the United States will adopt a first-to-file rule, or at least a modified first-to-file rule. Before doing so, however, the United States will likely insist that other major industrial countries enact changes in their laws to favor true international protection of patentable subject matter.

The adoption of the first-to-file rule in the United States may have only a relatively small effect on the drug discovery field, especially for large corporate entities and others involved in the global marketplace, because they already have significant incentives to file patent applications as quickly as possible. The adoption of the first-to-file rule in the United States more likely might have a significant effect on individual inventors or small corporations who may be interested almost entirely in the U.S. market or who do not have adequate resources for quickly developing inventions or filing patent applications. Such individuals and small corporations are generally at a significant disadvantage in any interference proceeding simply because of the cost involved. Such individual inventors and small corporations may not, therefore, be as deeply affected in a practical sense by a first-to-file rule as one might first imagine.

2.3 Absolute Novelty

In most countries, except the United States, a public disclosure of an invention before filing a patent application precludes obtaining patent protection for the invention. This is in contrast to the United States, where an applicant has 1 yr after publication, public use, or offer of sale of the subject matter of the invention in which to file a patent application. The effect of such a public disclosure is generally the same whether it is made by the inventor or by another (13). Thus, if protection outside the United States is desired, a patent application must be filed in at least one Paris Convention country (see section 5.1 below) before the public disclosure, followed by the filing of the corresponding applications in other countries within the convention

year. Public disclosure within the convention year does not adversely affect any later filed applications filed within the convention year.

Valuable patent rights can be lost because of early disclosure of the patentable technology. Such loss can be especially damaging to a company or organization involved in drug discovery because of the extensive market for drug and drug-related technology. Because of required public disclosure related to the FDA approval process, the patent rights associated with drug discovery are especially at risk through premature disclosure. Disclosure of technical information should be closely monitored and controlled as part of a comprehensive intellectual property program. All employees, including research, medical, technical, and business personnel, should be carefully educated in regard to the confidential nature of technical information and the consequences of premature disclosure. An essential component of the program is an evaluation procedure for all articles, abstracts, seminars, or presentations before actual submission or presentation. In addition to preventing premature disclosures, such an evaluation program can aid in educating personnel on the importance of protecting confidential information.

An intellectual property committee responsible for reviewing and approving all disclosures containing technical information, including FDA submissions, is highly recommended. In cases for which disclosure is a potential problem, the committee should, if possible, delay publication until the appropriate patent applications are filed or recommend against publication. To avoid delays in FDA submissions and scientific or technical publications, such submissions or publications should be reviewed by the committee as early as possible, to allow for sufficient time to prepare and file any necessary patent applications (14). Due to the importance of FDA submissions and the amount of technical data involved, it may be desirable to have at least one individual responsible for FDA matters included on the committee to ensure proper coordination between the functions.

The need for monitoring and controlling technical information does not end with the filing of the initial patent application. Disclosures relating to an invention claimed in an earlier patent application may also contain information concerning new inventions or improvements of the earlier claimed invention that may be the subject of later filed applications. In addition, control of the disclosure of inventions contained in a patent application may allow for filing patent application in countries requiring absolute novelty after expiration of the convention year, should that become necessary or desirable. Failures to file such applications within the convention year may be intentional (i.e., too expensive or perceived lack of technical merit) or accidental. If funds become available, or technical merit is established, or the accident discovered, such applications may be filed after the convention year if there has not been a public disclosure. Any patent filed after the convention year, however, cannot rely on the earlier priority date; its effective filing date will be the actual filing date in the specific country. Loss of the priority date can be significant because additional prior art may be available against the application.

3 REQUIREMENTS FOR PATENTS

To obtain a patent on an invention in the United States, the inventor or inventors must, as the initial step, file a patent application describing the invention in such terms as to teach one of ordinary skill in the art how to make and use the invention and claiming the subject matter that the inventor (or inventors) regards as the invention. The subject matter of the claimed invention must be within the statutory classes of patentable inventions. In addition, the claimed invention must have utility and be both new and nonobvious. The requirements for patentability (especially as to what constitutes patentable subject matter) can vary considerably throughout the world. This section addresses the requirements for patentability in the United States and, to a much lesser extent, variations encountered in a few representative countries. The actual patenting procedure in the U.S. PTO also will be briefly discussed.

3.1 Patentable Subject Matter in the United States

In the United States, patentable subject matter includes "any new and useful process, machine, manufacture, or composition of matter, or any new and useful improvement thereof" (15). An invention must be claimed so as to fit within one of the four statutory classes of inventions: process, machine, manufacture, and composition of matter. A process is essentially the means to achieve a desired end, e.g., a method to synthesize a drug or a method of using a drug to treat a specific condition. The other patentable classes are basically the end products themselves. These four classifications are broad and generally encompass the vast majority of technological advances. Examples of generally nonpatentable subject matter include laws of nature or abstract ideas, products of nature, algorithms (a physical process using an algorithm can, however, be patented (16)), printed materials, and business methods.

The subject matter of most inventions clearly falls within one of the four statutory classes. But for cases where the issue of patentable subject matter is raised, the line between what is patentable and nonpatentable often cannot be clearly drawn and must be evaluated on a case-by-case basis.

Consider "products of nature": compounds occurring in nature normally cannot be patented. So a naturally occurring drug collected from, for example, a particular plant species is not generally patentable. However, if through human intervention the naturally occurring drug is produced in a purer or more concentrated form not naturally occurring, the new form of the drug may be patentable. Even if the actual drug is not patentable, a new and unobvious use for that drug may be patentable. Or the combination of the drug with other active ingredients may be patentable. Likewise, a new method of preparing, concentrating, or purifying the drug (even if the drug is exactly the same as the naturally occurring drug) may also be patentable.

Patentable pharmaceutical inventions generally and broadly include drugs, diagnostics, intermediates, drug formulations, dosage forms, methods of treatments, kits containing a drug or diagnostic, methods of preparing the drug or diagnostic, and the like. More recently, microorganisms, plasmids, cell lines, DNA, animals, and other biological materials have been found patentable if they are the result of human intervention or manipulation. Initially, the PTO resisted granting patents on living organisms on the basis that the claimed invention was a product of nature. The U.S. Supreme Court in the landmark case of *Diamond v. Chakrabarty* (17) held that new life-forms (i.e., bacteria altered genetically to digest crude oil) can be patentable subject matter. In 1987, the PTO formally issued a notice indicating that it "considers nonnaturally occurring nonhuman multicellular living organisms, including animals, to be patentable subject matter" (18). It is now clearly established that nonnaturally occurring biological materials, including microorganisms, plants, and animals, can be protected by patents in the United States (19).

In addition to fitting into one of the statutory classes, a patentable invention must also possess utility (i.e., it must provide some useful function to society). The invention must be operable and accomplish some function that is not clearly illegal (20). A chemical compound for which the only known use is to make another compound, which does not have a known use, is not patentable; if, however, the final product is useful, then the starting material is also useful and has sufficient utility for patentability (21). The patent specification must disclose at least one nontrivial utility for the invention. Thus at least one practical utility for a new composition of matter (e.g., a new drug) must be disclosed. Where possible, however, it is generally recommended that several utilities are disclosed to reduce the risk that the PTO will find the invention lacking utility. Composition of matter claims covering the drug will generally protect all uses of the drug, even ones not disclosed in the patent application and ones discovered after the patent issues. The utility of the drug does not have to be patentable in its own right. Nor does the utility have to be developed or discovered by the inventor of the composition of matter; the inventor merely has to disclose, and sometime provide proof of, the utility.

Generally, if the utility disclosed in the patent specification is easily understood and is consistent with known scientific laws, the PTO will not question it. If, however, the disclosed utility clearly conflicts with general scientific principles or is incredible on its face (e.g., a perpetual motion machine), the PTO will presume the invention lacks utility and will require strong evidence supporting operability (22). Thus, for example, it is likely that an invention asserting, as the only utility, a complete cure for leukemia, other cancer, or AIDS will require an especially strong showing of effectiveness (23).

For inventions involving pharmaceuticals and methods of treatment, the PTO often requires a relatively high level of proof for the disclosed utility. A utility likely to be deemed incorrect or unbelievable by one skilled in the relevant art in view of the contemporary knowledge of that art will require adequate proof. The proof required can generally be based on clinical data, *in vivo* data, *in vitro* data, or combinations thereof, where such data would convince one skilled in the art. The data may be included in the patent specification as filed or provided (or, if appropriate, supplemented) in a later submitted declaration or affidavit (24).

The data necessary to support utility will, of course, vary as the relevant art advances. For example, proving the effectiveness of a new drug, which is also the first of a new class of drugs for a particular disease, will require more convincing evidence than a later, but still new and nonobvious, drug of the same class. The PTO has recently indicated that

> if the utility relied on is directed *solely* to the treatment of humans, evidence of utility, if required, must generally be clinical evidence . . . although animal tests may be adequate where the art would accept these as appropriately correlated with human utility or where animal tests are coupled with other evidence, including clinical evidence and a structural similarity to compounds marketed commercially for the same indicated uses. If there is no assertion of human utility or if there is an assertion of animal utility, operativeness for use on standard test animals is adequate for patent purposes (24).

Thus the data required to show utility for human use are generally of the amount and type that those skilled in the art would consider acceptable for extrapolation to *in vivo* human effectiveness. Clinical data, while not required, will generally be preferred and, where available, should normally be provided. For the PTO to require clinical testing in all cases of pharmaceutical inventions would have, however, a decidedly detrimental effect on the industry

and its research efforts and, most likely, would be inconsistent with the overall goals of the patent system.

3.2 Patentable Subject Matter Outside the United States

Patentable subject matter in many countries (especially for health-related and biotechnology inventions) is often significantly restricted compared with the United States. Most countries do not allow plants or animals to be patented. Both the United States and Japan currently allow genetically engineered animals to be protected by patent. The patentability of genetically engineered animals is currently being considered in Europe (25). Many countries do not allow pharmaceuticals or methods of medical treatment to be patented. Each country will, of course, have its own specific limitations and exceptions for patentable subject matter (26). It is not possible in the present chapter to provide an even limited discussion of such patentable subject matter. Moreover, any details provided could very well be out of date in a relatively short time. However, a few examples from selected countries (27) are helpful to illustrate the variations in patentable subject matter.

1. *Australia.* Medicines that are mixtures of known ingredients are generally not patentable.
2. *Canada.* Plants and methods of medical treatment are generally not patentable.
3. *France.* Surgical or therapeutic treatment of humans and animals or diagnostic methods for humans and animals are generally not patentable (however, the first use of a known composition or substance for carrying out these methods may be patentable); plants and animals and biological processes for producing them (except microbiological

processes and products) are generally not patentable.

4. *Germany*. Plants, animals, and biological processes for producing plants or animals (except microbiological processes and products) are not patentable; surgical, therapeutic, and diagnostic methods applied to humans or animals are generally not patentable, although the products used in these processes may be patentable.

5. *Italy*. Plants and animals as well as the methods of producing them (except microbiological processes) are generally not patentable; surgical, therapeutic, and diagnostic methods applied to humans and animals are generally not patentable, although compositions for carrying out these methods may be; pharmaceuticals are patentable, but the compounding of medicine in a pharmacy is not.

6. *Japan*. Generally similar to patentable subject matter in the United States.

7. *Sweden*. Methods for treating humans and animals are generally not patentable, although products used in these methods may be patentable; plants and animals and processes (except microbiological processes and products) for producing them are generally not patentable.

8. *UK*. Animals and plants and nonmicrobiological processes for producing them are generally not patentable; surgical, therepeutic, and diagnostic methods for humans and animals are generally not patentable, although compositions for use in such methods may be patentable.

Applicants interested in seeking worldwide protection for inventions, especially for the drug discovery and biotechnology industries, must take these differences in patentable subject matter into account. Even in jurisdictions where specific classes of inventions cannot be patented, it is often possible to claim the invention in a manner so as to be within patentable subject matter. For example, many countries that do not allow drugs to be patented may allow claims directed to a method of making the drug. Likewise, many countries that do not allow patent claims directed at methods for medical treatment of humans may allow claims directed to devices or compositions for carrying out the treatment processes. Generally, locally accredited patent counsel in the relevant country is retained to aid in the prosecution of the application because of the need for knowledge and understanding of substantive and procedural patent law in the relevant country. One of the tasks of such counsel is to adapt the legal definition of the invention to local law and practice, especially in regard to patentable subject matter.

3.3 Patent Specification

The specification is that part of a patent application in which the inventor describes and discloses his or her invention in detail. In the United States, the specification "shall contain a written description of the invention, and of the manner and process of making and using it, in such full, clear, concise, and exact terms as to enable any person skilled in the art to which it pertains, or with which it is most nearly connected, to make and use the same, and shall set forth the best mode contemplated by the inventor of carrying out his [or her] invention" (28). Furthermore, the specification "shall conclude with one or more claims particularly pointing out and distinctly claiming the subject matter the applicant regards as his [or her] invention" (29). Thus the specification must meet four general requirements: (*1*) provide a written description, (*2*) provide sufficient detail to teach persons of ordinary skill in the art how to make and use the invention, (*3*) reveal the best mode of making and using the invention known by the inventor at the time the application is filed, and (4) provide at least one claim covering the applicant's invention. Each of these requirements will be discussed in turn below. Almost without exception, the requirements for a legally sufficient specification in other countries are less stringent than in the United States. Thus a patent application that is legally sufficient in the United States is usually sufficient for filing in other countries with only relatively minor modifications to conform it to specific national regulations and practices of the relevant country (30).

3.3.1 WRITTEN DESCRIPTION. The claimed invention must be the invention described in the specification. In other words, the claims must be "supported" by the specification as originally filed. Thus the claims cannot encompass or contain more or different elements, steps, or compositions than are described in the specification. The claims cannot be amended or new claims added during prosecution of the patent application in the PTO unless the portion added is found within or supported by the specification as originally filed. The test for whether amended or new claims are supported is generally "whether one skilled in the art, familiar with the practice of the art at the time of the filing date, could reasonably have found the 'later' claimed invention in the specification as [originally] filed" (31).

Although new matter cannot be introduced into the specification or claims by amendment during prosecution (32), not all additions to the specification constitute new matter. For example, an applicant can generally supplement the specification by relying on well-known principles, prior art, and "inherency" (33). New matter, however, can be added by filing a CIP application claiming a priority date of the earlier filed application for the subject matter

disclosed in the original application. The effective filing date for the newly added subject matter (i.e., the new matter) is the actual filing date of the CIP application. Nonetheless, it is generally recommended that the specification as originally filed be as complete as possible.

Care should be taken in preparing the patent specification to consider fully the ramifications of the invention and the possibility of extending or expanding the scope of the invention. Thus, if a specific new drug is developed, consideration should be given to structural and functional analogs. For example, in many cases, the effectiveness of a drug will not be significantly affected by replacing a methyl group with an alkyl group containing, for example, two to six carbon atoms. Such variations, if allowed by the technology and the prior art, can considerably expand the scope of the claimed invention and the scope of protection afforded by the patent (34).

3.3.2 ENABLEMENT. In the United States, the specification, as filed, must teach one of ordinary skill in the art how to make and use the invention without undue experimentation. Enablement is essentially what the inventor gives to the public in exchange for the 17-yr exclusive right afforded by the patent. The public must be able to understand the invention based on the specification to build on the invention and develop new technology. Furthermore, the public is entitled to a complete description of the invention and the manner of making and using it so that the public can practice the invention after the patent expires. A specification that fails to teach one of ordinary skill in the art how to make and use the invention is not legally sufficient.

The enablement requirement does not mandate that each and every detail of the invention be included or that the specification be in the form of a detailed "cookbook" with every step specified to the last detail (35). Rather, the skilled artisan must be able to practice the invention without "undue experimentation." Generally, "a considerable amount of experimentation is permissible, if it is merely routine, or if the specification ... provides a reasonable amount of guidance with respect to the direction in which the experimentation should proceed" (36). Although the acceptable amount of experimentation will vary from case to case, the factors normally considered by the PTO and the courts in determining the level of permissible experimentation include (1) quantity of experimentation required, (2) amount of direction or guidance provided by the specification, (3) presence or absence of working examples, (4) nature of the invention, (5) state of the prior art, (6) relative skill of workers in the art, (7) predictability or unpredictability of the art, and (8) breadth of the claims (37). The level of acceptable experimentation will vary as the state of the art advances and the level of skill in the art increases.

Working examples are one factor in determining whether the specification is enabling. They are not required if the specification otherwise teaches one skilled in the art how to practice the invention without undue experimentation. However, in appropriate cases and if drafted with sufficient detail, such examples provide a relatively easy and straightforward way in which to make the specification enabling. So-called paper examples (i.e., examples describing work that has not actually been carried out (38)) can be used to satisfy the enablement requirement if the level of predictability for the art and invention is sufficiently high.

Pharmaceutical patents, especially those involving microorganisms or other biological material, can raise significant enablement issues. These issues arise whether the microorganism or other biological material is simply used in an invention sought to be patented or is itself the subject matter sought to be patented. If the microorganism is known and readily available or can be prepared using a procedure described in the specification, the enablement requirement is fulfilled. Otherwise, the applicant may need to take additional steps to comply with the enablement requirement. In such cases, this requirement can normally be satisfied by the deposit of a microorganism or other biological material in a depository meeting PTO requirements. The deposit must be made in "a depository affording permanence of the deposit and ready accessibility thereto by the public if a patent is granted" (24). Once the patent is granted, all restrictions on the availability of the deposit must be irrevocably removed. The PTO has indicated that "permanent availability" is

satisfied if the depository is contractually obligated to store the deposit for a reasonable time after expiration of the enforceable life of the patent. The [PTO] will not insist on any particular period after expiration of the enforceable life of the patent. The enforceable life of the patent for this purpose is considered to be seventeen years plus six (6) years to cover the statute of limitations. Any deposit which is made under the Budapest Treaty will be for a term acceptable to the [PTO], unless the thirty years from the date of deposit will expire before the end of the enforceable life of the patent. With this one exception, any deposit made under the Budapest Treaty will meet all of the requirements for a suitable deposit except that assurances must also be provided that all restrictions on the availability to the public of the deposited microorganism or other biological material will be irrevocably removed upon the granting of the patent (24).

The submitter will generally have a continuing responsibility to replace the deposit during the enforceable life of the patent should the deposit become nonviable or otherwise unavailable from the depository.

The Budapest Treaty enables an applicant to make a deposit of a microorganism or other biological material in a single "international cell depository authority" and thereby satisfy the enabling requirements of the signatory nations to the treaty (and, generally, nonsignatory countries as well) (39). Where a deposit is required and patent protection outside the United States will be sought, a deposit under the Budapest Treaty will generally be recommended, because the applicant can minimize the number of deposits required. Deposits made under the Budapest Treaty are generally available to certain "certified parties" 18 months after the priority date (i.e., after the patent application is published) (40). For purposes of U.S. patent law, deposits can be made outside of the Budapest Treaty so long as the conditions required by the PTO are ensured. Under U.S. law, deposits are generally not required to be released to the public until the patent issues. Should the applicant later determine that protection outside the United States will be sought, a non–Budapest Treaty deposit can generally be converted to a Budapest Treaty deposit. The major depository in the United States is the American Type Cell Culture Collection (ATCC) in Rockville, Maryland. The ATCC is an "international cell depository authority" under the Budapest Treaty; the ATCC also accepts non–Budapest Treaty deposits.

Deposits can also provide a convenient mechanism whereby the patent owner can monitor individuals and organizations obtaining samples of the deposit during the life of the patent. Most depositories will provide the submitter with notice of sample requests (in some cases a relatively small fee may be required). Such information can be helpful in enforcing patent rights. Especially in cases where the deposited material is patented, the patent holder may wish to consider a simple "letter license" allowing the requester to use the deposited material only in a certain manner (e.g., research purposes only) and requiring the requester to report any commercial uses of, or derived from, the deposited material.

3.3.3 BEST MODE. The specification must "set forth the best mode contemplated by the inventor of carrying out his [or her] invention" (28). The inventor cannot hide or conceal the best physical mode of making or using the invention. The purpose of this requirement "is to restrain inventors from applying for patents while at the same time concealing from the public preferred enbodiments of their inventions" (41). Questions of failure to meet the best mode requirements are rarely raised during prosecution of a patent in the PTO. Best mode issues are more often raised during interference proceedings or during litigation to enforce the patent.

The inventor must disclose the best mode known to him or her at the time the application was filed. If the inventor was aware of a better mode at the time of filing the application but did not disclose it, the entire patent is invalid and no claims are enforceable. However, a better mode of carrying out the invention discovered after the filing date need not be disclosed (42). Inventors should be carefully advised about the importance of the best mode requirement and of the necessity of informing patent counsel of any improvements made or considered before the actual filing date (43). Of particular concern is the time period between preparation of the application and its filing date; any potential improvements made during this period must be carefully evaluated to determine whether they must be included in the specification to satisfy the best mode requirement. Any improvements made after the application is filed (especially those made shortly after the filing date) should be carefully documented in case it ever becomes necessary to prove they were made after the filing date.

Generally, the best mode requirement focuses on the inventor's state of mind at the time the application was filed. It is the best mode contemplated by the inventor, not anyone else, for carrying out the invention. It is generally immaterial whether the failure to include the best mode in the specification was intentional or accidental. The subjective test is whether the inventor knew of a better mode at the time of the filing date, and if so, whether it is *adequately* disclosed in the specification (44). In some cases, deposit of biological materials may also be required to satisfy the best mode requirement. It is possible to include the best mode in the specification but to describe the best mode so poorly as to effectively conceal it. Because the potential penalty for failure to meet the best mode requirement is invalidity of the entire patent, considerable care should be taken to identify the best mode contemplated by the inventor and to describe it carefully and fully.

3.3.4 CLAIMS. The specification must "conclude with one or more claims particularly pointing out and distinctly claiming the subject matter which the applicant regards as his [or her] invention" (29). Claims are the numbered paragraphs (each only one sentence long) at the end of the patent specification. The claims define the metes and bounds of the exclusive right granted by the patent. Each claim defines a separate right to exclude others from making, using, or selling embodiments coming within the scope of the specific claim.

The claims are critically important. They require careful drafting, preferably by highly qualified and experienced patent counsel, to cover the invention as broadly and comprehensively as appropriate. Normally the claims should be drafted as broadly as the prior art and the specification allow. Allowable claim scope will, of course, depend in large part on the state of the art. Inventions in a crowded art (i.e., technolo-

gy with a relatively large amount of closely related prior art) can generally only be claimed relatively narrowly. Inventions for which there is relatively little prior art can be claimed more broadly. Generally, one attempts to draft one or more independent claims that describe the invention as broadly as the prior art will allow and then narrower, dependent claims specific to preferred embodiments, with dependent claims of intermediate scope in between. A dependent claim refers to an earlier claim and incorporates by reference all the limitations of the earlier claim and adds additional limitations. Thus the scope of the claimed invention generally varies from the broader independent claim or claims to the narrower, more restricted dependent claims. Should a court later find, for example, that the broader claims are obvious over the prior art, the narrower claims, with added limitations or elements, may still be valid and enforceable.

Normally it is also preferred that the invention be claimed so as to fit into as many of the statutory classifications as possible. For example, for a newly discovered drug, one might attempt to claim a method of making the drug, the drug itself, formulations containing the drug, and a method of using the drug to treat one or more conditions. For a new diagnostic, one might attempt to claim a method of making the diagnostic, the diagnostic itself, a method of using the diagnostic, and a kit containing the diagnostic. Other aspects of claims are discussed below.

3.4 Invention Must Be New and Unobvious

In the United States, an invention to be patentable must be both new (45) and unobvious (2) over the prior art. Generally, the prior art is the body of existing technological information (i.e., the state of the art) against which the invention is evaluated. Prior art may include other patents from anywhere in the world; printed publications from anywhere in the world; U.S. patent applications that eventually issue as patents; public use or offer for sale of the subject matter embodying the invention in the United States; and, depending on the circumstances, unpublished and unpatented research activities of others in the United States. These types of prior art are defined in § 102 of the Patent Statute.

U.S. patents are effective as prior art in the United States as of their filing dates. Patents from other countries, as well as publications from anywhere in the world, are effective as prior art in the United States as of their actual publication dates. Admissions by the inventor as to the content or status of the prior art, even if later shown to be incorrect, are also part of the prior art for that invention. Care should be taken, therefore, to ensure that admissions against interest are not made in the patent application or during prosecution of the application before the PTO. Unless it is absolutely clear that a given document qualifies legally as prior art against the invention, it should not be referred to as "prior art" or otherwise admitted to be "prior art."

3.4.1 NOVELTY UNDER 35 U.S.C. § 102. The determination of novelty of an invention is generally straightforward: the issue is whether the invention is old or new. If a single prior art reference shows identically every element of the claimed invention (i.e., anticipation), the invention is not novel and, therefore, not patentable. The anticipating reference must, however, be enabling. In other words, it must teach one of ordinary skill in the art how to practice the invention. Thus the inclusion of only the name or chemical structure of a compound in a reference, without providing a method of making the compound, will generally not be considered to have anticipated a later patent claiming that compound (46). On the other hand, an anticipating prior art reference is not required to provide a use or utility for a compound (47). Thus a reference that teaches how to make a specific compound but does not disclose a use will still prevent a later inventor, who discovers a use, from claiming the compound itself (48). The later inventor may be able to claim the use or a process taking advantage of a newly discovered property of the compound, if such use or process is new and nonobvious. In some cases, especially where new uses have been discovered, the effective amount required or the mode of administration of, for example, a drug may provide sufficient novelty for patentability.

An invention may also not be patentable under § 102 if certain events (so-called statutory bars) occur more than 1 yr before the patent application is filed in the PTO. The statutory bars are designed to encourage the inventor to file his or her patent application in a timely manner. For example, a written description of the invention, a public use, or offer of sale of the subject matter of the invention in the United States more than 1 yr before the filing date of the application bars the invention from being patented. An inventor has, therefore, a 1-yr grace period after such a public disclosure in which to file a patent application in the United States.

Most countries other than the United States require absolute novelty. A written description, public use, or offer of sale that actually discloses the invention would, in most cases, prevent the inventor from obtaining patent protection outside of the United States. If worldwide patent protection is important, as is likely in almost all drug-related inventions, one should file a patent application covering the invention before any public disclosure occurs. Any potential public disclosures should be carefully screened and, where appropriate, controlled to ensure that valuable patent rights are not lost.

3.4.2 OBVIOUSNESS UNDER 35 U.S.C. § 103.

Even if the invention is novel under § 102, the invention may not be patentable under § 103 if "the differences between the subject matter sought to be patented and the prior art are such that the subject matter as a whole would have been obvious at the time the invention was made to a person having ordinary skill in the art to which the subject matter pertains" (2). The determination of obviousness under § 103 is considerably more difficult than the determination of novelty under § 102. Obviousness is determined using a three-part inquiry: (1) a determination of the scope and content of the prior art, (2) a determination of the differences between the prior art and the claimed invention, and (3) a determination of the level of ordinary skill in the art (49).

Relevant and applicable prior art is that which is pertinent to a determination of obviousness of the claimed invention under § 103. Prior art for determining obviousness is not limited to the narrow technical area of the invention. The relevant prior art is normally found in the general technical field (or fields) to which the claimed invention is directed as well as analogous fields to which one of ordinary skill in that field or fields would reasonably turn or use to solve the problem. Factors used to evaluate the level of ordinary skill often include (1) educational level of the inventor, (2) nature of problems generally encountered in the art, (3) solutions provided by the prior art for these problems, (4) rate of innovation in the art, (5) level of sophistication of the art, and (6) educational level of active workers in the art (50). These factors, when applied to the drug discovery and development field, suggest a high level of ordinary skill in this art.

In addition, so-called secondary considerations or objective indices of nonobviousness are often used in determining whether an invention is obvious (49). Secondary considerations that are used in support of a showing of nonobviousness and patentability include, for example, commercial success, a long-standing problem that resisted solution until the invention was made, failure of others to solve the problem, unexpected results, copying of the invention by others in the art, and initial skepticism in the art concerning the success or value of the invention. Such secondary considerations provide evidence about how others in the art viewed the advance provided by the claimed invention. They are often used in arguments presented to the PTO by the applicant in support of patentability. For such secondary considerations to be useful in establishing patentability, there must be a direct relationship between the secondary factor and the merits of the claimed invention. Therefore, to be useful in demonstrating nonobviousness, commercial success should be predominately the result of the benefits and merits of the invention rather than, for example, advertising or marketing considerations. Independent and essentially simultaneous development of the invention by others in the art to solve the same or very similar problem is one secondary consideration that supports the conclusion that the invention is obvious.

Against this factual background of the three-pronged test and secondary considerations (if any), the obviousness or nonobviousness of the invention is determined. The decision maker must step back in time and determine whether a person of ordinary skill would have found the invention as a whole obvious at the time the invention was made. The Court of Appeals for the Federal Circuit has offered the following guidelines for this determination:

> [T]he following tenets of patent law ... must be adhered to when applying § 103: (1) the claimed invention must be

considered as a whole ... [because] though the difference between [the] claimed invention and prior art may seem slight, it may also have been the key to advancement of the art ...; (2) the references must be considered as a whole and suggest the desirability and thus the obviousness of making the combination; (3) the references must be viewed without the benefit of hindsight vision afforded by the claimed invention; [and] (4) "ought to be tried" is not the standard with which obviousness is determined (51).

In the PTO, obviousness rejections are usually based on the combination of two or more prior art references. However, to support an obviousness rejection, the prior art references must do more than simply provide the elements of the claimed invention when combined. The references must also provide the motivation for the person of ordinary skill to combine the references in a way so as to achieve the claimed invention (52).

The standard for determining obviousness is not the same as "obvious to try." Thus a claim cannot be properly rejected on obviousness grounds simply because all the parameters or numerous possibilities in the prior art reference could be varied or tried to arrive at the successful combination of the claimed invention, unless the references also provided directions to the successful combination. Nor can a claim be properly rejected because it might be obvious to try a new technology or approach that offers promise for solving a particular problem unless the prior art provides more than general guidance as to the form of the invention or methods to achieve it (53). Nor can a claim be properly rejected using hindsight to reconstruct the invention from the prior art using applicant's own patent specification (54).

Once a case of *prima facie* obviousness is made out, the burden shifts to the applicant to rebut obviousness by showing that the invention had unexpected or surprising results (55). Unexpected results for a drug or drug formulation can include properties superior to those of the prior art compound including, for example, greater pharmaceutical activity than would have been predicted from the prior art, greater effectiveness, reduced toxicity or side effects, effectiveness at lower dosage, greater site-specific activity, and the like as well as properties that the prior art compound does not have. The unexpected results can be included in the patent application itself or presented by affidavit or declaration during prosecution of the patent application. If such unexpected results cannot be shown in cases of *prima facia* obviousness, the invention is not patentable. On the other hand, if a case of *prima facie* obviousness is not made out, it is not necessary to offer rebuttal evidence in the form of unexpected or surprising results for patentability.

Composition of Matter Claims Prior art compounds that are structurally similar to the claimed compound or drug may render the claimed compound obvious and, therefore, unpatentable. But "[a]n assumed similarity based on a comparison of formulae must give way to evidence that the assumption is erroneous" (56). Recently, the Court of Appeals for the Federal Circuit reaffirmed this standard for *prima facie* obviousness as applied to composition of matter claims:

This court ... reaffirms that structural similarity between claimed and prior art subject matter, proved by combining references or otherwise, where the prior art gives reasons or motivation to make the claimed compositions, creates a *prima facie* case of obviousness, and that the burden (and opportunity) then falls on an applicant to rebut the *prima facie* case. Such rebuttal or argument can consist of a comparison of test data showing that the claimed composition possesses unexpectedly superior properties or properties that the prior art does not have (57).

The court also affirmed that *prima facie* obviousness does not require, given structural similarity, the same or similar utility between the claimed compositions and the prior art composition (57).

Structural similarity to support a case of *prima facie* obviousness is often found in cases of homologous series of compounds, isomers, stereoisomers, esters and corresponding free acids, and the like. Bioisosterism, which may be of particular interest to the medicinal and pharmaceutical researcher, can also give rise to *prima facie* obviousness for both a compound and for methods of using such compounds (58). Bioisosterism recognizes that substitution of an atom or group of atoms for another atom or group of atoms having similar size, shape, and electron density generally provides compounds having similar biological activity. For example, the Court of Appeals for the Federal Circuit found that the use of amitriptyline for treating depression was obvious in view of the closely related antidepressant imipramine. Imipramine differs structurally from amitriptyline by replacement of the unsaturated carbon in the center ring of amitriptyline with a nitrogen atom. Another prior art reference showed that chloropromazine (a phenothiazine derivative) and chloroprothixene (a 9-aminoalkylene-thioxanthene derivative) had similar biological properties. Chloropromazine and chloroprothixene differ in the same manner as imipramine and amitriptyline (i.e., an unsaturated carbon versus nitrogen in the central ring structure) and are also structurally related, but not as closely as imipramine, to amitriptyline. In fact, this prior art reference "concluded that, when the nitrogen atom located in the central ring of the phenothiazine compound is interchanged with an unsaturated carbon atom as in the corresponding 9-aminoalkylene-thioxanthene compound, the

pharmacological properties of the thioxanthene derivatives resemble very strongly the properties of the corresponding phenothiazines" (59).

As indicated above, an applicant has the opportunity to rebut the case of *prima facie* obviousness by presenting evidence showing unexpected or surprising results. In cases for which it is known that the compound to be claimed is structurally similar to known compounds, it is generally preferred that the data supporting patentability be included in the application as filed. Even if the *prima facie* case against the compound cannot be overcome, it may be possible in some cases to obtain at least some patent protection by claiming a method of making the compound or a method of using the compound.

Process Claims There are generally two types of process or method claims: (*1*) claims directed to a method of synthesizing or otherwise transforming a chemical or biological material and (*2*) claims directed to a method of using particular compounds or materials to achieve a desired result. The same basic obviousness standard is generally applied to process claims as is applied to other claims, including composition of matter claims. The Court of Appeals for the Federal Circuit in *In re Durden* held that the use of novel starting materials and/or the production of novel products (even if the products are patentable in their own right) in a known process for making a compound may make the process new but does not necessarily make it unobvious (60). The PTO interpreted *In re Durden* as effectively holding that an old process could never become unobvious through the use of novel starting materials and/or the creation of novel products. More recently, the Court of Appeals for the Federal Circuit suggested that *In re Durden* merely "refused to adopt an unvarying rule that the fact that nonobvious starting materials and nonobvious products are involved *ipso facto* makes the process obvious" and added:

> The materials used in a claimed process, as well as the results obtained therefrom, must be considered along with the specific nature of the process, and the fact that new or old, obvious or nonobvious, materials are used or result from the process are only factors to be considered, rather than conclusive indicators of the obviousness or nonobviousness of a claimed process (61).

The patentability of process claims, whether method of making or method of using, should be determined in the same way as any other claim, i.e., by applying § 103 to determine whether the invention as a whole is obvious or unobvious.

3.5 Procedure for Obtaining Patents in the U.S. PTO

Obtaining a patent in the United States involves an *ex parte* procedure solely between the inventor or the inventor's assignee and the PTO (62). The proceedings between the applicant and the PTO are conducted in writing. The proceedings themselves and the written record of the proceedings, often called the file or prosecution history, are carried out and maintained in secret. If and when the patent actually issues, the secrecy of the proceeding ends and the entire written record is open to the public. Should a patent not issue, the record will, in most cases, be maintained in secret (63). Thus, in most cases and assuming corresponding patent applications were not filed in other countries, an abandoned U.S. patent application will remain secret and the information contained therein may be maintained as a trade secret. If a corresponding patent application has been filed elsewhere in the world, however, retention of any trade secrets contained therein is possible only until the application is published (normally 18 months after the priority date).

For invention developed in the United States, the patenting process generally begins with filing a patent application that meets the statutory requirements of the PTO. A flow chart generally illustrating the U.S. patenting procedure is shown in Figure 3.1. Once an application is filed in the United States, the applicant or assignee has 12 months in which to file patent applica-

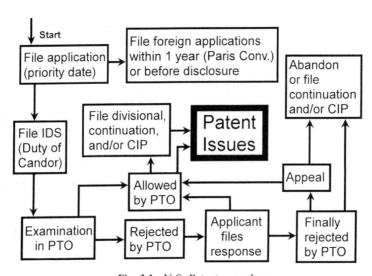

Fig. 3.1 U.S. Patent procedure.

tions throughout the rest of the world. Normally, the PTO will not have undertaken the initial examination of the application before the expiration of the 12-month period. Thus one normally does not have the benefit of the PTO's initial patentability review before decisions must be made concerning filings elsewhere.

The applicant can attempt to speed up the PTO process by filing a petition with the PTO to have the application declared "special" (64). If special status is granted, the PTO provides expedited examination of the application. Speeding up the examination process may be beneficial in making decisions concerning patent applications outside the United States and, if the patentability analysis is favorable, in seeking outside funding. On the other hand, in many cases it may not be desirable to speed up the examination process. Generally, it will be preferred that a patent issue as far along in the FDA approval process as possible, to receive the maximum benefit and protection during the time a product can actually be produced and sold. Thus, in many instances, it may be in the applicant's best interest to prolong the examination process rather than speed it up.

Because the proceedings in the PTO are *ex parte* in nature, the applicant has a "duty of candor" to be forthcoming in dealing with the PTO throughout the prosecution of the patent application. This duty of candor includes providing the PTO with all information that may be material to the examination of applicant's patent application (e.g., potential prior art) of which the applicant is aware. The duty of candor does not require the applicant to carry out a literature or prior art search. However, if the applicant or the applicant's representative is aware of relevant prior art, it must be disclosed. Normally, such relevant prior art is provided to the PTO in an Information Disclosure Statement (IDS). The duty to disclose relevant prior art continues throughout the prosecution of the applica-

tion. Therefore, if the applicant later becomes aware of relevant prior art, including prior art found by patent offices outside the United States during prosecution of the corresponding applications filed in other countries, that information should be provided to the PTO. Failure to comply with this duty of candor can result in any patent issuing from the application being held unenforceable.

Upon receipt of a patent application, the PTO assigns the application a serial number and filing date. Shortly thereafter and if disclosure of the content of the application would not be detrimental to the national security, the PTO issues a foreign filing license that allows the application to be filed in other countries (65). Thereafter, patent applications based on the U.S. patent application can be filed elsewhere in the world.

In some instances, the first response the applicant has from the PTO is a restriction requirement. The filing fee entitles the applicant to examination of one invention (e.g., a drug, a method of making a drug, and a method of using a drug may be considered separate inventions). If the application claims more than one invention, the PTO can issue a restriction requirement, thereby separating the claims into groups corresponding to the various inventions and requiring the applicant to choose (i.e., elect) one of the groups of claims for examination. The other, nonselected inventions can be refiled as divisional applications while relying on the priority date of the original application. Such divisional applications must be filed before the original application is abandoned or issues as a patent. Divisional applications potentially allow the application to obtain several patents in series on the same basic concept and, thereby, extend patent protection beyond the 17-year term of the first patent to issue. This can be especially important in the drug discovery and development area because of the length of the FDA approval process. Thus applicants should attempt to claim their invention in as many ways as possible (e.g., composition of matter claims, method of making claims, method of using or treating claims) to encourage the PTO to issue a restriction requirement.

If an applicant, on his or her own, files separate applications covering separate but related inventions, the PTO may reject the claims in one application over claims in the other application. Such an "obviousness type double patenting" rejection can generally be overcome by filing a terminal disclaimer (66) whereby the claims in the second patent to issue would expire at the same time as the claims in the first patent to issue. The PTO cannot require such a terminal disclaimer if it requires the separation of the inventions via a restriction requirement.

A patent examiner at the PTO examines the patent application to determine if it meets the statutory requirements. This includes a search by the examiner of the prior art (primarily directed to U.S. patents). Using the prior art uncovered in the search and information submitted by the applicant, the examiner evaluates the claims and determines whether the claimed invention is novel and nonobvious. Although rare, especially in drug discovery and biotechnology areas, the examiner may find the claims as submitted to be patentable. The patent would, on payment of the appropriate issue fees, then proceed to issuance.

More likely, the examiner will initially find at least some of the claims to be anticipated or obvious over the prior art and will inform the applicant of this finding in an Office Action, along with the rationale for the rejection or rejections. The applicant has a limited time (normally 3 months (67)) in which to respond to the Office Action. The applicant can choose, especially if the examiner's arguments appear persuasive, to abandon the application and, if possible, retain the invention as a trade secret. The applicant can attempt to amend some or all of the claims to overcome the rejections and/or present arguments demonstrating why the examiner has improperly rejected the claims. The applicant can also present, if appropriate, additional information or data, including information relating to secondary considerations, demonstrating the novel and nonobvious nature of the invention. Such information or data are normally presented in an affidavit or declaration.

The examiner, on reconsideration of the claims in light of the applicant's response (and any supporting information or data) can repeat the rejections, submit new rejections based on other prior art or reasoning, or withdraw the rejections wholly or in part. If the examiner withdraws all the rejections and allows the claims, the patent will issue on payment of the issue fee. If the examiner allows some claims but continues the rejection of other claims, the applicant has several options. The applicant could contest the rejection of the claims once again in the pending application. Or the rejected claims could be canceled and the application passed to issue with the allowed claims. After a final rejection, any rejected claims can be appealed to the Board of Patent Appeals and Interferences in the PTO. It is often preferred in cases having both allowed and rejected claims to allow a patent to issue with the allowed claims and file a continuation application with the rejected claims before the parent application actually issues. If the claims in the continuation application are again finally rejected, the appeal would only involve the rejected claims. By effectively separating the allowed claims from the rejected claims, the risk that the Board of Patent Appeals and Interferences will undermine the decision on patentability of the already allowed claims on appeal of the rejected claims is significantly reduced.

If the applicant is not successful in overcoming the examiner's rejections and the examiner makes the rejections final, several options remain. Again, the applicant may simply abandon the application and, if possible, retain the invention as a trade secret. Or the applicant can refile the application as a divisional, continuation, or CIP application and continue prosecution in the PTO. Or the applicant may appeal the examiner's rejection to the Board of Patent Appeals and Interferences within PTO. If not satisfied with the Board's decision, the applicant may appeal that decision either to the Court of Appeals for the Federal Circuit based on the record before the PTO or to a federal district court for a *de novo* review. If the examiner's position is overturned, the Court of Appeals for the Federal Circuit or the district court can order the PTO to issue the patent. Appeal to either the Court of Appeals for the Federal Circuit or a federal district court destroys the secrecy of the application as well as that of the record of the proceedings within the PTO and, thus, destroys any trade secrets that may have been contained therein.

3.6 Interference Proceedings

With the first-to-invent system in the United States, it is sometimes necessary to determine which of two or more inventors (or groups of inventors) first invented the subject matter that is claimed in common by the parties. Interferences are the proceedings within the PTO for making such determinations. These proceedings, which are overseen by senior examiners within the PTO, are ultimately decided by the Board of Patent Appeals and Interferences in the PTO. The party who first conceives an invention and first reduces it to practice will normally be awarded priority and will be awarded the U.S. patent (68). This is not the case, however, if another party, who reduced the invention to practice at a later date, can prove that he or she was the first to conceive the inven-

tion and proceeded diligently to reduce it to practice from a time before the other party's date of conception. The diligence of the first to reduce the invention to practice is normally immaterial in the priority contest.

Patent interferences are possible between two or more copending applications or between a pending application and a recently issued patent (69). In the case of copending applications, an applicant will often be notified by the examiner that his or her application appears to be in allowable condition but that prosecution is being suspended for consideration of the potential declaration of an interference. In cases involving a pending application and an issued patent, the examiner may cite the issued patent as a reference and suggest that the applicant may wish to "copy" claims from the patent to provoke an interference, or the applicant may become aware of the issued patent and attempt to amend his or her application (i.e., "copy" claims) to contain claims from the issued patent to provoke an interference. In the case of a pending application and an issued patent, claims from the issued patent must be copied by the applicant within 1 yr of the issue date of the patent to provoke an interference. Moreover, if the applicant has an effective filing date less than 3 months after the effective filing date of the issued patent, a significantly reduced showing is generally required by the applicant to justify the interference (70). If the PTO determines that both parties have allowable claims directed to the same subject matter, a formal Declaration of Interference is issued.

An interference is a complex, multistage, *inter partes* procedure designed to determine which party has priority with respect to the patentable subject matter that is disclosed and claimed by two or more inventors. The interference normally proceeds through the following stages: (*1*) declaration of interference by the PTO, (*2*) motion period, (3) filing of preliminary statements, (3) discovery, (4) testimony period, (5) final hearing, (6) decision by Board of Patent Appeals and Interferences, and (7) appeal and court review. Each of these stages are governed by complex procedural and substantive rules with many potential pitfalls for the unwary. Failure to follow these rules carefully can result in adverse rulings or, ultimately, judgment against the party violating them.

The party with the earlier priority date is designated the senior party and is presumed to be the first inventor. The other party is designated the junior party and has the burden of proving an earlier date of invention, generally by a preponderance of the evidence. If, however, the junior party's application was filed after the issuance of the senior party's patent, an earlier invention date must be proven beyond a reasonable doubt. Throughout the interference proceeding, the senior party retains significant procedural and substantive advantages.

Once an interference has been declared by the PTO the parties are given an opportunity to redefine the interfering subject matter (i.e., the counts of the interference that are similar in form to patent claims) and, if possible, to assert an earlier effective filing date based on a related U.S. patent application or a corresponding patent application in another country. In redefining the interfering subject matter, each party will generally seek to amend the counts in a manner more favorable to itself (i.e., consistent with and supported by his or her evidence concerning conception and reduction to practice). The parties, if appropriate, may also raise issues that are not directly related to the dates of conception or reduction to practice. For example, one party may allege that the other party derived the interfering subject matter from someone else or that the other party's application has deficiencies that render the interfering subject matter unpatentable to

that party. Either party can also argue that the subject matter in question is simply not patentable to anyone (i.e., effectively that neither party is entitled to a patent) (71). Generally, however, the most significant issues relate to establishing the respective dates of conception and reduction to practice and, where appropriate, diligence in reducing the invention to practice.

Once the PTO has declared the interference, each party must file a preliminary statement by a date set by the PTO. Facts alleged in the preliminary statement must be proved later in the proceedings. The preliminary statement must provide the dates of invention each party will rely on. A party intending to rely on an invention date earlier than his or her filing date must allege the earlier invention date and identify facts supporting the earlier date in the preliminary statement. The parties are held strictly in their proofs to any dates alleged in the preliminary statement. Thus a party able to introduce evidence showing an invention date earlier than alleged in the preliminary statement will still be held to the alleged date. The preliminary statement, therefore, should be carefully prepared and only allege dates and facts that the party can prove by clear and convincing evidence. A party relying on dates of conception and actual reduction to practice for the invention date must generally prove such dates by corroborated evidence. The testimony of an inventor or co-inventor must be corroborated as it relates to priority of invention.

The preliminary statements are placed under seal and provided to the opposing party only at a later time set by the PTO. In the initial stages of the proceeding, neither party is aware of the alleged invention date of the opposing party or if the opposing party has even alleged an invention date earlier than its filing date. An inventor from outside the United States is generally not allowed to establish an invention date earlier than his or her priority date because the acts of conception or actual reduction to practice must occur in the United States. After filing the preliminary statements, the parties generally undertake discovery and testimony to develop their cases. Once all evidence periods have expired, each party presents the formal record of evidence on which it wishes to rely. After the parties have submitted formal briefs enumerating their legal arguments and, where appropriate, rebuttal arguments, and after any oral arguments, the interference is decided by a board of three senior PTO examiners. The losing party may appeal the decision to the Court of Appeals for the Federal Circuit based on the interference record or bring a *de novo* civil action in an appropriate federal district court.

Conception generally is considered to occur when the inventor forms a definite perception of the complete invention sufficient to allow one of ordinary skill in the art to understand the invention and reduce it to practice without further inventive steps. Reduction to practice can be either constructive (i.e., by filing a patent application meeting the statutory requirements) or actual (i.e., by making and testing the invention to demonstrate that it yields the desired result). Therefore, to achieve an actual reduction to practice for a pharmaceutical, there must be both an available process for making the chemical compound (i.e., the drug) and testing to establish its utility. To be useful in an interference proceeding, such evidence generally must be corroborated by one or more persons who are not inventors. Circumstantial evidence can also be used to help establish an actual reduction to practice. Often the best corroborative evidence is provided by laboratory notebooks used to record ideas and experiments associated with the invention. Preferably, laboratory notebooks should be signed and dated daily by the investigators actually doing the work and diligently witnessed in writing by at least one non-inven-

tor co-worker who has read and understood the record. The witness should be able to understand the significance of the experiments being witnessed. Generally, the witness should not be actively involved in the work, so as to reduce the risk that the witness will later be found to be a co-inventor. If a witness is later determined to be a co-inventor, he or she cannot corroborate the work. For particularly important work, two witnesses should be considered so that even if one witness is effectively disqualified (e.g., one witness is later found to be a co-inventor), there still remains a corroborating witness. Without independent corroborating evidence of the events surrounding the invention, including conception and the reduction to practice and, possibly, diligence, a junior party will most likely lose the priority contest even if he or she was the first to invent. Should a party need to prove diligence, a corroborated written record showing almost continuous activity from a time before the other party's date of conception up to the time of that party's own reduction to practice is generally required. If a party fails to work on the project for several successive weeks without adequate explanation, such inactivity will often be sufficient to destroy the case for diligence. The activity of the inventor in developing another invention does not normally constitute an adequate excuse for such a period of inactivity.

A comprehensive intellectual property program should, therefore, accord special attention both to implementing acceptable record-keeping procedures (including procedures for witnessing notebooks and other records of invention in a timely manner) and to ensuring that these record-keeping procedures are followed. Once again, the intellectual property committee is the logical focus for this task.

Interferences are long, costly, and complex procedures that are laden with procedural pitfalls for both the senior party and, especially, junior party. The senior party is heavily favored to be awarded the right to a patent on the contested invention (72). Based on the advantage of the senior party in such interference proceedings, patent applications should be filed in the United States as quickly as possible to increase the probability of achieving senior status in any interference that may be declared.

3.7 Correction of Patents

Issued patents are often found to contain errors of varying degrees. Minor errors (e.g., clerical or typographical errors and erroneous inclusion or exclusion of an inventor), if made without deceptive intent, can usually be corrected through a Certificate of Correction issued by the PTO at the request of the inventor or assignee (73). Generally, a mistake is not minor if its correction would materially affect the scope or meaning of the patent claims.

Patents that are wholly or partly inoperative or invalid may, in some cases, be corrected by reissuing the patent. Reissue patents are generally sought because (*1*) the claims in the original patent are either too narrow or too broad, (*2*) the specification contains inaccuracies or errors, (*3*) priority from a patent application in another country was not claimed or was claimed improperly, or (*4*) reference to a prior copending application was not included or was improperly made.

To obtain a reissue patent, the patent owner must establish that (*1*) the patent is considered "wholly or partly inoperative or invalid" because of a "defective specification or drawing" or because the inventor claimed "more or less than he [or she] had a right to claim," (*2*) the defect arose "through error without any deceptive intention," (*3*) new matter is not introduced into the specification, and (*4*) the claims in the reissue application meet the legal requirements for patentability (74). An appli-

cation for a reissue patent that contains claims enlarging the scope of the original patent must be filed within 2 years of the date of grant of the original patent. The term of a reissue patent is the unexpired portion of the original patent; a reissue patent cannot extend the duration of the original patent. An infringer may have a personal defense of intervening rights to continue an otherwise infringing activity if the activity or preparation for the activity took place before the grant of the reissue patent (75). The reissue process is sometimes used to "clean up" a patent prior to embarking on litigation to enforce that patent.

A patent owner or any third party can seek a review of an issued patent by the PTO on the basis of prior art not considered by the PTO during the original examination (76). Such a reexamination procedure, although technically not a mechanism for correcting a patent, allows the PTO to determine the correctness of the original patent grant in light of the newly presented prior art. A third party requesting reexamination has a limited, but potentially significant, opportunity to present written arguments against patentability in response to the applicant's initial statement concerning patentability. The original patent is not presumed valid during the reexamination proceeding. The PTO can reaffirm the original grant, substitute a new grant by allowing new or amended claims, or withdraw the original grant.

The legal presumption of validity of the patent is not strengthened by the successful completion of the reexamination proceeding. However, the practical effect of the reexamination proceeding may considerably strengthen the patent in the eyes of a judge or jury in later litigation. Courts and juries will generally look with particular favor on a patent that has twice been found patentable by the PTO (i.e., once during the original prosecution in the PTO and then again during the reexamination proceeding). On the other hand, the reexamination proceeding provides an accused infringer the possibility of invalidating a patent outside of the court system at a considerably reduced cost. An accused infringer should, of course, carefully consider the risks and implications of the PTO upholding the patent grant through the reexamination process before embarking on such a process due to the limited involvement of the accused infringer in the process and the strengthened validity resulting if the PTO finds the original grant sustained. Considering the potential risk to third parties that the patent might actually be strengthened and considering their limited involvement in the reexamination process, it is not generally recommended that third parties request reexamination, unless the prior art is believed, to a high level of certainty, to render the patent invalid (77).

4 ENFORCEMENT OF PATENTS

Enforcement of patents is limited both geographically and temporally. Generally, a patent can be enforced only within the country in which it was granted. There is one exception to the general principle that a U.S. patent does not provide legal protection against acts outside its geographical borders. In 1988, Congress amended the U.S. Patent Statute to make the importation, use or sale of a nonpatented product in the United States an act of infringement, if the nonpatented product was made outside the United States by a process patented in the United States (78). (There is also comparable law in many other countries.) Thus a patent covering a new and novel process for producing known products or drugs can no longer be circumvented by manufacturing it outside the United States and then importing the product or drug into the United States. (The patentee cannot, of course, use its patent to prevent the use of that

process overseas or the importation of products produced by that process into other countries.)

A patent can be enforced only against acts occurring during its term (79). In the United States, the normal patent term is 17 yr from the grant of the patent. In most other countries, the patent term is 20 yr as measured from the priority date. Patents can lapse earlier than the standard term by failure to pay a required maintenance fee or tax. In the United States, maintenance fees are required to keep the patent in force after 4, 8, and 12 yr as measured from the grant date of the patent. Failure to pay any of the three required maintenance fees will result in the lapse of the patent (80).

4.1 Patent Infringement

In the United States, patent infringement is a federal cause of action. To enforce a patent, the patent holder normally brings suit against the alleged infringer in a federal district court. When speaking of infringement, it is the claims of the patent that are infringed. The claims set the legal bounds of the technical area in which the patent holder can prevent others from making, using, or selling the patented invention; in other words, the claims define the metes and bounds of the exclusive right granted by the patent. Each claim defines a separate right; some claims may be infringed while others are not. Claims also define the bounds outside of which others can operate without infringing the patent. In the case of ambiguous claim terms, the patent specification or disclosure, including drawings and other claim language, if any, can be used to interpret the claim term.

The terms *comprising, consisting essentially*, and *consisting* are used in patent claims to link the preamble and the elements of the invention; these "terms of art" have special meanings in patent claims and can dramatically affect the scope or coverage of a patent claim. For example, a claim directed to a "composition of matter *comprising* compound X" would be infringed by a formulation containing compound X regardless of the presence of other components; an infringing composition must contain the listed element and can contain any other elements. A claim directed to a "composition of matter *consisting essentially* of compound X and compound Y" would be infringed by a formulation containing both compounds X and Y and other components that do not materially affect the basic and novel characteristic of the invention. A claim directed to a "composition of matter *consisting* of compound X and compound Y" would be infringed by a formulation containing only compounds X and Y (and normal impurities and the like); an infringing composition in this case must have only the listed elements and no others.

The U.S. Patent Statute provides that "[w]hoever without authority makes, uses or sells any patented invention, within the United States during the term of the patent therefor, infringes the patent" (81). This provision may be enforced against a direct infringer who makes, uses, or sells the patented invention without the permission of the patent holder. In the United States, patent infringement can occur either by literal infringement or under the doctrine of equivalents. Literal infringement of a patent requires that each and every material limitation or element of a claim of the relevant patent be found in the composition, device, or process as claimed. If there is no literal infringement, infringement may still be found under the doctrine of equivalents. The U.S. Supreme Court has held that infringement may occur under the doctrine of equivalents where the accused composition, device, or process performs "substantially the same function, in substantially the same way, to achieve the same result" as the composition, device, or process defined in the patent claim (82).

The doctrine of equivalents gives a court the ability effectively to expand the scope of a patent claim beyond the literal language of the claim. Otherwise, a party who copies a patent's inventive concept but avoids actual infringement by some trivial or obvious change would avoid legal infringement. The doctrine of equivalents is a flexible concept. Pioneer patents will normally be entitled to a broader range of equivalents than patents claiming a relatively small advance over the prior art. As a technology develops and matures (i.e., becoming a "crowded art"), claims generally will be entitled to a smaller range of equivalents.

Infringement cannot be found, however, under the doctrine of equivalents when changes or "amendments" to the claims or arguments that were made during prosecution of the application before the PTO are contrary to, or inconsistent with, the broader interpretation of the claim necessary to cover the accused composition, device, or process. In other words, a patentee cannot generally take a position when determining infringement contrary to the position taken during the prosecution of the patent. Furthermore, a composition, device, or process cannot infringe a patent under the doctrine of equivalents when the broader interpretation of the patent claims necessary to cover the accused device or process would also cover "prior art" (i.e., the state of the technology before the filing of the patent application) (83).

It is also an act of infringement actively to induce another to carry out the infringing act: "Whoever actively induces infringement of a patent shall be liable as an infringer" (84). In addition, it is an act of infringement to contribute to the infringement of others under certain circumstances: "Whoever sells a component of a patented machine, manufacture, combination or composition, or a material or apparatus for use in practicing a patented process, constituting a material part of the invention, knowing the same to be especially made or especially adapted for use in an infringement of such patent, and not a staple article or commodity of commerce suitable for substantial non-infringing use, shall be liable as a contributory infringer'' (85). The establishment of both active inducement and contributory infringement requires knowledge or awareness of the infringement of the patent by the infringer. As opposed to the case of direct infringement, a truly "innocent infringer" cannot be liable for either actively inducing infringement or for contributory infringement.

For a composition of matter claim covering a drug, the manufacturer who prepares the drug using any process, the drugstore that sells it, and the patient who takes it may each be liable as direct infringers; the doctor who prescribes it may be liable by actively inducing infringement by the patient. For a claim covering a process for making a specific drug, both the manufacturer who makes the drug in the United States using the patented process and the manufacturer who makes the drug outside the United States using the patented process and sells the drug in the United States would be liable as infringers. Manufacturing the drug by a different process would not, of course, infringe the process claim (assuming the process used and the patented process are not equivalent under the doctrine of equivalents). For a claim covering a method of treatment using a specific drug, the ultimate user might be liable as a direct infringer; the manufacturer, druggist, and doctor might be liable if they actively induce infringement by the patient. For a claim covering a process of making a specific drug that employs an ingredient capable of use only in the process, the users of the process may be liable as direct infringers and the manufacturer of the ingredient who sells it to the users of the process may be liable as a contributory infringer. Thus, from the patent holder's viewpoint, it is desirable to have as many different types of claims as possible in the patent to protect against infringement.

4.2 Defenses to Infringement

In a patent infringement suit, the alleged infringer may assert that the accused product or process does not infringe the patent claims either literally or under the doctrine of equivalents. The burden is on the patentee to show that the claims cover the alleged infringing device or process. The alleged infringer may also attempt to show that the patentee is estopped from expanding the claims under the doctrine of equivalents sufficiently to cover the alleged infringing device or process either because of admissions or arguments presented during the prosecution of the patent before the PTO or because the broader reading of the claims would encompass and cover prior art devices or processes. Noninfringement of the patent claims by the accused device or process is frequently raised as a defense in patent infringement suits.

The validity of the patent can also be raised as a defense. Patents are presumed valid. Thus the alleged infringer must prove the patent is invalid by a clear and convincing standard of proof. Validity generally involves three components: novelty, utility, and nonobviousness. For a given claim, if the court finds that a claim lacks any one of the three components, that claim is invalid and cannot be infringed by the alleged infringer or anyone else. In other words, a holding by court that a patent claim is invalid (assuming that holding is not overturned on appeal) prevents the patentee from asserting the specific claim against anyone. Other claims in the patent may, however, remain valid and enforceable.

The validity of a patent is often attacked by a challenger presenting prior art that, in the challenger's opinion, anticipates the patent claims or renders them obvious. If the prior art offered by the challenger is the same as, or essentially equivalent to, that considered by the PTO during examination of the patent, the challenger will have a difficult time showing that the patent is not valid; in effect, the challenger must convince the judge or jury that the PTO failed to do its job properly in granting the patent. If the challenger can present prior art that was not before the PTO examiner and especially if the new prior art is more relevant to the invention than the prior art before the examiner, the challenger will have an easier time, because he or she will not have to convince the judge or jury that the PTO failed to perform its duties properly. In important cases, the challenger may be willing to go to great lengths to find additional prior art.

A challenger may also attempt to invalidate a patent by showing a sale or offer of sale of the invention more than 1 yr before the effective filing date of the patent application. In other cases, a challenger may also attempt to invalidate a patent by showing that the specification is not enabling or that it fails to disclose the best mode of carrying out the invention known by the inventor at the time the application was filed.

The challenger may also assert that the patentee acted improperly before the PTO in obtaining the patent. This inequitable conduct or fraud defense is raised in many patent infringement suits. The process of obtaining a patent is an *ex parte* proceeding between the applicant and the PTO. Because representations made by the applicant are generally accepted at face value, the courts have established a relatively high standard of candor and conduct for the applicant in the dealings with the PTO. A challenger asserting inequitable conduct will attempt to prove that the applicant was not entirely forthcoming during the *ex parte* proceedings before the PTO. Inequitable conduct might include, e.g., an applicant failing to bring relevant and material prior art of which the applicant is aware to the

attention of the PTO, attempting to "bury" an especially relevant prior art document in a large collection of seemingly less relevant prior art, falsifying data, or otherwise misleading the PTO. The challenger must show by clear and convincing evidence that the alleged mischaracterization or other inequitable conduct was "material" and that the applicant acted with the required intent to mislead or deceive the PTO.

The materiality and intent requirements of inequitable conduct are interrelated. For example, a high level of materiality can create an inference that the conduct was willful, and a specific showing of willfulness can reduce the level of materiality required. Most often, information is considered material if there is a reasonable likelihood that a reasonable examiner would have considered it important in deciding whether to allow the patent. The necessary "intent," which can be shown by circumstantial evidence, is usually characterized as an intent to deceive the PTO. Simple negligence or an erroneous judgment made in good faith will generally not support a finding of the necessary intent (86). Gross negligence may support a finding of the required intent. A specific showing of wrongful intent clearly provides the necessary intent (87). In contrast to invalidity based on the other criteria discussed, a finding of unenforceability based on inequitable conduct affects the entire patent, not just the claims to which the inequitable conduct may specifically relate.

There is no general "experimental use" exemption or defense against a charge of infringement (88). There is, however, the so-called clinical trial exemption, which is of special interest to the drug discovery and development industry. This clinical trial exemption generally provides that it is not infringement to make, use, or sell a patented invention "solely for uses reasonably related to the development and submission of information under a Federal law which regulates the manufacture, use, or sale of drugs or veterinary biological products" (89). Thus, a third party may use certain patented drug-related devices, compositions, or processes during the life of the patent to develop data and information reasonably necessary for use in, e.g., the FDA approval process. This exemption is generally intended to allow a manufacturer to obtain FDA approval during the life of the patent to be able to offer a generic drug as quickly as possible after the patent on the drug expires. If the manufacturer is forced to delay clinical trials and similar data-generating activities until the patent term expires, FDA approval would be delayed until well after the end of the patent term, thereby effectively extending the patent term and depriving the public of the alternative product during such period. This provision and the patent term extension provision for drug-related inventions are generally designed to insure that the patentee obtains the full measure of protection normally offered by a patent, but no more.

4.3 Remedies for Infringement

If a patent claim is found infringed and not invalid, the court "shall award . . . damages adequate to compensate for the infringement but in no event less than a reasonable royalty . . . together with interest and costs" (90). The purpose of such compensatory damages is to return to the patentee the value of the loss associated with the unauthorized use of the patented item or process. The minimum recoverable damages award is a "reasonable royalty," which is generally defined as the amount a reasonable person who wished to obtain a license to make, use, or sell a patented device or process would be willing to pay and still make a reasonable profit. Several methods are commonly used to estimate a reasonable royalty. Where nonexclusive licenses have been issued, the prevailing royalty

rate provides a good basis for a reasonable royalty. Where the patentee or exclusive licensee is exploiting the patent and lost or diverted sales can be demonstrated that, but for the infringement, would have gone to the patentee or exclusive licensee, lost profits (rather than a reasonable royalty) might be a reasonable estimate of damages. Damages are usually not based on the infringer's profits. Nonetheless, the infringer's profits can be a factor in determining damages or a reasonable royalty.

Infringement can range from unknowing or accidental to deliberate or reckless disregard of the patentee's legal rights. For "willful infringement," damages can be increased up to three times the actual damages (90) (i.e., a reasonable royalty) and may, in exceptional cases, include attorney fees awarded at the discretion of the court (91). Willful infringement can be found where an infringer knew of the patent and lacked a reasonable legal justification for the infringing actions. The potential infringer with notice of the patent has an affirmative duty to determine whether any of its actions would constitute infringement. This duty can generally be discharged by obtaining competent legal advice concerning the potential infringement. A failure to seek such advice, however, may not by itself be sufficient for a finding of willful infringement, nor will obtaining such advice automatically prevent a finding of willful infringement. The awards of up to triple damages in the case of willful infringement, and attorney fees in exceptional cases, are generally designed to deter infringement and encourage would-be infringers to evaluate their actions carefully in light of the claims of relevant patents.

In addition to money awards, the court may grant an injunction to "prevent the violation of any rights secured by patent, on such terms as the court deems reasonable" (92). Preliminary injunctions by which the alleged infringer is required or forbidden to do certain specified acts before a full trial on the merits of the case are rarely granted. Generally, the patentee is required to make a "clear showing" that the patent is valid and infringed before a preliminary injunction will be granted (93). Such a showing is often difficult to make before a full trial on the merit, as the alleged infringer is likely to dispute vigorously the validity and/or infringement issues at trial. To obtain a preliminary injunction, the patentee must generally show (1) a reasonable likelihood of success on the merits, (2) irreparable harm to the patentee if the injunction is not granted, (3) hardships favoring the patentee, and (4) that the public interest will be favored by granting the injunction.

In contrast to preliminary injunctions, permanent injunctions are routinely granted after a trial court has found the patent not invalid and infringed. Such injunctions generally forbid the infringer from continuing the infringing acts during the remaining term of the patent.

To enforce a patent, the patent holder may bring suit against the alleged infringer in a federal district court located "in the judicial district where the defendant resides, or where the defendant has committed acts of infringement and has a regular and established place of business" (94). The courts have interpreted the word *res-ides* to include any judicial district where the defendant is subject to personal jurisdiction (95).

A trial by jury can be requested in suits for infringement. In many cases, judges and juries do not have sufficiently strong technical backgrounds to understand and appreciate easily the complex technical issues normally involved in patent cases. The complexity of the technical issues and the often unpredictable nature of juries give rise to considerable uncertainty as to the outcome of the trial. Crowded federal court dockets can mean considerable delays in getting one's day (or, as is commonly the case in patent litigation, weeks or months)

in court. Even if a favorable judgment is obtained, it is likely that the losing party will appeal to the Court of Appeals for the Federal Circuit, thereby prolonging the case and significantly increasing the costs to both parties.

These legal proceedings, which can last years, can seriously disrupt business planning and strategy as well as divert human and economic resources away from the drug discovery and development process. The extremely high cost of litigation generally and especially in complex patent cases, coupled with the unpredictability of the outcome, the considerable time periods involved, and the likelihood of appeals resulting in even further delays, may increase the desire of both parties to reach an acceptable settlement before or even during trial. A settlement reached on reasonable business terms can, in many cases, provide a more favorable and satisfactory outcome for both parties.

In many cases, alternative dispute resolution processes (e.g., negotiation, mediation, arbitration, minitrial, rent-a-judge, summary jury trial, neutral expert fact-finding, and the like) can offer significant benefits over traditional litigation for resolving patent-related disputes, including infringement (96). Such benefits include, e.g., faster resolution of the disputed issues, the ability to tailor the process to the needs of the parties, the ability to select fact-finders or decision makers with the educational and technical backgrounds suitable for the technology, generally lower cost, increased predictability of outcome, and a finite and definite resolution of the dispute. Alternative dispute resolution processes are likely to be used with increasing frequency in patent-related cases.

5 WORLDWIDE PATENT PROTECTION

As the marketplace for the products from drug discovery and development has become global in nature, worldwide patent protection has become increasingly important. Seeking patent protection in many countries throughout the world can be extremely expensive. The cost of obtaining patent protection should be weighed against the benefits derived from patent protection on a country-by-country basis. The countries most often chosen for patenting purposes include the United States, Canada, the European Community (usually designating at least Germany, France, the UK, Italy, and Sweden), Australia, and Japan. In the case of some specific products or processes and marketing considerations, other countries may be as important, if not more important, than those just listed. Pharmaceutical companies, for example, may wish to file patent applications in most or all countries where they (or their subsidiaries, affiliates, or licensees) are likely to produce and/or market a new drug.

In most cases, it is simply too expensive to attempt to file patent applications in a majority of the countries of the world, much less in every country. The evaluation of where to file should be undertaken on a case-by-case basis taking into account the technology itself and the marketplace. In many cases, it may be possible to obtain significant patent protection without seeking patent coverage in a large number of countries. For example, if there are interrelated markets, a patent in one country often can offer practical and effective protection (but not legal, enforceable protection) against infringing acts in another country or countries. Thus, e.g., a competitor may be discouraged from offering a drug in Canada, if that drug cannot be offered in the United States because of the existence of a blocking U.S. patent. In effect, the United States and Canada (and to an increasing extent Mexico) form a single North American market (97). Taking such market considerations into account throughout the world, it may be possible, depending on the specific technology, to obtain practical worldwide patent protection through patents in only a relatively few countries.

5.1 International Agreements

Having determined where to file, one faces the task of filing patent applications in the appropriate countries. International agreements have made this process much easier. Although it is possible to file separate patent applications in each of the countries selected, this procedure is rarely used. Rather, the procedures of various international intellectual property treaties are used to simplify this administrative task considerably. The principal international treaty governing patents is the Paris Convention for the Protection of Industrial Property (98), which has approximately 113 signatory member nations. A patent application filed in any member nation creates a priority date for applications filed within 12 months (i.e., the convention year) in other convention nations. Thus an applicant can file a patent application in the United States and then file separate patent applications in other member countries within the ensuing 12 months. Such applications have an effective filing date that is the same as the filing date of the U.S. application (99). For non–Paris Convention countries (e.g., Taiwan), patent applications must be filed directly in the national patent offices. Patent applications in non–Paris Convention countries must rely on their actual filing date in the particular country. The filing procedure using the Paris Convention still requires a separate application to be filed in every country in which protection is sought and is, therefore, still unwieldy if a large number of countries are selected.

The European Patent Convention (EPC) (100) allows for the filing of a single patent application designating selected member European countries that, following prosecution before and issuance by the

European Patent Office, becomes effective as national patents in the designated countries. Currently, 17 European nations (listed in Table 3.1) are members of the EPC. A patent issued by EPC is not a true European patent; rather, it is a grant of separate national patents in the member countries designated by the applicant, each of which is enforceable under the laws of the country in which it was granted. Although applications can be filed in individual countries, the use of the single EPC application has been widely accepted as a convenient and less expensive mechanism to obtain coverage when seeking patent protection in 4 or more of the European-member countries. If protection is desired in only a few member countries (i.e., 3 or less), national applications in the individual countries may be a less expensive alternative.

The Patent Cooperation Treaty (PCT) (101), since its adoption in 1978, has become an increasingly important and useful mechanism to obtain patent protection throughout the world. Currently, the PCT has about 69 member states, including the United States, Canada, Japan, Australia, and most European countries. The member states are listed in Table 3.2. About 20 additional countries are considering becoming PCT members. The PCT allows the filing of a single international application that has the same effect as if separate applications were filed in each designated country. The PCT does not create an international patent and does not modify the substantive requirements for patentability in the member countries. It simply reduces the effort and resources necessary to file the patent application initially in multiple countries at the same time, thus proving an effective mechanism for filing international applications (especially as the convention year draws to a close and it becomes necessary to file applications very quickly).

Typical practice for an applicant based in the United States might involve filing an application in the U.S. PTO, and then filing applications in desired countries throughout the world within the convention year. Alternatively, the procedures offered by the EPC and/or PCT could be used for foreign filing. Filing a PCT application directly in the local national patent office (provided it is a PCT-receiving office) while designating most, if not all, of the PCT countries is increasingly becoming the preferred practice both in the United States and the remainder of the world. In the United States, this procedure would involve filing a PCT application in the U.S. PTO that designates the desired PCT countries. Due to the increasing importance of role of the PCT in obtaining patent protection, it is important to have at least a basic understanding of PCT procedures to capitalize on the advantages it offers.

Table 3.1 Members of the European Patent Convention (as of mid-1994)

EPC Member States

Austria
Belgium
Denmark
France
Germany
Greece
Ireland
Italy
Liechtenstein
Luxembourg
Monaco
Netherlands
Portugal
Spain
Sweden
Switzerland
United Kingdom

Table 3.2   Contracting States of the Patent Cooperation Treaty (as of mid-1994) Listed by Regions

	PCT Contracting States
Africa	Benin, Burkina Faso, Cameroon, Central African Republic, Chad, Congo, Cote d'Ivoire, Gabon, Guinea, Kenya, Madagascar, Malawi, Mali, Mauritania, Niger, Senegal, Sudan, and Togo
Americas	Barbados, Brazil, Canada, Trinidad and Tobago, and the United States of America
Asia/Pacific	Australia, China, Democratic People's Republic of Korea, Georgia, Japan, Kazakhstan, Kyrgyzstan, Mongolia, New Zealand, Republic of Korea, Sri Lanka, Tajikistan, Uzbekistan, Viet Nam, and Lithvania
Europe	Austria, Belarus, Belgium, Bulgaria, Czech Republic, Denmark, Finland, France, Germany, Greece, Hungary, Ireland, Italy, Latvia, Liechtenstein, Luxembourg, Monaco, Netherlands, Norway, Poland, Portugal, Republic of Moldova, Romania, Russian Federation, Slovakia, Slovenia, Spain, Sweden, Switzerland, Ukraine, and United Kingdom

5.2 PCT Patent Practice

A single PCT application can be filed in a PCT-receiving office (the U.S. PTO is one such receiving office) designating all or only certain member states. For example, a U.S. applicant could file a PCT patent application in the English language in the U.S. PTO and designate the appropriate PCT member states (102) in which protection is desired. A flow chart generally illustrating typical PCT procedure is shown in Figure 3.2. Once the PCT application is filed, an international search is performed by the International Search Authority—through a national patent office or intergovernment alliance (e.g., the U.S. PTO or the European Patent Office). The application is published 18 months after the effective filing date (i.e., the priority date). Therefore, 18 months after the priority date any trade secrets or other technical information contained in the application are disclosed to the public.

The PCT also provides for an optional international preliminary examination related to the patentability of the claimed invention. Although the results of the preliminary examination are not binding on individual member states, the results of preliminary examination as well as the international search report can offer significant insight and assistance for an applicant in determining the likelihood of ultimately obtaining patent protection and, thus, whether to proceed with the application in the individual designated states.

The applicant must elect whether or not

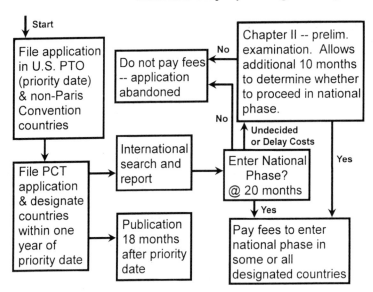

Fig. 3.2 PCT practice.

to go forward in some or all of the designated countries (i.e., enter the national stage in the elected countries) within a certain time period after the priority date. Normally, this election must be made within 20 months of the priority date. The election can be delayed a further 10 months by entering so-called Chapter II proceedings and payment of an additional fee. By delaying the final selection of the elected countries up to 30 months after the priority date, the applicant can postpone significant fees associated with entering the national stages, including the costs associated with preparing the required foreign translations. This delay may, at least in some cases, allow the applicant to have a better understanding of the patentability, marketability, and/or commercial potential of the invention. If the viability or importance of the invention has decreased, the number of countries where the invention will be pursued can be appropriately reduced (even to zero) for a significant cost savings. The PCT process, therefore, allows additional time to consider the appropriate countries in which to pursue patent protection. It is important to remember when considering the PCT process that, although the number

of PCT countries in which patent protection is sought can be reduced, the PCT countries in which the national stage can be entered is limited to those listed or selected in the original PCT filing.

After the PCT application has been searched and published, it is transferred to the patent offices of the individual nations designated by the applicant for entry into the national stage. In the national stage, the individual countries proceed to grant or reject the application in accordance with their specific domestic laws.

5.3 Other Aspects of Patent Laws in Other Countries

The U.S. patent system differs in a number of ways from other national patent systems. Some of these differences are discussed above, including patentable subject matter, priority of invention, and absolute novelty. Applicants evaluating whether and where to seek patent protection throughout the world should also be aware of working requirements and compulsory licensing requirements that are included in various forms in the patent laws of many countries.

Applicants should also be aware of, and perhaps use in appropriate cases, opposition proceedings in certain countries whereby anyone, including competitors, can oppose the granting of a patent and, thereby, become involved in the patenting process.

In the United States there is no requirement to use a patented invention. The patent holder, if he or she so chooses, may prevent others from making, using, or selling the invention during the entire term of the patent regardless of whether the patent holder practices or uses the invention. In contrast, many other countries have working requirements and/or compulsory license provisions.

A typical working provision provides that a patentee can lose patent rights if (1) the patentee does not use the invention or discovery within the relevant country within a fixed time period (usually 1 to 4 yr) after the grant of the patent or (2) the patentee ceases the use of the invention or discovery for a fixed time period (usually 1 to 3 yr consecutively) unless the patentee can justify the cause of the inaction. Thus in many countries the patent owner must either use the invention or run the risk of losing certain rights otherwise granted by the patent. A sufficient use must be determined on a case-by-case basis in light of each specific country's working provision. Use or manufacture on a commercial scale is sufficient in literally all cases to satisfy such working provisions. Where commercial use is not possible, production on a more limited scale with offers of sale of the product may be acceptable. Such uses should be carefully documented in the event the working of the invention is contested and must be proven. Where it is not possible to use the invention on even a limited scale, it may be possible to satisfy the working provision by offering licenses to parties within the country who would be reasonably interested in such licenses or by advertising the availability of such licenses in appropriate local or regional media. In

most cases, the working of the invention by a licensee satisfies the working requirement. In some cases, and especially when countries have entered into agreements granting reciprocal rights, working in another country may satisfy the working requirement. Generally, the greater the demand for the patented invention within the country, the more difficult it will be to justify manufacture outside the country.

In addition, in many countries, if the invention is not adequately worked within the country or if the public interest so requires, the law provides for and requires the patent holder to grant licenses under the patent on application. Generally, such compulsory licenses are not available until 4 yr after the filing of the application or 3 yr after the grant of the patent, whichever is later. In many countries, compulsory licenses can be granted, regardless of any working requirement, when it is in the public interest. Inventions relating to food products, pharmaceuticals, and health-related products can fall within this public interest provision. In general, the royalty for such a compulsory license is agreed on by the parties. Should the parties not reach agreement as to an acceptable royalty, the compulsory licensing provisions generally provide that the royalty will be determined by the government. In general, the royalty set by the government to be paid by a domestic organization to a foreign patent holder is likely to be lower than the royalty determined in an arms-length negotiation between the licensor and licensee.

Both the working requirements and compulsory license provisions vary considerably from country to country. Thus the laws of each relevant country must be reviewed to determine the potential effects of such provisions on specific inventions and patents. Such effects should also be taken into account in determining where to seek patent protection. Even in cases for which it is unlikely that the working requirement can be satisfied and that compulsory licenses might be required, it is still generally advisable to seek patent protection. It is possible that no one will actually seek such a compulsory license. Even if a compulsory license is sought, the patent owner may be able to object on the grounds that the delay in working was unavoidable for economic reasons and thereby frustrate or delay the grant of a compulsory license for an extended period of time. The granting of a compulsory license might, of course, provide a reasonable return in the form of royalty payments. Any royalty may be better than letting a competitor freely practice the invention. Finally, especially if the grant of the compulsory license is contested, the patent holder will generally have a number of years in which to develop the market for himself or herself before the compulsory license is finalized. A competitor coming into the market at that later time may find the market more difficult to penetrate.

The prosecution of a U.S. patent application is conducted in secrecy. Third parties are generally unaware that a patent application has even been filed, much less what, if any, claims will be granted until the patent actually issues. This is not the case in nearly all other countries. In most countries, a patent application is published 18 months after the priority date. Furthermore, in many countries, once the patent application has been allowed by a national patent office, it is published for pre-grant opposition.

In general, such pre-grant oppositions give third parties an opportunity to bring additional prior art or other factors affecting the grant of the patent to the attention of the pertinent national patent office before the patent actually issues. Oppositions generally must be filed within a fixed time (normally 1 to 12 months) after publication for opposition. Once filed, however, the opposition proceeding may take several years and include a lengthy appeal process from the national patent office's decision.

In many cases, the opposition procedure has made it even more expensive to obtain patents, especially important patents, in such countries as Japan and many European countries (e.g., Germany, the Netherlands, and the Scandinavian countries). In many countries, the patent is not granted or issued and is not enforceable until the opposition proceedings are complete and the national patent office actually issues the patent. In Europe, this potential problem has been alleviated to some degree by the advent of the EPC. Although the EPC has a 9-month period in which an opposition can be brought, the opposition does not forestall the issuance of the individual national patents that, once issued, are immediately enforceable against a third-party infringer who may be opposing the patent grant in the European Patent Office. There is some movement globally to prevent or at least reduce the ability of a competitor to stall interminably the issuance of key patents until late in the patent term (usually 20 years as measured from the priority date). Of course, the desirability of curtailing oppositions and their effect will depend on which side of the fence one is on. For a competitor, delaying or even preventing the grant of such a patent may be important.

In the United States, the reexamination proceeding allows a limited form of opposition for issued patents. During a reexamination, the claims of an issued patent are examined in light of prior art that was not considered by the PTO in the original prosecution. The involvement of third parties in reexamination proceedings is, however, strictly limited. The reexamination process is discussed in more detail in section 3.7 above.

6 TRADEMARKS

Although laws regulating and protecting trademarks were mainly developed in the

20th century, trademarks have been in use in one form or another (e.g., artisan's "potter's marks") for at least 4000 yr (103). The motivation for placing such a "potter's mark" on products probably arose from the artisan's pride in his or her work and the desire of individual artisans to take credit for what each had produced. For them, their marks were a means of identifying and distinguishing their products from similar works by other artisans. That concept still remains the primary function of trademarks and generally is the basis for trademark law and protection throughout the world.

Trademarks are the words, names, slogans, pictures, or other symbols that are used to identify the source or origin of goods. Similarly, service marks are the words, names, slogans, pictures, or other symbols that are used to identify and distinguish services. Trademarks and service marks are generally governed by the same legal principles. Throughout this section, references to *trademarks* or *marks* will generally include and apply to both trademarks and service marks. Trademarks perform four basic functions: (*1*) identify one seller's goods and distinguish them from the goods of others, (*2*) indicate a common source of goods, (*3*) indicate a certain level of quality of the goods, and (*4*) assist in selling the goods (e.g., advertising). Trademarks do not protect the underlying goods. That is the role of patents or trade secrets.

The capacity to identify and distinguish the goods of one party from those of another is an essential prerequisite and function for a trademark. Contemporary trademark laws generally do not recognize property rights in a trademark per se. Rather, the "property" in which a trademark owner may claim a legitimate and protectable interest is the goodwill of the business symbolized by the trademark. It is the value of that goodwill that establishes the value and worth of the trademark. Thus

a competitor should be precluded from misappropriating another's goodwill by using the trademark that symbolizes that goodwill.

In the United States, the Lanham Act (104) provides the framework for registration of trademarks in the PTO and for claims for infringement of federally registered trademarks as well as related claims for specific acts of unfair competition committed "in commerce." The Trademark Counterfeiting Act of 1984 provided several new remedies against parties who counterfeit federally registered trademarks, including *ex parte* seizures and criminal sanctions. The Lanham Act was further amended by the Trademark Law Revision Act of 1988, which established, for the first time, a procedure for applying to register a trademark based not on actual use in interstate commerce but rather on a bona fide intent to use a mark.

6.1 Trademarks as Marketing Tools

Trademarks are uniquely suited to facilitate the marketing of drugs. The value of a trademark is measured by the goodwill that is generated from sales of products using that trademark. Goodwill, however, depends on the consumer's favorable perception of the goods. If the customer is satisfied with the product, he or she is likely to form a favorable impression as to products bearing the same trademark and may look for the same mark when purchasing similar products in the future (i.e., brand loyalty). Such brand loyalty is difficult to establish when products are essentially interchangeable and compete mainly through price. Generally, however, it is relatively easy to establish brand loyalty for drugs and other health-related products, especially when they are patented. During the patent term for a new drug, the consumer's selection of alternate medication may be limited or nonexistent. Consequently, patent protection can aid in the creation of brand loyalty that may continue after the patent expires. Furthermore, successful medications act positively and directly on the patient; they heal, relieve pain, lower blood pressure, ease breathing, or otherwise improve the health and comfort of the patient. Each successful use may result in a positive psychological reinforcement as to the importance and value of that particular medication. That value can translate directly into goodwill. If that goodwill can be successfully linked to a trademark in the mind of the consumer or prescribing doctor, the marketing potential for that trademark can be significantly increased.

Unlike a patent, the duration of a trademark is not limited to a fixed term. Hence, a trademark can be a valuable tool to help protect and maintain a market long after patent protection has expired. Individuals accustomed to buying a trademarked product during the life of a patent (when the patent owner may be the only one offering the product) will likely continue to seek that same product after the expiration of the patent. Such product and brand loyalty, along with its associated goodwill (if carefully developed and nurtured) can represent a significant obstacle for market entry and/or penetration by others even after the patent expires. Efforts to establish and promote the trademark undertaken during the exclusive period offered by the patent may pay dividends well into the future. Thus, in addition to seeking patent protection, drug companies should at the earliest stages develop marketing strategies to maximize and link the potential goodwill of a new drug with a particular trademark. Although generic drugs offered after the drug patent expires may cost less, many patients will request, and doctors prescribe, the trusted product they used in the past and can identify by trademark.

6.2 Selection of Trademarks

Before bringing a new drug to the marketplace, careful consideration should be given to the selection of its trademark. Normally, a trademark that will not only identify and distinguish the drug in the marketplace but also will secure a market advantage for the original manufacturer will be preferred. Some words, however, can be more successfully developed as trademarks than others because of their distinctiveness. There is a "spectrum of distinctiveness" for potential trademarks. At one end is the arbitrary or fanciful word, in the middle are suggestive or descriptive words relating to the product or its characteristics, and at the other end is the generic name of the product itself. An arbitrary or fanciful word is ideally suited for use as a trademark. A generic name cannot be used as a trademark for the product that it describes. Such a generic name, however, might function as a trademark for other, unrelated products. Thus words such as *mustang*, *jaguar*, and *cougar* can function as trademarks for automobiles, notwithstanding their recognized meanings. For a new drug, however, it may be preferable to coin a new term or word as opposed to appropriating an existing word.

A suggestive term (i.e., one that suggests but does not directly describe something associated with the goods or services) may function as a trademark without further evidence of the public's recognition of its status as a trademark. A descriptive term (i.e., one that directly describes something associated with the goods or services) cannot function as a trademark until and unless it is established that, in addition to its descriptive meaning, it has also acquired a "secondary meaning" (i.e., a new meaning attached to the term relating to its use as a trademark that identifies and distinguishes the goods or services of a particular manufacturer or merchant) (105).

For example, generic names of animals such as mustang, jaguar, and cougar are successful as trademarks for cars because such names have connotative meanings that *suggest* that the characteristics associated with these animals might also be found in the cars themselves (e.g., speed, agility, and power). However, if instead of merely suggesting the qualities or characteristics of a product, a word actually *describes* the qualities or characteristics, then it cannot be recognized as a trademark by the PTO until it has been shown to have acquired secondary meaning. Of course, some terms may be so descriptive that they could never be appropriated as trademarks for one particular company. Thus, *coupe*, *sedan*, *convertible*, and *fastback* are not likely candidates for acquiring secondary meaning and trademark status for automobiles, as they clearly describe types of automobiles. Such terms should be free to be used by all. Other descriptive terms, however, may become legitimate trademarks by acquiring secondary meaning.

Whether a particular term is suggestive or descriptive is a gray area in trademark law. In attempting to distinguish between suggestive and descriptive terms, the PTO has indicated that

> Suggestive marks are those which require imagination, thought or perception to reach a conclusion as to the nature of the goods or services. Thus a suggestive term differs from a descriptive term, which immediately tells something about the goods or services. Suggestive marks, like fanciful and arbitrary marks, are register-able on the Principal Register without proof of secondary meaning. . . . A mark is considered merely descriptive if it describes an ingredient, quality, characteristic, function, feature, purpose or use of the specified goods or services. . . . The great variation in facts from case to case prevents the formulation of specific rules for specific fact situations. Each case must be decided on its own merits (106).

The acquisition of secondary meaning for a descriptive mark usually requires a calculated effort by the mark's user to establish in the public's mind a specific relationship or recognition between the mark and the particular goods or service. Thus the mark's user can attempt through marketing techniques to form an association in the relevant marketplace between the mark and the specific goods or services for which the mark is used. For example, Owens-Corning Fiberglas Corporation employed an advertising and marketing campaign (using the Pink Panther cartoon character) for its pink-colored insulation to establish that color as an identification of its insulation. This effort to strengthen the public's recognition and association of the desired mark with the product was so successful that Owens-Corning was able to establish secondary meaning and obtain a federal trademark registration for the color pink for its insulation products (107). Proof of secondary meaning, however, is not always easy to acquire. Recently, the Court of Appeals for the Federal Circuit held that several million dollars of advertising and many millions of dollars of sales under a particular term were insufficient to prove that the term has acquired secondary meaning in the marketplace (85). The court stressed the need for consumer surveys to measure whether the sales and advertising have been successful in creating secondary meaning for a particular mark.

Descriptive and suggestive terms are generally not good candidates as trademarks for drugs. Because a new drug often represents a new discovery, it is useful to select or develop a new word or name to identify the product to the public. The selection process of a new trademark for a new drug (or any new product) must, however, take into account the fact that the Lanham Act prohibits certain items from ever being registered as trademarks (109). Registered trademarks cannot include, e.g., "immoral, deceptive, or scandalous" matter, state or national flags or similar insignia, names of living individuals (except by written consent) or a deceased U.S. president during the life of his widow (except by written consent), "merely descriptive or deceptively misdescriptive" names, "primarily geographically descriptive or deceptively misdescriptive" names, or surnames. The selection process should also take into account, especially if registrations in other countries are desired, the possible meaning of any potential mark in other countries and languages. For example, an arbitrary and fanciful word in the English language may have a different (perhaps negative, scandalous, or bizarre) meaning in another country or language.

A mark cannot be registered "which so resembles a mark registered in the Patent and Trademark Office, or a mark or trade name previously used in the United States by another and not abandoned, as to be likely, when used on or in connection with the goods of the applicant, to cause confusion, or to cause mistake, or to deceive" (110). Once a tentative choice of one or more potential trademarks is made, it is prudent, if not essential, to conduct a trademark search to protect the expected investment in the chosen mark. Normally, an initial computer search of the records in the PTO should be made to locate any similar marks that are registered or for which registration is pending before the PTO. This search of the PTO files is a relatively fast and inexpensive procedure by which possibly insurmountable problems (e.g., so-called knock-out marks that likely prevent registration) can be identified (111). If similar marks are not found in the PTO search, a more comprehensive search, including databases containing state and local common law marks, is generally undertaken to provide additional security that the mark in question is available for adoption. Generally, an outside search agency conducts the search using databases containing registered and unregistered names and marks in use throughout the United States. If no closely similar marks are found (or, in some cases, if such marks are used on very different types of goods), one may proceed to register the new mark in the PTO and, if appropriate, seek registrations in other countries as well.

6.3 Registration Process

In the United States, trademark rights arise from use of a mark, rather than from its registration in the PTO (112). However, registration in the PTO provides significant advantages to a trademark owner. Furthermore, marks can now be registered based only on a bona fide intent to use the mark with a particular product. Under the new intent-to-use filing provisions, however, it is still necessary to establish actual commercial use of the mark before the actual registration will issue. One important benefit of the intent-to-use process is the recognition of the date of filing of an intent-to-use application as the priority date, on which trademark rights begin, rather than the date the mark is first used commercially on the product. The intent-to-use provisions can be especially useful in marketing a new drug, because they provide a method for obtaining protection for a trademark before the drug actually enters the marketplace.

A trademark application must include both the mark for which registration is sought and a description of the goods on which it is to be used. Once an application for registration of a mark has been filed in the PTO, the examination process is essentially the same whether the application is based on actual use or intent to use. A trademark examiner in the PTO reviews the application to determine whether it meets the statutory requirements. The examiner may issue a refusal to register the mark based on a failure to meet one or more of the statutory requirements. The applicant is given an opportunity to present arguments or to amend the application to overcome these objections. If the examiner finds the application to be in order, the mark will be published for opposition in the PTO's *Official Gazette*. Anyone who believes he or she may be injured by the registration of the mark may file a Notice of Opposition within 30 days of the date of publication, unless an extension of time is granted.

If an opposition is not filed, an application based on actual use will mature into an issued registration or an intent-to-use application will be allowed. For an allowed intent-to-use application, the applicant has 6 months within which to establish actual use of the mark. If actual use of the mark is not established within this 6-month period, the applicant may request, on payment of required fees, further extensions of time (in 6-month increments up to a total of 24 months). If after 24 months from the date of allowance, actual use of the mark in commerce has not been made, the application will be deemed abandoned. Thereafter, a new application for registration of the same mark may be filed, but the earlier priority date will be lost.

The initial term of a registered mark is 10 yr. Between the 5th and 6th yr of the initial term, the registrant must file an affidavit or declaration stating that the mark is still in use with the goods specified in the registration. Failure to file this affidavit or declaration will result in the cancellation of the registration. If the registrant files an affidavit or declaration confirming, in addition to the mark still being in use, that it has been in continuous use for the preceding 5 yr, the registration becomes "incontestable" (113).

Trademark rights arise mainly from use and not from the registration of the mark. However, registration of a mark in the PTO provides the mark's owner many significant procedural advantages. First, a certificate of registration of a mark on the principal register constitutes "*prima facie* evidence of the validity of the registration . . . and the registrant's exclusive right to use the registered mark in commerce on or in connection with the goods and services specified in the certificate" (114). The registrant's rights are not limited geographically to the locations in the United States where the mark has actually been used. The registrant's "exclusive" rights extend throughout the United States (and territories and possessions). Moreover, if the registration has become "incontestable" based on the consecutive 5 yr of continuous use after registration, then the registrant's "exclusive rights" are incontestable except on certain limited grounds specified in the Lanham Act (115) and the incontestable registration constitutes "conclusive evidence" of the registrant's "exclusive rights" in the registered mark (116). The registration is also "constructive notice of the registrant's claim of ownership" throughout the United States. Constructive notice means that, after a mark has been registered, others have legal notice of the registrant's trademark rights even if they are not aware of the registration (117). Constructive notice prevents later users of a mark from relying on the common law defense of "good faith" adoption of the mark. To take advantage of this constructive notice provision, the registrant must use the mark with the proper registration notation (118).

These procedural advantages are of considerable importance should the registrant attempt to enforce the trademark rights in court. The federal courts, rather than state courts, have original jurisdiction over causes of action arising from federally registered marks (119). Furthermore, a registrant may claim a priority date earlier than the date of first use based on an intent-to-use application. The ability to claim an earlier priority date may be critical in a contest between rival claimants of the same or similar marks. A single day of priority over a junior party has been held sufficient to sustain a senior party's rights and require the junior party to discontinue further use of the mark (120).

Registration also provides a relatively simple mechanism to prevent importation of goods bearing a counterfeit or infringing copy of the mark into the United States. Upon the filing of a certified copy of a trademark registration with the U.S. Customs Service and payment of the required fee, the Customs Service will undertake to prevent entry into the United States of products bearing an infringing copy of the registrant's mark (121). The presumed ability to determine infringement (i.e., that the alleged infringing mark is confusingly similar to the registered mark) by direct visual inspection allows for the simplified procedure.

Finally, registration of a trademark entitles the registrant to both injunctive and monetary relief for trademark infringement. Under the Lanham Act, monetary relief can include (1) the profits that an infringer has earned by marketing products under the infringing trademark and (2) any damages that have been sustained by the registrant from the infringement (122). Moreover, "[i]n assessing profits [of the infringer] the plaintiff [registrant] shall be required to prove defendant's sales only; defendant must prove all elements of costs or deduction claimed" (122). Similarly, the court may increase the award of damages to the registrant by three times the amount of damages proven at trial, and in exceptional cases, the court may award attorney fees to the prevailing party (122). The court may also order "that all labels, signs, prints, packages, wrappers, receptacles, and advertisements in the possession of the defendant bearing the registered mark . . . shall be delivered up and destroyed" (123).

In an action for trademark infringement,

the issue is whether a mark used by the defendant with particular goods is likely to cause confusion, mistake, or deception of the public. Generally, the best evidence of likelihood of confusion is that which shows substantial actual confusion. However, actual confusion is not necessary to prove infringement of a federally registered trademark: "It has been said that the most successful form of copying is to employ enough points of similarity to confuse the public with enough points of difference to confuse the courts" (124). The registration of a trademark in the PTO considerably strengthens trademark rights and makes them easier to enforce.

6.4 Oppositions and Cancellations

Once the mark is published in the *Official Gazette*, anyone believing that he or she will be injured by the issuance of the registration may file a Notice of Opposition within 30 days. In addition, anyone who believes he or she may be injured by maintenance of a registration on the Principal Register may file a Petition for Cancellation of that registration. Once either a Notice of Opposition or Petition for Cancellation are filed, the application is transferred to the Trademark Trial and Appeal Board for a determination of the merits of the opposition or cancellation request. Opposition and cancellation proceedings are, in many ways, procedurally similar to a court trial. The only issues before the Board, however, are whether an applicant should be allowed to register the mark or whether a registrant can maintain the registration for the mark. Either party can appeal the Board's decision to the Court of Appeals for the Federal Circuit on the record established before the Board or to a federal district court for a *de novo* review of the Board's decision.

6.5 Preserving Trademark Rights through Proper Use

Trademark rights can be diminished and even destroyed through improper use. A trademark should be used as an adjective modifying the generic name of a product. The trademark owner should never use the trademark as the name of the product itself. The trademark owner should also attempt to prevent others from doing so.

Once established, the trademark must be protected and its usage carefully monitored and controlled. A trademark (even if arbitrary or fanciful when first coined) can be lost if it becomes a descriptive or generic name for the product itself and thus fails to identify the particular product offered by the trademark owner. The original "aspirin" trademark lost its status as a trademark in the United States when it lost its distinctiveness in identifying the particular Bayer Company product. The general public came to regard this term as identifying the type of drug rather than distinguishing the product of the Bayer Company. Consequently, the term *aspirin* was held to have fallen into the public domain in the United States and not the exclusive property of the Bayer Company (125).

In addition to proper use in its own advertising and marketing, the trademark owner should police the use of the mark by others. For example, the trademark owner may wish to subscribe to a service that will search various media databases on a routine basis for improper uses of the mark. Or the trademark owner can carry out the search on its own. When improper uses are found, a letter or other notification can be sent to the user explaining and requesting proper usage. Depending on the degree of misuse and the importance of the mark, other mechanisms, including, e.g., advertising and marketing campaigns, might be used. Documentation of such policing should be maintained in the event

it becomes necessary during litigation or cancellation proceedings to prove that the trademark owner acted in a proper and prudent manner to protect the trademark.

When used, the mark should be set apart, preferably in bold type, from the other words around it. If the mark has not been registered in the PTO, it should be followed whenever possible by the designation ™; if it has been registered, it should be followed by the proper registration notice:

[A] registrant of a mark registered in the Patent and Trademark Office, may give notice that his mark is registered by displaying with the mark the words "Registered in U.S. Patent and Trademark Office" or "Reg. U.S. Pat. & Tm. Off." or the letter R enclosed within a circle, thus ®; and in any suit for infringement under this Act by such a registrant failing to give such notice of registration, no profits and no damages shall be recovered under the provisions of this Act unless the defendant had actual notice of the registration (126).

6.6 Worldwide Trademark Rights

It is impossible here to discuss in any detail the plethora of laws of other countries regarding the establishment and protection of trademark rights, but a few comments may be in order. As noted above, when selecting a trademark it is prudent to verify whether the desired mark has some meaning in another language or sounds similar to a word in another language. In a few instances, trademark owners have discovered to their chagrin that an English or made-up word used as a trademark is so similar to a foreign word having a negative or otherwise inappropriate connotation that it is impossible to use the trademark in some countries. It is far better to discover such problems before significant resources are expended to develop the goodwill associated with that mark.

In the global marketplace, trademark protection normally will be required throughout the world. However, like patent protection, trademark protection is limited geographically. Determining the appropriate countries in which to seek trademark protection should be an integral part of the intellectual property strategy. Due to the generally lower cost of obtaining trademark protection, it may be advantageous to obtain such protection in more countries than in which one might seek patent protection. As a rule of thumb, trademark protection should be perfected, at a minimum, in every country in which patent protection is sought. Similarly, if licensing in other countries is contemplated, registration of the mark in those countries is advised. Licensees are likely to be interested in both the patent and trademark rights. It may also be appropriate to obtain trademark registrations in those countries having potentially significant markets even though patent protection will not be sought or licenses will not be granted. It is prudent to ensure that a well-known drug can be exported into various countries under its trademark and that an unrelated company does not acquire the rights to market a drug or other health-related product under that trademark.

When and to what extent trademark rights should be acquired in countries throughout the world must necessarily be determined on a case-by-case basis. Therefore, when a drug is ready to be announced to the public under a particular trademark, even if it is not anticipated that sales under the mark will begin for quite some time, the strategy for establishing trademark rights in other countries should generally already be in place. Unfortunately, it is not uncommon for unrelated parties, upon learning that a new product will be marketed under a particular mark, to attempt to register the mark in at least some foreign countries in advance of the originator of the mark. The unrelated party then could, e.g., hold the mark for ransom or transfer the rights to the mark to a local company for marketing similar products in that country under the mark. Although redress may, in some instances, be achieved through the courts in the appropriate foreign countries, this can be expensive and may involve many years of litigation. Thus, in considering the development of trademark rights for new drugs in other countries, an "ounce of prevention" may be worth considerably more than several "pounds of cure."

6.7 Other Rights under the Lanham Act

The Lanham Act in § 43(a) also creates a federal cause of action for "false designation of origin and false description of goods" (127). Courts have construed § 43(a) as regulating any act or representation that might cause the purchasing public mistakenly to believe that a product originating from one manufacturer or merchant originated from some other manufacturer or merchant; § 43(a) now forms the basis of the federal law of unfair competition.

Under § 43(a), some characteristics of a product can be protected from imitation by others. Thus, e.g., the color, shape, and size of pills have been held to be protectable. A court allowed a drug company, even after the patent on the drug expired, to market the particular drug exclusively in capsules of a particular color, shape, and size (128). Other drug companies could, of course, market generic forms of the drug after the patent had expired, but not in the format in which the public had come to know and recognize the product. Thus the exclusive right to market a drug in capsules of the same color, shape, and size that the public has come to associate with "the authentic product" can be a protectable property interest and a valuable marketing tool. Section 43(a) is not restricted to registered trademarks. Rather it embraces the broad panoply of "trade dress" for a product (i.e., the total visual combination of elements in which a product or service is packaged and offered to the public). The development of valuable rights that may be protected under this section depends primarily on how the product is marketed and presented to the public.

The protection offered by § 43(a) was expanded further by the Trademark Revision Act of 1988 to cover false representations made in regard to another's goods. Section 43(a) provides that any person who

> in commercial advertising or promotion, misrepresents the nature, characteristics, qualities, or geographical origins of his or her *or another person's* goods or services or commercial activities, shall be liable in a civil action by any person who believes that he or she is or is likely to be damaged by the act (129).

Thus false or misleading statements about one's own goods or another's goods can give rise to a cause of action.

7 TRADE SECRETS

Information that has value because it is not generally known, including business and technical, patentable and nonpatentable information, can be protected as a trade secret against discovery by improper means or through breach of confidence. To be protected as a trade secret, the information must in fact be "secret," i.e., not generally known by the industry. The duration of a trade secret is the length of time the information is kept secret. Public disclosure of the information by the trade secret owner or anyone else results in the loss of the protection offered by the trade secret.

The practical role of trade secrets in the drug development and discovery industry may, of course, be significantly limited by the public disclosure of information and data required by the FDA approval process as well as the large number of groups working in this area who may independently discover the secret. Information or data that the FDA publicly discloses or otherwise makes available to the public loses its status as a trade secret. Where trade secret protection is not available due to the inability to maintain secrecy, patent protection may be the only viable form of protection available.

Although trade secret law may provide only limited and short-term protection for technical and business information in the drug discovery and development area, such protection can be a valuable component of an overall intellectual property strategy. Trade secret protection can be especially important in protecting technology at its earliest stages of development (e.g., before publication of a patent application or release of data and information by the FDA). Of course, trade secrets can be used to protect technical or business information that is not disclosed to the FDA (or, if disclosed, not released to the public by the FDA) or to the public through, e.g., published patent applications or other publications. In such cases, trade secrets can provide a viable alternative and/or adjunct to obtaining patent protection, especially when the patentability of an invention is in doubt. Like patents and trademarks, trade secrets and general technical know-how can be sold outright or licensed.

Relying too heavily on trade secret protection to protect intellectual property, however, has significant limitations and risks. The cornerstone of a trade secret is secrecy. Once secrecy is lost (regardless of how it is lost), the protection afforded by trade secret law is lost and competitors are free to use the technology. To reiterate, the duration of a trade secret is the length of time the information is kept secret. Even if secrecy is maintained, the technology can be used by others as long as it is discovered in a fair and honest manner (e.g., independent discovery or reverse engineering). Thus it may be proper, e.g., for a competitor to analyze a new drug and, based on the information obtained, seek FDA approval to market the drug (assuming there are no blocking patents and the drug sample was obtained properly). Public disclosure of the information by the trade secret owner or others (even by one who improperly obtained and/or disclosed the information) effectively terminates the protection offered by the trade secret. Therefore, the scope of protection available and risks associated with trade secrets must be carefully considered and evaluated, and procedures must be defined and implemented to protect and maintain the required secrecy before significant reliance is placed on trade secret protection as an alternative to patent protection. This is especially true for the drug discovery and development industry, where detailed technical disclosures to the FDA are generally required. Ideally, patent protection and trade secret protection should be carefully coordinated to provide maximum protection.

7.1 Trade Secret Definition

Trade secret protection in the United States is generally governed by state law; thus its definition can vary from state to state. One common definition provides that a trade secret consists "of any formula, pattern, device, or compilation of information which is used in one's business, and which gives him an opportunity to obtain an advantage over competitors who do not know or use it" (130). Another definition, which a significant number of states have adopted in some version, is provided by the Uniform Trade Secrets Act: "[I]nformation, including a formula, pattern, compilation, program, device, method, technique, or process that: (i) derives independent economic value, actual or potential, from

not being generally known to, and not being readily ascertainable by proper means by, other persons who can obtain economic value from its disclosure or use, and (ii) is the subject of efforts that are reasonable under the circumstances to maintain its secrecy" (131). Therefore, trade secrets generally can, e.g., include formulas for chemical compounds and drugs; processes for manufacturing, treating, and preserving materials; patterns and designs for a machine or device; computer software; business strategies and plans; customers lists; and similar business and technical information having economic value.

7.2 Requirements for Trade Secret Protection

For a protectable trade secret to exist, generally it must meet four interrelated criteria: (1) it must be the proper subject matter for a trade secret (i.e., it must fall within the type of information protectable as a trade secret), (2) it must not generally be known in the trade (i.e., it must be a secret), (3) it must be of commercial value to the holder, and (4) it must be treated and maintained as a secret. Although the trade secret must be secret, novelty in the patent sense is not required. Thus an obvious improvement in a drug manufacturing process, which could not be protected by a patent, could be retained as a trade secret so long as it is not known to others in the industry (assuming the other criteria are met). The third requirement, commercial value, is generally met if knowledge or use of the trade secret by the holder provides some competitive advantage. The fourth criterion essentially requires that the trade secret holder treat the information in an appropriate manner, i.e., reasonable measures must be taken to keep and maintain the information as a secret. The efforts to maintain secrecy will vary with the information and the financial resources of the organization. At a minimum, such reasonable efforts should include limiting access to the information to key employees who have a need to know, having employees sign confidentiality agreements, and alerting employees about the status of the sensitive information that is considered to be a trade secret (e.g., appropriate labeling of documents as "confidential," storing such documents in a secure manner, and marking process areas that are off-limits). Disclosure to outsiders should be limited to that necessary for business reasons and should be carefully controlled; such disclosure generally should be through confidentiality agreements.

In addition to the general criteria above, courts have used a number of specific factors in determining the existence of a trade secret. Some of these factors include (1) the extent to which the information is known outside of one's business, (2) the extent to which it is known by employees and others involved in the business, (3) the extent of measures taken to guard the secrecy of the information, (4) the value of the information to the trade secret holder and potentially to competitors, (5) the amount of effort or money expended in developing the information, and (6) the ease or difficulty with which the information could be properly acquired or duplicated by others (130).

In setting up a program to protect trade secrets, these factors should be carefully considered to maximize the probability of a court later finding that a protectable trade secret does in fact exist. For example, documents containing trade secrets should be labeled "confidential" or with a similar notation. Overuse of a "confidential" stamp, however, should be avoided. If all documents are routinely labeled "confidential" without regard to the trade secret content, a court might later determine that employees were not properly informed of the trade secrets or that trade secrets were treated no differently from other information. Moreover, if all documents are marked "confidential," employees may not treat the trade secrets with the appropriate care, thereby increasing the risk that actual secrecy will be lost. In some instances, several classifications of information with varying degrees of control might be appropriate.

It is generally desirable to have a comprehensive and documented program for protection of trade secrets. This program can be invaluable in maintaining a competitive advantage in the marketplace as well as providing a means to demonstrate to a court that protectable trade secrets existed and were treated in the appropriate manner. Such a program should have a mechanism for identifying trade secrets and then protecting and maintaining them. This trade secret program can form an integral component of an overall security program to maintain patentable inventions as secrets until the appropriate patent applications are filed. Such a program can be implemented through the intellectual property committee responsible for general intellectual property matters.

7.3 Enforcement of Trade Secrets

Trade secrets generally protect only against wrongful disclosure or discovery of information by competitors or others. Thus one might have a cause of action, e.g., against an employee who leaks information to a competitor, against a competitor who discovers a trade secret through improper industrial espionage (e.g., by bribing an employee to disclose a trade secret or by breaking into a computer system or facility), or against one who improperly obtains and/or uses a trade secret (e.g., misrepresentation or breach of an implied or express confidentiality agreement). In addition, in an appropriate case, one might bring suit to prevent the improper disclosure of a trade secret (132). For example, a key employee who resigns to join a competitor might be enjoined from disclosing trade secrets of his or her former employer to the new employer.

Not all means of discovering a trade secret are actionable. For example, it is acceptable to learn of the trade secret by independent discovery, by reverse engineering, or by evaluation of products or data available publicly. Thus, for example, a trade secret holder would not have a cause of action against a competitor who independently discovers the trade secret. In addition, one who properly obtains the trade secret without any obligation to maintain the trade secret in confidence is free to use it and, if desired, disclose it to the public, thereby destroying the original trade secret status. Indeed, one who independently and properly discovers an invention held as trade secret by another may be able to obtain a patent covering the invention. In such a case, the potential rights of the patentee and the trade secret holder relative to each other appear to remain an unresolved question (133).

Remedies for misappropriation of a trade secret can include actual and punitive damages as well as injunctive relief. An injunction may only prevent the wrongdoer from using the trade secret information for a fixed length of time. Some courts will limit the length of the injunction to the estimated time it would take a hypothetical competitor to discover the trade secret by reverse engineering or other proper means (a so-called lead-time injunction). Only the wrongdoer may be prevented from using the trade secret. Other competitors as well as the general public are generally free to use the trade secret to the extent that it has been publicly disclosed.

Although trade secrets potentially offer protection for an unlimited duration (i.e., so long as secrecy is maintained), in practice the time of protection is often relatively brief. One estimate is that most trade secrets have an average life expectancy of

about 3 years (134). Due to the intense competition, employee mobility, and FDA disclosure requirements, the lifetime of an average trade secret in the drug discovery and development industry may be even shorter.

Even within such a short time span, however, trade secrets remain a useful adjunct to patent protection. For example, trade secret protection can be used to protect an invention before filing a patent application and while the application is pending before the PTO. Trade secrets may also be used to protect later improvements in patented processes or materials that do not, in themselves, warrant filing separate patent applications.

7.4 Relationship of Trade Secrets and Patents

Trade secret and patent protection have coexisted in the United States for more than 200 yr. The U.S. Supreme Court in 1974 made it clear that federal patent law does not preempt state trade secret law (135). Nonetheless, the disclosure requirement of patent law and the secrecy requirement of trade secret law are often in conflict. The Patent Statute requires a patent specification to teach one of ordinary skill in the art how to make and use the invention and to disclose the best mode of carrying out the invention known to the inventor as of the application filing date. Any trade secrets disclosed in the patent specification lose their status as trade secrets once the patent application is made public (published or issued as a patent). Failure to disclose a trade secret in an application for which the trade secret is necessary for enablement or best mode considerations will result in an invalid patent.

Although the issue is easily stated, it is considerably more difficult in practice to determine which trade secrets relating to an invention must be disclosed. Clearly an applicant should not attempt to obtain patent protection for an invention while seeking to keep the commercial embodiment (the best mode) as a trade secret. Yet, as noted, the best mode requirement relates to the applicant's knowledge at the time the application is filed. Improvements made before the filing date may be required to be included in the original application. Such improvements made after the filing date, even if they constitute a better method of practicing the invention, can be retained as trade secrets. Improvements made after the filing date of the original application may, however, have to be disclosed in any subsequent continuation or CIP applications (42).

Generally, it is not necessary to disclose trade secrets that are related to the invention but are not required for its operation or are not related to the best mode of operation known to the applicant as of the filing date of the patent application. Of course, by not disclosing related trade secrets in a patent application, one runs the significant risk that a court may later hold the patent invalid or unenforceable for failure to provide an enabling specification or to disclose the best mode. In a close case, it may be preferable to err on the side of disclosing more than the required minimum. After all, trade secrets, for the most part, have only a limited lifetime, especially if disclosed in submissions to the FDA or other federal agencies.

7.5 Freedom of Information Act

So-called sunshine-type laws, including state and federal Freedom of Information Acts (FOIAs) and state right-to-know laws, can significantly impact the ability of pharmaceutical and drug discovery companies to retain the secrecy required for viable trade secrets. The general purpose of these laws is to increase the openness of governmental processes and decision making. Yet release of information by the government under FOIAs can destroy valuable trade secrets rights. Some of the information submitted to government agencies will be routinely released to the public as part of the functioning of the agencies. Other information may be released based on specific requests by members of the public.

The federal FOIA mandates disclosure of official information of the administrative agencies of the federal executive branch (including, e.g., FDA and EPA) unless the information falls within one of nine statutory exemptions (136). FOIA provides that "[e]ach agency, upon any request for records which (A) reasonably describes such records, and (B) is made in accordance with published rules stating the time, place, and fees (if any), and procedures to be followed, shall make the records promptly available to any person." Thus any member of the public, including, e.g., domestic or foreign competitors, can obtain records through the FOIA. Such records can include drug-related submissions to FDA and identifications of new chemical compounds submitted to EPA.

Under FOIA, the burden of proof for withholding information is on the government agency having possession of the information. Potentially, a government agency can rely on two FOIA exemptions to withhold trade secret–type information. FOIA exemption 3 generally allows an agency to withhold information exempted from disclosure by another statute, "provided such statute (A) requires that the matters be withheld from the public in such a manner as to leave no discretion on the issue, or (B) establishes particular criteria for withholding or refers to particular types of matters to be withheld" (137). This provision, taken together with the Trade Secrets Act (138), may provide a basis for exempting trade secrets from disclosure under FOIA. Exemption 4 provides that the disclosure requirements of the FOIA do not apply to "trade secrets and commercial or financial information obtained from a person and privileged or confidential" (139). On their face, these exemptions appear to provide considerable protection against public disclosure for trade secrets disclosed to government agencies such as FDA and EPA. However, the courts, especially the U.S. Court of Appeals for the District of Columbia, have tended to read these exemptions narrowly. Furthermore, the U.S. Supreme Court has held that FOIA exemptions are permissive rather than mandatory:

> FOIA by itself protects the submitters' interest in confidentiality only to the extent that this interest is endorsed by the agency collecting the information. Enlarged access to governmental information undoubtedly cuts against the privacy concerns of nongovernmental entities, and as a matter of policy some balancing and accommodation may well be desirable. We simply hold here that Congress did not design the FOIA Exemptions to be mandatory bars to disclosure (140).

Therefore, an agency retains the discretion to disclose information that falls within the exemptions. Agencies may tend to grant more liberal disclosure simply to avoid lawsuits by requesters seeking to compel disclosure (141).

The North American Free Trade Agreement (NAFTA) may also significantly affect trade secrets that are disclosed to the FDA or other regulatory agencies for product approval (96). The full effect of NAFTA on trade secrets and their potential disclosure under FOIA must await the adoption of statutes and regulations implementing the Treaty. Drug discovery organizations would be well advised to keep abreast of developments associated with, or resulting from, NAFTA that relate to trade secrets in general and, more specifically, to

the FDA's drug approval procedures. Where appropriate, such organizations should modify their treatment of trade secret information accordingly.

The details and nuances of the current law governing FOIA disclosures are beyond the scope of this chapter. But any submitter of information and data, especially information and data involving drug discovery and development relating to the public health, should realize (and perhaps even expect) that government agencies may at some time release that information or data either to the public at large or to individuals or organizations that submit specific requests. This possibility increases the importance and significance of patent protection, if appropriate, relative to trade secret protection. The intellectual property strategy devised for the drug discovery and development organization should take this factor into account.

7.6 Trade Secret Protection outside the United States

It is impossible here to discuss in any detail the protection afforded to trade secrets in other countries. Moreover, any details provided could be out of date in a relatively short time as new cases are decided or new statutes are adopted. A few general comments, however, may be in order.

Protection for trade secrets in other countries varies dramatically, ranging from essentially none or very little up to, and even exceeding, the level of protection provided in the United States. Therefore, local counsel in the relevant country should be consulted in the event that trade secret or related issues arise. A few examples for selected countries, however, can be helpful to illustrate the scope of variations for the protection for trade secrets (142).

1. *Australia.* In Australia, trade secret protection is based on common law

(both English and Australian). The subject matter of the trade secret must relate to a trade. Portions of the trade secret may be known, but the overall result must not be known or achievable based on information known to the public. Protection can be based on breach of an express or implied contract or breach of a confidential relationship. Remedies can include injunctions (preliminary or permanent); damages; profits; and in appropriate cases, destruction of property embodying the trade secret.

2. *France.* Trade secret protection per se does not exist in France. However, the combined protection afforded to manufacturing secrets, commercial secrets, and "know-how" is similar to trade secret protection. Manufacturing secrets must actually be used, or be ready for immediate use, in industry; thus ongoing research and development information or data may not qualify as a manufacturing secret. To qualify as a manufacturing secret, the information must not be known by others in France (143). Protection is also afforded to know-how; technical information that will ultimately be used in industry may be protected as know-how. Commercial secrets include commercial and financial information. Remedies for improper use include damages, injunctions, and specific performance.

3. *Germany.* In Germany, protection is generally afforded to "industrial and commercial secrets" that relate to a business enterprise. The information must not be generally known or available and the holder of the information must intend to maintain its secrecy. Remedies include damages, criminal sanctions, and injunctions.

4. *Italy.* Legal protection is generally afforded to commercial and industrial secrets. To be protected, the secret must meet the following requirements: (*1*) it must not be known or readily available to competitors or others in Italy, (*2*) there must be an objective, justifiable economic reason for maintaining secrecy, and (*3*) the holder must have taken adequate steps to maintain secrecy. Manufacturing secrets must be connected with a manufacturing or production activity; commercial secrets relate to other activities of the organization. Remedies include damages, injunctions, declaratory relief, and removal of the effects of unfair competition.

5. *Japan.* In Japan there is generally no protection afforded trade secrets. However, expressed contracts or agreements not to disclose specific information will generally be enforced. Remedies for violating such agreements include damages and injunctive relief.

6. Mexico. Currently, the protection afforded trade secrets in Mexico is relatively limited and weak. The situation is likely to change because of the recent adoption of NAFTA (96). NAFTA, covering the United States, Canada, and Mexico, requires each country, at a minimum, to provide "adequate and effective protection and enforcement of" intellectual property rights, specifically including trade secret rights. The actual effect of NAFTA must, of course, await its actual implementation in the member countries.

7. *United Kingdom.* Although there appears to be no generally accepted definition of trade secrets in the UK, protection is generally afforded to commercial, industrial, and scientific information that is not generally known and that is capable of industrial or commercial application, where the holder has acted in a manner consistent with an intent to keep the information secret. Remedies include injunction, damages, accounting of profits, and inspection of the defen-

dant's premises for materials relating to the trade secret.

Even in countries that do not afford significant protection through laws directly covering trade secrets, protection may be possible through contracts or agreements to protect confidential information disclosed to other parties. Preferably and wherever possible, any required disclosure of the trade secrets or other confidential information to third parties (e.g., to employees, potential business partners, vendors, and the like)—whether in the United States or elsewhere—should be made using confidentiality or secrecy agreements between the parties. Improper disclosure of such trade secrets or information likely would be a breach of contract. In countries not recognizing trade secrets or offering little trade secret protection, redress for improper disclosure of a trade secret could be sought under contract law. In countries offering significant protection for trade secrets, redress could be sought under contract law and/or trade secret law.

Trade secret holders interested in using their trade secrets throughout the world must protect the secrecy of the relevant information in each and every country in which it is used. The loss of secrecy anywhere in the world can affect, and often destroy, the trade secret around the world. Perhaps even higher safeguards should be maintained in countries that do not offer adequate trade secret protection, because such countries might provide ideal havens for individuals or organizations seeking to discover trade secrets for their own use or for sale to others. Even where redress may be obtained in local courts for improper use of disclosure of a trade secret, such litigation can be expensive, and it is unlikely that a damage award could be obtained that would reasonably compensate the trade secret holder for loss of his or her trade secret throughout the world.

8 OTHER FORMS OF PROTECTION

Other forms of protection for intellectual property that are available in the United States include copyrights, statutory invention registrations, and design patents. These methods of protecting intellectual property generally have only limited applicability to drug discovery and related technology. Copyrights, for example, protect a work of authorship; they do not protect inventions such as new drugs, diagnostic assays, or methods of treatment. Thus, although the copyright owner may prevent others from making copies of, e.g., a published article, manual, pamphlet, or computer program, he or she cannot prevent others from using the ideas or data contained therein. Copyrights can be useful in drug discovery by protecting printed materials such as advertising, manuals, pamphlets, computer programs, and the like. For instance, a computer program useful in DNA sequencing can be protected by copyright even though the ideas contained in the computer program and the actual DNA sequences determined using the program cannot be protected by copyright. A copyright is created once the work of authorship is produced in any tangible form. Although not required, registering the copyright in the Copyright Office of the Library of Congress provides certain advantages should it become necessary to enforce the copyright (144).

Limited protection can also be provided by the statutory invention registration (SIR) program administered by the PTO (145). This procedure provides for a patent-like document that officially and affirmatively places the invention in the public domain for defensive purposes. The SIR is essentially a defensive publication that can be used when the inventor does not wish to obtain patent rights, yet wishes to be free of any later patents by others claiming the same invention. The SIR is treated in the same manner as a patent for defensive purposes, i.e., both as prior art and as establishing a constructive reduction to practice in interference proceedings. The SIR cannot be used to prevent others from making, using, or selling the disclosed invention or inventions. The publication of the invention in a trade publication or other media has essentially the same defensive effect as a SIR. However, the effective date of a publication is generally the actual date of publication; for the SIR, the effective date is the filing date (146). The SIR procedure is often used to disclose work done at federal research agencies for which agency does not wish to seek patent protection. Anyone, however, can use the SIR procedure. The SIR program should be considered as an alternative to publication in a technical journal when one has determined not to seek patent protection for a specific invention but wishes to prevent others from obtaining patents covering that invention (147).

Design patents can be used to protect the ornamental design or aspect of a useful product (148). A design patent grants the holder the exclusive right to exclude others from making, using, and selling designs closely resembling the patented design. To be eligible for protection in this manner, the design must be novel, nonobvious, and ornamental. For example, a design patent could cover an ornamental packaging design for a drug or diagnostic kit or an ornamental design for a pill or capsule. The term of a design patent is 14 years from the date of grant. Thus, where possible and appropriate (e.g., for a unique pill or capsule design), trademark protection may be preferred because its duration is generally limited only by continued use. Design patents do not have claims like utility patents. Rather, a design patent contains one or more drawings that defines the scope of protection. The drawings are compared with the appearance of an alleged infringing product. Infringement is found "if, in the eye of an ordinary observer, giving such attention as a purchaser usually gives, two designs are substantially the same, if the resemblance is such as to deceive such an observer, inducing him to purchase one supposing it to be the other, the first one patented is infringed by the other" (149). Generally, design patents are governed by the same rules for validity as utility patents. However, they cover different aspects of a given product: a utility patent relates to the functional aspects, whereas a design patent relates only to the ornamental aspects of an article. Thus it is possible to have a utility patent and a design patent covering the same product. For a drug manufacturer, design patents might be used to help establish brand loyalty and recognition in a manner similar to trademarks.

9 CONCLUSION

Careful use of the intellectual property system, especially the patent system, in the United States and elsewhere in the world can enable those in the drug discovery and biotechnology industry to protect the fruits of their labor. By making effective use of the legal protection afforded by the intellectual property laws, a drug developer can protect its investment, enhance the value of its technology, and earn a profit sufficient to allow further research into improving existing drugs and therapies as well as developing new drugs and therapies. Indeed, by providing such protection, the intellectual property system seeks to encourage the development of new and useful technologies and products. For any industry, attention to the protection of intellectual property at the earliest stages of its development is of the utmost importance. This is especially true for the drug discovery and biotechnology industry because of the rapidly developing nature of the technology and the FDA submission requirements. The appointment of an intellectual property committee that oversees the protection process and offers overall guidance in the development of the intellectual property strategy on a continuing basis is highly recommended. The organization and the intellectual property committee should work closely with qualified legal counsel, preferably patent counsel skilled in the relevant technology, to fashion internal mechanisms for protecting the technology and for seeking the appropriate legal protection. In this manner, one can strive to obtain the legal protection that the particular technology demands and deserves.

ACKNOWLEDGMENTS

The authors would like to thank the following individuals for many helpful comments and suggestions and for assistance in preparation of this manuscript: Francis A. Even, Morgan L. Fitch Jr., Robert J. Fox, James P. Krueger, Greg H. Leitich, Timothy E. Levstik, R. Steven Pinkstaff, Andrew J. Schaefer, James J. Schumann, Stephanie L. Seidman, and Chen Wang. Errors and omissions remain the responsibility of the authors.

REFERENCES

1. For following up on specific points, more detail is available in several excellent treatises devoted to intellectual property. See, e.g., D. Chisum, *Patents* (1994); I. P. Cooper, *Biotechnology and the Law* (1993); J. Rosenstock, *The Law of Chemical and Pharmaceutical Invention* (1993); P. Rosenberg, *Patent Law Fundamentals* (1989); S. Ladas, *Patents, Trademarks and Related Rights: National and International Protection* (1975); E. B. Lipscomb, *Lipscomb's Walker on Patents* (3d ed.; 1986); M. F. Jager, *Trade Secret Law*, (1994); R.M. Milgrim, *Milgrim on Trade Secrets* (1993); J. T. McCarthy, *McCarthy on Trademarks and Unfair Competition*. (3d ed.; 1994); L. Altman, *Callmann on Unfair Competition, Trademarks and Monopolies* (4th ed.; 1993).

2. 35 U.S.C.A. § 103 (West Supp. 1993).

3. Charles Warren, Deputy Director of the U.S. PTO, personal communication (June 14, 1993). The size of the Biotechnology Examining Group has grown from about 67 examiners in 1988 (its first year) to about 173 examiners in mid-1993.

4. Congress has attempted to alleviate this problem somewhat with the Orphan Drug Act which provides, with some limitations, an exclusive 7-year right to market a drug for treatment of a disease affecting less than 200,000 individuals or for which there is "no reasonable expectation" that the developmental costs of the drug can be recovered through sales in the United States. 21 U.S.C.A. §§ 360aa-360ee (West Supp. 1993).

5. In the United States, patent applications must be filed in the name of the inventors. Inventors may assign their rights in the patent application and any patents which may issue therefrom to third parties (i.e., assignees). In many other countries, patent applications may be filed in the name of the assignee.

6. 35 U.S.C.A. § 112 (West 1984).

7. An export license is generally required to export technology developed in the United States. 35 U.S.C.A. § 184 (West Supp. 1993); 37 C.F.R. § 5.13 (1992); see also 22 C.F.R. parts 120-130 (1993) (International Traffic in Arms Regulations of the Department of State); 15 C.F.R. part 700 (1993) (Export Administration Regulations of the Department of Commerce); 10 C.F.R. part 810 (1993) (Foreign Atomic Energy Activities Regulations of the Department of Energy). Thus, a patent application for an invention made in the United States generally cannot first be filed in another country with a lesser enabling requirement unless the appropriate foreign filing license is obtained.

8. U.S. Const., art. I, § 8, cl. 8.

9. A patent does not give the patentee the right to practice the patented invention; the patent only allows the patent holder to prevent others from practicing the invention. A patentee's use of the invention may be blocked by other patents. A patentee can only practice the invention if not prevented by other patents.

10. 35 U.S.C.A. § 156 (West Supp. 1993).

11. Generally, most countries provide an exception to the first-to-file rule in cases of derivation (i.e., where the first to file learns of the invention from the inventor who files second).

12. 35 U.S.C.A. § 102(g) (West 1984).

13. A notable exception to this general rule' is found

in Canada. Generally an inventor has a 1-year grace period from the date of a public disclosure in which to file a Canadian application if the public disclosure is made by the inventor or by a person who obtained the information from the inventor. There is no grace period (i.e., absolute novelty applies) if the disclosure is made by someone other than the inventor who did not obtain the information from the inventor. A.J. Jacobs, *Patents Throughout the World* C-3 (1993).

14. The FDA submission will generally not be released to the public upon receipt. Rather, at some later time the FDA may make the information publicly available. However, one should not rely on the FDA delaying disclosure if valuable patent rights are at stake. See also Subsection 7.5.

15. 35 U.S.C.A. § 101 (West 1984).

16. See, e.g., *Arrhythmia Research Technology, Inc. v. Corazonix Corp.*, 958 F.2d 1053 (Fed. Cir. 1992) (method and apparatus claims relating to the analysis of electrocardiographic signals employing an algorithm were patentable).

17. *Diamond v. Chakrabarty*, 447 U.S. 303 (1980).

18. Donald J. Quigg, "Notice: Animals-Patentability" (April 7, 1987) (notice issued by Assistant Secretary and Commissioner of Patents and Trademarks). This PTO Notice reaffirmed that an "article of manufacture or composition of matter will not be considered patentable unless given a new form, quality, properties or combination not present in the original article existing in nature." The PTO Notice also added that a "claim directed to or including within its scope a human being will not be considered to be patentable subject matter."

19. See, e.g., *Ex parte Hibberd*, 227 U.S.P.Q. 443 (Bd. Pat. App. & Int. 1985) (corn plant with increased level of tryptophan was patentable); U.S. Patent No. 4,736,866 (April 12, 1988) (first animal patent; transgenic mouse with cancer causing gene made at Harvard University); U.S. Patent No. 5,183,949 (Feb. 2, 1993) (rabbit infected with HIV-1 virus).

20. An invention which can be used for both "useful" and illegal or fraudulent purposes may be patented. Only an invention which could *only* be used for an illegal or fraudulent purpose would be rendered unpatentable because of the utility requirement. For example, a process for making tobacco *only appear* to be of higher quality or grade and having no other function or utility (i.e., the sole utility being to deceive the public) was not patentable because of lack of utility. *Rickard v. Du Bon*, 103 F. 868 (2d Cir. 1900).

21. See *Brenner v. Manson*, 383 U.S. 519, 528-36 (1966).

22. See, e.g., *In re Langer*, 503 F.2d 1380, 1391 (C.C.P.A. 1974); *In re Newman*, 763 F.2d 407 (Fed. Cir. 1985); *Newman v. Quigg*, 877 F.2d 1575 (Fed. Cir. 1989), cert. denied, 495 U.S. 932 (1990).

23. See, e.g., *In re Jolles*, 628 F.2d 1322 (C.C.P.A. 1980); *Ex parte Kranz*, 19 U.S.P.Q.2d 1216 (Bd. Pat. App. & Int. 1991); *Ex parte Balzarini*, 21 U.S.P.Q.2d 1892 (Bd. Pat. App. & Int. 1991).

24. See generally U.S. PTO, *Manual of Patent Examining Procedure*, § 608.01(p) (5th ed.; 1993).

25. A European Patent Convention (EPC) patent issued on the Harvard mouse (see U.S. Patent No. 4,736,866, note 19 supra) in May 1992. The patent was first refused by the European Patent Office (EPO) Examining Division. After a decision of the EPO Appeal Board reversing the initial refusal and remission to the Examining Division, the patent was finally granted. The EPO Appeal Board concluded that animals, in general, can be patented. The EPC post-grant opposition period for the patent ended on February 13, 1993, after a record 16 oppositions were filed. The oppositions are currently undergoing examination. The status of the patent, and the resolution of the patentability of animals in general in Europe, must await completion of the opposition proceedings and any appeals therefrom. The opposition and appeal process is likely to take several years, if not longer. Moreover, it is not clear at this time, assuming the EPC patent survives the opposition process, just how the individual member countries will respond to the patenting of genetically-engineered animals. See generally Hepworth Lawrence Bryer & Bizley, "The Patentability of Higher Life Forms in Europe: An Update" 10 *PageView* (May 1993) (newsletter published by British law firm).

26. For a detailed description of patent laws and procedures in countries throughout the world, see A.J. Jacobs, *Patents Throughout the World* (1993).

27. The countries discussed here, along with the United States, are those which are usually recommended for global filings. See Section 5.

28. 35 U.S.C.A. § 112 (first paragraph) (West 1984)

29. 35 U.S.C.A. § 112 (second paragraph) (West 1984).

30. See, e.g., Helfgott, "A 'Global' Patent Application," 74 J. Pat. & Trademark Off. Soc. 26 (1992).

31. *Texas Instruments v. International Trade Commission*, 871 F.2d 1054, 1062 (Fed. Cir. 1989).

32. 35 U.S.C.A. § 132 (West 1984).

33. See, e.g., *In re Wands*, 858 F.2d 731 (Fed. Cir. 1988); *Kennecott Corp. v. Kyocera International*,

Inc., 835 F.2d 1419 (Fed. Cir. 1987), cert. denied, 486 U.S. 1008 (1988).

34. Such variations may fall within the scope of a claim under the doctrine of equivalents. See Subsection 4.1. It is, however, easier to prove literal infringement. Moreover, an original claim of properly expanded scope may have its own scope expanded, based on the doctrine of equivalents.

35. *In re Gay*, 309 F.2d 769, 774 (C.C.P.A. 1962) ("Not every last detail is to be described, else patent specifications would turn into production specifications, which they were never meant to be.").

36. *In re Jackson*, 217 U.S.P.Q. 804, 807 (Bd. Pat. App. & Int. 1986).

37. *Ex parte Forman*, 230 U.S.P.Q. 546, 547 (Bd. Pat. App. & Int. 1986); *In re Wands*, 858 F.2d 731, 737 (Fed. Cir. 1988).

38. Past tense, which might imply that the work was actually carried out, should not be used for paper examples. It should be clear from the text that the work described was not carried out.

39. Budapest Treaty on the International Recognition of Microorganisms for the Purposes of Patent Procedure of April 28, 1977, reprinted in A.J. Jacobs, *Patents Throughout the World*, App. C4(a) (1993). Currently, 24 nations (including, for example, the United States, Japan, Australia, and most European countries) are contracting states of the Budapest Treaty.

40. The "certified parties" entitled to obtain a deposit under the Budapest Treaty are determined by the laws and regulations of the country or countries in which a patent application is filed. See Rule 11, Regulations Under the Budapest Treaty on the International Recognition of Microorganisms for the Purposes of Patent Procedure of April 28, 1977, reprinted in A.J. Jacobs, *Patents Throughout the World*, App. C4(b) (1993).

41. *DeGeorge v. Bernier*, 768 F.2d 1318, 1324 (Fed. Cir. 1985).

42. Recently lower courts have found that improvements made after the filing date of an original application may have to be disclosed in any subsequent continuation or CIP applications. *Transco Products Inc. v. Performance Contracting Inc.*, 821 F. Supp. 537, 548-550 (N.D. Ill. 1993); *Applied Material, Inc. v. Advanced Semiconductor Materials of America Inc.*, No. C-91-20061-RMW (N.D. Cal. April 26, 1994) (best mode must be updated in CIP application). As applied to CIP applications, such a rule seems reasonable. It is likely, however, that the Court of Appeals for the Federal Circuit will be called upon to determine whether such a rule generally applies to all continuation applications. See also Subsection 7.4.

43. Many countries do not have a specific best mode requirement. Thus, an application filed by a foreign inventor based on the application filed in the home country potentially may not disclose the best mode. Foreign inventors are advised to supplement their United State patent application to include the best mode known as of the priority date. Otherwise, enforcement of such patents in the United States may present significant best mode problems.

44. *Spectra-Physics, Inc. v. Coherent, Inc.*, 827 F.2d 1524, 1536 (Fed. Cir.), cert. denied, 484 U.S. 954 (1987).

45. 35 U.S.C.A. § 102 (West 1984).

46. If the method of making the compound is clearly within the skill in the art, such a reference could place the compound within the public domain. In such a case, the reference could anticipate a claim to the compound.

47. *In re Schoenwald*, 964 F.2d 1122 (Fed. Cir. 1992).

48. *In re Spada*, 911 F.2d 705 (Fed. Cir. 1990).

49. *Graham v. John Deere Co.*, 383 U.S. 1, 17-18 (1966).

50. *Environmental Designs, Ltd. v. Union Oil Co.*, 713 F.2d 693, 696-697 (Fed. Cir. 1983), cert. denied, 464 U.S. 1043 (1984).

51. *Hodosh v. Block Drug Co.*, 786 F.2d 1136, 1143 n.5 (Fed. Cir.) (citations omitted), cert. denied, 479 U.S. 827 (1986).

52. See, e.g., *In re Dow Chem. Co.*, 837 F.2d 469, 473 (Fed. Cir. 1988).

53. *In re O'Farrell*, 853 F.2d 894, 903 (Fed. Cir. 1988).

54. See, e.g., *Graham v. John Deere Co.*, 383 U.S. at 36 (courts should "resist the temptation to read into the prior art the teachings of the invention in issue"); *Uniroyal, Inc. v. Rudkin-Wiley Corp.*, 837 F.2d 1044, 1051 (Fed. Cir.), cert. denied, 488 U.S. 825 (1988); *W.L. Gore & Assoc., Inc. v. Garlock, Inc.*, 721 F.2d 1540, 1553 (Fed. Cir. 1983), cert. denied, 469 U.S. 851 (1984).

55. *In re Grabiak*, 769 F.2d 729, 731 (Fed. Cir. 1985); *In re Dillon*, 919 F.2d 688, 692 (Fed. Cir. 1990) (in banc), cert. denied, 111 S.Ct. 1682 (1991).

56. *In re Papesch*, 315 F.2d 381, 391 (C.C.P.A. 1963).

57. *In re Dillon*, 919 F.2d at 692-693.

58. See, e.g., *In re Merck & Co.*, 800 F.2d 1091,

1096-1098 (Fed. Cir. 1986) ("bioisosterism was commonly used by medicinal chemists prior to 1959 in an effort to design and predict drug activity"); *Imperial Chemical Industries v. Danbury Pharmacal*, 777 F. Supp. 330, 368-373 (D. Del. 1991) (bioisosterism theory used to invalidate a patent claim directed to use of atenolol for treatment of hypertension under 35 U.S.C. § 103), aff'd, 972 F.2d 1354 (Fed. Cir. 1992).

59. *In re Merck & Co.*, 800 F.2d at 1094-1095.

60. *In re Durden*, 763 F.2d 1406 (Fed. Cir. 1985).

61. *In re Dillon*, 919 F.2d at 695 (dicta).

62. The inventor or assignee is normally represented by a patent agent or attorney in proceedings before the PTO. Patent agents and attorneys are admitted to practice before the PTO upon passing the PTO bar examination. The inventor may, however, represent himself or herself.

63. The written record of an abandoned application is open for public inspection if a later United States patent formally relies upon, or is formally related to, the abandoned application.

64. 37 C.F.R. § 1.102 (1992). An application can be advanced out of turn for examination if the Commissioner of Patents and Trademarks believes advancement is justified. Suitable reasons for advancement include, for example, applicant's health or age or that "the invention will materially enhance the quality of the environment or materially contribute to the development or conservation of energy resources." A more significant showing will generally be required for advancement based on other reasons.

65. 35 U.S.C.A. § 184 (West Supp. 1993); 37 C.F.R. §§ 5.11-5.25 (1992). Unless the PTO notifies the applicant otherwise, the applicant can file foreign applications 6 months after the United States filing date without a foreign filing license.

66. 35 U.S.C.A. § 253 (West 1984); 37 C.F.R. § 1.321 (1992).

67. Up to 3 additional months for responding generally can be obtained by payment of an extension fee.

68. Such a party, however, could lose priority if that party "abandoned, suppressed, or concealed" the invention. 35 U.S.C.A. § 102(g) (West 1984). For example, if the first party to conceive and reduce the invention to practice decided to keep the invention a trade secret and was only spurred to file an application upon learning of another's invention of the same subject matter, the first party's priority could be extinguished by its failure to file its patent application in a timely manner.

69. On occasion the PTO may inadvertently issue two patents that claim the same subject matter. In such cases, the PTO does not have jurisdiction to institute an interference proceeding. If one of the patentees brings an appropriate civil action in a federal district court, the court could determine which patentee is entitled to a patent claiming the subject matter.

70. In such cases, the PTO will normally accept an affidavit or declaration filed by the applicant that alleges a basis upon which applicant is entitled to a judgment relative to the patentee. If applicant's effective filing date is more than 3 months after the effective filing date of the patentee, the PTO will generally demand evidence and arguments as to why the applicant is prima facie entitled to judgment relative to the patentee. 37 C.F.R. § 1.606 (1992).

71. A party who cannot prove an earlier filing date may prefer that no one obtain a patent so he or she can practice the invention without restriction. See, e.g., *Perkin v. Kwon*, 886 F.2d 325 (Fed. Cir. 1989). Such a party (i.e., one who knows that priority cannot be proven) could also seek a favorable license (especially while the preliminary statements remain sealed) and thereby, at least to some degree, benefit from the protection offered by the other party's patent (if granted by the PTO). The other party may be willing to make concessions in the terms of such an agreement since it would effectively terminate the interference and eliminate the risk of losing the priority contest.

72. In recently reported interference proceedings, the senior and junior parties prevailed in about 60 and 29 percent of the cases, respectively, with the remainder resulting in split decisions. For proceedings decided by the Board, the senior and junior parties prevailed in about 47 and 38 percent of the cases, respectively, with the remainder being split decisions. Of the 530 interferences during this period, only about 24 percent proceeded to a decision by the Board. Calvert & Sofocleous, "Interference Statistics for Fiscal Years 1986 to 1988," 71 J. Pat. & Trademark Off. Soc. 399 (1989).

73. 35 U.S.C.A. §§ 254-256 (West 1984).

74. 35 U.S.C.A. § 251 (West 1984); 37 C.F.R. §§ 1.171-1.179 (1992).

75. 35 U.S.C.A. § 252 (West 1984).

76. 35 U.S.C.A. §§ 301-307 (West 1984 & Supp. 1993).

77. One exception to this general rule is where a third party is precluded from entering a market by a blocking patent which, in the opinion of the third party, is invalid based on prior art not considered by the PTO. By requesting a reexamination, the third party would hope to invalidate

the patent and clear the path for its entry into the market. If unsuccessful, the third party may wish to move on to other business opportunities.

78. 35 U.S.C.A. § 271(g) (West Supp. 1993).

79. A suit alleging infringement during the term of a patent can generally be brought after the patent expires. Damages cannot, however, be recovered for infringing acts occurring more than 6 years prior to filing the complaint. 35 U.S.C.A. § 286 (West 1984).

80. A lapsed patent can be reinstated if it is shown that the delay in paying the maintenance fee was "unintentional" (if within 24 months of the 6-month grace period) or "unavoidable" (at any time after the 6-month grace period). 35 U.S.C.A. § 41(c)(1) (West Supp. 1993). Persons who made, purchased, or used the invention after the lapse of the patent and before the actual payment of the missed maintenance fee may continue to use, or to sell to others to be used or sold, the specific items made, purchased, or used during the time the patent was not in force. A court may also allow for continuedmanufacture, use, or sale of the invention "to the extent and under such terms as the court deems equitable for the protection of investments made or business commenced" during the time the patent had lapsed. 35 U.S.C.A. § 41(c)(2) (West 1984).

81. 35 U.S.C.A. § 271(a) (West 1984).

82. *Graver Tank & Manufacturing Co. v. Linde Air Products Co.*, 339 U.S. 605, 608 (1950).

83. See, e.g., *Wilson Sporting Goods Co. v. David Geoffrey & Assoc.*, 904 F.2d 677, 684-685 (Fed. Cir.), cert. denied, 111 S.Ct. 537 (1990).

84. 35 U.S.C.A. § 271(b) (West 1984).

85. 35 U.S.C.A. § 271(c) (West 1984).

86. However, such intent may be sufficient for a finding of willful infringement if the materiality of the particular prior art is especially high. See, e.g., *N.V. Akzo v. E.I. Du Pont de Nemours*, 810 F.2d 1148, 1153 (Fed. Cir. 1987).

87. See, e.g., *Kingsdown Medical Consultants Ltd. v. Hollister Inc.*, 863 F.2d 867, 876 (Fed. Cir. 1988), cert. denied, 490 U.S. 1067 (1989); *Atlas Powder Co. v. E.I. Du Pont de Nemours*, 750 F.2d 1569, 1578 (Fed. Cir. 1984).

88. A very limited "experimental use" exception permits otherwise infringing acts if the acts are "for amusement, to satisfy idle curiosity or for strictly philosophical inquiry." *Roche Products, Inc. v. Bolar Pharmaceutical Co.*, 733 F.2d 858, 863 (Fed. Cir. 1984). Commercial activities are very unlikely to fall within this exception.

89. 35 U.S.C.A. § 271(e) (West Supp. 1993). This exemption specifically excludes from its coverage "a new animal drug or veterinary biological product . . . which is primarily manufactured using recombinant DNA, recombinant RNA, hybridoma technology, or other processes involving site specific genetic manipulation techniques."

90. 35 U.S.C.A. § 284 (West 1984).

91. 35 U.S.C.A. § 285 (West 1984). An award of attorney fees might be appropriate for an especially willful and egregious infringer or against a patentee who litigated in bad faith or committed fraud during the prosection of the patent in the PTO. See, e.g., *Machinery Corp. of Am. v. Gullfiber AB"*, 774 F.2d 467, 472-473 (Fed. Cir. 1985).

92. 35 U.S.C.A. § 283 (West 1984).

93. *Atlas Powder Co. v. Ireco Chemicals.*, 773 F.2d 1230 (Fed. Cir. 1985).

94. 28 U.S.C.A. § 1400(b) (West 1976).

95. *VE Holding Corp. v. Johnson Gas Appliance Co.*, 917 F.2d 1574 (Fed. Cir. 1990), cert. denied, 111 S.Ct. 1315 (1991).

96. See, e.g., Brunda, "Resolution of Patent Disputes by Non-litigation Procedures," 15 AIPLA Q.J. 73 (1987); Arnold, "Alternative Dispute Resolution in Intellectual Property Cases," 9(1) *AIPLA Selected Legal Papers* 289 (July 1991).

97. The recently adopted North American Free Trade Agreement (NAFTA) between the United States, Canada, and Mexico will continue the trend towards such a single North American market. See generally R.M. Milgrim, 2 *Milgrim on Trade Secrets* § 9.07 (1993); Paul, Hastings, Janofsky & Walker, *North American Free Trade Agreement: Summary and Analysis* (1993).

98. Paris Convention of March 20, 1883, as revised at Stockholm on July 14, 1967, reprinted in A.J. Jacobs, *Patents Throughout the World*, App. B1(d) (1993) (Stockholm text; earlier revisions are also included in Appendix B).

99. Applications generally can be filed in Paris Convention countries after the 12 month period if there has been no public disclosure. However, the priority date of the earlier filed application cannot be claimed.

100. European Patent Convention of October 5, 1973 (as amended to 1979), reprinted in A.J. Jacobs, *Patents Throughout the World*, App. B3(a) (1993).

101. Patent Cooperation Treaty of June 19, 1970 (as amended in 1985), reprinted in A.J. Jacobs, *Patents Throughout the World*, App. B2(a) (1993).

102. For the European countries, an applicant can

designate a single EPC application (which in turns designates the desired member states) or separate national applications in the individual European countries.

103. F.I. Schechter, *The Historical Foundations of the Law Relating to Trademarks* (1925). See also Diamond, "The Historical Development of Trademarks," 65 Trademark Rep. 265 (1975).

104. 15 U.S.C.A. §§ 1051-1127 (West 1963, 1976, 1982 & Supp. 1993).

105. Secondary meaning is "acquired when the name and the business become synonymous in the public mind; and [it] submerges the primary meaning of the name . . . in favor of its meaning as a word identifying that business." *Visser v. Macres*, 137 U.S.P.Q. 492,494 (Cal. Dist. Ct. App. 1963).

106. U.S. PTO, *Trademark Manual of Examining Procedure* §§ 1209.01(a) & (b) (2d ed.; 1993) (citations omitted).

107. *In re Owens-Corning Fiberglas Corp.* 774 F.2d 1116 (Fed. Cir. 1985).

108. *Braun Inc. v. Dynamic Corp. of Am.*, 975 F.2d 815, 826-827 (Fed. Cir. 1992).

109. 15 U.S.C.A. § 1052 (West 1976 & Supp. 1993).

110. 15 U.S.C.A. § 1052(d) (West Supp. 1993).

111. If such a knock-out mark is found, one can abandon that mark and attempt to find another, more suitable mark or, in some cases, attempt to obtain the rights to the mark from the registrant.

112. Thus, registration of a mark is not necessary. A common law trademark can be created by using the mark in commerce. Generally, such a common law trademark affords protection to its owner only in the geographical area of actual use.

113. 15 U.S.C.A. §§ 1065 & 1115 (West Supp. 1993).

114. 15 U.S.C.A. § 1057(b) (West Supp. 1993).

115. 15 U.S.C.A. § 1065 (West Supp. 1993).

116. 15 U.S.C.A. § 1115 (West Supp. 1993).

117. 15 U.S.C.A. § 1072 (West 1963).

118. See 15 U.S.C.A. § 1111 (West Supp. 1993) (relevant portion quoted in text at note 126 infra).

119. 15 U.S.C.A. § 1121 (West Supp. 1993).

120. *Walt Disney Productions v. Kusan, Inc.*, 204 U.S.P.Q. 284 (C.D. Cal. 1979).

121. 15 U.S.C.A. § 1124 (West 1976).

122. 15 U.S.C.A. § 1117 (West Supp. 1993). The registrant is also entitled to recover the "costs" of the litigation against an infringer.

123. 15 U.S.C.A. § 1118 (West Supp. 1993).

124. *Baker v. Master Printers Union*, 34 F. Supp. 808, 811 (D.N.J. 1940).

125. *Bayer Co. v. United Drug Co.*, 272 F. 505 (2d Cir. 1921).

126. 15 U.S.C.A. § 1111 (West Supp. 1993).

127. 15 U.S.C.A. § 1125(a) (West Supp. 1993).

128. *Ciba-Geigy Corp. v. Bolar Pharmaceutical Co.*, 547 F. Supp. 1095 (D.N.J. 1982), aff'd, 719 F.2d 56 (3d Cir. 1983), cert. denied, 471 U.S. 1137 (1984).

129. 15 U.S.C.A. § 1125(a)(1)(B) (West Supp. 1993) (emphasis added).

130. Restatement (First) of Torts, § 757 cmt. b (1939).

131. Uniform Trade Secrets Act, § 1(4) (1985). As of 1992, the Uniform Trade Secrets Act was adopted in some version in about 37 states and the District of Columbia.

132. Uniform Trade Secrets Act, § 2 (1985).

133. See, e.g., Robbins, "The Rights of the First Inventor-Trade Secret User as Against Those of the Second Inventor-Patentee (Part I)," 61 J. Pat. Off. Soc. 574 (1979); Jorda, "The Rights of the First Inventor-Trade Secret User as Against Those of the Second Inventor-Patentee (Part II)," 61 J. Pat. Off. Soc. 593 (1979).

134. Jorda, supra note 133, at 597. Of course, some trade secrets may have a considerable longer life. For example, the original formula for Coca-Cola® has remained a trade secret for well over 100 years.

135. *Kewanee Oil Co. v. Bicron Corp.*, 416 U.S. 470 (1974).

136. 5 U.S.C.A. § 552 (West 1977 & Supp. 1993). Virtually every state has adopted a corresponding state version of FOIA.

137. 5 U.S.C.A. § 552(b)(3) (West 1977).

138. 18 U.S.C.A. § 1905 (West Supp. 1993).

139. 5 U.S.C.A. § 552(b)(4) (West 1977).

140. *Chrysler Corp. v. Brown*, 441 U.S. 281, 293 (1979).

141. A trade secret owner may seek, through a so-called "reverse FOIA" suit, to enjoin an agency from releasing information containing trade secrets. See generally R.M. Milgrim, 1 *Milgrim on Trade Secrets* § 6.02A[3] (1993).

142. The specific information on trade secrets which follows for countries outside the United States is generally taken from R.M. Milgrim, 4 *Milgrim on Trade Secrets* App. R, R-49 (1993) (reprinting Prasinos, "International Legal Protection of Computer Programs," 26 Idea 173 (1984)). The trade secret laws of these countries have likely changed, perhaps significantly, since the publi-

cation of this article. Nonetheless, this information illustrates the variability expected in trade secret law throughout the world. Clearly one should seek guidance from local counsel in the relevant country before attempting to enforce a trade secret in that country.

143. Some countries (e.g., France and Italy) allow trade secret protection for information which is not known within their national boundaries even if it is known in other countries. In this age of rapid communication and computer databases, it is increasingly unlikely that information which is known elsewhere in the world can effectively remain a secret for any significant length of time in a given country (especially in the highly industrialized countries). Generally, the more valuable the information, the quicker its spread throughout the world once it becomes known in one part of the world.

144. See, e.g., 17 U.S.C.A. §§ 411-412 (West Supp. 1993).

145. 35 U.S.C.A. § 157 (West Supp. 1993).

146. Essentially the same effect can be obtained with an issued patent by simply not enforcing the patent or filing a disclaimer whereby the patent is dedicated to the public. 35 U.S.C.A. § 253 (West 1984); 37 C.F.R. § 1.321(a) (1992). Such dedication to the public does not effect the defensive aspects of the patent.

147. The time lag between submission and actual publication date in a technical journal, especially in a peer-reviewed journal, can be significant. Such delays may allow for another inventor to file a patent application covering the invention before the actual publication date and ultimately obtain patent protection.

148. 35 U.S.C.A. §§ 171-173 (West 1984).

149. *Gorham Co. v. White*, 81 U.S. (14 Wall.) 511, 528 (1871).

CHAPTER FOUR

Information Science in Drug Discovery

Y. LIN CHANG and
LINDA M. KLUG

Marion Merrell Dow Inc.
Kansas City, Missouri, USA

CONTENTS

1 Introduction, 104
2 Development of Information Retrieval
  Technology, 104
  2.1 On-line vendors and databases, 105
  2.2 Databases for PCs and CD-ROMs, 105
  2.3 Informal retrieval packages, 105
  2.4 Database management software for PCs, 105
  2.5 Database management software for in-house
    mainframes, 106
  2.6 Others, 106
3 Information Needs in Phases of Drug
  Discovery, 106
  3.1 Initiation of research projects, 106
  3.2 Synthesis of target compounds, 107
  3.3 Isolation, characterization, and structural
    determination, 107
  3.4 Patent filing, 108
  3.5 Optimization of the lead compound, 108
  3.6 Product development, 109
  3.7 Chemical development, 109
  3.8 In- and out-licensing opportunities, 109
4 Benefit of Information Sciences to Drug
  Process, 110
5 Conclusion, 110

Burger's Medicinal Chemistry and Drug Discovery,
Fifth Edition, Volume 1: Principles and Practice,
Edited by Manfred E. Wolff.
ISBN 0-471-57556-9 © 1995 John Wiley & Sons, Inc.

1 INTRODUCTION

In the last few decades, pharmaceutical research has become more competitive as well as expansive. It has been estimated that it takes 10–12 years and well over $200 million to develop a new drug fully from synthesis to launch, and it can fail at any stage along the way. Now, the entire industry is going through various cycles of reorganization, directional assessment, redesign, quality improvement, and benchmarking throughout drug discovery and development in an intensive effort to shorten R&D cycle time so that a drug can be brought to market as soon as possible while it is still under patent protection. Most pharmaceutical companies have invested a lot of money and resources in state-of-the-art technologies to modernize the drug discovery effort, such as Cray super computers for rational drug design. However, one of the best ways to ensure the success in drug discovery and development is to utilize the enormous amount of knowledge that has been accumulated in the past effectively, to plan ahead carefully and make informed decisions in every stage of the research and development cycle. This information can be specific data generated by research scientists, published literature, patent information, regulatory information, and even business information for competitive intelligence and enabling technologies. Unfortunately, as critical as it is, the amount of information is growing so rapidly that the information explosion is more than a catch phrase to describe the proliferation of technical information in recent years. Information is more abundant and more specialized than ever before, whereas the drug discovery process has become increasingly complex. Thus, the use of information science in managing the vast wealth of information and tailoring it to specific needs of individual scientists, specific projects or the entire research area has become an important facet of drug discovery.

This chapter discusses the diversity of the information needs in different phases of drug discovery. It is not intended to examine all the databases available in the industry, but rather to give enough information and sufficient examples to demonstrate the various information technologies available as tools for drug discovery as well as to emphasize the importance of information science in drug discovery.

2 DEVELOPMENT OF INFORMATION RETRIEVAL TECHNOLOGY

For many years, primary sources of information have been delivered in traditional ways, such as books, journals, patents, encyclopedias, handbooks, dictionaries, and literature abstracting and indexing services. However, powerful information systems, advanced computer graphics hardware and software have been developed in the last few decades. As a result, information is now available in various forms of electronic media. On-line databases are provided by vendors through telecommunication links, and there are many databases for personal computers, CD-ROMs, and in-house mainframes. The access to these different types of databases has been greatly enhanced by telecommunication networks, local area networks, and distributed system technology. This capability to share and exchange information across laboratories, sites, and even continents, has added tremendous value for most pharmaceutical companies that are competing in a global environment. At the same time, system software and application software have proliferated, thus providing information scientists and bench scientists various useful tools to access different types of information from their desktops. The following are some examples in each important category.

2.1 On-Line Vendors and Databases

On-line retrieval systems have been available since the 1970s. An user can directly search a computerized database on a remote computer using a terminal and a modem via a telecommunication link. Some well-known on-line vendors include Dialog, BRS, STN, Orbit, Data-Star, National Library of Medicine, etc. These vendors provide a wide variety of databases containing information in a number of areas including chemistry, medicine, engineering, regulatory information and news. These databases can be bibliographic in format such as CA File, BIOSIS, and Medline; full-text such as CJACS and CJWILEY; reaction information such as CASREACT; numeric data such as RTECS and SPECINFO; sequences such as GENBANK; and news such as SCRIP (or PHIND, Pharmaceutical Industry Database). Many vendors offer directories and database indexes to help users locate the relevant databases. Also, many databases now have a thesaurus on line or menu-driven systems to assist end user searching.

2.2 Databases for PCs and CD-ROMs

There are a number of databases now available for personal computers and CD-ROMs. They are affordable, easy to maintain and, with proper networking, they can be an important source for sharing information and providing desktop access for bench scientists. Unique products include a CD-ROM database for MSDS (Material Safety Data Sheets), Current Facts in Chemistry from Beilstein on CD-ROM, a PC-based Pharmaprojects, CIPSLINE PC (structural databases selected from Drugs of the Future and the Drug Data Report) and ESPACE, a patent imaging product on CD-ROM, from Micropatents.

2.3 Information Retrieval Packages

Most pharmaceutical companies have gone through a major initiative to provide personal computers in their research facilities since computers have become an important tool for drug discovery. A number of front-end packages are available which offer automatic log-on procedures and guided search menus, as well as capabilities to upload queries and download citations to edit. These are designed to help end users such as bench chemists do their own searching without significant training in information retrieval. Recently, many packages such as STN Express, ChemTalk, Molkick, etc., have developed graphic interfaces to draw, upload, search and display structures and reactions. Some are designed to handle 3-dimensional visualization and searching such as Alchemy, while others, such as PC-Gene, are used for sequence/homology searches.

2.4 Database Management Software for PCs

Like the development of front-end packages for information retrieval, there are now quite a few software packages available for research scientists to create their personal or project databases for storing, retrieving, searching, displaying and printing information such as references, substances, or reactions. Software for reference databases include Pro-Cite, Reference Manager, Personal File Systems, Papyrus, etc. These packages enable users to download citations from on-line databases in order to create their own collection of literature tailored to their subjects of interest. Other available software, such as Chembase or ISIS Base, offers the capability to create graphic databases for compounds and reactions that enable chemists in the pharmaceutical industry to store structural information and search graphically on their personal computers.

2.5 Database Management Software for In-House Mainframes

This is one of the most exciting developments in the pharmaceutical industry as far as information science is concerned. The principal information needs of chemists in the drug discovery area center around a substance and its structure, preparations, reactions, physiochemical properties, biological properties, and toxicity. In terms of the drug design effort, the chemical structures of compounds and their relationship to biological activities form the core of proprietary information that many pharmaceutical companies are attempting to centralize and disseminate in support of the drug discovery process. The software that has been unique and commonly used in the industry is MACCS (Molecule ACCess System) and REACCS (REaction ACCess System) from MDL Information Systems. MACCS provides capabilities to build proprietary and commercial databases of substances with easy-to-use point-and-click graphic interfaces for structural querying, viewing, and reporting of data. It also offers interfaces to relational databases for biological, inventory information, etc. There are a growing number of commercial databases available for use on the MACCS software which are designed to facilitate the structure–activity relationship and modeling studies in rational drug design. These include Standard Drug File (SDF), MACCS Drug Data Report (MDDR), Comprehensive Medicinal Chemistry (CMC-3D), Fine Chemical Directory (FCD-3D), etc. Recently, there are a few more new exciting products in this area, such as Unity from Tripos and Chem-X from Chemical Design.

REACCS, as a tool for synthetic and development chemists, provides chemists with powerful and flexible search capabilities for reaction searching in a variety of commercial databases such as Theilheimer's Synthetic Methods of Organic Chemistry, Current Chemical Reactions, or ChemInform. REACCS also enables users to create corporate proprietary reaction databases. Other databases in REACCS format, such as Xenobiotic Metabolism, are used to provide access on metabolic information related to compounds. Other new products in this area are Protecting Groups and MOS (Methods in Organic Synthesis) from Synopsis.

A new generation of software from MDL Information Systems, called ISIS, is beginning to be used within the pharmaceutical industry. ISIS, the Integrated Scientific Information System, is an integrated, distributed system that can potentially integrate the workstations, databases, and computer platforms throughout a company's entire research organization. However, it remains to be seen whether ISIS or other similar products will replace the existing chemical information systems in the decade to come.

2.6 Others

There are still many other different software now available to assist research scientists in handling information in various types of applications. SANDRA (Structure and Reference Analyzer), for example, is a PC software that generates reference pointers to the Beilstein Handbook by drawing the chemical structure of a compound. AutoNom, another example of PC software from the Beilstein Institute, converts structures to IUPAC names.

3 INFORMATION NEEDS IN PHASES OF DRUG DISCOVERY

3.1 Initiation of Research Projects

The progression in the birth of a new drug starts at the initiation of a research project.

Once a therapeutic interest within a company is established, the project team begins with a broad retrospective review of all current and past knowledge of the disease and its treatment. This includes the biochemistry of the disease, mechanism of action of known drugs, pharmacology for its treatment, as well as the chemistry and structure–activity relationships of presently available agents. This requires a major search in the published and patent literature. Once the new state-of-the-art review is completed, a SDI (Selective Dissemination of Information) profile is usually set up in several major on-line databases for future reference so the project team can continue to be informed, on a regular basis, of any new findings or new patent applications by competitors. This current awareness service is very essential for any on-going projects.

Sometimes, ideas are generated by evaluating the biological activity in relation to the chemical structure of current drugs. Besides finding structures in CAS Registry File, chemists can search in-house commercial databases such as SDF, MDDR or CMC as well as the company's proprietary structural file in order to find a potential link in certain structural entities to the desired biological activity or undesired toxicities. With many 3D-searching capabilities in the mainframe, it is also possible to systematically develop ideas on possible pharmacophores from these compounds with proven therapeutic uses.

3.2 Synthesis of Target Compounds

Once a desired structure is conceived, there are several steps that should be taken before chemists begin their bench work. First of all, a novelty search of this structure is very crucial, to ensure the patentability in the future. Usually, structural searches begin in the CAS Registry File, which contains more than 12 million substances reported in the literature from 1957. If the exact compound is not found, a substructural search is done to retrieve its related compounds. Generally, queries are broadened as often as needed to ensure their comprehensiveness. The same structural searches are executed in the Beilstein database on-line to cover the literature prior to 1957. Sometimes if the project is very critical and extremely competitive, a Markush-type structural search is performed in the Derwent patent files using fragmentation codes and the Markush DARC topological search system, or the CAS MARPAT file to determine whether a compound has been described as a member of a generic class of substances in a patent. If the compound is deemed to be novel, the next thing is to plot a synthetic plan from commercially available starting materials. Besides searching the on-line chemistry files for preparative papers of similar compounds, reaction searches can be very helpful. There are several reaction databases available with the in-house REACCS system and on-line systems such as STN. Reaction searches can be done by either defining products, reactants, reagents, or intermediates. Reaction searches, especially on REACCS, have become a very useful tool for synthetic planning. They provide chemists with easy access to the proven reaction technology and novel transformations reported in the literature. During the strategic planning process, searches can also be performed to look for commercially available chemical reagents or intermediates in the FCD file on REACCS, or other similar files on-line. Another available computer program, called LHASA (Logic and Heuristics Applied to Synthetic Analysis), can also be used to generate a synthetic plan by working backward from target compounds by retrosynthetic analysis.

3.3 Isolation, Characterization, and Structural Determination

During the phase of synthetic preparations,

chemists are constantly dealing with problems in the isolation, characterization, and structural determination of products and intermediates. Searches in the chemical literature for work-ups, physiochemical properties, NMR, IR or mass spectral data, chromatographic separation techniques, etc., can be very helpful. There are many databases on-line available for this purpose, such as CA File, Analytical Abstracts, SpecInfo, and Cambridge Crystallographic Database. When questions arise in the potential toxicity of compounds, MSDS sources and other toxicity databases or databanks are available on-line or on CD-ROM for retrieving this type of information.

3.4 Patent Filing

After target compounds are synthesized and preliminary biological tests indicate the desired potential of therapeutic action, a patent needs to be filed as soon as possible to ensure the patent protection for the intellectual property and the extensive research and development effort down the road. In fact, patent applications for all of the countries where there is potential market should be filed. Prior to the filing, an exhaustive patent search is needed to find out whether the compound of interest or its close analogs have been described in the prior art. The results of the search are used to establish the broadest possible claim scope for the invention in order to obtain the strongest patent protection possible. Once a drug has been introduced, new synthetic methods, therapeutic utilities and dosage forms under consideration are evaluated for their patentability, and additional patent applications are filed to protect them. The patent literature is followed carefully to identify potential competitors or infringers. There are many databases on-line that provide information about patents. Chemical Abstracts, the

Derwent World Patents Index, the French Patent Office's Pharmsearch, and the IFI/ Plenum CLAIMS Uniterm and Comprehensive databases provide indexing of chemical structures in patents, whereas bibliographical, legal status, and textual data are available from databases such as INPADOC, PATFULL, GPAT, and JAPIO.

When new products or processes are planned, it is essential to search for patents that might be infringed upon. When a third party patent covering the proposed new product or process is discovered, additional searching may be needed in order to determine whether the patent is valid and in force. Decisions as to whether the company should offer to license the patents or challenge their validity are made on the basis of these patent status and patent validity searches. Patentability and validity searching are very specialized and complex; therefore they are performed by information specialists, rather than end users.

3.5 Optimization of the Lead Compound

The next phase of research effort is generally focused on the optimization of the lead compound in order to find the best compound with the most desired biological response and minimum side effects for development. This is usually done by systematic evaluation of structural activity relationship (SAR) and/or modeling studies. This type of study is facilitated now by the in-house database management software that offers interface and spreadsheet functions to study 2D and/or 3D structures in relation to the specific biological test data. Again, MACCS and a few other database management software packages offer the capability to track structures and numerous biological activities across the research areas, information systems, and sites. This type of searching is generally performed by the chemists and biologists themselves. The need for the information support is in the on-going training and support of end users.

3.6 Product Development

When one or two lead compounds are chosen to become clinical candidates, information services continue to be crucial to the success of the development. A drug's activity depends on many factors, including route of administration, metabolic transformation and toxicities, etc. It requires the team effort of multidisciplinary areas, such as analytical science, pharmacokinetics, drug metabolism, pharmacy research, and clinical research. All of these efforts lead to the filing of regulatory submissions. During this time, continued dissemination of information on the drug's development across the functions is very important. Also, in compliance with regulatory requirements, published literature on the clinical candidates must be tracked and reported regularly for any early warning of unwanted toxicities or adverse reactions. Another important source of proprietary information in this stage is internal reports. Information services are needed to provide ready access for all the reports on the work done on the compound regardless of time and place, since the full-scale development of a compound may take a span of several years. The management of this vast amount of information is undoubtedly critical.

3.7 Chemical Development

When compounds enter the development stage, a larger amount of supply is con-stantly in demand to provide samples for development research and clinical studies. A group of development chemists are assigned to study possible alternative routes for synthesis to increase the overall yields, reduce synthetic steps, utilize cheaper starting materials and intermediates, or use milder reaction conditions. Again, reaction and structural searching of REACCS commercial databases and on-line databases provide a useful tool in generating better synthetic plans from the literature. Many companies have also found it useful to establish in-house proprietary reaction databases to avoid duplication of synthetic work as a compound progresses through the scale-up process.

3.8 In- and Out- Licensing Opportunities

During the progression of phases of drug discovery, research projects may come to a stop due to some unexpected difficulties in development, or undesired side effects, or changed market competition. Many pharmaceutical companies are exploring licensing and external partnership opportunities as options to handle the compounds in these projects. Information services can be useful for locating expertise and providing analysis and competitive intelligence as well as for evaluating other companies' patent port-folios. There are many databases or programs which are tailored to fulfill the need in this area. For example, a program called Science Models is designed to provide this type of information by an algorithm in linking and mapping research concepts and institutes via cocitation in the literature. Other novel databases available now are BEST North America and BEST Europe which contain unique information on the expertise and inventions in the major universities and research parks in Europe and North America.

4 BENEFIT OF INFORMATION SCIENCES TO DRUG PROCESS

To summarize, the major benefits are

- Time savings
  Computer-aided searching of literature in electronic media saves time for research scientists. Thus, efficiency and productivity is enhanced.
- Eliminating duplicate efforts
  The flow and the exchange of information is streamlined via better information management throughout the discovery cycle. With better communication among research groups, duplicate efforts can be reduced.
- Shortening the time line of drug discovery
  Improved efficiency and productivity, better communication, and timely informed decisions contribute to shortening discovery cycle time.
- Preventing patent infringement
  Keeping scientists informed in the patent literature safeguards the legal protection of inventions.
- Better strategic planning
  Information sciences can offer services and tools which help keep executives, project leaders, and research scientists keenly aware of new competitive developments in the competition, thus allowing better planning in the research strategic direction.

5 CONCLUSION

The significance of information sciences in the different phases of drug discovery from the conception of a new drug through its early development has been discussed. The benefits of information services and tools for information retrieval and management is clearly demonstrated. However, research scientists and top management in the drug discovery area need to be educated and trained to take full advantage of information sciences. They need more knowledge of what information services can provide in order to ask better questions and make a better interpretation of information which is provided to them.

With this knowledge, it should become clear that effective use of information can significantly improve a company's drug discovery efforts.

REFERENCES

1. M. Grayson, ed., *Information Retrieval in Chemistry and Chemical Patent Law*, Wiley-Interscience, New York, 1983.
2. H. G. Grabowski and J. M. Vernon, *Studies on Drug Substitution, Patent Policy and Innovation in the Pharmaceutical Industry*, NTIS, National Science Foundation, Washington D.C., 1983, PB85-109700/XAB.
3. H. D. Brown, *J. Chem. Inf. Comput. Sci.*, **24**, 155–158 (1984).
4. E. S. Simmons and F. C. Rosenthal, *World Patent Information*, **7**, 33–67 (1985).
5. S. E. French, *Chemtech*, 106 (1987).
6. K. B. Ward, *Final rept., March 1, 1988–April 14, 1989*, NTIS, Naval Research Lab., Washington, D.C., Dec. 10, 1990, AD-A256 419/3/SAB.
7. I. Chithelen, *Forbes*, 154–155 (June 1989).
8. T. Busch, M. Blunck, A. Mullen, and E. Muller, *Proc. Intl. Chem. Inf. Conf.*, 159–176 (1990).
9. P. Gund, *Proc. Intl. Chem. Inf. Conf.* 312–317 (1990).
10. P. Blake and M. J. Ratcliffe, *Drug Inf. J.*, **25**, 13–18 (1991).
11. S. R. Heller, *J. Chem. Inf. Comput. Sci.*, **31**, 430–432 (1991).
12. R. S. Rapaka, A. Makriyannis, M. J. Kuhar, *Engineering Technologies and New Directions in Drug Abuse Research*, NTIS, National Institute on Drug Abuse, United States, 1991, PB92-155449/XAB.
13. Discovery and Development of Therapeutic Drugs Against Lethal Human RNA Viruses: A Multidisciplinary Assault, NTIS, Tempe Cancer Research Inst., Arizona, March 17, 1992, AD-A251 561/7/XAB.
14. W. A. Warr and C. Suhr, *Chemical Information Management*, 1992. Published by VCH at Weinheim.

PART II
PRODUCT DEVELOPMENT ISSUES

Drug Absorption, Distribution and Elimination

LESLIE Z. BENET and
BEATRICE Y. T. PEROTTI

Department of Pharmacy, University of California
San Francisco, California, USA

CONTENTS

1 Overview of Product Development Issues, 114

2 Defining Drug Absorption, Disposition and Elimination Using Pharmacokinetics, 114

3 Important Pharmacokinetic Parameters Used in Defining Drug Disposition, 115
   3.1 Clearance, 116
   3.2 Bioavailability, 119
   3.3 Volume of distribution, 120

4 Important Pharmacokinetic Parameters Used in Therapeutics, 121
   4.1 Dosing rate, 121
   4.2 Dose adjustment, 122
   4.3 Dosing interval, 122
   4.4 Loading dose, 125

5 How is Pharmacokinetics Used in the Development Process?, 126
   5.1 Pre-clinical development, 126
   5.2 Pharmacokinetics in initial phase I human studies, 126
   5.3 Pharmacokinetics in phases II and III studies, 127
   5.4 Late phase I pharmacokinetic studies, 127
   5.5 Pharmacokinetics in phase IV, 128

6. Applications in Areas Other Than Drug Discovery, 128

Burger's Medicinal Chemistry and Drug Discovery,
Fifth Edition, Volume 1: Principles and Practice,
Edited by Manfred E. Wolff.
ISBN 0-471-57556-9   © 1995 John Wiley & Sons, Inc.

1 OVERVIEW OF PRODUCT DEVELOPMENT ISSUES

Although many compounds come through drug discovery every year, only a rare few can actually make their way through product development and pass the scrutiny of the United States Food and Drug Administration (U.S. FDA). With some ups and downs in marketing, these newly approved pharmaceutical products eventually land on the shelves in pharmacies where they are dispensed to patients upon presentation of the proper prescriptions.

Why are so many compounds "killed" in the product development stage? Since the bottom line question in drug development asks, "Is this drug safe and effective in the human body?" many of these compounds simply do not prove to be safe and effective in the human body.

In order to answer this safety and efficacy question satisfactorily, development scientists must address issues from many areas. Some of the common questions are: What route of administration will be used to deliver the drug? How much of the drug gets into the systemic circulation and to the site of action? Where in the body will the drug distribute? How long does the drug remain intact in the body? How does the drug get eliminated from the body? Is the administered compound metabolized into other entities? Is the pharmacological effect derived from the administered compound, or/and from metabolites? How much drug in the body is needed to elicit the pharmacological effect? Can patients develop allergic or toxic reactions toward the administered compound or its metabolites? How much drug in the body is needed to initiate such adverse reactions? What is the mechanism for such allergic reactions? Are these reactions reversible? Is the drug or the metabolites carcinogenic, teratogenic, or mutagenic? If so, what is the underlying mechanism?

2 DEFINING DRUG ABSORPTION, DISPOSITION AND ELIMINATION USING PHARMACOKINETICS

Initial progress in product development rests heavily on a thorough understanding of the absorption, distribution and elimination characteristics of a drug. Absorption, distribution and elimination processes begin when a dose is administered, and may govern the appearance of any therapeutic effect (Fig. 5.1). Pharmacokinetics is used to quantitate these processes. Apart from its usefulness in explaining the safety and toxicity assessment data which will be discussed later in the chapter, pharmacokinetic analysis is used primarily to design appropriate dosing regimens, and also to quantitatively define drug disposition (2).

The term pharmacokinetics can be defined as what the body does to the drug. The parallel term, pharmacodynamics, can be defined as what the drug does to the body. A fundamental hypothesis of pharmacokinetics is that a relationship exists between a pharmacologic or toxic effect of a drug and the concentration of the drug in a readily accessible site of the body (e.g., blood). This hypothesis has been documented for many drugs (3, 4), although for some drugs no clear relationship has been found between pharmacologic effect and plasma or blood concentrations.

This chapter will focus on the conceptual approach to pharmacokinetics, its use as a tool in therapeutics and in defining drug disposition. The more common mathematical modeling-exponential equation-data analysis approach to pharmacokinetics will not be discussed here. These mathematical techniques are necessary so as to be able to determine the important pharmacokinetic parameters that are to be discussed; however, for medicinal chemists who need to interact with other pharmaceutical scientists in the drug development process, a conceptual approach to pharmacokinetics

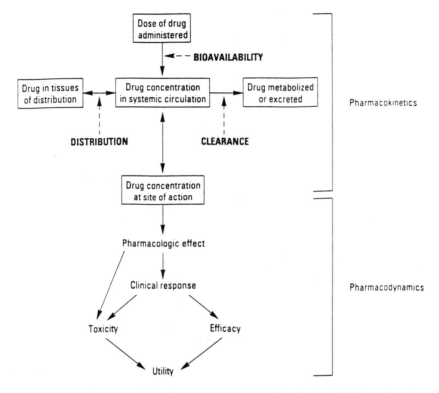

Fig. 5.1 A schematic representation of the dose-response relationship of a drug (1). Reproduced courtesy of the author and Appleton & Lange.

will be more useful. Nevertheless, to even gain a conceptual understanding of pharmacokinetics and its application to drug development, some basic simple equations, as discussed in this chapter, are necessary. This approach should allow the medicinal chemist to appreciate why modification of a drug molecule may lead to important changes in drug disposition.

3 IMPORTANT PHARMACOKINETIC PARAMETERS USED IN DEFINING DRUG DISPOSITION

Among the many pharmacokinetic parameters (Table 5.1) that can be determined

Table 5.1 Ten Critical Pharmacokinetic and Pharmacodynamic Parameters in Drug Development in Order of Importance[a]

1. Clearance
2. Effective concentration range
3. Extent of availability
4. Fraction of the available dose excreted unchanged
5. Blood/Plasma concentration ratio
6. Half-life
7. Toxic concentrations
8. Extent of protein binding
9. Volume of distribution
10. Rate of availability

[a]Ref. 5. Reproduced courtesy of L.Z. Benet and Plenum Press.

when defining a new drug substance, clearance (CL) is the most important for defining drug disposition. Bioavailability (F) and volume of distribution (V) are also of primary importance when pharmacokinetics are used to define drug disposition.

3.1 Clearance

Clearance (CL) is the measure of the ability of the body to eliminate a drug. Initially, clearance will be looked at from a physiological point of view. Figure 5.2 depicts how a drug is removed from the systemic circulation when it passes through an eliminating organ. The rate of presentation of a drug to a drug elimination organ is the product of organ blood flow (Q) and the concentration of drug in the arterial blood entering the organ (C_A). The rate of exit of a drug from the drug eliminating organ is the product of the organ blood flow (Q) and the concentration of the drug in the venous blood leaving the organ (C_V). By mass balance, the rate of elimination (or extraction) of a drug by a drug eliminating organ is the difference between the rate of presentation and the rate of exit.

$$\text{Rate of presentation} = Q \cdot C_A \quad (5.1)$$

$$\text{Rate of exit} = Q \cdot C_V \quad (5.2)$$

$$\text{Rate of elimination} = Q \cdot C_A - Q \cdot C_V$$
$$= Q \cdot (C_A - C_V) \quad (5.3)$$

Extraction ratio (ER) of an organ can be defined as the ratio of the rate of elimination to the rate of presentation.

$$\text{Extraction ratio} = (\text{Rate of elimination}/$$
$$\text{Rate of presentation}) \quad (5.4a)$$

$$ER = Q \cdot (C_A - C_V)/Q \cdot C_A$$
$$ER = (C_A - C_V)/C_A \quad (5.4b)$$

The maximum possible extraction ratio is 1.0 when no drug emerges into the venous blood upon presentation to the eliminating organ (i.e., $C_V = 0$). The lowest possible extraction ratio is zero when all the drug passing through the potential drug eliminating organ appears in the venous blood (i.e., $C_V = C_A$). Drugs with an extraction ratio of more than 0.7 are by convention considered as high extraction ratio drugs, while those with an extraction ratio of less than 0.3 are considered as low extraction ratio drugs.

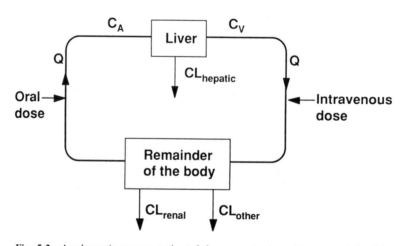

Fig. 5.2 A schematic representation of the concentration–clearance relationship.

The product of organ blood flow and extraction ratio of an organ represents a rate at which a certain volume of blood is completely cleared of a drug. This expression defines the organ clearance (CL_{organ}) of a drug.

$$CL_{organ} = Q \cdot ER = Q \cdot (C_A - C_V)/C_A \quad (5.5)$$

From equations 5.3 and 5.5, one can see that clearance is a proportionality constant between rate of elimination and the arterial drug concentration.

At steady state, by definition, rate in equals rate out. Rate in is given by the dosing rate ($Dose/\tau$, i.e., dose divided by dosing interval τ) multiplied by the drug availability (F), whereas rate out is the rate of elimination (clearance multiplied by the systemic concentration (C)).

$$\text{Rate In} = \text{Rate Out} \quad (5.6)$$

$$F \cdot Dose/\tau = CL \cdot C \quad (5.7)$$

When equation 5.7 is integrated over time from zero to infinity, equation 5.8 results.

$$F \cdot Dose = CL \cdot AUC \quad (5.8)$$

where AUC is the area under the concentration time curve, and F is the fraction of dose available to the systemic circulation (see Bioavailability in section 3.2).

Clearance may be calculated as the available dose divided by the area under the systemic drug concentration curve.

$$CL = F \cdot Dose/AUC \quad (5.9)$$

The maximum value for organ clearance is limited by the blood flow to the organ, i.e., extraction ratio is 1. The average blood flow to the kidneys and the liver is approximately 66 L/h and 81 L/h, respectively. Clearance can occur in many sites in the body and is generally additive. Elimination of a drug may occur as a result of processes occurring in the liver, the kidney, and other organs. The total systemic clearance will be the sum of the individual organ clearances.

$$CL_{total} = CL_{hepatic} + CL_{renal} + CL_{other} \quad (5.10)$$

Among the many organs that are capable of eliminating drugs, the liver, in general, has the highest metabolic capability. Drug molecules in blood are bound to blood cells and plasma proteins such as albumin and alpha$_1$-acid glycoprotein. Yet only unbound drug molecules can pass through hepatic membranes into hepatocytes where they are metabolized by hepatic enzymes or transported into the bile. Thus in order to be eliminated, drug molecules must partition out of the red blood cells, and dissociate from plasma proteins to become unbound or free drug molecules. Because unbound drug molecules are free to partition into and out of blood cells and hepatocytes, there is an equilibrium of free drug concentration between the blood cells, the plasma, and the hepatocytes. The ratio between unbound drug concentration and total drug concentration constitutes the fraction unbound (f_u).

Fraction unbound = Unbound drug concentration/Total drug concentration

$$f_u = C_u/C \quad (5.11)$$

Since an equilibrium exists between the unbound drug molecules in the blood cells and the plasma, the rate of elimination of unbound drugs is the same in the whole blood as in the plasma at steady state. Thus,

$$CL_p \cdot C_p = CL_b \cdot C_b = CL_u \cdot C_u \quad (5.12)$$

where the subscripts p, b, and u refer to plasma, blood and unbound, respectively.

From the material presented so far, one may intuitively imagine that hepatic drug clearance will be influenced by hepatic blood flow, fraction unbound, and intrinsic clearance; that is, the intrinsic ability of the organ to clear unbound drug. The simplest model that describes hepatic clearance in terms of these physiologic parameters is the well-stirred model (6). Assuming instantaneous and complete mixing, the well-stirred model states that hepatic clearance (with respect to blood concentration) is

$$CL_{hep} = Q_{hep} \cdot f_u \cdot CL_{int}/(Q_{hep} + f_u \cdot CL_{int})$$

$$(5.13)$$

Note that f_u is calculated from unbound and total concentration in whole blood.

Equation 5.5 advises that hepatic clearance is the product of hepatic blood flow and hepatic extraction ratio. Therefore, as shown in equation 5.13, hepatic extraction ratio is

$$ER_{hep} = f_u \cdot CL_{int}/(Q_{hep} + f_u \cdot CL_{int})$$

$$(5.14)$$

Examining equations 5.13 and 5.14, one finds that for drugs with a high extraction ratio (i.e., ER approaches 1.0), $f_u \cdot CL_{int}$ is much greater than Q_{hep}, and clearance approaches Q_{hep}. In other words, the clearance for a high extraction ratio drug, imipramine for example, is perfusion rate limited. For drugs with a low extraction ratio (i.e., ER approaches zero), Q_{hep} is much greater than $f_u \cdot CL_{int}$, and clearance is approximated by $f_u \cdot CL_{int}$. An example of a low extraction ratio drug is acetaminophen.

The intrinsic ability of an organ to clear a drug is directly proportional to the activity of the metabolic enzymes in the organ. Such metabolic processes, both *in vitro* and *in vivo*, are characterized by Michaelis-Menten kinetics:

$$\text{Rate of metabolism} = V_{MAX} \cdot C/(K_M + C)$$

$$(5.15)$$

in which V_{MAX}, the maximum rate at which metabolism can proceed, is propor-

tional to the total concentration of enzyme. K_M is the Michaelis-Menten constant corresponding to the drug concentration which yields 1/2 of the maximum rate of metabolism. Dividing both sides of equation 5.15 by the systemic concentration (C) yields:

$$\text{Rate of metabolism}/C = CL_{metabolism}$$

$$= V_{MAX}/(K_M + C) \quad (5.16)$$

Since identification of a saturable process only occurs for low extraction ratio compounds (i.e., $CL_{metabolism} = f_u \cdot CL_{int}$), the relationship between classical enzyme kinetics and pharmacokinetics is revealed:

$$f_u \cdot CL_{int} = V_{MAX}/(K_M + C) \quad (5.17)$$

As V_{MAX} and K_M can be obtained from *in vitro* metabolism experiments, development scientists may reasonably predict the *in vivo* clearance parameter of a low or intermediate extraction ratio drug from *in vitro* data, using equations 5.13 and 5.17. By using appropriate scaling factors, the *in vivo* clearance parameter in humans can be approximated from *in vitro* metabolism data from other species (7, 8).

The kidneys are also important drug eliminating organs. Renal clearance (CL_r) is a proportionality term between urinary excretion rate and systemic concentration. Integrating equation 5.18a over time from zero to infinity, renal clearance is the ratio of the total amount of drug excreted unchanged to the area under the systemic concentration curve. The total amount of drug excreted unchanged can be measured experimentally or can be calculated from the dose if the fraction of the available dose excreted unchanged (f_e) is known.

$$CL_r = \text{Urinary excretion rate}/C \quad (5.18a)$$

$$= \text{Total amount of drug excreted}$$

$$\text{unchanged}/AUC \quad (5.18b)$$

$$= f_e \cdot F \cdot Dose/AUC \quad (5.18c)$$

It is obvious above that the conceptual approach to clearance requires measurements of blood concentrations. Yet, bioanalytical measurements are often carried out in plasma due to the ease of sample handling. However, measuring the blood to plasma ratio allows one to convert clearance values determined in plasma, to their corresponding blood values using equation 5.12.

3.2 Bioavailability

The bioavailability of a drug product via various routes of administration is defined as the fraction of unchanged drug that is absorbed intact and then reaches the site of action; or the systemic circulation following administration by any route. For an intravenous dose of a drug, bioavailability is defined as unity. For drug administered by other routes of administration, bioavailability is often less than unity. Incomplete bioavailability may be due to a number of factors that can be subdivided into categories of dosage-form effects, membrane effects and site of administration effects. Obviously, the route of administration that offers maximum bioavailability is the direct input at the site of action for which the drug is developed. This arrangement may be difficult to achieve because the site of action is not known for some disease states, and in other cases, the site of action is completely inaccessible even when the drug is placed into the bloodstream. The most commonly used route is oral administration. However, orally administered drugs may decompose in the fluids of the gastrointestinal lumen, or be metabolized as they pass through the gastrointestinal membrane. In addition, once a drug passes into the hepatic portal vein, it may be cleared by the liver before entering into the general circulation. The loss of drug as it passes through drug eliminating organs for the first time is known as the first pass effect.

The fraction of an oral dose available to the systemic circulation considering both absorption and the first pass effect, can be found by comparing the ratio of AUCs following oral and intravenous dosing.

$$F = AUC_{oral}/AUC_{i.v.} \qquad (5.19)$$

If an assumption is made that all of a drug dose is absorbed through the gastrointestinal tract intact, and that the only extraction takes place at the liver, then the maximum bioavailability (F_{max}) is

$$F_{max} = 1 - ER_{hep} \qquad (5.20)$$

From equations 5.5 and 5.20, one can derive the following relationship for F_{max}:

$$F_{max} = 1 - (CL_{hep}/Q_{hep}) \qquad (5.21)$$

For high extraction ratio drugs, where CL_{hep} approaches Q_{hep}, F_{max} will be small. For low extraction ratio drugs, Q_{hep} is much greater than CL_{hep}, and F_{max} will approximate one.

Recently, bioavailability and clearance data obtained from a cross-over study of cyclosporine kinetics before and after rifampin dosing, revealed a new understanding of drug metabolism and disposition of this compound (9). Healthy volunteers were given cyclosporine, intravenously and orally, before and after their CYP3A (P450 3A) enzymes were induced by rifampin. As expected, the blood clearance of cyclosporine increased from 0.31 to 0.42 L/h/kg due to the induction of the drug's metabolizing enzymes (i.e., an increase in V_{MAX} in equation 5.15). There was no change in volume of distribution, but there was a dramatic decrease in bioavailability from 27% to 10% in these individuals.

A decrease in bioavailability is to be expected, because cyclosporine undergoes some first-pass metabolism as it goes through the liver following oral dosing. But if one predicts on the basis of pharmacokinetics what the maximum bioavailability (as calculated by Eq. 5.21) would be before and after rifampin dosing, the maximum bioavailability would decrease from 77% to 68%. Thus, there would be an expected cyclosporine bioavailability decrease of approximately 12% just on the basis of the clearance changes resulting from inducing CYP3A enzymes in the liver. In fact, there was a bioavailability decrease of 60%. Furthermore, bioavailability was significantly less than would be predicted at maximum. While some of that lower bioavailability was due to formulation effects, the discrepancy between the theoretical maximum bioavailability and the achievable bioavailability of cyclosporine remained a question.

However, on the basis of new findings during the last several years about the high prevalence of CYP3A isozymes in the gut, significant metabolism of cyclosporine in the gut as well as in the liver was speculated. This hypothesis can consistently explain the *significantly lower* bioavailability than would be predicted even if all of the drug could be absorbed into the blood stream. This finding, particularly quantification of the magnitude of gut metabolism (more than 2/3s of the total metabolism for an oral dose of cyclosporine occurs in the gut), would not have been realized had pharmacokinetics not been utilized in the analysis of the given data.

3.3 Volume of Distribution

The volume of distribution (V) relates the amount of drug in the body to the concentration of drug in the blood or plasma, depending upon the fluid measured. At its simplest, this relationship is defined by equation 5.22:

$$V = \text{Amount of drug in body}/C \quad (5.22)$$

For a normal 70-kg man, the plasma volume is 3 L, the blood volume is 5.5 L, the extracellular fluid outside the plasma is 12 L and the total body water is approximately 42 L. However, many classical drugs exhibit volumes of distribution far in excess of these known fluid volumes. The volume of distribution for digoxin is about 700 L, which is approximately 10 times greater than the total body volume of a 70-kg man. This example serves to emphasize that the volume of distribution does not represent a real volume. Rather, it is an apparent volume which should be considered as the size of the pool of body fluids that would be required if the drug were equally distributed throughout all portions of the body. In fact, the relatively hydrophobic digoxin has a high apparent volume of distribution because it distributes predominantly into muscle and adipose tissue, leaving only a very small amount of drug in the plasma in which the concentration of drug is measured.

At equilibrium, the distribution of a drug within the body depends upon binding to blood cells, plasma proteins, and tissue components. Only the unbound drug is capable of entering and leaving the plasma and tissue compartments. A memory aid for this relationship can be summarized by the expression:

$$V = V_{\mathrm{p}} + V_{\mathrm{TW}} \cdot f_{\mathrm{u}}/f_{\mathrm{u,T}} \quad (5.23)$$

where V_{p} is the volume of plasma, V_{TW} is the aqueous volume outside the plasma, f_{u} is the fraction unbound in plasma, and $f_{\mathrm{u,T}}$ is the fraction unbound in tissue. Thus, a drug that has a high degree of binding to plasma proteins (i.e., low f_{u}) will generally exhibit a small volume of distribution. Unlike plasma protein binding, tissue binding of a drug cannot be measured directly. Generally, this parameter is assumed to be constant unless indicated otherwise.

In equation 5.22, the body is considered as a single homogeneous pool of body fluids as described above for digoxin. For most drugs, however, two or three distinct pools of distribution space appear to exist. This condition results in a time-dependent decrease in the measurable blood or plasma concentration, which reflects distribution into other body pools independent of the body's ability to eliminate the drug. Figure 5.3 describes mean serum IFN-α concentrations after a 40 min intravenous infusion as well as after intramuscular and subcutaneous injections of the same dose. Note the logarithmic biphasic nature of the mean plasma concentration time curve following the intravenous infusion. This biphasic nature represents both the distribution and elimination processes.

Generally, comparisons of volume of distribution are made using a parameter designated as the volume of distribution at steady state (V_{SS}), which reflects the sum of the volumes of all the pools into which the drug may distribute. V_{SS} can be calculated from the area under the moment curve ($AUMC$) and the area under the curve (AUC) as defined by Benet and Galeazzi (11):

$$V_{SS} = Dose_{i.v.} \cdot AUMC/AUC^2 \quad (5.24)$$

$AUMC$ can be calculated from areas under a plot of concentration $\cdot$ time vs time. Both AUC and $AUMC$ may be calculated from the coefficients and exponents of the equations utilized to described the multicompartment nature of drug kinetics as depicted in Figure 5.3. These concepts will be revisited following a discussion of half-life.

4 IMPORTANT PHARMACOKINETIC PARAMETERS USED IN THERAPEUTICS

In addition to the three parameters, clearance (CL), bioavailability (F), and volume of distribution (V) discussed previously, a fourth parameter, half-life ($t_{1/2}$), is also crucial in therapeutics. The decreasing order of importance of these four parameters are clearance, bioavailability, half-life and volume. Clearance defines the dosing rate, bioavailability defines dose adjustment, and half-life defines the dosing interval. Volume of distribution defines the loading dose.

4.1 Dosing Rate

As discussed in equation 5.6 in section 3.1, rate of presentation equals rate of exit at steady state. Whereas rate of presentation is the product of bioavailability and dosing rate, rate of exit is the product of clearance and average (steady state) concentration. By replacing the average concentration with the target concentration, the dosing rate can be computed with known values of bioavailability and clearance.

$$\text{Rate in} = \text{Rate out} \quad (5.6)$$

Bioavailability $\times$ Dosing rate $=$ Clearance

$\times$ Average concentration $\quad (5.7a)$

$$F \cdot \text{Dosing rate} = CL \cdot C_{\text{target}} \quad (5.7b)$$

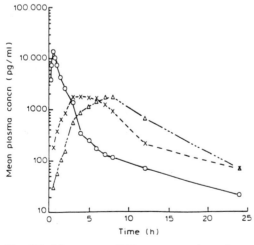

Fig. 5.3 Mean serum IFN-α concentrations after a single 36×10^6 U dose as an intravenous infusion ($\bigcirc$) or an intramuscular ($\times$) or subcutaneous ($\triangle$) injection (10). Reproduced courtesy of the author and *Clin. Pharmacol. Ther.*

4.2 Dose Adjustment

There is often a therapeutic concentration range of drug in the blood that is necessary to elicit a clinical effect without causing drug toxicity. The boundaries of this range are set by the minimum effective concentration (MEC) and the minimum toxic concentration (MTC). For example, in order to maintain a steady rate of presentation of 100 mg/min, one can either administer a completely bioavailable i.v. infusion at 100 mg/min, or a sustained release oral dosage form with 50% bioavailability at 200 mg/min. As shown in equations 5.7a and 5.7b, the actual dosing rate depends on the bioavailability of the dosage form. For proper dosing adjustment, the bioavailability (F) of a given dosage form stands as a must-know parameter in therapeutics.

4.3 Dosing Interval

Half-life ($t_{1/2}$) is an extremely useful kinetic parameter in terms of therapeutics, since this parameter, together with therapeutic index, helps define the dosing interval at which drugs should be administered. By definition, half-life is the time required for 50% of the drug remaining in the body to be eliminated. In three and one third half-lives, 90% of the dose would have been eliminated. Table 5.2 shows the percentage of dose lost in different numbers of half-lives. If the dosing interval is long relative to the half-life, large fluctuations in drug concentration will occur. On the other hand, if the dosing interval is short relative to half-life, significant accumulation will occur. The half-life parameter also allows one to predict drug accumulation within the body and quantifies the approach to plateau that occurs with multiple dosing and constant rates of infusion. Conventionally, three and one third half-lives are used as the time required to achieve steady state under constant infusion. The concentration

Table 5.2   Percentages of Dose Lost as a Function of Number of Half-Lives

Number of Half-Lives	Dose Lost, %
1	50
2	75
3	87.5
3.3	90
4	93.8
5	96.9

level achieved after this time is already 90% of the steady state concentration, and clinically, it is difficult to distinguish a 10% difference in concentrations.

After determining the extent of oral drug bioavailability, half-life is probably the next most important parameter in terms of deciding the appropriateness of a drug for further development. Drugs with very short half-lives create problems in maintaining steady-state concentrations in the therapeutic range. Thus, a successful drug product with a short half-life will require a dosage form which allows a relatively constant prolonged input. Drugs with a very long half-life are favored in terms of efficacy considerations; however, this long half-life may be a negative characteristic in terms of toxicity considerations. Figure 5.4 illustrates the importance of half-life in defining the dosing interval.

This figure depicts the relationship between the frequency of theophylline dosing and the plasma concentration time course when a steady-state theophylline plasma level of 15 μg/mL is desired. The smoothly rising curve shows the plasma concentrations achieved with an intravenous infusion of 43.2 mg/h to a patient exhibiting an average theophylline clearance of 0.69 mL/min/kg. The steady-state theophylline plasma level achieved is midway within the therapeutic concentration range of 10–20 μg/mL. The figure also depicts the time courses for 8-hourly administration of

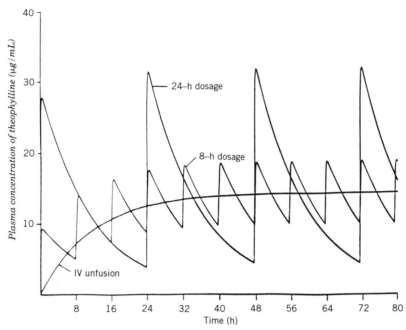

Fig. 5.4 Relationship between frequency of dosing and maximum and minimum plasma concentrations when a steady-state plasma level of 15 μg/mL is desired. The time course of plasma concentrations for 43.2 mg/h intravenous infusion, an 8-hourly 340 mg oral dose, and a 24 hourly 1020 mg oral dose are depicted. Reproduced courtesy of the author and Appleton & Lange.

340 mg and 24-hourly administration of 1020 mg, assuming that these doses are administered in an immediate release dosage form. In each case the mean steady-state concentration is 15 μg/mL. However, the peak to trough ratio and the concentrations achieved with the once daily dosing (i.e., 1020 mg) of a rapidly released formulation would result in concentrations in the toxic range, exceeding 20 μg/mL for certain periods of time, as well as concentrations expected to not yield efficacy, i.e., less than 10 μg/mL, for significant periods during each dosing interval. In contrast, the 8-hourly dosing, which is approximately equivalent to the half-life of theophylline, shows a 2-fold range in peak to trough, and theophylline levels stay within the therapeutic plasma concentration range.

Although half-life is a very important parameter in therapeutics for defining the dosing interval, half-life can be a very misleading parameter when one is attempt-ing to use pharmacokinetics as a tool in defining drug disposition. As depicted in equation 5.29, half-life varies as a function of the two physiologic-related parameters, volume and clearance.

$$t_{1/2} = 0.693 \cdot V/CL \qquad (5.29)$$

Half-life has little value as an indicator of the processes involved in either drug elimination or distribution. Yet, early studies of drug pharmacokinetics in disease states have relied on drug half-life as the sole measure of alterations in drug disposition. Disease states can affect the physiologically related parameters, volume of distribution and clearance; thus, the derived parameter, half-life, will not necessarily reflect the expected change in drug elimination.

As clearance decreases, due to a disease process, half-life would be expected to increase. However, this reciprocal relationship is exact only when the disease does not change the volume of distribution. For example, as Klotz and co-workers have shown, the increase in half-life of diazepam with age does not result from a decrease in clearance but rather due to an increase in volume as the patient ages (12). Clearance, a measure of the body's ability to eliminate the drug, does not significantly decrease with age for diazepam. However, when volume increases, less drug is in the blood flowing to the liver, and elimination can occur only for those drug molecules which come in contact with the liver. Thus the time that the drug remains in the body is increased. Another example of how half-life is not a good predictor of mechanisms of elimination is given by studies with the oral antihypoglycemic, tolbutamide. The half-life of tolbutamide decreases in patients with acute viral hepatitis; that is, the drug appears to be eliminated faster by a diseased liver, the exact opposite from what one might expect. Here, the disease appears to decrease protein binding in both plasma and tissues, causing no change in volume of distribution but an increase in free fraction in the plasma which results in an increase in total clearance, and subsequently a decrease in half-life (13).

Equation 5.29 describes the half-life relationship for a drug that appears to follow one-compartment body kinetics; that is, when the body is considered to be a single homogeneous pool of body fluids. However, many drugs appear to exhibit multiple distribution pools, and therefore may have multiple half-lives (as was depicted in Figure 5.3 for IFN-α). Drugs with multiple half-lives are usually reported in the literature as "distribution" and "terminal elimination" half-lives. Defining the "relevant" half-life in such situations has been addressed by Benet and co-workers (2, 14, 15).

Consider the situation in which a drug is best described by a two-pool model, as has been suggested for IFN-α by Wills et al.

(10). The data in the Wills manuscript were recalculated to represent the equation describing the concentration (ng/mL) of the drug following a 228 μg dose of IFN-α as a function to time (h) as given in equation 5.30.

$$C = 14.13e^{-1.04t} + 0.545e^{-0.136t} \quad (5.30)$$

The disposition constants in the exponents of equation 5.30 correspond to half-lives of 0.667 h (40 min) and 5.1 h. In the interferon literature, the 5.1 h half-life is generally referred to as the mean elimination half-life, while the 40 min half-life, if mentioned at all, is generally referred to as a distribution half-life. These representations may not be accurate: The relevance of a particular half-life may be defined in terms of the fraction of the clearance that is related to each half-life. Note in equation 5.8 that clearance is inversely related to area under the drug concentration time curve (AUC). When the equation describing the time-course of drug concentrations requires more than one exponential term, this circumstance can be represented by equation 5.31. For an n-compartment pharmacokinetic model:

$$C = L_1e^{-\lambda_1 t} + L_2e^{-\lambda_2 t} + \cdots + L_ne^{-\lambda_n t} \quad (5.31)$$

AUC can be calculated as the ratio of coefficients and exponents as in equation 5.32.

$$AUC = L_1/\lambda_1 + L_2/\lambda_2 + \cdots + L_n/\lambda_n \quad (5.32)$$

Calculating AUC for IFN-α as described in equation 5.30 yields:

$$AUC(\text{ng} \cdot \text{h} \cdot \text{mL}^{-1}) = 13.59 + 4.01$$
$$(77\%) \quad (23\%)$$

Note that 77% of the AUC relates to the coefficient and exponent for the 40 min half-life, which suggests that the 5.1 h half-life is in fact a minor contributor to the prediction of steady-state concentrations of *IFN*-α. The importance of these fractional areas can be observed if equation 5.7 is rearranged to predict steady state concentrations (C_{SS}):

$$C_{SS} = F \cdot Dose/(\tau \cdot CL) \qquad (5.7c)$$

Now since *CL* can be defined as given in equation 5.9 as the relationship between an available single dose and *AUC*, equation 5.7c becomes:

$$C_{SS} = F \cdot Dose \cdot AUC/(\tau \cdot F \cdot Dose)$$
$$(5.33)$$

Thus, the ability to correctly predict C_{SS} is dependent upon the accuracy of the measurement of AUC. If the 5.1 h half-life for IFN-α is ignored, the data of Wills et al. suggests that the value for AUC, and therefore the steady-state concentration, will be underestimated by only 23%, since this longer half-life represents a relatively small fraction of the total IFN-α clearance (10). This error in drug concentrations could probably be ignored with confidence, since a 23% difference may often be within analytical error for protein drugs, as well as within the day to day variability in a particular patient.

The above calculations assume that drug concentrations are important in defining the efficacy or toxicity of IFN-α. If this is true, the clinician can safely ignore the 5.1 h half-life in patients with normal elimination characteristics, since little change in steady-state drug levels will be observed. However, it may be that the response, particularly toxicity, is related to the amount of drug in the body, rather than the systemic concentration. The amount in the body at steady-state (A_{SS}) is the product of the systemic concentration and the steady-state volume of distribution:

$$A_{SS} = C_{SS} \cdot V_{SS} \qquad (5.34)$$

As can be seen from equation 5.24, the

accurate calculation of V_{SS} requires an understanding of how AUMC relates to the fractional area of each half-life. The complications of this relationship will not be discussed in this introductory chapter but the correct estimation of V_{SS} is always significantly affected by the terminal half-life.

More recently, Benet has described so-called multiple dosing half-lives, the half-life for a drug which is equivalent to the dosing interval to choose so that plasma concentrations (eq. 5.35) or amounts of drug in the body (eq. 5.36) will show a 50% drop during a dosing interval at steady state. These parameters are defined in terms of the mean residence time in the central compartment (*MRTC*) and the mean residence time in the body (*MRT*).

$$t_{1/2_{MD}}^{\text{plasma}} = 0.693\,MRTC \qquad (5.35)$$

$$t_{1/2_{MD}}^{\text{amount}} = 0.693\,MRT \qquad (5.36)$$

MRTC in a one compartment body model is the inverse of the rate constant for elimination. In a multiple compartment model, where the multiple dosing plasma half-life is useful, MRTC is given by the volume of the central compartment where drug concentrations are measured divided by clearance. MRT in equation 5.36 is the ratio of AUMC/AUC.

4.4 Loading Dose

For drugs with long half-lives, the time to reach steady state is substantial. In these instances, it may be desirable to administer a loading dose that promptly raises the concentration of drug in plasma to the projected steady state value. In theory, only the amount of the loading dose needs to be computed, not the rate of its administration. To a first approximation, this is true. The amount of drug required to achieve a given steady state concentration in the plasma is the amount of drug that must be in the body when the desired steady state is reached. For intermittent dosage schemes, the amount is that at the average concentration. The volume of distribution is the proportionality factor that relates the total amount of drug in the body to the concentration in the plasma. If a loading dose is administered to achieve the desired steady-state concentration, then:

Loading dose = Amount in the body at

$$\text{steady state} = C_{p,ss} \cdot V_{ss} \qquad (5.37)$$

For most drugs, the loading dose can be given as a single dose by the chosen route of administration. However, for drugs that follow complicated multi-compartment pharmacokinetics, such as a two-compartment model, the distribution phase cannot be ignored in the calculation of the loading dose. If the rate of absorption is rapid relative to distribution (this circumstance is always true for intravenous bolus administration), the concentration of drug in plasma that results from an appropriate loading dose can initially be considerably higher than desired. Severe toxicity may occur, albeit transiently. This may be particularly important, for example, in the administration of antiarrhythmic drugs, where an almost immediate toxic response is obtained when plasma concentrations exceed a particular level. Thus, while the estimation of the amount of the loading dose may be quite correct, the rate of administration can be crucial in preventing excessive drug concentrations, and slow administration of an intravenous drug (over minutes rather than seconds) is almost always wise.

5 HOW IS PHARMACOKINETICS USED IN THE DEVELOPMENT PROCESS?

5.1 Pre-Clinical Development

The pharmacokinetics of a new molecular entity must be defined in the animal species used in pre-clinical drug development. This information serves as a portion of the required data necessary for submission of an IND (investigational new drug) application. Generally, the absorption, distribution, metabolism and excretion of a new molecular entity is characterized in a small animal such as a rodent (usually the rat) and in a large animal (usually the dog and/or monkey). The drug should be characterized in terms of its clearance, volume of distribution, bioavailability and half-life. In addition, the linearity of the drug pharmacokinetics over the doses anticipated for use in toxicology studies, must be determined. Where non-linearities are observed, the Michaelis-Menten parameters are characterized. This pre-clinical pharmacokinetic data may be utilized in an initial prediction of the disposition characteristics in man. Theoretically, intrinsic clearance or clearance and volume of distribution may be scaled up from the pre-clinical animal species to predict parameters in man. At this time, these approaches have not been as successful as one would hope. With the rapid development in the understanding of the metabolic isozymes involved in drug metabolism, and their conservation of characteristics across animal species, it is anticipated that scale-up procedures from animal data may be more readily utilized in the future.

5.2 Pharmacokinetics in Initial Phase I Human Studies

Phase I human studies are designed to evaluate the absorption, distribution, metabolism and excretion characteristics of a new molecular entity in humans. Except for potentially toxic drugs, as used in life-threatening diseases such as cancer and AIDS, phase I studies are usually undertaken in healthy volunteers. Here, the pharmacokinetic characteristics of the drug are defined as in the pre-clinical studies. As described previously, the extent of availability following oral dosing and the half-life of the drug are two of the critical parameters utilized by the drug industry in making decisions as to whether further study of the drug is justified. For example, if first-pass elimination of a drug is extensive, as defined by equation 5.21, the drug manufacturer must make a decision as to whether it is economically feasible to pursue further studies of this drug in man. If the drug is unique in its pharmacodynamic characteristics, or is useful in treating life-threatening conditions, where intravenous dosing will be acceptable to the medical community, then companies may pursue further development even though they may anticipate that oral bioavailability may be low and consequently highly variable from patient to patient. Similarly, as discussed previously, drugs with very short half-lives will only be useful if a controlled release dosage form of the drug can be developed so as to maintain necessary systemic concentrations without excessive dosing throughout the day. As described earlier in the section on pre-clinical development, phase I studies are also useful to determine whether a drug exhibits non-linear kinetics and whether clearance may change during multiple dosing either as a result of induction or inhibition of elimination pathways. Another important part of phase I evaluation is the effect of meals on drug bioavailability, both in terms of the extent and the rate of availability. The studies carried out in initial phase I evaluation are utilized to predict the appropriate dose and the drug disposition characteristics which might be expected in patient populations.

5.3 Pharmacokinetics in Phases II and III Studies

Once the drug disposition characteristics of a new molecular entity are defined, the drug must also be evaluated in the patient populations which will receive the drug. Phase II studies, the first studies in patients, are designed to select the appropriate dosage and conditions to be utilized in the pivotal multicenter large scale clinical studies (phase III) required to prove safety and efficacy. Phases II and III studies do not routinely involve detailed studies designed to characterize the drug's pharmacokinetics. Rather, on the basis of the information gained in the phase I studies, investigators predict the systemic concentration time course which would be observed in patients receiving the drug. Generally, a few plasma samples are taken during phases II or III studies which are then utilized in a "population pharmacokinetic model" to determine whether the characteristics of the drug in the patient population differ from that determined in healthy volunteers. This knowledge, of course, is important to accurately predict the appropriate dosage regimen to be administered to the patient population, and to define the labeling for the dosage form to be marketed in the future.

5.4 Late Phase I Pharmacokinetic Studies

Once a drug sponsor has obtained information in patient populations via phase III studies that a drug is safe and effective, a number of so-called phase I studies are then carried out to complete the pharmacokinetic package of information to be supplied to regulatory agencies. These studies include evaluating the effects of disease states on the drug pharmacokinetics. For example, the effect of decreased renal function, the effect of hepatic disease, the effects of age and gender, and the evaluation of potential interactions with other drugs which the patients may be taking are carried out during late phase I studies. These studies are characterized as phase I since they are usually carried out in subjects who do not have the disease for which the drug is being prescribed, but rather have a particular characteristic which the regulatory agencies and the company wish to have evaluated.

Often, the final dosage form to be marketed by the drug manufacturer is not exactly coincident with the dosage form which was utilized in the efficacy and safety studies in phase III patient populations. Thus, the drug sponsor must carry out a bioequivalence study between these dosage forms to assure the regulatory agencies that the product to be marketed is equivalent, in terms of the active ingredients, to the dosage form used in the pivotal phase III studies proving efficacy and safety.

5.5 Pharmacokinetics in Phase IV

Phase IV constitutes studies that are carried out following regulatory approval and commercial sales of the product. In some cases, regulatory agencies may request the pharmaceutical manufacturer to carry out a drug interaction or a disease interaction study following approval of the drug for marketing. These studies are utilized to assure that the labeling and the dosage recommendations under particular conditions are accurate. In addition, the pharmaceutical manufacturer may need to change the manufacturing processes for the dosage form after the drug is on the market. Under these conditions, bioequivalence studies would be required by the regulatory agencies to assure that the new product is equivalent to that previously marketed by the company.

6 APPLICATIONS IN AREAS OTHER THAN DRUG DISCOVERY

In addition to the wide application of pharmacokinetics in the drug discovery process and in clinical pharmacology, pharmacokinetics has been found to be extremely useful in environmental science also. In toxicological studies such as pesticide exposure, water contaminants exposure and air-borne carcinogens exposure, pharmacokinetics becomes a valuable tool in evaluating the safety level of such compounds in humans or domestic animals.

REFERENCES

1. L. Z. Benet in B. G. Katzung, ed., *Basic and Clinical Pharmacology*, Appleton & Lange, Norwalk, Conn., 1992, pp. 35–48.
2. L. Z. Benet, *Eur. J. Resp. Dis.*, **65**, 45–61 (1984).
3. L. Z. Benet, J. R. Mitchell, and L. B. Sheiner in A. G. Gilman, T. W. Rall, A. S. Nies, and P. Taylor, Eds., *Goodman and Gilman's The Pharmacological Basis of Therapeutics*, Pergamon Press Inc., Elmsford, N.Y., 1990, pp. 3–32.
4. L. Z. Benet and R. L. Williams in Ref. 3, 1990, pp. 1650–1735.
5. L. Z. Benet in A. Yacobi, J. P. Skelly, V. P. Shah, and L. Z. Benet, Eds., *Integration of Pharmacokinetics, Pharmacodynamics and Toxicokinetics in Rational Drug Development*, Plenum Press, New York, 1993, pp. 115–123.
6. K. S. Pang and M. Rowland, *J. Pharmacokinet. Biopharm.*, **5**, 625–653 (1977).
7. H. Boxenbaum, *J. Pharmacokinet. Biopharm.*, **8**, 165–170 (1980).
8. J. Mordenti, S. A. Chen, J. A. Moore, B. L. Ferraiolo, and J. D. Green, *Pharm. Research*, **8**, 1351–1359 (1991).
9. M. F. Hebert, J. P. Roberts, T. Prueksaritanont, and L. Z. Benet, *Clin. Pharmacol. Ther.*, **52**, 453–457 (1992).
10. R. J. Wills, S. Dennis, H. E. Spiegel, D. M. Gibson, and P. I. Nadler, *Clin. Pharmacol. Ther.*, **35**, 722–727 (1984).
11. L. Z. Benet and R. L. Galeazzi, *J. Pharm. Sci.*, **68**, 1071–1074 (1979).
12. U. Klotz, G. R. Avant, A. Hoyumpa, S. Schenker, and G. R. Wilkinson, *J. Clin. Invest.*, **55**, 347–359 (1975).
13. R. L. Williams, T. F. Blaschke, P. J. Meffin, K. L. Melmon, and M. Rowland, *Clin. Pharmacol. Ther.*, **21**, 301–309 (1977).
14. B. L. Ferraiolo and L. Z. Benet in R. T. Borchard, A. J. Repta, and V. J. Stella, Eds., *Directed Drug Delivery: The Multi-disciplinary Problem*, Humana Press, Clifton, N.J., 1985, pp. 13–33.
15. C. A. Gloff and L. Z. Benet, *Advanced Drug Delivery Reviews*, **4**, 359–386 (1990).

CHAPTER SIX

Drug Metabolism

BERNARD TESTA

Institut de Chimie Thérapeutique, Ecole de
Pharmacie, Université de Lausanne
Lausanne, Switzerland

CONTENTS

1 Introduction,   130
  1.1 Definitions and concepts, 131
  1.2 Types of metabolic reactions affecting
    xenobiotics, 131
  1.3 Specificities and selectivities in xenobiotic
    metabolism, 132
  1.4 Pharmacodynamic consequences of xenobiotic
    metabolism, 133
  1.5 Biological factors affecting drug
    metabolism, 133
2 Functionalization Reactions,   134
  2.1 Introduction, 134
  2.2 Enzymes catalyzing functionalization
    reactions, 134
    2.2.1 Oxidoreductases, 134
    2.2.2 Hydrolases, 137
  2.3 Oxidation and reduction of carbon atoms, 137
    2.3.1 sp^3-Carbon atoms, 137
    2.3.2 sp^2- and sp-Carbon atoms, 140
  2.4 Oxidation and reduction of nitrogen
    atoms, 141
  2.5 Oxidation and reduction of sulfur and other
    atoms, 143
  2.6 Oxidative cleavage reactions, 146
  2.7 Hydration and hydrolysis, 147
3 Conjugation Reactions,   147
  3.1 Introduction, 147
  3.2 Methylation, 148
    3.2.1 Introduction, 148
    3.2.2 Methylation reactions, 148
  3.3 Sulfation, 150
    3.3.1 Introduction, 150
    3.3.2 Sulfation reactions, 150
  3.4 Glucuronidation and glucosidation, 152

Burger's Medicinal Chemistry and Drug Discovery,
Fifth Edition, Volume 1: Principles and Practice,
Edited by Manfred E. Wolff.
ISBN 0-471-57556-9 © 1995 John Wiley & Sons, Inc.

3.4.1 Introduction, 152
3.4.2 Glucuronidation reactions, 152
3.4.3 Glucosidation reactions, 156
3.5 Acetylation and acylation, 156
   3.5.1 Acetylation reactions, 156
   3.5.2 Other acylation reactions, 157
3.6 Conjugation with coenzyme A and subsequent reactions, 158
   3.6.1 Conjugation with coenzyme A, 158
   3.6.2 Formation of amino acid conjugates, 159
   3.6.3 Formation of hybrid lipids and sterol esters, 160
   3.6.4 Chiral inversion of arylpropionic acids, 161
   3.6.5 β-Oxidation and 2-carbon chain elongation, 161
3.7 Conjugation and redox reactions of glutathione, 163
   3.7.1 Introduction, 163
   3.7.2 Glutathione reactions, 164
3.8 Other conjugation reactions, 167
4 The Significance of Drug Metabolism in Medicinal Chemistry, 168
4.1 Structure-metabolism relationships, 168
   4.1.1 Metabolic schemes, 168
   4.1.2 The influence of configurational factors, 170
   4.1.3 Quantitative structure–metabolism relationships: the influence of electronic factors and lipophilicity, 170
4.2 Metabolism and drug design, 171
   4.2.1 Modulation of drug metabolism by structural variations, 171
   4.2.2 Principles of prodrug design, 172
   4.2.3 Examples of prodrugs and chemical delivery systems, 174
4.3 The concept of toxophoric groups, 177
5 Concluding Remarks, 178

1 INTRODUCTION

Xenobiotic metabolism, which includes drug metabolism, has become an important pharmacological science with particular relevance to biology, therapeutics, and toxicology. Drug metabolism also is of great importance in medicinal chemistry, because it influences in qualitative, quantitative, and kinetic terms the deactivation, activation, detoxication, and toxication of the vast majority of drugs. As a result, medici-nal chemists engaged in drug discovery (lead finding and optimization) must be able to integrate metabolic considerations into drug design. To do so, however, requires a fair or even good knowledge of xenobiotic metabolism.

This chapter presents knowledge and understanding rather than encyclopedic information. Readers wanting to go further in the study of xenobiotic metabolism should consult available references (1–3).

1.1 Definitions and Concepts

Drugs are but one category of the many xenobiotics (Table 6.1) that enter the body but have no nutritional or physiological value. The study of the disposition (or fate) of xenobiotics in living systems includes the consideration of their absorption into the organism, how and where they are distributed and stored, the chemical and biochemical transformations they may undergo, and how and by what route(s) they are finally excreted and returned to the environment. The word metabolism has acquired two meanings: it is synonymous with (*1*) disposition (i.e., the sum of the processes affecting the fate of a chemical substance in the body) and (*2*) biotransformation as understood in this chapter (5).

In pharmacology, one speaks of pharmacodynamic effects to indicate what a drug does to the body and pharmacokinetic effects to indicate what the body does to a drug; these two aspects of the behavior of xenobiotics are strongly interdependent. Pharmacokinetic effects will obviously have a decisive influence on the intensity and duration of pharmacodynamic effects, while metabolism will generate new chemical entities (metabolites) that may have distinct pharmacodynamic properties of their own. Conversely, by its own pharmacodynamic effects, a compound may affect the state of the organism (e.g., hemodynamic changes and enzyme activities) and hence its capacity to handle xenobiotics. Only a systemic approach can help one appreciate the global nature of this interdependence (6).

1.2 Types of Metabolic Reactions Affecting Xenobiotics

A first discrimination that can be made among metabolic reactions is based on the nature of their catalysts. Reactions of xenobiotic metabolism, like other biochemical reactions, are catalyzed by enzymes. However, while the vast majority of reactions of xenobiotic metabolism are indeed enzymatic ones, some nonenzymatic reactions are also well documented. This is due to the fact that a variety of xenobiotics have been found to be labile enough to react nonenzymatically under biological conditions of pH and temperature (7). But there is more. In a normal enzymatic reaction, metabolic intermediates exist en route to the product(s) and do not leave the catalytic site. However, many exceptions to this rule are known: the metabolic intermediate leaves the active site and reacts with water, an endogenous molecule or macromole-

---

Table 6.1   Major Categories of Xenobiotics[a]

Drugs
Food constituents devoid of physiological roles
Food additives (preservatives, coloring and flavoring agents, antioxidants, etc.)
Chemicals of leisure, pleasure, and abuse (ethanol, coffee and tobacco constituents, hallucinogens, etc.)
Agrochemicals (fertilizers, insecticides, herbicides, etc.)
Industrial and technical chemicals (solvents, dyes, monomers, polymers, etc.)
Pollutants of natural origin (radon, sulfur dioxide, hydrocarbons, etc.)
Pollutants produced by microbial contamination (e.g., aflatoxins)
Pollutants produced by physical or chemical transformation of natural compounds (polycyclic aromatic hydrocarbons from burning, Maillard reaction products from heating, etc.)

---

[a]Modified from Ref. 4.

cule, or a xenobiotic. Such reactions are also nonenzymatic but are better designated as postenzymatic reactions (7).

The metabolism of drugs and other xenobiotics is typically a biphasic process in which the compound first undergoes a functionalization reaction (phase I reaction) of oxidation, reduction, or hydrolysis. This introduces or unveils a functional group such as a hydroxyl or amino suitable for linkage with an endogenous molecule or moiety in the second metabolic step known as a conjugation reaction (phase II reaction). In a number of cases, phase I metabolites may be excreted before conjugation, while many xenobiotics can be directly conjugated. And what is more, functionalization reactions may follow some conjugation reactions, e.g., some conjugates are hydrolyzed and/or oxidized before their excretion.

Xenobiotic biotransformation thus produces two types of metabolites: functionalization products and conjugates. However, with the growth of knowledge, biochemists and pharmacologists have progressively come to recognize the existence of a third class of metabolites: xenobiotic-macromolecule adducts, also called macromolecular conjugates (8). Such peculiar metabolites are formed when a xenobiotic binds covalently to a biological macromolecule, usually following metabolic activation (i.e., postenzymatically). Both functionalization products and conjugates have been found to bind covalently to biological macromolecules, the reaction often being toxicologically relevant.

1.3 Specificities and Selectivities in Xenobiotic Metabolism

The words *selectivity* and *specificity* may not have identical meanings in chemistry and biochemistry. In this chapter, the *specificity* of an enzyme will be taken to mean an ensemble of properties, the description of which makes it possible to specify the enzyme's behavior. In contrast, the term *selectivity* will be applied to metabolic processes, indicating that a given metabolic reaction or pathway is able to select some substrates or products from a larger set. In other words, the selectivity of a metabolic reaction is the detectable expression of the specificity of an enzyme. Such definitions may not be universally accepted, but they have the merit of clarity.

What, then, are the various types of selectivities (or specificities) encountered in xenobiotic metabolism? What characterizes an enzyme from a catalytic viewpoint is first its chemospecificity, i.e., its specificity in terms of the type(s) of reaction it catalyzes. When two or more substrates are metabolized at different rates by a single enzyme under identical conditions, substrate selectivity is observed. In such a definition, the nature of the product(s) and their isomeric relationship are not considered. Substrate selectivity is distinct from product selectivity, which is observed when two or more metabolites are formed at different rates by a single enzyme from a single substrate. Thus substrate-selective reactions discriminate between different compounds, whereas product-selective reactions discriminate between different groups or positions in a given compound.

The substrates being metabolized at different rates may share various types of relationships. Chemically, they may be very or slightly different (e.g., analogs), in which case the term *substrate selectivity* is used in a narrow sense. Alternatively, the substrates may be isomers such as positional isomers (regioisomers) or stereoisomers, resulting in substrate regioselectivity or substrate stereoselectivity. Substrate enantioselectivity is a particular case of the latter.

Products formed at different rates in product-selective reactions may also share various types of relationships. Thus they may be analogs, regioisomers, or stereoisomers, resulting in *product selectivity* (narrow sense), product regioselectivity, or product stereoselectivity (e.g., product enantioselectivity). Note that the product selectivity displayed by two distinct substrates in a given metabolic reaction may be different; in other words, the product selectivity may be substrate selective. The term *substrate-product selectivity* can be used to describe such complex cases, which are conceivable for any type of selectivity but have been reported mainly for stereoselectivity.

1.4 Pharmacodynamic Consequences of Xenobiotic Metabolism

The major function of xenobiotic metabolism can be seen as the elimination of physiologically useless compounds, some of which may be harmful; witness the tens of thousands of toxins produced by plants. The function of toxin inactivation justifies the designation of detoxication originally given to reactions of xenobiotic metabolism. However, the possible pharmacological consequences of biotransformation are not restricted to detoxication. In the simple case of a xenobiotic having a single metabolite, four possibilities exist:

1. Both the xenobiotic and its metabolite are devoid of biological effects (at least in the concentration or dose range investigated); such a situation has no place in medicinal chemistry.
2. Only the xenobiotic elicits biological effects, a situation that in medicinal chemistry is typical of but not unique to soft drugs.
3. Both the xenobiotic and its metabolite are biologically active, the two activities being comparable or different either qualitatively or quantitatively.
4. The observed biological activity is caused exclusively by the metabolite, a

situation that in medicinal chemistry is typical of prodrugs.

When a drug or another xenobiotic is transformed into a toxic metabolite, the reaction is one of toxication (9). Such a metabolite may act or react in a number of ways to elicit a variety of toxic responses at different biological levels (10, 11). However, it is essential to stress that the occurrence of a reaction of toxication (i.e., toxicity at the molecular level) does *not* necessarily imply toxicity at the levels of organs and organisms, as discussed in section 4.3.

1.5 Biological Factors Affecting Drug Metabolism

A variety of physiological and pathological factors influence xenobiotic metabolism and may thus affect the wanted and unwanted activities of drugs. It is customary to distinguish between interindividual and intraindividual factors, depending on whether they vary between or within given organisms or individuals, respectively (Table 6.2).

The interindividual factors by definition remain constant during the life span of an organism or individual. Species differences in xenobiotic metabolism are important in

Table 6.2 Biological Factors Affecting Xenobiotic Metabolism

Interindividual Factors	Intraindividual Factors
Animal species	Age
Genetic factors	Biological rhythms
Sex	Pregnancy
	Stress
	Nutritional factors
	Enzyme induction
	Enzyme inhibition
	Diseases

the extrapolation of animal data to humans (12–14). Genetic differences result from the fact that some xenobiotic-metabolizing enzymes are defective in a number of individuals (15). The consequences of these genetic polymorphisms include an impaired metabolism of the drugs that are substrates of such enzymes, with a marked risk of overdose or therapeutic failure in affected individuals. This is the realm of pharmacogenetics. Sex is also a factor of significance in a number of cases, being related to hormonal influences on enzyme activities.

Intraindividual factors express physiological changes or pathological states affecting, e.g., the hormonal balance and immunological reactions of individuals. The age of a person may markedly influence his or her ability to metabolize drugs, especially at the extremes of life. The influence of biological rhythms on pharmacokinetics and pharmacodynamics is the object of chromopharmacology (16). Pregnancy affects drug metabolism due to the profound hormonal and physiological changes in the woman, but the intrinsic activity of the placenta must not be forgotten (17). Much information is available on the influence of disease, but relatively few rationalizations and explanatory mechanisms have been proposed (18).

Nutritional factors such as diet, nutrients, and starvation influence xenobiotic metabolism. As far as drug therapy and toxicology are concerned, factors of even greater significance are enzyme induction and enzyme inhibition (19–21). Enzyme inducers act by increasing the concentration and hence activity of some enzymes or isozymes, while inhibitors decrease the activity of some enzymes or isozymes by reversible inhibition or irreversible inactivation. Enzyme induction and enzyme inhibition by coadministered drugs are two of the major causes of drug–drug interactions. Many examples are known of drugs inhibiting the metabolism of other drugs and thus intensifying and prolonging their effects. In contrast, enzyme induction is frequently accompanied by a decrease in efficacy.

2 FUNCTIONALIZATION REACTIONS

2.1 Introduction

Functionalization reactions comprise oxidations (electron removal, dehydrogenation, and oxygenation), reductions (addition of electrons, hydrogenation, and removal of oxygen), and hydrations–dehydrations (hydrolysis and addition or removal of water). The reactions of oxidations and reductions are catalyzed by a large variety of oxidoreductases, while various hydrolases catalyze hydrations. A large majority of enzymes recognized to be involved in xenobiotic functionalization are briefly reviewed in section 2.2 (22), and metabolic reactions and pathways are also addressed in section 2. Catalytic mechanisms, however, fall outside the scope of this chapter and will not be discussed.

2.2 Enzymes Catalyzing Functionalization Reactions

2.2.1 OXIDOREDUCTASES. Alcohol dehydrogenases (ADH; alcohol:NAD$^+$ oxidoreductase; EC 1.1.1.1) are zinc enzymes found in the cytosol of the mammalian liver and in various extrahepatic tissues. Mammalian liver alcohol dehydrogenases (LADHs) are dimeric enzymes. The human enzymes belong to three different classes: class I, comprising the various isozymes that are homodimers or heterodimers of the α, β, and γ subunits (e.g., the $\alpha\alpha$, $\beta_1\beta_1$, $\alpha\beta_2$ and $\beta_1\gamma$ isozymes); class II, comprising the $\pi\pi$ enzyme; and class III, comprising the $\chi\chi$ enzyme (23).

Enzymes categorized as aldehyde reductases include alcohol dehydrogenase (NADP$^+$) [aldehyde reductase (NADH);

alcohol:NADP$^+$ oxidoreductase; EC 1.1.1.2], aldehyde reductase [alditol:NAD-(P$^+$) 1-oxidoreductase; aldose reductase; EC 1.1.1.21], and many others of lesser relevance (24). Aldehyde reductases are widely distributed in nature and occur in a considerable number of mammalian tissues. Their subcellular location is primarily cytosolic and in some instances also mitochondrial. The so-called ketone reductases include α- and β-hydroxysteroid dehydrogenases (e.g., EC 1.1.1.50 and EC 1.1.1.51), various prostaglandin ketoreductases (e.g., prostaglandin F synthase, EC 1.1.1.188; prostaglandin E2 9-reductase, EC 1.1.1.189), and many others that are comparable to aldehyde reductases. One group of particular importance is the carbonyl reductases (NADPH) (EC 1.1.1.184). Furthermore, the many similarities (including some marked overlap in substrate specificity) between monomeric, NADPH-dependent aldehyde reductase (AKR1), aldose reductase (AKR2), and carbonyl reductase (AKR3) have led to their designation as aldoketo reductases (AKRs) (25).

Other reductases that play a role in drug metabolism include glutathione reductase (NADPH:oxidized-glutathione oxidoreductase; EC 1.6.4.2) and quinone reductase (NAD(P)H:(quinone acceptor) oxidoreductase; DT-diaphorase; EC 1.6.99.2).

Aldehyde dehydrogenases (ALDHs; aldehyde:NAD(P)$^+$ oxidoreductases; EC 1.2.1.3 and EC 1.2.1.5) exist in multiple forms in the cytosol, mitochondria, and microsomes of various mammalian tissues. It has been proposed that aldehyde dehydrogenases form a superfamily of related enzymes consisting of class 1 ALDHs (cytosolic), class 2 ALDHs (mitochondrial), and class 3 ALDHs (tumor-associated and other isozymes). In all three major classes, constitutive and inducible isozymes exist (26).

Dihydrodiol dehydrogenases (*trans*-1,2-dihydrobenzene-1,2-diol:NADP$^+$ oxidore-

ductase; EC 1.3.1.20) are cytosolic enzymes, several of which have been characterized. Although the isozymes are able to use NAD$^+$, the preferred cofactor is NADP$^+$. Other oxidoreductases that play a major or less important role in drug metabolism are hemoglobin; monoamine oxidases (EC 1.4.3.4; MAO-A and MAO-B), which are essentially mitochondrial enzymes; the cytosolic molybdenum hydroxylases (xanthine oxidase, EC 1.1.3.22; xanthine dehydrogenase, EC 1.1.1.204; and aldehyde oxidase, EC 1.2.3.1); and the broad group of copper-containing amine oxidases (EC 1.4.3.6) (27–30).

Monooxygenation reactions are of major significance in drug metabolism and are mediated by various enzymes that differ markedly in their structure and properties. Among these, the most important as far as xenobiotic metabolism is concerned are the cytochromes P450 (EC 1.14.14.1, also EC 1.14.15.1, 1.14.15.3, 1.14.15.4, 1.14.15.5, 1.14.15.6), a large group of enzymes belonging to heme-coupled monooxygenases (31, 32). The cytochrome P450 (CYP) enzymes are encoded by the *CYP* gene superfamily and are classified in families and subfamilies (Table 6.3). The cytochrome P450 is perhaps the major drug-metabolizing enzyme system, playing a key role in detoxication and toxication, and is of additional significance in medicinal chemistry because several CYP enzymes are drug targets, e.g., TX synthase (CYP5) and aromatase (CYP19). Other monoxygenases of importance are the flavin-containing monooxygenases (dimethylaniline monooxygenase (*N*-oxide-forming); EC 1.14.13.8) and dopamine β-hydroxylase (dopamine β-monooxygenase; EC 1.14.17.1).

Various peroxidases are progressively being recognized as important enzymes in drug metabolism. Several cytochrome P450 enzymes have been shown to have peroxidase activity (33). Prostaglandin-endoperoxide synthase (EC 1.14.99.1) is able to

Table 6.3 The Human *CYP* Gene Superfamily[a]

Families (P450)	Subfamilies (P450)	Representative Gene Products (*CYP*)
1 (mammalian aryl hydrocarbon hydroxylases; xenobiotic metabolism inducible by polycyclic aromatic hydrocarbons)	1A	1A1, 1A2
2 (mammalian; xenobiotic and steroid metabolism; constitutive and xenobiotic-inducible)	2A	2A6, 2A7
	2B (includes phenobarbital-inducible forms)	2B6
	2C (constitutive forms; includes sex-specific forms)	2C8, 2C9, 2C10, 2C18, 2C19
	2D	2D6
	2E (ethanol inducible)	2E1
	2F	2F1
3 (mammalian; xenobiotic and steroid metabolism; steroid-inducible)	3A	3A3, 3A4, 3A5
4 (mammalian fatty acid ω- and (ω-1)-hydroxylases; peroxisome proliferator inducible)	4A	4A9, 4A11
	4B	4B1
	4F	4F2
5 (TXA synthase)		5
7 (mammalian cholesterol 7α-hydroxylase		7
11 (mammalian mitochondrial steroid hydroxylases)	11A (cholesterol side-chain cleavage)	11A1
	11B (steroid 11β-hydroxylases)	11B1, 11B2
17 (mammalian steroid 17α-hydroxylase)		17
19 (mammalian steroid aromatase)		19
21 (mammalian steroid 21-hydroxylases)	21A	21A2
27 (mammalian steroid hydroxylase; mitochondrial)		27

[a]From Ref. 32.

use a number of xenobiotics as cofactors in a reaction of cooxidation (34). And finally, a variety of other peroxidases may oxidize drugs, e.g., catalase (EC 1.11.1.6) and myeloperoxidase (donor:hydrogen-peroxide oxidoreductase; EC 1.11.1.7) (35).

2.2.2 HYDROLASES. Hydrolases constitute a complex ensemble of enzymes, many of which are known or suspected to be involved in xenobiotic metabolism. Relevant enzymes among the serine hydrolases include carboxylesterases (carboxylic-ester hydrolase; EC 3.1.1.1), arylesterases (arylester hydrolase; EC 3.1.1.2), cholinesterase (acylcholine acylhydrolase; EC 3.1.1.8), and a number of serine endopeptidases (EC 3.4.21). The roles of arylsulfatases (EC 3.1.6.1), aryldialkylphosphatases (EC 3.1.8.1), β-glucuronidases (EC 3.2.1.31), and epoxide hydrolases (EC 3.3.2.3) are worth noting. Some cysteine endopeptidases (EC 3.4.22), aspartic endopeptidases (EC 3.4.23), and metalloendopeptidases (EC 3.4.24) are also of potential interest.

2.3 Oxidation and Reduction of Carbon Atoms

When examining reactions of carbon oxidation (oxygenations and dehydrogenations) and carbon reduction (hydrogenations), it is convenient from a mechanistic viewpoint to distinguish between sp^3-, sp^2- and sp-carbon atoms.

2.3.1 sp^3-CARBON ATOMS. Reactions of oxidation and reduction of sp^3-carbon atoms are schematized in Figure 6.1 and will be discussed sequentially below. In the simplest cases, a nonactivated carbon atom in an alkyl group undergoes cytochrome P450-catalyzed hydroxylation, the terminal and penultimate positions being the preferred but not exclusive sites of attack (reactions 1-A and 1-B, respectively). Dehydrogenation by dehydrogenases can then

yield a carbonyl derivative (reactions 1-C and 1-E), which is either an aldehyde or a ketone. Note that reactions 1-C and 1-E act not only on metabolites but also on xenobiotic alcohols and are reversible (i.e., reactions 1-D and 1-F), because dehydrogenases catalyze the reactions in both directions. And while a ketone is seldom oxidized further, aldehydes are good substrates of aldehyde dehydrogenases or other enzymes and lead irreversibly to carboxylic acid metabolites (reaction 1-G). A classical example is that of ethanol, which in the body exists in redox equilibrium with acetaldehyde; this metabolite is rapidly and irreversibly oxidized to acetic acid.

Recent evidence indicates that for a number of substrates, the oxidation of primary and secondary alcohols and of aldehydes can also be catalyzed by cytochrome P450. A typical example is the C(10)-demethylation of androgens and analogues catalyzed by aromatase (CYP19). A special case of carbon oxidation, recognized only recently and of underestimated significance, is desaturation of a dimethylene unit by cytochrome P450 to produce an olefinic group (reaction 2). An interesting example is provided by testosterone, which among many cytochrome P450-catalyzed reactions undergoes allylic hydroxylation to 6β-hydroxytestosterone and desaturation to 6,7-dehydrotestosterone (36) (Fig. 6.2).

There is a known regioselectivity in cytochrome P450–catalyzed hydroxylations for carbon atoms adjacent (α) to an unsaturated system (reaction 3) or an heteroatom such as N, O, or S (reaction 4-A) (see Fig. 6.1). In the former cases, hydroxylation can easily be followed by dehydrogenation (not shown). In the latter cases, however, the hydroxylated metabolite is usually unstable and undergoes a rapid, post-enzymatic cleavage of a hydrolytic nature (reaction 4-B). Depending on the substrate, this pathway produces a secondary or primary amine, an alcohol or phenol, or

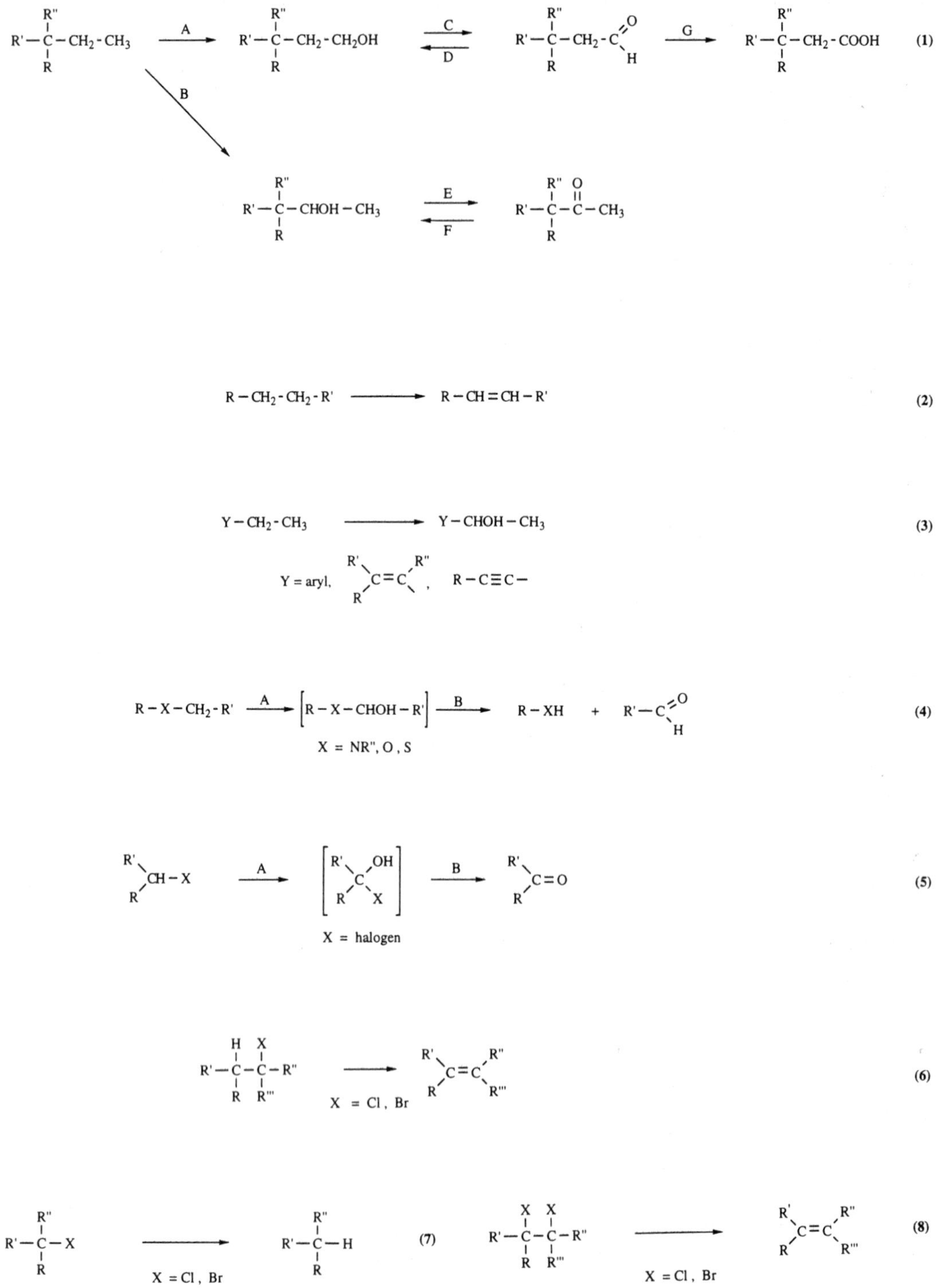

Fig. 6.1 Major reactions of functionalization involving an sp^3-carbon in substrate molecules. The reactions shown here are mainly oxidations (oxygenations and dehydrogenations) and reductions (hydrogenations) plus some postenzymatic reactions of hydrolytic cleavage.

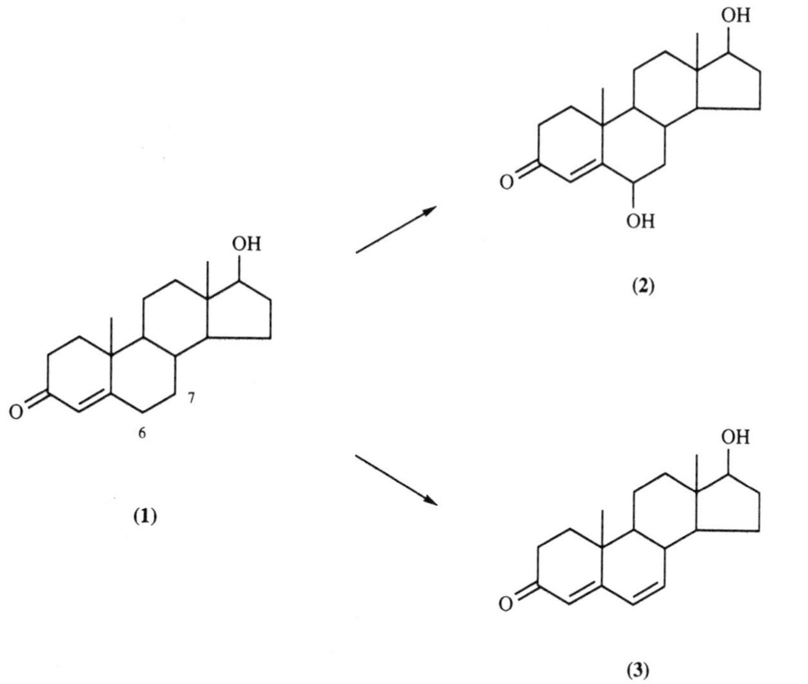

OH

(2)

OH

7

6

(1)

OH

(3)

Fig. 6.2 Testosterone (**1**), 6β-hydroxytestosterone (**2**), and 6,7 dehydrotestosterone (**3**).

a thiol, while the alkyl group is cleaved as an aldehyde or a ketone. Reactions 4 constitute a frequent pathway as far as drug metabolism is concerned, because the pathway underlies some well-known metabolic reactions of N–C cleavage (discussed in section 2.6). Note that the actual mechanism of such reactions is usually more complex than shown here and may involve intermediate oxidation of the heteroatom.

Aliphatic carbon atoms bearing one or more halogen atoms (mainly chlorine or bromine) can be similarly metabolized by hydroxylation and loss of HX to dehalogenated products (reaction 5-A and 5-B) (see Fig. 6.1 and Section 2.6). Dehalogenation reactions can also proceed reductively or without change in the state of oxidation. The latter reactions are dehydrohalogenations (usually dehydrochlorination or dehydrobromination) occurring nonenzymatically (reaction 6). Reductive dehalogenations involve replacement of a halogen by a hydrogen (reaction 7), or *vic*-bisdehalogenation (reaction 8). Some radical species formed as intermediates may have toxicological significance.

Halothan offers a telling example of the metabolic fate of halogenated compounds of medicinal interest. Indeed, this agent undergoes two major pathways: oxidative dehalogenation, leading to trifluoroacetic acid and reduction, producing a reactive radical (Fig. 6.3).

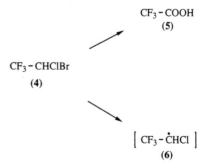

CF_3-COOH
(5)

CF_3-CHClBr
(4)

$\left[CF_3$-$\overset{\cdot}{C}HCl \right]$
(6)

Fig. 6.3 Halothan (**4**), trifluoroacetic acid (**5**), and a reactive radical (**6**).

2.3.2 sp^2 AND sp-CARBON ATOMS. Reactions at sp^2-carbons are characterized by their own pathways, catalytic mechanisms, and products (Fig. 6.4). Thus the oxidation of aromatic rings generates a wealth of (usually stable) metabolites. Their common precursor is often a reactive epoxide (reaction 1-A), which can be either hydrolyzed by epoxide hydrolase (reaction 1-B) to a dihydrodiol or rearranged under proton catalysis to the phenol (reaction 1-C). Dehydrogenation of dihydrodiols by dihydrodiol dehydrogenase restores aromaticity on production of a catechol metabolite (reaction 1-D). The further oxidation of phenols and phenolic metabolites is also possible; the rate of reaction and the nature of the products depend on the ring and on the nature and position of its substituents. Catechols are thus commonly formed by reaction 1-E, and hydroquinones also are sometimes produced (reaction 1-F).

Catechols and hydroquinones have the potential to undergo further oxidation to

quinones (reactions 1-G and 1-I). Such reactions occur by two single-electron steps and can be either enzymatic or nonenzymatic (i.e., resulting from autoxidation and yielding as by-product the superoxide anion radical $O_2^{\bullet -}$). The intermediate in this reaction is a semiquinone. Both quinones and semiquinones are reactive, in particular toward biomolecules, and have been implicated in many reactions of toxication. For example, the high toxicity of benzene for bone marrow is believed to be due to the oxidation of catechol and hydroquinone catalyzed by myeloperoxidase.

The oxidation of diphenols to quinones is reversible (reactions 1-H and 1-J); a variety of cellular reductants are able to mediate the reduction of quinones either by a two-electron mechanism or by two single-electron steps. The two-electron reduction can be catalyzed by carbonyl reductase and quinone reductase, while cytochrome P450 and some flavoproteins act by single-elec-

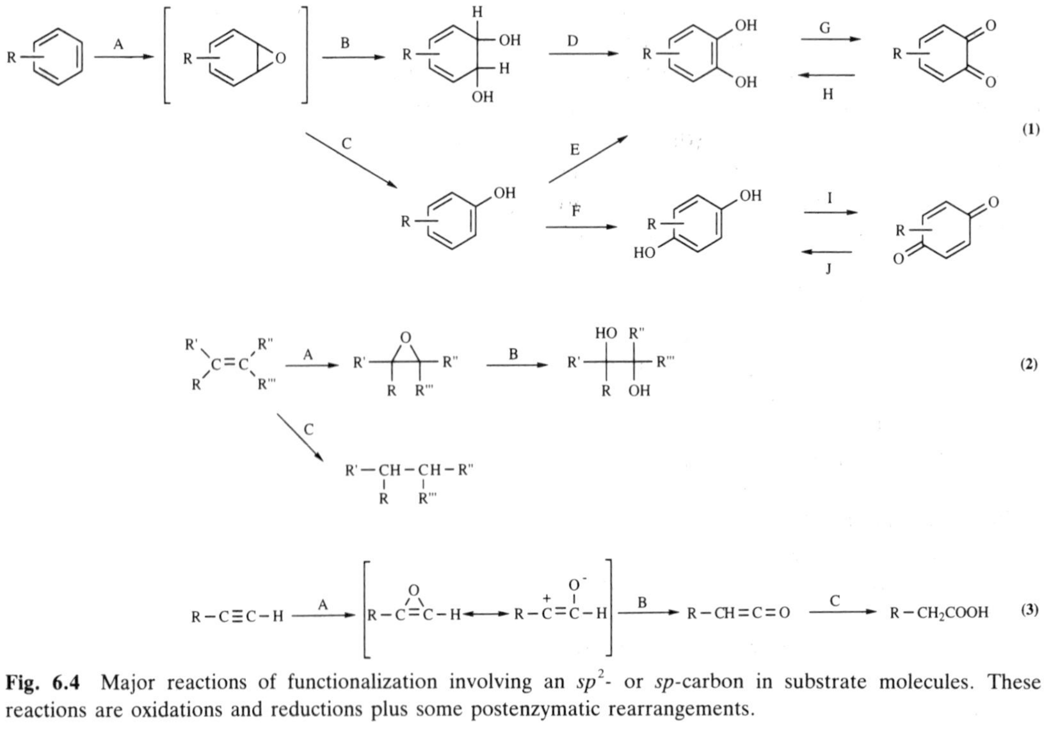

Fig. 6.4 Major reactions of functionalization involving an sp^2- or sp-carbon in substrate molecules. These reactions are oxidations and reductions plus some postenzymatic rearrangements.

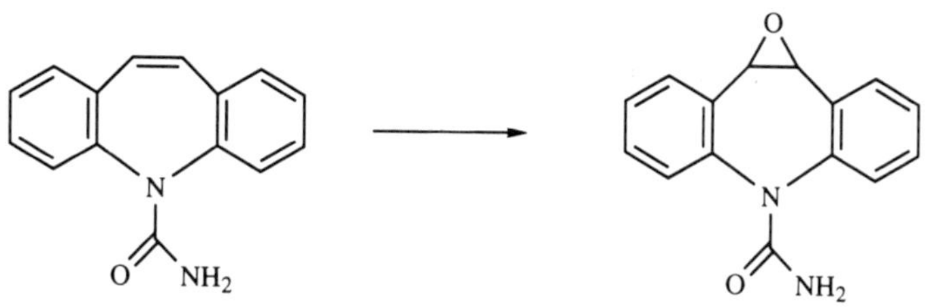

Fig. 6.5 Carbamazepine (**7**) and its 10,11-epoxide (**8**).

tron transfers. The nonenzymatic reduction of quinones can occur, e.g., in the presence of $O_2^{\bullet-}$ or some thiols such as glutathione.

Olefinic bonds in xenobiotic molecules can also be targets of cytochrome P450–catalyzed epoxidation (reaction 2-A in Fig 6.4). In contrast to arene oxides, the resulting epoxides are fairly stable and have often been isolated and characterized. But like arene oxides, they are substrates of epoxide hydrolase and yield dihydrodiols (reaction 2-B). This is exemplified by carbamazepine whose 10,11-epoxide is a major and pharmacologically active metabolite in humans and is further metabolized to the inactive dihydrodiol (37) (Fig. 6.5).

Reduction of olefinic groups (reaction 2-C) is documented for a few drugs bearing an α,β-ketoalkene function. The reaction is thought to be catalyzed by various NAD(P)H oxidoreductases. Acetylenic bonds are also targets for cytochrome P450–catalyzed oxidation. Oxygenation of the triple bond (reaction 3-A) yields an intermediate that, depending on the substrate, can react in a number of ways, e.g., binding covalently to the enzyme or forming a highly reactive ketene whose hydration produces a substituted acetic acid (reactions 3-B and 3-C).

2.4 Oxidation and Reduction of Nitrogen Atoms

The main metabolic reactions of oxidation and reduction of nitrogen atoms in organic molecules are summarized in Figure 6.6. The functional groups involved are amines and amides and their oxygenated metabolites as well as 1,4-dihydropyridines, hydrazines, and azo compounds. In many cases, the reactions can be catalyzed by cytochrome P450 and/or flavin-containing monooxygenases.

Nitrogen oxygenation is an (apparently) straightforward metabolic reaction of tertiary amines (reaction 1-A), be they aliphatic or aromatic. Numerous drugs undergo this reaction, and the resulting N-oxide metabolite is more polar and hydrophilic than the parent compound. Identical considerations apply to pyridines and analogous aromatic azaheterocycles (reaction 2-A). Note that these reactions are reversible; cytochrome P450 and other reductases are able to deoxygenate N-oxides back to the amine (i.e., reactions 1-B and 2-B).

Secondary and primary amines also undergo N-oxygenation, the first isolable metabolites being hydroxylamines (reactions 3-A and 4-A, respectively). Again, reversibility is documented (reactions 3-B and 4-B). These compounds can be aliphatic or aromatic amines, but they can also be secondary or primary amides (i.e., R = acyl), while tertiary amides appear resistant to N-oxygenation. The oxidation of secondary amines and amides usually stops at the hydroxylamine–hydroxylamide level, but formation of short-lived nitroxides (not shown) has been reported.

As opposed to secondary amines and amides, primary amines and amides can be

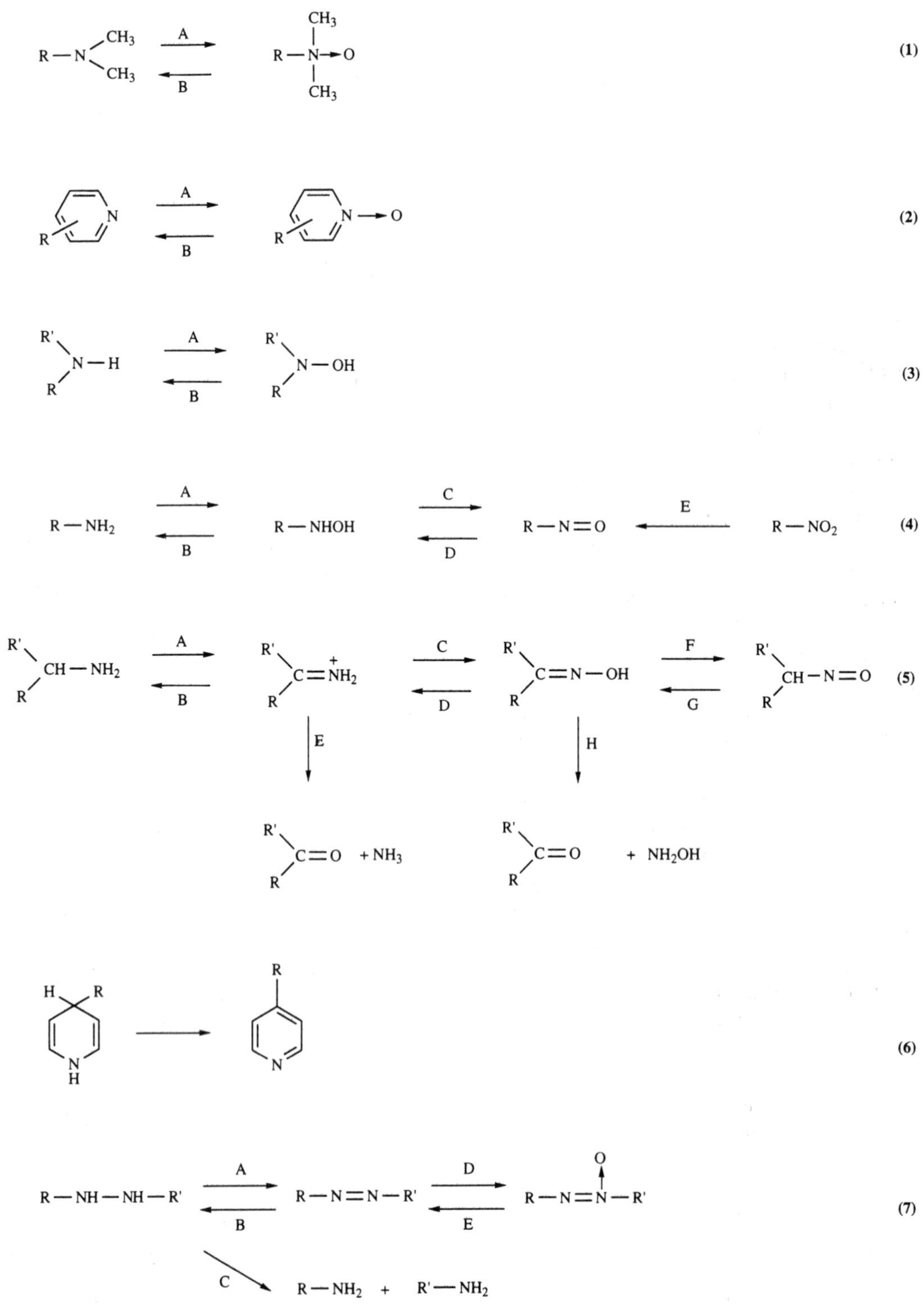

(1)

(2)

(3)

$$R-NH_2 \underset{B}{\overset{A}{\rightleftarrows}} R-NHOH \underset{D}{\overset{C}{\rightleftarrows}} R-N=O \overset{E}{\longleftarrow} R-NO_2 \quad (4)$$

(5)

(6)

$$R-NH-NH-R' \underset{B}{\overset{A}{\rightleftarrows}} R-N=N-R' \underset{E}{\overset{D}{\rightleftarrows}} R-N=\overset{O}{\underset{}{N}}-R' \quad (7)$$

$$\overset{C}{\searrow} \quad R-NH_2 \; + \; R'-NH_2$$

Fig. 6.6 Major reactions of functionalization involving nitrogen atoms in substrate molecules. The reactions shown here are mainly oxidations and reductions (deoxygenations and hydrogenations).

oxidized to nitroso metabolites (reaction 4-C), but further oxidation of the latter compounds to nitro compounds does not seem to occur *in vivo*. In contrast, automatic nitro compounds can be reduced to primary amines via reactions 4-E, 4-D, and finally 4-B. This is the case of numerous chemotherapeutic drugs such as metronidazole, a reactive nitro anion radical being the first (and therapeutically active) intermediate (Fig. 6.7).

Note that primary aliphatic amines that have a hydrogen on the α-carbon can display additional metabolic reactions as shown in reactions 5. Indeed, *N*-oxidation can also yield imines (reaction 5-A), whose degree of oxidation is equivalent to that of hydroxylamines. Imines can be further oxidized to oximes (reaction 5-C), which are in equilibrium with their nitroso tautomer (reactions 5-F and 5-G). 1,4-Dihydropyridines, and particularly calcium channel blockers such as nivaldipide (**10**), are effectively oxidized by cytochrome P450. The reaction is one of aromatization (reaction 6), yielding the corresponding pyridine.

Dinitrogen moieties are also targets of oxidoreductases. Depending on their substituents, hydrazines are oxidized to azo compounds (reaction 7-A), some of which can be oxygenated to azoxy compounds (reaction 1-D). Another important pathway of hydrazines is their reductive cleavage to primary amines (reaction 7-C). Reactions 7-A and 7-D are reversible, the corresponding reductions (reactions 7-B and 7-E) being mediated by cytochrome P450 and other reductases. A toxicologically significant pathway thus exists for the reduction of some aromatic azo compounds to potentially toxic primary aromatic amines (reactions 7-B and 7-C).

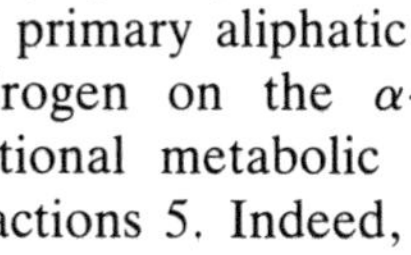

2.5 Oxidation and Reduction of Sulfur and Other Atoms

The major redox reactions occurring at sulfur atoms in organic compounds are summarized in Figure 6.8. Thiol compounds can be oxidized to sulfenic acids (reaction 1-A), then to sulfinic acids (reaction 1-E), and finally to sulfonic acids (reaction 1-F). Depending on the substrate, the pathway is mediated by cytochrome P450 and/or flavin-containing monooxygenases. Another route of oxidation of thiols is to disulfides either directly (reaction 1-C via thiyl radicals) or by dehydration between a thiol and a sulfenic acid (reaction 1-B). However, the understanding of sulfur biochemistry is largely incomplete, and much remains to be understood in reactions 1. This is particularly true for reactions of reduction. Although reaction 1-C is well known to be reversible (i.e., reaction 1-D), the case of reaction 1-A is unclear, and reduction of sulfinic and sulfonic acids appears unlikely.

The metabolism of sulfides (thioethers) is rather straightforward. Besides reactions of *S*-dealkylation discussed in section 2.3.1, these compounds can also be oxygenated by monooxygenases to sulfoxides (reaction 2-A) and then to sulfones (reaction 2-C).

CH$_2$CH$_2$OH

O$_2$N, N, CH$_3$

N

(9)

NO$_2$

H

CH$_3$OOC, COOCH(CH$_3$)$_2$

CH$_3$, N, CH$_3$

H

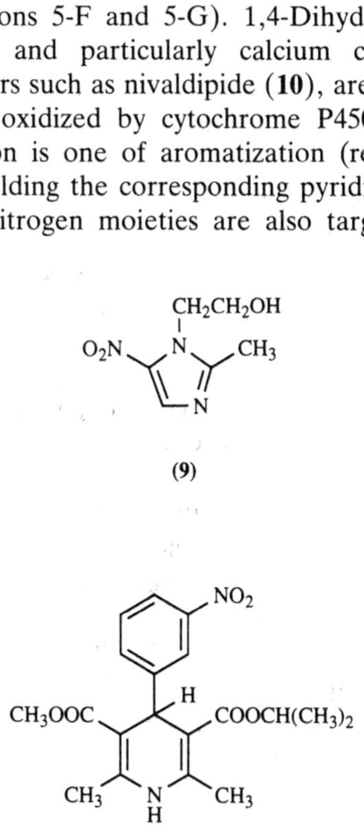

(10)

Fig. 6.7 Metronidazole (**9**) and nivaldipide (**10**).

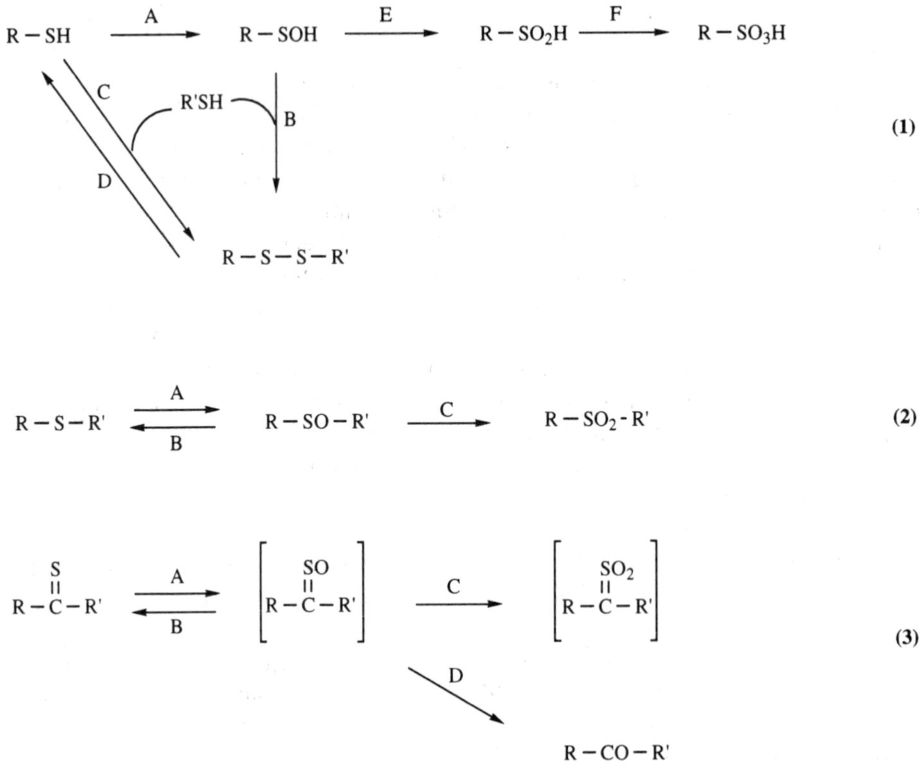

$$R-SH \xrightarrow{A} R-SOH \xrightarrow{E} R-SO_2H \xrightarrow{F} R-SO_3H \tag{1}$$

(with side reactions C, D, B and R'SH leading to $R-S-S-R'$)

$$R-S-R' \underset{B}{\overset{A}{\rightleftarrows}} R-SO-R' \xrightarrow{C} R-SO_2-R' \tag{2}$$

$$\underset{R-C-R'}{\overset{S}{\overset{\|}{}}} \underset{B}{\overset{A}{\rightleftarrows}} \left[\underset{R-C-R'}{\overset{SO}{\overset{\|}{}}}\right] \xrightarrow{C} \left[\underset{R-C-R'}{\overset{SO_2}{\overset{\|}{}}}\right] \tag{3}$$

$$\xrightarrow{D} R-CO-R'$$

Fig. 6.8 Major reactions of oxidation and reduction involving sulfur atoms in organic compounds.

Here it is known with confidence that reaction 2-A is indeed reversible, as documented by many examples of reduction of sulfoxides (reaction 2-B), but the reduction of sulfones has never been found to occur.

Thiocarbonyl compounds are also substrates of monooxygenases, forming S-monoxides (sulfines, reaction 3-A) and then S-dioxides (sulfenes, reaction 3-C). As a rule, these metabolites cannot be identified as such due to their reactivity. Thus S-monoxides rearrange to the corresponding carbonyl by expulsing a sulfur atom (reaction 3-D). This reaction is known as oxidative desulfuration and occurs in thioamides and thioureas (e.g., thiopental). As for the S-dioxides, they react rapidly with nucleophiles and particularly with nucleophilic sites in biological macromolecules. This covalent binding results in the formation of adducts of toxicological sig-

nificance. Such a mechanism is believed to account for the carcinogenicity of a number of thioamides.

Some other elements besides carbon, nitrogen, and sulfur can undergo metabolic redox reactions. The direct oxidation of oxygen atoms in phenols and alcohols is well documented for some substrates, yielding, for example, quinones and ketones. Such reactions can be catalyzed in particular by cytochrome P450 and various peroxidases. A classic example is that of the antiinflammatory drug paracetamol (acetaminophen), a minor fraction of which is oxidized by cytochrome P450 to the highly reactive and toxic quinone imine (Fig. 6.9).

Other elements of lesser quantitative importance in medicinal chemistry that can enter redox reactions include silicium, phosphorus, arsenic, and selenium (Fig.

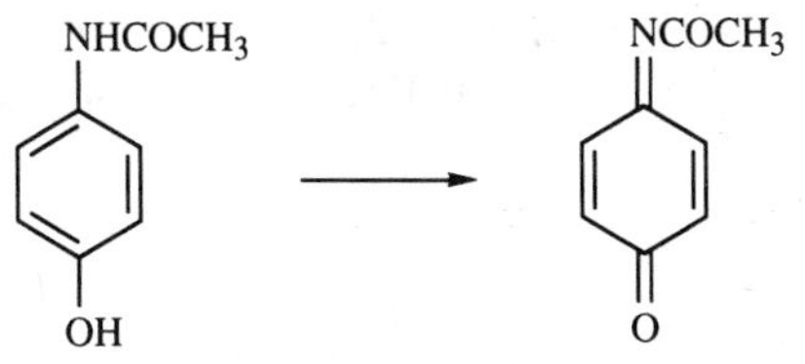

NHCOCH₃

OH

(11)

NCOCH₃

O

(12)

Fig. 6.9 Paracetamol (**11**) and its toxic quinone imine metabolite (**12**).

6.10). Note however that the enzymology and mechanisms of these reactions are insufficiently understood. For example, a few silanes have been shown to yield silanols *in vivo* (reaction 1). The same applies to some phosphines, which can be oxygenated to phosphine oxides by monooxygenases (reaction 2).

Arsenicals have received some attention due to their therapeutic significance. Both

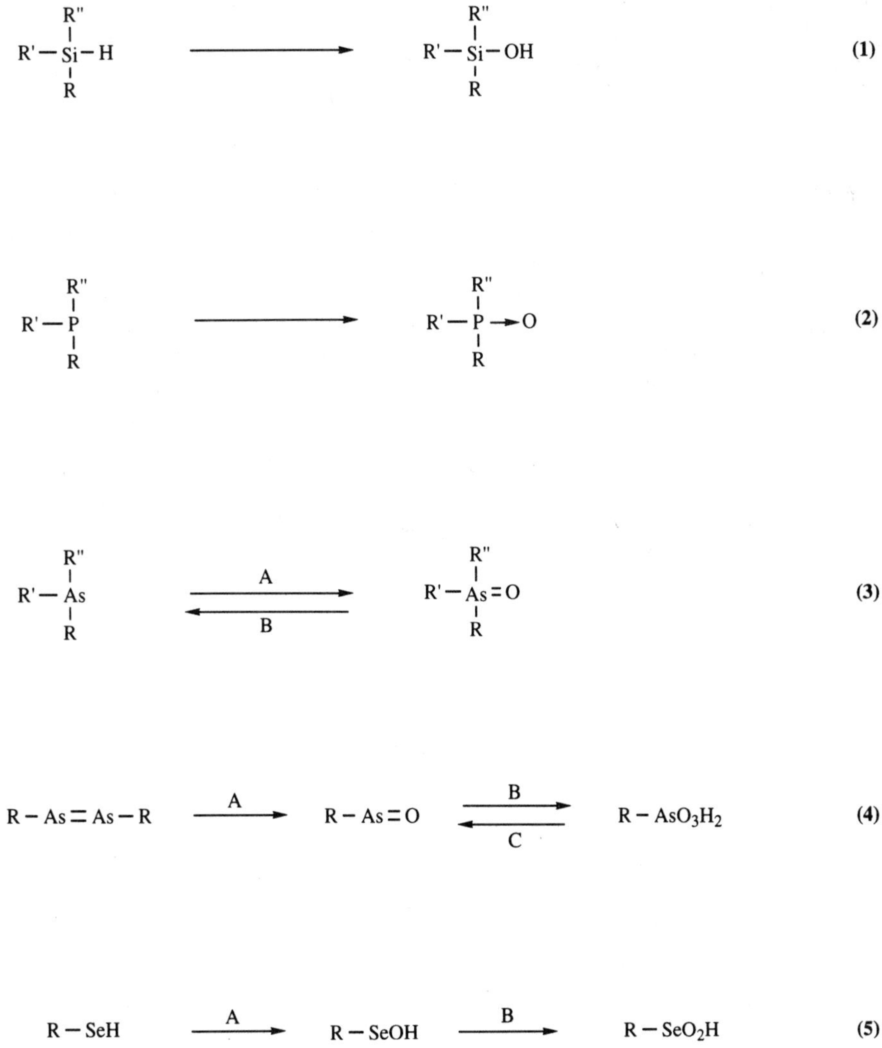

R' — Si — H   ⟶   R' — Si — OH   (1)

R' — P   ⟶   R' — P → O   (2)

R' — As   ⟶   R' — As = O   (3)

R — As ≡ As — R   ⟶   R — As = O   ⟶   R — AsO₃H₂   (4)

R — SeH   ⟶   R — SeOH   ⟶   R — SeO₂H   (5)

Fig. 6.10 Some selected reactions of oxidation and reduction involving silicon, phosphorus, arsenic, and selenium in xenobiotic compounds.

inorganic and organic arsenic compounds display an As(III)–As(V) redox equilibrium in the body. This is illustrated with the arsine–arsine oxide and arsenoxide–arsonic acid equilibria (reactions 3-A and 3-B and reactions 4-B and 4-C, respectively). Another reaction of interest is the oxidation of arseno compounds to arsenoxides (reaction 4-A), which is important in the bioactivation of a number of chemotherapeutic arsenicals.

The biochemistry of organoselenium compounds is now becoming a rich source of interest. For example, a few selenols have been seen to be oxidized to selenenic acids (reaction 5-A) and then to seleninic acids (reaction 5-B).

2.6 Oxidative Cleavage Reactions

A number of oxidative reactions presented in the previous sections yield metabolic intermediates of usually poor stability that undergo postenzymatic cleavage of a C–X bond (X being an heteroatom). As briefly mentioned in section 2.3.1, reactions 4-A and 4-B in Figure 6.1 represent important metabolic pathways that affect many drugs. When X = N (by far the most frequent case), the metabolic reactions are known as N-demethylations, N-dealkylations or deaminations, depending on the moiety being cleaved. Consider for example the anorectic drug fenfluramine, which is N-deethylated to norfenfluramine—an active metabolite—and deaminated to (m-trifluoromethyl)phenylacetone—an inactive metabolite that is further oxidized to m-trifluoromethylbenzoic acid (Fig. 6.11).

When X = O or S in reactions 4 in Figure 6.1, the metabolic reactions are known as O-dealkylations or S-dealkylations, respectively. O-Demethylations are a typical case of the former reaction. And when X = halogen in reactions 5-A and 5-B (Fig. 6.1), loss of halogen can also occur and is known as oxidative dehalogenation.

The reactions of oxidative C–X cleavage discussed above result from carbon hydroxylation and are catalyzed by cytochrome P450. However, reactions of N-

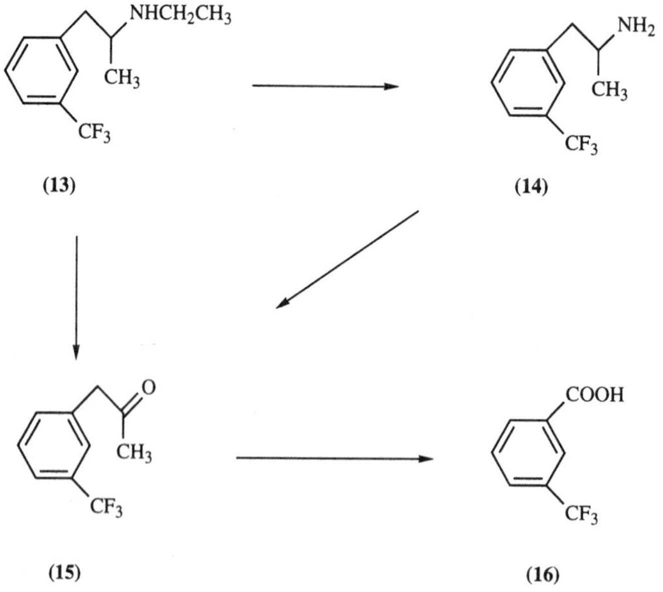

Fig. 6.11 Fenfluramine (**13**), norfenfluramine (**14**), (m-trifluoromethyl)phenylacetone (**15**), and m-trifluoromethylbenzoic acid (**16**).

oxidation followed by hydrolytic C–N cleavage can also be catalyzed by cytochrome P450 (e.g., reactions 5-E and 5-H in Fig. 6.6). The sequence of reactions 5-A and 5-E in Figure 6.6 is of particular interest, because it is the mechanism by which monoamine oxidase deaminates endogenous and exogenous amines.

2.7 Hydration and Hydrolysis

Hydrolases catalyze the addition of a molecule of water to a variety of functional moieties. Thus epoxide hydrolase hydrates epoxides to yield *trans*-dihydrodiols (reaction 1-B in Fig. 6.4). This reaction is documented for many arene oxides, particularly metabolites of aromatic compounds and epoxides of olefins. Here a molecule of water has been added to the substrate without loss of a molecular fragment, hence the use of the term *hydration* sometimes found in the literature.

Reactions of hydrolytic cleavage (hydrolysis) are shown in Figure 6.12. They are frequent for organic esters (reaction 1), inorganic esters such as nitrates (reaction 2) and sulfates (reaction 3), and amides (reaction 4). These reactions are catalyzed by esterases, peptidases, or other enzymes, but nonenzymatic hydrolysis is also known to occur for sufficiently labile compounds under biological conditions of pH and temperature. Acetylsalicylic acid, glycerol trinitrate, and lidocaine are three representative examples of drugs undergoing extensive cleavage of the organic ester, inorganic ester, and amide group, respectively. The reaction is of particular significance in the activation of ester prodrugs (Section 4).

3 CONJUGATION REACTIONS

3.1 Introduction

As defined in Section 1.3, reactions of conjugation (also but infelicitously known as phase II reactions) result in the covalent binding of an endogenous molecule or moiety to the substrate. Such reactions are of critical significance in the metabolism of endogenous compounds; witness the impressive battery of enzymes that have evolved to catalyze them. Conjugation is also of great importance in the biotransformation of xenobiotics, involving unchanged compounds or metabolites thereof (38).

Reactions of conjugation are characterized by a number of criteria:

1. They are catalyzed by enzymes known as transferases.
2. They involve a cofactor that binds to the enzyme in the close proximity of the substrate and carries the endogenous molecule or moiety to be transferred.
3. This endogenous molecule or moiety is highly polar (hydrophilic), and its size is comparable with that of the substrate.

$$R-COO-R' \longrightarrow R-COOH + R'-OH \qquad (1)$$

$$R-ONO_2 \longrightarrow R-OH + HNO_3 \qquad (2)$$

$$R-OSO_3H \longrightarrow R-OH + H_2SO_4 \qquad (3)$$

$$R-CONHR' \longrightarrow R-COOH + R'-NH_2 \qquad (4)$$

Fig. 6.12 Major reactions of hydrolysis involving esters (organic and inorganic) and amides.

It is important from a biochemical and practical viewpoint, however, to note that these criteria are neither sufficient nor necessary to define conjugations reactions. They are not sufficient, since in reactions of hydrogenation (i.e., typical reactions of functionalization) the hydride is also transferred from a cofactor (NADPH or NADH). And they are not necessary, since all the above criteria suffer from important exceptions discussed below. As a result of this fuzziness, reactions of hydration may be classified as conjugations, as favored by some authors.

3.2 Methylation

3.2.1 INTRODUCTION. Reactions of methylation imply the transfer of a methyl group from the cofactor S-adenosyl-L-methionine (**17**, SAM) (Fig. 6.13) to the substrate. A number of methyltransferases are able to methylate small molecules (39). Thus reactions of methylation fulfill only two of the three criteria defined above, since the methyl group is hydrophobic and small compared with the substrate. The main enzyme responsible for O-methylation is catechol O-methyltransferase (EC 2.1.1.6; COMT) which is mainly cytosolic but also exists in membrane-bound form. Several

enzymes catalyze reactions of xenobiotic N-methylation with different substrate specificities, e.g., nicotinamide N-methyltransferase (EC 2.1.1.1), histamine methyltransferase (EC 2.1.1.8), phenylethanolamine N-methyltransferase (noradrenaline N-methyltransferase; EC 2.1.1.28), and nonspecific amine N-methyltransferase (arylamine N-methyltransferase, tryptamine N-methyltransferase; EC 2.1.1.49), of which some isozymes have been characterized. Reactions of xenobiotic S-methylation are mediated by the membrane-bound thiol methyltransferase (EC 2.1.1.9) and the cytosolic thiopurine methyltransferase (EC 2.1.1.67) (38).

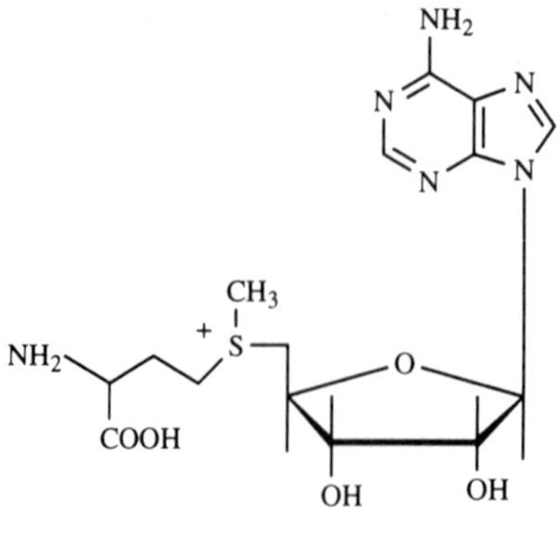

The above classification of enzymes makes explicit the three types of functionalities undergoing biomethylation, namely hydroxyl (phenolic), amino, and thiol groups. Before discussing and exemplifying these reactions, it is worth noting that the methyl group in S-adenosylmethionine is bound to a sulfonium center, giving it a marked electrophilic character and explaining its reactivity. Interestingly, the positive charge is also transferred during some N-methylations.

3.2.2 METHYLATION REACTIONS. Figure 6.14 summarizes the main reactions of methylation seen in drug metabolism. O-methylation is a common reaction of compounds containing a catechol moiety (reaction 1), with a usual regioselectivity for the *meta* position. The substrates can be xenobiotics and particularly drugs, of which L-DOPA is a classic example. More frequently, however, O-methylation occurs as a late event in the metabolism of aryl groups, after they have been oxidized to catechols as shown in reactions 1 in Figure 6.4. This sequence was seen, e.g., in the metabolism of the antiinflammatory drug diclofenac (**18**), which in humans yielded 3'-hydroxy-4'-methoxy-diclofenac as a major metabolite with a long plasma half-life (40) (Fig. 6.15).

(**17**)

Fig. 6.13 S-Adenosyl-L-methionine.

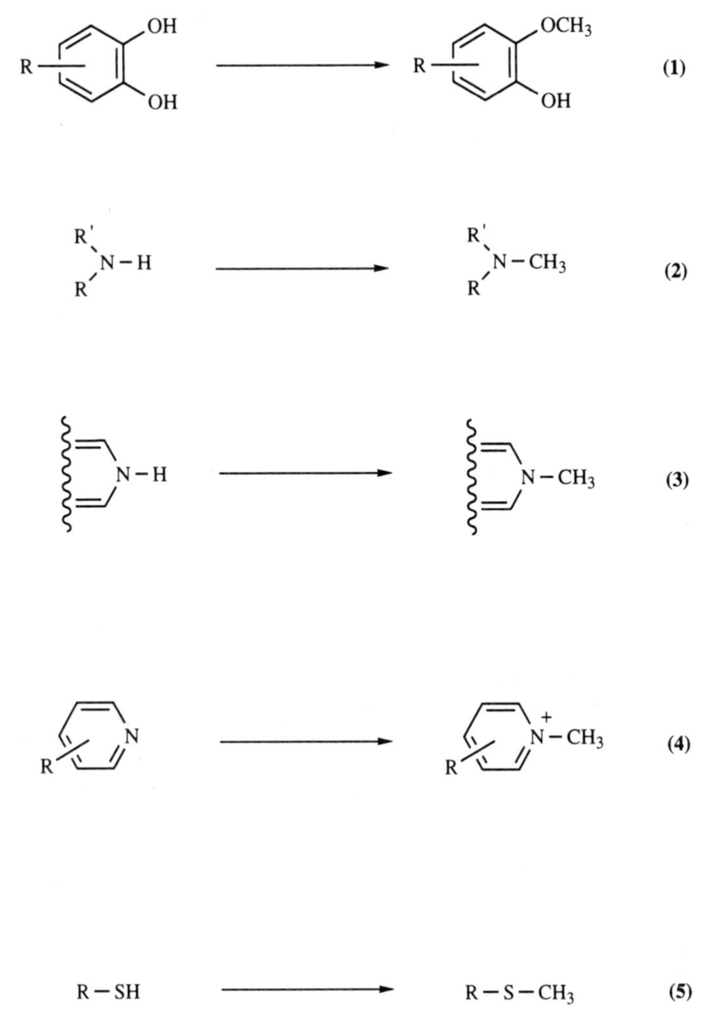

Fig. 6.14 Major reactions of methylation involving catechols, various amines, and thiols.

Three basic types of reactions of *N*-methylation have been recognized (reactions 2–4). A number of primary amines (e.g., amphetamine) and secondary amines (e.g., tetrahydroisoquinolines) have been shown to be *in vitro* substrates of amine *N*-methyltransferase, whereas some phenylethanolamines and analogues are methylated by phenylethanolamine *N*-methyltransferase (reaction 2). However, such reactions are seldom significant *in vivo*, presumably due to effective oxidative *N*-demethylation. A comparable situation involves pyrrol-type nitrogen atoms (reac-

tion 3), as exemplified by imidazole and histamine (41). A therapeutically relevant example is that of theophylline (**19**) whose *N*(9)-methylation is masked by *N*-demethylation in human adults, but not newborns.

N-Methylation of pyridine-type nitrogen atoms (reaction 4) appears to be of greater *in vivo* pharmacological significance than reactions 2 and 3 for two reasons. First, the resulting metabolites, being quaternary amines, are more stable than tertiary or secondary amines toward *N*-demethylation. And second, these metabolites also are

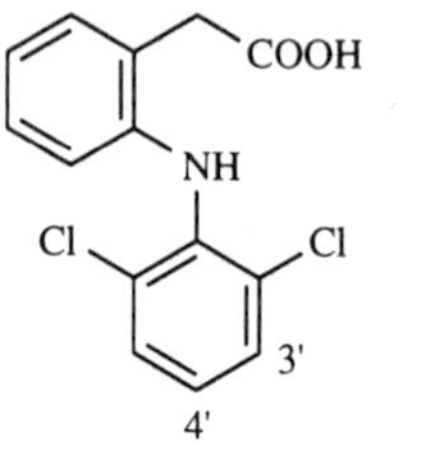

Fig. 6.15 Diclofenac (**18**), theophylline (**19**), nicotinamide (**20**), and 6-mercaptopurine (**21**).

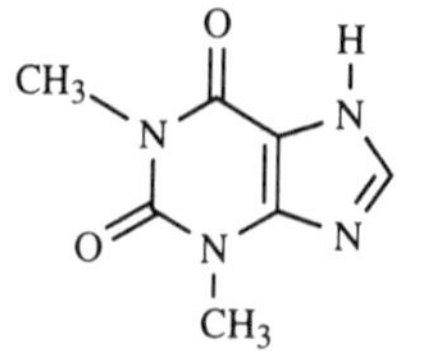

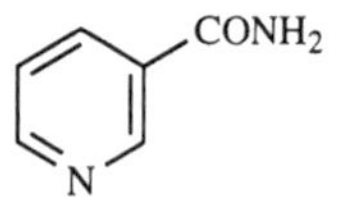

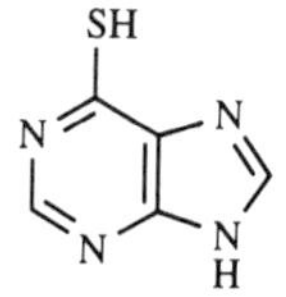

more polar than the parent compounds, in contrast to the products of reactions 2 and 3. Good substrates are nicotinamide (**20**), pyridine, and a number of monocyclic and bicyclic derivatives (41).

S-Methylation of thiol groups (reaction 5) is documented for such drugs as 6-mercaptopurine (**21**) and captopril (42). Other substrates are metabolites (mainly thiophenols) resulting from the S–C cleavage of (aromatic) glutathione and cysteine conjugates (see sections 2.6 and 3.7). Once formed, such methylthio metabolites can be further processed to sulfoxides and sulfones before excretion (i.e., reactions 2-A and 2-C in Fig. 6.8).

3.3 Sulfation

3.3.1. INTRODUCTION. Reactions of sulfation consist in a sulfate being transferred from the cofactor 3′-phosphoadenosine 5′-phosphosulfate (PAPS; **22**) to the substrate

under catalysis by the sulfotransferase (Fig. 6.16). The three criteria of conjugation (see Section 3.1) are met in these reactions. Sulfotransferases, which catalyze a variety of physiological reactions, are soluble enzymes that include aryl sulfotransferase (phenol sulfotransferase; EC 2.8.2.1), alcohol sulfotransferase (hydroxysteroid sulfotransferase; EC 2.8.2.2), amine sulfotransferase (arylamine sulfotransferase; EC 2.8.2.3), estrone sulfotransferase (EC 2.8.2.4), tyrosine-ester sulfotransferase (EC 2.8.2.9), steroid sulfotransferase (EC 2.8.2.15), and cortisol sulfotransferase (glucocorticosteroid sulfotransferase; EC 2.8.2.18). Among these enzymes, the former three are of particular significance in the sulfation of xenobiotics (38, 43).

The sulfate moiety in PAPS is linked to a phosphate group by an anhydride bridge whose cleavage is exothermic and supplies enthalpy to the reaction. The leaving SO_3^- moiety is electrophilic and will bind to an nucleophilic –OH or –NH– site in the substrate, forming an ester sulfate or a sulfamate (Fig. 6.17). Some of these conjugates are unstable under biological conditions and will form electrophilic intermediates of considerable toxicological significance.

3.3.2. SULFATION REACTIONS. Sulfoconjugation of alcohols (reaction 1 in Fig. 6.17) leads to metabolites of different stabilities.

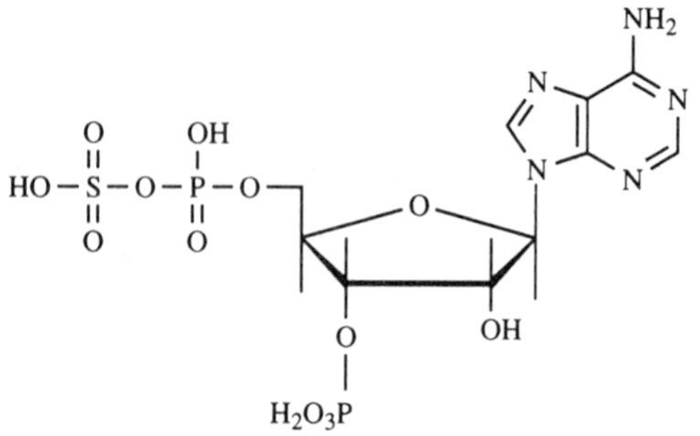

Fig. 6.16 3′-Phosphoadenosine 5′-phosphosulfate.

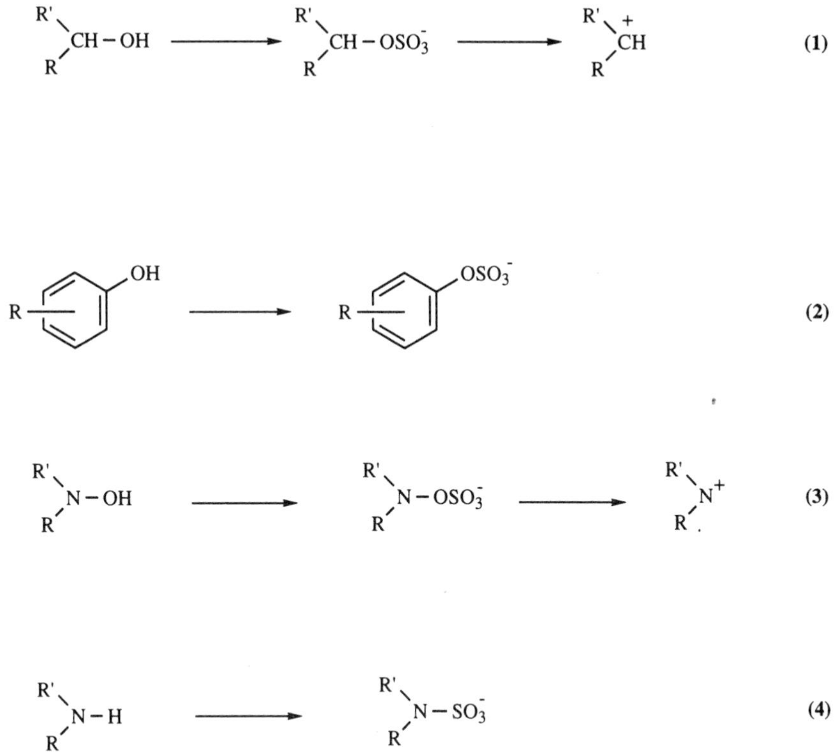

Fig. 6.17 Major reactions of sulfation involving primary and secondary alcohols, phenols, hydroxylamines and hydroxylamides, and amines.

Endogenous hydroxysteroids (i.e., cyclic secondary alcohols) form relatively stable sulfates, while some secondary alcohol metabolites of allylbenzenes (e.g., safrole and estragole) form highly genotoxic carbocations (44). Primary alcohols (e.g., methanol and ethanol) also can form sulfates, whose alkylating capacity is well known (45). Similarly, polycyclic hydroxymethylarenes yield reactive sulfates believed to account for their carcinogenicity.

In contrast to alcohols, phenols form stable sulfate esters (reaction 2). The reaction is usually of high affinity (i.e., rapid), but the limited availability of PAPS restricts the amounts of conjugate being produced. Typical drugs undergoing limited sulfation include paracetamol (**11**) and diflunisal (**23**, Fig. 6.18).

Aromatic hydroxylamines and hydroxyl-amides are good substrates for some sulfotransferases and yield unstable sulfate esters (reaction 3). Indeed, heterolytic N–O cleavage produces a highly electrophilic nitrenium ion. This is a mechanism believed to account for part or all of the cytotoxicity of arylamines and arylamides (e.g., phenacetin). In contrast, significantly more stable products are obtained on N-sulfoconjugation of amines (reaction 4). Alicyclic amines, and primary and secondary alkyl- and arylamines can all yield sulfamates (46). The significance of these reactions in humans is still poorly understood.

An intriguing reaction of conjugation occurs for minoxidil (**24**), a hypotensive agent that also produces hair growth. This drug is an N-oxide, and the actual active form responsible for the different therapeu-

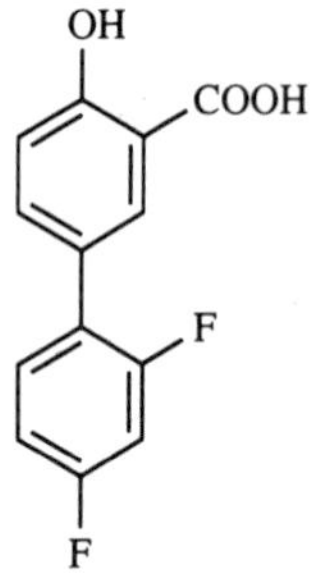

Fig. 6.18 Diflunisal (**23**), minoxidil (**24**) and its *N,O*-sulfate ester (**25**).

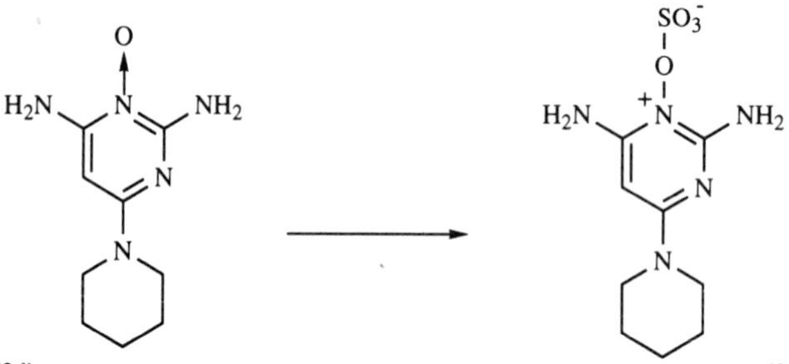

tic effects is the *N,O*-sulfate ester (**25**) (47).

3.4 Glucuronidation and Glucosidation

3.4.1 INTRODUCTION. Glucuronidation involves the transfer to the substrate of a molecule of glucuronic acid from the cofactor uridine-5′-diphospho-α-D-glucuronic acid (UDPGA; **26**) (Fig. 6.19). The enzyme catalyzing this reaction is known as glucuronyltransferase (UDP-glucuronosyltransferase; EC 2.4.1.17, UDPGT) and consists in a number of products of the *UGT* gene superfamily. According to a recent nomenclature, the human UDPGT isozymes are the products of two gene families (*UGT*1 and *UGT*2) and include UGT1*1 and UGT1*4 (bilirubin UDPGTs), UGT1*6, UGT2B4, UGT2B7 (catechol estrogen UDPGT), UGT2B8) (estriol UDPGT), UGT2B9 and UGT2B10

(48–50). In addition to glucuronidation, this section briefly discusses glucosidation, a minor metabolic reaction seen for a few drugs. Candidate enzymes catalyzing this reaction could be phenol β-glucosyltransferase (EC 2.4.1.35), arylamine glucosyltransferase (EC 2.4.1.71), and nicotinate glucosyltransferase (EC 2.4.1.196).

3.4.2 GLUCURONIDATION REACTIONS. Glucuronic acid exists in UDPGA in the 1α configuration, but the products of conjugation are β-glucuronides. This is because the mechanism of the reaction is nucleophilic substitution with inversion of configuration. Indeed, and as shown in Figure 6.20, all functional groups able to undergo glucuronidation are nucleophiles, a common characteristic they share despite their great chemical variety. As a consequence of this diversity, the products of glucuronidation are classified as *O*-, *N*-, *S*-, and *C*-glucuronides.

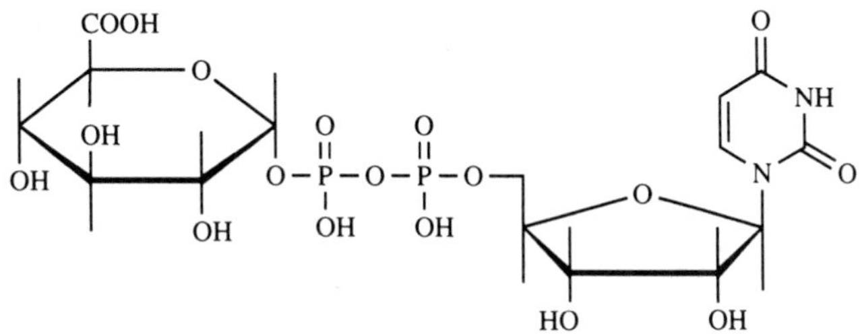

(26)

Fig. 6.19 Uridine-5′-diphospho-α-D-glucuronic acid.

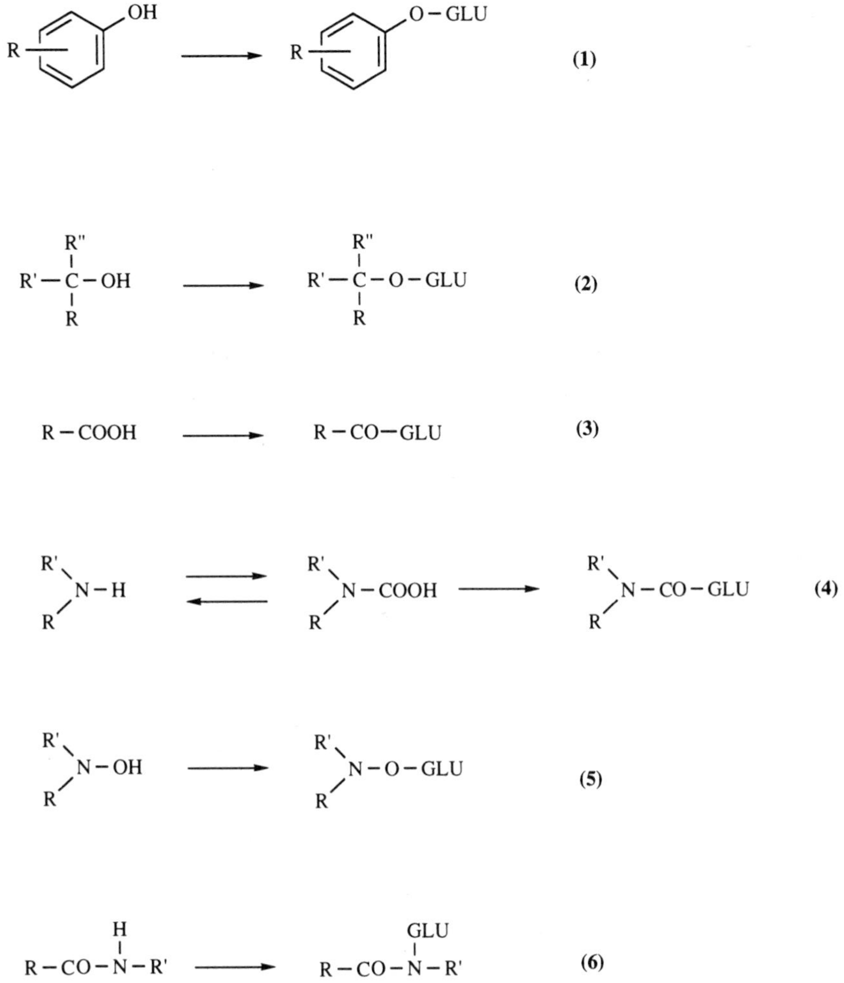

Fig. 6.20 Major reactions of glucuronidation involving phenols, alcohols, carboxylic acids, carbamic acids, hydroxylamines and hydroxylamides, carboxamides, sulfonamides, various amines, thiols, dithiocarboxylic acids, and 1,3-dicarbonyl compounds.

$$R-SO_2-\overset{\overset{\text{H}}{|}}{N}-R' \longrightarrow R-SO_2-\overset{\overset{\text{GLU}}{|}}{N}-R' \qquad (7)$$

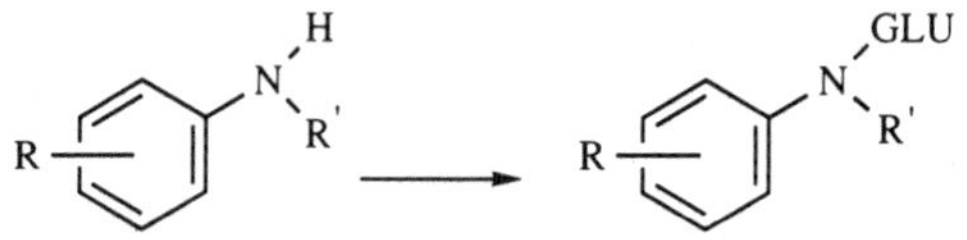

$$\qquad (8)$$

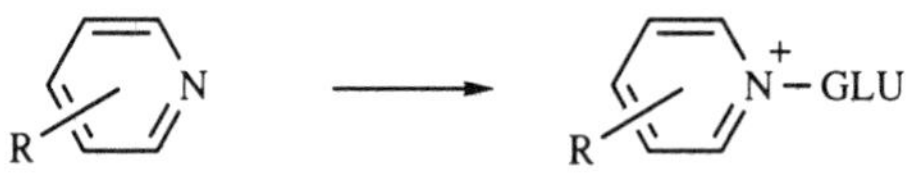

$$\qquad (9)$$

$$\overset{R'}{\underset{R}{>}}N-H \longrightarrow \overset{R'}{\underset{R}{>}}N-GLU \qquad (10)$$

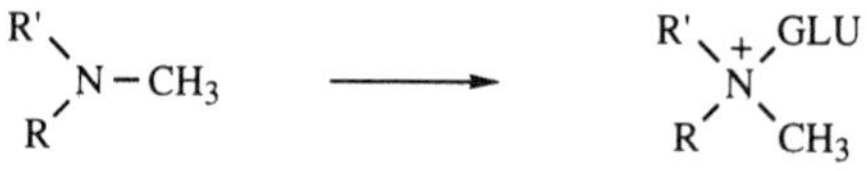

$$\overset{R'}{\underset{R}{>}}N-CH_3 \longrightarrow \overset{R'}{\underset{R}{>}}\overset{+}{N}\overset{GLU}{\underset{CH_3}{}} \qquad (11)$$

$$R-SH \longrightarrow R-S-GLU \qquad (12)$$

$$R-CSSH \longrightarrow R-CS-S-GLU \qquad (13)$$

$$R-CO-CH_2-CO-R' \longrightarrow R-CO-\overset{\overset{\text{GLU}}{|}}{CH}-CO-R' \qquad (14)$$

GLU =

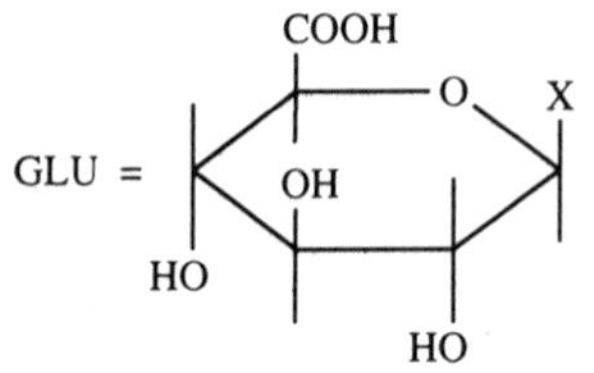

Fig. 6.20   (*Continued*)

Reactions of *O*-glucuronidation are shown in reactions 1–5 in Figure 6.20. A frequent metabolic reaction of phenolic xenobiotics or metabolites is their glucuronidation to yield polar metabolites excreted in urine and/or bile. *O*-Glucuronidation is often in competition with *O*-sulfation (section 3.3); the latter reaction predominates at low doses, and the former, at high doses. In biochemical terms, glucuronidation is a reaction of low affinity and high capacity, whereas sulfation displays high affinity and low capacity. A typical drug that undergoes extensive glucuronidation is paracetamol (**11**). Another major group of substrates are alcohols, be they primary, secondary, or tertiary (reaction 2). Medicinal examples include chloramphenicol and oxazepam. Another important example is that of morphine, which is conjugated on its phenolic and secondary alcohol groups to form the 3-*O*-glucuronide (a weak opiate antagonist) and the 6-*O*-glucuronide (a strong opiate agonist), respectively (51).

An important pathway of *O*-glucuronidation is the formation of acyl-glucuronides (reaction 3). Substrates are arylacetic acids (e.g., diclofenac; **18**) and aliphatic acids (e.g., valproic acid, **27**, Fig. 6.21). Aromatic acids are seldom substrates, a noteworthy exception being diflunisal (**23**) which yields both the acyl and phenolic glucuronides. The significance of acyl glucuronides has long been underestimated, perhaps because of analytical difficulties. Indeed, these metabolites are quite reactive; they rearrange to positional isomers and bind covalently to plasmatic and, it seems, tissue proteins (52). Thus acyl glucuronide formation cannot be viewed solely as a reaction of inactivation and detoxication.

A special class of acyl glucuronides is the carbamoyl glucuronides. An increasing number of primary and secondary amines are found to yield this type of conjugate, while as expected, the intermediate car-

Fig. 6.21 Valproic acid (**27**), carvedilol (**28**), phenytoin (**29**), and sulfadimethoxine (**30**).

bamic acids are not stable enough to be characterized. Carvedilol (**28**) is one drug exemplifying the reaction, in addition to forming an *O*-glucuronide on its alcohol group and a carbazole *N*-linked glucuronide (see below) (53). Much remains to be understood on the chemical and biochemical reactivity of carbamoyl glucuronides.

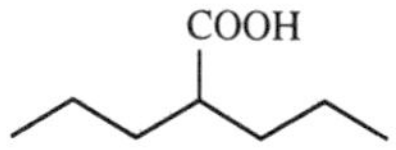

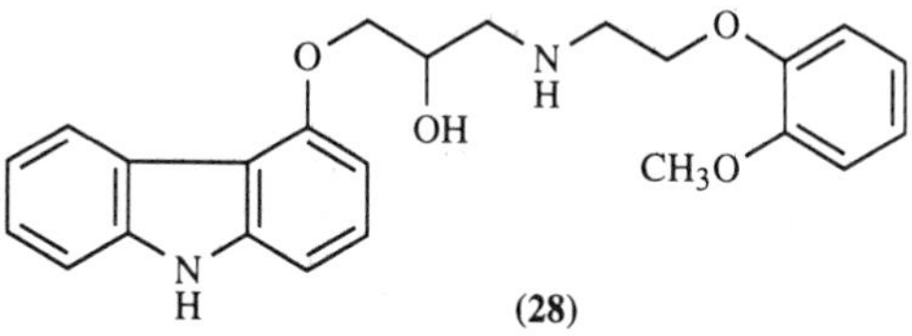

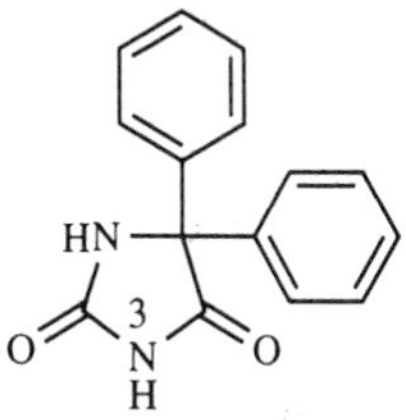

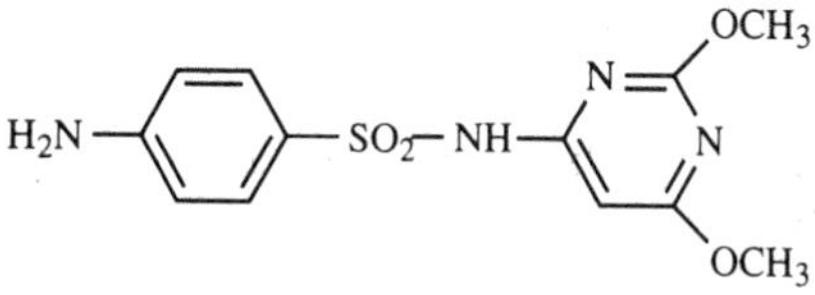

Hydroxylamines and hydroxylamides may also form *O*-glucuronides (reaction 5). Thus a few drugs and a number of aromatic amines are known to be *N*-hydroxylated and then *O*-glucuronidated. The glucuronidation of N-OH groups competes with *O*-sulfation, but the reactivity of *N*–*O*-glucuronides to undergo heterolytic cleavage and form nitrenium ions does not appear to be well characterized.

Second in importance to *O*-glucuronides are the *N*-glucuronides, which are formed by reactions 6–11 in Figure 6.20, i.e., amides (reactions 6–7), amines of medium basicity (reactions 8–9), and basic amines (reactions 10–11). The *N*-glucuronidation of carboxamides (reaction 6) is exemplified by carbamazepine (**7**) and phenytoin (**29**). In the latter case, *N*-glucuronidation was found to occur at N(3). The reaction has special significance for sulfonamides (reaction 7) and particularly antibacterial sulfanilamides such as sulfadimethoxine (**30**), because it produces highly water-soluble metabolites that show no risk of crystallizing in the kidneys.

N-Glucuronidation of aromatic amines (reaction 8) has been observed in a few cases only (e.g., conjugation of the carbazole nitrogen in carvedilol (**28**)). Similarly, there are a number of observations that pyridine-type nitrogens and primary and secondary basic amines can be *N*-glucuronidated (reactions 9 and 10, respectively). As far as human drug metabolism is concerned, another reaction of significance is the *N*-glucuronidation of lipophilic, basic tertiary amines that contain one or two methyl groups (reaction 11) (54). More and more drugs of this type—and many do exist (e.g., antihistamines and neuroleptics)—are found to undergo this reaction to a marked extent in humans, e.g. cyproheptadine (**31**, Fig. 6.22).

Third in importance are the *S*-glucuronides formed from aliphatic and aromatic thiols (reaction 12) and from dithiocarboxylic acids (reaction 13) such as diethyldithiocarbamic acid, a metabolite of disulfiram. As for *C*-glucuronidation (reaction 14), this reaction has been seen in humans for 1,3-dicarbonyl drugs such as phenylbutazone and sulfinpyrazone (**32**).

3.4.3 GLUCOSIDATION REACTION. A few drugs have been observed to be conjugated

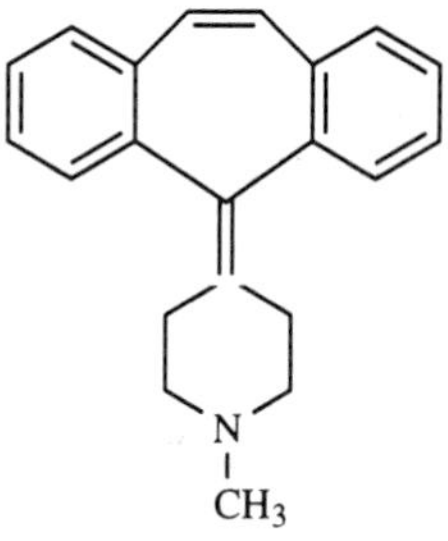

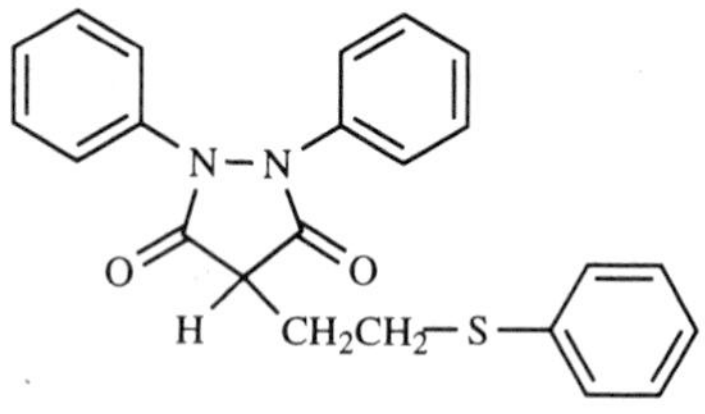

Fig. 6.22 Cyproheptadine (**31**) and sulfinpyrazone (**32**).

to glucose in mammals (55). This is usually a minor pathway in some cases for which glucuronidation is possible. An interesting medicinal example is that of some barbiturates, such as phenobarbital, which yield the *N*-glucosides.

3.5 Acetylation and Acylation

All reactions discussed in this section involve the transfer of an acyl moiety to an acceptor group. In most cases, an acetyl is the acyl moiety being transferred, while the acceptor group may be an amino or hydroxyl function.

3.5.1 ACETYLATION REACTIONS. The major enzyme system catalyzing reactions of acetylation is arylamine *N*-acetyltransferase (arylamine acetylase; EC 2.3.1.5; NAT). Two enzymes have been characterized (NAT1 and NAT2), the latter as two closely related isoforms (NAT2A and

NAT2B) whose levels are considerably reduced in the liver of slow acetylators (56, 57). The cofactor of *N*-acetyltransferase is acetylcoenzyme A (CoA–S–Ac), where the acetyl moiety is bound by a thioester linkage (Fig. 6.23).

Two other activities, aromatic-hydroxylamine *O*-acetyltransferase (EC 2.3.1.56) and *N*-hydroxyarylamine *O*-acetyltransferase (EC 2.3.1.118), are also involved in the acetylation of aromatic amines and hydroxylamines (see below). Other acetyltransferases exist, e.g., diamine *N*-acetyltransferase (putrescine acetyltransferase; EC 2.3.1.57) and aralkylamine *N*-acetyltransferase (serotonin acetyltransferase; EC 2.3.1.87), but their involvement in xenobiotic metabolism does not appear to be documented.

The substrates of acetylation as schematized in Figure 6.24 are mainly amines of medium basicity. Very few basic amines (primary or secondary) of medicinal interest have been reported to form *N*-acetylated metabolites (reaction 1) and when so the yields were low. In contrast, a large variety of primary aromatic amines are *N*-acetylated (reaction 2). Thus several drugs such as sulfonamides and *para*-aminosalicylic acid (PAS) (**35**) are acetylated to large extents as well as various carcinogenic amines such as benzidine (Fig. 6.25).

Arylhydroxylamines can also be acetylated, but the reaction is one of *O*-acetylation (reaction 3-A). This is the reaction formally catalyzed by EC 2.3.1.118 with acetyl-CoA acting as the acetyl donor; the *N*-hydroxy metabolites of a number of arylamines are known substrates. The same conjugates can be formed by intramolecular *N,O*-acetyl transfer, when an arylhydroxamic acid (an *N*-aryl-*N*-hydroxyacetamide) is substrate of, e.g., EC 2.3.1.56 (reaction 3-B). In addition, such an arylhydroxamic acid can transfer its acetyl moiety to an acetyltransferase, which can then acetylate an arylamine or an arylhydroxylamine (intermolecular *N,N*- or *N,O*-acetyl transfer). Because *N*-acetyltransferase (EC 2.3.1.5) can catalyze these various reactions, there is some doubt as to the individuality of EC 2.3.1.56 and EC 2.3.1.118 in mammals (58).

Besides amines, other nitrogen-containing functionalities undergo *N*-acetylation; hydrazines and hydrazides are particularly good substrates (reaction 4). Medicinal examples include isoniazid (**35**) and hydralazine (**36**).

3.5.2 OTHER ACYLATION REACTIONS. A limited number of studies have shown *N*-formylation to be a significant route of conjugation for some arylalkylamines and arylamines and particularly polycyclic aromatic amines. There is evidence to indicate that the reaction is catalyzed by arylformamidase (EC 3.5.1.9) in the presence of *N*-formyl-L-kynurenine.

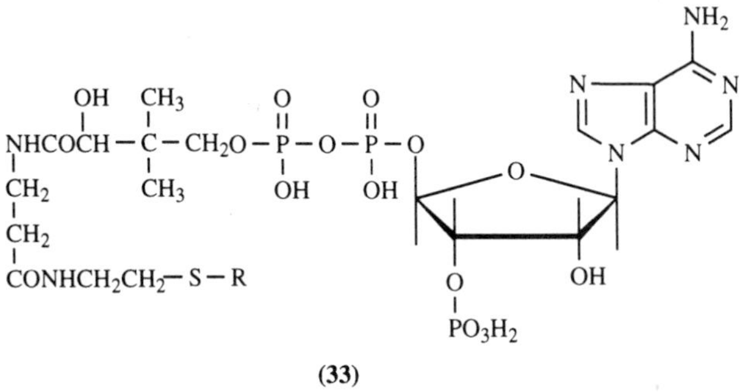

$$\underset{\text{(33)}}{\text{NHCOCH}\overset{\displaystyle\underset{|}{\text{OH}}}{\underset{|}{\text{CH}_2}}\overset{\displaystyle\underset{|}{\text{CH}_3}}{\underset{|}{\text{C}}}\text{CH}_2\text{O}-\overset{\displaystyle\overset{O}{\|}}{\underset{|}{\text{P}}}-\text{O}-\overset{\displaystyle\overset{O}{\|}}{\underset{|}{\text{P}}}-\text{O}}$$

Fig. 6.23 Acetylcoenzyme A (**33**); R = acetyl.

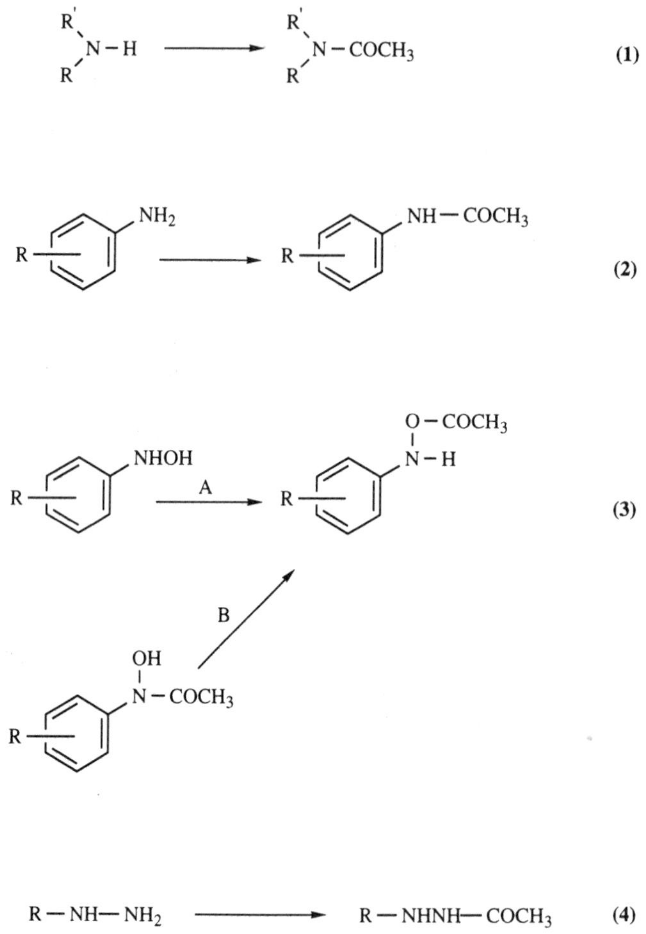
R'
N-H
R'
R'
N-COCH3
R'
(1)
NH2
R
R
NH-COCH3
(2)
NHOH
R
A
R
O-COCH3
N-H
(3)
B
OH
N-COCH3
R
R-NH-NH2
R-NHNH-COCH3
(4)

Fig. 6.24 Major reactions of acetylation involving aliphatic amines, aromatic amines, arylhydroxylamines, hydrazines, and hydrazides.

A different type of reaction is represented by the conjugation of xenobiotic alcohols with fatty acids, yielding highly lipophilic metabolites that accumulate in tissues. Thus ethanol and haloethanols form esters with, e.g., palmitic acid, oleic acid, linoleic acid, and linolenic acid; enzymes catalyzing such reactions are cholesteryl ester synthase (EC 3.1.1.13) and fatty-acyl-ethyl-ester synthase (EC 3.1.1.67) (59). Larger xenobiotics such as tetrahydrocannabinols and codeine are also acylated with fatty acids, possibly by sterol *O*-acyltransferase (EC 2.3.1.26).

3.6 Conjugation with Coenzyme-A and Subsequent Reactions

3.6.1 CONJUGATION WITH COENZYME-A. The reactions described in this section all have in common the fact that they involve xenobiotic carboxylic acids forming an acyl-CoA metabolic intermediate (**33**; R = xenobiotic acyl moiety). The reaction requires ATP and is catalyzed by various acyl-CoA synthetases of overlapping substrate specificity, e.g., acetate-CoA ligase (acetyl-CoA synthetase; EC 6.2.1.1), butyrate-CoA ligase (fatty acid thiokinase

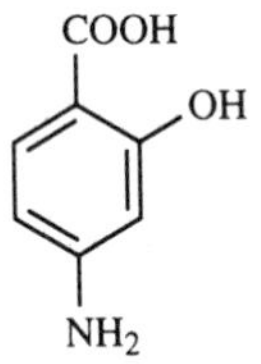

COOH

OH

NH$_2$

(34)

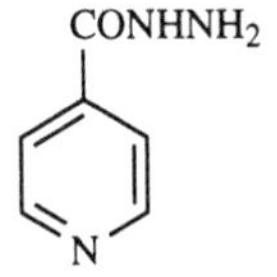

CONHNH$_2$

N

(35)

NHNH$_2$

N

N

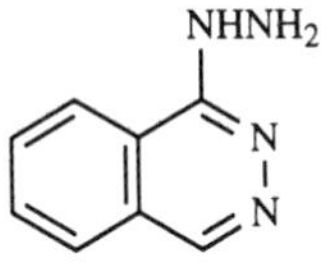

(36)

Fig. 6.25 *para*-Aminosalicylic acid (**34**), isoniazid (**35**), and hydralazine (**36**).

Table 6.4 Metabolic Consequences of the Conjugation of Xenobiotic Acids to Coenzyme-A (CoA–SH)

R–COOH → R–CO–S–CoA → •
- Hydrolysis
- Formation of amino acid conjugates
- Formation of hybrid triglycerides
- Formation of phospholipids
- Formation of cholesteryl esters
- Formation of bile acid esters
- Formation of acyl-carnitines
- Protein acylation
- Unidirectional chiral inversion of arylpropionic acids
- Dehydrogenation and β-oxidation
- 2-Carbon chain elongation

(medium chain); EC 6.2.1.2), long-chain fatty acid–CoA ligase (fatty acid thiokinase (long chain); acyl-CoA synthetase; EC 6.2.1.3), benzoate-CoA ligase (EC 6.2.1.25), and phenylacetate-CoA ligase (EC 6.2.1.30).

The acyl-CoA conjugates thus formed are seldom excreted, but they can be isolated and characterized relatively easily in *in vitro* studies. They may also be hydrolyzed back to the parent acid by thiolester hydrolases (EC 3.1.2). In a number of cases, such conjugates have pharmacodynamic effects and may even represent the active forms of some drugs, e.g., hypolipidemic agents. In the present context, the interest of acyl-CoA conjugates is

their further transformation by a considerable variety of pathways (Table 6.4) (60). The most significant routes are discussed below.

3.6.2 FORMATION OF AMINO ACID CONJUGATES. Amino acid conjugation is a major route for a significant number of xenobiotic acids and involves the formation of an amide bond between the xenobiotic acyl-CoA and the amino acid. Glycine is the amino acid most frequently used for conjugation (reaction 1 in Fig. 6.26), while a few glutamine conjugates have been characterized in humans (reaction 2). The enzymes catalyzing these transfer reactions are various *N*-acyltransferases, e.g., glycine *N*-acyltransferase (EC 2.3.1.13), glutamine *N*-phenylacetyltransferase (EC 2.3.1.14), glutamine *N*-acyltransferase (EC 2.3.1.68), and glycine *N*-benzoyltransferase (EC 2.3.1.71). In addition, other amino acids can be used for conjugation in various animal species, e.g., alanine and taurine, as well as some dipeptides (38).

The xenobiotic acids undergoing amino acid conjugation are mainly substituted benzoic acids. In humans, e.g., hippuric acid and salicyluric acid are the major

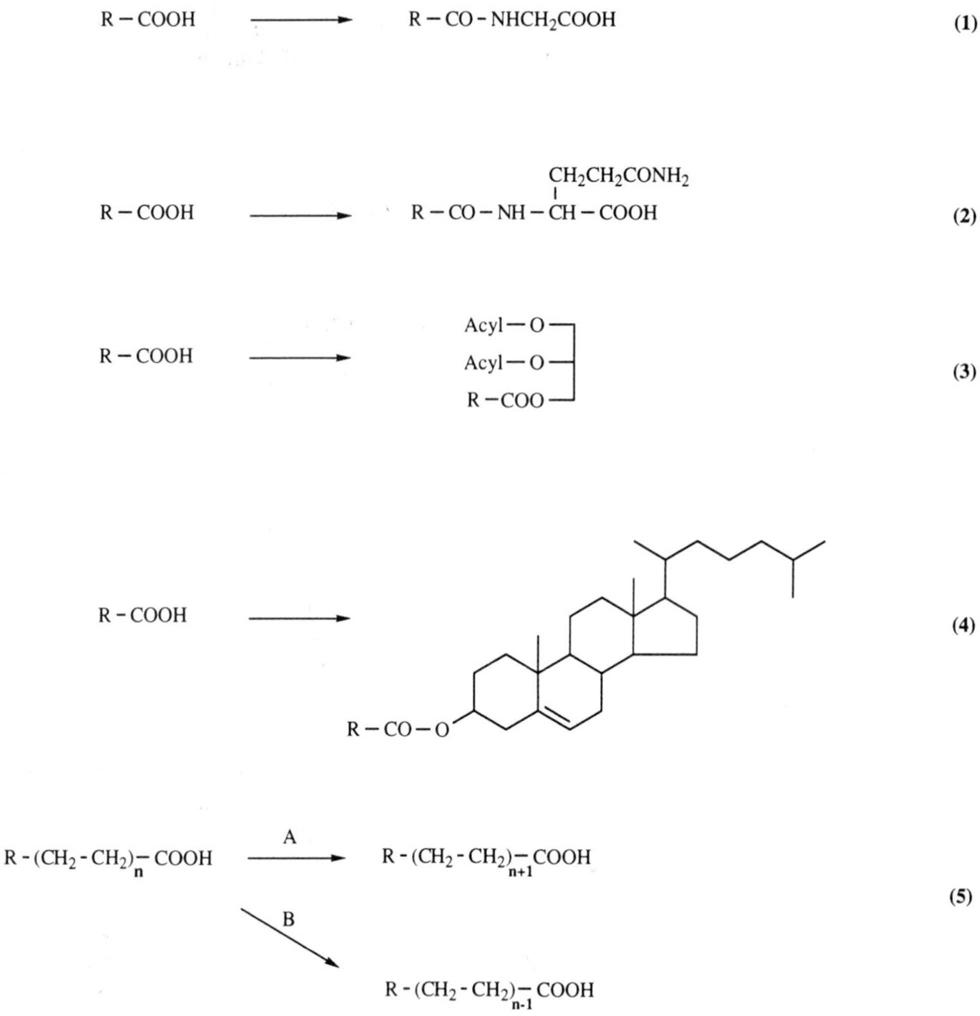

$$R-COOH \longrightarrow R-CO-NHCH_2COOH \tag{1}$$

$$R-COOH \longrightarrow R-CO-NH-\underset{\underset{CH_2CH_2CONH_2}{|}}{CH}-COOH \tag{2}$$

$$R-COOH \longrightarrow \left. \begin{array}{l} Acyl-O- \\ Acyl-O- \\ R-COO- \end{array} \right] \tag{3}$$

$$R-COOH \longrightarrow R-CO-O-[\text{cholesteryl}] \tag{4}$$

$$R-(CH_2-CH_2)_n-COOH \xrightarrow{A} R-(CH_2-CH_2)_{n+1}-COOH$$
$$\xrightarrow{B} R-(CH_2-CH_2)_{n-1}-COOH \tag{5}$$

Fig. 6.26 Metabolic reactions involving acyl-CoA intermediates of xenobiotic acids, namely conjugations and 2-carbon chain lengthening or shortening. Other products of β-oxidation are shown in Figure 6.30.

metabolites of benzoic acid and salicylic acid, respectively (Fig. 6.27). Similarly, *m*-trifluoromethylbenzoic acid (**16**), a major metabolite of fenfluramine (**13**), is excreted as the glycine conjugate. Phenylacetic acid derivatives can yield glycine and glutamine conjugates. Some aliphatic acids give glycine or taurine conjugates.

3.6.3 FORMATION OF HYBRID LIPIDS AND STEROL ESTERS. The incorporation of xeno-biotic acids into lipids is of rather recent characterization and forms highly lipophilic metabolites that may burden the body as long-retained residues. In the majority of cases, triacylglycerol analogs (reaction 3 in Fig. 6.26) or cholesterol esters (reaction 4) are formed. The enzymes catalyzing such reactions are *O*-acyltransferases, including diacylglycerol *O*-acyltransferase (EC 2.3.1.20), 2-acylglycerol *O*-acyltransferase (EC 2.3.1.22), and sterol *O*-acyltransferase

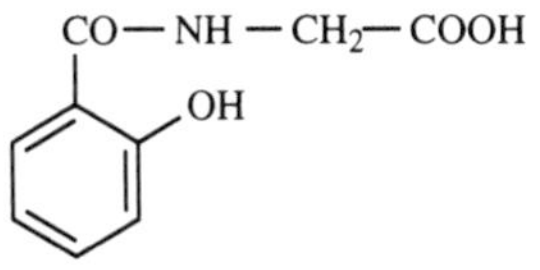

CO — NH — CH$_2$— COOH

OH

(37)

Fig. 6.27 Salicyluric acid (**37**).

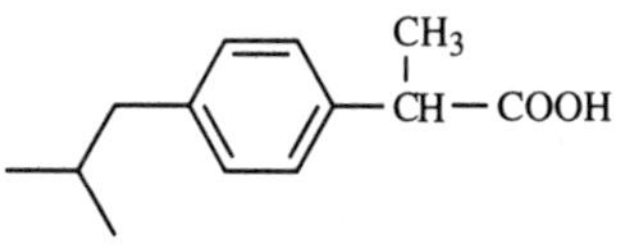

CH$_3$

CH — COOH

(38)

Fig. 6.28 Ibuprofen (**38**).

(cholesterol acyltransferase; sterol-ester synthase; EC 2.3.1.26; ACAT). Some phospholipid analogs as well as some esters to the 3-hydroxy group of biliary acids have also been characterized (61, 62).

The number of drugs and other xenobiotics that are currently known to form glyceryl or cholesteryl esters is comparatively limited but should increase due to increased awareness of researchers. One telling example is that of ibuprofen, a much used antiinflammatory drug whose (*R*) enantiomer forms hybrid triglycerides detectable in rat liver and adipose tissue (Fig. 6.28).

3.6.4 CHIRAL INVERSION OF ARYLPROPIONIC ACIDS. Ibuprofen (**38**) and other arylpropionic acids (i.e., profens) are chiral drugs existing as the (+)-(*S*) eutomer and the (−)-(*R*) distomer. These compounds undergo an intriguing metabolic reaction such that the (*R*) enantiomer is converted to the (*S*) enantiomer, while the reverse reaction does not occur or only negligibly.

This unidirectional chiral inversion is thus a reaction of bioactivation, and its mechanism is now reasonably well understood (Fig. 6.29) (63). The initial step in the reaction is the substrate stereoselective formation of an acyl-CoA conjugate with the (*R*) form but not with the (*S*) form. This conjugate then undergoes a reaction of epimerization possibly catalyzed by methylmalonyl-CoA epimerase (EC 5.1.99.1), resulting in a mixture of the (*R*)-profenoyl- and (*S*)-profenoyl-CoA conjugates. The latter can then be hydrolyzed (Fig. 6.29) or undergo other reactions such as hybrid triglyceride formation (see Section 3.6.3).

3.6.5 β-OXIDATION AND 2-CARBON CHAIN ELONGATION. In some cases, acyl-CoA conjugates formed from xenobiotic acids can also enter the physiological pathways of fatty acids catabolism or anabolism. A few examples are known of xenobiotic alkanoic and arylalkanoic acids undergoing two-carbon chain elongation, or two-, four- or

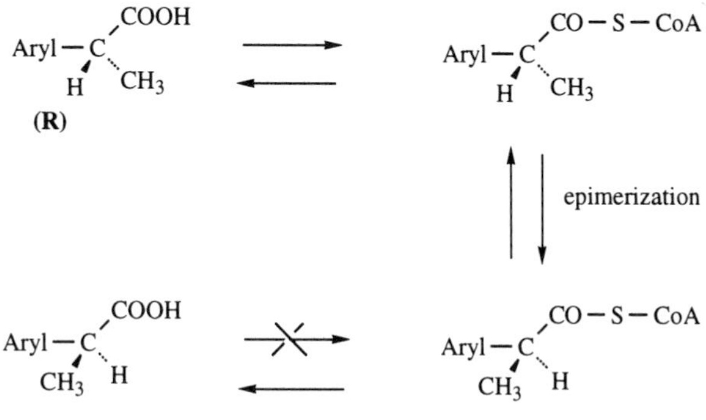

Aryl — C
COOH
H CH$_3$
(**R**)

Aryl — C
CO — S — CoA
H CH$_3$

epimerization

Aryl — C
COOH
CH$_3$ H
(**S**)

Aryl — C
CO — S — CoA
CH$_3$ H

Fig. 6.29 Mechanism of unidirectional chiral inversion of profens.

even six-carbon chain shortening (reactions 5-A and 5-B in Fig. 6.26). In addition, intermediate metabolites of β-oxidation may also be seen, as illustrated by valproic acid (27). Approximately 50 metabolites of

this drug have been characterized; they are formed by β-oxidation, glucuronidation, and/or cytochrome P450–catalyzed dehydrogenation or oxygenation. Figure 6.30 shows the β-oxidation of valproic acid seen

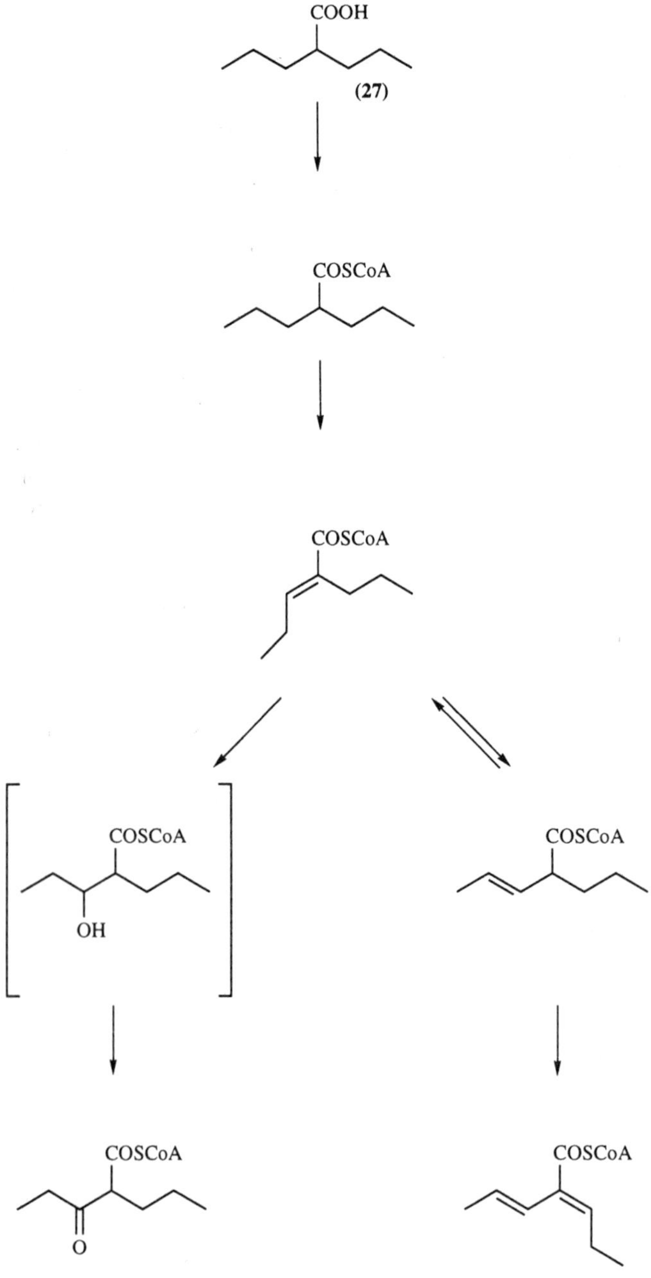

Fig. 6.30 Mitochondrial β-oxidation of valproic acid.

in mitochondrial preparations (64, 65). The resulting metabolites have also been found in unconjugated form in the urine of humans or animals dosed with the drug.

3.7 Conjugation and Redox Reactions of Glutathione

3.7.1 INTRODUCTION. Glutathione (GSH) (39) is a thiol-containing tripeptide of capital significance in the detoxication and toxication of drugs and other xenobiotics (Fig. 6.31) (66). In the body, it exists in a redox equilibrium between the reduced form (GSH) and an oxidized form (GS–SG). The metabolism of glutathione (i.e., its synthesis, redox equilibrium and degradation) is quite complex and involves a number of enzymes (67).

Glutathione reacts in a variety of manners. First, the nucleophilic properties of the thiol (or rather thiolate) group make it an effective conjugating agent, as emphasized in this section. Second, and depending on its redox state, glutathione can act as a reducing or oxidizing agent (e.g., reducing quinones, organic nitrates, peroxides, and free radicals or oxidizing superoxide). Another dichotomy exists in the reactions of glutathione, because these can be enzymatic (e.g., conjugations catalyzed by

glutathione S-transferases and peroxide reductions catalyzed by glutathione peroxidase) or nonenzymatic (e.g., some conjugations and various redox reactions).

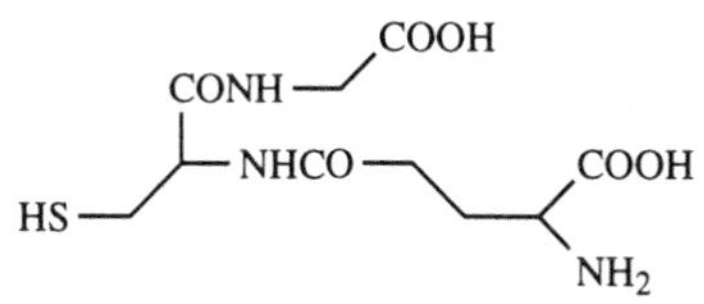

The glutathione S-transferases (EC 2.5.1.18; GSTs) are multifunctional proteins coded by a multigene family and act as enzymes and binding proteins. These enzymes are mainly localized in the cytosol as homodimers and heterodimers; there are four classes of these enzymes in mammals. The human enzymes comprise the following dimers: A1-1, A1-2, A2-2, and A3-3 (α class); M1a-1a, M1a-1b, M1b-1b, M1a-2, M2-2, and M3-3 (μ class); P1-1 (π-class); T1-1 (θ class); and a microsomal enzyme (MIC) (68). The GST A1-2, A2-2, and P1-1 display selenium-independent glutathione peroxidase activity, a property that also characterizes the selenium-containing enzyme glutathione peroxidase (EC 1.11.1.9). The GST A1-1 and A1-2 are also known as ligandin when they act as binding or carrier proteins, a property also displayed by M1a-1a and M1b-1b. In the latter function, these enzymes bind and transport a number of active endogenous compounds (e.g., bilirubin, cholic acid, steroid and thyroid hormones, and hematin) as well as some exogenous dyes and carcinogens.

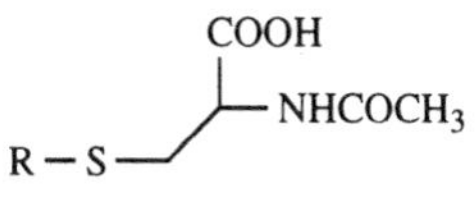

The nucleophilic character of glutathione depends on its thiol group ($pKa = 9.0$) in its neutral form and even more on the thiolate form. In fact, an essential component of the catalytic mechanism of glutathione transferase is the marked increase in acidity ($pKa = 6.6$) experienced by the thiol group on binding of glutathione to the active site of the enzyme (69). As a result, GSTs transfer glutathione to a large variety of electrophilic groups, depending on the nature of the substrate, the reactions can be categorized as nucleophilic substitutions or nucleophilic additions. And with compounds of sufficient reactivity, these reactions can also occur nonenzymatically (7, 70).

Once formed, glutathione conjugates

Fig. 6.31 Glutathione (39) and N-acetylcysteine conjugates (40).

(R-SG) are seldom excreted as such (they are best characterized *in vitro* or in the bile of laboratory animals), but usually undergo further biotransformation before urinary or fecal excretion. Cleavage of the glutamyl moiety by glutamyl transpeptidase (EC 2.3.2.2) and of the cysteinyl moiety by cysteinylglycine dipeptidase (EC 3.4.13.6) or aminopeptidase M (EC 3.4.11.2) leaves a cysteine conjugate (R-S-Cys), which is further *N*-acetylated by cysteine-*S*-conjugate *N*-acetyltransferase (EC 2.3.1.80) to yield an *N*-acetylcysteine conjugate (**40**; R-S-CysAc). The latter type of conjugates are known as mercapturic acids, a name that clearly indicates that they were first characterized in urine. This, however, does not imply that the degradation of unexcreted glutathione conjugates must stop at this stage, as cysteine conjugates can be substrates of cysteine-*S*-conjugate β-lyase (EC 4.4.1.13) and yield thiols (R-SH). These, in turn, can rearrange as discussed below or be *S*-methylated and then *S*-oxygenated to yield thiomethyl conjugates (R-S-Me), sulfoxides (R-SO-Me), and sulfones (R-SO$_2$-Me).

3.7.2 GLUTATHIONE REACTIONS. The major reactions of glutathione, both conjugations and redox reactions, are summarized in Figure 6.32. Reactions 1 and 2 are nucleophilic additions and substitutions to sp^3-carbons, respectively, while reactions 3 to 8 are nucleophilic substitutions or additions at sp^2-carbons, sometimes accompanied by a redox reaction. Reactions at nitrogen or sulfur atoms are shown in reactions 9 to 11. The first reaction in Figure 6.32 is nucleophilic addition to epoxides (reaction 1-A) to yield a nonaromatic conjugate. This is followed by several metabolic steps (reaction 1-B) leading to an aromatic mercapturic acid. This is a frequent reaction of metabolically produced arene oxides (section 2.3.2), as documented for naphthalene and numerous drugs and xenobiotics that contain a phenyl

moiety. Note that the same reaction can also occur readily for epoxides of olefins (not shown in Fig. 6.32).

An important pathway of substitution at sp^3-carbons is that represented by reaction 2-A, followed by the production of mercapturic acids (reactions 2-B). Various electron-withdrawing leaving groups (X in reaction 2) may be involved that are either of xenobiotic (e.g., halogens) or metabolic origin (e.g., a sulfate group). Such a reaction occurs for example at the –CHCl$_2$ group of chloramphenicol and at the NCH$_2$CH$_2$Cl group of anticancer alkylating agents.

The reactions at sp^2-carbons are quite varied and complex. Addition at activated olefinic groups (e.g., β,γ-unsaturated carbonyls) is shown in reaction 3. A typical substrate is acrolein (CH$_2$=CH–CHO). Quinones (*ortho*- and *para*-) and quinone imines react with glutathione by two distinct and competitive routes, namely nucleophilic addition to form a conjugate (reaction 4-A) and reduction to the hydroquinone or aminophenol (reaction 4-B) (71). A typical example is provided by the toxic quinone imine metabolite (**12**) of paracetamol (**11**). Because, in most cases, quinones and quinone imines are the result of the biooxidation of hydroquinones and aminophenols, respectively, their reduction by GSH can be seen as a futile cycle that consumes reduced glutathione. The conjugates produced by reaction 4-A may undergo reoxidation to *S*-glutathionylquinones or *S*-glutathionylquinone imines of considerable reactivity. These quinone or quinone imine thioethers are known to undergo further GSH conjugation and reoxidation (72).

Haloalkenes are a special group of substrates of GS-transferases, since they may react with GSH either by substitution (reaction 5-A) or by addition (reaction 5-B). Formation of mercapturic acids occurs as for other glutathione conjugates, but in this case, S–C cleavage of the *S*-cysteinyl

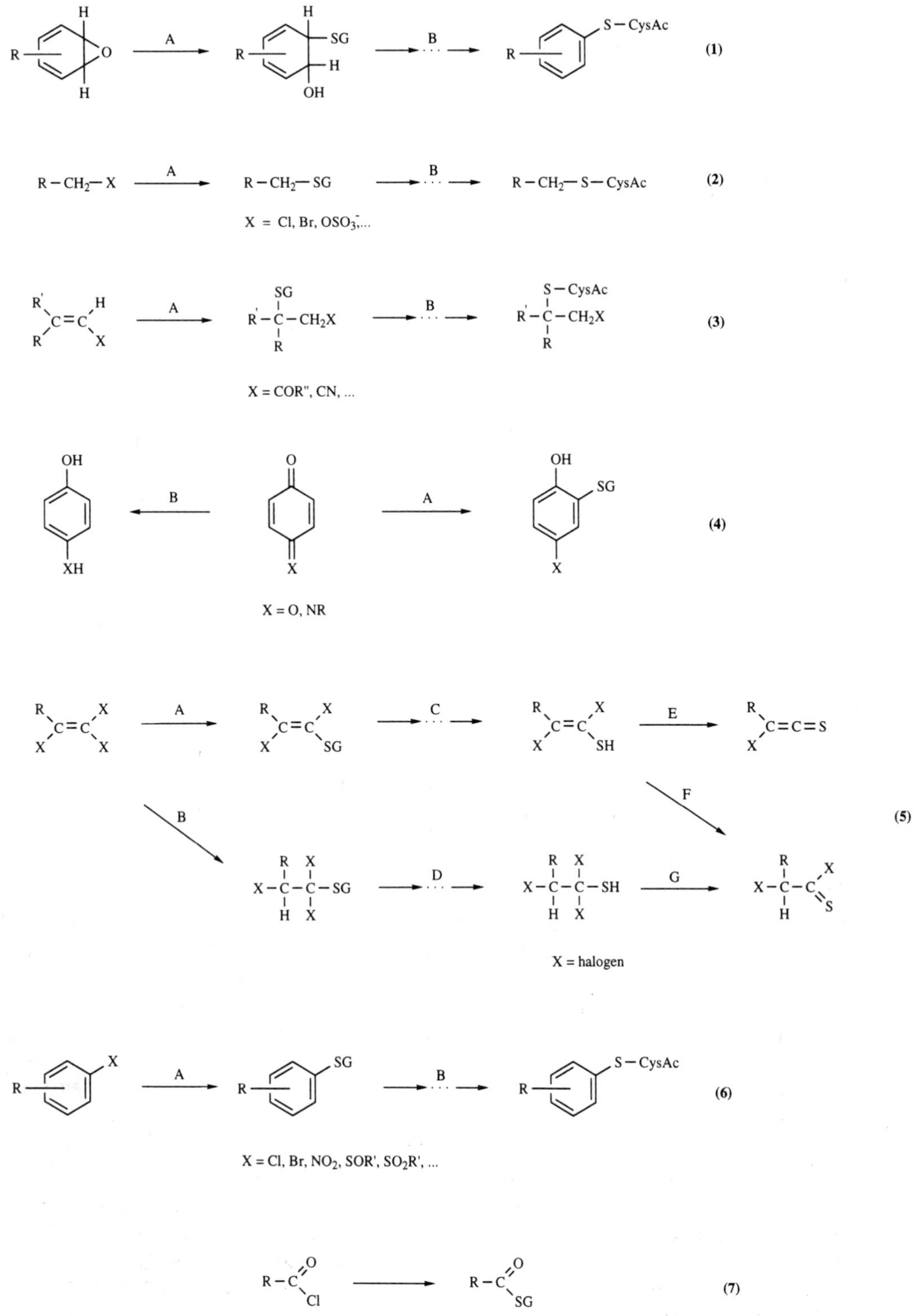

Fig. 6.32 Major reactions of conjugation of glutathione, sometimes accompanied by a redox reaction.

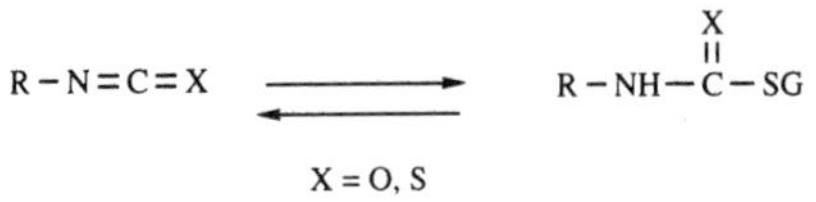

$$R-N=C=X \quad \longrightarrow \quad R-NH-\overset{\overset{\displaystyle X}{\|}}{C}-SG \qquad (8)$$

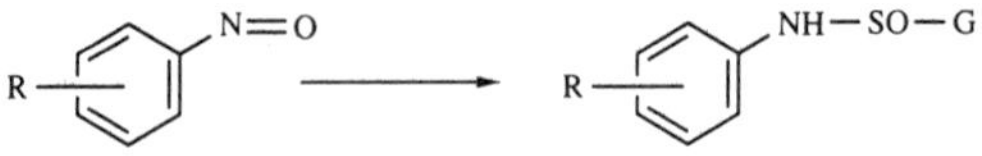

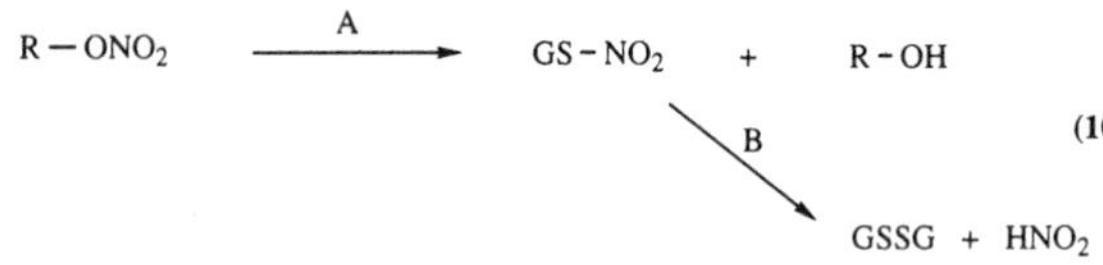

$$X = O, S$$

$$R \text{—} N=O \quad \longrightarrow \quad R \text{—} NH-SO-G \qquad (9)$$

$$R-ONO_2 \quad \overset{A}{\longrightarrow} \quad GS-NO_2 \quad + \quad R-OH \qquad (10)$$

$$\overset{B}{\searrow}$$

$$GSSG + HNO_2$$

$$R-SH \quad \rightleftharpoons \quad R-S-S-G \qquad (11)$$

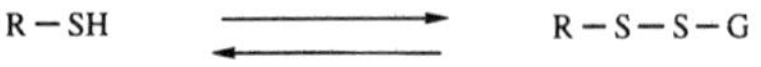

Fig. 6.32 (*Continued*)

conjugates by the renal β-lyase (reactions 5-C and 5-D) yields thiols of significant toxicity, as they rearrange by hydrohalide expulsion to form highly reactive thioketenes (reaction 5-E) and/or thioacyl halides (reactions 5-F and 5-G) (73).

With good leaving groups, nucleophilic aromatic substitution reactions also occur at aromatic rings that contain additional electron-withdrawing substituents and/or heteroatoms (reaction 6-A). As for the detoxication of acyl halides with glutathione (reaction 7), a good example is provided by phosgene (O=CCl$_2$), an extremely toxic metabolite of chloroform, which is inactivated to the diglutathionyl conjugate O=C(SG)$_2$.

The addition of glutathione to isocyanates and isothiocyanates has received some attention in recent years due in particular to its reversible character (reaction 8) (74). Substrates of the reaction are xenobiotics such as the infamous toxin methyl isocyanate, whose glutathione

conjugate behaves as a transport form able to carbamoylate various macromolecules, enzymes, and membranes structures. The reaction is also of interest from a medicinal viewpoint, because anticancer agents such as methylformamide appear to work by undergoing activation to isocyanates and then to the glutathione conjugate.

The reaction of N-oxygenated drugs and metabolites with glutathione also may have toxicological and medicinal implications. Thus the addition of GSH to nitrosoarenes forms sulfinamides (reaction 9) that have been postulated to contribute to the idiosyncratic toxicity of a few drugs such as sulfonamides (75). As for organic nitrate esters such as nitroglycerine and isosorbide dinitrate, the mechanism of their vasodilating action is now believed to result from their reduction to nitric oxide (NO). Thiols, and particularly glutathione, play an important role in this activation. In the first step, a thionitrate is formed (reaction 10-A) whose N-reduction may occur by more than one route. For example, a GSH-dependent reduction may yield nitrite (reaction 10-B), which undergoes further reduction to NO; S-nitrosoglutathione (GS–NO) has also been postulated as an intermediate (76).

The formation of mixed disulfides between GSH and a xenobiotic thiol (reaction 11) has been observed in a few cases, e.g., with captopril. Finally, glutathione and other endogenous thiols (including albumin) are able to inactivate free radicals (e.g., $R^\bullet$, $HO^\bullet$, $HOO^\bullet$, $ROO^\bullet$) and have thus a critical role to play in cellular protection (77). The reactions involved are highly complex and not completely understood; the simplest ones are

$$GSH + X^\bullet \rightarrow GS^\bullet + XH$$
$$GS^\bullet + GS^\bullet \rightarrow GSSG$$
$$GS^\bullet + O_2 \rightarrow GS-OO^\bullet$$
$$GS-OO^\bullet + GSH \rightarrow GS-OOH + GS^\bullet$$

3.8 Other Conjugation Reactions

Sections 3.2 to 3.7 present the most common and important routes of xenobiotic conjugation but, by far, not the only ones. A number of other routes have been reported, the importance of which is at present restricted to a few exogenous substrates or that have received only limited attention (78, 79). In the present section, two pathways of pharmacodynamic significance will be discussed: phosphorylation and carbonyl conjugation (Fig. 6.33). In both cases, the xenobiotic substrates belong to narrowly defined chemical classes.

Reactions of phosphorylation are of great significance in the processing of endogenous compounds and macromolecules. It is, therefore, astonishing that relatively few xenobiotics are substrates of phosphotransferases (e.g., EC 2.7.1) to form phosphate esters (reaction 1 in Fig. 6.33). The phosphorylation of phenol is a curiosity observed by some workers. In contrast, a number of antiviral nucleoside analogs are known to yield the mono-, di- and triphosphates *in vitro* and *in vivo*, e.g., zidovudine (AZT) (**41**), 2',3'-dideoxycytidine, and 9-(1,3-dihydroxy-2-propoxymethyl)-guanine (Fig. 6.34). These conjugates are active forms of the drugs, which are particularly incorporated in the DNA of virus-infected cells (80).

The second pathway of conjugation is the reaction of hydrazines with endogenous carbonyls (reaction 2) (81). This reaction occurs nonenzymatically and involves a variety of carbonyl compounds, namely aldehydes (mainly acetaldehyde) and ketones (e.g., acetone, pyruvic acid $CH_3-CO-COOH$, and α-ketoglutaric acid $HOOC-CH_2CH_2-CO-COOH$). The products thus formed are hydrazones, which may be excreted as such or undergo further transformation. Isoniazid (**35**) and

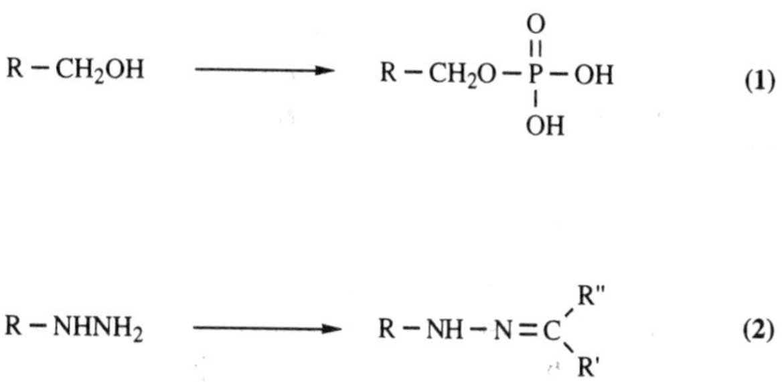

$$R-CH_2OH \longrightarrow R-CH_2O-\overset{\overset{\displaystyle O}{\|}}{\underset{\underset{\displaystyle OH}{|}}{P}}-OH \qquad (1)$$

$$R-NHNH_2 \longrightarrow R-NH-N=C\overset{\displaystyle R''}{\underset{\displaystyle R'}{}} \qquad (2)$$

Fig. 6.33 Additional reactions of conjugation discussed in section 3.8, namely formation of phosphate esters and hydrazones.

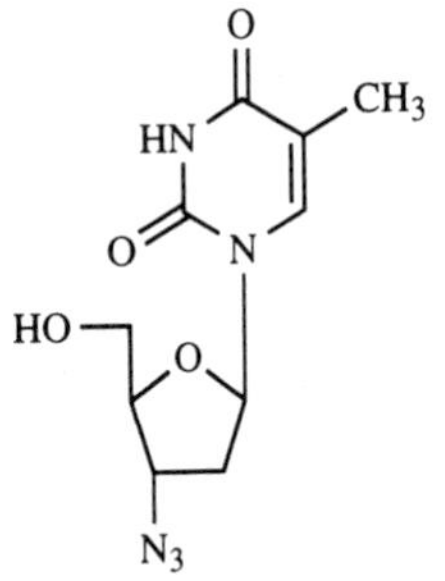

(41)

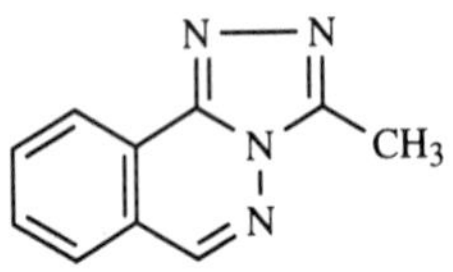

(42)

Fig. 6.34 Zidovudine (**41**) and methyltriazolophthalazine (**45**).

hydralazine (**36**) are two drugs that form hydrazones in the body. For example, the reaction of hydralazine with acetaldehyde or acetone is a reversible one, meaning that the hydrazones are hydrolyzed under biological conditions of pH and temperature. In addition, the hydrazone of hydralazine with acetaldehyde or pyruvic acid undergoes an irreversible reaction of cyclization to another metabolite, methyltriazolophthalazine (**42**).

4 THE SIGNIFICANCE OF DRUG METABOLISM IN MEDICINAL CHEMISTRY

In drug research and development, metabolism is of pivotal importance because of the interconnectedness between pharmacokinetic and pharmacodynamic processes. Early in the testing of a promising com-

pound, metabolic studies should be initiated to identify the metabolites, the pathways by which they are formed and the enzymes involved, and to postulate metabolic intermediates. Based on these findings, the metabolites can be synthesized and tested for their own pharmacological and toxicological effects. In preclinical and early clinical studies, many pharmacokinetic data must be obtained and relevant criteria must be satisfied before a drug candidate can enter large-scale clinical trials (82). As a result of these demands, the metabolic and pharmacokinetic registration files of a new drug may well be larger than the pharmacological and toxicological registration files.

4.1 Structure–Metabolism Relationships

4.1.1 METABOLIC SCHEMES. The approach followed in this chapter is an analytical one, meaning that the focus is on metabolic reactions, the target groups they affect, and the enzymes by which they are catalyzed. This fragmented information provides the foundations of drug metabolism but fails to give the synthetic view needed for a broad and meaningful understanding. Two steps are required to approach such an end: (*1*) the elaboration of metabolic schemes in which the competitive and sequential reactions undergone by a given drug are ordered and (*2*) the assessment of the various biological factors (see Table 6.2) that influence such schemes quantitatively and qualitatively. As an example of a metabolic scheme, Figure 6.35 presents the biotransformation of propranolol in humans (83). In this comprehensive study, more than 90% of the dose was accounted for and existed mainly in products of oxidation and conjugation. The missing 10% of the dose may represent other minor and presumably quite numerous metabolites, e.g., those resulting from ring hydroxylation at other positions or from the pro-

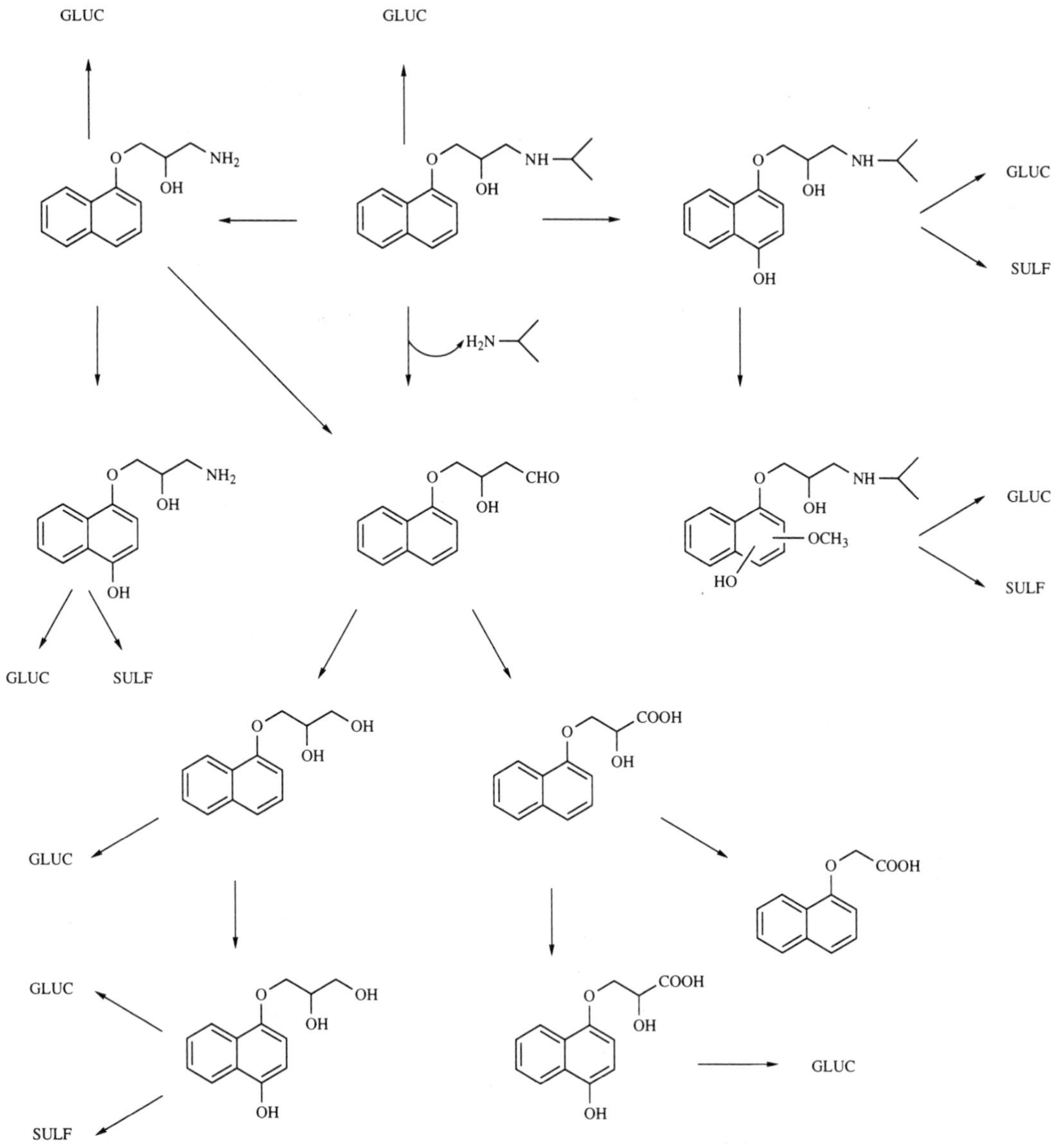

Fig. 6.35 The metabolism of propranolol in humans, accounting for more than 90% of the dose. GLUC, glucuronide(s); SULF, sulfate(s) (83).

gressive breakdown of glutathione conjugates.

While medicinal chemists are not usually expected to display a deep knowledge of the biological factors that influence drug metabolism, they will find it quite useful to understand structure–metabolism relationships sufficiently to be able to predict

reasonable metabolic schemes. A qualitative prediction of the biotransformation of a novel xenobiotic must be based on (1) an identification of all target groups and sites of metabolic attack, (2) a listing of all possible metabolic reactions able to affect these groups and sites, and (3) an estimate of the product regioselectivity of these reactions (see section 1.3). This is the information summarized in Sections 2 and 3.

Given this information, there has been a marked interest in expert systems that would be able to predict metabolic schemes for any molecular structure. A few such systems exist that make correct qualitative predictions for a number of metabolites, but they also indicate false positives and false negatives. The problems associated with the development of such expert systems lie perhaps not so much in logic and software as in the enormous amount of relevant information that must be compiled to create the necessary databases. Updating and validation are also critical aspects. The author is not aware of any independent, neutral, and comprehensive evaluation of the existing systems.

4.1.2 THE INFLUENCE OF CONFIGURATIONAL FACTORS. In addition to the three elements of prediction noted above, some molecular factors (such as configuration, electronic structure, and lipophilicity) influence the metabolism of drugs. As discussed, their significance is obvious only when comparing several substrates of a given enzyme.

The influence of stereochemical factors in xenobiotic metabolism is a well-known and abundantly documented phenomenon (84–86). Thus substrate enantioselective biotransformation is the rule for a great many chiral drugs and ranges from practically complete to moderate, with only a few proven examples of nonselectivity. Product stereoselectivity is also a common phenomenon in drug metabolism. In many prochiral or chiral drugs, the methylene group is frequently a center of prochirality; the enzymatic reaction discriminates between the two enantiotopic or diastereotopic hydrogens. An example of this phenomenon is provided by debrisoquine (**43**), a drug whose major metabolic pathway in humans is 4-hydroxylation (Fig. 6.36). The re-

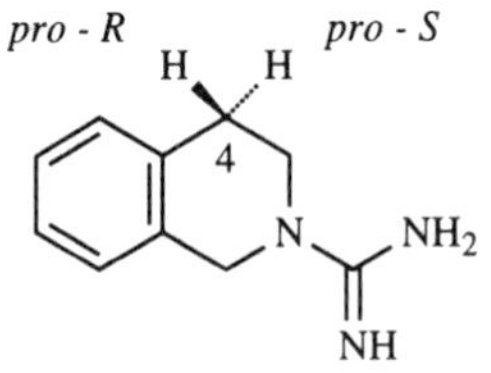

(43)

Fig. 6.36 Debrisoquine (**43**).

action, which has been extensively investigated in connection with its genetic polymorphism, leads to the enantioselective formation of (+)-(S)-4-hydroxydebrisoquine in extensive hydroxylators (enantiomeric excess 96% to 99.5%); loss of enantioselectivity is seen in poor hydroxylators (87).

It is thus clear that substrate and product stereoselectivities are the rules in the metabolism of stereoisomeric and stereotopic drugs. But if the phenomenon is to be expected per se, it remains difficult at present, except perhaps for closely related analogs, to predict which enantiomer will be the preferred substrate of a given metabolic reaction or which enantiomeric metabolite of a prochiral drug will predominate. This situation exists because the stereoselectivities depend as much on molecular factors of the substrate as on enzymatic factors (e.g., the stereoelectronic architecture of the catalytic site in the various isozymes involved). In fact, substrate and product stereoselectivities are determined by the binding mode(s) of the substrate and by the resulting topography of the enzyme–substrate complex. No tool short of molecular modeling can help us in predicting stereoselectivities.

4.1.3 QUANTITATIVE STRUCTURE-METABOLISM RELATIONSHIPS: THE INFLUENCE OF ELECTRONIC FACTORS AND LIPOPHILICITY. Many physicochemical and structural parameters have found applications in quantitative structure–activity relationships, in particular those quantitating electronic properties and lipophilicity. Stereoelectronic properties may influence the binding of substrates to enzymatic active sites in the same manner as they influence the binding of ligands to receptors. Of specific interest in the present context is the influence of electronic factors on the cleavage and formation of covalent bonds characteristic of a biotransformation reaction (i.e., the catalytic step). Correlations between electronic parameters and catalytic parameters obtained from *in vitro* studies (e.g., V_{max} or k_{cat}) allow a rationalization of substrate selectivity and some insight into reaction mechanism. In contrast, correlations between lipophilicity and metabolic parameters are interpreted to mean that binding and/or transport processes influence the reaction. Lipophilicity was shown to account for variations in metabolism in many series of compounds either *in vitro* or *in vivo*. Many *in vivo* metabolic studies have also demonstrated a dependence of biotransformation on lipophilicity, suggesting a predominant role for transport and partitioning processes.

In most cases, however, the extrapolative power of the correlations is doubtful, restricting the value of the correlations to the explored property space and to the chemical series investigated. The contributions of quantitative structure–metabolism relationships to drug design thus appear limited at present but are not devoid of promises. In particular, three-dimensional QSAR (3D-QSAR) methods allow more information to be extracted from metabolic studies of congeners; as such, they represent an important step toward a quantitative prediction of the substrate or inhibitor properties of novel compounds. The technique known as comparative molecular field analysis (CoMFA) is a powerful one that has, e.g., been applied to the MAO-mediated toxication of MPTP analogs (88).

4.2 Metabolism and Drug Design

4.2.1 MODULATION OF DRUG METABOLISM BY STRUCTURAL VARIATIONS. Many examples of the structure–metabolism relationships discussed above involve overall molecular properties such as configuration, conformation, electronic distribution, and lipophilicity. An alternative means of modulating metabolism is by structural modifications of the substrate at its target site, a direct approach whose outcome is often more predictable than that of altering molecular properties of structural changes not involving the reaction center. Globally, structural variations at the reaction center can aim either at decreasing or even suppressing biotransformation, or at promoting it by introducing labile groups. Metabolic switching is a combination of the two goals; the aim is to block metabolism in one part of the molecule and to promote it in another.

Inertness toward biotransformation can often be observed for highly hydrophilic or lipophilic compounds. But high polarity and high lipophilicity tend to be avoided by drug designers because they may result in poor bioavailability and slow excretion, respectively. However, metabolic stabilization can be achieved more conveniently by replacing a labile group with another, less or nonreactive moiety, provided this change is not detrimental to pharmacological activity (89). Classic examples include

- Introducing an *N-t*-butyl group to prevent *N*-dealkylation.
- Inactivating aromatic rings toward oxidation by substituting them with strongly electron-withdrawing groups (e.g., CF_3, SO_2NH_2, SO_3^-).
- Replacing a labile ester linkage with an amide group.
- Protecting the labile moiety by steric shielding.

Metabolic stabilization may offer the following advantages:

- Longer half-lives.
- Decreased possibilities of drug interactions.
- Decreased inter- and intrapatient variability.
- Decreased species differences.
- Decreased number and significance of active metabolites.

Nevertheless, drawbacks cannot be ignored, e.g., too long half-lives and a risk of accumulation. In contrast to metabolic stabilization, metabolic switching is a versatile means of deflecting metabolism away from toxic products to enhance the formation of therapeutically active metabolites and/or to obtain a suitable pharmacokinetic behavior.

Metabolic promotion can be achieved by introducing into a lead compound a functional group of predictable metabolic reactivity, for example, an ester linkage. This concept enjoys considerable success in the design of prodrugs (see below). Another approach rendered possible by metabolic promotion is the design of "soft" drugs (90). The concept of soft drugs—which are defined as "biologically active compounds (drugs) characterized by a predictable *in vivo* metabolism to non-toxic moieties, after they have achieved their therapeutic role" (90)—has led to valuable therapeutic innovations such as β-blockers with ultrashort duration of action. Examples of the latter are ((arylcarbonyl)oxy)propanolamines and esmolol (**44**) (Fig. 6.37).

In both cases, esterase-mediated hydrolysis produces metabolites that are inactive as a result of, respectively, the loss of the side-chain or a high polarity of the para-substituent.

For the sake of fairness, it must also be mentioned that the design of soft drugs is not without limitations. While emphasis is placed on the predictability of their metabolism, this predictability is qualitative more than quantitative due to the many biological factors that influence their biotransformation. A similar limitation also applies to many prodrugs, as discussed below.

4.2.2 PRINCIPLES OF PRODRUG DESIGN. Prodrugs are defined as therapeutic agents that are inactive per se but are predictably transformed into active metabolites (91). As such, prodrugs must be contrasted with soft drugs, which are active per se and yield inactive metabolites. And in a more global perspective, prodrugs and soft drugs appear as the two extremes of a continuum of possibilities, by which both the parent compound and the metabolite(s) contribute by a large or small proportion to the observed therapeutic response.

Prodrug design aims at overcoming a number of barriers to a drug's usefulness (Table 6.5). Based on these and other considerations, the major objectives of prodrug design can be listed as follows:

- Improved formulation (e.g., increased hydrosolubility).
- Improved chemical stability.
- Improved patient acceptance and compliance.

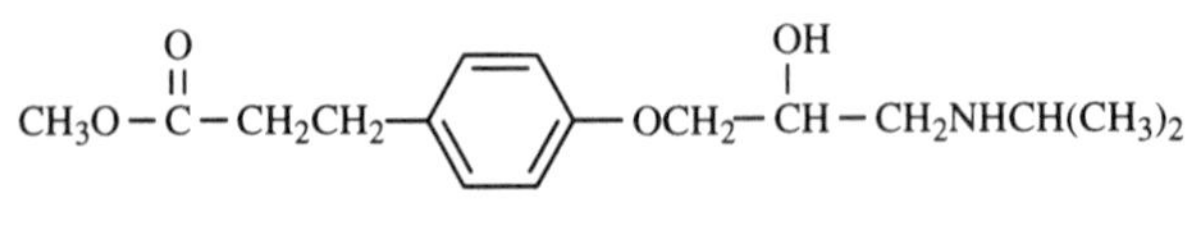

$$CH_3O-\overset{\overset{\displaystyle O}{\|}}{C}-CH_2CH_2-\underset{}{\boxed{}}-OCH_2-\overset{\overset{\displaystyle OH}{|}}{CH}-CH_2NHCH(CH_3)_2$$

(**44**)

Fig. 6.37 Esmolol (**44**).

Table 6.5 Prodrugs: A Concept to Overcome Barriers to Drug's Usefulness[a]

Pharmaceutical barriers
  Insufficient chemical stability
  Poor solubility
  Unacceptable taste or odor
  Irritation or pain

Pharmacokinetic barriers
  Insufficient oral absorption
  Marked presystemic metabolism
  Short duration of action
  Unfavorable distribution in the body

Pharmacodynamic barriers
  Toxicity

[a]Modified from Ref. 92.

- Improved bioavailability.
- Prolonged duration of action.
- Improved organ selectivity.
- Decreased side effects.
- Marketing considerations and "me-too" drugs.

The successes of prodrug design are many, and a large variety of such compounds have proven their therapeutic value. When discussing this multidisciplinary field of medicinal chemistry, several complementary viewpoints can be adopted: a chemical classification, the nature of activation (enzymatic or nonenzymatic), the tissue selectivity, the possible production of toxic metabolites, and the gain in therapeutic benefit (Table 6.6).

In a chemical perspective, it may be convenient to distinguish between carrier-linked prodrugs (i.e., drugs linked to a carrier moiety by a labile bridge) and bioprecursors, which do not contain a carrier group and are activated by the metabolic creation of a functional group (93). A special group of carrier-linked prodrugs are the site-specific chemical delivery systems (90, 94). Macromolecular prodrugs are syn-

Table 6.6 Complementary Viewpoints When Discussing Prodrugs

Chemical classification (overlapping classes)
  Bioprecursors
  Classical carrier-linked prodrugs
  Site-specific chemical delivery systems
  Macromolecular prodrugs
  Drug–antibody conjugates

Mechanisms of activation (may operate simultaneously)
  Enzymatic
    biological variability
    difficult optimization
  Nonenzymatic
    no biological variability
    easier optimization

Tissue–organ selectivity
  Caused by tissue-selective activation of classical prodrugs
  Produced by site-specific chemical delivery systems

Toxic potential
  Of a metabolic intermediate (for bioprecursors)
  Of the carrier moiety or a metabolite thereof

Gain in therapeutic benefit
  Post hoc design (prodrugs of established drugs)
    The gain ranges from modest (for some carrier-linked prodrugs) to marked (for some site-specific chemical delivery systems)
  Ad hoc design (a labile group is an initial specification)
    The gain is usually marked

thetic conjugates of drugs covalently bound (either directly or via a spacer) to proteins, polypeptides, polysaccharides, and other biodegradable polymers (95). A special case is provided by drugs coupled to monoclonal antibodies.

Prodrug activation occurs enzymatically, nonenzymatically, or sequentially (an enzymatic step followed by a nonenzymatic rearrangement). As much as possible, it is desirable to reduce biological variability, hence the particular interest of nonenzymatic reactions of hydrolysis or intramolecular catalysis. The problem of tissue or organ selectivity (targeting) is another important aspect of prodrug design. Many unsuccessful and a few successful attempts have been made to achieve organ-selective activation of prodrugs, and a few examples will be mentioned in the next section. A promising approach appears to be the site-specific chemical delivery systems.

The toxic potential of metabolic intermediates, of the carrier moiety, or of a fragment thereof should never be neglected. For example, some problems may be associated with formaldehyde-releasing prodrugs such as *N*- and *O*-acyloxymethyl derivatives or Mannich bases (see below). Similarly, arylacetylenes assayed as potential bioprecursors of antiinflammatory arylacetic acids proved to be highly toxic due to the formation of intermediate ketenes (see pathway 3 in Fig. 6.4).

4.2.3 EXAMPLES OF PRODRUGS AND CHEMICAL DELIVERY SYSTEMS. Bioprecursors are prodrugs that are activated by oxidation, reduction, or nonredox reactions (e.g., hydrolytic ring opening), without the release of a (nonexistent) carrier group. An example is Δ^1-pyrroline, which is converted to 2-pyrrolidinone and to γ-aminobutyric acid (GABA). Both cyclic precursors are more lipophilic than GABA and have better brain-penetrating properties, a promising feature in the design of bioprecursors of GABA-ergic drugs. Bioprecursors avoid potential toxicity problems caused by the carrier moiety, but here attention must be given to metabolic intermediates (see previous section).

Numerous carrier-linked prodrugs have been prepared from drugs that contain an adequate functional group. Although not comprehensive, a list of usual and less usual carrier groups is given here for three types of functional groups that are frequent sites of derivatization to prodrugs.

Drugs containing an alcoholic or phenolic group (R–OH) can be conveniently modified to the following esters or labile ethers:

- Esters of simple or functionalized aliphatic carboxylic acids, i.e., R–O–CO–R'.
- Esters of carbamic acids: R–O–CO–NR'R''.
- Esters of amino acids (e.g., lysine): R–O–CO–CH(NH$_2$)R'.
- Esters of ring-substituted aromatic acids: R–O–CO–aryl.
- Esters of derivatized phosphoric acids: R–O–PO(OR')(OR'').
- (Acyloxy)methyl or (acyloxy)ethyl ethers: R–O–CH$_2$–O–CO–R' or R–O–CH(CH$_3$)–O–CO–R'.
- (Alkoxycarbonyloxy)methyl or (alkoxycarbonyloxy)ethyl ethers: R–O–CH$_2$–O–CO–O–R' or R–O–CH(CH$_3$)–O–CO–O–R'.
- *O*-Glycosides.

Drugs containing a carboxylic group (R–COOH) can form a variety of esters and amides, and their structure–metabolism relationships are documented in many studies. Prodrugs of carboxylic acids include the following:

- Esters of simple alcohols or phenols: R–CO–O–R'.
- Esters of alcohols containing an amino or amido function: R–CO–O–(CH$_2$)$_n$–NR'R'', R–CO–O–(CH$_2$)$_n$–CO–NR'R'', or R–CO–O–(CH$_2$)$_n$–NH–COR'.
- (Acyloxy)methyl or (acyloxy)ethyl esters of the type R–CO–O–CH$_2$–O–CO–R' or R–CO–O–CH(CH$_3$)–O–CO–R'.
- Hybrid glycerides formed from diacyl-

glycerols: $R-CO-O-CH(CH_2-O-CO-R')_2$.

- Esters of diacylaminopropan-2-ols: $R-CO-O-CH(CH_2-NH-COR')_2$.
- *N,N*-Dialkyl hydroxylamine derivatives: $R-CO-O-NR'R''$.
- Amides of amino acids (e.g., glycine): $R-CO-NH-CH(R')-COOH$.

Another type of prodrugs of carboxylic acids deserves mention, namely 5-substituted (2-oxo-1,3-dioxol-4-yl)methyl esters whose activation avoids biological variability (96). Indeed, these compounds break down chemically under physiological conditions of pH and temperature as shown in Figure 6.38 (reaction 1).

Acetals appear as a versatile group of prodrugs of carbonyl compounds or of metabolites thereof. If, for example, an aldehyde is produced, it will be rapidly dehydrogenated to a carboxylic acid. As shown in Figure 6.38, the first activation step is an oxidation catalyzed by cyto-

chrome P450 (reaction 2-A), followed by breakdown steps to an aldehyde (reactions 2-B and 2-C). The latter can be reduced reversibly to an alcohol and irreversibly to the acid, as demonstrated by the formation of the target valproic acid (**27**) from 2-propylpentanal acetals (97). Acetals also appear as prodrugs of ketones worthy of further investigation.

Drugs containing an NH group ($RR'N-H$, i.e., amides, imides, and amines) are amenable to modification to a variety of prodrugs (98):

- Amides formed from simple or functionalized acyl groups: $RR'N-CO-R''$.
- Amides cleaved by intramolecular catalysis (with accompanying cyclization of the carrier moiety).
- Alkyl carbamates: $RR'N-CO-O-R''$.
- (Acyloxy)alkyl carbamates: $RR'N-CO-O-CH(R'')-O-CO-R'''$.
- (Phosphoryloxy)methyl carbamates: $RR'N-CO-O-CH_2-O-PO_3H_2$.

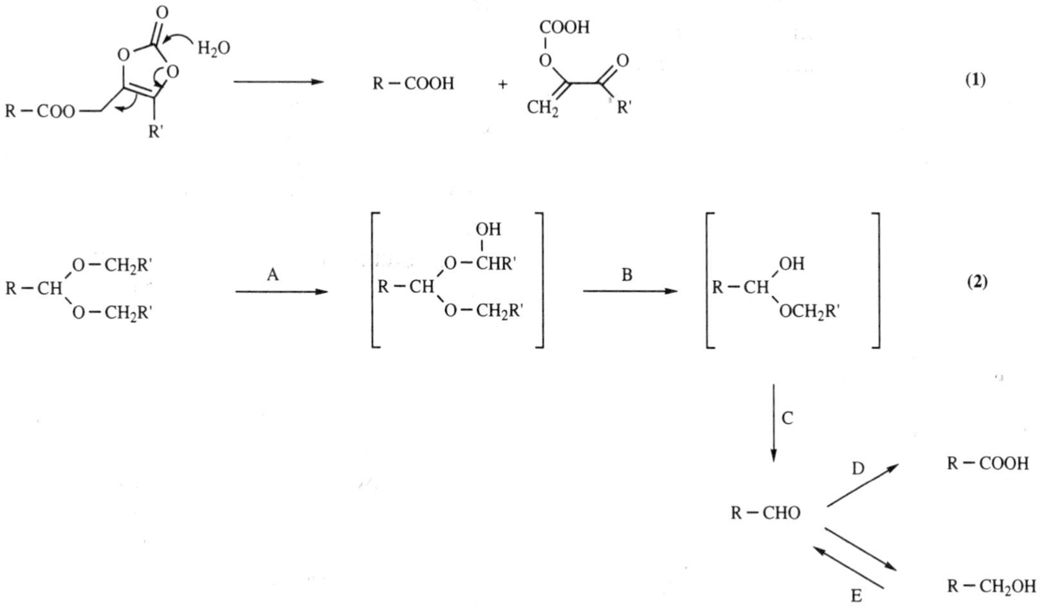

(1)

(2)

Fig. 6.38 Mechanism of nonenzymatic breakdown of (2-oxo-1,3-dioxol-4-yl)methyl esters (reaction 1) (96) and cytochrome P450–mediated oxidation of acetals to an aldehyde, which may then be reduced reversibly to an alcohol and oxidized irreversibly to an acid (97).

- *N*-(Acyloxy)methyl or *N*-(acyloxy)ethyl derivatives: $RR'N–CH_2–O–CO–R''$ or $RR'N–CH(CH_3)–O–CO–R''$.
- *N*-Mannich bases: $RR'N–CH_2–NR''R'''$.
- *N*-(*N,N*-Dialkylamino)methylene derivatives of primary amines: $RN=CH–NR'R''$.
- *N*-α-Hydroxyalkyl derivatives of peptides (reaction 1 in Fig. 6.39).
- Imidazolidinone derivatives of peptides (reaction 2 in Fig. 6.39).
- Oxazolidines of ephedrines and other 1-hydroxy-2-aminoethane congeners.

The reactivity of these prodrugs varies considerably. While several of them are activated nonenzymatically (e.g., Mannich bases), others undergo enzymatic hydrolysis followed by chemical breakdown (e.g., carbamic acids formed from carbamates).

Another type of prodrug is the ring-opened derivatives of heterocyclic drugs, e.g., hydantoins and benzodiazepines. These prodrugs are activated by a nonenzymatic cyclization accompanied by the release of a leaving group whose chemical properties influence the rate of reaction.

As mentioned earlier, tissue or organ selectivity is one of the goals of prodrug design. For example, much effort is being made toward dermal delivery (99) and

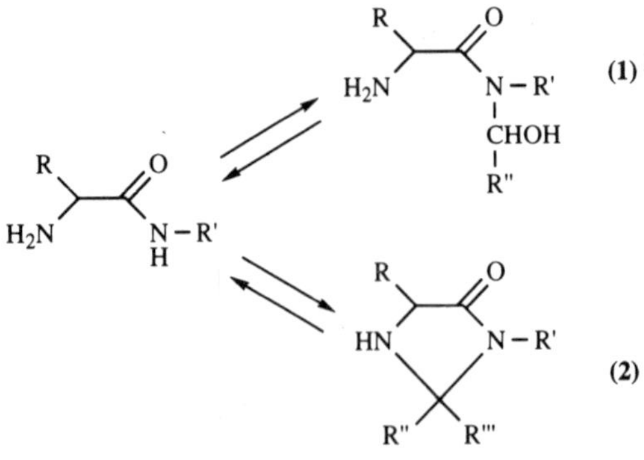

Fig. 6.39 Two types of peptide prodrugs. 1, *N*-α-hydroxyalkyl derivatives; 2, imidazolidinone derivatives.

brain penetration (94). In this context, site-specific chemical delivery systems may appear as the magic bullets of drug design, their selectivity being based on some enzymatic or physicochemical peculiarities characteristic of a given tissue or organ. For example, the selective presence of cysteine conjugate β-lyase in the kidney suggests that this enzyme might be exploited for delivery of sulfhydryl drugs to this organ (100). To date, the most elaborate and versatile chemical delivery systems are the brain-selective dihydropyridine carriers (90, 94). Figure 6.40 illustrates the example of an *N*-methyldihydropyridine carrier. This moiety undergoes enzymatic aromatization to a pyridinium derivative, which is polar and which, when formed in the brain, remains trapped there and upon hydrolysis yields the active drug. A large variety of drugs (e.g., neuropharmacological agents, steroid hormones, and chemotherapeutic agents) have been coupled to dihydropyridine carriers, resulting in improved and sustained brain delivery.

The gain in therapeutic benefit provided by prodrugs is not consistent. Depending on both the drug and its prodrug, the therapeutic gain, when it can be characterized, may be marked or modest. But as suggested in Table 6.6, a trend is apparent when comparing *post hoc* and *ad hoc* designed prodrugs. *Post hoc* design implies well-accepted drugs that are endowed with useful qualities but display some unwanted property that a prodrug form should ameliorate. The gain in such cases is usually modest yet real, but it may be marked if good targeting is achieved.

In contrast, an *ad hoc* design implies active compounds that suffer from some severe drawback (e.g., high hydrophilicity restricting bioavailability) that prevents therapeutic use. Here, a prodrug form may prove necessary, and its design will be integrated into the iterative process of lead optimization. A high therapeutic gain is obviously expected.

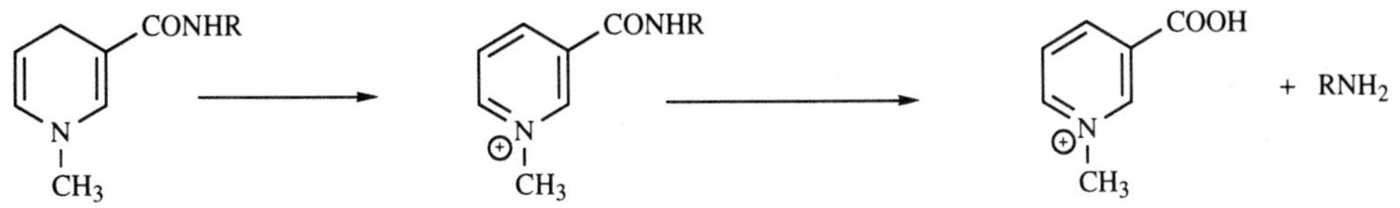

Fig. 6.40 Site-specific chemical delivery systems exemplified by an *N*-methyldihydropyridine carrier that delivers the drug (RNH_2) to the brain (90, 94).

4.3 The Concept of Toxophoric Groups

Biotransformation to reactive metabolic intermediates is one of the major mechanisms by which drugs exert toxic effects, particularly chronic toxicity. Other causes of (often acute) toxicity include all unwanted or exaggerated pharmacological responses. These various pharmacokinetic and pharmacodynamic mechanisms can be studied by structure–toxicity relationship methods (101) and are thus amenable to rational corrective steps within the framework of drug design.

For a reaction of toxication to occur at all, a proper moiety must be present, which has been termed a toxogenic, toxicophoric, or toxophoric group (102, 103). Major reactions of functionalization by which toxophoric groups are activated include oxidation to electrophilic intermediates or reduction to nucleophilic radicals (which may be followed by oxygen reduction). The electrophilic or nucleophilic intermediates may then react with bio(macro)molecules, producing critical or noncritical lesions. The toxic potential of radicals is particularly noteworthy. Of more recent awareness is the fact that a number of reactions of conjugation may also lead to toxic metabolites, either reactive ones or long-retained residues.

A drug designer worthy of the name must be conversant with toxication reactions and toxophoric groups, which include

- Some aromatic systems that can be oxidized to epoxides, quinones, or quinonimines (reactions 1 in Fig. 6.4).

- Ethynyl moieties activated by cytochrome P450 (reactions 3 in Fig. 6.4).
- Some halogenated alkyl groups that can undergo reductive dehalogenation (reaction 7 in Fig. 6.1).
- Nitroarenes that can be reduced to nitro anion radicals, nitrosoarenes, nitroxides, and hydroxylamines (reactions 4 in Fig. 6.6).
- Some aromatic amides that can be activated to nitrenium ions (reaction 3 in Fig. 6.6, followed by reactions 3 in Fig. 6.17).
- Some thiocarbonyl derivatives, particularly thioamides, that can be oxidized to *S,S*-dioxide (sulfene) metabolites (reaction 3 in Fig. 6.8).
- Thiols that can form mixed disulfides (reactions 1 in Fig. 6.8).
- Some carboxylic acids that can form reactive acylglucuronides (reaction 3 in Fig. 6.20).
- Some carboxylic acids that can form highly lipophilic conjugates (reactions 3 and 4 in Fig. 6.26).

However, it would be wrong to conclude from the above that the presence of a toxophoric group *necessarily* implies toxicity. Reality is far less gloomy, as only *potential* toxicity is indicated. In other words, the occurrence of a reaction of toxication is by no means a sufficient condition for toxicity, a sobering and often underemphasized fact. Given the presence of a toxophoric group in a compound, a number of factors will operate to render the latter either toxic or nontoxic:

1. Molecular properties of the substrate, which will increase or decrease its affinity and reactivity toward toxication or detoxication pathways.

2. Metabolic reactions of toxication are always accompanied by competitive and/or sequential reactions of detoxication that compete with the formation of the toxic metabolite and/or inactivate it. A profusion of biological factors control the relative effectiveness of these competitive and sequential pathways (see Table 6.2).

3. The reactivity and half-life of a reactive metabolite condition its sites of action and determine whether it will reach sensitive sites (11).

4. Dose, rate, and route of entry into the organism are all factors of known significance.

5. Above all, there exist essential mechanisms of survival value that operate to repair molecular lesions, remove them immunologically, and/or regenerate the lesioned sites.

In conclusion, the presence of a toxophoric group is by far not a sufficient condition for observable toxicity. Nor is it a necessary condition, because other mechanisms of toxicity exist.

5 CONCLUDING REMARKS

The overview of xenobiotic metabolism presented here will appear to many to be either too short or too long. This chapter is indeed too long for those organic chemists whose passion lies in the elegance of synthetic pathways and in the complexities of molecular architecture irrespective of the utility of the compounds obtained. And it may perhaps appear too short to the medicinal chemists, biochemists, and pharmacologists who are eager to learn all there is to know about the infinitely complex interactions between living organisms and xenobiotics. For such scientists, this chapter is a summary and an invitation to further studies.

REFERENCES

1. B. Testa, *The Metabolism of Drugs and Other Xenobiotics—Biochemistry of Redox Reactions*, Academic Press, Inc., London, in press.

2. B. Testa and J. M. Mayer, *The Metabolism of Drugs and Other Xenobiotics—Biochemistry of Hydration and Conjugation Reactions*, Academic Press, Inc., London, in press.

3. J. Caldwell and B. Testa, eds., *The Metabolism of Drugs and Other Xenobiotics—Biological Regulations and Consequences*, Academic Press, Inc., London, in press.

4. B. Testa in B. Testa, ed., *Advances in Drug Research*, Vol. 13, Academic Press, Inc., London, 1984, pp. 1–58.

5. F. J. Di Carlo, *Drug Metab. Rev.*, **13**, 1–4 (1982).

6. B. Testa, *Trends Pharmacol. Sci.*, **8**, 381–383 (1987).

7. B. Testa, *Drug. Metab. Rev.*, **13**, 25–50 (1982).

8. J. Caldwell, *Drug Metab. Rev.*, **13**, 745–777 (1982).

9. H. G. Neumann in Ref. 4, Vol. 15, 1986, pp. 1–28.

10. J. A. Timbrell, *Principles of Biochemical Toxicology*, 2nd ed., Taylor & Francis, London, 1991.

11. J. R. Gillette, *Drug Metab. Rev.*, **14**, 9–33 (1983).

12. J. Caldwell, A. Weil, and Y. Tanaka in R. Kato, R. W. Estabrook, and M. N. Cayen, eds., *Xenobiotic Metabolism and Disposition*, Taylor & Francis, London, 1989, pp. 217–224.

13. W. R. Chappell and J. Mordenti in Ref. 4, Vol. 20, 1991, pp. 1–116.

14. D. A. Smith, *Drug Metab. Rev.*, **23**, 355–373 (1991).

15. U. A. Meyer, U. M. Zanger, D. Grant, and M. Blum in Ref. 4, Vol. 19, 1990, pp. 197–241.

16. P. M. Bélanger in Ref. 4, Vol. 24, 1993, pp. 1–80.

17. M. Pasanen and O. Pelkonen, *Drug Metab. Rev.*, **21**, 427–461 (1990).

18. P. Jenner and B. Testa in P. Jenner and B. Testa, eds., *Concepts in Drug Metabolism*, Part B, Marcel Dekker, Inc., New York, 1981, pp. 423–513.

19. M. Barry and J. Feely, *Pharmacol. Therap.*, **48**, 71–94 (1990).

20. M. Murray and G. F. Reidy, *Pharmacol. Rev.*, **42**, 85–101 (1990).

21. B. Testa and P. Jenner, *Drug Metab. Rev.*, **12**, 1–117 (1981).

22. International Union of Biochemistry and Molecular Biology. *Enzyme Nomenclature 1992*. Academic Press, Inc., San Diego, 1992.

23. G. K. Chambers, *Gen. Pharmacol.*, **21**, 267–272 (1990).

24. R. L. Felsted and N. R. Bachur, *Drug Metab. Rev.*, **11**, 1–60 (1980).

25. H. P. Wirth and B. Wermuth, *FEBS Lett.*, **187**, 280–282 (1985).

26. R. Lindahl, *Crit. Rev. Biochem. Molec. Biol.*, **27**, 283–335 (1992).

27. P. A. Cossum, *Biopharm. Drug Dispos.*, **9**, 321–336 (1988).

28. E. Kyburz, *Drug News Perspect.*, **3**, 592–599 (1990).

29. C. Beedham, *Drug Metab. Rev.*, **16**, 119–156 (1985).

30. B. A. Callingham, A. Holt, and J. Elliott, *Biochem. Soc. Transact.*, **19**, 228–233 (1991).

31. F. J. Gonzalez, *Pharmacol. Therap.*, **45**, 1–38 (1990).

32. D. R. Nelson, T. Kamataki, D. J. Waxman, F. P. Guengerich, R. W. Estabrook, R. Feyereisen, F. J. Gonzalez, M. J. Coon, I. C. Gunsalus, O. Gotoh, K. Okuda, and D. W. Nebert, *DNA Cell Biol.*, **12**, 1–51 (1993).

33. C. E. Castro, *Pharmacol. Therap.*, **10**, 171–189 (1980).

34. T. E. Eling and J. F. Curtis, *Pharmacol. Therap.*, **53**, 261–273 (1992).

35. J. P. Uetrecht, *Drug Metab. Rev.*, **24**, 299–366 (1992).

36. K. R. Korzekwa, W. F. Trager, K. Nagata, A. Parkinson, and J. R. Gillette, *Drug Metab. Dispos.*, **18**, 974–979 (1990).

37. B. Rambeck, T. May, and U. Juergens, *Therap. Drug Monit.*, **9**, 298–303 (1987).

38. G. J. Mulder, ed., *Conjugation Reactions in Drug Metabolism*, Taylor & Francis, London, 1990.

39. M. Fujioka, *Int. J. Biochem.*, **24**, 1917–1924 (1992).

40. J. W. Faigle, I. Böttcher, J. Godbillon, H. P. Kriemler, E. Schlumpf, W. Schneider, A. Schweizer, H. Stierlin, and T. Winkler, *Xenobiotica* **18**, 1191–1197 (1988).

41. P. A. Crooks, C. S. Godin, L. A. Damani, S. S. Ansher, and W. B. Jakoby, *Biochem. Pharmacol.*, **37**, 1673–1677 (1988).

42. R. M. Weinshilboum, *Pharmacol. Therap.*, **43**, 77–90 (1989).

43. C. N. Falany, *Trends Pharmacol. Sci.*, **12**, 255–259 (1991).

44. R. S. Tsai, P. A. Carrupt, B. Testa, and J. Caldwell, *Chem. Res. Toxicol.*, **7**, 73–76 (1994).

45. J. E. Manautou and G. P. Carlson, *Xenobiotica*, **22**, 1309–1319 (1992).

46. K. Iwasaki, T. Shiraga, K. Noda, K. Tada, and H. Noguchi, *Xenobiotica*, **16**, 651–659 (1986).

47. K. D. Meisheri, G. A. Johnson, and L. Puddington, *Biochem. Pharmacol.*, **45**, 271–279 (1993).

48. B. Burchell, D. W. Nebert, D. R. Nelson, K. W. Bock, T. Iyanagi, P. L. M. Jansen, D. Lancet, G. J. Mulder, J. R. Chowdhury, G. Siest, T. R. Tephly, and P. I. Mackenzie, *DNA Cell Biol.*, **10**, 487–494 (1991).

49. J. O. Miners and P. I. Mackenzie, *Pharmacol. Therap.*, **51**, 347–369 (1991).

50. G. J. Mulder, *Annu. Rev. Pharmacol. Toxic.*, **32**, 25–49 (1992).

51. P. A. Carrupt, B. Testa, A. Bechalany, N. El Tayar, P. Descas, and D. Perrissoud, *J. Med. Chem.*, **34**, 1272–1275 (1991).

52. H. Spahn-Langguth and L. Z. Benet, *Drug Metab. Rev.*, **24**, 5–48 (1992).

53. W. H. Schaefer, A. Goalwin, F. Dixon, B. Hwang, L. Killmer, and G. Kuo, *Biol. Mass Spectrom.*, **21**, 179–188 (1992).

54. H. Luo, E. M. Hawes, G. McKay, E. D. Korchinski, and K. K. Midha, *Xenobiotica*, **21**, 1281–1288 (1991).

55. B. K. Tang, *Pharmacol. Therap.*, **46**, 53–56 (1990).

56. D. A. Price Evans, *Pharmacol. Therap.*, **42**, 157–234 (1989).

57. D. M. Grant, M. Blum, and U. A. Meyer, *Xenobiotica*, **22**, 1073–1081 (1992).

58. S. S. Mattano, S. Land, C. M. King, and W. W. Weber, *Molec. Pharmacol.*, **35**, 599–609 (1989).

59. H. K. Bhat and G. A. S. Ansari, *Chem. Res. Toxicol.*, **3**, 311–317 (1990).

60. K. Waku, *Biochim. Biophys. Acta*, **1124**, 101–111 (1992).

61. J. Caldwell and B. G. Lake, eds., *Biochem. Soc. Trans.*, **13**, 847–862 (1985).

62. P. F. Dodds, *Life Sci.*, **49**, 629–649 (1991).

63. J. M. Mayer, *Acta Pharm. Nord.*, **2**, 197–216 (1990).

64. S. M. Bjorge and T. A. Baillie, *Drug Metab. Dispos.*, **19**, 823–829 (1991).

65. J. Hulsman, *Pharm. Weekbl.* [*Sci.*], **14**, 98–100 (1992).

66. D. J. Reed, *Annu. Rev. Pharmacol. Toxicol.*, **30**, 603–631 (1990).

67. A. Meister, *J. Biol. Chem.*, **263**, 17205–17208 (1988).

68. S. Tsuchida and K. Sato, *Crit. Rev. Biochem. Molec. Biol.*, **27**, 337–384 (1992).

69. G. F. Graminski, Y. Kubo, and R. N. Armstrong, *Biochemistry*, **28**, 3562–3568 (1989).

70. B. Ketterer, *Drug Metab. Rev.*, **13**, 161–187 (1982).

71. P. J. O'Brien, *Chem. Biol. Int.*, **80**, 1–41 (1991).

72. T. J. Monks and S. S. Lau, *Crit. Rev. Toxicol.*, **22**, 243–270 (1992).

73. W. Dekant, S. Vamvakas, and M. W. Anders, *Drug. Metab. Rev.*, **20**, 43–83 (1989).

74. T. A. Baillie and J. G. Slatter, *Acc. Chem. Res.*, **24**, 264–270 (1991).

75. A. E. Cribb, M. Miller, J. S. Leeder, J. Hill, and S. P. Spielberg, *Drug Metab. Dispos.*, **19**, 900–906 (1991).

76. S. R. Kenkare and L. Z. Benet, *Biochem. Pharmacol.*, **46**, 279–284 (1993).

77. D. Ross, *Pharmacol. Therap.*, **37**, 231–249 (1988).

78. P. Jenner and B. Testa, *Xenobiotica*, **8**, 1–25 (1978).

79. B. Testa in D. J. Benford, J. W. Bridges, and G. G. Gibson, eds., *Drug Metabolism—From Molecules to Man.* Taylor & Francis, London, 1987, pp. 563–580.

80. E. De Clercq in Ref. 4, Vol. 17, 1988, pp. 1–59.

81. J. P. O'Donnell, *Drug Metab. Rev.*, **13**, 123–159 (1982).

82. L. P. Balant, H. Roseboom, and R. M. Guntert-Remy in Ref. 4, Vol. 19, 1990, pp. 1–138.

83. T. Walle, U. K. Walle, and L. S. Olanoff, *Drug Metab. Dispos.*, **13**, 204–209 (1985).

84. P. Jenner and B. Testa, *Drug Metab. Rev.*, **2**, 117–184 (1973).

85. B. Testa and J. M. Mayer in E. Jucker, ed., *Progress in Drug Research*, Vol. **32**, Birkhäuser, Basel, 1988, pp. 249–303.

86. F. Jamali, R. Mehvar, and F. M. Pasutto, *J. Pharm. Sci.*, **78**, 695–715 (1989).

87. M. Eichelbaum, L. Bertilsson, A. Küpfer, E. Steiner, and C. O. Meese, *Br. J. Clin. Pharmacol.*, **25**, 505–508 (1988).

88. C. Altomare, P. A. Carrupt, P. Gaillard, N. El Tayar, B. Testa, and A. Carotti, *Chem. Res. Toxicol.*, **5**, 366–375 (1992).

89. E. J. Ariëns and A. M. Simonis in J. A. Keverling Buisman, ed., *Strategy in Drug Research*, Elsevier, Amsterdam, The Netherlands, 1982, pp. 165–178.

90. N. Bodor in Ref. 4, Vol. 13, 1984, pp. 255–331.

91. D. G. Waller and C. F. George, *Br. J. Clin. Pharmacol.*, **28**, 497–507 (1989).

92. V. J. Stella, W. N. A. Charman, and V. H. Naringrekar, *Drugs*, **29**, 455–473 (1985).

93. C. G. Wermuth in G. Jolles and K. R. H. Wooldridge, eds., *Drug Design: Fact or Fantasy?*, Academic Press, Inc., London, 1984, pp. 47–72.

94. N. Bodor, *Ann. N. Y. Acad. Sci.*, **507**, 289–306 (1987).

95. R. Duncan, *Anti-Canc. Drugs*, **3**, 175–210 (1992).

96. W. S. Saari, W. Halczenko, D. W. Cochran, M. R. Dobrinska, W. C. Vincek, D. C. Titus, S. L. Gaul, and C. S. Sweet, *J. Med. Chem.*, **27**, 713–717 (1984).

97. D. Vicchio and P. S. Callery, *Drug Metab. Dispos.*, **17**, 513–517 (1989).

98. I. H. Pitman, *Med. Res. Rev.*, **1**, 189–214 (1981).

99. S. Y. Chan and A. Li Wan Po, *Int. J. Pharmaceut.*, **55**, 1–16 (1989).

100. I. Y. Hwang and A. A. Elfarra, *J. Pharmacol. Exp. Therap.*, **251**, 448–454 (1989).

101. D. E. Hathway, *Molecular Aspects of Toxicity*, Royal Society of Chemistry, London, 1984.

102. E. J. Ariëns, *Drug Metab. Rev.*, **15**, 425–504 (1984).

103. P. J. van Bladeren, *Trends Pharmacol. Sci.*, **9**, 295–299 (1988).

CHAPTER SEVEN

Drug Allergy

CHARLES W. PARKER

Department of Medicine
Washington University School of Medicine
St. Louis, Missouri, USA

CONTENTS

1 Introduction, 182
2 Mechanism of Sensitization, 182
  2.1 Lymphocyte stimulation, 182
  2.2 Responses to different classes of therapeutic agents, 184
  2.3 The role of the macromolecular carrier, 185
    2.3.1 The nature of the bond, 185
    2.3.2 The basis for protein carrier action, 186
    2.3.3 Other macromolecules, 186
    2.3.4 Evidence in human drug allergy, 188
    2.3.5 Site of conjugation, 189
3 Hypersensitivity Reactions to Drugs, 190
  3.1 General mechanisms, 190
  3.2 Classification, 190
  3.3 Types of hypersensitivity response, 191
    3.3.1 Anaphylaxis, 191
    3.3.2 Serum sickness, 193
    3.3.3 Selective organ damage, 194
  3.4 Drug reactions suspected to be allergic, 198
  3.5 Drug reactions simulating allergy, 204
4 Immunologic Assays for Drug Allergy, 207
  4.1 Assays for humoral immunity, 207
  4.2 Assays for cellular immunity, 209
5 Penicillin Allergy, 209
6 Evaluation of Drugs for Allergenicity, 213
  6.1 Evaluation of the protein reactivity of the drug and its metabolites, 213
    6.1.1 Evaluation for direct protein reactivity *in vitro*, 213
    6.1.2 Evaluation for protein reactivity *in vivo*, 213
  6.2 Direct immunologic evaluation, 214

Burger's Medicinal Chemistry and Drug Discovery,
Fifth Edition, Volume 1: Principles and Practice,
Edited by Manfred E. Wolff.
ISBN 0-471-57556-9 © 1995 John Wiley & Sons, Inc.

6.3 Simplified approaches to immunological
    analysis and their limitations, 214
    6.3.1 Attempts at obtaining hapten-protein
          conjugates without identifying the
          chemical reaction involved in their
          formation, 215
    6.3.2 "Artificial" conjugates, 215
    6.3.3 Metabolic activation *in vitro*, 215
    6.3.4 Utilization of the drug itself, 215
6.4 Screening for nonspecific activation of
    immunologic effector mechanisms, 216
6.5 Initial evaluation of drugs in humans, 216
7 Possible Future Directions, 216
7.1 Drug development, 216
7.2 HLA phenotyping, 216
7.3 Utilization of univalent haptens and haptens
    attached to metabolizable carriers, 216

1 INTRODUCTION

Adverse reactions to drugs are a common and important medical problem. As many as 5% of medical hospital admissions are due to drug reactions and at least 15% of hospitalized patients experience at least one adverse drug reaction (1). Allergic or possibly allergic reactions to drugs are variously estimated to constitute 3% to 25% of all adverse drug reactions (2). By definition, allergic drug reactions involve specific immunologic processes and are initiated by sensitized lymphocytes or antibodies. Therefore, allergic reactions differ mechanistically from adverse drug reactions due to overdosage, normal pharmacologic side effects, pharmacologic idiosyncrasy, nonspecific release of pharmacologic effector molecules, or interactions between drugs (3). Manifestations of drug allergy include anaphylaxis, serum sickness, hemolytic anemia, thrombocytopenia, granulocytopenia, dermatitis, hepatitis, nephritis, and pneumonitis. Although allergy is not the most common cause of untoward drug symptoms, it is often involved in the most serious reactions. Differentiation of allergic responses from other types of drug toxicity is frequently not easy since many of the symptoms overlap. The most definitive

criterion is the direct demonstration of altered immunologic reactivity directed toward the drug or its metabolites. Even this approach has its limitations since immunologic responses to drugs can occur in the absence of allergic symptoms.

2 MECHANISM OF SENSITIZATION

2.1 Lymphocyte Stimulation

Immunologic responses are the result of stimulation of lymphocytes by antigens. There are many different subpopulations of antigen-sensitive lymphocytes, each with a predetermined capability of responding to one or a circumscribed group of antigens (4, 5). The response is initiated through specific receptors for antigen on the cell surface. When a critical number of receptor sites become occupied, the cells are stimulated to replicate, greatly expanding the antigen-sensitive cell population. Two major classes of lymphocytes participate in the response: thymus derived or T lymphocytes and bone marrow directed B lymphocytes. Both classes contain receptors for antigen which are split in germ line DNA into segments (V, D, and J) which will later be brought together in a large number of different combinations. This arrangement creates the diversity needed to encompass the many possible antigens that may be encountered.

T lymphocytes are primarily responsible for cell-mediated immunity, including delayed hypersensitivity, graft versus host responses, and the most important form of lymphocyte-medicated cytotoxicity. T lymphocytes also carry immunologic memory and perform helper functions that aid in the differentiation of antibody-producing cells. There are also suppressor T lymphocytes that act by inhibiting the continuation of the immune response. The receptors for antigen on T cells are heterodimeric proteins (6) which primarily recognize peptide fragments of proteins rather than intact proteins. The peptides are presented to T cells by either dendritic cells, B cells or macrophages in the context of major histocompatibility complex (MHC) proteins. T cells produce many of their effects by releasing lymphokines (various interleukins and interferons) (7). Lymphokines are soluble proteins which act on other cells including B cells through specific receptors. Through these lymphokines, T cells help regulate antibody synthesis by B cells. Direct interactions of T cells with B cells are also important. T cells can be subdivided on the basis of their function, lymphokine production, the MHC antigens they recognize and surface proteins they display. For example, T cells promoting antibody synthesis by B cells typically are CD4 antigen positive and recognize antigen fragments bound to class II (human HLA, DR, DP, DQ) proteins. They can be further divided into type I T helper cells (Th1) cells, which secrete interleukin 2, interferon-γ and other lymphokines and type II T helper cells, (Th2 cells), which secrete interleukins 4, 5, 10 and 13. Th1 cell activity is important in the early antibody response and most forms of cellular immunity. Th2 cell activity is important in maturation of the antibody

response and especially in IgE antibody production (8). Th1 and Th2 cells themselves are regulated by lymphokines; IL-2 and IL-4 act as growth factors for Th1 and Th2 cells respectively. Th1 and Th2 cells reciprocally regulate one another through their lymphokines. The balance between these subsets is important in the overall pattern of immunologic activity and the nature and frequency of allergic manifestations. T cells producing cytotoxicity and suppression are primarily CD8+, CD4−, and recognize class I MHC antigens.

Once T cells have matured lymphocytes derived from bone marrow, or B lymphocytes, they express immunoglobulins on their surfaces. In response to antigen, they give rise to antibody-secreting cells (plasma cells). Antibodies (or immunoglobulins) are of 5 different classes, distinguishable on the basis of molecular size, antigenic markers, biologic function, and number of polypeptide chains. (For a review of antibody structure and function, see reference 5). Quantitatively, the most prominent immunoglobulin class is immunoglobulin G (IgG), which is a protein having a molecular weight of 150,000 daltons, and present in serum at concentrations ranging from 600 to 1000 μg/mL. IgG molecules are composed of two heavy and two light polypeptide chains. There are two combining sites for antigen, each formed by a pair of heavy and light chains. Alternative RNA splicing is used to create secreted and membrane bound forms of the immunoglobulins. The membrane forms are used for intracellular signaling by B cells. The secreted forms are distributed in the blood, interstitial fluid and on other immunocytes where they passively sensitize cells to react with antigen. As discussed below, IgE molecules are present in low concentration in serum but are important from the point of view of morbidity and mortality in drug reactions because of their very important role in anaphylactic sensitivity. IgG antibodies, on the other hand, though capable of producing certain types of allergic responses, at times appear to inhibit IgE-mediated responses. Thus the presence or absence of allergic symptoms may depend not only on the absolute amounts of antibody in the different immunoglobulin classes but also on the ratio of the different classes to one another.

In the absence of previous exposure to antigen, the first demonstrable antibodies or sensitized lymphocytes appear after about 4 or 5 days, depending on the sensitivity of the assay. The response rapidly increases in intensity, reaching a maximum after 2 or 3 weeks (9). In the absence of further exposure to antigen, the intensity of the response eventually decreases, and evidence of sensitization may disappear altogether. During the early phases of the response, there is a shift from a predominantly IgM response to a largely IgG response later. The antibodies are heterogeneous not only with respect to immunoglobulin class but also in their binding affinity for antigen, a variation that covers at least a 10,000-fold range. As the response evolves, the average affinity of the antibody for antigen increases. This effect is generally viewed as a thermodynamically-driven cell selection process. Much of the increase in antibody affinity involves antibody molecules that have been altered by somatic mutation during the ongoing immune response. As the level of antigen falls, the cells that are best adapted to bind the limited quantities of antigen available (i.e., the cells with the highest affinity for antigen) are selectively stimulated with the result that high affinity antibody molecules are secreted. Other cells that had been stimulated originally at high antigen concentrations are less able to proliferate, and their products become less prominent as the response proceeds. While immune reactivity tends to decrease with time, the induced immune reactivity may

persist for many years resulting in an accelerated response when the allergen is reintroduced.

It is apparent that the immune response is a complex process involving the formation of antibodies in different immunoglobulin classes as well as suppressor and effector lymphocytes. A further degree of complexity is added by the change in antibody affinity at different stages of the response. When variations in how drugs are administered and metabolized and individual differences in immune reactivity are also considered, it is not surprising that not everyone reacts to a drug in the same way.

2.2 Responses to Different Classes of Therapeutic Agents

The flexibility of the immune system in terms of the variety of foreign epitopes that are capable of producing a response, is staggering; some estimates extend into the millions. Proteins and to a lesser extent carbohydrates are effective stimulators of antibody formation. More recently, it has been recognized that lipopolysaccharides, nucleic acids, and even relatively small molecular weight polypeptides have the capability of inducing antibody formation, although often special efforts, such as their administration in an immunologic adjuvant, may be necessary to produce a response (9). Some of the important variables affecting immunogenicity include degree of antigenic foreignness, structural complexity, molecular size, and rate of biodegradability. Immune responses complicate the use of hormones, antibodies, or enzymes from foreign species in the treatment of human disease. Virtually everyone develops allergic symptoms when large quantities of foreign serum proteins are administered. The immune apparatus is also capable of forming antibodies in response to a wide variety of small molecular weight organic chemicals of pharmacologic value. However, allergic symptoms to these agents are much less frequent than they are to proteins, the usual incidence being well below 1% for a single course of treatment. On the other hand, benzylpenicillin, which has a molecular weight of less than 400 daltons, produces allergic symptoms in 1% to 10% of treated individuals and may even cause death. The high sensitizing capacity of penicillin is due to its unusual degree of chemical reactivity, permitting it to form stable bonds with proteins and other macromolecules *in vivo* (10).

The importance of covalent conjugation with protein in antibody formation to organic molecules was originally demonstrated by Landsteiner, based on an apparent correlation between potential protein reactivity (as measured *in vitro* by an ability to conjugate to the amino group on aniline) and sensitizing capacity *in vivo* (11). Eisen confirmed and extended these observations. He utilized a homologous series of polynitrobenzenes that differ in protein reactivity, but once reacted, form identical substituents on protein (12). He further showed that topically applied nitrohalobenzenes with protein reactivity *in vitro* did indeed combine with cutaneous proteins *in vivo*. Subsequent studies in human penicillin hypersensitivity in the early 1960s established the applicability of this principle to drug allergy in humans. The antibodies present in the serum of individuals receiving penicillin were not directed towards penicillin itself, but to breakdown products of penicillin capable of existing in stable linkage to protein, especially the penicilloyl group. This finding was demonstrated independently by a group which included Herman Eisen, Alain de Weck, Milton Kern, Jack Shapiro, and Charles Parker (10, 13–16) as well as Bernard Levine and his colleagues (17–20).

2.3 The Role of the Macromolecular Carrier

2.3.1 THE NATURE OF THE BOND. The term "hapten" has been used to describe a substance that is not immunogenic of itself but becomes immunogenic after conjugation to a macromolecule. The promotion of hapten immunogenicity by a macromolecule requires that a stable bond be formed. The necessary stability is provided by covalent, coordination, and multiple salt linkages, whereas the reversible, ionic, and hydrophobic interactions most drugs undergo with albumin and other serum proteins are apparently ineffective. Examples of the many simple chemicals with the required reactivity to form covalent bonds with proteins are acid chlorides, anhydrides, diazonium salts, isocyanates and halonitrobenzenes. Some of these agents are potent sensitizers in chemical industries.

As a rule, reactions leading to sensitization take place with functional amino acid residues of the protein (amino acids capable of assuming a charge on their side chains such as lysyl, tyrosyl, cysteinyl, or histidyl). In conjugating with a functional group of a protein, the chemical undergoes structural modification that may be extensive or, more often, is limited to the deletion of a small portion of its molecule. The bond that is formed is nonionic and is stable because the two reactants share electrons. Heavy metals such as nickel and chromium form coordination complexes with proteins, explaining the ability of these substances to produce contact dermatitis (21). Multiple salt linkages are probably involved in the ability of methylated serum albumins to promote the immunogenicity of polynucleotides.

Polynucleotides are polyanionic and ordinarily nonimmunogenic of themselves, but become immunogenic when they are electrostatically complexed to oppositely charged proteins (22). The energy of the

individual ionic bonds in the polynu-
cleotide-protein complex is small, but the
summation of binding energies at multiple
points on the same macromolecule results
in a much more stable complex. In view of
the ability of several different types of
linkage to promote a response, it appears
that the most important criterion is the
overall stability of the hapten-protein complex rather than any special chemical properties of the bonds themselves (23).

2.3.2 THE BASIS FOR PROTEIN CARRIER
ACTION. In the formation of antibodies to
a hapten it appears that the more immunogenic the carrier, the better the response
(4). On the other hand, endogenous macromolecules, to which there is normally
immunologic tolerance, must also be able
to promote a response, since this is the only
mechanism available when an immune response is stimulated by a drug *in vivo*. Of
course, the endogenous macromolecule is
structurally altered as it reacts with the
drug, helping to break tolerance (23). The
immunogenicity of haptens conjugated to
endogenous proteins has been directly
demonstrated by preparing the conjugates
in vitro and showing that injected animals
produce antihapten antibodies. This procedure has been used on numerous occasions to prepare antisera for the radioimmunoassay of small molecular weight
drugs, beginning with the radioimmunoassay of digitoxin (25).

Based on what is now known about
sensitization of T cells, the most straightforward mechanism for inducing drug allergy is when the drug or its metabolite
reacts with amino acid residues or a protein
in the blood or tissues. The altered protein
is taken up and partially degraded in antigen presenting cells to peptides, some of
which contain conjugated metabolites (26).
Receptors on T cells recognize the metabolite and nearby amino acid residues in the
peptide and a unique response is initiated.
Protein molecules containing the metabo-

lite also react directly with B cells and, in
the presence of appropriate lymphokines
from stimulated T cells, antibody synthesis
is initiated.

2.3.3 OTHER MACROMOLECULES. In addition to proteins, other endogenous macromolecules might act as carriers of hapten
immunogenicity. A variety of macromolecules might conceivably perform this function, since even nonmetabolizable polymers
appear to be capable of inducing antihapten antibody formation, provided an appropriate dose range is used. Under conditions
of repeated or continuing immunization,
haptens conjugated to highly purified polysaccharides and nucleic acids stimulate an
immune response. For example, penicilloylated dextrans and raffinose have been
reported to induce hapten-specific delayed
hypersensitivity responses in guinea pigs in
the absence of antipenicilloyl antibodies,
suggesting an unusually selective immune
response in which cellular but not humoral
immunity was being stimulated (27). More
frequently, polysaccharides induce antibody formation with little or no associated
cellular immunity. Indeed, a number of
polysaccharides are capable of inducing
antibody formation by B cells in the absence of effective T cell function (T independent antigens) (28).

DNA is another nonproteinaceous
macromolecule that appears to serve as an
effective carrier for immunization to haptens, since 2, 4, 6 trinitrophenyl (TNP)
residues substituted on deoxyguanosine
groups in DNA stimulate the formation of
anti-TNP antibodies (29). The hapten linkage to the macromolecule is quite stable,
and the possibility of endogenous breakdown with cross-conjugation to protein
appears minimal; thus, a direct role for the
polynucleotide in the antihapten response
appears likely. But again it must be kept in
mind that under ordinary conditions of
drug use *in vivo*, drugs probably conjugate
much more readily to proteins than to

other macromolecules. In situations in which chemically reactive haptens have been labeled with radioactive isotopes and studied for binding to macromolecules *in vivo*, proteins have contained most or all of the bound radioactivity. Moreover, delayed hypersensitivity responses involving penicilloyl and polynitrophenyl hapten sometimes show partial specificity for endogenous proteins in the circulation (e.g., serum albumin) or the skin, suggesting that these proteins have been part of the original immunizing complex (12, 30). Once the antihapten response is underway, however, other macromolecules containing bound hapten may also contribute to the response. Indeed, as discussed below, once antihapten molecules become available, the hapten itself may play the role of an immunologic carrier and help to break tolerance to a previously nonimmunogenic or poorly immunogenic macromolecule (23).

In addition to soluble macromolecules, the possible role of insoluble tissue constituents or vehicles such as the oils that are sometimes used to delay drug absorption, must be considered in the induction of haptenic responses. A role for cell-bound hapten seems particularly plausible, since cells containing bound hapten molecules are quite effective stimulators of cellular immune responses. Theoretically, a similar response might also occur in certain vehicles or following the binding of the drug to fragments of the cells in areas of local tissue necrosis. Kinsky and his colleagues have shown that small molecular weight phospholipids substituted with DNP and incorporated in liposomes stimulate the formation of antihapten antibodies (31).

The ability of hapten-protein conjugates to serve as immunogens does not entirely exclude the possibility that under special circumstances unconjugated haptens might initiate an immune response. This circumstance is of practical as well as theoretical interest, since if unconjugated drugs are capable of immunization, immunological detection systems should be directed toward the drugs themselves as well as toward potentially immunogenic metabolites. Unconjugated 2,4-dinitrophenyl (DNP) amino acids, and p-azobenzene arsonates have been reported to induce immune responses. In the response to p-azobenzene arsonates, delayed cutaneous hypersensitivity is induced, but little or no serum antibody detectable with azobenzene arsonate conjugates is demonstrable (32).

In interpreting these observations, the possibility must be considered that the hapten contains impurities or is metabolized *in vivo*. The absence of antibody to azobenzene arsonate is not inconsistent with the possibility of *in vivo* metabolism, since a major structural alteration in the molecule leading to conjugation to protein might so alter it structurally that the antibodies it produces would not recognize the original azobenzene arsonate molecule. Thus antibodies might be present but not detected in the azobenzene arsonate assay system. The difficulty in interpreting immunization results with small molecular weight haptens is exemplified in the studies of Frey and his colleagues with DNP amino acids (33). They have found that although delayed hypersensitivity responses were elicited in guinea pigs by sizable quantities of these agents, different preparations of the same apparently pure DNP amino acids varied markedly in their sensitizing capabilities. They have suggested that some DNP amino acid preparations might contain small amounts of ordinarily undetectable contaminants that were responsible for the immunization.

Thus the available evidence that small molecular weight haptens are immunogenic of themselves is not convincing. Even if the possibility of immunization is accepted, since administration in adjuvant was necessary to produce a response, the likelihood that this procedure is an important mechanism for sensitization to drugs in humans is small. Some years ago the study of the specificity of the antibody response in human beings with penicillin allergy had showed that the great majority of the antibodies were specific for penicilloyl and other penicillin breakdown products rather than penicillin itself, strongly suggesting the importance of protein conjugation (34, 35). As discussed below, the penicilloyl group is the major product formed when penicillin forms a covalent bond with a protein.

2.3.4 EVIDENCE IN HUMAN DRUG ALLERGY. In view of the importance of conjugation to protein in immunization, one would predict that drugs that combine readily with proteins under physiologic conditions would be the most immunogenic. This condition certainly appears to be true of penicillin, which not only is subject to direct aminolysis by protein lysyl groups but also gives rise to a variety of breakdown products with protein reactivity, including penicillenic acid and penicilloic acid (see below). A role for contaminants has been suggested in aspirin sensitivity, where aspiroyl anhydrides contaminating commercial aspirin preparations have been shown to be capable of producing an immune response in guinea pigs and antiaspiroyl antibodies have been demonstrated in human sera, although most acute reactions to aspirin appear to involve other mechanisms (36). Most drugs do not have direct protein reactivity, and it is necessary to assume that a reactive metabolite is formed *in vivo*. The possibility that a drug might be metabolized *in vivo* to a reactive intermediate capable of reacting with proteins, is well substantiated. Possible pathways are discussed in Section 3.4 of the chapter.

A requirement for metabolic processing of a drug permitting conjugation with protein can explain a number of otherwise puzzling features of drug allergy—its generally low incidence, the marked variation in frequency, and the frequent localization of clinical manifestations in a single organ system. Localization of allergic manifestations can occur if the enzymatic reaction leading to conjugation is primarily localized in a given organ. This situation would provide a higher concentration of antigen in that tissue, making it the major target in a hypersensitivity response. Alternatively, the conjugation of hapten with an organ-specific protein might produce an immunologic response with specificity for the protein as well as the hapten, creating a situation in which autoimmune tissue could occur (37).

Direct verification in humans that metabolites of drugs are directly involved in human allergy is limited. In thrombocytopenia precipitated by acetaminophen, an antibody to a sulfate conjugate of the drug appears to be implicated rather than the drug itself (38). Tentative or strongly suggestive identification of possible active metabolites has also been made in reactions to mesantoin, phenylbutazone, phenacetin, amidopyrine, halothane, hydralazine and procainamide. In most circumstances the formation of such intermediates and their reaction with protein can only be inferred. This condition is probably not surprising, since identification of the presumed protein-reactive metabolites formed *in vivo* is not easy:

1. The metabolic degradation of drugs involves multiple enzymatic pathways, and a single drug may produce many metabolites.

2. Focusing just on known major metabolic products may not be sufficient, since microgram amounts of highly reactive derivatives may be able to induce an immune response.

3. Difficulties in identifying antigenic precursors are compounded by the protein reactivity of these substances, which makes them difficult to isolate from tissue and body fluids.

4. The average levels of substitution on circulating proteins or tissue fluid may

be too low to permit detection by conventional analytical methods.

5. The most reactive metabolites are more likely to produce direct toxicity instead of allergy because they react inside rather than outside the cell.

Despite the strong evidence that protein reactivity is critically involved in human drug allergy, the notion persists in the literature that relatively loose attachments of drugs with cells or soluble macromolecules may occasionally lead to allergy (39). Most of this speculation is concerned with drug dependent reactions affecting formed elements of the blood and is discussed below under that topic.

2.3.5 SITE OF CONJUGATION. In considering the fate of an unusually reactive metabolite formed within a cell, there is an apparent analogy to cutaneous sensitization to chromium, which is a significant industrial problem in the cement and metal industries. The topical application of hexavalent chromium, which does not combine readily with proteins, results in sensitization, whereas trivalent chromium, which has protein reactivity, is nonimmunogenic (40–42). Yet hexavalent chromium induces antibodies to trivalent chromium. This action can be explained if it is assumed that only the hexavalent form of the metal penetrates the epidermis effectively. Once the appropriate area of the skin is reached, reduction to trivalent chromium occurs, followed by conjugation to protein and induction of an immune response. On the other hand, trivalent chromium reacts with proteins in superficial areas of the skin and never gets deep enough to produce sensitization. If a reactive metabolite is implicated, an organ such as the liver, which is especially active in metabolizing drugs, is probably often involved. Depending on the reactivity of the metabolite and the proteins it interacts with, the liver may or may

not become a major site of allergic tissue damage.

Attempts to determine the site of the lymphocytes' first encounter with the antigen suggest two major possibilities:

1. Lymphocytes may be sensitized in the target tissue itself. There is a recirculating lymphocyte pool that wanders through various tissues. During local exposure to antigen there is a selective localization of antigen-sensitive lymphocytes. Sensitization occurs wherever the local concentration of appropriately displayed antigen reaches a critical level. In kidneys perfused with allogeneic thoracic duct lymphocytes, local sensitization can occur within 5 to 12 hours (43). In the normal *in vivo* setting, these cells probably migrate back to lymphoid tissue, undergo proliferation and differentiation, then release their antibodies or rejoin the recirculating lymphocyte pool as sensitized lymphocytes. This arrangement results in generalized sensitivity and cytotoxic changes in the kidney and other areas containing the antigen.

2. Reactive metabolites or soluble hapten-protein conjugates produced elsewhere may penetrate into lymphoid tissue, producing an immune response that ultimately becomes generalized, as described for the local sensitization model. Alternatively, in sensitization of the skin, dermal dendritic cells are known to take antigens locally and migrate to regional lymph nodes where they act as antigen presenting cells.

As discussed below, lymphoid cells themselves are capable of forming reactive metabolites either through pathways shared with organs such as the liver or pathways that are especially well developed in leukocytes. The formation of metabolites in the lymphoid tissue itself may represent a particularly efficient form of sensitization. Once sensitization has occurred, other organs may become the primary focus for tissue damage because they also contain antigen.

3 HYPERSENSITIVITY REACTIONS TO DRUGS

3.1 General Mechanisms

Once antibodies and sensitized lymphocytes have been produced, the stage is set for the production of allergic symptoms. Often manifestations of hypersensitivity are not elicited until the drug has been readministered, reflecting a need for a fresh source of antigen to achieve the critical threshold for allergic symptoms. On the other hand, manifestations of allergy may occur during the initial course of drug administration or even some days after the drug has been discontinued. In this case, the delay is due to the time needed to accumulate quantities of antibody (or sensitized lymphocytes) large enough to achieve an appropriate antigen-antibody ratio and overall concentration (5).

To elicit symptoms of immediate hypersensitivity, the antigen must have multiple combining sites (be multivalent), permitting it to form cross-links or bridges between antibody molecules (14, 44–46). Bridging of soluble antibody molecules is needed for them to react with complement and release cytoactive peptides, a response that is important in mounting an inflammatory response. Bridging between cell-bound antibody molecules or antigen receptors on lymphocytes produces the conformational change in the cell membrane required for activation of mediator release or cell replication.

Since small molecular weight drugs are ordinarily univalent, even if the unaltered drug is reactive with the antibody, the eliciting of an anaphylactic response normally would require the drug to conjugate with endogenous macromolecules. In solution, this response would probably require that single protein molecules be substituted multiple times, although on cell surfaces a mixture of proteins substituted one at a time might be sufficient. In either case, this circumstance would entail the formation of the same types of multivalent protein conjugate involved in initiation of the immune response at the time of the rechallenge. Thus in the elicitation of symptoms of hypersensitivity and in the induction of the immune response originally, there is the same requirement for haptens to conjugate to protein. Drugs that conjugate slowly to proteins through the formation of reactive metabolites can produce manifestations of hypersensitivity; however, rapidly evolving responses are unlikely.

3.2 Classification

Hypersensitivity symptoms are classified as humoral or cellular, depending on whether antibodies or sensitized lymphocytes are primarily responsible for the response. In general, anaphylaxis, serum sickness, urticaria, Arthus reactions, glomerulonephritis, and reactions involving the formed elements of the blood, are considered to be antibody-mediated responses, whereas eczematous dermatitis and some forms of drug fever and organ-specific cytotoxicity are thought to be mediated by sensitized lymphocytes. Keep in mind, however, that the normal immune response involves the production of both cellular and humoral immunity and that symptomatic manifestations of the two forms of hypersensitivity can and do occur together. In addition, there are many drug reactions that at the moment cannot be easily classified as antibody- or cell-mediated or even as definitely immunologic in etiology.

3.3 Types of Hypersensitivity Response

3.3.1 ANAPHYLAXIS. Systemic anaphylaxis is is an acute, often life-threatening allergic reaction in which hypotension, bronchospasm, angioedema, urticaria, diffuse erythema, pruritus, laryngeal, pharyngeal, or epiglottal edema, cardiac arrhythmias, nausea and vomiting, dyspnea, and hyperperistalsis occur, either in combination or as isolated manifestations. Symptoms are more frequently produced by intravenous or intramuscular drug administration, although in highly sensitive persons oral, percutaneous, vaginal, or even respiratory exposure may produce the response. Typically, the reaction develops within seconds to minutes, reaching a maximum within 5–20 min. The reaction characteristically occurs during the institution of a new course of treatment with a previously used drug. There may or may not have been allergic symptoms during earlier exposure to the drug. Death, when it occurs, is usually due to hypotension, laryngeal edema, cardiac arrest, or bronchospasm. Early recognition and the use of epinephrine and other supportive measurements may be life-saving. Once the initial phase is over, symptoms usually subside rapidly, even in the absence of therapy.

Yunginger recently reported a list of drugs associated with anaphylactic reactions (47). Of the various life-threatening reactions to drugs in which antibodies have been clearly implicated, penicillin appears to be the most common causative agent. However, even penicillin does not produce anaphylaxis very often. At one time, it was estimated that penicillin-induced anaphylaxis caused up to 500 deaths per year in this country (10); however, greater awareness of the problem, routine skin testing at some centers in high risk groups and possible improvement in penicillin preparations have lowered the present mortality. Serious reactions appear to occur in no more than 1 in 10,000 injections. Non-fatal anaphylactic reactions to penicillin are probably considerably more common than generally recognized. Mild reactions may be undiagnosed unless the patient is examined at regular intervals during the first 30 minutes after administration of the drug. Anaphylactic deaths from oral penicillin are much less common than deaths following parenteral injections of the drug (48), possibly because of the slower absorption, differences in preparations, or destruction of antigen in the intestinal tract (23).

Protein or polysaccharide antigens associated with anaphylaxis include: foreign antisera, allergen extracts, hormones, enzymes, venoms and heparin. Sensitization to foreign proteins is readily produced and may even occur when the difference from the native protein is only a single amino acid or the native protein is aggregated (49).

Non-proteinaceous drugs, other than penicillin, that produce severe acute systemic reactions include opiates (particularly heroin), organic iodides used in radioopaque contrast media, local and general anesthetics, dextran, aspirin, heparin, streptomycin, sulfonamides, clindamycin, nitrofurantoin, sulfites, chemotherapeutic agents, organic mercurials, sulfobromophthalein (BSP), dehydrocholate sodium (Decholin), karaya gum, fluorescein, Congo red, vitamin B_{12}, tetracylines, triphenylmethane dyes, chlorpropamide, and cephalosporins (23, 37, 47, 50–53). However, as discussed below, some of these reactions may not be immunologically mediated. Acute anaphylactic reactions during general anesthesia are difficult to recognize (54). Causative agents include succinylcholine and thiopental. As with penicillin, prior exposure is necessary for a reaction to occur and repeated exposures increase the risk. Not all the reactions associated with drug injections necessarily involve the drugs themselves. Latex used in rubber gloves, syringe barrels and ports for administration of intravenous solutions contains potent antigens which may produce severe reactions (55). Reactions may also occur to chemicals such as ethylene oxide used to sterilize tubing for intravenous infusions and dialysis. Preservatives in drug solutions have also been implicated. For example, sulfites which are widely used as food and drug preservatives have been shown to produce reactions. In one report, six individuals with asthma who had had life-threatening bronchospastic reactions after restaurant meals later showed a similar reaction on double-blind challenge with metabisulfite (56). Sulfites have since been implicated in a variety of reactions to solutions containing sulfite as a preservative (57).

Anaphylactic sensitivity is largely or entirely mediated by IgE antibody. Systemic sensitization is almost always accompanied by reactivity in the skin, and local skin testing provides a convenient and relatively safe means of detecting this particular form of allergy.

IgE antibodies sensitize by attaching to the surface of basophils and mast cells in a reversible reaction involving high affinity receptors. When the antibody molecules are cross-linked by antigen, the cells release histamine, leukotrienes, kinin activator enzymes, heparin, and other components (58). The response probably requires an influx of calcium, as well as alterations in cyclic nucleotides and possibly the formation of labile hydroxylated fatty acids. Complement does not participate in the reaction, in contrast to its critical role in vascular inflammation induced by serum sickness. Some of the mediators of hypersensitivity such as histamine are preformed, whereas others like SRS (leukotrienes C and D) are generated at the time of the stimulus (58, 59).

The mechanism of most acute life-threatening reactions to drugs in human beings is not well established (70). The post mortem changes of acute anaphylaxis usually are not diagnostic of themselves

(60, 61). With the majority of drugs that produce such responses, appropriate immunologic studies have not been carried out. Attempts at retrospective studies such as measurements of plasma histamine have been of limited value because of histamine's short plasma half-life. However, measurements of tryptase (62), a protease secreted by activated mast cells, are potentially useful for samples obtained within several hours. Studies of complement fragments and PGD_2 and its metabolites may also be useful (61). Demonstrating that allergic mediators are increased in body fluids or tissue does not necessarily prove that an immunologic reaction has been involved. As discussed below, some of the reactions may involve activation of complement or nonspecific release of immunologic mediators such as histamine, so that although immunologic sensitization is not involved, the final common pathway is the same as in acute immunologic reactions. Nor are the mediators involved in responses that are definitely anaphylactic, such as those produced by penicillin, clearly elucidated. Histamine has direct effects on smooth muscle tone and vascular permeability and could be responsible for the urticaria, bronchospasm, hypotension, and increased intestinal peristalsis that are part of the syndrome of acute systemic anaphylaxis. Histamine is released in increased amounts in some patients with bee venom induced anaphylaxis (63). However, several other vasoactive substances, bradykinin, proteases, leukotrienes and the prostaglandins, produce similar manifestations and quite conceivably contribute to anaphylactic symptoms (58, 64, 65). Complement and coagulation activation may also be involved as secondary manifestations after the acute mediator release phase is completed (63). The site of mediator formation also is unclear. One might speculate that mast cells in blood vessel walls or circulating basophils are the major sources of the mediators that produce systemic hypotension, whereas mast cells present locally in lung, skin, and other tissues are responsible for the local organ manifestations of acute mediator release.

β-Adrenergic agents such as epinephrine rapidly relieve anaphylactic symptoms. They act on at least two levels by interfering with mediator release and by antagonizing the action of the mediators on end organ receptors such as bronchial smooth muscle. On the basis of studies in rat peritoneal mast cells, it is known that catecholamines exert their effect on histamine release through alterations in intracellular cyclic AMP concentrations (66).

As discussed briefly earlier, antigens that elicit hypersensitivity responses must (in nearly all instances) have multiple combination sites, permitting them to combine with two antibody molecules at the same time, forming a bridge. This multiplicity is also true in the anaphylactic response. Univalent haptens, as free drugs or unconjugated drug metabolites, fail to elicit allergic responses and may even be used to block such responses (15). This finding helps explain why the incidence of anaphylactic or serum sickness reactions to drugs is low. When drug-induced anaphylaxis does occur, the drug almost always has a high degree of chemical reactivity, enabling it to react rapidly with proteins in serum and tissue to form multivalent conjugates. Penicillin has this property, helping explain its unusual propensity to produce anaphylaxis.

Fortunately very few drugs have sufficient protein reactivity to form significant amounts of antigen within the relatively short time required to produce an anaphylactic reaction. Another factor limiting the anaphylactic response is the presence, ordinarily in great excess, of unreacted drug, which inhibits the allergic response, depending on its structural similarity to the actual immunogen (15). In addition, large numbers of IgG antibody molecules may be present that do not bind to the mast cell but compete with cell-bound IgE for antigen. Thus anaphylactic reactions to small molecular weight drugs are unusual for a number of reasons.

However, there is a rare situation in which a univalent hapten elicits rather than inhibits an immediate allergic response. This reversal can occur with haptens, which have large organic substituents, well separated from the haptenic group (37). A possible explanation is that the extra organic group interacts nonspecifically with antibody and other proteins, whereas the haptenic group reacts specifically, leading to an aggregate containing both specific and nonspecific bonds. Under these circumstances bridging between antibody molecules can take place, just as it does with multivalent haptens.

Anaphylaxis also is possible with drugs that readily polymerize or contain macromolecular contaminants. Theoretically, physical aggregation in the form of an insoluble precipitate or micelles may provide a functionally multivalent antigen (23). Nuclear magnetic resonance studies have shown that benzyl penicillin molecules self-associate in aqueous solution, probably because of benzyl side chains (67). Reversible or irreversible reactions of the drug with cell surfaces constitute a possible mechanism for allergic reactivity, as appears to be true in quinidine-induced thrombocytopenia (see below).

3.3.2 SERUM SICKNESS. Serum sickness is another systemic allergic reaction produced by antibodies, in this case, by circulating antibodies complexed to antigen. Among the more common manifestations are fever, rash, lymphadenopathy, arthritis, edema, nephritis, and neuritis. Urticarial and maculopapular rashes are frequent and while usually generalized may be present locally at the site of an earlier injection of antigen. The term was originally applied to foreign serum reactions, but drugs are now the most frequent cause. Drugs that produce serum sickness include the penicillins, the sulfonamides, the thiouracils, diphenylhydantoin, aminosalicylic acid, the cholecystographic dyes, the thiazides, and streptomycin (37, 50, 68).

The common feature of antigens that produce this syndrome is that they remain in the circulation for prolonged periods; thus when antibody first appears, intravascular antigen is still present, permitting the formation of circulating antigen-antibody complexes. The production of serum sickness symptoms by penicillin is due to the drug's ability to conjugate readily to serum proteins *in vivo* without markedly altering their metabolic half-life. This mechanism also presumably applies to other drugs that produce serum sickness, although direct evidence is not available. During the initial course of therapy with a drug, symptoms of serum sickness develop after a latent period of 6 days or more, representing the time needed to synthesize appreciable amounts of antibody (69). On reexposure, symptoms may appear within 12–48 h, representing the time needed for the drug to conjugate to serum proteins, precipitate an anamnestic antibody response (in some cases), and provide a critical concentration of circulating immune complexes. With long-acting penicillin or sulfonamides, symptoms of serum sickness may first appear as long as 3 weeks after the last dose of the drug. Allergic symptoms usually last for a few days to a week; however, in association with diphenylhydantoin, long-acting penicillin or sulfonamide therapy, they may persist for several weeks. If necessary, control of allergic symptoms can be accomplished using a combination of a corticosteroid and antihistamine, especially the former. Residual organ damage is rare.

As in the anaphylactic response, cross-linking of antibody by multivalent antigen is needed to generate and inflammatory response. The antibodies involved appear to be largely of the IgG class. However, in penicillin hypersensitivity, persons with IgE antibodies have an increased likelihood of development of serum sickness, suggesting that IgE antibodies contribute to the response (34). There is evidence that histamine alters the vascular endothelial surface in rabbits, favoring the deposition of immune complexes (69) and providing a possible explanation for the association. Immune complexes containing IgG vary in their ability to mediate inflammation, depending on their IgG antibody subclass representation, overall size, and the ratio of antigen to antibody.

When antibodies are first released into the circulation, complexes formed in great antigen excess are obtained. These complexes do not fix complement and fail to produce allergic symptoms. As more antibody is synthesized, immune complexes of the appropriate size (moderate antigen excess) are formed and complement is activated. Components of complement actually become incorporated into the immune complex in the Fc portion of the antibody molecule. The presence of complement makes the complexes sticky, and they adhere to the walls of small blood vessels. Complement activation also leads to the release of chemotactic peptides, which stimulate leukocyte infiltration into the area. As leukocytes accumulate, they bind and ingest the immune complexes, then release their lysosomal contents extracellularly. Among the substances released are cathepsins, prostaglandins, cytokines, kinin-generating enzymes, superoxide ion, platelet activating factor and other agents that contribute to the response. Vascular damage is more marked in small blood vessels in the kidney, joints, and skin, helping explain the localization of symptoms in these areas. As still more antibody is formed, complexes are formed in antibody excess, complement is no longer fixed and allergic symptoms subside.

3.3.3 SELECTIVE ORGAN DAMAGE. In addition to anaphylaxis and serum sickness, which are systemic allergic drug reactions, immunologic reactions to drugs may result in damage to individual organs. Possible target sites include the liver, skin, kidneys, lungs, heart, muscle, peripheral nerves, and formed elements of the blood (70). Three general mechanisms for organ localization are possible:

1. In generalized allergic reactions such as serum sickness, occasionally the clinical manifestations may be limited to a single organ simulating an organ-directed response as a possible mechanism. Antigen–antibody complexes are formed in the fluid phase, then react with complement and secondarily localize on the cell surface, damaging the cell as an innocent bystander.

2. The drug may react chemically with the tissue, introducing haptenic groups on the cell surface and making the tissue susceptible to antibody- or lymphocyte-mediated cytotoxicity. Direct toxicity due to chemically reactive drug metabolites present locally may contribute to tissue damage.

3. Reactions of organ-specific proteins by hapten may render them immunogenic, resulting in organ-directed autoimmunity. Alternatively the drug may nonspecifically damage cells, releasing sequestered tissue constituents, resulting in an immune response.

In many of the examples of selective organ damage due to allergic drug reactions, it can be assumed that the antigen is formed and conjugated locally in that organ. Subcutaneous immunization with trinitrophenyl groups attached to liver protein in guinea pigs results in generalized sensitization but little or no liver damage. But when the immunogen is introduced into the liver via the mesenteric liver, severe hepatitis is produced (71). This example illustrates the importance of localized allergen in the target organ in producing local reactions. The most effective localization of antigen in terms of rendering the target system susceptible to damage would be the formation of conjugates on the cell surface, giving antibodies or sensitized lymphocytes free access to the antigen (72). The role of antibodies to intracellular constituents is less clear. Although most individuals with antimitochondrial and nuclear antibodies have a degree of continuing tissue damage, the means by which this damage is accomplished has never been clearly elucidated. Antibodies do not readily penetrate into intact cells, and when they do, they are largely catabolized, making the basis for cytotoxicity uncertain. Possibly some sort of synergistic mechanism is operating whereby antibodies to cell surface antigens also are present and cause enough cell damage to enable antibodies with specificity for cytoplasmic or nuclear constituents to enter the cell. Also possible is the issue that secreted antigens might combine with antibody and complement in the extracellular compartment and damage nearby cells. Once a significant level of cell damage has occurred, a vicious cycle might be set up in which partially damaged cells release additional antigens from their interior. These antigens would combine with antibody, adding new antigen-antibody complexes to those already present. Eventually the cell might become sufficiently permeable to permit free access of antibody to the cell interior and a response of sufficient intensity to destroy the cell. These are all possible mechanisms; however, the reactions that are best understood involve cell surface antigens, particularly those on cells normally present in the peripheral blood.

Hemolytic Anemia. Penicillin-induced hemolytic anemia is an example of an immunodestructive response involving hapten-substituted erythrocytes. It is seen occasionally in individuals receiving high dose penicillin therapy (73, 74). Normal erythrocytes are readily substituted with penicillin derivatives, particularly penicilloyl groups when they are exposed to the drug *in vitro*. At sustained high penicillin blood levels during penicillin treatment for diseases such as bacterial endocarditis, the circulating red cells become substantially substituted with penicillin haptens. Penicillin induces antibodies which react with these red cells. If the right kind of antihapten antibody is present, there is accelerated red cell destruction, probably through the participation of complement. If the bone marrow cannot compensate, anemia develops. The presence of antibody on the surface of the red cell can be demonstrated with anti-immunoglobulin (Coombs) reagents. After the cessation of drug therapy, clinical improvement occurs rapidly, since newly synthesized erythrocytes have not reacted with penicillin and survive normally. Penicillin-induced hemolytic anemia usually occurs as an isolated manifestation of penicillin allergy.

Other pharmacologic agents that produce immune hemolytic anemia include nomifesin, quinine, quinidine, dipyrone, *p*-aminosalicylic acid, mephenytoin, stibophen, cephalothin, Fuadin[R], and phenacetin (37). In some of these responses the mechanism of red cell destruction is probably similar to that in penicillin-induced reactions, but further studies are needed. α-Methyldopa and mefenamic acid produce an autoimmune hemolytic anemia in which the antibodies are directed toward native antigens on the red cell surface and the drugs do not appear to be as involved as haptens in the reaction.

Granulocytopenia. Immunologically mediated granulocytopenia is produced by aminopyrine, phenylbutazone, the sulfonamides, the phenothiazines, the thiouracils, the anticonvulsants, chloramphenicol, tolbutamide, and many other drugs (75, 76). Often the leukopenia redevelops rapidly after the drug is readministered, indicating peripheral destruction of leukocytes. In addition, leukocyte precursors in the bone marrow may be abnormal in number or morphology, suggesting a maturation arrest

or exhaustion of the marrow in face of continuing leukocyte destruction (76). The former possibility is suggested by a well studied case of amidopyrine-induced agranulocytosis. Preincubation of the patient's peripheral leukocytes with their own serum and the drug in combination, inhibited granulocyte colony formation (77), strongly supporting a possible effect at the precursor cell level.

Formerly, amidopyrine was the commonest cause of drug-induced immune agranulocytosis. With decreased usage of this drug, the phenothiazines and thiouracils are probably the major causes of this condition, at least in this country. Following cessation of drug therapy, improvement may be expected within 1–2 weeks, provided death due to infection is forestalled during the interim. As in drug-induced thrombocytopenia, readministration of the drug in low dosage, with recrudescence of agranulocytosis, has been used to substantiate the role of the drug in leukocyte depression.

The involvement of serum antibodies in these reactions is evident from successful passive-transfer (person to person) experiments in which the passive administration of serum or plasma and drug, results in rapid leukocyte destruction. Moeschlin and Wagner (78) found that serum from a patient who had had amidopyrine agranulocytosis and had received a further dose of the drug, 3 h previously, produced acute agranulocytosis in two normal recipients. Agglutination of normal leukocytes has been demonstrated in the presence of the drug in the sera of a number of patients with amidopyrine and sulfonamide agranulocytosis, as well as in scattered instances involving other drugs. Usually, however, the patient's serum is not effective unless the drug was readministered to the patient within several hours before the sample was taken, presumably because of a requirement for metabolic processing of the drug before it can react with antibody.

The supposition of the immune nature of

granulocytopenic reactions to antithyroid agents such as propylthiouracil and methimazole is supported by a preliminary report that cellular immunity to these drugs was present in 5 of 6 patients with reactions 2 months to 10 years previously (79).

Thrombocytopenia. The most common causes of immunologically mediated thrombocytopenia are quinine, quinidine, meprobamate, chlorothiazide, the thiouracils, chloramphenicol, and the sulfonamides; however, a variety of other drugs also produce this complication (80). In the past, allylisopropylacetylcarbamide (Sedormid) has been an important cause (37, 81). Not surprisingly, bleeding is the most important symptom, although rash, fever, and other manifestations of allergy can occur. In sensitized persons who are challenged with the drug, there is a rapid fall in blood platelets within minutes to hours after initial exposure. Manifestations of bleeding may be preceded by fever and chills. Less commonly, thrombocytopenia does not recur until therapeutic quantities of the drug have been given for at least several days (81). In many subjects the rapidity of the fall of the platelet count following drug readministration is consistent with accelerated destruction of platelets in the peripheral circulation, as opposed to decreased synthesis and release of platelets from the bone marrow; the latter may also occur to a limited extent.

The immunologic nature of the reaction has been demonstrated both by passive transfer and by *in vitro* studies, primarily in thrombocytopenia produced by Sedormid, quinine, and quinidine (81, 82). The sera of affected patients contain antibodies that produce platelet lysis or agglutination, depending on whether complement is present. Altered platelet release reactions or delayed clot retraction may also be seen (81). The drug as well as the antibody must be present for these changes to occur, indicating that the specificity of the antibody is directed toward the drug or the drug-platelet complex rather than the platelet

per se. Most of the antibodies that have been characterized are members of the IgG class. In quinidine sensitivity the cells may be made susceptible to injury by a reversible reaction of the drug with platelets (60). Quinidine has been shown to bind to platelets and affect their susceptibility to aggregation. It is assumed that a similar combination between antibody and the hapten-platelet complex takes place *in vivo*, rendering platelets unusually susceptible to complement-mediated lysis or phagocytosis.

As noted earlier, a sulfate-containing metabolite of acetaminophen has been reported to be responsible for sensitization in a patient with thrombocytopenia induced by the drug, as evidenced by the ability of the sulfate to sensitize normal platelets to the patient's serum *in vivo*. However, this conclusion should be regarded as provisional because it was not shown that platelets from human subjects taking the drug actually contained this particular metabolite on their surface, as might be expected if this were the basis for sensitization *in vivo*.

The pathogenesis of many of these reactions remains controversial. Most drugs, inducing antibodies that destroy granulocytes, red cells or platelets, affect one of the cell types selectively. *In vitro* reactions typically require that the drug be present, however, in contrast to penicillin-induced hemolytic anemias, the sensitization of the cell is reversible by washing and the presence of excess hapten does not block the reaction (39, 84). Sera from individuals with hemolytic anemia may contain antibodies to surface proteins such as Rh, whereas with thrombocytopenia, antibodies to various platelet glycoproteins may be seen. One might speculate that the drug is interacting with cell surface proteins, altering their conformation and converting them to autoantigens. If this interaction is true, it is surprising that there is so much inconsistency in the target protein in affected individuals. The drug may be inducing an antihapten response in the usual way by conjugation with nontarget cell proteins and once having done so, acting as a carrier to induce responsiveness to a target cell protein. Conceivably, a combinatorial antigenic determinant contributed both by the drug and the target protein, is involved. Perhaps the drug is sequestered in a hydrophobic pocket of the protein and remains there as the protein is processed and presented to T cells, even though there is not a covalent bond between the two.

Immunologically-mediated destruction of leukocytes, erythrocytes, and platelets must be distinguished from direct cytotoxicity resulting in diminution of cell formation or life span. Special problems in interpretation arise with inherited abnormalities of metabolism in which otherwise unimportant enzymatic defects render a portion of the population susceptible to certain drugs. One example is congenital glucose-6-phosphate dehydrogenase deficiency, which is seen in 15% of African-Americans in this country. In this condition, the administration of analgesics, antimalarials, sulfonamides, and a variety of other agents produces an acute hemolytic anemia. Considering the various cytotoxic drugs now being used in the chemotherapy of malignancy and autoimmune disease, many more cases of drug-induced granulocytopenia, anemia, or thrombocytopenia are due to direct cytotoxicity than to an immune mechanism.

Dermatitis. Drugs produce virtually every known cutaneous reaction, including petechial, maculopapular, bullous, nodular, eczematous, urticarial, erythematous, fixed, lytic, and photosensitive eruptions. The appearance of an eruption generally is not sufficiently characteristic to implicate one particular drug or to distinguish a drug-induced eruption from dermatitis due to other causes. Many drugs (e.g., penicillin and the sulfonamides) are capable of producing a variety of cutaneous lesions. Cutaneous manifestations due to a given drug may change in character from day to day, sometimes beginning as an insignificant maculopapular eruption and progressing to a hemorrhagic or exfoliative lesion if exposure to the drug is continued or the drug readministered. Some drugs produce cutaneous changes that are primarily of only one or two types and may be sufficiently distinctive to suggest the diagnosis. Examples include the acneiform and bullous eruptions produced by iodides and bromides, and fixed drug eruptions due to phenolphthalein and other drugs (86). There are two mechanisms of photosensitive drug reaction—phototoxicity, which occurs on first exposure when adequate amounts of light and drug are present, and photoallergy, which involves an allergic response to a hapten produced by light.

The occurrence of dermatitis in a patient receiving a pharmacologic agent should always raise the possibility of drug allergy. Manifestations in the skin frequently accompany visceral drug reactions and may provide a valuable clue to the diagnosis. Involvement of the skin also frequently occurs as an isolated manifestation.

3.4 Drug Reactions Suspected to be Allergic

Hepatitis. The role of allergy in drug-induced inflammation of the liver, kidney, lungs, and small blood vessels is not well-delineated. Very frequently some form of direct toxicity appears to be involved, as suggested by a high reaction incidence, rapid induction of symptoms in the absence of known previous exposure, a more or less consistent dose dependency, and an inability to demonstrate marked fluctuations in sensitivity in serial studies of the same individual. In most forms of drug-induced hepatic toxicity, for example, some form of direct cellular damage is probably involved. On the other hand, some drugs probably do produce hepatic damage by an immune mechanism. In hepatitis induced by anticonvulsants, aminosalicylates, sulfonamides, and phenothiazines, there is frequently fever, skin rash, eosinophilia, leukopenia, infiltration of the liver with eosinophils, lymphocytes, or plasmacytes, lymphadenopathy, and recrudescence of symptoms on reexposure to low doses of the drug (87–90). Moreover, hepatic damage may be completely absent in other patients receiving the drug; the onset of hepatitis on initial exposure is delayed (suggesting a period needed for sensitization); and some individuals who have previously failed to tolerate the drug can take the drug in full dosage at later times. These features all suggest an allergic reaction. Extrahepatic manifestations are present though less frequently in hepatic reactions to halothane, methoxyflurane, phenylbutazone, zoxazolamine, iproniazid, indomethacin, isoniazid, chlorpropamide, erythromycin estolate, methyldopa (90), allopurinol, nitrofurantoins and oxyphenisatin, raising the possibility that allergy is involved in some of these reactions as well. Halothane reactions are typically associated with fever and the risk is markedly increased if the drug is used repeatedly over a several month period, strongly suggesting an immune ethiology.

Direct evidence for an immunologic reaction in most forms of drug-induced liver disease is either limited or lacking entirely, but this lack of evidence is probably partly because of limitations in the data. A number of laboratories have reported that lymphocytes from patients with hepatitis induced by isoniazid, aminosalicylate, or halothane are stimulated by the appropriate drug in vitro (91, 92). Although the responses are small, the evidence with isoniazid and p-aminosalicylate is good enough to support an argument in favor of an allergic etiology. Reported responses in vitro with halothane initially were controversial because of a number of inconclusive or negative studies (93–95). However, there is now rather convincing

evidence that halothane induced hepatitis in humans is due to an oxidative trifluoracetyl metabolite acting as a hapten (96, 97). Microsomes from rats treated with halothane in vivo readily produce the metabolite which in turn rapidly reacts with protein. Hepatic proteins substituted with the hapten were recognized by antibodies in the sera of individuals who have had clinically significant halothane reactions but not sera where no reaction had occurred. Interestingly, the antibody specificities were apparently directed toward proteins carrying the hapten as well as the hapten itself. This occurrence is probably due in part to the small size of the hapten which leaves a portion of antibody combining region available to react with amino acid residues. Studies with 2, 4 dinitrophenyl substituted (DNP) polypeptides have shown that highly purified anti-DNP antibodies may also bind to adjacent amino acid residues on the peptides (98). The dual specificities for halothane and hepatic proteins may help to target the liver as the site of allergic inflammation. In vitro studies have shown that diphenylhydantoin can be converted by microsomes into a chemically reactive metabolite, probably an amine oxide by an arylhydrocarbon inducible cytochrome P450 enzyme (99). As discussed below, evidence is available that oxidative enzymes in the liver or leukocytes are capable of converting hydralazine and procainamide to reactive metabolites (97).

Evidence for serum antibody responses to other hepatotoxic drugs is largely lacking, although lymphocyte transformation responses are sometimes seen (see below). Even when an allergic reaction can be strongly suspected on circumstantial or direct immunologic grounds, the structure of the antigenic determinants is not known, and the reason for the localization of allergic manifestations to the liver is not elucidated (70). A number of possible mechanisms might be considered; for example, in view of the importance of the liver microsomal cytochrome P-450 system in the oxidative degradation of drugs (100), one might suspect that antigen activation could occur through oxidized drug metabolites. Another enzyme that might be involved in drug reactions with proteins is transglutaminase, which has been shown to catalyze the conjugation of isoniazid through its hydrazide group to protein *in vitro* (101). Other drugs bearing free amino or hydrazine groups such as hydralazine and p-aminosalicylic acid probably undergo the same reaction.

Vasculitis. In patients with serum sickness, drug fever, drug-induced lupus erythematosus, and drug-induced syndromes with damage to visceral organs, inflammation of small blood vessels often occurs (102). Pathologically, the vascular changes are usually classified as hypersensitivity vasculitis, polyarteritis nodosa, or lymphocytic vasculitis, although patterns simulating temporal arteritis (103) or allergic granulomatosis have been reported in response to sulfonamides. The damage is predominantly in the smaller vessels and ranges in degree from mild cellular infiltration to acute necrosis (104). Mild vasculitis such as that seen in serum sickness may not produce local symptoms or gross pathological changes. When severe inflammatory changes and necrosis are present, vessels in many organs are usually involved, particularly those in the skin and kidneys. Apart from petechial skin lesions, proteinuria, hematuria, and manifestations of renal failure, symptoms often include fever, gastrointestinal bleeding, dermatitis, arthralgia, and edema, and less frequently myositis, coronary arteritis, and pneumonitis (104–106). Death is due primarily to renal failure.

It is important to consider drug allergy in any form of acute or chronic vasculitis, but even when drugs have been used, their role in the vasculitis may not be completely clear. A history compatible with drug allergy has been obtained in seven of 30 patients with pathological changes of "allergic vasculitis" studied by McCombs et al. (105). The drugs most frequently suspected to cause vasculitis are the penicillins, the sulfonamides, the promazines, the hydantoins, thiouracil, the tetracyclines, the thiazides, quinidine, phenylbutazone, busulfan, iproniazid, allopurinol, the iodides, and methamphetamine. At least some of the drugs that cause acute vasculitis appear to be capable of causing a more chronic form of vascular inflammation, provided drug administration is continued for many weeks or more; examples include hydralazine and the thiouracils (107, 108).

In one patient with arteritis during propylthiouracil therapy, an exacerbation of symptoms followed readministration of the drug on three separate occasions leaving no doubt about the causative role of the drug (108). However, when the vessel involvement is chronic and drug exposure has been limited rather than continuous, the role of drug allergy becomes open to serious question. There is no experimental evidence that a short exposure to an antigen can produce a chronic vasculitis in which fresh lesions continue to appear many months after the exogenous source of antigen has been withdrawn. On at least three occasions, an unsuccessful attempt has been made to implicate penicillin allergy in patients with chronic vasculitis and a history of exposure to penicillin at or near the onset of the illness. Possibly, the exposure to penicillin has been coincidental in these cases. One established cause of polyarteritis is infection with hepatitis B antigen, which may help explain the increased incidence of vasculitis associated with amphetamine abuse (87).

Nephritis. Most examples of drug-induced renal disease appear to be on a direct toxic basis. Even drugs such as cephalothins, which do produce immunologically mediated renal disease, also damage the kidney by direct toxicity, sometimes making interpretation difficult.

Because antigen-antibody complexes localize nonspecifically in the glomerulus, the most common allergic drug reaction in the kidney is serum sickness. Although proteinuria, microscopic hematuria, and alterations in renal function do occur; however, they are usually mild and subside completely once treatment is stopped. More severe glomerular involvement, apparently on an immunologic basis, occurs in association with drug induced generalized vasculitis, but this effect is a rare complication of drug therapy. A variety of drugs, most notably penicilamine, penicillin, captopril, organic mercurials, gold, and tridione, have been reported to cause the nephrotic syndrome, again presumably on an immune basis (70, 109). The characteristic pathologic change is a membranous glomerulopathy. A similar condition can be induced experimentally in appropriate rat strains (110) by injections of mercuric chloride. In this animal model, inflammation is associated with the local accumulation of antibodies to laminin, a connective tissue protein. The mercurial may be reacting directly with laminin and by altering its structure breaking immune tolerance to the protein. Renal lesions produced by penicillin and penicillamine have been shown by immunofluorescence to contain IgG and complement, strongly suggesting an immune etiology (109). Drug-induced membranous nephritis in humans is frequently associated with the HLA-DR3 antigen phenotype, consistent with an immune pathogenesis (110).

Drugs also produce interstitial inflammation of the kidney. Penicillin-induced interstitial nephritis has been suggested as a possible example of cellular or humoral immunity involving this organ (111, 112). This nephritis is a rare complication of high dose penicillin (particularly methicillin) or cephalothin therapy. Rash, fever, and eosinophilia are sometimes present, raising the possibility of allergy. The condition is characterized by increasing renal dysfunction with proteinemia, which may progress to full-blown renal failure and death if the condition is not recognized and the drug is withdrawn.

Immunopathological studies suggesting an immunologic basis for this disorder have been reported (111, 112). Pathologically, there has been infiltration of interstitial and tubular areas of the kidney with mononuclear cells, changes similar to those seen in cellular immune responses in other organs. Penicillin antigens, immunoglobulin, and complement have been demonstrated by immunofluorescence on the surface of renal tubular cells of affected individuals. In addition, the serum of one patient contained antibodies reactive with tubular basement membrane in a normal kidney that had not been exposed to penicillin (112). The presence of the antitubular basement antibodies has suggested a drug-induced autoimmune reaction in which renal tubular cells exposed to high concentrations of penicillin have become chemically altered and release their tubular antigens, resulting in an autoimmune response and local tissue damage (70).

Drug-induced interstitial nephritis has also been observed in conjunction with sulfonamides, nonsteroidal antiinflammatory agents, furosemide, cimetidine or thiazide therapy (112, 113), but there is no convincing evidence for drug allergy, and even the association itself can be questioned (70). Whether drug allergy is involved in the nephritis associated with analgesic abuse remains to be established. A major culprit is phenacetin (114), and at least two metabolites of phenacetin, p-phenetidine and 2-OH-p-phenetidine, are immunogenic in guinea pigs, as indicated by delayed skin reactions and lymphocyte stimulation responses (115). But it remains to be demonstrated convincingly that chronic nephritis can be produced by phenacetin or its metabolites in experimental animals or that human beings with renal damage are allergic to the drug.

Antinuclear Antibodies and Lupus-like Syndromes. A clinical syndrome resembling systemic lupus erythematosus (SLE) has been observed during treatment with hydralazine, procainamide (116–118), isoniazid, oral contraceptive pills, griseofulvin, methyldopa, tetracycline, thiouracil, antimalarials, practolol, and anticonvulsant agents (119–121).

The sera of patients with this syndrome contains antinuclear antibodies, occasionally with a positive lupus erythematosus cell reaction as well (119). Clinical manifestations include polyarthritis, serositis, fever, lymphadenopathy, dermatitis, and leukopenia. A common feature of drug-induced lupus is that the drugs involved had been used over at least 6–8 weeks before symptoms appeared. As a rule the symptoms subside slowly after the drug is withdrawn. Not infrequently antinuclear antibodies are observed in the absence of overt clinical symptoms.

The mechanism of the antinuclear antibody production is not well understood. Not everyone is in agreement, but it seems likely that at least some of these drugs produce a lupus-like syndrome *de novo* rather than activating latent SLE:

1. Hydralazine and isoniazid produce immunologic and pathologic changes resembling SLE in laboratory animals (122).
2. More than 50% of persons receiving procainamide in substantial dosage for several months or more develop clinical or laboratory manifestations of lupus (118, 123).
3. The clinical patterns differ in that in lupus induced by hydralazine and procainamide involvement of males is more frequent, and anemia, leukopenia, and nervous system, cutaneous, and renal involvement are less frequent than in the spontaneously occurring disease (124, 125).
4. In a prospective study of patients going on procainamide therapy, most of the individuals developing antinuclear antibodies during treatment had had negative serological reactions originally (126).
5. The specificity of the antibodies differs in that antibodies reacting with native (double-stranded DNA) are much more frequent in spontaneous than in drug-induced SLE. Moreover, antibodies in drug-induced SLE are especially likely to react with histones.

Just how the antinuclear antibodies are produced remains to be elucidated. Most of the drugs convincingly associated with drug-induced lupus have a hydrazine or arylamine functional group. Patients with hydralazine-induced lupus have antibodies that react with diazotized hydralazine, coupled to red cells, and their lymphocytes undergo a weak but possibly significant response in the presence of the drug, suggesting that hydralazine allergy is present (124). Hydralazine is probably capable of affecting DNA structure *in vitro* (118), and the photochemical reaction of DNA with procainamide has been reported to make it more antigenic than native or photoxidized DNA (127), raising the possibility that these drugs react with and antigenically alter DNA. As mentioned briefly earlier, conceivably the usual relationship between the immunologic carrier and the hapten is reversed in this situation. If both hapten protein and hapten DNA conjugates were formed, the more immunogenic protein conjugates might be expected to initiate an immune response. As antibodies to the hapten developed, the hapten might then serve as an immunogenic carrier favoring the development of an immune response to the normally poorly immunogenic DNA. Alternatively, since a number of the drugs that produce lupus-like syndromes are nitrogen-containing compounds with one or two benzene rings, antibodies formed in response to one of these drugs might fortuitously cross-react with one or more of the nucleic acid bases in DNA (97, 128). In support of the second possibility, conjugates of hydralazine (or a hydralazine metabolite) to serum albumin induced antibodies in rabbits that react with DNA as well as to the hapten (129). Presumably conjugation to DNA does not occur in this situation. Slow acetylators are more susceptible to hydralazine induced SLE (128). Slow acetylators metabolize less of the drug by acetylation but compensate by oxidizing a greater portion of the drug.

The metabolic activation of procainamide and hydralazine has been studied *in vitro* (97, 130, 131). Hydralazine is oxidized to a chemically reactive intermediate by rat liver microsomes. Procainamide is converted to hydroxylamine and nitroso derivatives by rat and human hepatic microsomal P-450 enzymes in the presence of NADPH. However, when rat livers were perfused with procainamide these metabolites could not be detected in the perfusate. On the other hand, activated monocytes and neutrophils both have produced these metabolites suggesting that metabolic conversion can occur outside the liver in lymphoid tissues. The activity in monocytes is particularly interesting in view of their role as antigen presenting cells. Hydralazine is also metabolized by activated monocytes and neutrophils. Myeloperoxidase is probably the major enzyme involved in metabolizing these drugs in leukocytes. Dapsone, sulfonamides, isoniazid, carbamazepine, chloramphenicol, propylthiouracil and phenytoin also are metabolized by these cells.

A related but apparently distinct clinical syndrome is produced by venocuran, which is a mixture of pharmacologically active substances used in the treatment of venous diseases in Europe (132). Affected individuals develop symptoms very similar to those in drug-induced lupus, including fever, myalgia, arthralgia, pleuritis, and pericarditis, but the serum contains antimitochondrial rather than antinuclear antibodies.

Another very interesting reaction to a drug simulating a spontaneously occurring connective tissue disorder has been seen in response to practolol, which for a brief period, was in clinical use as a selective β-blocking agent (133). In addition to cutaneous and musculoskeletal manifestations and a lupus-like syndrome, some of the affected individuals have developed keratoconjunctival manifestations similar to those seen in Sjogren's syndrome, an autoimmune disorder affecting the eyes, salivary glands, and joints. A portion also has had antinuclear antibodies in their sera, providing a possible link with drug-induced lupus. Metabolic studies in hamsters have shown that a metabolite of practolol formed by liver microsomes could bind irreversibly to proteins (134). Antibodies in the sera of affected patients bound to metabolites produced in an *in vitro* mixed function oxygenase system (135).

Although Symmers (106) has stated that there is no evidence that polymyositis is caused by drug allergy, in several patients observed personally there was a very suggestive relationship between penicillin therapy and onset of this disease. No attempt was made, however, to produce an exacerbation of symptoms by readministration of penicillin. Several patients have been described in whom thrombotic thrombocytopenic purpura appeared to be caused by drug allergy, but in no instance was a causal relationship established. A more convincing relationship has existed between penicillamine treatment and myasthenia gravis (136).

Pneumonitis. The role of allergy in most forms of drug-induced pulmonary disease is unclear. Eosinophilic pneumonitis, apparently on an allergic basis, has been reported in response to sulfonamides, aminosalicylic acid, penicillin, cromoglycate, mephenesin, and azathioprine (102). Hilar adenopathy and acute asthmatic reactions may also be caused by drug allergy. A role for allergy in pulmonary reactions to nitrofurantoin also seems very possible, although further studies are needed. Nitrofurantoin produces acute inflammation of the lung with fever, cough, diffuse pulmonary infiltration of an edematous nature, pleural effusion, hilar adenopathy, or asthma (137, 138). Symptomatic improvement usually occurs a few hours to days after withdrawal of the drug. An allergic etiology is suggested by the frequent presence of eosinophilia, rash, and rapid recurrence of symptoms after rechallenge with the drug. In addition, there are several reports of lymphocyte responses to the drug *in vitro*. Nitrofurantoin has also been reported to produce chronic pulmonary fibrosis.

Fibrotic reactions to busulfan, methotrexate, and cyclophosphamide probably have a nonallergic basis. Several cases of diffuse alveolitis or full-blown Goodpasture's syndrome with accompanying glomerulonephritis have been reported in patients receiving penicillamine (139). Allergy has been suspected, but more studies are needed.

3.5 Drug Reactions Simulating Allergy

Many acute life-threatening reactions to drugs have an uncertain etiology. Although the possibility of acute anaphylaxis is difficult to exclude, most reactions of this kind probably occur on a nonallergic basis. Some may be due to the nonspecific release of vasoactive amines or some other form of pharmacologic hypersensitivity. Iodinated dyes and opiates release histamine nonspecifically by a direct effect on rat mast cells, although in each case relatively high concentrations of the drug are required (140, 141). Another possible cause of iodinated dye reactions is activation of complement (142–145). This might result in the formation of histamine-releasing peptides (anaphylatoxins) or other peptides exerting

direct effects on blood vessels. The coagulation, fibrolytic and kinin systems also may be activated by dye infusions. One important factor in reactions to contrast agents may be their hypertonicity. Newer more polar and less hypertonic agents give a considerately lower frequency of serious reactions. While more expensive, the newer agents are being used increasingly, particularly in allergic individuals in whom the risk of a severe reaction is increased. Premedication with antiallergic medications also reduces the frequency of reactions.

In large urban areas in this country acute pulmonary edema due to the intravenous or intranasal demonstration of heroin and its congeners has become an important cause of death in young adults and teenagers (146, 147). The possibility of an anaphylactic mechanism is suggested by the rapidity of the response and the presence of circulating antibodies to morphine in the serum of addicts and laboratory animals repeatedly injected with the drug (148). However, the clinical picture is mainly one of acute respiratory depression and pulmonary edema rather than acute circulatory failure or bronchospasm, making the role of allergy in the reaction unlikely. Moreover, the reaction is seen during an initial exposure to the drug, and the intravenous injection of heroin or morphine has been reported to increase blood histamine levels in immunized dogs (149), suggesting the nonspecific release of pharmacologic mediators of hypersensitivity. Apparently no one has carefully studied morphine addicts for IgE-mediated allergy to opiates.

In susceptible individuals, aspirin produces rhinitis, acute bronchospasm, urticaria, or even very rarely sudden death. A few of these reactions appear to represent IgE-mediated reactions to aspiroyl groups, probably attributable to the presence of aspiroyl anhydrides in commercial aspirin (150). However, the majority are probably due to an ability of aspirin to nonspecifically release histamine and other pharmacological mediators of immediate hypersensitivity including leukotrienes. Some individuals with aspirin sensitivity have a history of vasomotor rhinitis and asthma, often present for many years before difficulties with aspirin are identified (151). When individuals with adult onset idiopathic asthma who do not have known aspirin sensitivity are challenged with aspirin, approximately 10% experience an acute exacerbation of their respiratory symptoms (152). When sinusitis and nasal polyps are present, aspirin intolerance is more frequent (153). Organic chemicals such as tartrazine, a yellow dye used as a food and drug additive, and other nonsteroidal anti-inflammatory agents (antipyrine, mefenamic acid, or indomethacin), which do not resemble aspirin structurally, also cause reactions in these patients (152). Most of these agents interfere with prostaglandin biosynthesis, suggesting a possible basis for their action. With inhibition of the cyclooxygenase pathway more arachidonic acid may be available for the lipoxygenase pathway and indeed evidence is emerging that 5-lipoxygenase metabolites are involved in the reaction (154). An occasional individual with aspirin sensitivity reports a family history of a similar condition, apparently inherited as a Mendelian recessive characteristic (155). Aspirin also causes symptomatic exacerbations in individuals with urticaria, regardless of the underlying cause. As a rule, respiratory symptoms are absent, indicating a site or possibly even a mechanism of action different from that associated with aspirin-sensitive asthma.

An inhibitor of coagulation factor VIII has been described in association with penicillin therapy (156). The inhibitor is an immunoglobulin, suggesting that it is an antibody with specificity either for factor VIII alone or for both factor VIII and penicillin. The second possibility is suggested by a recent study in which soluble penicillin blocked the anti-factor VIII activity of the immunoglobulin, whereas insolubilized penicillin removed it entirely, as might be expected for an antipenicillin antibody with fortuitous cross-reactivity for factor VIII (156). However, further investigation is needed, since in an earlier study penicillin was weakly inhibitory at best (157).

Another rare but interesting drug reaction for which an immunologic origin has been suggested is the lymphadenopathy (158) associated with anticonvulsant therapy in association with long-term diphenylhydantoin or mephenytoin therapy or, less commonly, with other drugs. The reaction ranges from a transient serum sickness type of response to a chronic lymphoproliferative syndrome resembling a lymphoma. Lymphoproliferation is often associated with more transient symptoms suggestive of allergy. Rarely, the lymphoid involvement progresses even after the drug is withdrawn (159), and death due to lymphoma can occur. Whether this type of death represents the fortuitous development of a lymphoma during drug therapy, the failure of normal negative feedback mechanism during an intense immune stimulus, or an interference of the drugs with normal immunologic surveillance remains to be established (160). Since diphenylhydantoin has been reported to suppress lymphocyte transformation, it conceivably is interfering with immunoprotective mechanisms against malignancy (161). A possibly related clinical syndrome is angioimmunoblastic lymphadenapathy which is characterized clinically by hyperglobulinemia, lymphadenopathy, splenomegaly, hepatomegaly, and autoimmune hemolytic anemia, and pathologically, by immunoblastic infiltration and neovasculation (162). Drugs appear to be a precipitating factor in some individuals with this condition. This condition may start as an ordinary allergic drug reaction in which normal regulatory mechanisms for controlling the reaction fail to function properly. Overproduction of interleukin 6, a lymphokine that produces fever and stimulates B cell growth and differentiation to plasma cells, may be important in the pathogenesis of this condition (163).

The role of allergy in drug-induced aplastic anemia is also unclear. In the past, the commonest cause of drug-induced aplastic anemia was chloramphenicol. Other drugs producing this complication are various sulfonamides, gold, quinacrine (50), phenylbutazone, anticonvulsants, various cytotoxic agents and a variety of organic solvents including benzene and materials used as insecticides and pesticides (75). Chloramphenicol, the principal causative agent, may produce bone marrow hypoplasia when given in large doses, but there is some doubt that this effect is relevant to blood changes seen in some patients receiving much smaller doses. Antibodies have been produced to reduced chloramphenicol by binding it in azo linkage to proteins and immunizing animals (164), but there is no convincing evidence that similar antibodies are produced under natural conditions of exposure to the unconjugated drug in humans. Other than the observation that aplasia to chloramphenicol usually occurs in a patient who has been exposed to the drug on multiple occasions, there is little to suggest allergy. Nonetheless, toxic metabolites of chloramphenicol produced by metabolic activation may well be involved as inhibitors of stem cells in this condition, so sharing of metabolic pathways with those involved in drug allergy appears possible.

Drugs may affect the immune system by altering immune regulation rather than by participating directly in allergic reactions. Many immunoregulatory drugs have been identified and some of them are used therapeutically for this purpose. Drugs not normally thought of as immunoregulatory agents may act in this manner. For example, while the mechanism is unknown, chronic treatment with dilantin is sometimes associated with decreased IgA production. The selectivity of the effect and its persistence after the drug is withdrawn suggest that a permanent regulatory disorder has been induced perhaps through effects of the drug on B cell precursors. Penicillamine is another immunogenic drug which has immunomodulatory activities (128). Hydrazine and other strong nucleophiles may act in part by inactivating complement protein C4 (a susceptible esterase) reducing clearance of immune complexes and exacerbating immune complex diseases. Captopril, an angiotensin-converting enzyme inhibitor produces a maculopapular rash that appears to be dose-related. In view of its kininase activity, the rash is probably often due to reduced kinin degradation (120A) although allergy also can occur.

Underlying diseases and concurrent drug therapy may affect allergic drug reactions. There are striking increases in the frequency of reactions to sulfonamide (and other drugs) in AIDS, to ampicillin in infectious mononucleosis, and to gold (and other drugs) in lupus (63, 70). The predilection to drug reactions in AIDS is due to their increased use and the immunodysregulation associated with HIV infection of T cells. Intestinal, liver and renal diseases affecting drug absorption, metabolism, excretion and protein binding obviously may alter the frequency of drug reactions. By inducing or suppressing enzyme systems metabolizing drugs or competing with drug transport pathways, drugs affect one another's metabolism and the likelihood of allergy. If activation of leukocytes is important in some forms of drug allergy as suggested by studies of procainamide and hydralazine, stimulation of the immune system by infection or immunization may affect the likelihood of a response. Allergic drug reactions are commonly thought to be less frequent in young children or elderly patients but this was not verified in a cooperative study on cutaneous reactions (166).

4 IMMUNOLOGIC ASSAYS FOR DRUG ALLERGY

Despite certain characteristic pathological, clinical, and epidemiologic features, the only definitive way of proving that the reaction to a drug is immunologic is to demonstrate that there is altered immunologic reactivity. This research requires systematic immunologic studies. Although a good deal is known about the mechanism of drug allergy, practical immunologic detection systems rarely are available. This unavailability is due not to a lack of suitable immunological methods but to a general scarcity of information on responsible antigenic determinants in drug allergy. First, there is no assurance that the drug itself will closely resemble the actual antigenic determinant. Moreover, many immunologic assay systems require that the candidate haptens be identified and rendered multivalent by attachment to soluble or insoluble macromolecular carriers before one can realistically expect to obtain a positive response. Only in penicillin hypersensitivity is detailed information available both about the mechanism of formation of antigen and the most suitable assay systems for analysis, and even here, there are still significant gaps. Obviously much more work is needed in the identification of antigenic determinants in drug allergy before reliable assays can be developed.

In the meantime, fragmentary evidence that a drug might be producing an immune response based on studies in a single immunologic assay system in a limited number of patients or animals should be interpreted with caution. Obviously a drug might produce an immune response as an ancillary manifestation when the actual cause of the tissue damage has been a somewhat more direct form of toxicity.

One must show not only that there are immunologic alterations but also that there is a reasonably consistent relationship between altered immunological reactivity and symptoms. And since the immune process is a dynamic one changing with time after initiation of the immune response, it can not be assumed that retrospective testing will always be successful. In addition, even during symptoms of hypersensitivity there may be phases of the response in which altered immunologic reactivity is not demonstrable. For example, in human penicillin hypersensitivity during serum sickness type responses, it is frequently not possible to demonstrate positive immediate skin reactions, probably because the antigen-antibody complexes evolved in the production of allergic tissue damage are already formed and there is no available additional antibody for combination with antigen. Despite these limitations, carefully conducted immunologic studies are crucial in obtaining a better understanding of drug allergy.

4.1 Assays for Humoral Immunity

Demonstration of IgE antibodies is prima facie evidence for anaphylactic sensitivity and a substantial risk of serious reactions if the drug is readministered. Skin testing for immediate hypersensitivity has been the most widely used clinical approach to the demonstration of IgE antibodies both in humans and in experimental animals. Test materials that may be used for immediate skin testing include the drug itself, a suspected reactive metabolite of the drug, or a conjugate containing the suspected determinant itself attached at multiple sites to a protein or polyamino acid carrier by previous reaction *in vitro*.

Since IgE antibodies circulate in low concentrations, they are difficult to detect in serum by direct binding assays. The most successful approach has been to attach the antigen to an insoluble particle, react the particle with the serum under evaluation, and quantitate the amount of IgE antibody taken up by the particle with a labeled second antibody specific for human IgE (167). IgG, IgM, and other antibodies also bind to the antigen on the particle but do not react with the anti-IgE antibody. Serum assays for IgE antibodies give comparable results to direct skin testing.

In general hemagglutination, in which red cells substituted with haptenic groups are clumped by antihapten antibody, is a sensitive detection system for IgM, IgG, and IgA antibodies. In some hemagglutination system as little as 1 ng of IgM antibody per milliliter of serum can be detected (168). IgG is not detected as readily in routine hemagglutination procedures, but special techniques such as the use of antihuman gamma globulin can be employed to increase the sensitivity of the system. Changes in the hemagglutination titer in the presence of monospecific antibodies to gamma globulins help identify the type of antibodies present. Rigorous controls are required to ensure specificity. Not only should little or no reactivity be demonstrable with control sera, but it should be possible to inhibit hapten-specific hemagglutination reactions by homologous univalent hapten at concentrations in the 1–100 μM range. Inhibition at 10–100 mM concentrations is much less significant and is likely to be either nonspecific or due to trace contaminants in the inhibitor solution.

In radioactive binding measurements involving antibodies (radioimmunoassays), a drug or a suspected antigenic metabolite of a drug may be labeled and evaluated for binding reactivity with the patient's serum. Alternatively, a hapten that is attached to a labeled protein may be used to study binding. Enzymes as well as radioactive markers may be used for labeling. One of the most convenient assay procedures involves the incubation of serum or gamma globulin fraction with radioactive antigen, followed by precipitation of the gamma globulin with ammonium sulfate at 40–50% of saturation. Any molecules of antigen that are bound to the antibody coprecipitate with the gamma globulin and, assuming the free antigen is soluble, and appropriate controls are done, a measure of specific binding activity may be identified. Antihuman immunoglobulins specific for individual immunoglobulin classes may also be used to precipitate the antibody, providing a measure of antibody class distribution. Hapten inhibition of precipitation of radioactivity should be easily demonstrable and can be used to evaluate immunological cross-reactivity. Radioimmunoassays are capable of detecting as little as 1 ng of antibody per milliliter of serum (168), depending in part on antibody affinity and antigen specific activity (9). Unless antigen of high specific activity is available, however, significant levels of serum antibody activity may easily be missed.

Even though IgG and IgM antibodies are relatively easy to measure, it may be much more important, depending on the drug, to determine the IgE antibody titer. In penicillin allergy at least the existence of IgG and IgM antibodies does not necessarily prove that allergic symptoms will be produced on reexposure to the drug. Previous studies suggest that virtually everyone treated with sizable quantities of penicillin develops a serum antibody response, but no more than 5% develop allergic symptoms during a subsequent course of therapy (34). When IgE antibodies are present the risk is much higher, although even here not everyone develops allergic symptoms. Thus an IgM or IgG antibody response indicates that the immune system has been stimulated but does not necessarily establish that the patient is at risk as far as future therapy is concerned. However, for drugs that immunize less frequently, the presence of IgG or IgM antibodies may have greater significance.

4.2 Assays for Cellular Immunity

Another laboratory approach to the diagnosis of drug allergy involves an attempt to stimulate circulating lymphocytes in tissue culture, either with the drug itself or with a multivalent hapten protein conjugate of a metabolite of the drug. What is usually measured is incorporation of radioactive thymidine into intracellular macromolecules, which is considered to be a measure of DNA synthesis. In antigen-stimulated cells, there is a two to tenfold increase in thymidine incorporation after 3–7 days in tissue culture. Lymphocyte stimulation is also accompanied by the appearance of large lymphoblasts and the release of biologically active products of lymphocyte metabolism (lymphokines). Lymphokines are proteins or glycoproteins that modulate immune processes. Their detection can be a useful index of immunologic stimulation since spontaneous production is normally low or absent.

Most of the reported examples of lymphocyte stimulation in drug allergy have involved unconjugated drugs (136). As a rule, a range of drug concentrations have been used and the response is shown to be dose dependent (70, 169). Since all the available evidence indicates that haptens must be multivalent (bound to a macromolecular carrier or cell membrane) to produce a lymphocyte response, it seems possible for some drugs that one or more of the cell types present in the leukocyte suspension is capable of converting the drug to a complete antigen in tissue culture. Studies with hydralazine and procainamide and leukocytes have already been discussed. Moreover, human peripheral blood mononuclear cells have been shown to metabolize benzo-(a)-pyrene, forming many of the same metabolites that are produced in liver (170). A number of drugs have been reported to stimulate lymphocytes under circumstances in which drug allergy is suspected. These include aspirin, cromoglycate, isoniazid, chlorpropamide, gold, nitrofurantoin, p-aminosalicylic acid, halothane, and penicillin (70, 171, 172). As discussed earlier, it may well be that some of the active metabolites involved in sensitization to drugs are actually being formed in the lymph nodes or spleen (169) during immune responses *in vivo*. The most effective approach to demonstrating cellular immunity *in vitro* may be to use preformed microsome or leukocyte drug metabolites in lymphocyte transformation assays (173), not relying on the production of metabolites in the culture.

Cellular immunity may also be evaluated by bioassay by testing for delayed cutaneous sensitivity. The drug may be injected intradermally or may be placed on the surface of the skin as a patch test. The reaction reaches a maximum at 24–48 h and may include erythema, induration, and vesiculation. When the drug is applied on the surface of the skin it may be necessary to find a suitable vehicle to promote its penetration through the outer layers of the epidermis. The quantity of drug used must be carefully titrated to avoid concentrations that nonspecifically irritate normal skin.

In lieu of direct evidence of altered immune reactivity to drugs, evidence that the immune system is activated may be sought using various immunologic markers. However, demonstrating that immune reactivity is increased does not prove that the drug itself is necessarily responsible.

5 PENICILLIN ALLERGY

In addition to its importance medically, penicillin allergy is the most extensively studied and best understood example of human allergy; thus it is discussed in some detail.

The specificity of antibodies formed in penicillin allergy has been studied by immediate and delayed skin testing, hemagglutination inhibition, radioimmunoprecipitation or absorption, histamine release from peripheral blood leukocytes, fluorescence polarization, and bacteriophage neutralization (20, 34, 174, 175). One of the most impressive features of penicillin allergy is the multiplicity of antigenic determinants involved. Virtually everyone who is treated with penicillin develops an immune response to the penicilloyl group, but in addition antibodies are sometimes demonstrable to penicillenate (or its oxidation products), penicillamine, penamaldoyl, penicilloaldehyde, and polymers of 6-aminopenicillanic acid (15, 16, 20, 174, 176, 177). The complexity of the response is not particularly surprising, considering the unusual properties of the penicillin molecule and its ability to rearrange and conjugate to protein in a variety of ways. Moreover, since benzylpenicillin gives rise to at least 10 decomposition products under mild conditions *in vitro* (178), it seems possible that not all of the possible penicillin antigens have been identified (23). Indeed unconjugated penicillin and penicilloic acid occasionally elicit immediate skin responses in individuals in whom allergy to penicilloyl and other known penicillin haptens is not demonstrable: this fact is consistent with the possibility of unrecognized antigenic determinants. All the penicillin determinants that have been identified have the capability of forming covalent bonds with proteins, thus providing additional support for the macromolecular carrier concept of hapten immunization already discussed in detail. Some the penicillin haptens cross-react immunologically with one another; others, like the penicillinate molecule, appear to represent entirely distinct antigenic determinants.

In the attachment of penicilloyl groups to proteins, the β-lactam ring of the penicillin is opened and its carbonyl moiety forms an amide linkage with amino groups on the protein. There are two possible mechanisms for formation of protein-bound

penicilloyl groups: (1) direct aminolysis of penicillin by the protein, and (2) rearrangement of penicillin to penicillenic acid, a highly reactive acid anhydride, which then reacts rapidly with protein amino and sulfhydryl groups (37). In the penicillenate rearrangement, a mixture of penicilloyl diastereoisomers is formed, whereas in the direct aminolysis reaction D-α-configuration of the parent penicillin is retained.

Initially, the penicillenate rearrangement was presumed to be the principal pathway by which protein-bound penicilloyl was formed *in vivo*. This view was apparently supported both by the presence of penicillenate in therapeutic preparations of penicillin and by its high level of chemical reactivity in comparison with the parent penicillin. However, subsequent observations indicated that the direct conjugation reaction is also important: (1) the specificity of antipenicilloyl antibodies in human serum was largely directed toward the D-α-penicilloyl group, rather than a mixture of its penicilloyl diastereoisomers (34, 37), and (2) acid-stable penicillins, which rearranged very slowly to penicillenic acid in neutral solution, coupled readily to serum proteins under physiological conditions *in vitro* and were comparable in their immunogenicity to benzylpenicillin in experimental animals (178, 179). Schwartz (181) and Yamana and his colleagues (182) later showed that other functional groups of proteins catalyze the direct aminolysis reaction, helping explain why aminolysis of penicillin by proteins has been faster than studies with model monofunctional amines otherwise have indicated.

The observations above make it unlikely that a truly nonallergic penicillin will be developed (23). All bacteriologically active penicillins appear to undergo the direct aminolysis reaction. Indeed, penicillin may exert its antibacterial action by acylating a transpeptidase involved in bacterial cell wall synthesis (183, 184). If this acylating a transpeptidase is how penicillin works, attempts to prepare a penicillin without protein reactivity are self-defeating, since its antibiotic activity would also be lost. Moreover, even if the aminolysis reaction were to be eliminated, there are other pathways for forming antigens that might continue to operate or even might be accelerated. However, this situation does not mean that attempts to find penicillins with lower degrees of immunogenicity should not be made. Quantitative differences in penicillin allergenicity may and probably do exist; thus the screening of new penicillins with this possibility in mind should be continued.

Even if the intrinsic immunogenicity of penicillin can not be eliminated, the effort to minimize the contamination of penicillin solutions by proteins, polymers, and potentially allergenic penicillin breakdown products should be possible. Benzylpenicillin is prepared by fermentation, creating the possibility that proteins from the original fermentation mixture will contaminate the final product. In addition, semisynthetic penicillins may contain bacterial enzymes used to remove the original penicillin side chain prior to reacylation.

Protein contamination has not been the only potential problem. Large molecular weight penicillin (or cephalothin) polymers have formed in poorly buffered penicillin solutions, particularly after storage for several days or more (185). The possible role of high molecular weight contaminants was first suggested by hemagglutination inhibition studies conducted in 1964, which indicated that allergic reactivity was frequently present to a polymer of 6-aminopenicillanic acid (16). Several groups subsequently reported that large molecular weight impurities are present in commercial penicillins (186–188). In addition to macromolecular contaminants, it is important to consider the possible role of small molecular weight penicillin breakdown products that may be introduced at the time of manufacture, during storage, or in solu-

tions of penicillin at the time of therapy, particularly if the pH is not adequately controlled (21). Indeed, under favorable conditions both penicillin and 6-aminopenicillanic acid have had the capability of polymerizing to themselves after the drug has been manufactured (187). In a minority of patients with recent penicillin anaphylaxis, small molecular weight, multivalent penicillin degradation products such as penicillenate disulfide have produced immediate skin responses, suggesting that these substances may also play a role in life-threatening reactions to penicillin (15, 47, 177).

Obviously more investigation is needed to elucidate the relative importance of these various large and small molecular weight contaminants in allergic reactions to penicillin and other drugs. High standards of penicillin manufacture and utilization appear desirable to keep contamination to a minimum, provided the increase in cost of the product can be kept within reasonable bounds. This approach appears to have paid dividends. Serious reactions to penicillin appear to be less frequent than in the past, and improved procedures in preparing penicillins for clinical use may be part of the reason.

The most effective and practical method of detecting the form of penicillin allergy likely to be associated with anaphylaxis is by immediate skin testing. Testing is carried out with a combination of test materials including penicilloyl-polylysine, penicillin, penilloic, and penicilloic acid. If the history suggests a high degree of sensitivity, considerable caution is needed in testing, particularly with penicillin and penicilloic acid. Penicilloyl-polylysine is a preformed multivalent conjugate of penicilloyl on a polymer of lysine. Parker and colleagues had originated this technique in an effort to minimize the danger of sensitization that would have been incurred if penicilloyl proteins had been used for testing (34). Useful *in vitro* assays for penicillin antibodies also have been available but probably do not cover as broad a spectrum as comprehensive skin testing.

In patients with a history of penicillin allergy, the incidence of positive skin responses to penicillin antigens depends on when the testing is performed. Two or three months after the allergic episode, up to 90% of patients exhibit positive responses to penicilloyl-polylysine (175). During allergic symptoms, however, the incidence of positive reactions is considerably less, probably because most of the antibody is complexed to antigen. If the diagnosis of penicillin allergy is in doubt, confirmation can be obtained by retesting later. In patients with a history of penicillin allergy more than 5 years previously, only about 25% exhibit cutaneous reactivity to penicilloyl-polylysine. This loss of reactivity with time helps explain why individuals with a history of penicillin allergy 5–10 years previously usually fail to experience a second reaction when penicillin is readministered. In the past, new penicillins have been administered to small groups of subjects with a history of benzylpenicillin allergy to evaluate allergic cross-reactivity. When no reactions had been seen, the erroneous conclusion was drawn that there was little or no cross-reactivity.

Numerous studies have shown that if skin testing is carefully performed and no allergic reactivity is demonstrated, the risk of a reaction to subsequent penicillin treatment is low regardless of the history (61). If positive skin tests are obtained, it is normally best to use another drug. In the face of a life-threatening illness where penicillin is clearly the drug of choice, desensitization is often possible but this is a specialized procedure requiring considerable care.

Antibodies to structurally complex haptens such as the benzylpenicilloyl group vary in their degree of adaptation to different portions of the hapten molecule. Part of the specificity of the antibody is directed toward the alkyl side chain of lysine, which is the amino acid to which most of the penicilloyl on the protein is attached. The antibodies vary in their overall affinity for the hapten molecules as well as in the extent to which they cross-react with penicillins with different side chains. All penicillins contain the 6-aminopenicillanic acid nucleus and are, therefore, potentially cross-reactive immunologically. Benzylpenicilloyl–polylysine and 2,6-dimethoxybenzylpenicilloyl–polylysine (the polylysines from penicillin G and methicillin, respectively) are almost equivalent as elicitors of cutaneous allergic responses in some patients with benzylpenicillin allergy, but in others the cross-reactivity is minimal (189, 190). Thus the extent of adaptation to the 6-aminopenicillanic nucleus and the R group at the 6-amino position varies considerably.

Cephalosporins also have chemical reactivity for proteins and the capability of sensitizing, although the bond formed is less stable than the penicilloylamide bond. Variation in allergic cross-reactivity is also seen with the cephalothins, about 30% (191) or greater (192) of patients with allergy to penicillin G exhibiting significant skin reactivity to cephalothin or cephaloridine, and several instances of cephalothin-induced anaphylaxis having been recorded. Penicillins and cephalothins differ not only in the nature of the R group but also in the structure of the sulfur containing ring. Chemical routes for forming antigenic determinants are less well defined than they are for the penicillins (128). One factor is that aminolysis of cephalosporins leads to formation of unstable intermediates which decompose to penaldates and penamaldates.

Allergic cross-reactivity probably is not solely a function of the degree of structural similarity between two penicillins (189). The particular antigenic determinant responsible for the allergy and the extent to which it is formed *in vivo* by the second penicillin may also be important. In view of the difficulty in predicting how much cross-reactivity might be present, the empirical use of cephalothins or penicillins with different side chains in individuals with a history of benzylpenicillin allergy is difficult to justify. Unless skin testing is carried out, allergic cross-reactivity cannot be excluded.

In addition to the penicillins and cephalothins, cross-sensitivity may also exist between aminoglycosides (streptomycin, kanamycin, neomycin, and gentamicin), or p-aminobenzene derivatives (sulfonamides, sulfonylureas, procaine, procainamide, thiazides, and carbonic anhydrase inhibitors) (70). There has been speculation that the cross-reactivity of the aminoglycoside antibiotics may be due to the formation of a common metabolite, neosamine (193). Often it is possible to find a drug that is so different structurally that the possibility of allergic cross-reactivity is absent or minimal. For example, antibodies to procaine-type local anesthetics, which contain the p-aminophenyl group, do not appear to cross-react immunologically with lidocaine and other local anesthetics that lack this group (52).

6 EVALUATION OF DRUGS FOR ALLERGENICITY

6.1 Evaluation of the Protein Reactivity of the Drug and its Metabolites

In evaluating a drug as a potential allergen in people, its chemical properties, mode of synthesis, and metabolism must be considered.

6.1.1 EVALUATION FOR DIRECT PROTEIN REACTIVITY *IN VITRO*. First the drug should be thoroughly reviewed in terms of purity, chemical properties, stability, possible contaminants, and metabolism *in vivo*. Protein reactivity can often be predicted on the basis of chemical structure and may also be evaluated directly with purified proteins *in vitro*, varying the temperature and pH so that reactions that go slowly under physiologic conditions are favored. This type of analysis is greatly facilitated if a radioactive drug is available. However, it is not enough simply to show binding. The linkage of the drug to the protein should be stable to prolonged dialysis and extraction with organic solvents, and reactivity should be demonstrable with at least one of the amino acid residues normally present in mammalian proteins. Obviously any drug that readily forms stable bonds with proteins under physiological conditions *in vitro* is potentially hazardous as a sensitizer.

Contaminants with protein reactivity also need to be considered. The preparation of drugs by organic synthesis may necessitate the use of highly reactive precursors that are difficult to remove in the later stages of purification. By ordinary chemical standards 99% purity is often considered to be acceptable, but keep in mind that drugs are often used in gram amounts, and that microgram quantities of a reactive contaminant may be enough to produce an immune response. Trace contaminants can often be detected if sizable quantities of the drug are subjected to chromatographic analysis. Thin layer, high pressure liquid, and gas chromatographic techniques are particularly useful because of their high resolving power. In addition, as discussed in connection with penicillin hypersensitivity, drugs that are prepared biosynthetically may be contaminated by proteins and other macromolecules, and this possibility must be evaluated. If possible, known or suspected metabolites that might have protein reactivity should also be prepared and evaluated.

6.1.2 EVALUATION FOR PROTEIN REACTIVITY *IN VIVO*. Whole animals or tissue slices may be used with radiolabeled drugs, drug contaminants, or drug metabolites in an effort to show metabolic activation leading to conjugation of soluble or cell-bound proteins. This technique is not as easy an experimental approach as it might seem: the conjugation may be inefficient; difficulties may arise in distinguishing covalent from noncovalent binding; and the structure of protein-bound metabolites may be impossible to identify. Moreover, small amounts of conjugated drug may not be immunologically significant. Once characterized antisera have become available (see below), however, the distribution and relative quantity of antigen in various tissues can be determined directly, providing a more refined approach to analysis.

6.2 Direct Immunologic Evaluation

Suspected antigenic precursors and the conjugates formed by their reaction with proteins are prepared and evaluated in parallel with the drug itself for immunogenicity in experimental animals. As a rule the materials are emulsified in complete Freund's adjuvant and administered subcutaneously or intradermally to guinea pigs and rabbits or both (9). Percutaneous sensitization may also be attempted. Since animals vary in their ability to respond immunologically, the use of a sizable number of animals in each group is desirable. Useful animal species include monkeys, mice, rats, rabbits, and guinea pigs. The animals are screened for hypersensitivity by delayed and immediate skin testing *in vivo*, again using both conjugates and reactive metabolites for analysis, and using as controls animals injected with adjuvant alone or with unconjugated proteins. Serum antibody and lymphocyte transformation measurements also are carried out, and attempts are made to passively transfer immediate hypersensitivity by injecting serum locally in the skin of unimmunized animals. If hypersensitivity responses are elicited, pathologic evaluation may be useful in helping establish that a typical histologic pattern is being elicited.

Even if attempts at immunization with the drug and its metabolites are unsuccessful, the protein conjugates should be immunogenic, providing a starting point for further investigation. After sera containing antibodies have been identified, they are carefully studied in regard to antibody specificity and titer. As discussed in the section on immunologic analysis, specificity is evaluated by comparing the ability of various univalent haptens to inhibit the antigen-antibody reaction. Once antisera have been characterized, they can be used to evaluate the immunologic cross-reactivity of various haptens and to study the sensitivity and specificity of different immunologic detection systems. In this way one accumulates a panel of antigen and antibody preparations encompassing all the major candidates as antigens. When sensitive and specific reagents and test systems are available, samples from human beings exposed to the drug can be analyzed for similar reactivities. In this setting, a negative reaction has some meaning, since the reagents have already been shown to be effective in detecting allergy in experimental animals.

6.3 Simplified Approaches to Immunological Analysis and Their Limitations

Short of the tentative identification of possible antigenic determinants and the preparation and immunologic characterization of appropriate conjugates, reactive precursors, and univalent haptens, diagnostic procedures in drug allergy are usually unsuccessful. Nonetheless, describing some less complex approaches, while keeping in mind their limitations, may be worthwhile.

6.3.1 ATTEMPTS AT OBTAINING HAPTEN-PRO-
TEIN CONJUGATES WITHOUT IDENTIFYING THE
CHEMICAL REACTION INVOLVED IN THEIR FOR-
MATION (37). Leftwich used serum proteins
from patients receiving substantial doses of
sulfonamides for skin testing, on the assumption that the hapten might have
reacted sufficiently with serum proteins *in
vivo* to elicit responses in subjects with
sulfonamide allergy (194). Although he
reported the production of wheal and
erythema responses by certain sera, others
were unable to confirm this observation
(195). In a somewhat similar approach, the
serum and urine of human subjects ingesting acetaminophen were shown to sensitize
platelets to an antiserum from a patient
with thrombocytopenia induced by the
drug, even though the drug itself failed to
do so. As noted in the discussion of thrombocytopenia, the sensitizing substance was
later identified as acetaminophen sulfate
(38).

6.3.2 "ARTIFICIAL" CONJUGATES. Frequently
drugs have been attached to proteins by
"artificial" means; for instance, using a
type of covalent bond that would not be
expected to form *in vivo*. For example,
Wedum conjugated sulfonamides to proteins using an azo linkage (196). Apparently the conjugates formed were not of value
in the study of sulfonamide allergy in
humans (195). However, in an azo conjugate of hydralazine, the red cells proved to
be useful in the detection of antibodies to
hydralazine in human sera (124). Obviously
there is not a priori reason for immunologic
similarity to exist between the substituent
on the artificial conjugate and the actual
antigenic determinant; thus a negative result is considerably less significant than a
positive one.

6.3.3 METABOLIC ACTIVATION *IN VITRO*. As
discussed above, intact cells or subcellular
fractions from blood, liver or other organs

may be used in attempts to metabolically
activate drugs *in vitro* and obtain conjugated protein preparations. This method is
an important approach which is being increasingly utilized.

6.3.4 UTILIZATION OF THE DRUG ITSELF. As
discussed in relation to diagnostic methods,
another approach is to employ the drug
itself under conditions where a positive
response is known to sometimes occur.

1. Elicitation of immediate hypersensitivity
   responses by direct skin testing is sometimes possible with penicillin and a few
   other drugs; however, with most drugs
   this type of analysis is fruitless. IgE
   antibodies may be present but remain
   undetected because the drug does not
   conjugate effectively to proteins or cells
   during the time restrictions on the assay.

2. An ability to demonstrate delayed or
   contact cutaneous hypersensitivity is
   considerably more frequent, although
   rigorous specificity controls are needed
   to rule out nonspecific irritancy. Even
   though cell-mediated rather than
   humorally-mediated immunity is measured, if a drug produces a delayed
   cutaneous hypersensitivity response with
   any degree of consistency, its effectiveness as a sensitizer is established and
   other types of allergic reaction probably
   can be anticipated.

3. Radiolabeled drugs occasionally can be
   shown to bind to gamma globulins in
   selected human or animal sera, presumably because serum antibodies are
   present. However, rigorous controls are
   needed to exclude nonspecific binding,
   particularly in the presence of altered
   gamma globulin levels. As with the
   artificial conjugates, since the actual
   antigenic determinant may differ considerably from the drug structurally, a
   negative result is of little or no value.

4. Lymphocyte transformation responses

are sometimes elicited by drugs, although the responses are small and controls are needed to be certain that a nonspecific pharmacologic effect of the drug is not involved.

6.4 Screening for Nonspecific Activation of Immunologic Effector Mechanisms

Drugs should also be studied for nonspecific activation of immunologic effector mechanisms. A variety of positively charged drugs and radioopaque dyes nonspecifically stimulate histamine release from mast cells and basophils, providing a possible explanation for acute systemic reactions to these agents. A number of agents including polysaccharides and lipopolysaccharides activate the alternative complement pathway, suggesting another possible mechanism for acute systemic reactions. Incubation of isolated mast cells or sera containing fresh complement with drugs may be useful in identifying these and similar reactivities, although the most important ones will probably be detected during acute animal toxicity studies *in vivo*.

6.5 Initial Evaluation of Drugs in Man

Even extensive immunologic screening studies in animals can not entirely exclude the possibility of serious allergic reactions in humans once clinical testing is underway. Numerous examples can be cited in which a drug that had passed seemingly rigorous screening requirements in experimental animals proved unacceptable for human use. Obviously patients must be monitored carefully during the early stages of human use with this possibility in mind. In addition, the possibility of unusual reactions appearing for the first time after a drug is released for general use must be recognized at all times. Manifestations of drug allergy

are sufficiently protean that a high index of suspicion is needed.

7 POSSIBLE FUTURE DIRECTIONS

There is no real prospect that allergic drug reactions will ever be eliminated entirely. However, some interesting approaches have been or may be applied in the future, and these approaches could help to keep serious complications to a minimum.

7.1 Drug Development

As more of the important metabolites in drug allergy become identified, a rational approach to the development of less immunogenic congeners with similar pharmacologic actions will be available.

7.2 Serologic, Enzymatic and Genetic Analyses

Genetic influences on drug metabolism and immune responsiveness is well-established. In the near future, some attention will undoubtedly be given to the usefulness of HLA phenotyping or genotyping prospectively and related analytic approaches for drug metabolizing enzymes in the identification of the subjects most at risk for serious drug reactions.

7.3 Utilization of Univalent Haptens and Haptens Attached to Metabolizable Carriers

From work with experimental animals there is evidence to indicate that the induction of immunity to a hapten-protein conjugate can be diminished by preinjection with univalent hapten or multivalent hapten in stable combination with a poorly metabolizable polymer such as poly-D-lysine (197, 198). Moreover, at the time of allergic symptoms the hapten itself will normally be inhibitory, provided it is univalent and not reactive with proteins (14, 15, 47). Systemic anaphylaxis is one of the reactions that can be inhibited. De-Weck and Girard have shown that the systemic administration of a univalent penicilloyl derivative is associated with diminished skin reactivity and allergic symptoms (199). Clearly, if only penicilloyl allergy is present, it may be possible to prevent or arrest the allergic response. Whether these approaches will ever be utilized regularly remains to be seen, since the possibility of rare but serious reactions to the reagents themselves or to antibodies of other specificities must be considered.

REFERENCES

1. National Academy of Sciences, *Report of the International Conference on Adverse Reactions Reporting Systems*, Washington, D.C., 1971.

2. K. P. Mathews, *J. Allergy Clin. Immunol*, **74**, 558 (1984).

3. C. W. Parker, "Drug Allergy," in C. W. Parker, Ed., *Clinical Immunology*, 2 vols., W. B. Saunders, Philadelphia, Pa., 1980, p. 1219.

4. P. A. H. Moss, W. M. C. Rosenberg, and J. I. Bell, *Annu. Rev. Immunol.* **10**, 71 (1992).

5. E. D. Day, Ed., *Advanced Immunochemistry*, 2nd ed., Wiley-Liss, New York, 1990.

6. F. R. Carbone, and M. J. Bevan, "Major Histocompatibility Complex Control of T Cell Recognition," in W. E. Paul, Ed., *Fundamental Immunology*, Raven Press, Philadelphia, Pa., 1988, p. 541.

7. C. W. Parker, "Allergic Mediators," in P. E. Korenblat and H. J. Wedner, Eds., *Allergy Theory and Practice*, 2nd ed., W. B. Saunders, Philadelphia, Pa., 1992, p. 81.

8. T. R. Mosmann and R. L. Coffman, *Adv. in Immunol.*, **46**, 111 (1989).

9. C. W. Parker, *Radioimmunoassay of Biologically Active Compounds*, Prentice-Hall Inc., Englewood Cliffs, N.J., 1976.

10. C. W. Parker, *Am. J. Med.*, **34**, 747 (1863).

11. K. Landsteiner, *The Specificity of Serological Reactions*, Harvard University Press, Cambridge, Mass., 1945.

12. H. N. Eisen, "Hypersensitivity to Simple Chemicals," in H. S. Lawrence, Ed., *Cellular and Humoral Aspects of the Hypersensitive States*, Hoeber, New York, 1959, p. 89.

13. C. W. Parker, M. Kern, and H. N. Eisen, *J. Lab. Clin. Med.*, **58**, 948 (1961).

14. C. W. Parker, A. L. de Weck, M. Kern, and H. N. Eisen, *J. Exp. Med.*, **115**, 803 (1962).

15. C. W. Parker, J. Shapiro, M. Kern, and H. N. Eisen, *J. Exp. Med.*, **115**, 821 (1962).

16. J. A. Thiel, S. Mitchell, and C. W. Parker, *J. Allergy*, **35**, 399 (1964).

17. B. B. Levine, *Fed. Proc.*, **24**, 45 (1965).

18. B. B. Levine, "Immunochemical Mechanisms of Drug Allergy," in P. A. Miescher and H. J. Muller-Eberhard, Eds., *Textbook of Immunopathology*, Vol. 1, Grune & Stratton, New York, 1968, p. 260.

19. B. B. Levine and Z. Ovary, *J. Exp. Med.*, **114**, 875 (1961).

20. B. B. Levine, A. P. Redmond, M. J. Fellner, H. E. Voss, and V. Levytska, *J. Clin. Invest.*, **45**, 1895 (1966).

21. R. M. Adams, *Occupational Contact Dermatitis*, Lippincott, Philadelphia, Pa., 1969, p. 159.

22. O. J. Plescia, W. Braun, S. Imperato, E. Cora-Block, L. Jaroskova, and C. Schimbor, "Methylated Serum Albumin as a Carrier for Oligo- and Poly-nucleotides," in O. J. Plescia and W. Braun, Eds., *Nucleic Acids in Immunology*, Springer-Verlag, New York, 1968, p. 5.

23. C. W. Parker, "Allergic Drug Responses. Mechanisms and Unsolved Problems," in L. Goldberg, Ed., *Critical Reviews in Toxicology*, Vol. 1, Issue 3, CRC Press, Cleveland, Ohio, 1972, p. 261.

24. C. W. Parker, "Mechanisms of Penicillin Allergy," in H. L. Joachim, Ed., *Pathobiology Annual*, Appleton-Century-Crofts, New York, 1972, p. 405.

25. G. C. Oliver, Jr., B. M. Parker, D. L. Brasfield, and C. W. Parker, *J. Clin. Invest.*, **47**, 1035 (1968).

26. J. A. Berzofsky and I. J. Berkower, "Immunogenicity and Antigen Structure," in W. E. Paul, Ed., *Fundamental Immunology*, Raven Press, Philadelphia, Pa., 1988, p. 169.

27. C. H. Schneider and A. L. de Weck, *Immunochemistry*, **4**, 331 (1967).

28. P. W. Kincade and J. M. Gimble, "B. Lymphocytes," in W. E. Paul, Ed., *Fundamental Immunology*, Raven Press, Philadelphia, Pa., 1988, p. 41.

29. E. W. Voss, Jr., K. Corley, and L. H. Huang, *Immunochemistry*, **6**, 361 (1967).

30. M. R. Vickers and E. S. K. Assem, *Immunology*, **26**, 425 (1974).

31. K. Uemura, R. A. Nicolotti, H. R. Six, and S. C. Kinsky, *Biochemistry*, **13**, 1572 (1974).

32. S. Leskowitz, V. E. Jones, and S. J. Zak, *J. Exp. Med.*, **123**, 229 (1966).

33. J. R. Frey, A. L. de Weck, H. T. Geleick, and W. Lergier, *J. Exp. Med.*, **130**, 1123 (1969).

34. C. W. Parker, *Fed. Proc.*, **24**, 51 (1965).

35. C. W. Parker, *Ann. N. Y. Acad. Sci.*, **123**, 55 (1965).

36. P. Minden and R. S. Farr, *Arthritis Rheum.*, **10**, 299 (1967).

37. C. W. Parker, "Drug Reactions," in M. Samter and H. L. Alexander, Eds., *Immunological Diseases*, Little, Brown, Boston, Mass., 1965, p. 663.

38. E. V. Eisner and N. T. Shahidi, *New Engl. J. Med.*, **287**, 376 (1972).

39. A. Salama and C. Mueller-Eckhardt, *Seminars in Hematology*, **29**, 54 (1992).

40. J. W. H. Mali, W. J. Van Kooten, and F. C. J. Van Neer, *J. Invest. Dermatol.*, **41**, 111 (1963).

41. M. H. Samitz and S. Katz, *J. Invest. Dermatol.*, **42**, 35 (1964).

42. H. A. Cohen, *J. Invest. Dermatol.*, **38**, 13 (1962).

43. S. Strober and J. L. Gowans, *J. Exp. Med.*, **122**, 347 (1965).

44. F. S. Farrah, M. Kern, and H. N. Eisen, *J. Exp. Med.*, **112**, 1211 (1960).

45. C. W. Parker, M. Kern, and H. N. Eisen, *J. Exp. Med.*, **115**, 789 (1962).

46. D. H. Campbell and G. E. McCasland, *J. Immunol.*, **48**, 315 (1944).

47. J. W. Yunginger, *Ann. Allergy*, **69**, 87 (1992).

48. D. Krapin, *New Engl. J. Med.*, **267**, 820 (1962).

49. L. C. Grammer, B. E. Metzger, and R. Patterson, *JAMA*, **251**, 1459 (1984).

50. H. L. Alexander, *Reactions with Drug Therapy*, Saunders, Philadelphia, Pa., 1955.

51. K. P. Mathews, *Am. J. Med.*, **44**, 310 (1967).

52. R. D. DeWarte, "Drug Allergy," in R. Patterson, Ed., *Allergic Diseases Diagnosis and Management*, Lippincott., Philadelphia, Pa., 1985, p. 505.

53. J. Poothullil, A. Shimizu, R. P. Day, and J. Dolovich, *Ann. Intern. Med.*, **82**, 58 (1975).

54. K. Binkley, A. Cheema, G. Sussman, G. Moudgil, M. O'Connor, S. Evans, and J. Dolovich, *J. Allergy Clin. Immunol.*, **89**, 768 (1992).

55. D. Jaeger, D. Kleinhans, A. B. Czuppon, and X. Baur, *J. Allergy Clin. Immunol.*, **89**, 759 (1992).

56. D. D. Stevenson and R. A. Simon, *J. Allergy Clin. Immunol.*, **68**, 26 (1981).

57. R. A. Simon, *J. Allergy Clin. Immunol.*, **74**, 623 (1984).

58. T. J. Sullivan and C. W. Parker, *Am. J. Pathol.*, **85**, 437 (1976).

59. C. W. Parker, "Mediators: Release and Function," in W. E. Paul, Ed., *Fundamental Immunology*, Raven Press, Philadelphia, Pa., 1984, p. 697.

60. L. P. James and K. F. Austen, *New Engl. J. Med.*, **270**, 597 (1964).

61. C. Delage and N. S. Drey, *J. Forensic Sci.*, **17**, 525 (1972).

62. D. Laroche, M-C. Vergnaud, B. Sillard, H. Soufarapis, and H. Bricard, *Anesthesiology*, **75**, 945 (1991).

63. P. L. Smith, A. Kagey-Sobotka, E. R. Bleecker, R. Traystman, A. P. Kaplan, H. Gralnick, M. D. Valentine, S. Permutt, and L. M. Lichtenstein, *J. Clin. Invest.*, **66**, 1072 (1980).

64. T. J. Sullivan, "Drug Allergy", in E. Middleton, C. E. Reed, E. F. Ellis, N. F. Adkinson, and J. W. Yunginger, Eds., *Allergy: Principles and Practice*, Vol. II, C.V. Mosby Company, St. Louis, Mo., 1988, Chapt. 65, p. 1523.

65. T. J. Sullivan, *J. Allergy Clin. Immunol.*, **74**, 594 (1984).

66. C. W. Parker, H. J. Wedner, and T. J. Sullivan, "Cyclic AMP and the Immune Response," in P. Greengard and G. A. Robison, Eds., *Advances in Cyclic Nucleotide Research*, Vol. 4, Raven Press, New York, 1974, p. 1.

67. J. F. Scholand, J. I. Tennenbaum, and G. J. Cerilli, *J. Am. Med. Assoc.*, **206**, 130 (1968).

68. L. Meyler and A. Herxheimer, *Side Effects of Drugs*, Vol. 7, Excerpta Medica, Amsterdam, 1972.

69. W. T. Kniker, and C. G. Cochrane, *J. Exp. Med.*, **127**, 119 (1968).

70. C. W. Parker, *New Engl. J. Med.*, **292**, 511, 732, 957 (1975).

71. H. Nishimoto, K. Mori, and Y. Mizoguchi, *Int. Arch. Allergy Appl. Immunol.*, **95**, 221 (1991).

72. A. I. de Weck, *Symp. Med. Hoechst.*, **22**, 199 (1988).

73. P. P. Vanarsdel, Jr. and B. C. Gilliland, *J. Lab. Clin. Med.*, **65**, 277 (1965).

74. L. D. Petz and H. H. Fudenberg, *New Engl. J. Med.*, **274**, 171 (1966).

75. C. M. Huguley, Jr., *DM*, (Oct. 1963).

76. S. Moeschlin, "Agranulocytosis Due to Sensitivity to Drugs," in M. L. Rosenheim and R.

Moulton, Eds., *Sensitivity Reactions to Drugs*, Blackwell Scientific Publications, Oxford, UK., 1958, p. 77.

77. A. J. Barrett, E. Weller, N. Rozengurt, P. Longhurst, and J. G. Humble, *Brit. Med. J.*, **2**, 850 (1976).

78. S. Moeschlin and K. Wagner, *Acta Haematol.*, **8**, 29 (1952).

79. J. Wall, S. Fang, S. Ingbar, and L. Braverman, *Clin. Res.*, **25**, 516A (1977).

80. D. P. Stites, J. D. Stobo, and J. V. Wells, Eds., *Basic & Clinical Immunology*, 6th ed., Appleton & Lange, Norwalk, Conn., 1987, p. 414.

81. J. F. Ackroyd, *Proc. Roy. Soc. Med.*, **55**, 30 (1962).

82. N. R. Shulman, *J. Exp. Med.*, **107**, 665 (1958).

83. D. Deykin and L. J. Hellerstein, *J. Clin. Invest.* **51**, 3142 (1972).

84. A. Salama, S. Santoso, and C. Mueller-Eckhardt, *Brit. J. Haemat.*, **78**, 535 (1991).

85. W. B. Sherman and W. R. Kessler, *Allergy in Pediatric Practice*, Mosby, St. Louis, Mo., 1957.

86. V. N. Sehgal and O. P. Gangwani, *Intrn. J. Derm.*, **26**, 67 (1987).

87. D. G. Simpson and J. H. Walker, *Am. J. Med.*, **29**, 297 (1960).

88. S. Zelman, *Am. J. Med.*, **27**, 708 (1959).

89. C. A. Dujovne, C. H. Chan, and H. J. Zimmerman, *New Engl. J. Med.*, **277**, 785 (1967).

90. H. J. Zimmerman, "Drug-Induced Hepatic Injury," in M. Samter and C. W. Parker, Eds., *International Encyclopedia of Pharmacology and Therapeutics*, *Section 75: Hypersensitivity to Drugs*, Vol. 1, Pergamon Press, Oxford, UK., 1972, p. 299.

91. B. N. Halpern, "Antibodies Produced by Drugs and Methods for Their Detection," in M. Samter and C. W. Parker, Eds., *International Encyclopedia of Pharmacology and Therapeutics*, *Section 75: Hypersensitivity to Drugs*, Vol. 1, Pergamon Press, Oxford, UK., 1972, p. 113.

92. F. Paronetto and H. Popper, *New Engl. J. Med.*, **283**, 277 (1970).

93. G. E. Davies and J. E. Holmes, *Brit. J. Anaesth.*, **44**, 941 (1972).

94. D. L. Bruce and F. Raymon, *New Engl. J. Med.*, **286**, 1218 (1972).

95. C. W. Parker, *Arthritis, Rheumat.*, **24**, 1030 (1981).

96. L. R. Pohl, H. Satoh, D. D. Christ, and J. G. Kenna, *Ann. Rev. Pharm.*, **28**, 376 (1988).

97. J. Uetrecht, *Crit. Rev. in Toxicology*, **20**, 213 (1990).

98. C. W. Parker, S. Godt, and M. C. Johnson, *Biochemistry*, **5**, 2314 (1966).

99. C. Pantarotto, M. Arboix, P. Sezzano, and R. Abruzzi, *Biochem. Pharmacol.*, **31**, 1501 (1982).

100. H. Remmer and R. Schuppel, "The Formation of Antigenic Determinants," in M. Samter and C. W. Parker, Eds., *International Encyclopedia of Pharmacology and Therapeutics, Section 75: Hypersensitivity to Drugs*, Vol. 1, Pergamon Press, Oxford, UK., 1972, p. 67.

101. L. Lorand, L. K. Campbell, and B. J. Robertson, *Biochemistry*, **11**, 434 (1972).

102. O. P. Sharma, *Ann. Intern. Med.*, **78**, 616 (1973).

103. H. G. Grieble and G. G. Jackson, *New Engl. J. Med.*, **258**, 1 (1958).

104. P. M. Zeek, *New Engl. J. Med.*, **248**, 764 (1953).

105. R. P. McCombs, J. F. Patterson, and H. E. MacMahon, *New Engl. J. Med.*, **255**, 251 (1956).

106. W. St. C. Symmers, *Proc. Roy. Soc. Med.*, **55**, 20 (1962).

107. G. A. Rose and H. Spencer, *Quart. J. Med.*, **26**, 43 (1957).

108. R. V. McCormick, *J. Am. Med. Assoc.*, **144**, 1453 (1950).

109. P. A. Bacon, C. R. Tribe, J. C. Mackenzie, J. V. Jones, R. H. Cumming, and B. Amer, *Quart. J. Med.*, **45**, 661 (1976).

110. J. Aten, A. Veninga, J. A. Bruijn, F. A. Prins, E. DeHeer, and J. J. Weening, *Clin. Immunol. and Immunopath.*, **63**, 89 (1992).

111. D. S. Baldwin, B. B. Levine, R. T. McCluskey, and G. R. Gallo, *New Engl. J. Med.*, **279**, 1245 (1968).

112. W. A. Border, D. H. Lehmann, J. D. Egan, H. J. Sass, J. E. Gode, and C. B. Wilson, *New Engl. J. Med.*, **291**, 381 (1974).

113. S. G. Adler, A. H. Cohen, and W. A. Border, *Amer. Jr. Kidney Dis.*, **5**, 75 (1985).

114. A. F. Macklon, A. W. Craft, M. Thompson, and D. N. S. Kerr, *Brit. Med. J.*, **1**, 597 (1974).

115. J. R. Frey, H. Geleick, A. Geczy, and A. L. de Weck, *Int. Arch. Allergy*, **46**, 571 (1974).

116. H. M. Perry, Jr. and H. A. Schroeder, *J. Am. Med. Assoc.*, **154**, 670 (1954).

117. E. L. Dubois, *Medicine* (Baltimore), **48**, 217 (1969).

118. E. M. Tan, *Fed. Proc.*, **33**, 1894 (1974).

119. D. Alarcon-Segovia, E. Fishbein, and V. M. Betancourt, *Clin. Exp. Immunol.*, **5**, 429 (1969).

120. G. G. Bole, Jr., M. H. Friedlaender, and C. K. Smith, *Lancet*, **1**, 323 (1969).

121. C. W. Parker, *Pharm. Rev.*, **85**, 94 (1982).

122. A. Cannat and M. Seligmann, *Clin. Exp. Immunol.*, **3**, 99 (1968).

123. A. S. Russell and M. Ziff, *Clin. Exp. Immunol.*, **3**, 901 (1968).

124. B. H. Hahn, G. C. Sharp, W. S. Irvin, O. S. Kantor, C. A. Garoner, M. K. Bagby, H. M. Perry, and C. K. Osterland, *Ann. Intern. Med.*, **76**, 365 (1972).

125. H. L. Holley, *J. Chronic Dis.*, **17**, 1 (1964).

126. S. E. Blomgren, J. J. Condemi, M. C. Bignall, and J. H. Vaughan, *New Engl. J. Med.*, **281**, 64 (1969).

127. S. E. Blomgren and J. H. Vaughan, *Arthritis Rheum.*, **11**, 470 (1968).

128. H. E. Amos and B. K. Park, "Understanding Immunotoxic Drug Reactions," in J. Dean and Co-Eds., *Immunotoxicology and Immunopharmacology*, Raven Press, New York, New York, 1985, p. 207.

129. Y. Yamauchi, A. Litwin, L. Adams, H. Zimmer, and E. V. Hess, *J. Clin. Invest.*, **56**, 958 (1975).

130. J. P. Uetrecht, R. W. Freeman, and R. L. Woosley, *Arth. & Rheumat.*, **24**, 994 (1981).

131. A. H. Hofstra, L. C. Matassa, and J. P. Uetrecht, *J. Rheumat.*, **18**, 1673 (1991).

132. P. J. Grob, J. W. Muller-Schoop, M. A. Hacki, and H. I. Joller-Jemelka, *Lancet*, **2**, 144 (1975).

133. R. H. Felix, F. A. Ive, and M. G. C. Dahl, *Brit. Med. J.*, **4**, 321 (1974).

134. T. C. Orton and C. Lowery, *J. Pharmacol. Exp. Ther.*, **219**, 207 (1981).

135. H. E. Amox, B. G. Lake, and J. Artis, *Brit. Med. J.*, **1**, 402 (1978).

136. P. A. Berg, P. T. Daniel, J. Holzschuh, and N. Brattig, *DMW*, **113**, 65 (1988).

137. E. C. Rosenow, III, *Ann. Intern. Med.*, **77**, 977 (1972).

138. H. R. Pearsall, J. Ewalt, M. S. Tsoi, S. Sumida, D. Backus, R. H. Winterbauer, D. R. Webb, and H. Jones, *J. Lab. Clin. Med.*, **83**, 728 (1974).

139. C. J. Eastmond, *Brit. Med. J.*, **1**, 1506 (1976).

140. S. D. Rockhoff, R. Brasch, C. Kuhn, and M. Chraplyvy, *Invest. Radiol.*, **5**, 503 (1970).

141. R. C. Brasch, S. D. Rockoff, C. Kuhn, and M. Chraplyvy, *Invest. Radiol.*, **5**, 510 (1970).

142. C. M. Arroyave, K. N. Bhat, and R. Crown, *J. Immunol.*, **117**, 1866 (1976).

143. J. E. Erffmeyer, R. L. Siegle, and P. Lieberman, *J. Allergy Clin. Immunol.*, **75**, 401 (1985).

144. W. H. Bush and D. P. Swanson, *Amer. J. Roent.*, **153**, 1153 (1991).

145. J. Ring, "Mechanisms of Pseudo-Allergic Reactions to Drugs", in R. W. Estanbrook, E. Lindenlaub, and A. L. de Weck, Eds., *Toxicological and Immunological Aspects of Drug Metabolism and Environmental Chemicals*, F. K. Schattauer Verlag, New York, 1987, p. 569.

146. J. D. Sapira, *Am. J. Med.*, **45**, 555 (1968).

147. P. H. Abelson, *Science*, **168**, 1289 (1970).

148. J. J. Ryan, C. W. Parker, and R. C. Williams, *J. Lab. Clin. Med.*, **80**, 155 (1972).

149. R. E. Brashear, M. T. Kelly, and A. C. White, *J. Lab. Clin. Med.*, **83**, 451 (1974).

150. A. L. de Weck, *Int. Arch. Allergy Appl. Immunol.*, **41**, 393 (1971).

151. M. Samter and R. F. Beers, Jr., *Ann. Intern. Med.*, **68**, 975 (1968).

152. J. R. McDonald, D. A. Mathison, and D. D. Stevenson, *J. Allergy Clin. Immunol.*, **50**, 198 (1972).

153. P. P. Van Arsdel, *Ann. of Allergy*, **57**, 305 (1986).

154. J. P. Arm, H. P. O'Hickey, R. J. Hawksworth, C. Y. Fon, A. E. Crea, D. W. Spur, and P. H. Lee, *Am. Rev. Resp. Dis.*, **142**, 1112 (1990).

155. R. F. Lockey, D. L. Ruchnagel, and N. A. Vanselow, *Ann. Intern. Med.*, **78**, 57 (1973).

156. K. G. Klein, J. D. Parkin, and F. Madaras, *Clin. Exp. Immunol.*, **26**, 155 (1976).

157. D. Green, *Brit. J. Haematoll.*, **15**, 57 (1968).

158. S. L. Saltzstein and L. V. Ackerman, *Cancer*, **12**, 164 (1959).

159. R. A. Garms, J. A. Neal, and F. G. Conrad, *Ann. Intern. Med.*, **69**, 557 (1968).

160. T. C. Sorrell, I. J. Forbes, F. R. Burness, and R. H. C. Rischbieth, *Lancet*, **2**, 1233 (1971).

161. A. A. MacKinney and H. E. Booker, *Arch. Intern. Med.*, **129**, 988 (1972).

162. G. Frizzera, E. M. Moran, and H. Rappaport, *Am. J. Med.*, **59**, 803 (1975).

163. J. Van Snick, *Ann. Rev. Immunol.*, **8**, 253 (1990).

164. R. N. Hamburger, *Science*, **152**, 1 (1966).

165. J. K. Wilkin, J. J. Hammond, and W. M. Kirkendall, *Arch. Dermatol.*, **116**, 902 (1980).

166. K. A. Arndt and H. Jick, *JAMA*, **235**, 913 (1976).

167. L. Wide and L. Juhlin, *Clin. Allergy*, **1**, 171 (1971).

168. J. R. Marrack, *Brit. Med. Bull.*, **19**, 178 (1963).

169. C. W. Parker, "Problems in Identification of Responsible Antigenic Determinants in Drug Allergy," in H. Jundgaard, P. Juul, and H. Kofod, Eds., *Drug Design and Adverse Reactions*, Academic Press, New York, 1977.

170. J. K. Selkirk, R. G. Croy, J. P. Whitlock, Jr., and H. V. Gelboin, *Cancer Res.*, **35**, 3651 (1975).

171. K. P. Mathews, P. M. Pan, and J. H. Wells, *Int. Arch. Allergy Appl. Immunol.*, **46**, 653 (1972).

172. A. L. Sheffer, R. E. Rocklin, and E. J. Goetzl, *New Engl. J. Med.*, **293**, 1220 (1975).

173. H. F. Merk, *Allergologie*, **11**, 57 (1988).

174. A. L. de Weck and G. Blum, *Int. Arch. Allergy Appl. Immunol.*, **27**, 221 (1965).

175. C. W. Parker, "Practical Aspects of Diagnosis and Treatment of Patients Who Are Hypersensitive to Drugs," in M. Samter and C. W. Parker, Eds., *International Encyclopedia of Pharmacology and Therapeutics, Section 75: Hypersensitivity to Drugs*, Vol. 1, Pergamon Press, Oxford, UK., 1972, p. 367.

176. R. H. Schwartz and J. H. Vaughan, *J. Am. Med. Assoc.*, **186**, 1151 (1963).

177. A. L. de Weck, C. H. Schneider, and J. Gutersohn, *Int. Arch. Allergy Appl. Immunol.*, **33**, 535 (1968).

178. D. A. Johnson and C. A. Panetta, *J. Org. Chem.*, **29**, 1826 (1964).

179. F. R. Batchelor, J. M. Dewdney, and D. Gazzard, *Nature*, **206**, 362 (1965).

180. M. A. Schwartz, *J. Pharm. Sci.*, **57**, 1209 (1968).

181. T. Yamana, A. Tsuji, E. Miyamoto, and E. Kiya, *J. Pharm. Pharmacol.*, **27**, 287 (1975).

182. C. H. Schneider and A. L. de Weck, *Nature*, **208**, 5055 (1965).

183. H. J. Rodgers, *Biochem. J.*, **103**, 90 (1967).

184. J. L. Strominger and D. J. Tipper, *Am. J. Med.*, **39**, 708 (1965).

185. J. M. Dewdney, H. Smith, and A. W. Wheeler, *Immunology*, **21**, 517 (1971).

186. E. T. Knudsen, O. P. W. Robinson, E. A. P. Croydon, and E. C. Tees, *Lancet*, **1**, 1184 (1967).

187. F. R. Batchelor, J. M. Dewdney, J. G. Feinberg, and R. D. Weston, *Lancet*, **1**, 1175 (1967).

188. G. T. Stewart, *Lancet*, **1**, 1177 (1967).

189. C. W. Parker and J. A. Thiel, *J. Lab. Clin. Med.*, **62**, 482 (1963).

190. R. G. Van Dellen, W. E. Walsh, and G. J. Gleich, *J. Allergy*, **45**, 121 (1970).

191. J. P. Girard, *Int. Arch. Allergy Appl. Immunol.*, **33**, 428 (1968).

192. E. S. K. Assem and M. R. Vickers, *Immunology*, **27**, 255 (1974).

193. V. Pirila and L. Pirila, *Acta Dermatol. Venereol. (Stockholm)*, **46**, 489 (1966).

194. W. B. Leftwich, *Bull. Hopkins Hosp.*, **74**, 26 (1944).

195. W. B. Sherman, *Am. J. Med.*, **3**, 586 (1947).

196. A. G. Wedum, *J. Infect. Dis.*, **70**, 173 (1942).

197. C. W. Parker, J. A. Thiel, and S. Mitchell, *J. Immunol.*, **94**, 289 (1965).

198. D. H. Katz, T. Hamaoka, and B. Benacerraf, *Proc. Nat. Acad. Sci. (USA)*, **70**, 2776 (1973).

199. A. L. de Weck and J. P. Girard, *Int. Arch. Allergy Appl. Immunol.*, **42**, 798 (1972).

CHAPTER EIGHT

The Application of Structural Concepts to the Prediction of the Carcinogenicity of Therapeutic Agents

HERBERT S. ROSENKRANZ

Department of Environmental and
    Occupational Health
Graduate School of Public Health
University of Pittsburgh
Pittsburgh, Pennsylvania, USA

and

GILLES KLOPMAN

Department of Chemistry
Case Western Reserve University
Cleveland, Ohio, USA

CONTENTS

1 Introduction, 223
2 CASE Methodology, 227
3 Results, 232
4 Conclusions, 246

1 INTRODUCTION

Application of SAR (structure–activity relationship) techniques has a tradition of use in the design of therapeutic drugs. However, since in that situation one is dealing primarily with large series of homologous

Burger's Medicinal Chemistry and Drug Discovery,
Fifth Edition, Volume 1: Principles and Practice,
Edited by Manfred E. Wolff.
ISBN 0-471-57556-9 © 1995 John Wiley & Sons, Inc.

chemicals, the SAR procedures that are effective have been designed largely to handle chemical congeners (i.e., molecules belonging to the same chemical class). Moreover, characteristic of the testing of the biological activity of therapeutic agents is the fact that a well-delineated activity is generally ascertained, e.g., minimal inhibitory activity toward bacteria or binding to a receptor or to the active site of an enzyme. The application of SAR techniques to problems in toxicology has been more recent. The main reason for the delay derives from the need to develop methods that can handle groups of noncongeneric chemicals. In addition, the application and validation of SAR methods to toxicological problems require the availability of reliable peer-reviewed databases that can be used as learning sets. The paucity of such experimental data is one of the major obstacles to the extension of SAR techniques to toxicology. Moreover, the biological endpoints measured (e.g., systemic toxicity, carcinogenicity) are generally more diffuse than those associated with other biological phenomena. In fact, biological effects such as carcinogenicity may result from multiple causes.

The availability of reliable SAR-based methods for predicting carcinogenicity would be especially useful in view of the cost (in excess of $2 million) and duration (2 to 3 yr) of the accepted animal cancer bioassay procedures. In the last two decades, to abbreviate the cancer assay proper and decrease the backlog of untested chemicals, a number of short-term tests have been developed to predict carcinogenicity (1, 2). Chief among these is the *Salmonella* mutagenicity assay. The use of this assay is based on the premise that the induction of cancer is initiated by a mutational event that results from an electrophilic attack on the cellular DNA (3). Indeed, this approach has received mechanistic support from the recent discoveries of the role of mutations in the activation of

protooncogenes and the inactivation of suppressor genes (4–12).

However, in parallel with these discoveries came the realization that, in spite of the development of a large number of short-term tests designed to detect DNA reactive–mutagenic molecules ("genotoxicants"), there are a number of rodent cancer-causing agents that are not detected as genotoxicants. Operationally these agents are classified as "nongenotoxic carcinogens" (13). They may act by a variety of alternate mechanisms; as yet there are no validated predictive short-term tests for detecting these mechanisms (14). The ability to predict the activity of such chemicals by SAR techniques would be most useful. Still, it should be noted that mutagenic carcinogens (i.e., "genotoxic" carcinogens) are considered by some to present a greater risk to humans than nongenotoxic carcinogens (14–20), because (1) the vast majority of recognized human carcinogens are mutagens (21–23), (2) mutagenic rodent carcinogens appear to be more potent than nongenotoxic ones (24, 25), and (3) mutagenic rodent carcinogens generally affect both genders and multiple species at multiple sites (13, 26) and, therefore, are more likely to affect humans as well.

In considering the development of SAR capabilities to predict cancer-causing agents, several factors must be taken into consideration. First, since the process of cancer causation can develop by a multiplicity of mechanisms, including nongenotoxic ones, it would be preferable to predict carcinogenicity directly rather than to predict mutagenicity, because the latter would indicate only a potential for a genotoxic carcinogen. Moreover, not all mutagens are carcinogens. In fact, among the chemicals tested by the U.S. National Toxicology Program (NTP), 25% of noncarcinogens are mutagens (13). This, therefore, requires the availability of SAR techniques that can handle not only noncongeneric databases but also biological phenomena that can occur by a multiplicity of mechanisms (e.g., genotoxic and nongenotoxic ones). On the other hand, the predictivity of SAR techniques also depends on the number of chemicals in the learning set as well as their informational content (27–30), i.e., the number of structural features that are represented in the learning set. Obviously, given the high cost and long duration of animal carcinogenicity assays, on the one hand, and the relatively low cost and rapidity of mutagenicity assays, on the other, mutagenicity databases can be expected to be much larger and more diverse than carcinogenicity databases. Indeed, it was estimated that in excess of 15,000 chemicals had been tested for mutagenicity in *Salmonella* by 1983 (31), while heretofore the carcinogenic potential of only approximately 340 chemicals have been reported using the rigorous protocol developed by the NTP (13).

Because mutagenicity assays are used as surrogates to predict carcinogenicity, which is a multistage progression that can also be caused by nonmutagenic events, and because the health effect of interest is the potential to cause cancer in humans, it would seem reasonable to apply SAR techniques directly, whenever feasible, to human carcinogenicity databases to predict cancers in humans. However, recognized human carcinogens and noncarcinogens constitute a small database (32, 33), insufficient for SAR modeling. Thus, out of necessity, one must use the rodent carcinogenicity databases that are available and assume that chemicals that cause cancer in rodents also have the potential for inducing cancer in humans (34). It must be mentioned, however, that because a considerable portion of the recognized rodent carcinogens cause cancer only at the maximum tolerated dose (MTD) and as humans are rarely, if ever, exposed to the MTD, the bioassay protocol has been criticized as being unrealistic. It has been suggested that the resulting cancers are often the conse-

quence of cell proliferation secondary to toxicity (35, 36). In spite of these reservations, the most reliable rodent carcinogenicity database available is that developed under the aegis of the NTP. Presently, it consists of approximately 340 chemicals (13). In addition, the compilation of Gold et al. (37–40) is also useful. It consists of test results on approximately 950 chemicals and includes information on carcinogenic potency. Moreover, due to the possibility of a greater risk to humans as a result of genotoxic mutagenic carcinogens, there is also interest in the ability to predict mutagens, using SAR techniques (41, 42). An obvious advantage of a validated SAR model is the fact that it can be applied to predict the activity of chemicals under consideration before they are even synthesized.

In this chapter, we describe our experience with an expert SAR method we developed (43–45) for the specific purpose of studying the structural basis of the mutagenicity, carcinogenicity, and other toxicological properties of chemicals. The output of this method can be used to predict the activity of untested chemicals as well to gain a mechanistic insight into the basis of these biological activities. It should be noted, however, that the approach described here is being adopted by others as well and that as such it is not unique or restricted. In addition, a consensus is emerging that the predictivity of these expert systems has probably reached close to its maximal effectiveness and that currently the deficits in predictivity are attributable to the paucity of reliable databases that can be used as learning sets.

The system we designed, known as the Computer-automated Structure Evaluation (CASE) is knowledge based (43–46). It is driven solely by the informational content of the learning set, i.e., the structures of the chemicals and their specific biological or toxicological activity. Unlike other approaches, the system is not hypothesis driven, i.e., it is not based on the assumption that a specified activity requires a specific spatial dimension or that it depends on a specific mechanism such as electrophilicity or nucleophilicity. This is unlike hypothesis-driven approaches. Thus, based on the electrophilic theory of carcinogenesis (3), Ashby and co-workers (13, 47–49) have devised the concept of "structural alerts" for genotoxicity. The working hypothesis of this approach is that cancer results from an electrophilic attack on the DNA. Accordingly, structural alerts are structures that are either intrinsically electrophilic or become so after metabolism. This approach requires a broad knowledge of metabolic capabilities that Ashby indeed possesses. It is to be noted that structural alerts go beyond the mere identification of functionalities that are mutagenic in *Salmonella*. They include recognition of new metabolic conversions, resulting in the generation of Michael-type chemicals capable of inducing cancer. Thus acrylates and related structures, which are not mutagenic in *Salmonella* but can form Michael-type reagents, are listed as structural alerts (48, 50). Thus the structural alerts are geared to the recognition of genotoxic carcinogens, and as such they are effective. In fact, the concordance between structural alerts and mutagenicity in *Salmonella* is high (87%) (13). However, as with *Salmonella* mutagenicity results there are chemicals that possess structural alerts but are not carcinogens (13). Moreover, structural alerts are not designed to recognize nongenotoxic carcinogens (51).

The concept of structural alerts has been successful for Ashby in recognizing genotoxic carcinogens, in view of his extensive knowledge of mechanisms of carcinogenicity and biotransformation pathways of carcinogens. Moreover, his extensive knowledge has allowed the recognition of new or additional structural determinants that are based on the knowledge and intuition of the human expert. This approach does not adhere to strict statistical requirements, which are the bases of other SAR approaches. In addition, the human knowledge and intuition that are involved in the recognition of the presence of a putative structural alert in a chemical of unknown carcinogenicity are not readily transmitted from the expert to others. Hence, the widespread applicability of this approach may be restricted to a select group of experts. (To circumvent this restriction, computer-based expert systems are being developed that can predict the metabolic conversion of chemicals and thus their potential carcinogenicity).

The reason for designing a system that differs from approaches that have been successful in the design of therapeutic agents is due mainly to the fact that for most toxicological actions, especially the systemic ones, (1) the exact site or the mechanism of action thereof is not known with certainty, (2) the same toxicological effects may result from different biological phenomena, and (3) the effect may be the result of a sequence of events. This is a different situation from, e.g., the action of a calcium channel blocker or an opiate agonist, both of which exert specific actions at specific sites involving spatial restrictions. The corollary to this approach requires that a given SAR model should be able to handle a variety of chemical classes that may cause the same toxicological effect by a variety of mechanisms. Moreover, the system must be able to handle and recognize chemical moieties that are much larger than the functionalities commonly visualized, for example, by chemists (e.g., amino, carboxylic acid, and benzene moieties). For optimal effectiveness, it should be able to recognize the type of molecular moieties that are bound to the active site of an enzyme or attached to a specific cell receptor. Because the approach is knowledge based and because it deals with biological effects (the basis of which may be unknown), the selected methodology should be completely automatic, i.e., it should be free of operator bias. Finally, as mentioned earlier, the results of the analyses should be readily usable for prediction as well as for mechanistic interpretation. We also wished to include the additional requirement that the resulting system be able to compare and relate the structural determinants associated with different databases such that in the design of new molecules it should be able to optimize beneficial (therapeutic) effects and decrease unwanted side effects (i.e., toxicity).

2 CASE METHODOLOGY

The CASE methodology has been described (41–46). Basically, CASE selects its own descriptors automatically from a learning set composed of active and inactive molecules. The descriptors are easily recognizable single, continuous structural fragments that are embedded in the complete molecule. These are obtained by fragmentation of each of the molecules in the learning set into all of the possible overlapping fragments of sizes 2 to 10 atoms, excluding the hydrogens. The descriptors consist of either activating (biophore) or inactivating (biophobe) fragments. Upon completion of these analyses, MULTI-CASE (the most recent improvement of the CASE program) (52), selects the most important of these fragments as a biophore, i.e., the functionality that is responsible for the experimentally observed activity of the molecules that contain it. MULTICASE then, using the molecules containing this biophore, will use them as a learning set to identify the chemical properties (i.e., structural fragments) or physical chemical properties (log P, solubility, and quantum mechanical) that modulate the activity of the initially identified biophore. This will result in a QSAR equation for this subset of

molecules. To illustrate these and other points, a database of mouse carcinogens will be considered here. Thus biophore 1 (CH=C–C.=C.–) shown in Table 8.1 is present in 16 molecules, of which 15 are active and 1 is marginally active. Thus presence of the biophore carries with it a 94% probability that a chemical is a mouse carcinogen ($p < 0.001$) (Fig. 8.1).

With respect to the QSAR portion of the program, the program augments the 16 molecules that contain this biophore with 2 molecules that contain expanded forms of biophore 1 (molecules 6 and 10 in Table 8.4). On the basis of this set of molecules, MULTICASE performs a QSAR analysis wherein the presence of biophore 1 carries with it 15.28 CASE activity units (Table 8.5). The program then identifies factors that modulate the activity of the biophore. These modulators may be structural and/or physical chemical in nature. The ones modifying biophore 1 are shown in Table 8.5. Based on the presence of these modifiers among the molecules in the subset (see Table 8.4), contribution to the QSAR activity is determined.

Thus because reserpine (see Fig. 8.1) contains biophore 1, it has a 94% probability of carcinogenicity. Moreover, the presence of that biophore contributes 15.28 CASE activity units. Also, the presence of modulator B (modulator 6 in Table 8.5) contributes 10.04 activity units. The water solubility of reserpine, another modulator, is calculated by the program according to a previously described method (53) and is −3.02 (see Table 8.4); according to the QSAR regression equation, it is to be multiplied by −3.84 (Table 8.5), i.e., the water solubility contribution is 11.7. Finally, to take into consideration the possibility of multiple biophores in larger molecules, the equation includes a term ln (number of biophores/molecular weight, where ln is the natural logarithm). Since reserpine contains only one biophore (see Table 8.4), this term becomes ln $1/608.7 = −6.411$,

Table 8.1   Major Biophores Associated with Potential for Carcinogenicity in Mice

Number	Fragment size = *** 1···2···3···4···5···6···7···8···9 List of Biophore Attributes[a,b]		Total	Inactive	Marginal	Active	Average Active
1	CH=CH–C.=C.–		16	0	1	15	61.0
2	O–C=CH–CH=		13	0	0	13	57.0
3	NH2–C=C–CH=		40	12	2	26	32.3
4	S–C=N–C=		4	0	0	4	63.0
5	NH2–NH–		23	3	0	20	48.0
6	NH–NH–		15	4	9	11	41.5
7	NH2–N–		7	0	0	7	60.1
8	CH2–CH2–N–CH2–CH2–		13	1	0	12	64.0
9	Cl–CH=		7	0	0	7	52.0
10	O–CH=		7	0	0	7	60.9
11	Cl–C–C–	⟨2–Cl⟩	12	3	0	9	57.0
12	CH2–N–CH2–	⟨2–NO⟩	5	0	0	5	74.0
13	CH2–CH2–CH2–CH–		7	1	0	6	46.0
14	Br–CH2–		8	2	0	6	46.0
15	Cl–C''–Cl		5	0	0	5	51.0
16	CH=CH–C=CH–CH=C–C=	⟨3–NH2⟩	5	0	0	5	62.0
17	Cl–C=C–C=C–C''–Cl	⟨4–Cl⟩	4	1	0	3	44.0
18	CH3–CO–NH–C=CH–	⟨4–CH=⟩	7	1	2	4	33.0
19	Cl–CH2–C=		4	1	0	3	36.0
20	CH=C.–CO–C.=		6	1	1	4	39.0
21	CH=C–CH=CH–C=CH–	⟨2–CH2⟩	12	2	0	10	61.0

[a]C., a carbon atom shared by two rings; ⟨2–Cl⟩, a chlorine atom attached to the second atom from the left.
    [b]There are some simple rules for interpreting the structural determinants; thus the fourth carbon from the left of biophore 13 is shown with an atom missing, i.e., in reality it is CH$_2$–CH$_2$–CH$_2$–CH–X, where X can represent any atom except hydrogen. On the other hand, for biophore 16, the third carbon from the left must be substituted by an amino group. Biophore 1 is shown embedded in reserpine and C.I. vat yellow 4 in Figures 8.1 and 8.2, respectively. Biophore 3 is shown embedded in 2,4-xylidine HCl in Figure 8.3, while biophore 11 is shown embedded in heptachlor in Figure 8.4.

which must be multiplied by −6.47 (see Table 8.5) to give a contribution of 41.45. Thus the projected activity of reserpine is 78 CASE units (this is also summarized in Fig. 8.1). The relationship between CASE activity units and metric units is

$$\text{CASE activity} = 14.1329 \times \log$$
$$(1/\text{mmole}/\text{kg}/\text{day}) + 44.1329$$

This equation was determined initially when cutoffs for carcinogens, marginal carcinogens, and noncarcinogens were set, before the SAR analyses. Hence, an activity of 78 CASE units is equal to 0.004 mmoles/kg/day or 2.45 mg/kg/day for the

TD$_{50}$ value, the dose at which 50% of the animals are tumor free (37, 54). This relationship between dose and CASE activity units is based on the designation as carcinogens of those molecules with TD$_{50}$ values below 10 mmoles/kg/day, while chemicals with TD$_{50}$ values in excess of 51 mmoles/kg/day are called noncarcinogenic and molecules with TD$_{50}$ values in the range of 10–51 mmole/kg/day are designated as marginally active.

If the data set is a congeneric one, the single biophore and associated modulators may explain the activity of all the molecules in the database and the program will exit. With noncongeneric databases, this will usually not occur, and there will be a

Table 8.2   Molecules That Contain the *o*-Substituted Aromatic Amine Moiety NH2–C=C–CH= [a]

Copies	Chemical	Carcinogenicity	Mutagenicity
2	3,3-Dimethylbenzidine.2HCl	A	+
2	3,3'-Dimethoxybenzidine.2HCl	A	+
1	1-Amino-2-methylanthraquinone	A	+
1	*o*-Anisidine HCl	A	+
1	4-Chloro-*m*-phenylenediamine	A	+
1	Cinnamyl anthranilate	A	−
1	*p*-Cresidine	A	+
1	2,4-Diaminoanisole sulfate	A	+
1	2,4-Diaminotoluene	A	+
2	4-Chloro-*o*-phenylenediamine	A	+
1	5-Nitro-*o*-anisidine	A	+
1	Phenazopyridine.HCl	A	+
1	*o*-Toluidine.HCl	A	+
1	2,4,5-Trimethylaniline	A	+
1	5-Chloro-*o*-toluidine	B	−
1	5-Nitro-*o*-toluidine	B	+
1	4-Chloro-*o*-toluidine.HCl	C	−
1	*m*-Cresidine	C	+
2	2,6-Dichloro-*p*-phenylenediamine	C	+
1	3-Amino-4-ethoxyacetanilide	D	+
1	2-Biphenylamine hydrochloride	D	+
1	2-Nitro-*p*-phenylenediamine	D	+
1	*o*-Anthranilic acid	NC	−
1	2-Chloro-*p*-phenylenediamine sulfate	NC	+
1	2,4-Dimethoxyaniline.HCl	NC	+
1	4-Nitroanthranilic acid	NC	+
2	4-Nitro-*o*-phenylenediamine	NC	+
1	2,5-Toluenediamine sulfate	NC	+
1	2-Amino-4-nitrophenol	D	+
1	2-Amino-5-nitrophenol	D	+

[a]The chemicals listed here were tested for carcinogenicity in rodents and mutagenicity in *Salmonella* by the U.S. National Toxicology Program (13). The chemicals containing this biophore are primarily mutagenic (genotoxic) carcinogens.

residue of molecules not explained by the single biophore and associated modulators. When this happens, the program will remove from consideration the molecules already explained by the previous biophore, and it will search for the next biophore (and associated modulators). The process is iterated until all of the molecules in the original database have been explained. In fact, this results in a multiple

CASE analysis, wherein the molecules in the database have been reclassified into logical subsets.

The resulting list of biophores (see Table 8.1) is then used to predict the activity of yet untested molecules. Thus, upon submission for evaluation, MULTICASE will determine if the unknown molecule contains a biophore. If it does not, the molecule will be assumed to be inactive (Fig. 8.5), unless

Table 8.3   Molecules Containing the Dichloroalkane Moiety $Cl-C\overset{\displaystyle Cl^{\,a}}{\underset{\displaystyle C}{\Big\backslash}}$

Copies	Chemical	Carcinogenicity	Mutagenicity
6	Chlordane	C	–
6	Heptachlor	C	–
17	Toxaphene	C	+
6	Aldrin	D	–
3	Dicofol	D	–
6	Dieldrin	E	–
6	Endrin	NC	–
6	Hexachloroethane	A	–
5	Photodieldrin	NC	+

[a]The chemicals listed here were tested for carcinogenicity in rodents and mutagenicity in *Salmonella* by the U.S. National Toxicology Program (13). The chemicals containing this moiety are primarily nonmutagenic (nongenotoxic) carcinogens.

Table 8.4   Distribution of Biophore 1 and Modifiers in a Subset of Chemicals

Number	Name	Number of Biophore 1	Modifier Number[a]	Water Solubility[b]	Molecular Weight
1	Benzo[a]pyrene	2		−5.09	252.3
2	Reserpine	1	6	−3.02	608.7
3	N-Hydroxy-2-acetylaminofluorene	2	6	−1.73	239.3
4	C.I. Vat yellow 4	4	4 × no. 1	−3.08	332.4
5	2-Acetylaminofluorene	2	6	−2.85	223.3
6	2-Amino-3,8-dimethylimidazo[4,		2 × no. 8	−1.66	213.2
7	2-Amino-3-methylimidazo[4,5-f]	1	8, 9	−1.19	198.3
8	3-Amino-1-methyl-5H-pyrido[4,3	1	5	−0.37	197.2
9	3-Amino-1,4-dimethyl-5H-pyrido	1	5	−0.81	211.3
10	Aflatoxin		3, 7	+0.56	312.3
11	3-Amino-9-ethylcarbazole	1		−1.67	210.3
12	2-Amino-3,4-dimethylimidazo[4,	1	7, 8	−1.62	212.3
13	2-Amino-3-methyl-9H-pyrido[2,3	1		−0.37	197.2
14	2-Amino-9H-pyrido(2,3-b)indole	2	9	+0.06	183.2
15	2-Aminodiphenylene oxide	1	3	−0.26	183.2
16	Carbazole	2	9	−0.51	167.2
17	Dibenz[a,h]anthracene	2		−5.80	278.4
18	7,12-Dimethylbenz[a]anthracene	1	5	−4.95	256.4

[a]Refers to modifiers listed in Table 8.5.
[b]Water solubility is calculated by the program according to the procedure of Klopman and co-workers (53). The values are expressed as log of g soluble/100 g water. That number is multiplied by the factor −3.8388, which was determined by the QSAR regression analysis (Table 8.5).

The molecule contains the Biophore

(1)

$$CH=CH$$
$$\diagdown$$
$$C.=C.$$
$$\diagup$$

*** 15 out of the known 16 molecules (94%) containing such Biophore are Mouse Carcinogens with an average activity of 61 (conf. level = 100%)

Constant is 15.3

** The following Modulators are also present:

(B) $CH=C—CH=CH—C.=C.—$ Activating 10.0

Water solubility   = −3.02;   WS contribution is   11.6

Ln Nr.Bi/Mol.Wt. = −6.41;   Nr.Bioph/MW contrib.is 41.5

** The probability that this molecule is a Mouse Carcinogen is 94.1% **

** The compound is predicted to be EXTREMELY active **

** The projected Mouse Carcinogenicity activity is 78.0 CASE units **

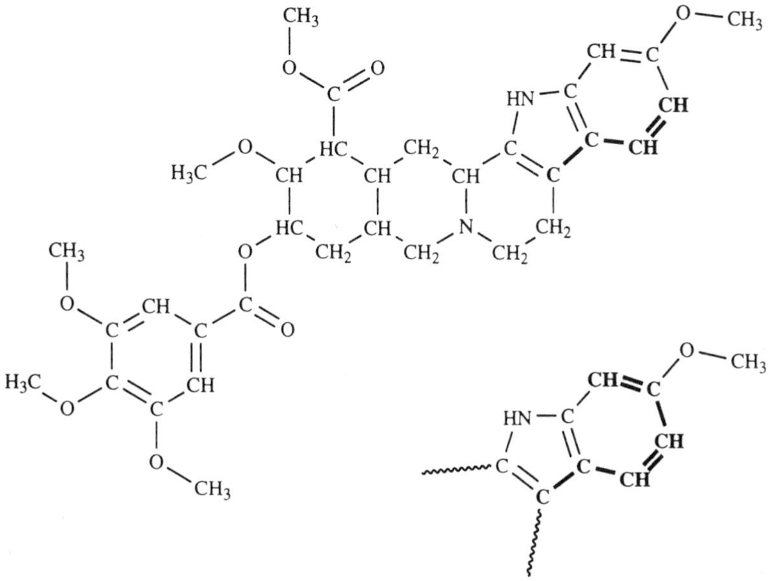

Fig. 8.1 MULTICASE prediction of the carcinogenicity in mice of reserpine (see text). A total of 78 CASE units correspond to a TD_{50} of 2.45 mg/kg/day. The biophore and activating modulator are shown in bold.

it contains a group that resembles chemically one of the biophores, in which case it will be flagged. When the molecule contains a biophore, the presence of modulators for that biophore will be investigated. MULTICASE will then make qualitative as well as quantitative predictions of the activity of the unknown molecule (see Fig. 8.1).

Obviously, while biophores are the determining structures, the modulators may influence the biological potential of the chemical. This is illustrated in Figures 8.1 and 8.2, which describe the MULTICASE predictions of the activity of chemicals that contain the same biophore 1 and, therefore, show the same overall probability of carcinogenicity (94.1%). However, in one instance, i.e., reserpine (see Fig. 8.1), the biological potency is *enhanced* by a modifier (B), and, in the other, C.I. vat yellow 4

The molecule contains the Biophore

(1)   CH=CH
                                   \
                                    C.=C.
                                   /

     *** 15 out of the known 16 molecules (94%) containing such Biophore are Mouse Carcinogens with an average activity of 61 (conf. level = 100%)

                                             Constant is   15.3

    ** The following Modulators are also present:

(C)   CH=C.—CO—C.=   Activating -33.7

         Water solubility   = -3.08;   WS contribution is   11.8

         Ln Nr.Bi/Mol.Wt. = -4.42;   Nr.Bioph/MW contrib.is   28.6

    ** The probability that this molecule is a Mouse Carcinogen is 94.1% **

    ** The compound is predicted to be MARGINALLY active **

    ** The projected Mouse Carcinogenicity activity is 22.0 CASE units **

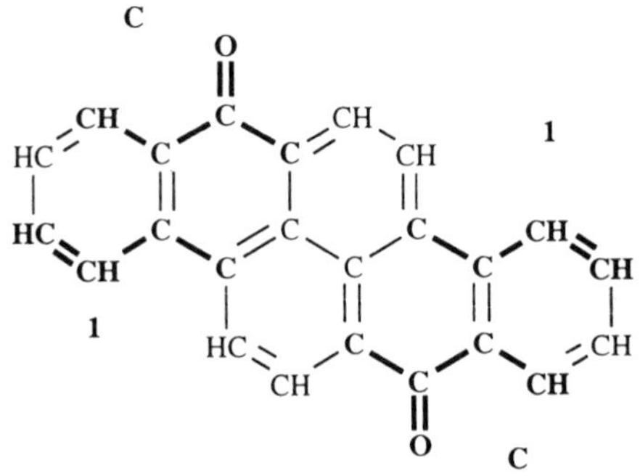

Fig. 8.2 MULTICASE prediction of the marginal carcinogenicity of C.I. vat yellow 4. This chemical contains the same biophore 1 (in bold) as reserpine (see Fig. 8.1). However, because of the presence of the inactivating modulator C (in bold), the activity is predicted to be marginal (22 CASE units) which corresponds to a TD_{50} of 12, 241 mg/kg/day.

(see Fig. 8.2), it is decreased (modifier C) such that while the molecule has a potential for activity (94.1%), the activity will be minimal, hence resulting in an overall prediction that is essentially negative (marginal activity).

3 RESULTS

Obviously, in light of the preceding description, the method described above crucially depends on the availability of reliable databases. Thus, for optimal effectiveness, the experimental protocol to obtain the experimental data for each chemical included in the learning set must be uniform, the test object (cell or animal species) must be defined (e.g., strains, sex, age, and weight), and the nature and purity of the test chemical must be ensured.

By necessity, therefore, the SAR approach is interdisciplinary. The research group must include individuals with expertise in the specific biological phenomenon under consideration, with respect to experimental conditions, the nature of the biological response, and knowledge about the mechanism leading to it. Moreover, the quality and accuracy of the protocol and the data generated must also be ensured. Since, in fact, the SAR program becomes an expert on the particular system under investigation, a human expert (e.g., a medicinal chemist) is needed to challenge

The molecule contains the Biophore:

(3)   NH2—C
                    $\backslash\backslash$
                      C—CH″

*** 26 out of the known 40 molecules (65%) containing such Biophore are Mouse Carcinogens with an average activity of 32 (conf. level = 99%)

                                        Constant is   58.2

** The following Modulators are also present:

(3)   NH2—C=C—CH=   Inactivating   −6.7
(A)   CH=C—CH—   ⟨2—CH3⟩ Activating   8.9
(B)   CH=CH—C=CH—C=   Inactivating −15.5
      Water solubility = 1.03;   WS contribution is   −3.2

** The probability that this molecule is a Mouse Carcinogen is 67.5% **
** The compound is predicted to be VERY active **
** The projected Mouse Carcinogenicity activity is 42.0 CASE units **

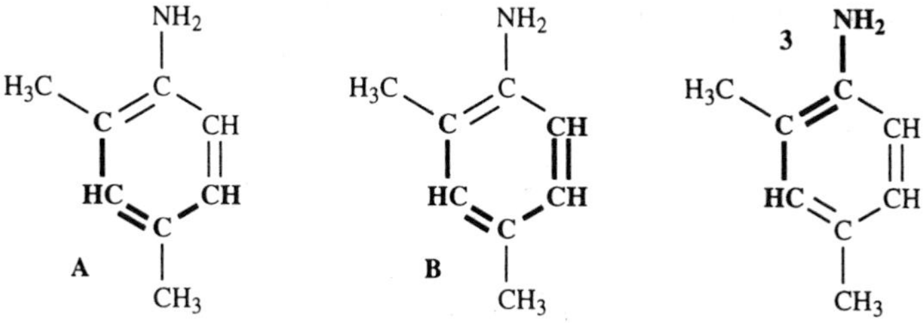

Fig. 8.3 MULTICASE prediction of the carcinogenicity in mice of 2,4-xylidene HCl. The probability of carcinogenicity is based on the presence of biophore 3 (in bold) (see Table 8.1). The high potency is due to the presence of the modulators (in bold). Biophore 3 is a typical biophore associated with mutagenic (genotoxic) carcinogens (see Table 8.2).

Table 8.5 Contribution of Biophore 1 and Its Modulators to Carcinogenic Potency[a]

	Biophore	CASE Units
	CH=CH–C.=C.–	15.28

	Modulators	
1.	CH=C.–CO–C.=	−8.42
2.	ln (no. of biophores/molecular weight)	−6.47[b]
3.	CH=C–C.=C.–	24.70
4.	water solubility	−3.84[c]
5.	CH3–C=C.–C.=	13.32
6.	CH=C–CH=CH–C.=C.–	10.04
7.	C.=CH–C=C.–	7.83
8.	C=N–C.=C.–	4.71
9.	NH–C.=CH–CH=CH–CH=C.–C.=CH–	3.55

[a]The distribution of the biophore and modulators among the molecules of the subset are given in Table 8.4. See the text for calculation of the predicted carcinogenic potency of a molecule.

[b]This number is multiplied by the ratio of the number of copies of biophore 1/molecular weight. The number of copies of biophore 1 and the molecular weights are listed in Table 8.4.

[c]This number is multiplied by the calculated water solubility (see Table 8.4).

The molecule contains the Biophore:

(11)

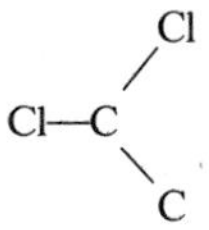

*** 9 out of the known 12 molecules (75%) containing such Biophore are Mouse Carcinogens with an average activity of 57 (conf. level = 95%)

	Constant is	50.8

The following Modulator(s) is/are also present:

(A)   CH″—CH—CH—C—   Activating   24.2
        Log partition coeff. =   7.76;   Log P contribution is   82.1
        Water solubility   = −3.92;   WS contribution is   −47.7
        Lg Nr.Bi/Mol.Wt. = −4.54;   Nr.Bioph/MW contrib.is   −40.5

The probability that this molecule is a Mouse Carcinogen is 71.4% **
** The compound is predicted to be EXTREMELY active **
** The projected Mouse Carcinogenicity activity is 69.9 CASE UNITS **

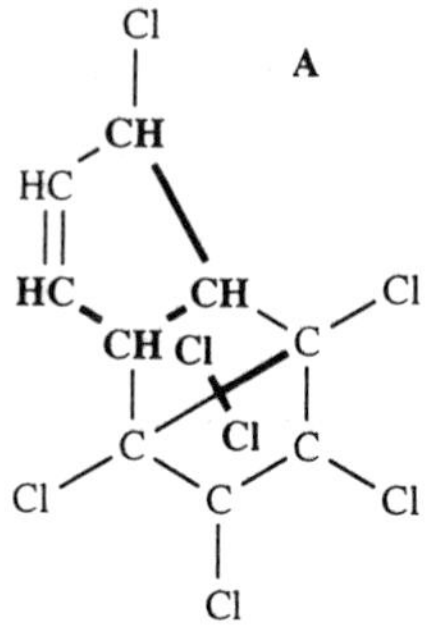

Fig. 8.4 MULTICASE prediction of the carcinogenicity of heptachlor. The probability of carcinogenicity is due to the presence of biophore 11 (in bold) (see Table 8.1), while the potency is also the result of modulators. Biophore 11 is a typical biophore associated with nonmutagenic (nongenotoxic) carcinogens (see Table 8.3).

** The molecule does not contain any known biophore**
it is therefore presumed to be INACTIVE

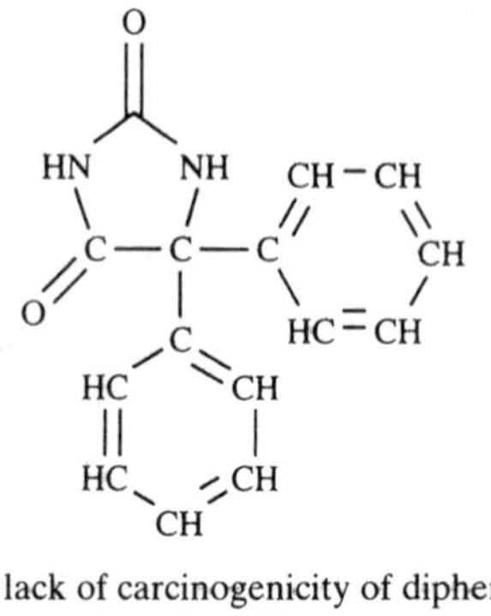

Fig. 8.5 MULTICASE prediction of the lack of carcinogenicity of diphenylhydantoin. This prediction is based on the fact that among the 253 unique fragments of size 2 to 10 atoms, there was no fragment that was identified as a biophore.

the SAR program, to validate the model that is derived, and to interpret it effectively.

In collaboration with others, we have been able to model successfully a number of toxicological endpoints (Table 8.6). Using such an array of predictive capabilities, we are able to project toxicological profiles not only of parent substances (Table 8.7) but also of their putative metabolites (Fig. 8.6).

For further illustrative purposes, we describe some of our findings with respect to the murine carcinogenicity database generated under the aegis of NTP (13) and those compiled by Gold et al. (37–40). As mentioned earlier, the program identifies the biophores associated with activity and then determines whether such structural determinants are found in untested molecules. In addition, the program can also document the origin of the identified biophores and biophobes, and this can be used in assessing the mechanism of carcinogenicity. Thus, biophore 3 in Table 8.1 is present in a number of other molecules that were tested for carcinogenicity (see Table 8.2) and that are mutagenic in nature; in fact, the presence of this aromatic amine moiety is a recognized structural alert for DNA reactivity (13, 73). Because this biophore is associated with genotoxicity (see Table 8.2) and because, e.g., 2,4-xylidine is predicted to be a mouse carcinogen (see Fig. 8.3), it may be further predicted that it will be a mutagenic

Table 8.6 Some Toxicological Activities Modeled with the CASE Program

Activity	Reference
Mutagenicity in *Salmonella*	41, 42, 55
Induction of SOS repair in *E. coli*	56–58
Antimutagens	99
Structural alerts for DNA reactivity	59, 60
Induction of sister chromatid exchanges	61
Induction of chromosomal aberrations	61
Induction of unscheduled DNA synthesis	100
Oncogenic cell transformation	[a]
Induction of micronuclei in rodents	62
Induction of somatic mutations in *Drosophila*	*
Cell toxicity	63
Sensory irritation in mice	*
Contact allergenicity	*
Pulmonary hyperreactivity	*
Reproductive toxicity (rabbits, rats, mice, and humans)	*
Maximum tolerated dose (mice, rats)	64
Induction of $\alpha 2\mu$ nephropathy in male rats	*
Inhibition of human cytochrome P4502D	*
Toxicity to minnows	65
Carcinogenicity to rodents	66–68
Microtox test	101
Induction of preneoplastic lesions	102
Binding to AHH receptor	69
Biodegradability	70

[a] An asterisk indicates unpublished results.

Table 8.7   Some Predicted Properties of Tamoxifen[a]

	Activity[b]	Prediction
1.	Mutagenicity in *Salmonella*	−
2.	Nitrosatable to a genotoxic phenyldiazonium ion	−
3.	Induction of chromosomal aberration	+
4.	Induction of sister-chromatid exchange	+
5.	Induction of unscheduled DNA synthesis	+
6.	Cell transformation of balb 3T3 cells	+
7.	Induction of somatic mutations and recombinations in *Drosophila*	+
8.	Induction of micronuclei in rodent bone marrow	+
9.	Cell toxicity (below 1 μM)	+
10.	Rodent carcinogen	+
11.	Maximum tolerated dose in rats (below 0.9 mmol/kg/day)	+
12.	Maximum tolerated dose in mouse (below 1.8 mmol/kg/day)	+
13.	Binding to AHH (TCDD) receptor	−
14.	Inhibition of human cytochrome P4502D	+
15.	Inducer of $\alpha 2\mu$-nephropathy in male rats	−
16.	Human developmental toxicant	+
17.	Mouse developmental toxicant	+
18.	Rat developmental toxicant	−
19.	Rabbit developmental toxicant	+
20.	Toxicity to minnow (LC$_{50}$ below 0.1 mmol/L)	+

[a]Tamoxifen [Z-(1-(4-(2-dimethylaminoethoxy)phenyl)1,2-disphenyl-1-butene] is widely used in the treatment of breast cancer. Tamoxifen is predicted to be a rodent carcinogen. This is, in fact, consistent with a recent report (71). While tamoxifen is not predicted to be a *Salmonella* mutagen, it is predicted to be genotoxic to eukaryote cells (assays 3, 4, and 5) and to whole animals (assays 7 and 8). This is consistent with the report (72) that this agent forms DNA-adducts as determined by the highly sensitive ^{32}P-postlabeling procedure (72). It should be noted that tamoxifen has a number of other toxicological potentials as well (e.g., developmental effects).
[b]References for these assays are given in Table 8.6.

(genotoxic) carcinogen. This has certain consequences with respect to possible risk to humans. On the other hand, biophore 11, which is present in heptachlor (see Fig. 8.4), is derived from a variety of molecules (see Table 8.3) that, although carcinogenic, are not associated with mutagenicity and may, therefore, derive their activity from a nonmutagenic mechanism. Hence molecules containing this biophore may be predicted to be nongenotoxic carcinogens.

As described earlier, MULTICASE, the latest version of the CASE program (52), identifies not only biophores but also modulators of the activity. This may be

invaluable in understanding the mechanistic basis of the action of a carcinogen.

It is to be noted that heretofore the predictions described have been qualitative ones, i.e., they are expressed as a probability of the test chemical being active or inactive. Obviously, a given chemical will either be 100% active of 100% inactive. However, if a database such as that compiled by Gold and co-workers is expressed in TD$_{50}$ values (37, 54) (i.e., in quantitative terms), then the QSAR option of the program comes into play. It allows the prediction of the probable potency of a molecule that is predicted to be active (see

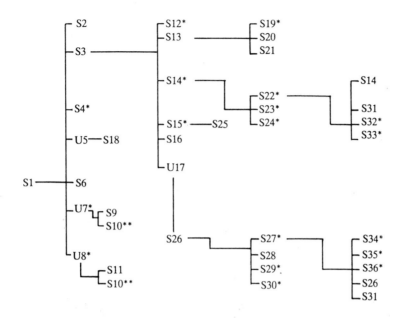

S2, S3, U7, U8	Obtained via P450 monooxygenase
S4, S12, S19, S22	Obtained via *N*-acetyltransferase
U5, S6, S16, U17,	
S20, S21, S23, S24,	Obtained via methyltransferase
S32, S33	
S13, S34	Obtained via glucuronyl transferase
S14, S35	Obtained via sulfotransferase
S15, S36	Obtained via alcohol dehydrogenase
S11, S18, S26	Obtained by spontaneous reaction
S9, S10	Obtained by spontaneous decomposition of hemiacetal/hemiketal
S25	Obtained via aldehyde dehydrogenase
S14, S26, S31	Obtained via amidase

Fig. 8.6 The potential biotransformation of omeprazole. This scheme was generated by the META program and indicated some of the possible metabolic pathways of omeprazole (S1). The structures associated with each metabolite are given in Fig. 8.7. META also indicates the enzymic or spontaneous reaction associated with each metabolite, which are shown here. *, chemicals predicted to be rodent carcinogens based on MULTICASE analysis of the NTP rodent carcinogenicity database; **, formaldehyde (S10), a known carcinogen, is too small for analysis by MULTICASE.

Figs. 8.1–8.4). This is due to the QSAR calculations described earlier (see Table 8.5). In turn, this allows an estimation of the carcinogenic potency of a molecule.

A number of analyses and reconstruction experiments have shown that, as expected, the SAR predictions are sensitive to the size of the learning set. Thus, within limits, for the usual learning set consisting of 200 to 400 *noncongeneric* chemicals, the larger the number of chemicals included in the learning set, the greater the predictive accuracy (27, 28, 74, 75). However, in view of the rationale used, the SAR model is also sensitive to the informational content of the learning set (28). Thus we have

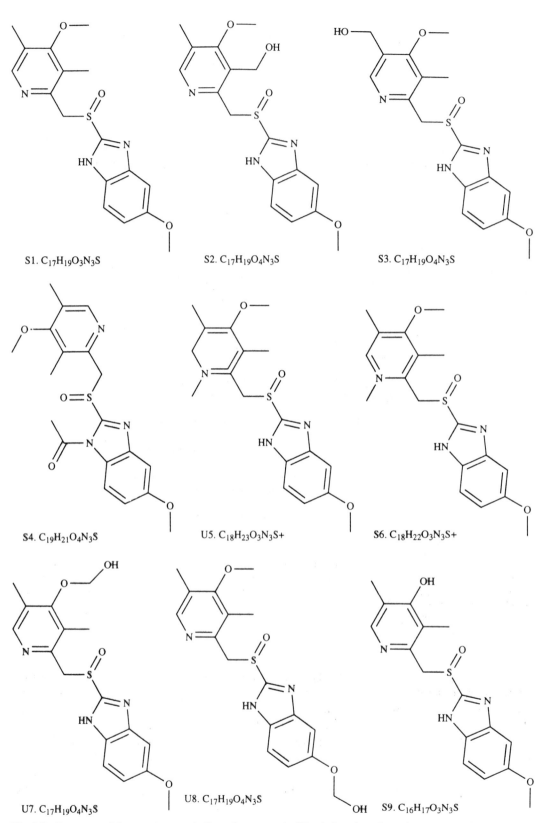

S1. $C_{17}H_{19}O_3N_3S$

S2. $C_{17}H_{19}O_4N_3S$

S3. $C_{17}H_{19}O_4N_3S$

S4. $C_{19}H_{21}O_4N_3S$

U5. $C_{18}H_{23}O_3N_3S+$

S6. $C_{18}H_{22}O_3N_3S+$

U7. $C_{17}H_{19}O_4N_3S$

U8. $C_{17}H_{19}O_4N_3S$

S9. $C_{16}H_{17}O_3N_3S$

Fig. 8.7 Structures of the putative metabolites of omeprazole. The designations Sn and Un refer to the metabolic scheme given in Figure 8.6.

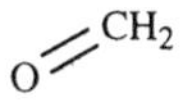

O=CH₂

S10 CH₂O

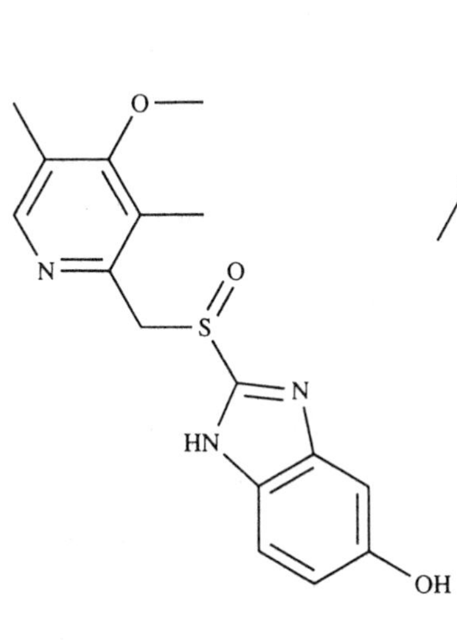

S11. $C_{16}H_{17}O_3N_3S$

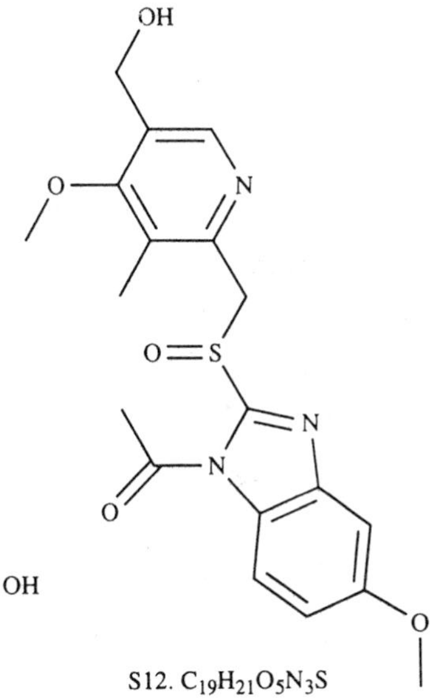

S12. $C_{19}H_{21}O_5N_3S$

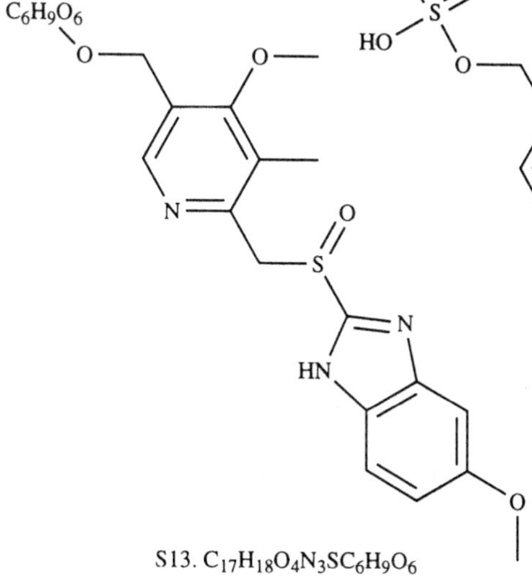

S13. $C_{17}H_{18}O_4N_3SC_6H_9O_6$

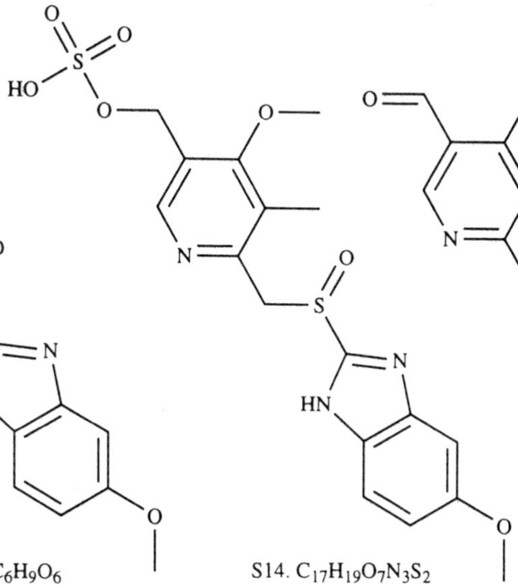

S14. $C_{17}H_{19}O_7N_3S_2$

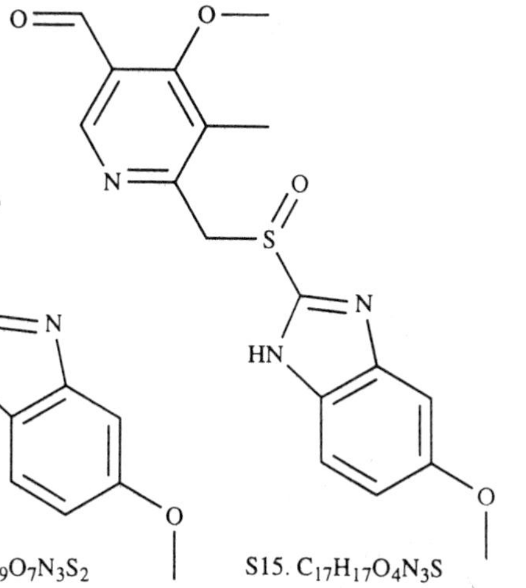

S15. $C_{17}H_{17}O_4N_3S$

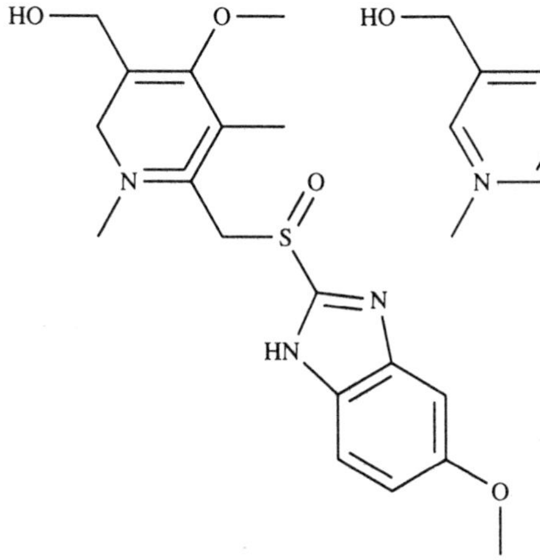

S16. $C_{18}H_{23}O_4N_3S+$

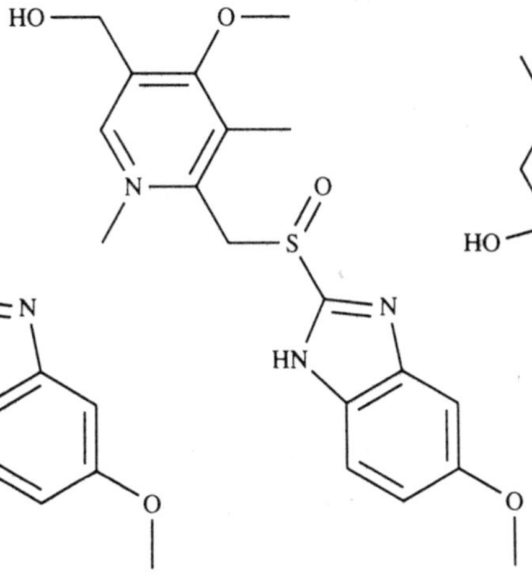

U17. $C_{18}H_{22}O_4N_3S+$

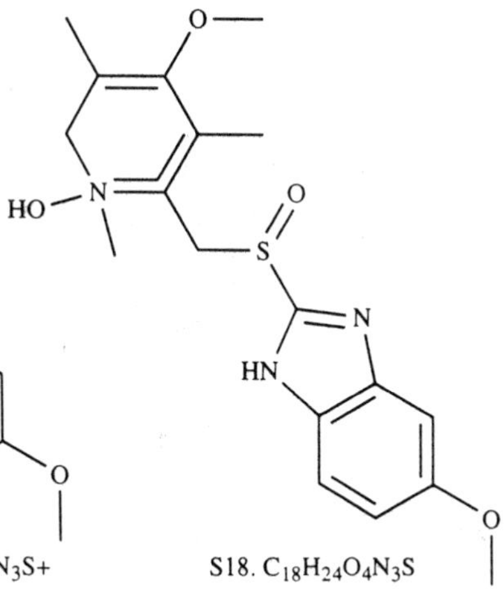

S18. $C_{18}H_{24}O_4N_3S$

Fig. 8.7 (*Continued*)

239

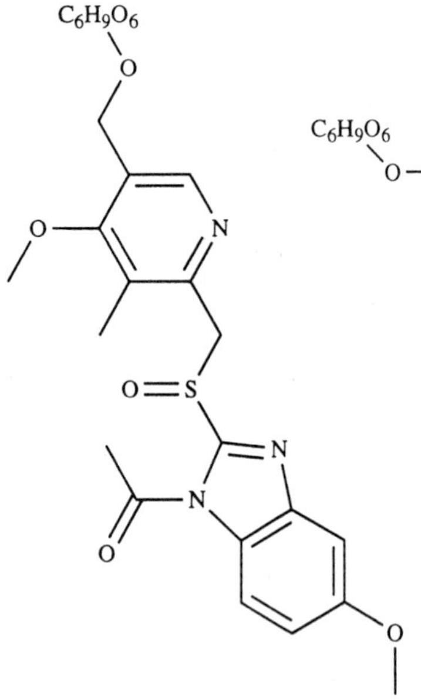

S19. $C_{19}H_{20}O_5N_3SC_6H_9O_6$

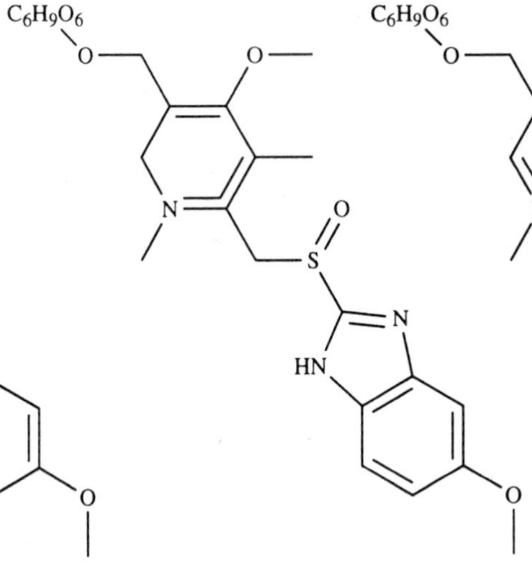

S20. $C_{18}H_{22}O_4N_3SC_6H_9O_6+$

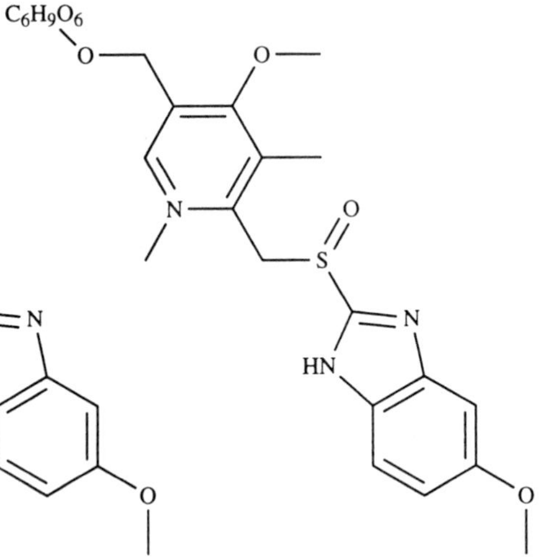

S21. $C_{18}H_{21}O_4N_3SC_6H_9O_6+$

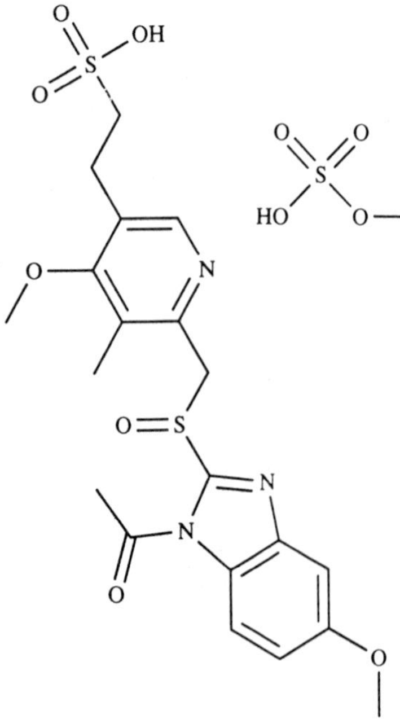

S22. $C_{19}H_{21}O_8N_3S_2$

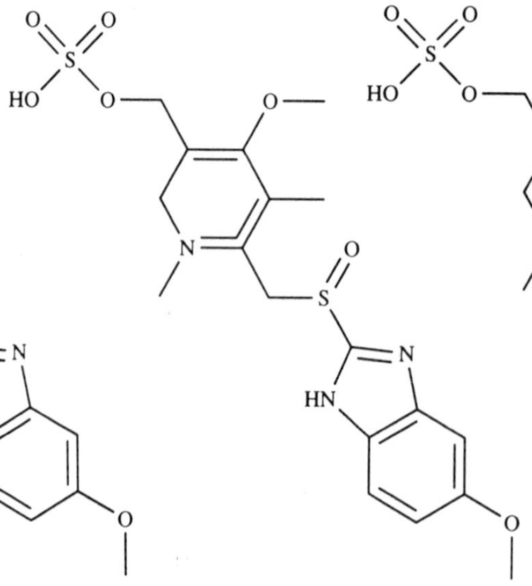

S23. $C_{18}H_{23}O_7N_3S_2+$

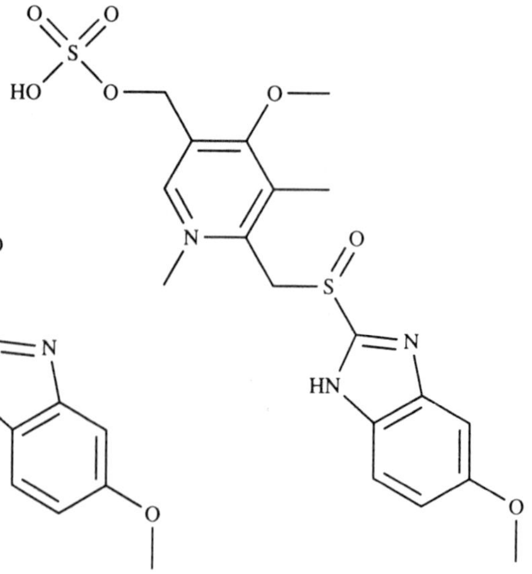

S24. $C_{18}H_{22}O_7N_3S_2+$

Fig. 8.7 (*Continued*)

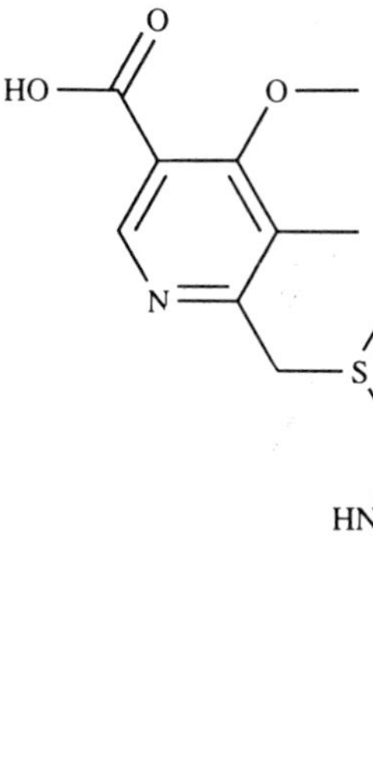

S25. $C_{17}H_{17}O_5N_3S$

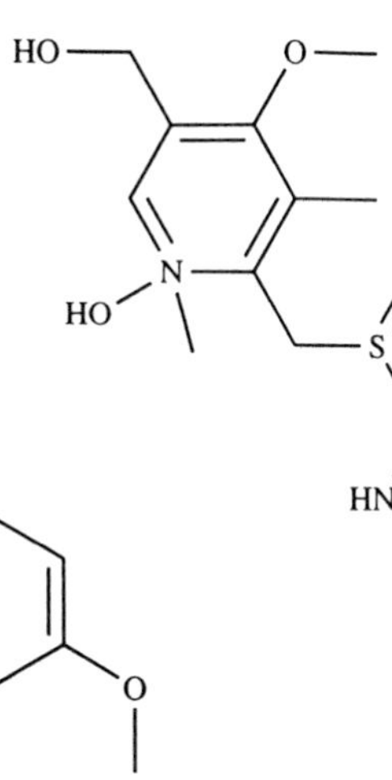

S26. $C_{18}H_{23}O_5N_3S$

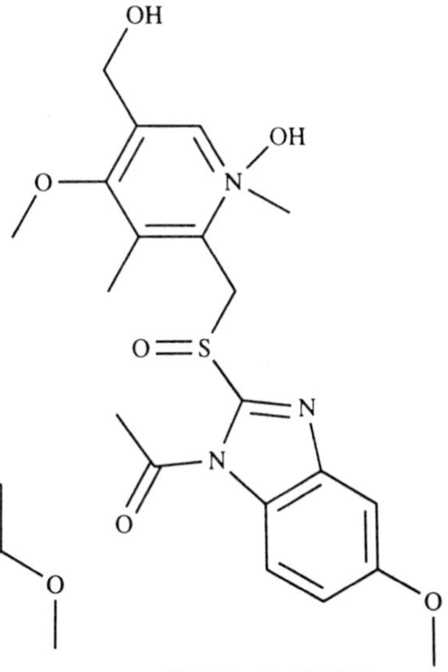

S27. $C_{20}H_{25}O_6N_3S$

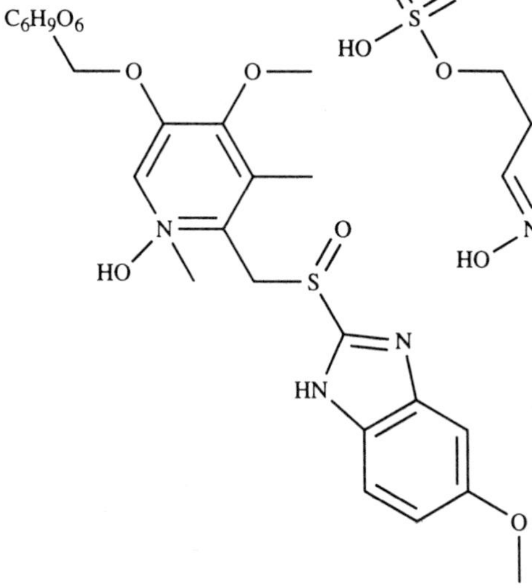

S28. $C_{18}H_{22}O_5N_3SC_6H_9O_6$

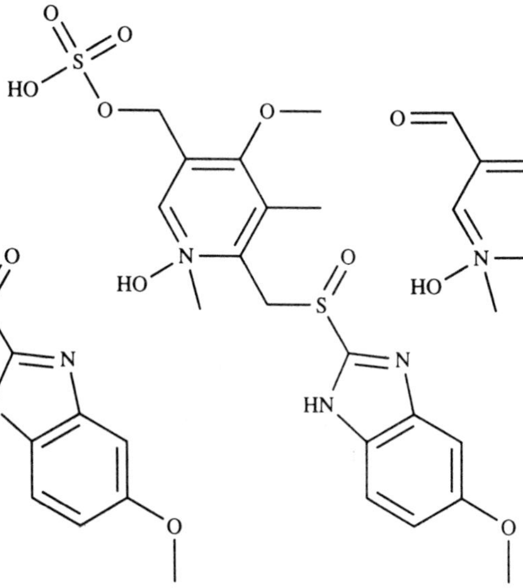

S29. $C_{18}H_{23}O_8N_3S$

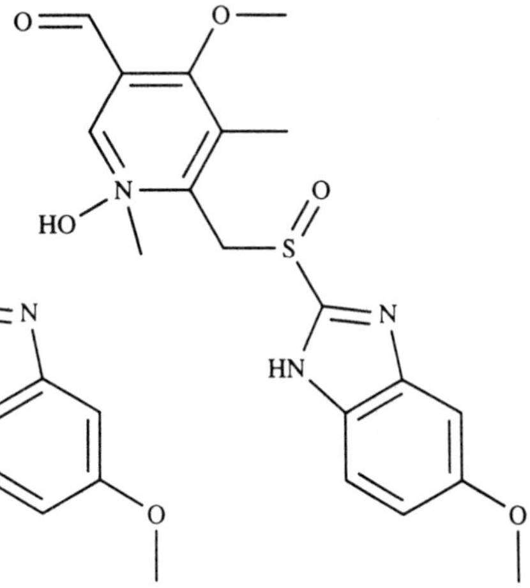

S30. $C_{18}H_{21}O_5N_3S$

Fig. 8.7 (*Continued*)

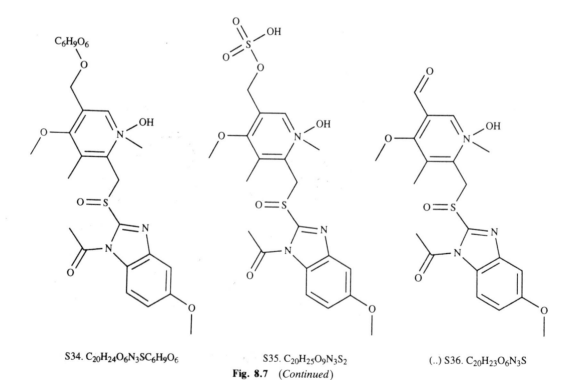

S31. $C_2H_4O_2$

S32. $C_{20}H_{25}O_8N_3S_2+$

S32. $C_{20}H_{24}O_8N_3S_2+$

S34. $C_{20}H_{24}O_6N_3SC_6H_9O_6$

S35. $C_{20}H_{25}O_9N_3S_2$

(..) S36. $C_{20}H_{23}O_6N_3S$

Fig. 8.7 (*Continued*)

found that lack of accuracy (i.e., decreased concordance between predictions and experimental results) may be due to the presence, among the fragments generated, of moieties that are "unknown" to the learning set (Fig. 8.8). This introduces a degree of uncertainty, since the unknown fragment could, e.g., be an unidentified biophore. Such a situation may result from the practice of including among the chemicals that have been tested structural analogs of agents that are already known to be active in the assay system (29). This, in fact, has occurred among the chemicals included with those tested for carcinogenicity in rodents during the early phase of the National Cancer Institute–National Toxicology Program cancer bioassays (76). To overcome this problem, we have developed a method for evaluating the informational content of databases, and then, using this information, we are able to develop databases with maximal informational content (29, 77, 78) (Table 8.8). In fact, we could thus demonstrate that the informational content of a database consisting of 200 chemicals chosen on the basis of structural diversity can be as informative

(i.e., predictive) as a database consisting of 800 chemicals chosen randomly (28).

Once a database has been analyzed by CASE, the method needs to be validated with respect to its ability to predict the activity of chemicals not included in the learning set. Practically, this is accomplished by randomly deleting from the learning set a number of chemicals for which experimental data are available and then determining the ability of the biophores and biophobes derived from the reduced learning set of predict the activity of the deleted chemicals. Furthermore, to evaluate the concordance between experimental and predictive results, we have developed an objective method for evaluating the significance of these predictions (79, 80). This method takes into consideration the prevalence of active chemicals in the learning set and the number of chemicals that are to be predicted.

Because the performance of CASE depends on the size of the learning set, the chemicals initially deleted for the purpose of the validation are reintegrated into the learning set, and the program is then run with a complete set of test results. There-

---

*** WARNING *** The following functionalities are UNKNOWN to me:
    *** NH2—CH—CH3
      ** The molecule does not contain any known biophore **
        it is therefore presumed to be INACTIVE
    ** However, the results may be INCONCLUSIVE due to the presence of
      UNKNOWN functionalities **

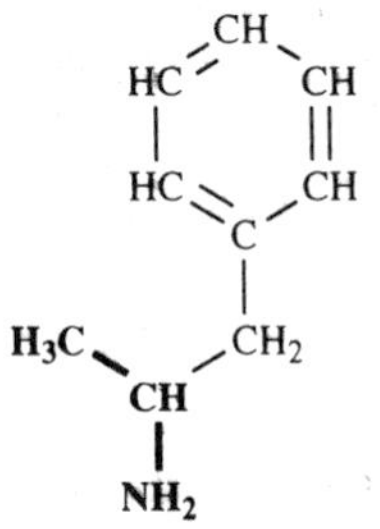

Fig. 8.8 MULTICASE prediction of the lack of carcinogenicity of amphetamine. This prediction is based on the finding that none of the 59 unique fragments derived from amphetamine is recognized as a biophore. However, one of the fragments (in bold) is "unknown" to the learning set. Because the unknown fragment might be a biophore, this introduces an element of uncertainty in the conclusion.

Table 8.8   Most Abundant Fragment Unknown to the Mouse Carcinogenicity Database[a]

Occurrence (Number)	Fragment	Example
61	N≡C–C=	o-Tolunitrile
56	NH–C″–CH3	Cimetidine
26	COH–C≡C–	o-Vanillin
24	NH2–CH–CH–	Isoleucine
23	N≡C–CH2–	Allyl cyanide
20	N–C–	Clotrimazle
19	S–CH=CH–	Sulfathiazole
18	OH–NH–	Bufexamac
17	NH–C″–CH2–	Tolazoline
17	NH2–CH–CH3	Amphetamine
15	N″–N=N–	Cefazolin
14	CO–CH2–CO–	Barbituric acid
13	CO–CH2–OH	Prednisone
13	COH–CH2–CH2–	Valeraldehyde
13	N–C–CH3	Budipine
13	N″–CH2–CH2–	Lofexidine
13	NH2–CH2–CH–	Octopamine
13	OH–N=CH–	Nifuroxine
12	CO–CH–CH=	Bromocriptine
12	CO–CH–Cl	Chloramphenicol
12	NH2–CH–NH–	Amiloride
12	OH–NH–C=	N-Phenylhydroxylamine
12	SH–CH2–	Cysteine
11	COH–CH=	Retinene
11	N–CO–C–	Loperamide
11	NH–CH=CH–	Thiouracil
11	NH2–CH–NH– ⟨2–NH2⟩	Amiloride
11	NH2–CH–NH2	Amiloride
11	NH2–CO–N–	Carbamazepine
10	CO–CO–CH2–	Mimosine
10	NO–NH–	1-Methyl-3-nitrosoguanidine
10	S–CH=N–	Thiamazole
10	SO2–O–CH–	2-Butyl methanesulfonate

[a]After MULTICASE identified the structural determinants associated with the induction of cancers in mice (see Table 8.1), these biophores were used to determine the proportion of chemicals, in a collection of 5400 agents representing the "universe of chemicals," which contained moieties unknown to the learning set (see Fig. 8.8). When the 5400 chemicals were screened, it was found that 19% of the predictions were accompanied by warnings of the presence of unknown moieties. The most abundant unknown moieties are listed here with an example of chemical that contains that moiety. Testing of agents containing such moieties and adding the results to the learning set would increase the accuracy of the predictions.

fore, the concordance between predicted and experimental results of the total database will be somewhat greater than that determined from the abridged dataset.

Finally, as mentioned earlier, the pro-gram also yields information related to the mechanistic basis of the biological phenomenon under investigation. Thus CASE allows the determination of whether the chemical under consideration is likely to be

Table 8.9 Overlaps between Structural Determinants of Carcinogenicity in Mice and Other Biological Activities

Biophore[a]		Salmonella	Cell Toxicity
Cl–CH2–		X	X
Br–CH2–		X	
NO–N–		X	
C''–O–C=			X
Cl–CH2–CH2–		X	X
NO–N–CH2–		X	
NO–N–CH3		X	
NH–C=N–	⟨2–S⟩		X
O–C=CH–	⟨2–NO2⟩	X	X
S–C=N–	⟨2–NH⟩		X
NO2–C=CH–	⟨2–O⟩	X	X
CH''–C=CH–C=		X	
CH=C–O–C=			X
CH=CH–C.=C.–			X
CH''–CH=C–CH=		X	X
CH=CH–C."–CH2–		X	
CH3–O–C=C–			X
NH2–C=CH–C.=		X	
Cl–CH2–CH2–N–		X	X
CO–C.=C–C=		X	
NH2–C=C–CH=	⟨3–CH3⟩		X
CH=C–CH=C–C=	⟨2–CH3⟩		X
NH2–C=C–CH=CH–	⟨3–O⟩		X
CH3–CO–NH–C=CH–	⟨4–CH=⟩		X
NH–NH–C=CH–CH=CH–			X
NH2–C=CH–CH=C–C=			X
Cl–C=CH–CH=C–NH2			X
Cl–CH2–CH2–N–CH2–CH2–		X	X
NO2–C=CH–CH=C–O–		X	X
CH=C–CH=CH–C=CH–	⟨2–CH2⟩		X
CH=CH–C=C–CH=CH–	⟨3–NH2⟩		X
CH=CH–C=CH–CH=C–	⟨3–CH2⟩		X
CH=CH–CH=C–C=CH–	⟨4–NH2⟩		X
CH=CH–CH=CH–C=C–	⟨5–NH2⟩		X
CH2–C=CH–CH=C–CH=CH–			X
Cl–C=CH–C=CH–C''–Cl			X
Cl–CH2–CH2–N–CH2–CH2–Cl		X	X
CH=CH–C=CH–CH=C–C=	⟨3–NH2⟩	X	X
NH2–C=CH–CH=C–CH=CH–	⟨5–C=⟩		X
O–CH2–O–C.=CH–C=CH–	⟨6–CH2⟩		X
O–C.=CH–CH=C–CH=C.–O–	⟨5–CH2⟩		X

[a]Some of the biophores identified as associated with carcinogenicity in mice were also found to be identical to or embedded in biophores associated with mutagenicity in *Salmonella* (42) or toxicity to cultured cells (63).

a genotoxic or nongenotoxic carcinogen (see Tables 8.2 and 8.3). These parameters have been associated with the extent of risk to humans (13–26). The mechanistic studies can be extended further by comparing the biophores and biophobes associated with carcinogenicity with those that have been identified as associated with other databases. The overlap between the databases can then be taken as a measure of a commonality of mechanisms (63–65, 81). Thus an analysis of the structural determinants associated with carcinogenicity in mice overlap with structural determinants associated with mutagenicity in *Salmonella*, while other structural determinants associated with carcinogenicity overlap with structural determinants shown to be associated with toxicity to cells (Table 8.9). This then provides direct evidence for the possibility that cancer causation may be derived by two independent mechanisms (81). In fact, this confirms current thoughts that carcinogenicity, in addition to being derived from a mutagenic event, can also occur as a result of cell proliferation that may be secondary to cell toxicity (35, 36, 51, 82–86).

As mentioned earlier, the current version of the program incorporates the ability to predict the metabolites of a parent chemical (META program). This is based on elaborating an expect system that has learned 665 enzymic-catalyzed and 286 spontaneous reactions (46). This capability permits the prediction of the toxicological profile not only of a parent molecule but also of its putative metabolites (see Figs. 8.6 and 8.7).

Currently, there is much controversy regarding the potential carcinogenicity of omeprazole (87) and the mechanism by which this occurs (88–97). To explore this, we used the META program in conjunction with MULTICASE. A number of potential metabolites and spontaneous transformation products were thus identified (see Figs. 8.6 and 8.7). It should be stressed that not

all of these will necessarily be generated in every tissue of every species. However, some of the metabolites (e.g., hydroxy-omeprazole (S12) and omeprazole acid (S25)) have indeed been identified (98).

Using the NTP rodent carcinogenicity database (13) MULTICASE identified a number of putative metabolites (indicated by an asterisk in Fig. 8.6) that possess the potential to induce tumors in rodents. Attempts to detect such metabolites in rodents and in humans receiving omeprazole for therapeutic reasons together with the determination of their biological properties might shed further clues on the basis of the reported carcinogenicity of that agent.

4 CONCLUSIONS

The application of SAR techniques to complex toxicological phenomena is now feasible. Given the long duration, high cost, and societal concerns with animal assays, the routine use of SAR techniques for toxicological assessment during the development of therapeutic agent deserves consideration.

ACKNOWLEDGMENTS

This investigation was supported by the U.S. Environmental Protection Agency (R818275) and the Center for Indoor Air Research.

REFERENCES

1. IARC, *Monographs on the Evaluation of the Carcinogenic Risk of Chemicals to Humans*, Suppl. **6**, International Agency for Research on Cancer, Lyon, France, 1988.

2. M. Hollstein, J. McCann, F. A. Angelosanto, and W. W. Nichols, *Mutat. Res.*, **65**, 133–226 (1979).

3. J. A. Miller and E. C. Miller in H. H. Hiatt, J. D. Watson, and J. A. Winsten, Eds., *Origins of*

Human Cancer, Cold Spring Harbor Laboratory, Cold Spring Harbor, N.Y., 1977, pp. 605–627.

4. S. H. Reynolds, S. J. Stowers, R. M. Patterson, R. R. Maronpot, S. A. Aaronson, and M. W. Anderson, *Science*, **237**, 1309–1316 (1987).

5. S. J. Stowers, R. R. Maronpot, S. H. Reynolds, and M. W. Anderson, *Environ. Health Perspect.*, **75**, 81–86 (1987).

6. M. W. Anderson, S. H. Reynolds, M. You, and R. M. Maronpot, *Environ. Health Perspect.*, **98**, 13–24 (1992).

7. C. C. Harris, *Cancer Res.*, **51**, 5023s–5044s (1991).

8. S. A. Aaronson, *Science*, **254**, 1146–1153 (1991).

9. M. Hollstein, D. Sidransky, B. Vogelstein, and C. C. Harris, *Science*, **253**, 49–53 (1991).

10. S. H. Reynolds, C. K. Anna, K. C. Brown, J. S. Wiest, E. J. Beattie, R. W. Pero, J. D. Iglehart, and M. W. Anderson, *Proc. Natl. Acad. Sci. U. S. A.*, **88**, 1085–1089 (1991).

11. D. Sidransky, A. Von Eschenbach, Y. C. Tsai, P. Jones, I. Summerhayes, F. Marshall, M. Paul, P. Green, S. R. Hamilton, P. Frost, and B. Vogelstein, *Science*, **252**, 706–709 (1991).

12. R. A. Weinberg, *Science*, **254**, 1138–1146 (1991).

13. J. Ashby and R. W. Tennant, *Mutat. Res.*, **257**, 229–306 (1991).

14. J. Ashby and R. S. Morrod, *Nature*, **352**, 185–186 (1991).

15. Health Council of the Netherlands, *Report of the Evaluation of the Carcinogenicity of Chemical Substances*, Government Printing Office, The Hague, 1980.

16. J. Ashby and I. F. H. Purchase, *Mutat. Res.*, **205**, 51–58 (1987).

17. G. M. Williams in B. E. Butterworth and T. J. Slaga, Eds., *Non-genotoxic Mechanisms in Carcinogenesis: Banbury Report 25*, Cold Spring Harbor Laboratory, Cold Spring Harbor, N. Y., 1987, pp. 367–380.

18. G. M. Williams, *Regul. Toxicol. Pharmacol.*, **12**, 30–40 (1990).

19. J. D. Wilson in C. C. Travis, Ed., *Biologically-based Methods for Cancer Risk Assessment*, Plenum Press, New York, 1989, p. 275–287.

20. M. E. Andersen, J. Higginson, D. Krewski, I. C. Munro, A. E. Pegg, H. S. Rosenkranz, K. R. Solomon, E. Weisburger, G. M. Williams, and G. N. Wogan, *Regul. Toxicol. Pharmacol.*, **12**, 2–12 (1990).

21. F. K. Ennever, T. J. Noonan, and H. S. Rosenkranz, *Mutagenesis*, **2**, 73–78 (1987).

22. H. Bartsch and C. Malaveille, *Cell Biol. Toxicol.*, **5**, 115–127 (1989).

23. M. D. Shelby, *Mutat. Res.*, **204**, 3–15 (1988).

24. H. S. Rosenkranz and F. K. Ennever, *Mutat. Res.*, **244**, 61–65 (1990).

25. S. Parodi, D. Malacarne, P. Romano, and M. Taningher, *Environ. Health Perspect.*, **95**, 199–204 (1991).

26. L. S. Gold, L. Bernstein, R. Magaw, and T. H. Slone, *Environ. Health Perspect.*, **81**, 211–219 (1989).

27. G. Klopman and H. S. Rosenkranz, *Environ. Health Perspect.*, **96**, 67–75 (1991).

28. H. S. Rosenkranz, N. Takihi, and G. Klopman, *Multagenesis*, **6**, 391–394 (1991).

29. N. Takihi, H. S. Rosenkranz, and G. Klopman, *Quality Assurance*, **2**, 232–243 (1993).

30. N. Takihi, Y. P. Zhang, G. Klopman, and H. S. Rosenkranz, *Mutagenesis*, **8**, 257–264 (1993).

31. National Academy of Sciences, *Identifying and Estimating the Genetic Impact of Chemical Mutagens*, National Academy Press, Washington, D.C., 1983.

32. IARC, *Monographs on the Evaluation of the Carcinogenic Risk of Chemicals to Humans*, Supp. 7, International Agency for Research on Cancer, Lyon, France, 1987.

33. H. Vainio, K. Hemminki, and J. Wilbourn, *Carcinogenesis*, **6**, 1653–1665 (1985).

34. J. Wilbourn, L. Haroun, E. Heseltine, J. Kaldor, C. Partensky, and H. Vainio, *Carcinogenesis*, **7**, 1853–1863 (1986).

35. B. N. Ames and L. S. Gold, *Proc. Natl. Acad. Sci. U. S. A.*, **87**, 7772–7776 (1990).

36. S. M. Cohen and L. B. Ellwein, *Science*, **249**, 1007–1011 (1990).

37. L. S. Gold, C. B. Sawyer, R. Magaw, G. M. Backman, M. deVeciana, R. Levinson, N. K. Hooper, W. R. Havender, L. Bernstein, R. Peto, M. C. Pike, and B. N. Ames, *Environ. Health Perspect.*, **58**, 9–319 (1984).

38. L. S. Gold, M. deVeciana, G. M. Backman, R. Magaw, P. Lopipero, M. Smith, M. Blumenthal, R. Levinson, L. Bernstein, and B. N. Ames, *Environ. Health Perspect.*, **67**, 161–200 (1986).

39. L. S. Gold, T. H. Slone, G. M. Backman, R. Magaw, M. DaCosta, P. Lopipero, M. Blumenthal, and B. N. Ames, *Environ. Health Perspect.*, **74**, 237–329 (1987).

40. L. S. Gold, T. H. Slone, G. M. Backman, S. Eisenberg, M. DaCosta, M. Wong, N. B. Manley, L. Rohrbach, and B. N. Ames, *Environ. Health Perspect.*, **84**, 215–286 (1990).

41. G. Klopman, M. R. Frierson, and H. S. Rosenkranz, *Mutat. Res.*, **228**, 1–50 (1990).

42. H. S. Rosenkranz and G. Klopman, *Mutat. Res.*, **228**, 51–80 (1990).

43. G. Klopman, *J. Amer. Chem. Soc.*, **106**, 7315–7321 (1984).

44. H. S. Rosenkranz, G. Klopman, V. Chankong, J. Pet-Edwards, and Y. Y. Haimes, *Environ. Mutagen.*, **6**, 231–258 (1984).

45. H. S. Rosenkranz in H. Vainio, P. Magee, D. McGregor, and A. J. McMichael, Eds., *Mechanisms of Carcinogenesis in Risk Identification*, No. **116**, International Agency for Research on Cancer, Lyon, France, 1992, pp. 271–277.

46. G. Klopman and H. S. Rosenkranz, *Mutat. Res.*, **305**, 33–46 (1994).

47. J. Ashby, *Environ. Mutagen*, **7**, 919–921 (1985).

48. J. Ashby, R. W. Tennant, E. Zeiger, and S. Stasiewicz, *Mutat. Res.*, **223**, 73–103 (1989).

49. J. Ashby and R. W. Tennant, *Mutat. Res.*, **204**, 17–115 (1988).

50. T. J. Warr, J. M. Parry, R. D. Callander, and J. Ashby, *Mutat. Res.*, **245**, 191–199 (1990).

51. H. Vainio, P. Magee, D. McGregor, and A. J. McMichael, Eds., *Mechanisms of Carcinogenesis in Risk Identification*, No. 116, International Agency for Research on Cancer, Lyon, France, 1992.

52. G. Klopman, *Quantitative Struct. Activity Relationships*, **11**, 176–184 (1992).

53. G. Klopman, S. Wang, and D. M. Balthasar, *J. Chem. Infor. Comput. Sci.*, **32**, 474–482 (1992).

54. R. Peto, M. C. Pike, L. Bernstein, L. S. Gold, and B. N. Ames, *Environ. Health Perspect.*, **58**, 1–8 (1984).

55. Y. P. Zhang, G. Klopman, and H. S. Rosenkranz, *Environ. Mol. Mutagen.*, **21**, 100–115 (1993).

56. H. S. Rosenkranz, G. Klopman, H. Ohshima, and H. Bartsch, *Mutat. Res.*, **230**, 9–27 (1990).

57. V. Mersch-Sundermann, G. Klopman, and H. S. Rosenkranz, *Mutat. Res.*, **265**, 61–73 (1992).

58. V. Mersch-Sundermann, H. S. Rosenkranz, and G. Klopman, *Mutagenesis*, **7**, 211–218 (1992).

59. H. S. Rosenkranz and G. Klopman, *Mutagenesis*, **5**, 333–361 (1990).

60. H. S. Rosenkranz and G. Klopman, *Mutagenesis*, **5**, 525–527 (1990).

61. H. S. Rosenkranz, F. K. Ennever, M. Dimayuga, and G. Klopman, *Environ. Mol. Mutagen.*, **16**, 149–177 (1990).

62. W.-L. Yang, G. Klopman, and H. S. Rosenkranz, *Mutat. Res.*, **272**, 111–124 (1992).

63. H. S. Rosenkranz, E. J. Matthews, and G. Klopman, *ATLA*, **20**, 549–562 (1992).

64. H. S. Rosenkranz and G. Klopman, *Environ. Mol. Mutagen.*, **21**, 193–206 (1993).

65. H. S. Rosenkranz, E. J. Matthews, and G. Klopman, *Ecotoxicol. Environ. Safety*, **25**, 296–299 (1993).

66. H. S. Rosenkranz and G. Klopman, *Mutat. Res.*, **228**, 105–124 (1990).

67. H.S. Rosenkranz and G. Klopman, *Teratogen. Carcinogen. Mutagen.*, **10**, 73–78 (1990).

68. H. S. Rosenkranz and G. Klopman in M. L. Mendelsohn and R. J. Albertini, Eds., *Mutation and the Environment, Part B: Metabolism, Testing Methods, and Chromosomes*, Wiley-Liss, New York, 1990, pp. 23–48.

69. U. Rannug, M. Sjogren, A. Rannug, M. Gillner, R. Toftgard, J.-A. Gustafsson, H. Rosenkranz, and G. Klopman, *Carcinogenesis*, **12**, 2007–2016 (1991).

70. G. Klopman, D. M. Balthasar, and H. S. Rosenkranz, *Environ. Toxicol. Chem.*, **12**, 231–240 (1993).

71. G. M. Williams, M. J. Iatropoulos, M. V. Djordjevic, and O. P. Kaltenberg, *Carcinogenesis*, **14**, 315–317 (1993).

72. I. N. H. White, F. de Matteis, A. Davies, L. L. Smith, C. Crofton-Sleigh, S. Venitt, A. Hewer, and D. H. Phillips, *Carcinogenesis*, **13**, 2197–2203 (1992).

73. J. Ashby and D. Patton, *Mutat. Res.*, **286**, 3–74 (1993).

74. H. S. Rosenkranz and G. Klopman in A. M. Goldberg, Ed., *Alternative Methods in Toxicology, Vol. 8: In Vitro Toxicology: New Technology*, Mary Ann Liebert, Inc., New York, 1991, pp. 145–162.

75. H. S. Rosenkranz and G. Klopman, *Quality Assurance*, **2**, 251–254 (1993).

76. D. B. Clayson and D. L. Arnold, *Mutat. Res.*, **257**, 91–106 (1991).

77. N. Takihi, Y. P. Zhang, G. Klopman, and H. S. Rosenkranz, *Mutagenesis*, **8**, 257–264 (1993).

78. N. Takihi, Y. P. Zhang, G. Klopman, and H. S. Rosenkranz, *Quality Assurance*, **2**, 255–264 (1993).

79. G. Klopman and H. S. Rosenkranz, *Mutat. Res.*, **253**, 237–240 (1991).

80. G. Klopman and H. S. Rosenkranz, *Mutat. Res.*, **272**, 59–71 (1992).

81. H. S. Rosenkranz and G. Klopman, *Mutat. Res.*, **303**, 83–89 (1993).

82. S. M. Cohen and L. B. Ellwein, *Cancer Res.*, **51**, 6493–6505 (1991).

83. B. E. Butterworth, *Mutat. Res.*, **239**, 117–132 (1990).

84. B. E. Butterworth, J. A. Popp, R. B. Conolly, and T. L. Goldsworthy in Ref. 51, pp. 279–305.

85. S. Preston-Martin, M. C. Pike, R. K. Ross, P. A. Jones, and B. E. Henderson, *Cancer Res.*, **50**, 7415–7421 (1990).

86. R. B. Conolly, *Comments Toxicol.*, **4**, 269–293 (1992).

87. L. Ekman, E. Hansson, N. Have, E. Carlsson, and C. Lundburg, *Scand. J. Gastroenterol.*, **20**, 53–69 (1985).

88. B. Burlinson, S. Morriss, D. G. Gatehouse, D. J. Tweats, and M. R. Jackson, *Mutagenesis*, **6**, 11–18 (1991).

89. C. Furihata, K. Hirose, and T. Matsushima, *Mutat. Res.*, **262**, 73–76 (1991).

90. H. J. Evans, *Mutat. Res.*, **264**, 87–88 (1991).

91. C. Furihata and T. Matsushima, *Mutat. Res.*, **264**, 89–91 (1991).

92. D. H. Phillips, A. Hewer, and M. R. Osborne, *Mutagenesis*, **7**, 277–283 (1992).

93. G. Sachs and D. Scott, *Mutagenesis*, **7**, 475–476 (1992).

94. D. H. Phillips, M. R. Osborne, and A. Hewer, *Mutagenesis*, **7**, 476–477 (1992).

95. S. P. Adams, R. D. Storer, J. G. Deluca, S. M. Galloway, and W. W. Nichols, *Mutagenesis*, **7**, 395–396 (1992).

96. H. S. Rosenkranz and G. Klopman, *Mutagenesis*, **5**, 381–384 (1991).

97. J. Ashby, *Mutat. Res.*, **272**, 1–7 (1992).

98. C. Cederberg, T. Andersson, and I. Skanberg, *Scand. J. Gastroenterol.*, **24**, 33–40 (1989).

99. S. DeFlora, H. S. Rosenkranz, and G. Klopman, *Mutagenesis*, **9**, 39–45 (1994).

100. Y. P. Zhang, A. van Praagh, G. Klopman, and H. S. Rosenkranz, *Mutagenesis*, **9**, 141–149 (1994).

101. J. Pangrekar, G. Klopman, and H.S. Rosenkranz, *Environm. Toxicol. Chem.*, **13**, 979–1001 (1994).

102. T. Sakai, G. Klopman, and H.S. Rosenkranz, *Terato. Carcinog. Mutag.*, in press, 1994.

CHAPTER NINE

From Discovery to Market: The Development of Pharmaceuticals

JAN I. DRAYER
JAMES P. BURNS

G. H. Besselaar Associates
Princeton, New Jersey, USA

CONTENTS

1 Introduction,   252
  1.1 Evolution of drug development, 253
    1.1.1 Regulatory environment, 253
    1.1.2 Scientific environment, 255
    1.1.3 Commercial environment, 256
  1.2 Costs of drug development, 257
2 The Drug Development Process,   258
  2.1 Chemistry, 259
    2.1.1 Preformulation, 261
    2.1.2 Product development/formulation, 261
    2.1.3 Phase 2 and phase 3 clinical
       supplies, 261
    2.1.4 Containers, 262
    2.1.5 Closures, 262
  2.2 Preclinical studies, 264
    2.2.1 Acute toxicity, 265
    2.2.2 Subacute toxicity studies, 265
    2.2.3 Chronic toxicity studies, 266
    2.2.4 Carcinogenicity studies, 266
    2.2.5 Mutagenicity studies, 267
    2.2.6 Reproduction studies, 267
    2.2.7 Special toxicity studies, 267
  2.3 Transition from preclinical to clinical, 268
  2.4 Planning the drug development process, 269
    2.4.1 Assumptions, 269
    2.4.2 Defining the development strategy, 271
    2.4.3 The drug development master plan, 272

Burger's Medicinal Chemistry and Drug Discovery,
Fifth Edition, Volume 1: Principles and Practice,
Edited by Manfred E. Wolff.
ISBN 0-471-57556-9   © 1995 John Wiley & Sons, Inc.

251

2.4.4 Critical components of the clinical part of the drug development master plan, 275

2.5 Clinical research; the conduct of clinical trials, 279

2.5.1 Phase 1 clinical research, 280

2.5.2 Phase 2 and phase 3 clinical research, 282

2.5.3 Periapproval clinical trial programs, 286

2.5.4 Development of the final protocol and case report forms, 286

2.5.5 Investigator selection, 288

2.5.6 Monitoring of studies, 290

2.5.7 Evaluation of adverse events in clinical trials, 291

2.5.8 Ethical considerations in clinical research, 292

2.5.9 Clinical trial reports, 295

2.5.10 When to stop the development of a drug, 295

2.5.11 Regulatory review during the conduct of clinical trials, 296

2.5.11.1 End of phase 2 and phase 3 conferences, 297

2.5.11.2 FDA interactions under subpart E, 297

2.5.11.3 Regulatory approval process, 298

2.5.11.4 Approval and launch, 299

1 INTRODUCTION

Through the early years of this century, most drugs or medicines that were sold to the public were little more than home remedies or extracts of various natural products including barks and flowers, that owed their activity more to the alcoholic content of the elixir than to the actual activity of the product. With the advent of modern drug discovery technology and the ability to synthesize chemicals with specific pharmacologic activities, drug development has evolved considerably from that point.

This chapter addresses the process of modern drug development from the point where a candidate drug has emerged from the drug discovery process, up through regulatory approval, and beyond into periapproval and post-marketing activities. Although the development of drugs is becom-

ing an increasingly global endeavor, the focus of this discussion is the U.S. Food and Drug Administration (FDA) and the associated steps in drug development necessary to satisfy the FDA, the regulatory body that holds the power of approval or disapproval for drugs on the U.S. market. The FDA also has statutory authority for approval of other therapeutic/diagnostic modalities such as biologics and devices; however, this chapter will focus exclusively on drug development even though there are many concepts of drug development that are applicable to both biologics and devices.

During drug development, not only does the FDA evaluate the scientific merit of the data presented in support of approval of a drug, but also the labeling or package insert which contains the directions for use of the approved drug. The labeling instructs physicians about the mechanism of action of the drug: the specific indication(s) approved for the drug; any special precautions that patients should be advised to take when using the drug; any safety issues that have arisen in animal or human testing with the drug that physicians and patients should be aware of; potential adverse effects and their incidence that have been known to occur in clinical studies and could therefore occur in clinical use; any potential for abuse or addiction; and dosing recommendations (see Table 9.1). The content of this labeling determines how the approved drug can be marketed and promoted. As such, labeling becomes a crucial document that can ultimately define the commercial success of the drug and the blueprint upon which drug development should be planned and executed. The evolution of that drug development process is the starting point of this chapter.

1.1 Evolution of Drug Development

Three factors have played a major role in shaping the evolution of drug development. They are: Regulatory Environment, Scientific Environment, and Industrial/Commercial Environment. Each of these en-

Table 9.1 Standard Sections of a Package Insert

- Description
- Clinical Pharmacology
- Indications and Usage
- Contraindications
- Warnings
- Precautions
- Adverse Reactions
- Drug Abuse and Dependence
- Overdosage
- Dosage and Administration
- How Supplied

vironments has had an impact, but not necessarily at the same time or to the same degree. They have evolved at their own pace.

1.1.1 REGULATORY ENVIRONMENT. During drug discovery, only general federal laws, regulations, or guidelines regarding environmental protection, animal care and scientific misconduct govern the basic research process. However, once a chemical becomes a candidate for development to ultimate commercialization, the company developing this product must be aware of the specific laws, regulations, and guidelines that are appropriate to the development of such products so that the results of the investigations conducted will be acceptable to the Food and Drug Administration (FDA) and health regulatory authorities in other countries as necessary.

The involvement of the Federal government in the regulation of drugs and the close relationship of this regulation of drugs with foods, dates back more than 100 years. At that time, the practice of medicine in the United States was generally limited to providing advice on the consumption of various herbs, spices, and other food substances that were taken to achieve the desired result; for instance, maintenance of good health or improved health. Because of this differentiation, the U.S. Department of Agriculture has been the federal agency that was initially responsible for monitoring the potential adverse health effects resulting from adulterated food products. Specifically, this responsibility fell to the Division of Chemistry within the Department of Agriculture and this department has been the entity which is the direct forerunner of the present Food and Drug Administration.

The regulation of drugs in the United States has largely been shaped by three major events. First, in the early 1900s, there were widespread abuses in the food industry, especially the meat packing industry. As a result of focus on meat packing by a number of "muckraking" journalists and the publication of a book in 1906 by Upton Sinclair entitled *The Jungle* (1), there was substantial outcry on the part of the public to reform the food industry. Coincidental with public outcry, the Division of Chemistry had performed a number of food product investigations and determined that a wide variety of harmful substances could be found in the food products. As a result, the Federal Government passed the Pure Food and Drugs Act of 1906. This law prohibited the mislabeling and adulteration of food and drugs sold in interstate commerce. Be aware that, at this time, little advertising of drugs had been aimed directly at physicians since any non-narcotic drug could be purchased without a physician's prescription.

The next major event that helped shape the regulatory environment was the "Elixir of Sulfanilamide Tragedy" of 1937. Up to this time, drugs were not required to be tested for safety or efficacy before being introduced into the market. The only requirement was that the drug not be adulterated and the required information instructing the physician or consumer about its use be contained on the label. Sulfanilamide had been one of the first miracle drugs to emerge from drug discovery during this century, showing great promise as an all-round antiinfective agent. The manufacturer of sulfanilamide, thinking that this drug in liquid form would make a good medicine for sore throat, proceeded to prepare an "elixir" of the drug in diethylene glycol, a highly toxic, common ingredient in automobile antifreeze. However, this toxicity was not recognized at the time. Because there was no required safety testing, this elixir was introduced onto the market with no safety tests having been conducted. Subsequently, 107 children were killed who had consumed the product. As a result, there was a nation-wide outcry for new and stricter legislation regulating the marketing of drugs.

Responding to this public outcry, the U.S. Congress passed the Food, Drug, and Cosmetic Act of 1938 (FD&C Act). This act and its many subsequent amendments, has been the controlling legislation for all foods and drugs. For the first time, the safety of drugs was now required to be tested prior to their introduction into the market. Under the FD&C Act of 1938, now all drug manufacturers had to submit a New Drug Application (NDA) to the FDA before introducing the drug in interstate commerce. This application required that a manufacturer list the drug's intended uses and provide the FDA with adequate scientific evidence that the new drug was safe for the intended uses. An NDA became effective 60 days after filing provided the FDA proposed no objections. If the government did not raise objections, the manufacturer was free to proceed with product introduction.

For the next 24 years, all drugs were approved essentially on safety with no statutory requirement to demonstrate efficacy. The regulatory environment of this period was much different than from today. The cost of regulatory compliance was relatively minor and the average regulatory review time was approximately 7 months. Interestingly, the main drug-related concern of the U.S. Congress during this period was the profits of companies, not the products of these companies.

The third defining event that prompted new drug regulations for the regulatory environment, was again a tragedy. In the early 1960s, a new drug, Thalidomide, was approved and used in Europe for nausea associated with pregnancy. By 1962, there was mounting evidence that pregnant women receiving Thalidomide were giving birth to children with severe deformities. Although this drug had not yet been approved in the U.S., the publicity surrounding the events in Europe and the possibility that this drug or a similar drug could be approved in the U.S., prompted the U.S. Congress to further strengthen the regulation of drugs. Thus, in 1962 the Kefauver-

Harris Amendments to the FD&C Act of 1938 were approved by the U.S. Congress. With these amendments, manufacturers now had to demonstrate proof of effectiveness of their products as well as proof of safety before marketing any new drug. The amendments also mandated that the FDA had to approve, rather than just review, an NDA before a drug could be marketed. A new regulatory document appeared on the scene at this time, the Investigational Exemption to a New Drug Application or IND. In order to meet the requirements of establishing the effectiveness of drugs, manufacturers were now required to conduct clinical studies of their drugs. This requirement necessitated the shipment of "investigational" drugs in interstate commerce which would be in violation of the FD&C Act. Thus, an exemption to this Act, an IND, was established to allow for the shipment of investigational drugs for the purpose of conducting clinical trials.

In addition to these three pivotal defining events of the regulatory environment, additional legislation and regulations have further defined the regulatory environment. These initiatives have included the passage of the Orphan Drug Act of 1983, which provided financial and commercial incentives to manufacturers of "Orphan Drugs" to bring these drugs to market for the limited population for which they were intended. These drugs are designed to treat diseases or conditions affecting less than 200,000 people in the United States.

The next major legislation was the Drug Price Competition and Patent Term Restoration Act of 1984. Under the provisions of this Act, pharmaceutical manufacturers could file what were termed abbreviated NDAs (ANDAs) to market generic versions of already approved drugs whose patent life had expired and which had been on the market for a sufficient period of time so that their marketing exclusivity (usually 5 years) had expired.

On its own initiative the FDA has also been attempting to improve and streamline the drug development and approval process. Thus, new regulations have been promulgated on February 22, 1985 affecting NDAs, and on March 19, 1987 affecting INDs. Additional regulations promulgated by the FDA and designed to get drugs on the market more quickly, have included: the Treatment IND regulations of 1987 (intended to provide promising investigational new drugs to desperately ill patients before general marketing begins); regulations of 1988 for Drugs intended to Treat Life-threatening and Severely Debilitating Illnesses (intended to facilitate the development, evaluation and marketing of such products especially where no satisfactory alternative therapy exists); and the Accelerated Approval Regulations of 1992 (intended to provide expedited marketing approval of drugs for patients suffering from life-threatening illnesses when the drugs provide meaningful therapeutic benefit compared to existing treatment).

Even though the FDA is both a scientific and a political agency, charged with protecting the public against unsafe and ineffective drugs, it also has a public health mission to promote the availability of drugs to meet perceived public health needs. Those needs are framed against three constituencies: the public, Congress, and the Executive Branch, of which the FDA is a part. Each of these constituencies can and will exert pressure on the FDA to satisfy various agendas. Decisions taken by the FDA try to balance the various competing needs of each constituency.

1.1.2 SCIENTIFIC ENVIRONMENT. From exploratory science to receptor-specific and molecule-specific research, the scientific environment surrounding the development of drugs has rapidly evolved over the last 30–40 years. Interestingly, over 90% of all the drugs in use in 1964 were unknown prior to 1938. By comparison, Reis-Arndt reported that about 490 new chemical entities were marketed in the seven major markets of the world or by the seven major drug producing companies in the world between 1976 and 1985 (2). These seven major drug producing countries are the United States, the United Kingdom, France, Italy, Germany, Switzerland, and Japan. Commenting on this information, Drews noted than an internal panel at Hoffmann-La Roche and some outside pharmacologists, looked at these drugs and tried to characterize them in the same way the FDA had done (3). The 3 categories used were: (a) drugs that really allowed or enabled novel treatment that had not been available previously; for example, drugs for diseases that probably had not been treatable up to that time; (b) drugs that represented some distinct advantage over existing therapy without really allowing for novel therapy; and (c) drugs that have provided modest increments of quality or therapeutic versatility compared to drugs that have already existed. This panel classified only 8 (1.5%) of these compounds as truly representing novel therapy, whereas 406 (83.5%) were classified as providing no significant novelty or improvement. These results, which show a tremendous degree of redundancy in drug research and development, should not be construed as a criticism of that effort. Redundant development of similar therapeutic entities has led to the approval of products that have provided therapeutic relief for that subgroup of patients for which a similar product did not provide the degree of relief necessary.

As the end of this century nears, scientific research has evolved to the point where research can now be focused at the molecular, cellular, and receptor level. This focus will allow for targeted research to improve the potential for causing a positive therapeutic effect while diminishing or eliminating the potential for unwanted effects. In addition, the ability to study disease mechanisms will be significantly improved so that drugs can go beyond providing symptomatic relief of serious diseases to actually preventing or stabilizing a disease condition. Also, research in the biotechnology area has much promise for attacking diseases of genetic defects. Thus, it appears that the pharmaceutical industry is poised for another golden era of pharmaceutical development toward the relief and elimination of diseases.

1.1.3 COMMERCIAL ENVIRONMENT. The U.S. pharmaceutical industry has evolved to the point where it is a major player in the U.S. and world economies. Not only is the pharmaceutical industry a leader in innovative development of pharmaceuticals but it also has a positive balance of trade with the rest of the world in terms of exporting their products. As the world shrinks as a trading market, it is only natural that more formal links be constituted among international partners in the development of products or among the far flung international entities of a single corporation. Thus, the day of independent development of drugs for Europe, for the U.S. and for other markets is gradually disappearing. Presently, the development of drugs is more on a global level so that one clinical development program will suffice for registration of a product in all appropriate markets worldwide. This universality demands strong project management and information links with the various elements of the developmental team worldwide, as well as extensive knowledge of the world regulatory environment to ensure compliance with all appropriate regulations. Lastly, universality requires special attention to marketing issues so as to successfully commercialize the product in its various markets. The increasing governmental demand to restrain cost on pharmaceuticals is requiring pharmaceutical companies to look very closely at their developmental costs in relation to the programs that they want to develop. The need for strict project and budget management has never been more apparent than in the pharmaceutical industry at this time.

As the industry moves towards the end of this century, more than likely there will be continued consolidation of the industry into several large companies with the smaller companies joining in these ventures or falling by the wayside. The emergence of the biotechnology industry is still evolving and will play a role in the evolution of mainstream pharmaceutical industries who are also developing their own biotechnology capabilities as well. Whether the biotechnology industry will live up to its full potential remains to be seen.

1.2 Costs of Drug Development

The development of pharmaceuticals is complex, lengthy, and expensive. The process includes many steps from the synthesis and scale-up of the product through animal testing to the testing of the compound in the target population of patients. Of each 5,000 chemical entities synthesized, it has been estimated that only 250 will reach animal testing, 5 will reach the level of clinical testing in healthy volunteers or patients and only one will ultimately reach the market place (4). Others have estimated that of all drugs that reach the first phase of clinical testing, approximately 10% will reach the market in one way or form. Unfortunately, which of the drugs in development will be successful cannot be predicted.

Data from DiMasi et al. have provided some insight into the areas where the pharmaceutical industry has spent research money (5). Between 1976 and 1990, 269 new chemical entities were approved by the Food and Drug Administration in the United States. Of these entities, 131 (49%) were defined as having little or no gain over existing products, 94 (35%) were classified as having a modest gain over existing therapies and 41 (15%) significantly improved existing treatments with only 3 drugs (1%) fulfilling the greatest therapeutic need: the treatment of AIDS. DiMasi has calculated that, on average, the clinical development of these drugs took from 2.7 to 6.4 years for the various therapeutic gain classifications, the shortest for drugs in the area of the greatest therapeutic need. The regulatory review for drugs in the four different categories ranged from 1.2 to 3.1 years.

Obviously, drug development carries a significant financial burden. It has been estimated that global research and development expenditures for pharmaceutical companies have reached 24 billion dollars (1990 dollars) with 30% of this amount spent on discovery and clinical evaluation of new drugs (6). According to DiMasi (5), the overall development of a new chemical entity costs approximately 114 million dollars (1987 dollars). In a recent report, the Office of Technology Assessment estimate that the average after tax cash requirement for drugs that reached the market in the 1980s, was 65 million dollars (1990 dollars) (4). These costs are out-of-pocket costs only and do not include capitalization or opportunity costs.

Undoubtedly, for a variety of reasons, the cost of the development of new chemical entities will increase. In view of the recent pressure on cost reductions in medical health–care worldwide, leading to significant reductions in the revenues from the sales of pharmaceuticals, the industry has no option but to focus its discovery and development activities on drugs that can be marketed globally; new entities that promise at least a modest gain over existing therapeutics, and on new treatment for diseases for which drugs are not available in the marketplace. Recently, various pharmaceutical executives have commented that the development of a pharmaceutical that will be the fifth drug in its class in the market place can not be tolerated in the future. Such comments seem appropriate in view of revenues listed for the numerous angiotensin–converting enzyme (ACE) inhibitors now available in the marketplace, for the treatment of hypertension. Revenues drop significantly with the order in which the drug reaches the market. A similar picture has been provided for the many calcium channel blockers that have reached the market to treat a variety of cardiovascular diseases including angina, cardiac arrhythmias and hypertension.

An urge to speed up the discovery, development and review processes for new drugs has been created with the purpose of extending the patent life of these drugs in the marketplace and hence, to gain the highest market share possible.

Unfortunately, the time from discovery to market of new pharmaceuticals is not expected to be reduced significantly, despite new technologies and computerization innovations in the entire process. Any time gained through modernization of the drug development process will be offset by more rigorous scientific demands on the evaluation of the product and increasing regulatory requirements. These constraints will result in more complex clinical trials and greater numbers of patients being exposed to assess the benefit/risk ratio of the new pharmaceutical.

Finally, the drug development process will likely be prolonged because of increasingly complex interactions between development partners, through mergers, joint ventures, co-development agreements, or outlicensing among pharmaceutical companies worldwide.

From the data presented, there is an increasing need within the pharmaceutical industry to focus its drug discovery and development on those drugs that meet the needs of the market (customers). Changing these processes can make them more time and cost efficient so that pharmaceutical products can be developed on a global basis. In fact, many companies already are changing the way they are structured and

have implemented many of the Total Quality Management principles that have helped other companies to become more cost efficient (7).

Anticipating that, once a new drug development candidate has surfaced, the regulatory requirements for the development of such a product have been determined, and the potential future market share has been assessed, the development plan for such a drug would be relatively straightforward and comparable between pharmaceutical companies worldwide. Unfortunately, this scenario is not the case. Drug development plans differ significantly with the culture, size and experience/expertise of each pharmaceutical company. The process is quite different for a large, well-established, centralized pharmaceutical company, with several new drug candidates under development and an established market in a selected number of therapeutic areas, than for a small start-up biotechnology company with limited financial resources and virtually no expertise in the development of new drugs (with many variants in between these extremes).

In this chapter, guidance will be provided on the drug development process in a structured manner, from late pre-clinical studies through market approval and beyond. The approach presented is based on the understanding of regulatory requirements and targeted on the needs of the consumer. The expectation is that the approach can be implemented by any company (large or small), on a local or worldwide scale and in its entirety or as separate, deliberate steps.

2 THE DRUG DEVELOPMENT PROCESS

The drug development process can arbitrarily be subdivided into 2 phases, early and late. The early phase of drug development includes parts of preclinical toxicology, IND preparation and the implementation of a relatively small number of Phase 1 and early Phase 2 clinical studies. At the end of this process, if a drug survives these early hurdles with no significant deficiencies, (e.g., preclinical toxicity, lack of efficacy, unacceptable tolerance) a drug should have more than a 50% chance of surviving a full fledged clinical development in the target patient population and of reaching marketing approval. This phase of drug development requires input from people with good knowledge of the company's vision and mission, the regulatory environment, and the scientific input from consultants, with limited input from marketing analysts.

The late phase of the drug development process includes long-term preclinical and clinical studies after which the data on the drug will be submitted to regulatory authorities for marketing approval. In the late phase, personnel involved are project managers and people with broad experience in clinical research, regulatory affairs and in marketing. These individuals are different from those involved with early drug development.

2.1 Chemistry

The various activities ongoing in the areas of chemistry, pre-clinical research, clinical research, and regulatory review during the early and late development phases are presented in Table 9.2.

Activities in each of these phases should be implemented following a specific plan with a predetermined budget, defined intermediate and final goals, and rewards. Commonly, most activities included in the early development phase will be performed by the pharmaceutical company, while late phase development activities are done more frequently by utilizing outside resources.

Table 9.3 lists the various disciplines and activities within these disciplines as they relate to the drug development process. These activities are performed under specific regulations and guidelines: Good Manufacturing Practices (GMP), Good Laboratory Practices (GLP), and Good Clinical Practices (GCP), respectively. Details for all these activities will be presented in this chapter.

Experienced personnel in the pharmaceutical industry's drug development process are in short supply because many compounds under development never reach the market. Also, for those compounds that do, the lengthy development process coupled with the relatively short amount of time spent by employees involved in the development process, ensures rapid personnel turnover which results in a continuing lack of experienced personnel. Conse-

Table 9.2   Activities Required Early and Late in the Development of a New Pharmaceutical

Early Development Phase	Late Development Phase
Dosage form development	Chronic toxicology
Pre-clinical pharmacology	Carcinogenicity studies
Sub-acute toxicology	Special toxicology
IND Filing	Final formulation
Selected Phase 1 studies	Long-term stability testing
Early Phase 2 studies	Late Phase 2 studies
	Phase 3 clinical trials
	NDA preparation
	Regulatory review process

Table 9.3 Overview of the Various Disciplines and Activities Involved in the Drug Development Process

Chemistry	Pre-Clinical	Clinical	Regulatory
Good manufacturing practices (GMP)	Good laboratory practices (GLP)	Good clinical practices (GCP)	Disease specific drug development Guidelines–Code of Federal Regulations (CFR)
Preformulation	Pharmacology Pharmacokinetics Pharmacodynamics	Phase 1	IND
Scale up	Metabolism	Early Phase 2	NDA
Choice of formulation	General toxicology Acute Sub-Acute	Late Phase 2	
Stability	Chronic Carcinogenicity studies Special toxicology Mutagenicity studies Reproduction studies	Phase 3 clinical trials	

quently, there are only a relatively few seasoned project champions who have had experience in the complete development of a variety of compounds and understand the differences in development philosophies among companies.

All this turmoil could change if companies would focus only on the early phase of the drug development process; a time during which critical decisions have to be made with regard to the continuation of the development of new pharmaceuticals. This phase of the process usually is of short duration. The longer and large-scale late phase of the drug development process, preferably, should be outsourced to contract research organizations. These organizations have broad expertise in how to perform chronic toxicology, carcinogenicity studies and large scale clinical research projects, in a timely and cost efficient manner, and according to one single standard acceptable to regulatory agencies worldwide. While the outsourcing of toxicology studies is a well-accepted part of drug development, the outsourcing of clinical research is a relatively recent phenom-

enon, especially for large-scale Phase 2 and Phase 3 clinical programs.

The scope of dosage form development of a pharmaceutical product usually develops well in advance of the implementation of a clinical program and will continue past the submission of an NDA (8). These sequential activities are: preformulation, dosage form development/scale-up, and commercialization. These activities typically occur in parallel with and simultaneous to the preparation of clinical supplies.

Typical pharmaceutical objectives in the preparation of investigational drug supplies are to produce products that are: stable, bioavailable, processable, and elegant. All products supplied for clinical use must be stable throughout the duration of clinical studies (8). Simple dosage forms are commonly used in Phase 1 (e.g., hand-filled capsules containing only a diluent or C-14 solution or suspension) to provide the relatively small amount of dosage form required. Stability requirements in these cases are minimal since these inpatient studies are of short duration (several days). However, by the time Phase 3 clinical studies are reached, the investigational drug will be a more sophisticated formulation that approaches the "final" commercial formulation. Stability data on investigational drug supplies assures the FDA that the drug product remains essentially unchanged during the duration of clinical studies and should therefore not contribute to any variability observed for clinical efficacy nor pose any safety problems.

Because particle size, polymorphism, pK_a, and solubility can often influence the bioavailability and enhance the activity of drugs, it is necessary to provide a quantitative indication that the drug is being absorbed and to what extent. This is typically done in Phase 1 metabolism studies where the bioavailability of solid dosage forms are compared to an IV injection, an oral solution, or a suspension form of the same drug.

For a drug to be processable, a reasonable technique for combining the drug with inactive excipients is required. These processes must insure that the required quantity of drug is consistently contained in each and every dosage unit produced so that any variability in clinical response can be attributed to human variability and not to variability in a dosage form (8). An "elegant" dosage form possesses uniform appearance with acceptable product characteristics, such as taste, tablet hardness, and capsule disintegration (8).

2.1.1 PREFORMULATION. Preformulation is a name given to the pharmaceutical activity where the candidate drugs' physical, chemical, and mechanical properties are characterized to provide a rationale for the selection of other ingredients to be used in a dosage form, and to provide guidance to the manufacturing processes that may be employed. The determination of the key pharmaceutical parameters at this early stage can also serve as a benchmark for the comparison test in the future for lots of the new drug substance (8). Monitoring of the

key parameters identified in the preformulation phase allows for a check on consistency of the bulk drug substance as dosage form development proceeds.

2.1.2 PRODUCT DEVELOPMENT/FORMULATION. The FDA has promulgated Current Good Manufacturing Practices (cGMP) regulations that have been codified in the Code of Federal Regulations (CFR). These regulations address controls that must be in place with respect to materials, manpower, methods, and machines used in the preparation of drug products for human use. These regulations have been further refined in the form of guidelines with respect to clinical trial supplies. Guidelines addressing clinical trial supplies have been promulgated by both the Pharmaceutical Manufacturers Association (PMA) and the FDA.

2.1.3 PHASE 1, 2, AND 3 CLINICAL SUPPLIES. Initial formulation efforts are usually directed at developing dosage forms for Phase 1 clinical trials. The identification of the dosage forms to be utilized, typically depends on several factors including: type and purpose of study, pharmaceutical preformulation profile, and estimated clinical dose range.

Phase 1 studies are often studies of a dose-ranging type which utilize an oral solid dosage form where multiple dosage strengths are administered. These simple formulations are often referred to as "loose filled lactose plus drug capsules" and are intended to provide the most expedient dosage form. Because Phase 1 dose-ranging studies often utilize a small fraction of the estimated dose, a major factor to be considered is the drug load (drug load is the ratio of the active drug to the total contents of dosage form). For example, a low drug load may pose homogeneity problems while a high drug load may pose flow problems or require an extra large capsule, especially if the drug substance is fluffy and has low bulk density (8). During this stage, dosage form development is typically focused on providing an appropriate final dosage form for the Phase 3 clinical trials.

The factors to be considered for dosage form development for Phase 3 studies include marketing preferences of the company and any special protection needed to maximize drug stability. Stability studies for final dosage form material, will be used to establish an appropriate expiration date (shelf life) and product storage requirements. Stability information on the drug substance before formulation is valuable in identifying characteristics of the intact molecule that can change under defined conditions of storage.

A program for stability assessment would typically include storage at ambient temperature and under stressed conditions. Stress conditions ordinarily include temperature (e.g., 5, 50, and 75°C); humidity, where appropriate (e.g., 75% RH or greater), and exposure to various wavelengths of electromagnetic radiation (UV and visible ranges), preferably in open containers, where applicable.

Using a "stability-indicating assay" to detect any degradation products as separate and distinct from each active ingredient is important. Such an assay is a quantitative analytical method that is based on the characteristic structural, chemical, or biological properties of each active ingredient of a drug product (9).

2.1.4 CONTAINERS. The container is the device that will hold the drug and that will probably be in direct contact with the drug. The immediate container is that which is in direct contact with the drug at all times. The closure is also considered part of the container. The container must not interact physically or chemically with the contents and must also be shown not to affect the strength, quality, or purity of the drug beyond official requirements or product specifications as submitted to the FDA.

The types of containers typically used for clinical supplies include (10):

- Light-resistant containers such as amber glass or opaque HDPE plastic.
- Well-closed containers which protect the contents from extraneous solids and from loss of the drug under ordinary or customary conditions of handling, shipment, storage, and distribution.
- Tight-containers protect the contents from contamination from extraneous liquids, solids, or vapors; from loss of the drug; and from efflorescence, deliquescence, or evaporation under ordinary or customary conditions of handling, shipment, storage, and distribution, and is capable of tight reclosure. Most bottles with screw-on caps are tight containers; most bottles with snap caps are not.
- Hermetic containers are impervious to air or any other gas under ordinary or customary conditions of handling, shipment, storage, and distribution (e.g., ampules).
- Single-unit containers are closed in such a manner that none of the contents may be removed without obvious destruction of the closure, and the contents are intended for use promptly after being opened.
- Single-dose containers are single-unit containers for articles intended for parental administration only. A single-dose container is labeled as such.
- Unit-dose containers are single-unit containers so designed that the contents are administered to the patient as a single dose.
- Multiple-unit containers are containers that permit withdrawal of successive portions of the contents without changing the strength, quality, or purity of the remaining portion.
- Multiple-dose containers are a multiple-unit container for articles intended for parental administration.

2.1.5 CLOSURES. A closure is an essential part of a container/closure system that is required to maintain the integrity of the drug product and to ensure its stability, safety, and effectiveness. Closures include screw-on, threaded, lug, crimp-on (crown), press-on (snap), and roll-on. All closures should include a liner-contact surface that is compatible with the drug product and capable of providing a tight seal.

Special closures include child-resistant closures and tamper-evident closures. Child-resistant closures are used to protect children from serious personal injury or illness resulting from handling, using, or ingesting a drug product considered to be hazardous to children. In order for a closure to be qualified as being child-resistant, it must pass test panels comprised of 200 children under the age of five (5) years, and 100 adults (10). Tamper-resistant packaging has an indicator or barrier to entry, which if breached or missing, can reasonably be expected to provide visible evidence to consumers that tampering has occurred.

In recent years, there has been an increased use of plastic containers for drug supplies because of the many advantages they offer. However, plastics can also have distinct disadvantages. Ingredients added to the plastic resin to perform a specific function during fabrication include plasticizers, lubricants, mold release agents, pigments, stabilizers, anti-oxidants, and binding or antistatic agents. These ingredients may be leached from the plastic into the drug product. Certain ingredients from the drug preparation may bind to the plastic or be adsorbed by it, and oxidation, degradation, or precipitation of the drug product may occur. It is also possible for a component of the drug product to migrate through the walls of the container, and oxygen, carbon-dioxide, or other gases may pass through the plastic into the drug system. Because of this hazard, certain tests, as noted below, are required to be conducted on the plastic substance to determine its suitability for use as a container for a drug product submitted to the FDA.

The U.S. Pharmacopeia/National Formulary (USP/NF) has investigative procedures for physical/chemical tests to be conducted for the evaluation of plastics to determine their suitability for drug containers. The tests are based on extraction of specified amounts of plastic by water and are needed to characterize or determine the presence of chemical impurities as a result of the manufacturing process. In addition, a number of physical and chemical techniques may be used to identify and characterize plastics. Some characteristics that are frequently considered are: IR spectrum (ATR), UV, thermal analysis, melt viscosity, molecular weight, molecular weight distribution, polymer linearity, degree of crystallinity, stiffness, softening temperature, film or sheet thickness, ash, and heavy metals. Additional testing of plastic containers may include the effect of moderate degrees of cold or heat, water vapor and light transmission, and the extent of degradation under exposure to heat and light. Biological testing should also be conducted when appropriate (11).

Samples of a drug that are selected for stability studies should be packaged in the container/closure system in which the drug is to be marketed or distributed. Because the drug may absorb toxic impurities from its container/closure system, or react with or be absorbed by the container/closure system, tests to define or control any of these possible problems should be performed. In addition, laboratory tests should be conducted when appropriate, to assure that contamination with micro-organisms or foreign matter will not occur through the container or closure.

Some substances used as label adhesives for drug containers, such as cements and lacquers, are typically not water-based. Because of this method, there is the possibility that the solvent used may allow for leaching of adhesive components into the drug. Therefore, appropriate testing should be conducted to determine whether adhesive and/or ink components migrate through the container.

Although most drugs are administered orally using a solid oral dosage form, there are drugs that are administered by means of an aerosol dosage form. In this case, the valve-closure system determines the rate and amount of drug delivered. Thus, the most critical part of an aerosol or pressurized package is the valve mechanism through which the content of the container is released. For aerosols, information pertaining to the materials of fabrication, specifications, spray characteristics, compatibility and stability of the product is particularly important. When metered-dose valves are used, full information is also necessary with respect to accuracy and precision of the dose delivered. For inhalation or oral dose aerosols, complete information about the actuator, including data showing it can deliver the medication in the proper particle size, is especially significant (11).

2.2 Preclinical Studies

Before the first introduction of a drug into humans, it is important to conduct preclinical studies to determine the pharmacological activity of the drug, to determine its safety profile, and to identify what parameters should be monitored for safety in clinical studies.

Pharmacology studies of a drug candidate are really an extension of the drug discovery process and help define and confirm the intended activity of the drug. These studies can also hopefully provide better insight into the mechanism of action of the drug so as to assist in designing clinical studies in the future. Initial preclinical pharmacology studies are a pharmacological screen which involves the use of *in vitro* and *in vivo* assays to determine the pharmacological activities of a drug and which of these activities are predominant. Once the general pharmacologic activity has been defined, pharmacological studies

are then conducted to further explore the activity of the drug in specific animal and *in vitro* models of disease states to quantitate, as best as possible, the activity of the drug versus other known compounds with similar pharmacologic activity. Pharmacological studies should be extensive enough to determine a dose response relationship, and a drug's duration and mechanism of action.

Information about a drug's absorption, distribution, metabolism, and excretion (ADME) characteristics are also developed in these early preclinical studies. Such studies typically use radioactive tracers to determine distribution of a drug in various organs and blood and also to determine the route and extent of excretion. These studies may also identify species-to-species drug effect differences that may affect later preclinical and clinical studies and their interpretation. Metabolites may also be identified in which the specific activity of the drug resides. Should this occur, the direction of drug development may focus more on the specific metabolite than the parent drug.

The FDA has also recently developed a policy dealing with drugs that are stereoisomeric. By FDA definition, "stereoisomers" include all isomers that differ only in the orientation of the atoms in space. Thus, it would include not only mirror image enantiomers, but also geometric (cis/trans) isomers and diastereoisomers (isomers of drugs with more than one chiral center that are not mirror images of one another).

Since diastereoisomers and geometric isomers are both chemically distinct and pharmacologically different, and are generally readily separated without chiral techniques, the FDA believes that they should be treated as separate drugs and developed accordingly.

In addition to the preclinical pharmacology studies that are conducted to support the proposed therapeutic action of the drug, preclinical toxicology studies are also conducted to ensure that the drug is safe for study in humans. While there are no specific guidelines for the conduct of pre-clinical pharmacology studies, the FDA has published guidelines for the conduct of preclinical toxicology studies. These guidelines define the types of studies that need be conducted to support the various phases of clinical testing up to and including marketing.

Animal studies are used as predictors of the safety of a product in people. Because a clinical program of study for a drug product will involve usually only several thousand patients, the chance of determining subtle, yet important toxic events is limited. Therefore, the use of animals becomes an important surrogate to assess the safety of products. Drugs are given at high doses to large numbers of animals assuring that a toxic effect will be noted, at least at the highest dose. These toxic findings then become the potential limiting safety of the product in future clinical studies. Results from these toxicology studies will determine an appropriate safe dose to be used in clinical studies and what clinical parameters to monitor for.

The types of toxicity studies that are normally conducted in a clinical development program, vary in relation to the type of drug and its intended use (e.g. short-term or chronic; oral or parenteral/ inhaled) and to the phases of clinical testing. In general, the length of the study and the numbers of animals in the study increases as the phases of clinical development increase.

2.2.1 ACUTE TOXICITY STUDIES. Acute toxicity studies are designed to determine the short-term effects of a drug when administered in a single dose or in multiple doses within 24 hours or less. Acute toxicity studies provide insights into a drug's activity, degree of toxicity, and overt toxic effects.

To determine acute toxicity, the investigational drug is administered to several species of animals at exaggerated doses by the route of administration proposed for clinical use. In addition, at least one other route of administration is typical for comparison purposes. The animals are observed for at least one week after the initial dosing for delayed toxic effects.

Acute toxicity is a gross measure of the toxicity of a product and has the potential for identifying that system or those systems, e.g., central nervous system (CNS) or cardiovascular system (CVS), that are the most sensitive to the toxic effects of the drug. Acute toxicity can also provide information related to potential overdose situations in clinical studies.

2.2.2 SUBACUTE TOXICITY STUDIES. Subacute toxicity studies are conducted in animals to observe the toxic effects from multi-dose administration of the drug at doses which are expected to cause some toxicity but are not lethal. The length of these studies will typically vary from 1 to 6 months. Such studies are conducted in two species, a rodent and a nonrodent. The rodent species of choice has usually been the rat or mouse. The non-rodent species of choice has usually been the dog. Additional species are acceptable as long as there is adequate historical information about the incidence of spontaneous lesions in the species chosen.

In conducting these studies, the test material is administered by the intended route of administration. If the drug is to be administered orally in clinical studies, the test material can be administered either admixed in the feed, in the drinking water, or given by oral gavage. The latter is the preferred route of administration as there is better control over the exact amount of material that is actually ingested by the animal. Using the other routes of administration, there is less precision per animal, but on average, all animals will ingest approximately the intended dosage for that dose group. Typically, 3 dose levels are chosen for these studies. There will also be a control group and, sometimes, a positive control group, i.e., a group receiving a compound whose toxicity profile is known for the species being studied. This procedure validates the test and gives a basis for comparison.

During the conduct of these studies, animals are observed for clinical signs of toxicity. In addition, blood and urine samples are taken periodically to monitor for changes in analytes that might presage later morphologic toxicity. These early predictors of toxicity could be used as monitors for potential safety problems in later clinical studies. At the conclusion of the study, the surviving animals are euthanasized and gross and histopathologic examination is performed on key tissues and organs. In addition, those animals that might have died during the course of the study would also have had a gross and microscopic pathologic examination of tissues conducted.

The results of these studies serve two purposes: They identify those doses that are obviously toxic to the animals and allow for proper choice of doses in later animal carcinogenicity studies, if required. The results also allow for an assessment of the safe dose to be chosen for clinical studies. The ratio of the safe dose to be chosen for clinical studies to the toxic dose observed in animal studies will be based on the therapeutic area for which the drug is intended. For example, if the drug is an anti-cancer agent, there is more reason to allow a lower benefit/risk ratio than in a drug intended for a less life-threatening disease.

2.2.3 CHRONIC TOXICITY STUDIES. For those drugs that are intended to be taken orally on a chronic basis, either regularly or as needed, the FDA requires that studies of at least one year duration, in a rodent and a non-rodent, be conducted to determine the chronic toxicity of the compound. Al-

though most other health regulatory bodies will only require studies of six months duration in animals to satisfy the chronic toxicity study requirement, the FDA has required studies of 12 months duration in the belief that there are certain latent effects that could only be observed in studies of this duration, e.g., toxicity changes in the eye. There are currently ongoing discussions among the major health authorities (e.g., FDA, EC, and Japan), to harmonize chronic toxicity requirements. Hopefully in the near future, studies of 6 months duration will satisfy chronic toxicity requirements for all health authorities including the FDA, except in certain situations where, because of the chemical class of the product, there is reason to believe that studies of longer duration may be required.

The observations conducted in these chronic toxicity studies are the same as conducted in the sub-chronic toxicity studies. In addition, opthalmological tests are usually performed during the study.

2.2.4 CARCINOGENICITY STUDIES. In addition to chronic toxicity studies, the FDA also requires that carcinogenicity studies be conducted on drugs intended for chronic use either daily or intermittently. The FDA might also require carcinogenicity studies to be conducted for a compound which has exhibited mutagenic activity or whose chemical structure makes it a suspected carcinogen.

Carcinogenicity studies are typically conducted in rats and mice and usually are of two years duration, which essentially is a life-time exposure. In these studies, the dosages used are at a level that are not expected to induce toxicity but rather allow for survival of the animals for the duration of the study. The focus of these studies is not toxicity but an evaluation of the carcinogenicity potential of the drug. As such, the measurements conducted during the in-life phase of the study are less than are normally conducted in a chronic toxicity study. The focus, rather, is on the postmortem examination of the animals who either have died during the course of the study or have been euthanasized after the completion of the study. Importantly in these studies, strains of animals need to be selected for which historical control information regarding the incidence of spontaneous tumors in these strains, has been well developed. Often, a company will include a positive control (known carcinogen) during the conduct of the study.

2.2.5 MUTAGENICITY STUDIES. Although mutagenicity testing has not displaced whole animal carcinogenicity testing, as had been hoped when these studies were first developed, mutagenicity testing continues to be used as a screening tool to identify those compounds which have mutagenic potential and, therefore, could have both teratogenetic and carcinogenic potential. These studies usually involve a battery of 3–5 *in vivo* and *in vitro* tests that are designed to determine if a compound can cause gene mutation, chromosomal damage, or primary DNA damage.

2.2.6 REPRODUCTION STUDIES. The FDA requires reproduction studies be conducted for any drugs to be used in women of child-bearing potential, regardless of whether the target population is or is not pregnant women. These studies are divided into three segments, each of which is designed to reveal drug effects during a specific stage of the reproductive process, including: male and female fertility; effects on the zygote; its implantation; embryotoxicity and fetal death; effects on parturition and the newborn; lactation and care of the young; and the teratogenetic potential of the drug.

The three segments of reproduction studies are the following: (1) Study of Fertility and General Reproductive Performance—this research generally involves studies in the male and female rat with emphasis placed upon drug effects on gonadal function, estrus cycles, mating behavior, conception rates, and early stages of gestation. Males are treated with drug sufficiently prior to mating (usually 60 to 80 days) to assure the absence of a potential drug effect on spermatogenesis. Females are treated for less time prior to mating (usually 2 weeks) and then exposed to treated males. Drug administration is continued for females through gestation and weaning. (2) Teratology – this research generally involves studies in at least 2 species, usually chosen from among the mouse, rat, or rabbit. The drug is typically administered to pregnant animals by oral gavage during the period of organogenesis, to measure the compound's embryotoxicity and/or teratogenetic effects. (3) Perinatal/ Postnatal study—this research evaluates the drug's effect during the last trimester of pregnancy through delivery and on into the early period of lactation. The drug is administered to pregnant animals during the final one-third of gestation and administration continues to the mothers through lactation to weaning. Important parameters evaluated include late fetal development, labor and delivery, lactation, neonatal viability, and growth of the newborn.

2.2.7 SPECIAL TOXICITY STUDIES. As a result of the findings in the general toxicity studies, a sponsor may choose or the FDA may request to conduct additional targeted toxicity studies to look specifically at one or more organs that were the target organ for toxicity in the earlier toxicity studies. This protocol might involve looking more closely at the tissue through the use of electron microscopy, more close monitoring of the functional capacity of organs during the period of drug administration or evaluation of the reversibility of toxic effects. The results of these studies will assist the sponsor in determining the design of clinical studies or whether clinical studies should be conducted at all.

2.3 Transition from Preclinical to Clinical

Based on the results derived from early preclinical studies, a company will make a decision as to whether to proceed with at least initial clinical studies in humans. If the decision is to proceed, then the results obtained during the preclinical phase must be compiled into reports suitable for submission to the FDA in an IND. The purpose of this initial IND filing is to satisfy the FDA that the drug is safe enough to be administered to humans under a proposed protocol that would be submitted along with the IND.

The FDA has published regulations relating to the composition and format of an IND. The general outline of an IND is seen in Table 9.4. Sponsors wishing to submit an

IND must follow these regulations. Information that is submited to an IND falls into three general areas: (1) chemistry, manufacturing, and control information (2) pharmacology and toxicology information and (3) clinical information. Clinical information includes a protocol section which describes the proposed clinical studies to be conducted; a section on previous human experience which describes any clinical information known about the product, either generated by studies conducted by the sponsor or from other sources; and a section giving the overall investigational plan. One other important piece of information provided in the IND is a document entitled "Investigator's Brochure." This document is provided to all investigators and to those committees known as Institutional Review Boards who, in addition to the FDA, have the responsibility for approving research for their own institutions or on behalf of investigators not doing research at an institution. The Investigator's Brochure contains the following information:

Table 9.4 Standard IND Sections

Cover Sheet
Table of Contents
Introductory Statement and
    General Investigational Plan
Investigator's Brochure
Protocol(s)
Chemistry, Manufacturing, and
    Control Information
Pharmacology and Toxicology
    Information
Previous Human Experience With
    The Investigational Drug
Additional Information
- Information on drug abuse and
    drug dependence potential
- dosimetry information for
    radioactive drugs

- A brief description of the drug substance in the formulation, including its structural formula, if known.

- A summary of the pharmacological and toxicological effects of the drug in animals and, to the extent known, in humans.

- A summary of the pharmacokinetics and biological disposition of the drug in animals, and, if known, in humans.

- A summary of information relating to safety and effectiveness in humans obtained from any prior clinical studies.

- A description of possible risks and side effects to be anticipated, on the basis of prior experience with the drug under investigation or with related drugs.

- Any precautions or special monitoring to

be done as part of the investigational use of the drug.

Because the IND is a "living document," it can be amended and updated as additional information becomes available either from preclinical or clinical studies or additional chemical development. As additional safety information becomes available, it may also be necessary to update the Investigator's Brochure to provide the most up–to–date safety information to investigators, Institutional Review Boards, and, ultimately, to patients.

The IND becomes the repository file for all information known about the drug which is the subject of the IND. Such information is considered proprietary and will not be released to the general public. Even the existence of an IND is considered confidential information.

As the development of the product continues, the sponsor of the IND has the obligation to report, at least on an annual basis, the status of the development of the product. There are also additional reporting requirements, with respect to safety information that becomes known to the sponsor: reporting of what are called "serious adverse experiences" (SAEs). The FDA definition of a serious adverse experience means: any experience that is fatal or life-threatening, is permanently disabling, requires or prolongs in-patient hospitalization or is a congenital anomaly, cancer, or overdose. With respect to results obtained from tests in laboratory animals, a serious adverse drug experience includes any experience suggesting a significant risk for human subjects, including any findings of mutagenicity, teratogenicity, or carcinogenicity. The requirement for prompt reporting of these serious adverse experiences allows the FDA to immediately review the situation to determine if the safety finding is consequential enough to put a hold on the clinical studies. Fatal or life-threatening serious adverse experiences must be reported in 3 working days. Others must be reported in 10 working days.

2.4 Planning the Drug Development Process

2.4.1 ASSUMPTIONS. Mandatory for each pharmaceutical candidate, should be a plan developed upfront, with precise statements of intermediate and ultimate goals, go or no-go decision points, and an analysis of the time and costs involved at each step. Only recently, pharmaceutical companies have identified the need for detailed upfront planning. However, the creation of such a plan is rather time consuming and requires dedicated input from a variety of disciplines. Thus, few companies currently follow this process or are about to implement this strategy. Even fewer companies have documented knowledge of the costs involved in each step of the development of a new drug.

Obviously, without knowledge of certain characteristics of the new drug development candidate a concise development plan can not be created. Also obvious is the fact that the more information that is available, the more complete the plan will be and the more certain the goals set forth in the plan will be met. The timing for the creation of a plan is optimal when most of the following basic, preferred assumptions have been met at the time of the design of a Drug Development Plan:

Chemistry

- A reasonable amount of drug is available
- The manufacturing of the new drug is possible at reasonable cost of large scale production
- Method for analysis of the drug and its

major metabolites in blood and urine is available

- Early stability testing has provided acceptable results

Pre-Clinical

- Reasonable evidence is available that the drug has the desired pharmacodynamic effects
- Absorption of the drug has been observed in animals
- The absorption, metabolism and excretion in these animals follow a metabolic path similar to that expected in man
- The drug has few active metabolites
- The kinetics of the new product in animals is acceptable for the indication to be pursued
- No significant safety concerns are apparent from mutagenicity, or acute or subacute toxicology testing

For example, consider that company "A" wants to develop an angiotensin II antagonist to be used for the treatment of patients with hypertension. In this case, it would be desirable to establish, prior to the creation of a development plan, that the product: has the fewest possible active metabolites; is absorbed when given orally; has a pharmacokinetic half-life likely allowing once-a-day administration; has demonstrated hypotensive activity in appropriate animal models with hypertension; and has shown an acceptable outcome in mutagenicity and acute toxicology studies. In addition, it would be most appropriate to have available a comparison of pharmacodynamic effects in animal models and results of other special pharmacologic studies between the antiotensin II antagonist and the currently marketed antihypertensive agents in the same class, such as ACE inhibitors. If the angiotensin II antagonist would produce only minimal reductions of blood pressure when compared to the ACE inhib-

itor, the marketing of this less effective product at the time that most ACE inhibitors may be available as inexpensive generic brands, would be most unfavorable.

This early planning process is more or less complex depending on the ultimate clinical use of the product. Specific activities of certain drugs can readily be assessed *in-vitro* or *in-vivo* models of disease (e.g., antibiotics or antihypertensives) while for other drugs, the clinical efficacy cannot be predicted since no relevant model may yet exist (e.g., drugs to be used in the treatment of memory disorders in Alzheimer's Disease). In the latter case, indirect end points may have to be used such as receptor binding, activity of the drug in tissue cultures, or specific pharmacodynamic models (e.g., aorta strip preparations).

Once some or all of the assumptions have been met, a team has to be established to define the desirable goal for the ultimate development of the product. Experts need to review all available data and assess, as much as possible, the clinical indication for the drug in the most precise wording possible. Prescribing information provided for similar drugs already approved and used in the market place may help to guide this process. For instance, the development of a new angiotensin II antagonist would likely need to lead to an indication comparable to that for ACE inhibitors. The indication and limitations of use should at least be comparable to or better than those described for ACE inhibitors. Considerations have to be given as to whether the new drug should be used in the same patient population, new patient populations, or should be given in combination with the same or other drugs. At the same time a decision should be made with regard to the significant areas of concern (i.e., serious adverse events that may occur during the treatment with this product). In this instance, the market potential of the angiotensin II antagonist would be limited if the product would cause angioedema, neutropenia, agranulocytosis, proteinuria or initial hypotension, to the same degree or worse than that described for ACE inhibitors. Similarly, if a new analgesic is considered for development, it is imperative the drug has not caused significant toxicologic effects in the liver or kidneys and that the drug is unlikely to cause significant ulceration and bleeding of the gastrointestinal tract.

For novel drugs, (e.g., biotechnology products) comparisons with other drugs in the market may not be possible (e.g., erythropoietin or rGCSF). However, appropriate experts and consultants can help in the assessment of the therapeutic need for such products and at least identify a number of preliminary requirements for the indication, including areas of concern. The examples described here may help to illustrate the thought processes required to create the proper drug development plan.

The current economic climate and the significant changes expected in the health care system in the future, will require companies to focus more on drugs that are: innovative therapeutics; those drugs with greater efficacy than currently available treatments; those drugs providing a reduced adverse event profile that improves the benefit/risk ratio when compared to available therapies; and those drugs providing health economic advantages. Therefore, if, at this stage of the early development of a drug, such benefits are highly unlikely to be achieved, consideration should be given to either look for other development candidates or specific goals should be set to prove the presence of any such benefits in the shortest possible time at the most reasonable cost.

In many cases, the fate of a new drug candidate with potentially beneficial efficacy based on early pharmacology studies, will be determined by the assessment of its safety in acute and sub-acute toxicology

studies and in early phase 1 studies in humans, specifically, in rising single and multiple rising dose tolerance studies.

2.4.2 DEFINING THE DRUG DEVELOPMENT STRATEGY. The first step during the development of a drug candidate is the creation of a desired package insert (labeling). As noted earlier, the labeling for the drug determines how the drug, once approved, can be marketed and promoted. A variety of people from within and outside the company needs to be involved in this process: chemists, clinical pharmacologists, toxicologists, regulatory affairs personnel, scientists in clinical research and outside scientific consultants. There is some disagreement about the need for marketing personnel to be involved at this early stage. If a company has a well defined overall strategy (e.g., a mission to become the prime leader in the development of cardiovascular drugs), any new drug that provides significant advantages with regard to safety and efficacy in the treatment of cardiovascular diseases should go through the strategic planning process. The input from marketing would become more advantageous at later stages of development, once the drug has been proven to be reasonably safe and effective in the first Phase 1 and early Phase 2 studies. In the case where such defined commitment is lacking, a preliminary market analysis of the therapeutic indication to be considered and assessment of the market potential, may be useful.

In evolving the clinical part of the development plan for a drug, consideration should be given not only to the scientific and marketing aspects of the drug, but also to the regulatory strategy which takes into account the various initiatives on the part of the FDA that allow for accelerated development and approval of certain products. Thus, if the candidate drug product is intended for an indication for which there is a limited patient population, this drug could be a candidate for approval under the Orphan Drug Act, if the patient population is less than 200,000 in the U.S. There are certain financial advantages for development of products granted Orphan Drug designation. Additionally, the sponsor of a drug approved under the Orphan Drug Act is granted 7 years of exclusive marketing of that drug for that indication.

For a drug which has the potential for multiple indications, it would be worthwhile to explore whether one or more of those indications would be eligible for accelerated development/approval under some of the new initiatives proposed and enacted by the FDA for drugs used to treat life-threatening and seriously debilitating diseases. If a drug is a viable candidate for accelerated development/approval, the possibility exists of securing regulatory approval with less than the normal number and size of clinical studies that are required for traditional drugs. In some instances, where a drug is approved under accelerated development/approval regulations, there are obligations taken on by the sponsor to conduct post-marketing studies to further explore the safety and efficacy of the product. Should these studies fail to confirm what was demonstrated in the smaller studies used to support approval, it is possible that the FDA could withdraw the product from the market.

In an effort to provide less expensive pharmaceuticals to the public, the U.S. Congress in 1984 passed the Drug Price Competition and Patent Term Restoration Act which allowed the approval of generic versions of already approved drugs whose patent protection had expired. A new vehicle for doing this, the Abbreviated New Drug Application (ANDA), was created by the FDA at the time of the passage of this act. An ANDA allowed sponsors of generic versions of already marketed drugs to secure approval of their product without the need to submit reports of nonclinical laboratory studies and reports of clinical in-

vestigations. The sponsor would only be required to submit chemistry and manufacturing controls information describing the synthesis of their product as well as reports of bioavailability/bioequivalence studies to show that their product is chemically comparable to the already approved product on the market.

The next phase in the creation of the development master plan can be started once the labeling, including the desired dosage form, the desired route of administration, the intended therapeutic indication, including acceptable contradictions, and the desirable pharmacologic effects of the drug, have been defined and agreed upon.

2.4.3. THE DRUG DEVELOPMENT MASTER PLAN. The drug development master plan includes all pre-clinical and clinical studies that need to be performed to complete the development of the drug. The plan includes timing of the implementation of such studies, time to completion, costs and critical go/no-go decision points. In addition, the plan should indicate the timing of interaction with regulatory authorities.

The detailed master plan only can be written once the strategy has been defined and the development team has a good knowledge of regulatory guidelines, requirements, and of relevant activities by competitor companies. The timing of the preparation of the detailed plan is most productive when all information required for filing of an IND is available or when the availability of the IND is known in the near future.

The scheduling of all these activities is needed in order to estimate the manpower and the budget for the entire program, from one decision point to the next and, or for each budget cycle as established within the company (e.g., calendar year). The ultimate goal is to prepare a plan that allows the delivery of top quality data on time and on budget.

Once the starting point of the plan has been determined (e.g., a date for the pre-IND meeting with regulatory authorities or for the submission of the IND) the next step would be to gain consensus on the best timing for reaching the end point (e.g., submissions for the expected approval of the NDA). The assertiveness with which this plan is to be established depends on outside and inside factors.

Table 9.5 provides a listing of major outside and inside factors that determine the speed of development of new pharmaceuticals.

Outside factors are determined mostly by the competition, the therapeutic need for development of the compound, and whether the product is to be developed for one country or globally. Other outside factors include the choice to develop the product in partnership with other companies or the need for reaching licensing agreements with other companies. Inside factors are determined by the company's

philosophy, strategic plan, the degree of conservatism, concurrent development activities with other compounds, the available manpower and the companies attitude towards outsourcing. Although it seems to be the tendency for most major companies to do the early phase development in-house and late phase development through outsourcing to contract research organizations, some innovative companies have emerged who, with a very small in-house staff, perform all work through outside resources. Likely, this trend will increase.

Some companies, for instance Japanese companies, prefer to pursue the first part of the development of their product in Japan and only once they are certain of a successful development of the product in their country, do they move the development abroad. However, recently some of the major pharmaceutical companies in Japan have started the development of new drugs on a worldwide basis: in Europe, the United States and in their home country.

A number of major pharmaceutical houses in the United States prefer to do the early development phase in the United States and perform late phase development internationally: in Europe, the U.S. and on occasion, in Australia and New Zealand. Current regulations in Japan make that country unfeasible in a pivotal worldwide development program for a drug, as the Japanese require a separate set of studies that are acceptable to the drug development culture in Japan and its regulatory authority. This status is not expected to change until more discussions have taken place with a tentative goal of reaching a more reasonable level of understanding and agreement on Good Clinical Practices (GCP). This agreement may govern clinical research worldwide in 1995 or beyond.

In contrast to some of the large companies in the U.S. or Europe, small firms, such as biotechnology companies with limited resources, have no option but to start the development on a relatively small scale

Table 9.5 Determinants of the Sequencing of Studies Required for the Development of New Pharmaceuticals

Outside Factors

- Therapeutic need for the drug
- Local or global development
- Partnership with other companies
- Licensing plans
- Competitive activities
- New scientific developments
- Changing regulatory requirements

Inside Factors

- The company's mission and culture
- The indication(s) to be pursued
- In-house experience
- Familiarity with regulations
- Budget and manpower
- Attitude towards outsourcing

in one country, usually the United States. Some of the larger biotechnology companies, specifically those who already have products in the market and thereby a defined source of revenues, may prefer parallel but shifted development in the U.S. and Europe.

Finally, some companies without reasonable manpower located in the U.S. or in Europe, have no option but to outsource the development in the area where they do not have a significant presence. The same strategy is true for many of the Japanese companies who do not have adequate resources in the U.S. or Europe to develop one or more of their products by themselves.

The timing of go/no-go decision points and the willingness to take a more risky development course, also is determined by the company's culture and philosophy. Is the company willing to pursue further development based on preliminary or interim results from studies or willing to continue development of a broad dose range well into Phase 2? Or is the company only willing to continue the late phase development once efficacy, the final dose range, and preliminary safety is fully determined? This choice obviously is determined by the financial stability of the company, the experience and expertise of the staff, and the comfort level they have with regard to local and global regulations.

The following example may illustrate some of the issues raised. It is quite understandable that company "A", who considered developing an angiotensin II antagonist and who had reason to believe that they could be the second or third company to bring such a drug to the market, be aggressive in its approach. A failure to have that drug approved on time may cause the drug to fail in the market place because any angiotensin II antagonist beyond number 5 in the market, would unlikely reach an acceptable level of revenues.

Similarly, in the development of antibiotics, where newer, more effective antibiotics follow older ones in relatively rapid fashion, it is imperative that the development process be completed as soon as possible. In contrast, development of novel drugs with new indications may require a more cautious approach and large scale studies may not be initiated in these cases until reasonable certainty has been obtained on the safety and efficacy of the product. Specifically, this approach is true for drugs where definitive efficacy data only can be obtained through complex and larger scale studies. This strategy would include drugs to be used in the improvement of memory disorders associated with Alzheimer's Disease.

Currently, some classes of new drugs are being developed which are in search of the disease for which they will provide benefit (12). This orientation seems to be true for PAF-antagonists, thromboxane synthetase inhibitors, thromboxane A_2 receptor antagonists and other novel compounds affecting specific mediators in the complex immune system. In such cases, a variety of early Phase 2 studies may need to be conducted to provide preliminary answers to the efficacy of the product in a number of diseases. Obviously, not all of these indications will be successful, and it may be difficult to establish a precise timeline for the late phase of development.

Also, changing requirements may have a significant impact on the strategy to be followed with regard to the scheduling of studies and definition of go/no-go decision points for certain drugs. Currently, most new drugs for the treatment of cardiac arrhythmias would require large scale long-term mortality studies before they will be allowed in the market. The same vigilance is true for positive inotropes in the treatment of congestive heart failure. Before the start of such expensive long-term mortality studies, it is imperative for the company to be certain of the pharmacokinetics and pharmacodynamics of the drug, potential drug interactions, the effect of food on the drug's absorption, and special effects that the drug may have in certain patient populations (e.g., the elderly, or patients with diabetes). This vigilance obviously will lengthen the total development phase.

Finally, unpredictable changes in the scientific or regulatory environment may have an effect on the strategy related to the development of new pharmaceuticals. Examples include companies who have chosen to delay or even cancel the development of positive inotropes in heart failure or antiarrhythmics because of the recent evidence of adverse morbidity related to treatment with such drugs and the hesitancy in the scientific world to accept new studies with drugs in these classes. The lack of proper guidelines for drugs to be developed in the treatment of memory disorders related to Alzheimer's Disease also have delayed the development of such drugs. Only after the regulatory authorities have agreed upon desired endpoints in studies with drugs for the treatment of memory disorders in Alzheimer's Disease (based on their experience with Tacrin), have other companies commenced or continued the development of such drugs. Keep in mind that regulators currently are discussing the viability of drugs that have been developed up to ten years ago, while pharmaceutical companies are planning the development of drugs that hopefully will reach the market five or ten years from this timepoint. Only continued and timely discussion between companies, scientists and regulatory authorities can help to bridge this gap.

2.4.4 CRITICAL COMPONENTS OF THE CLINICAL PART OF THE DRUG DEVELOPMENT MASTER PLAN. Critical components that determine the course for the development of a drug will be different depending on the class of drug, the indication to be pursued, the philosophy of the company, and other scientific, regulatory and environmental factors. Despite this complexity, critical components of the clinical development master plan need to be defined (Table 9.6). The plan has to have a clear starting point

Table 9.6 Critical Components of the Clinical Part of the Drug Development Plan

- Clear starting point and end point
- Go/no-go decision points
- Interactions with regulatory authorities
- Schedule of studies and study reports
- Budget
- Personnel requirements

and a clear endpoint. The starting point that would be most appropriate would be the date for a pre-IND meeting with the FDA, or the date of filing the IND. The endpoint could be the time of first proof of efficacy in humans (e.g., reasonable hypotensive action of an antihypertensive in patients after a few weeks of therapy) or the date of filing of an NDA.

Also, the development plan should include significant go/no-go decision points; for example, outcome of the pre-IND meeting; outcome of regulatory review after IND filing; the start of the first study in patients with the disease and the end of Phase 2 studies (better defined as the start of Phase 3), the outcome of an end of a Phase 2 meeting with the regulatory authorities; and finally, a go/no-go decision at the time of NDA filing.

These examples are not the only go/no-go points that can be chosen. Others may include the identification of a co-development or licensing partner, while not infrequently, reasons for decisions appear unexpectedly; for instance, formulation problems or the emergence of significant adverse events.

Figure 9.1 shows the outline of the clinical part of the development plan for a drug to be used in the treatment of hypertension and angina. In this plan a minimal number of critical Phase 1 studies are performed with a goal of starting large pivotal Phase 2 studies as soon as possible to assure that the drug is efficacious when given once daily. Following that goal, the Phase 3 program is planned.

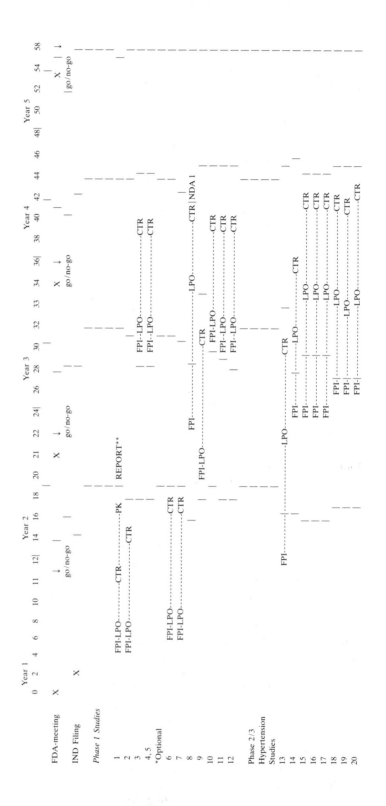

Fig. 9.1 A sample of the clinical part of the drug development plan for phases 1–5 for a calcium channel blocker in hypertension and angina. Company B AB-105. *Pending results of available data. **Worst case scenario. FPI = first patient in study. LPO = last patient out of study. CTR = clinical trial report. NDA 1 = hypertension NDA. NDA = angina NDA.

Phase 1. Study 1, Single and multiple dose tolerance study; Study 2, Food interaction study; Studies 3–5, Drug interaction studies; Study 6, Pharmacokinetic study in liver impairment; Study 7, Pharmacokinetic study in liver impairment; Study 8, Special pharmacodynamic study; Study 9, Pharmacokinetic study in the elderly; Study 10, Radiolabeled ADME study; Study 11, Dose proportionality study; and Study 12, Bioavailability of the final dosage form.

Phase 2/3 Hypertension. Study 13, Double blind, placebo-controlled dose finding study of one month duration in mild to moderate hypertension; Study 14, Double blind, placebo-controlled dose finding study with 24-hour blood pressure monitoring; Study 15, Double blind, placebo-controlled dose finding study of 3 month duration; Study 16, Double blind, placebo-controlled dose finding study on top of a diuretic; Study 17, Double blind, placebo-controlled efficacy study in the elderly; Study 18, Double blind, placebo-controlled efficacy study in moderate to severe hypertension; Study 19, Double blind, placebo-controlled efficacy study with non-invasive hemodynamics; and Study 20, Open label, placebo-controlled efficacy study in severe hypertension.

Phase 2/3 Angina. Study 21, Multiple dose open label titration study in patients with angina; Study 22, Double blind, placebo-controlled dose finding study; Study 23, Double blind, placebo-controlled dose finding study on top of selected other therapies for angina; Study 24, Open label hemodynamic study; Study 25, Double blind, placebo-controlled efficacy study; and Study 26, Double blind, placebo-controlled efficacy study with active control.

Note: Studies 15, 16, 17, 19, 22, 23, 24, 25 and 26 have a one year open extension.

Figure 9.2 presents a clinical development plan for a drug in the treatment of memory disorders associated with Alzheimer's Disease. In this case the endpoint is not the filing of the NDA, but the endpoint is to obtain adequate preliminary information to start a large scale Phase 2/3 study to demonstrate the safety and efficacy of the drug in patients with Alzheimer's Disease. In this case, preliminary Phase 1 information on the drug was obtained in volunteers without the disease, but of comparable age and gender to the patient population. At the same time, this plan included pharmacokinetic studies in patients with abnormal liver function, and in those with abnormal renal function, as well as drug interaction studies with drugs that are commonly given to patients with Alzheimer's Disease. Based on this plan, the proper dose, the dosing interval, the timing of dosing in relation to food intake as well as any necessary adjustments for dosing of the drug in patients with the disease due to abnormal organ function or to the presence of concurrent medication, could be established prior to the start of the large scale efficacy trials.

Preclinical factors that have to be considered in the preparation of the clinical plan include the availability of study drug, completion of relevant stability studies, completion of the appropriate toxicology and reproduction studies, and any other studies that are required in chemistry (See sections 2.1 and 2.2).

As noted earlier, the pharmaceutical industry still is struggling with the assessment of manpower requirements and costs for clinical development of new compounds. Only a few companies are able to properly assess these needs. In contrast, many contract research organizations, purely based on necessity and client demands, have been able to reasonably assess man-power and cost for clinical studies or

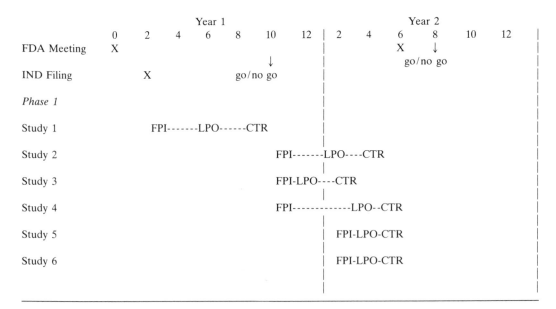

Fig. 9.2 A sample of the clinical part of the development plan for Phase 1 for a drug on the treatment of memory disorders in Alzheimer's Disease. Company B CD-101.

Study 1, Single Dose rising tolerance study in the elderly; Study 2, Multiple dose rising tolerance study in the elderly; Study 3, Effect of food study; Study 4, Single dose pharmacokinetics in renal impairment; Study 5, Drug interaction study; Study 6, Drug interaction study; FPI, First patient in study; LPO, Last patient out of study; and CTR, Clinical trial report.

entire clinical development plans. It is likely that the pharmaceutical industry will adopt the strategy to calculate financial and manpower needs at the time of completion of the clinical part of the development plan so that logical decisions can be made on how to spend research dollars and to distribute the available manpower. Alternatively, based on such calculations, the company will be able to make timely decisions with regard to the need for outsourcing.

2.5 Clinical Research; The Conduct of Clinical Trials

So far, a number of concepts as well as factors that determine the strategy and design of the clinical development of drugs, have been discussed. In the following section more specific information is provided with regard to clinical trials that need to be conducted during the development phase of a drug. These clinical trials can be categorized in different phases: 1, 2, 3, and 4. General characteristics of each of these phases are listed below.

PHASE 1. Phase 1 studies comprise the first trials of a new drug in humans, usually healthy volunteers. They are designed to provide a preliminary evaluation of drug safety, pharmacokinetics (absorption, distribution, metabolism and elimination) of the active ingredient(s), and identification of possible drug–drug and drug–food interactions. Phase 1 studies also include pharmacokinetic studies in volunteers with impaired renal or liver functions. Most Phase 1 studies are performed in specialized Phase 1 Units where subjects are closely monitored.

PHASE 2. In Phase 2, therapeutic studies are performed to demonstrate the pharmacodynamics of the new drug, and to assess its short-term safety in patients suffering from the intended disease or con-dition. The initial trials (Phase 2a) utilize a limited number of subjects, while later-stage trials (Phase 2b) study greater numbers and use well-controlled (i.e., placebo-controlled) comparative designs. Phase 2 studies also explore possible effective dose ranges and regimens and, if feasible, clarify dose-response relationship to guide the design of larger therapeutic (Phase 3) trials.

PHASE 3. The initial Phase 3 studies (Phase 3a) are intended to provide sufficient proof of efficacy and adequate safety of the new drug in a large number of patients prior to its registration with the FDA. These studies establish the short- and long-term safety/efficacy balance of the active ingredient and assess its therapeutic value. The profile of adverse drug experiences and the special features of the new drug are rigorously explored. Usually, Phase 3a studies are randomized and double-blind, however other designs may be employed (e.g., long-term safety studies). Phase 3 studies would be expected to mimic the conditions of the new drugs' intended clinical use, but often they do not because of restrictive enrollment criteria.

Later-staged Phase 3 studies (Phase 3b or "peri-approval" studies) are conducted after the NDA is submitted to the FDA, but prior to new drug's approval. Frequently in Phase 3b trials the new drug is compared with others already established as effective, or the studies are designed to complete or augment earlier trials (e.g., quality of life).

PHASE 4. Phase 4 studies typically are performed after the FDA grants marketing approval. Among other intentions, Phase 4 studies: continue documenting the safety of the drug; may reveal rare side-effects or unexpected interactions with other drugs; record the prescribing behavior of physicians (so-called "post marketing surveillance"); supplement (and in some cases support) the information initially provided to FDA for marketing approval; and further assess the drug's therapeutic value in special populations.

Note that although in general, the clinical trial phases are performed in chronological order, not all Phase 1 studies are necessarily completed before the start of Phase 2 and not all Phase 2 studies are completed before the start of Phase 3. In addition, recently, many clinical researchers have referred to Phase 2a as a small first study or studies in patients using the drug for the disease, often performed in Phase 1 institutions.

DiMasi described that, on average, Phase 1 of the clinical development of a drug takes approximately one year, Phase 2 approximately two years, and Phase 3, three years (5). These calculations are averages and the duration of these phases varies significantly for different classes of drugs.

2.5.1 PHASE 1 CLINICAL RESEARCH. Phase 1 trials are intended to determine the absorption, distribution, metabolism and excretion of the drug, including pharmacokinetics. Most Phase 1 trials are conducted in healthy volunteers, unless the potential effects of the drug may be harmful to these volunteers. In such cases, patients rather than volunteers are utilized; for instance, for drugs to be used in patients with cancer or AIDS. Also useful, may be the performance of Phase 1 trials directly in patients if, in such short trials, the preliminary efficacy of the drug can be tested; for example, drugs to be used in patients with hypertension, hyperlipidemia or diabetes.

Table 9.7 presents a list of typical Phase 1 studies.

Single and multiple rising dose tolerance studies usually are the first to be conducted with a new pharmaceutical. These studies usually are placebo-controlled and, for each dose level, six to twelve subjects are given active drug and two to four subjects a

Table 9.7 Typical Phase 1 Studies

1. Single rising dose tolerance
2. Multiple rising dose tolerance
3. Food interaction
4. Absorption, distribution, metabolism and excretion studies
5. Special population studies

   - elderly
   - post-menopausal
   - renally impaired
   - hepatic impaired
   - slow metabolizers

6. Drug interaction studies
7. Bioequivalence studies
8. Dose proportionality studies

placebo. The doses to be used in these studies depend on results from toxicology data in animals with a comparable metabolism of the drug to that in humans. The highest non-effect dose found in animals can be used to calculate the highest dose to be given in humans, while allowing for an acceptable safety ratio. Usually, a dose not higher than one-tenth to one-twentieth of the highest non-effect dose will be administered to volunteers (e.g., the highest non-effect dose of 50 milligrams per kg in dogs would translate to a highest dose of 250 milligrams of the drug given to humans, assuming a body weight of 50 kg.)

Single and multiple rising dose tolerance studies include extensive pharmacokinetics, requiring the availability of the proper assay for the drug, its active metabolites and, if possible, its stereoisomers. Multiple dose tolerance studies usually include pharmacokinetics after the first dose and following the last dose. These studies are of a duration to assure that a steady-state has been reached, usually after three to five half-lifes of the drug. Single and multiple rising dose tolerance studies are performed sequentially and one dose level at a time.

The next higher dose level will only be pursued after a full safety assessment of the previous dose has been made. Once mild but significant, adverse events (e.g., symptoms, laboratory abnormalities) have been observed, the maximum tolerated dose potentially having been reached, the study should be discontinued. Further Phase 1 and Phase 2 studies should be performed with a dose level lower than the maximum tolerated dose. If a maximum tolerated dose has not been reached and further increases in dose are not acceptable because they would exceed the noneffect dose in animals, further studies should be considered to demonstrate efficacy of the drug at that dose level. The results of such studies may provide a ratio of efficacy and safety in the target population, and this data can be used to establish the tolerance for the drug.

Food interaction studies should be done early, since it is important to establish the proper time relationship between food intake and the administration of the drug in Phase 2 and Phase 3 studies. Absorption, distribution, metabolism and excretion studies on the new chemical entity usually are done in a small healthy volunteer population (4–8 subjects) using a radiolabeled compound.

It is important to consider studies in subjects other than healthy volunteers early in the drug development process, especially when the drug is to be used in a target population that is different from the normal healthy volunteers commonly used in Phase 1 studies. Thus, for a drug to be used in the treatment of memory disorders associated with Alzheimer's Disease, it is essential to do pharmacokinetics in healthy elderly volunteers. If a drug is to be used to treat osteoporosis, the first Phase 1 studies also should be done in the elderly, including the post-menopausal female population. Consideration should be given to study pharmacokinetics of the drug in patients who have renal impairment, hepatic impairment, or abnormalities in the absorption of the drug (e.g., inflammatory bowel disease or other gastrointestinal diseases), if the drug is intended to be used in patients with such conditions. In these populations the pharmacokinetics may be quite different from that in healthy normal volunteers and the dosage and dosing interval may need to be adjusted accordingly. Evaluation of impaired patient populations needs to be properly addressed during Phase 1 rather than a chance encounter with this problem in larger patient populations studies during Phase 2 and 3, possibly resulting in significant adverse events due to improper dosing.

Recently, suggestions have been made by the regulatory authorities to include women (properly protected from pregnancies) in early Phase 1 studies and to consider performing pharmacokinetics in subjects who are shown to be slow metabolizers (13). It has been estimated that 9% of the American population may be slow metabolizers, and this statistic may significantly affect the metabolism and the safety profile of drugs in such patients.

Drug interaction studies should be done when, in the intended target population, the drug is to be used frequently with concomitant medications. Thus, if the drug is to be used in elderly patients with cardiovascular diseases, drug interactions with diuretics, anticoagulants, or aspirin should be considered. Similarly, if the drug is to be used in patients with diabetes, studies on the effect of the drug on glucose metabolism in the presence and absence of insulin or oral antidiabetic drugs, should be considered. Finally, drug interaction studies should be done if the new drug's absorption is expected to have an effect on the absorption of other drugs and vice–versa. Recently suggested has been a proposal to do a minimal number of drug level measurements during the large Phase 2 and 3 clinical trials to further study altered pharmacokinetics with the relationship between drug levels, drug effects and adverse events in the intended patient population and to limit the number of drug interaction studies in Phase 1.

Peck et al. (14) have strongly supported the need for careful assessment of the pharmacokinetics of each drug using toxicokinetic, pharmacokinetic, pharmacodynamic and population pharmacokinetic studies. These authors believe that the information obtained in such studies would provide essential information and guidance throughout the entire drug development process.

Bioequivalence studies usually are required when different dosage forms are being used in the early and the late phases of development. Powder-filled capsules are frequently used in Phase 1 and tablets in Phase 2 and 3. Thus, it may be necessary to show bioequivalence of these formulations in healthy normal volunteers. In addition, similarities in dissolution characteristics of both formulations have to be shown.

Most Phase 1 studies are done in healthy volunteers in groups of 8 volunteers to 12 volunteers per dose, and in a sequential study design except for bioequivalence studies and drug interaction studies where cross-over designs are more appropriate. The studies are performed while the volunteers are being observed, throughout the entire dosing interval, for adverse events and vital signs by experienced study staff. Concomitant medication, concomitant diseases, the use of caffeine, alcohol or smoking are usually not allowed during these studies. These measures are taken to study the effects of the drug in its purest setting and to assure that all observations or adverse events are not caused by factors other than the drug. It has been said that 1 in 10 serious adverse events will stop the development of most agents, at times already in Phase 1 studies (13). Although this approach has been well accepted, it is important to remember that because of the limitation of the design of these studies,

additional adverse events will be uncovered during studies in patients under more real life circumstances.

In total, the Phase 1 program for new drug entities includes 100 to 200 volunteers/patients, at a cost of approximately 2.5 million dollars (1987 dollars), and, on average, it takes one year before Phase 2 can be commenced.

Phase 1 studies need not always be conducted in the US if a drug has been extensively studied abroad, was previously used for other indications, has been already marketed, or is a new formulation of a known drug. In this case, a drug could directly be studied in Phase 2 and 3 trials.

Studies with drugs for the treatment of patients with severe diseases (e.g., cancer, AIDS), may not require testing in normal volunteers, because such drugs may be harmful to these volunteers without the chance for potential beneficial effects. Often these drugs are first evaluated in small patient populations with the disease, who are carefully observed for adverse effects as well as for potential beneficial events using surrogate or real endpoints.

2.5.2 PHASE 2 AND PHASE 3 CLINICAL RESEARCH. Phase 2 and 3 studies are conducted in patients with the targeted disease to demonstrate efficacy and safety of the drug and to provide the essential scientific information needed for the safe and effective use of the drug in clinical practice.

The protocols for Phase 2 and 3 studies usually are designed by the project team; for instance, relevant scientists, outside consultants, personnel from regulatory affairs, biostatistics, and data management and with some input from the marketing group. After a basic design for these studies has been drafted, it usually is most productive to have this design reviewed by the team and to discuss any revisions during a meeting with all team members present. A dedicated "protocol review day" to finalize the protocol and to start the process of case report form design is most efficient. This day allows for weighted decisions about the inclusion or exclusion of suggestions made by each team member and significantly shortens the protocol review time.

Most Phase 2 trials are designed for long-term multiple-dose exposure to the new pharmaceutical in patients with the disease. These trials usually are double-blind (single-blind when no other option is available), placebo-controlled and include multiple-dose levels. The dose range to be used in these trials depends on results of toxicology and Phase 1 trials. Usually, 3 to 4 doses and a placebo are used. It is relatively uncommon to use an active comparitor drug in these trials. However, where appropriate, this practice should be considered to evaluate potential differentiating factors between an established approved control agent and the new study drug. Studies including approved drugs as comparators during the later phases of development will likely become more prevalent. They already are required by authorities in France and Australia in order to establish pricing policies. In view of the ongoing healthcare system reforms, such studies also may become relevant for the acceptance of the new drug on formularies of medical institutions.

Most Phase 2 trials are of a parallel design. However, a crossover design may be useful, especially when complex dosage forms of the new drug are involved and the duration of treatment is relatively short (e.g., single dose analgesic studies in patients with dysmenorrhea or short term inhalation studies with bronchodilators in patients with asthma).

The duration of Phase 2 trials depends on the time of maximum effect. With some treatments (e.g., antihypertensive drugs) the maximum effect may not be reached until after 4–6 weeks of treatment. The duration also depends on the need for titration (e.g., the treatment of Parkinson's

disease or seizure disorders) and the availability of proper toxicology data to support long term administration of drug at this moment and time.

Phase 2 trials are performed in a relatively small patient population. While the focus of these studies is efficacy of the drug, preliminary safety data are gathered simultaneously. However, in some cases demonstrating efficacy of the new drug in small patient populations is impossible. In such cases, large Phase 2 studies are initiated immediately following completion of the relevant Phase 1 studies and these trials are then used as pivotal trials to demonstrate the efficacy of the drug. The size of such trials may be comparable to Phase 3 trials. Examples include multi-factorial design studies used in the evaluation of new anti-hypertensive agents and large trials to demonstrate efficacy of a drug to be used in the treatment of memory disorders in patients with Alzheimer's Disease. Depending on the safety profile for the drug, such large Phase 2 trials may have to start at a relatively low dose level and continue at higher doses once interim safety assessments have been done.

Most Phase 2 studies require anywhere between 20 to 80 patients per dose group, with exceptional trials needing more than 100 patients per group to demonstrate the efficacy of the product. The size of the study is determined by the endpoint selected and proper statistical power calculations.

In most cases, the early Phase 2 studies will include patients with the intended disease but who are otherwise free of concurrent diseases and concomitant medication. Therefore, in the evaluation of a new drug in the treatment of patients with hypertension, Phase 2 trials will include patients with mild to moderate hypertension who do not have significant renal impairment and have not had significant cardiovascular or cerebral vascular disease prior to the start of the study. However, a selection of relatively healthy patients is not always used. The evaluation of positive inotropes in the treatment of patients with heart failure could initially be done in patients with end-stage disease, so as to allow evaluation of beneficial effects over a relative short time period. Promising studies with drugs in the treatment of cancer may be done in patients for whom there is no alternative treatment. Assuming that the outcome in these patients in the absence of the new drug is not beneficial, any reasonable response may be considered as a preliminary sign of efficacy.

Trials with survival as the endpoint often include patients with concomitant diseases and medication (e.g., new treatments for patients with AIDS or for patients with cerebrovascular accidents). In such trials, it may not always be ethically acceptable to use placebo as a control. Therefore, other accepted therapies that are believed to be beneficial, multiple dosage levels of the new drug, or historical controls, may be used in the design of such trials. In other cases an uneven randomization of patients to placebo and active therapy may be a useful approach. However, when possible, Phase 2 trials should be placebo-controlled. In the past, small Phase 2 trials using open study designs often have led to improper conclusions with regard to potential benefits of the drug.

To include some form of rescue medication in placebo-controlled trials is quite acceptable; for instance, throughout the study, patients with angina would be allowed to take transdermal nitrates or patients with asthma would be allowed to take inhaled bronchodilators when needed, provided the usage of such medication is properly documented. In such studies, the difference in the amount of rescue medication used between the placebo and the active drug group may serve as an endpoint.

The endpoints to be used in clinical evaluation of new drugs should be clini-cally relevant, objectively measureable, adequately sensitive and specific to demonstrate efficacy of the drug, and, most importantly, acceptable to the regulatory authorities and scientists. In a number of diseases such endpoints are well defined; for example, laboratory measurements for the evaluation of antidiabetic and lipid lowering drugs; blood pressure for antihypertensive drugs; exercise testing used in the evaluation of drugs in the treatment of patients with congestive heart failure or angina; Holter monitoring in patients with arrhythmia; or measurements of changes in the size of benign or malignant tumors following therapy. However, some of these endpoints may not necessarily demonstrate a beneficial clinical outcome of treatment of the disease. Decreases in blood pressure during treatment with a diuretic with the potential of decreased potassium levels and adverse effects on glucose and lipid metabolism, may ultimately not improve the morbidity or mortality of such patients, and a decrease in the number of arrhythmias on the Holter monitor or in the frequency of angina is not necessarily predictive of long-term survival in such patients. Therefore, regulatory authorities and scientists seem to move towards measuring clinical endpoints such as morbidity or mortality in relevant diseases.

In the new guidelines for the evaluation of treatment of respiratory infections (e.g., acute exacerbations of chronic bronchitis or pneumonia) regulatory authorities have accepted significant improvement in the clinical status of a patient without the need to demonstrate the actual disappearance of the microorganism in all patient studies. This decision is based on the strong relation between the effect of the antibiotic on the microorganism and the clinical improvement of infected patients.

In many studies less defined endpoints may have to be used, such as severity and disability related to pain, stiffness of joints, symptomatic scores of shortness of breath and the use of rescue medication. Such endpoints often are reported by the patient in a diary or at the time of visit with the investigator. In such studies commonly the investigator provides an opinion on the improvement in the severity of the disease and symptoms reported by the patient or by the patient's caretaker.

Quality of Life measurements are included in a number of clinical trials, most commonly in Phase 3 or 4 trials. However, whenever Quality of Life questionnaires are being used, it is most important that such questionnaires have been validated for each specific patient population.

Changes in the scientific and regulatory environment with regard to the acceptability of surrogate endpoints, have significant effects on the strategy for the development of certain classes of drugs. According to Temple, the use of surrogate endpoints can lead to error in 3 different ways (13):

1. The relationship between surrogate endpoint and the clinical event may not be the intended causal relationship but may be coincidental or co-related to some third factor.
2. The risk benefit assessment of the drug may be wrong because the clinical benefit deriving from the effect on the surrogate is smaller than expected and may not outweigh the risk of the drug in general.
3. The surrogate endpoint only measures one effect of the drug, the property of the drug thought to be of value. However, drugs may have other effects that may be adverse although not as prominent and not as frequent.

Examples include anti-arrhythmics which lower the rate of ventricular premature beats and decrease rates of some serious arrhythmias but provoke or worsen other serious arrhythmias. Most recently, the usefulness of CD4 levels as a surrogate endpoint for drugs in the treatment of AIDS has been brought into question, with a renewed focus on clinical outcome.

Apart from endpoint measurements, Phase 2 and Phase 3 studies include relevant laboratory and EKG, EMG or EEG tests to assess the safety of a drug. It is also becoming more common to include some blood level measurements of the drug in Phase 2 and Phase 3 trials (14, 15). Blood level measurements would make it possible to demonstrate in the larger patient population a possible relationship between drug level and the effect, or between drug level and any observed adverse experiences. Some researchers favor the use of drug levels as measures of achieving the optimal dose of the medication in concentration response studies.

Most important is a good understanding about the effective dose range based on the results of Phase 2 trials, before starting the Phase 3 trials. In addition, adequate toxicology data, stability testing, manpower and budget are needed to perform Phase 3 trials.

The basic design for Phase 3 trials is not different from Phase 2 studies although Phase 3 trials often include fewer dose levels, more patients per dose and, when appropriate, an active comparator drug. Most of the Phase 3 trials are placebo-controlled, double-blind, randomized and of adequate size to show statistically significant efficacy and safety of the drug in the intended patient population. For certain drugs and indications this design of Phase 3 studies may not be adequate. In such cases more complex designs have to be used, including withdrawal studies, innovative survival studies, or large comparative studies. These studies often have been used in the assessment of treatment of a variety of cardiovascular diseases (e.g., GISSI trials, ISIS trials, SAVE, BHAT, Consensus, SOLVD, Cast).

Most Phase 3 trials and some Phase 2 trials have an open extension during which patients who responded adequately to treatment with the drug are allowed to continue this medication in an open-label fashion. This protocol allows the sponsor to evaluate long term safety and outcome in such patients, including interactions with any concomitant medication or concurrent diseases that may develop. Such extensions may well go beyond the date of filing of the NDA.

Additional information on considerations for the clinical evaluation of drugs can be found in a draft report prepared by the clinical pharmacology/clinical trial committee medical section of the science and technology division of the Pharmaceutical Manufacturer's Association. The draft of this report was presented on March 13, 1992 (16).

2.5.3 PERIAPPROVAL CLINICAL TRIAL PROGRAMS. Periapproval programs include:

- Phase 3b studies
- Post-Marketing Surveillance
- Phase 4 Programs
- R-to-OTC Switch Projects

Phase 3b. The time required for FDA review and approval of the NDA can be well spent by conducting additional studies to augment the database assembled during standard Phase 3 studies.

Phase 3b studies evaluate drugs under conditions that closely simulate actual clinical practice. Phase 3b studies include comparative trials that rigorously evaluate drug safety and efficacy. These trials provide high-quality clinical data invaluable for addressing medical, regulatory and marketing issues.

Post-Marketing Surveillance. Surveillance of drug performance in actual use yields many benefits. Combining epidemiology with trial design leads to powerful and useful Post Marketing Surveillance (PMS)

and Phase 4 studies. Population-based PMS programs conducted within the approved labeling can rapidly address specific safety, effectiveness, quality-of-life and cost-effectiveness issues.

Phase 4. Phase 4 clinical trials, generally smaller and more intensely monitored than large-scale PMS programs, offer another vehicle for expanding a product's database. Credible comparative safety and efficacy data along with quantitive data allowing for product differentiation, are hallmarks of Phase 4 studies.

Rx-to-OTC Switch Studies. Drugs once requiring prescription by physicians have increasingly been found safe enough for self-medication. However, large volumes of safety data derived from carefully designed and well-executed studies are generally required to lift regulatory restriction. Innovative program design, developed for post-marketing programs, are suitable for Rx-to-OTC switch safety studies.

As discussed previously, the need for health economy trials may be increasing, not only because of regulatory requirements, but also because of the fact that health care administrators may wish to obtain such data to make an assessment of the acceptability of approved drugs on the formulary of health care organizations. This situation is a recent development, and, in many cases, proper designs for such studies will have to be developed.

2.5.4 DEVELOPMENT OF THE FINAL PROTOCOL AND CASE REPORT FORM. Finalization of the draft protocol should include input from consultants, scientists, key investigators, regulators, statisticians and input from marketing. Additional input is required to finalize the protocol from: potential investigators who will implement the protocol; the data management group that will be involved in the design of case report forms and date entry of all study data; and, if appropriate, advocate groups for patients involved in the study. Advocate groups have become increasingly important in the evaluation of drugs in the treatment of serious diseases or those for which adequate therapies are not available such as AIDS, cancer, cystic fibrosis, and multiple sclerosis.

The design of the final protocol under discussion should be compared to designs of previous or planned future studies for a drug with the same indication. Where possible, protocols and case report forms should be standardized. This standardization will enhance the training of all involved in the clinical research on this drug and will make data management much easier and more consistent throughout the entire process.

All protocols used in clinical research, whether Phase 1, 2, 3 or peri-approval studies, should have a statistical analysis section describing the endpoints used and how sample size estimations have been defined. The statistical approach to analyzing the data must be carefully described by primary, secondary, and other endpoints along with any anticipated subgroup analyses and analysis of safety parameters. Interim analysis and procedures for unblinding must be addressed if they are to occur. A definition of an evaluable patient and/or a completed patient should be included in the protocol.

Most commonly an intent-to-treat analysis is being used in double-blind placebo-controlled, parallel or cross-over studies. Some regulatory authorities as well as scientists have expressed concern about using such excessive conservatism in the analysis of clinical trial results (17, 18). It is likely that additional, or other analyses will be used more frequently in the future.

The anticipation is that major design changes in the protocol will not occur at this stage. However, a careful final review of the protocol is intended to assure that the protocol is feasible, that patients will be available and that all tests required during patient visits can be performed within a reasonable timeframe.

Table 9.8 provides the listing of all standard sections that are included in a protocol.

Case report forms are created to permit accurate systematic collection of individual subject data. Case report forms should be designed to collect effectively all appropriate data required to meet study objectives, to permit investigators to record all data easily and clearly, to facilitate investigator's adherence to the protocol, rapid effective review of the study by the monitors and efficient data base generation. The case report forms are used to collect all data required by the protocol and intended for use in the ultimate clinical trial report. It has been observed that 65% of study costs are related to the amount of data collected in each trial (19). Therefore,

Table 9.8 Standard Sections of a Clinical Trial Protocol

Title Page
Protocol Outline (optimal)
Table of Contents
Flowchart of Events
Introduction and Rationale for Dose
Selection
Objective(s)
Study Design
Patient Selection
    Inclusion Criteria
    Exclusion Criteria
Study Periods
Study Medication
Concomitant Therapy
Safety and Efficacy Evaluations
    Safety
    Efficacy
Patient Withdrawal
Adverse Experiences
Data Analysis
Case Report Forms
Patient Confidentiality
Publication Policy

it is important to collect the minimal amount of data required to accurately evaluate the efficacy and safety of the product under development. Questions asked in the protocol or case report forms should be clear and easy to understand. They should not be repeated throughout the case report form unless changes in such parameters are expected during the study. In addition performing manual calculations of parameters at the time of collection is not helpful. Such calculations, whether they be body surface area, calendar time intervals, age, or derived variables for cardiac function, can more readily be obtained through computer analyses. Also important to note is that unnecessary information should not be obtained, specifically, routine analyses that have been performed historically in many trials in the past (e.g., chest X-rays, multiple ECGs, multiple complete physical examinations). Always review all data requested which will contribute to the evaluation of the drug. For instance, it is not worthwhile to include full physical examination of each subject in studies of dermatological products. In addition, it is not always useful to perform single or repeated ECGs in clinical trials. It may be worthwhile to perform selected laboratory tests only and not to use routine laboratory test batteries that do not reveal important information. Obviously, all this investigation is done to make the whole clinical research process more cost-efficient without losing proper efficacy or safety information on the drug.

Also, the design rules for case report forms are appropriate for patient diaries and other data collection forms that may be used during the conduct of the trial, including adverse event forms and forms needed to document drug accountability.

Once the case report forms have been finalized and agreed upon by all who will use them, including investigators, study staff, scientists, clinical research monitoring staff, data management, and regulatory affairs personnel, a quality control check should be done to assure that all evaluations described in the protocol are properly reflected on the case report forms.

2.5.5 INVESTIGATOR SELECTION. In Clinical Research, the Investigator and study staff are the central point for the collection of data on the efficacy and safety of a product. They work as a team with the sponsor, regulator and, most importantly, the patient, to obtain these data in a timely manner, with each party supporting the other parties needs (Fig. 9.3).

The basic qualifications of the investigator are listed in Table 9.9.

First of all, investigators and study staff have to have a good understanding and, preferably, experience in clinical research. They have to be able to show that they can perform all work related to the study according to good clinical practice (GCP) principles. They also have to be able and willing to follow local law and regulations with regard to clinical research and reporting of adverse experiences. In addition, they have to be willing to share with the monitors and the sponsor the source documentation so as to demonstrate the accuracy of the data. It is most important that the investigator has a qualified, experienced study staff, who usually will be more directly involved in the conduct of clinical research trials than the investigator himself or herself. The investigator and study staff have to have the appropriate facilities to perform the study, including not only those directly related to the routine evaluation done in a study but also facilities to perform any special tests needed in a particular protocol (exercise testing, MRIs, EEGs, etc). Most importantly the investigator and study staff must have time available to prepare for the study, to perform all tasks necessary for each patient visit and to be available at the time that the sponsor visits the site to monitor the study. The study staff has to be

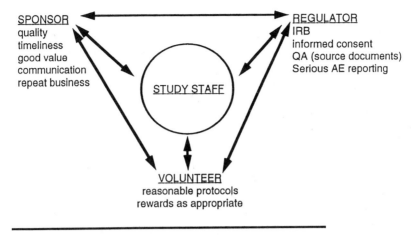

SPONSOR
quality
timeliness
good value
communication
repeat business

STUDY STAFF

REGULATOR
IRB
informed consent
QA (source documents)
Serious AE reporting

VOLUNTEER
reasonable protocols
rewards as appropriate

Fig. 9.3 A team approach to clinical research.

Table 9.9 Basic Qualifications of the Investigator

The ideal investigator has:

- Expertise in the therapeutic area
- Interest in participating in clinical research.
- A patient population from which adequate numbers of eligible subjects can be recruited on a timely basis.
- Willingness to comply with all protocol and regulatory requirements.
- Adequate facilities to conduct the study, store drug supplies and keep study documents securely.
- Willingness to accept quality assurance monitoring.
- Sufficient time to devote to this specialized practice of medicine.
- Trained study staff responsible for the day-to-day management of the trial.

responsive to answer any queries with regard to the data collected, including the adverse experiences in a timely manner. Therefore, it is important that the study staff understands up front how much time is involved in the trial, that any commitments made can be fulfilled and do not suffer from competitive activities. The study staff also has to have a facility to store the study drug and, preferably, a pharmacist to handle drug supplies for the trial.

Each investigator site will need Institutional Review Board (IRB) approval for the study and the IRB will need to be updated on the progress of the trial, on any changes in the current protocol and any serious adverse experiences that have occurred in any trial performed worldwide on the study drug.

Investigators are in the best position to know how satisfied their patients are with currently available treatments, that all protocol requirements can be met, and that patients and study staff are able to comply with all protocol requirements. Therefore, their input is mandatory in the planning of the timeline for the conduct of clinical trials.

Focus on pre-trial screening using the investigators' patient database is important. This screening is done most efficiently if the investigator has maintained a computerized database in which information is collected on each patient's disease, the severity of their condition, and a selected number of clinical trial criteria the patients meet, (e.g., age, body weight, use of concomitant treatment, concomitant diseases). Such data will help the investigators identify patient groups quickly, before the outset of the trial. If their local colleagues have similar data banks, and if they have established a network, they will have an increased capacity to run clinical trials even if their own patient pools are relatively small.

A creative supplement to networking is using advertisements to find patients with a certain disease, e.g., by asking potential patients to dial an 800 number for pre-screening of respondents. Then using a few straight-forward questions (e.g., covering age, gender, and a few protocol specific items), that the patient will know up-front whether he or she is a candidate for a particular clinical study. Centralized computerized screening programs now exist using interactive voice response systems (IVRS). Such a system also allows the investigator or study staff to place regularly a telephone call to a computer, and answer a number of specific questions to give the sponsor immediate on-time knowledge on the progress of the trial.

2.5.6　MONITORING OF STUDIES. Monitoring of clinical trials is essential to assure that investigators and study staff follow the protocol as intended and accurately report all data on the case report forms. Monitoring is done by specially trained staff who, in most cases, follow predefined monitoring conventions. These monitoring conventions are based on regulatory requirements pertaining to the study, the protocol and case report forms. The monitoring conventions describe exactly what monitors will look for when they visit the investigator site and what rules will be used to accept or to not accept the data (e.g.,

allowable range in time between visits, ranges in laboratory data).

To assure a scientifically and medically sound study, conducted in accordance with the principles of good clinical practice (GCP) and applicable law and regulation, the monitor has the following objectives during routine field monitoring:

- *Safety-related Issues.* To evaluate whether subjects' right, welfare and safety are being protected. To determine whether adverse experiences have been identified, recorded, and reported appropriately
- *Data-quality Issues.* To review case report form entries for completeness, accuracy and legibility. To assess protocol adherence and especially eligibility of subjects. To verify existence of subjects from source documents and study-related documents. To identify inconsistencies in the data, particularly efficacy data
- *Administrative/Compliance Issues.* Issues related to study files, contract with the investigator, payments to the investigator, enrollment rate, and accountability for study drug(s)

The frequency of monitoring visits depends on the requirements of the study, the size of the study, the phase of the study and any special requirements from the sponsor or regulatory authorities. Monitoring of Phase 1 usually is performed at time of dosing and at the end of the study. Phase 2 and 3 studies are usually monitored every 4 to 6 weeks on average, more frequently at the start of the study to assure protocol adherence and less frequently towards the end of the study. Peri-approval studies are less frequently monitored or not monitored at all.

For the conduct of the trial, it is important that immediate feedback on case report forms reviewed by the monitor is provided. This feedback can be done during the monitoring visit, but more efficiently, using express mail, fax, or remote data entry. Fax-based case report form submission is an extremely helpful way for investigators to get quick feedback on the quality of the case report forms. In this scenario, the investigator faxes the completed case report forms immediately to the sponsor, where they are displayed directly onto a computer screen, reviewed, and entered into a database. At the same time, the data are checked against the requirements for the study to see whether the data fall within pre-defined ranges. Errors or other data queries are highlighted on the screen and in the data file, and are immediately faxed back to the investigator for resolution.

Whether this communication is done through express mail or by automated faxing, remote monitoring of studies can be done almost on a real-time basis. At the same time, "just in time" case report form review provides instant information on the progress of the trial, on the enrollment rate of study participants and possible protocol violations. Depending on the needs of the study, problems can be resolved within a few days. In addition, this technique helps to improve safety monitoring and allows trend analysis of data in a more timely fashion. As a consequence, study visits become far more productive and useful when they occur.

Direct completion of the case report forms on the computer at the site is another possibility for monitoring, and there are two ways that this can be done: one-time remote data entry, where the data originally collected on paper case report forms are transcribed and entered into the database at the study site and then forwarded via electronic mail to the sponsor; or immediate on-site remote data entry, where the investigator enters the data directly into a computer while the patient is being examined, thus eliminating the need for tran-

scribing data. However, these solutions to case report form data entry become quite complex, specifically if an investigator is involved in many clinical trials for a number of different pharmaceutical companies, as this kind of technology has not yet been standardized across the industry to the point where investment in training and equipment would be reasonable.

2.5.7 EVALUATION OF ADVERSE EVENTS IN CLINICAL TRIALS. The evaluation of serious and non-serious adverse events are most important during clinical trials. They comprise basic information about the safety of the drug as ultimately used in the labeling for the product. A major task, for the investigator, study staff, the sponsor of the study, and regulatory authorities is to timely review these data and to provide interim assessments about the benefit/risk ratio of the new drug. For appropriate studies, establishing a special safety board to provide analyses of safety data for ongoing studies while all others involved maintain the blinding of the study is worthwhile. The board will evaluate all safety reports and, if appropriate, preliminary efficacy data obtained in pre-planned interim analyses and decide if the continuation of the trial is acceptable.

Most commonly, adverse experiences observed during treatment with the new drug, are compared to those observed in patients treated with placebo. Whenever possible, the adverse events should be evaluated as related to the time of the last dose, duration of therapy, and, when possible, drug levels to evaluate any causal relationship with the drug. The investigator will make a judgement regarding a causal relationship for each serious adverse experience. Also the investigator will evaluate any changes in routine laboratory parameters or ECG and decide if these changes are clinically important and related to the study drug.

A serious adverse experience (including

serious abnormal laboratory or ECG findings) is defined as any experience that is fatal, life-threatening, permanently disabling, requires or prolongs inpatient hospitalization, represents a significant hazard or is a congenital anomaly, cancer or overdose. Any serious adverse experience due to any cause which occurs after a patient has entered the study (including run-in or washout periods), whether or not related to the study drug, must be reported immediately to the sponsor of the study. In turn, the sponsor must ensure that all legal obligations for reporting of such adverse experiences to regulatory authorities are met.

An analysis of all adverse events will be used for the Integrated Safety Summary in the NDA and the preparation of the final safety information in the labeling. Evaluation of adverse events as related to the severity of the disease, age, gender and use of concomitant medication is commonly done.

Any patients who have withdrawn from the study have to be documented, including the reason for withdrawal. If many dropouts occur, whether or not related to adverse experiences, the analysis of the study may be impaired. The appearance of multiple drop outs also may be a reflection of improper study design or improper interpretation of the protocol by the investigator.

2.5.8 ETHICAL CONSIDERATIONS IN CLINICAL RESEARCH. Clinical investigators are faced with sometimes conflicting loyalties: to scientific integrity, to individual patients (with whom they may share long-standing relationships), to the general public, to parent institutions, and to their own careers.

Procedures for reporting and disciplining physicians who engage in fraud, either intentional or accidental, vary by country (20). The U.S. leads in the battle against fraudulent medical research—including re-search conducted in the form of clinical trials. Some of the most effective policing groups have traditionally included institutional review committees, professional medical associations, the Office of Research Integrity at the Public Health Service, the Subcommittee on Oversight and Investigations of the U.S. House of Representatives' Science and Technology Committee, the FDA (which conducts both routine and for-cause audits of clinical investigators), and, to some extent, sponsors of clinical trials. The most recent attempt to set general guidelines for identifying inappropriate behavior among researchers comes from the Office of Research Integrity (ORI) of the Public Health Service and is published sometime in 1993 as a "Notice of Proposed Rulemaking" (21).

Research misconduct is

- plagiarism
- fabrication or deliberate falsification of data, research procedures, or data analysis
- other deliberate misrepresentation in proposing, conducting, reporting or reviewing research

Between 1977 and 1983, the FDA conducted nearly 1000 routine data audits of clinical investigators. The most common findings of scientific misconduct and of varying degrees of seriousness and intent, were associated with: problems with patient consent (48% of all cases surveyed); inadequate drug accountability (34%); protocol nonadherence (23%); and inaccurate record-keeping (18%). Of these investigators, 11.5% were found to have "serious deficiencies" in their research practice. Slightly more than half of these investigators were able to clear their names on the basis of subsequent documentation. Forty-two investigators were disciplined—either declared ineligible to receive investigational new drugs, or were severely restricted in their use. Each disciplined investigator had inadequate or inaccurate records, and nearly all were found to have committed at least two violations. The most frequent problems were (in descending order): nonadherence to protocol; deliberate falsification of data (either by "fudging" or fabrication); failure to maintain adequate records of drug accountability; failure to obtain informed consent from patients; and failure to obtain IRB approval. Subsequent background checks of the disciplined investigators and a sample of the others who were audited, revealed few professional characteristics (institutional affiliation, length of bibliography, age, etc.) which distinguished one group from the other (22).

Australia and the UK have become more visibly aggressive in identifying scientific misconduct over the last several years. The centralized General Medical Council of the Association of British Pharmaceutical Industry (ABPI) gives the UK a distinct advantage in disciplining unethical researchers because it serves as a centralized clearing house for investigating fraud. The "scientific police" of the other European countries differ greatly in the stringency, procedures, and publicity with which they attack the problem, although "blacklists" of investigators are rumored to pass among pharmaceutical companies (23). Unofficial "anecdotal" information from higher-level officials in European pharmaceutical corporations suggest that between 0.4% and 7% of all data obtained are fraudulent (23).

The precise cause of misconduct in clinical research is difficult to decode. Some cases of fraud and negligence misconduct in clinical research are specific to the business of drug development. In an industry where time-to-market and cost effectiveness have become more like mantras than catchwords, it is not difficult to anticipate that some people may respond to accelerated timelines with haste—during protocol prep-aration and the recruitment and subsequent training of investigators. Impractical or overly-stringent procedural elements within protocols can be overlooked to the point where it would become impossible to get valid data from even the most expert and most ethical physician/researcher because they are not properly prepared. Under the pressure of unrealistic deadlines, often imposed, questionable data as it comes in from the field can be tempting to ignore.

Sponsors of trials should make very certain that "routine" clinical trials are still executed scientifically, and are monitored with care. If a company's internal project priorities lie outside a given investigator's studies, this disposition should not be translated to the investigator in language that suggests that detail does not matter, and that corners may be cut. Often implicit in this kind of behavior is the understanding that many investigators will eventually be transformed into customers, once a new drug is approved. It can therefore be tempting for a pharmaceutical company to ignore sloppy research methods during drug development, if an investigator can be expected to provide a large market for the product—once it is marketed (24).

The preponderance of investigated cases, however, seem to suggest that the misconduct of clinical researchers has more to do with human nature than it does with the idiosyncracies of the pharmaceutical industry. Among recently published studies on the issue, the most commonly cited causes of fraud, misconduct, and unethical behavior in clinical research are related to professional vanity, greed, and personal loyalty.

At times, there are financial incentives for some investigators to cut corners. When given the option of doing one study ethically, accurately, and responsibly and doing several studies (perhaps for different drug companies) with less fastidious methods, some investigators may be inclined to "bite off more than they can chew", in order to bring in more money (22).

Professional vanity is often cited as a prime cause of unethical clinical research. The infamous "publish or perish" requirements of certain academic institutions can drive physicians to turn out original, but less than exacting work, before anyone else does (25). In addition, it appears that some investigators would rather falsify data than risk "losing face" by admitting that they have been unable to recruit the required number of patients, or that they have not followed protocol (22).

Attention to the rights of patients has always been of significant concern to the sponsors and agents of clinical trials. Although the practice of recruiting subjects from among a researcher's students or other researchers has been widespread (and in some cases still is) in psychological and social research of "normals", such behavior is questionable both ethically and medically when testing drugs, when the collegial atmosphere at some academic institutions results in an inappropriate degree of informality and de-emphasis of risk involved, trouble and even death can occur (26).

In all but the rarest cases, the guidelines provided by the Food and Drug Administration, and the services of Institutional Review Boards responsible for permitting clinical trials, prevent large-scale unethical treatment of human subjects. However, the human aspects of clinical research can create very specific problems when an investigator must choose among several "goods": between compliance to protocol in the name of honest research and service to society, and treatment of patients with whom they have developed relationships; between risking a patient's life for a possible cure and maintaining life with a disease in remission; between immediate and long-term treatment, and numerous other clinical dilemmas (26).

A highly controversial series of examples of this dilemma are found in the continu-

ously publicized and politicized case of AIDS treatment and research. In a number of documented cases, patients desperate to have access to the only potentially effective treatment, have falsified information about their conditions and degree of compliance, sometimes conspiring with their physicians, in order to enter clinical trials for newly developed drugs, and to avoid being dropped from studies. Some groups of patients have managed to unblind studies by analyzing drugs given to them by investigators; others have engaged in cooperative fraud by pooling the medication they were given and redistributing it in order to increase their chances of obtaining active drug. Further exploration has indicated that "motivations of patients and doctors who falsify inclusion criteria are proportional to the seriousness of the disease, to the lack of availability of effective alternative therapies, and to the degree of publicity given to the results of the preliminary studies" (27).

Nearly every pharmaceutical company has a database of candidate investigators, but the FDA has not provided guidelines for the minimum requirements acceptable for physicians/investigators who conduct clinical trials, other than that they must be "qualified by training and experience as appropriate experts to investigate the drug." This broad suggestion does not begin to cover the intricate list of qualities which characterize reliable investigators (24). The sponsors of clinical trials should be pragmatic and cautious when enlisting the assistance of physicians/investigators who would be stretching their staff, resources, abilities and expertise beyond what can realistically be expected.

Investigators must learn how to balance between possible harm to an individual patient and possible greater benefit to science and the public at large. In the previously discussed scenario of entering subjects with chronic or life-threatening disease, physician-researchers must remember that they have "a higher moral obligation to test (drugs) critically than to prescribe (them) year-in, year-out with the support of custom or of wishful thinking" (26) or desperation.

2.5.9 CLINICAL TRIAL REPORTS. At the conclusion of each study a Clinical Trial Report is prepared. This report outlines the protocol, the methodology used, the statistical analysis, and the results, followed by a discussion. Table 9.10 provides the typical sections, following FDA guidelines, which are present in a Clinical Trial Report, including common addenda and data listings.

2.5.10 WHEN TO STOP THE DEVELOPMENT OF A DRUG. Discontinuing the development of a pharmaceutical is not an easy decision, especially if the drug has already entered the late phase of development and a lot of time and money already has been spent. However, as discussed earlier, critical decisions must be made at the time of each

Table 9.10 Standard Sections for a Clinical Trial Report

Report
Title
Introduction
Objective
Materials and Methods
  Study Design and Plan
  Study Population
  Study Drugs
  Effectiveness and Safety Data Recorded
  Statistical Methods
  Safety Analyses
Results
  Patients Studied
  Effectiveness
  Safety
Discussion
Conclusions
References
Addendum
Data Listings

go/no-go decision point in the drug development plan. The decision will depend upon the available data, on the efficacy of the drug, or lack thereof, and on all preclinical and clinical safety data obtained at that point in time. An assesment will have to be made of the benefit/risk ratio of the product and consequently the decision has to be made whether or not to continue its development. Many drugs are currently being used in the marketplace for which the pharmaceutical industries have had the temptation to stop the development. The recent approval of Tacrin is just such an example. A long time was taken for regulatory authorities, scientists and the sponsor to come to agreement on an acceptable benefit/risk ratio, and an approval for that drug. In this case, go/no-go decisions had to be made on the initiation of additional large clinical trials.

Particularly difficult is the assessment of the benefit/risk ratio of a drug early in Phase 1 when only limited safety data are available and, as for most drugs, evidence of efficacy is not available at that time. A clear decision has to be made as to whether any observed adverse events during Phase 1 studies are related to the drug or to other factors. In some cases abnormal liver function tests observed in normal volunteers during Phase 1 studies are related to alcohol abuse and not to the study drug. However, it has been estimated that 1 in 10 serious adverse events observed in Phase 1 trials has led to discontinuation of the development of a drug (13).

In early Phase 2 studies it may be difficult to assess the efficacy of the study drug because of the small sample size and different degrees of efficacy demonstrated between studies. In some cases, this discrepancy may be due to differences in the design of the protocol or in the location where the study is performed, rather than the study drug itself. Differences in medical practice between Europe and the United States and differences in the patient populations studied between investigators (e.g., differences in age, gender or race), all may cause the results of the studies to be different without necessarily bearing a direct relationship to the overall efficacy of the study drug. It seems wise that efficacy or lack of efficacy be demonstrated in at least two adequate studies before radical decisions, such as the discontinuation of the development of the drug are taken.

Other reasons for the discontinuation of a drug include the absence of desirable effects (e.g., a drug that was intended for once a day dosing failed to show efficacy over the full dosing period) or the presence of undesirable effects such as initial hypotension caused by a new antihypertensive drug. In addition, a decision may have to be made to discontinue the development of the drug based on changes in regulations and/or the environment. These changes can be related to changes in the regulatory guidelines, e.g., new requirements to provide long-term survival studies in certain drugs to be used in the treatment of congestive heart failure; disallowance of surrogate endpoints and hence new requirements for large, expensive clinical studies to show efficacy; or approval of other drug candidates in the same class. The approval of AZT in the treatment of AIDS may cause certain new drugs in the treatment of AIDS to be tested initially only in patients who failed on AZT and the new drug may not be effective in inducing an additional benefit. The same conclusion may be true for certain drugs in the treatment of memory disorders in patients with Alzheimer's Disease following approval of Tacrin.

Ongoing and planned changes in health care policy and health care management have an effect on the decision to continue or discontinue the development of drugs. Many companies will decide to develop fewer "me-too" products; that is, products that are similar to those already near to approval or in the market place. Such changes will require a much better assessment by the Industry of the true medical needs of the consumer-patient, and his assessment needs to be taken into account when decisions are made on the development of a new drug.

Finally, on occasion, drugs may need to be discontinued purely because of the fact that they are unlikely to raise adequate revenues even if approved. Although this decision seems acceptable for diseases for which there is a reasonable alternative drug treatment available, it is not acceptable for rare diseases, for example, orphan drug indications, or in cases where there is an urgent medical need.

The decision to discontinue the development of a product will become easier when goals for the development have been outlined in the product development plan and when continuation rules are clearly established at each go/no-go decision point. In such cases, the decision to discontinue the development will not come from top management, but from the entire team. An important task of the product champion and the project team is to be unbiased towards the results of all studies and not to pursue the development of a new drug for their own cause, but only when it is of benefit to the company and the intended patient population.

2.5.11 REGULATORY REVIEW DURING THE CONDUCT OF CLINICAL TRIALS. Once an IND is submitted to the FDA, there begins a process of dialogue that continues all during the drug development period. This dialogue is important to the sponsor not only to understand what the FDA will be requiring in the way of completed studies once a New Drug Application (NDA) is submitted for approval, but also for the FDA to understand the clinical program as it is unfolding and to comment on the evolution of that program as early as possible to prevent unnecessary conduct of studies that will not ultimately meet FDA needs.

The ability to establish a meaningful dialogue is sometimes difficult. The FDA has limited resources and does not like to engage in what is perceived as meaningless dialogue or exploratory dialogue that has no focus. However, the FDA does request that sponsors meet with them periodically at certain defined times to address the status of the program and to insure themselves and the sponsor that the program is headed in the proper direction.

2.5.11.1 End of Phase 2 and Phase 3 Conferences. Conferences with the FDA are typically held after the end of Phase 2 and Phase 3. The purpose of an End of Phase 2 meeting is to determine the safety of proceeding to Phase 3, to evaluate the Phase 3 plans and protocols and to identify any additional information necessary to support a marketing application (NDA) for the uses under investigation. While the End of Phase 2 meeting is designed primarily for holders of INDs involved with new molecular entities or major new uses of marketed drugs, a sponsor of any IND may request an End of Phase 2 meeting with the FDA. To be most useful to the sponsor, an End of Phase 2 meeting should be held before major commitments of effort and resources have been made to Phase 3.

Once the sponsor believes the requirements to support approval by the FDA for their product have been completed, they should arrange to discuss these results and the proposed NDA with the FDA. The primary purposes of this meeting are: to discuss any major unresolved problems; to identify those studies that the sponsor is relying on as adequate and well-controlled to establish the drug's effectiveness; to acquaint the reviewers at the FDA with the general information that would be submitted in the NDA (including pertinent technical information) to discuss appropriate methods for statistical analysis of the

data; and to discuss the best approach for the presentation and formatting of the data in the NDA.

In order to make the most efficient use of their limited resources, the FDA is requiring, more and more, that sponsors intending to submit NDAs, discuss at length all of the issues concerning the presentation and formatting of data in the proposed NDA so that these issues can be dealt with and disposed of prior to the actual submission of the NDA. The purpose of this approach is to ensure that when the NDA is submitted, there will be little or no need to go back to the sponsor to request additional analyses, request clarification of data submitted, or to request additional studies. That being the case, it is the FDA's hope that they will be more able to meet the statutory review time period of 6 months once an NDA is accepted for filing.

This new approach on the part of the FDA to "Refuse to File" NDAs that are felt to be deficient for review, requires more advance planning between the sponsor and FDA. This approach may cause delays in NDA submissions but should ultimately secure a more rapid review time so that the actual time to market may be shorter than anticipated.

2.5.11.2 FDA Interactions Under Subpart E. The interactions as outlined above are the case with the development of a typical drug product. However, there are other interactions that come into play if the drug product is a candidate for "Subpart E Designation." A drug can be eligible for Subpart E Designation if it is intended to treat persons with life-threatening and severely-debilitating illnesses especially where no satisfactory alternative therapy exists. For products intended to treat life-threatening or severely-debilitating illnesses, sponsors may request to meet with FDA reviewing officials early in the drug development process to review and reach agreement on the design of necessary pre-clinical and clinical studies. Where appropriate, the FDA will invite to such meetings, outside scientific consultants or advisory committee members. Instead of the usual End of Phase 2 and 3 meetings, meetings for products under Subpart E would include a Pre-Investigational New Drug (pre-IND) meeting and an End of Phase 1 meeting. The primary purpose of the pre-IND meeting is to review and reach agreement on the design of animal studies needed to initiate human testing. This meeting may also provide an opportunity for discussing the scope and design of Phase 1 testing and the best approach for presentation and formatting of data in the IND.

When data from Phase 1 clinical testing is available, the sponsor may again request a meeting with FDA reviewing officials. The primary purpose of this meeting is to review and reach agreement on the design of Phase 2 controlled clinical trials, with the goal that such testing will be adequate to provide sufficient data on the drug's safety and effectiveness to support a decision on its approvability for marketing.

The intent on the part of the FDA under Subpart E is to get promising drugs to market as quickly as possible. Thus, if sufficient information is generated in Phase 2 to make a decision about the efficacy of the product and the safety profile of the product, then the drug could be approved without the need to go to larger Phase 2 or Phase 3 trials. This approach also presumes that there may be a need for post-marketing studies to further define and confirm the initial results in Phase 2 on safety and efficacy.

2.5.11.3 Regulatory Approval Process. In order for a drug to be legally marketed in interstate commerce in the United States, it must be the subject of an approved New Drug Application (NDA). An NDA that is submitted to the FDA is a document that is typically 400 volumes to 700 volumes in size, with each volume containing approximately 400 pages. The NDA is made up of a number of sections (Table 9.11).

One major section is the Application Summary, one of the primary review documents. The Application Summary contains a number of detailed summaries including: a summary of the chemistry, manufacturing, and controls section of the application;

Table 9.11　Standard NDA Sections

Application Form
Index
Application Summary

- Proposed text of labeling
- Statement on pharmacologic class/scientific rationale and potential clinical benefits
- description of marketing history
- Summary of chemistry, manufacturing, and controls section
- Summary of pharmacology/toxicology section
- Summary of human pharmacokinetics and bioavailability section
- Summary of microbiology section (for anti-infective drugs only)
- Summary of clinical data section
- Risk/benefit discussion

Technical Sections

- Chemistry, manufacturing, and controls data
- Nonclinical pharmacology and toxicology data
- Human pharmacokinetics and bioavailability data
- Clinical data to include an integrated summary of effectiveness, an integrated summary of safety, and an integrated summary of benefits and risks
- Statistical data

Samples and Labeling
Case Report Forms and Tabulations

a summary of the nonclinical pharmacology and toxicology section of the application; a summary of the human pharmacokinetics and bioavailability section of the application; a summary of the microbiology section of the application (a requirement for antiinfective drugs only); a summary of the clinical data section of the application, including the results of statistical analyses of clinical trials; and a section which has a concluding discussion that presents the benefit and risk consideration of the drug, including a discussion of any proposed additional studies or surveillance the applicant intends to conduct post-marketing. The Application Summary will also include: the proposed text of the labeling for the drug (package insert), with annotations to the location of information in the summary and technical sections in the application that support the statement in the labeling; a statement identifying the pharmacologic class of the drug and a discussion of the scientific rationale for the drug, its intended use, and the potential clinical benefits of the drug product; a brief description of the marketing history, if any, of the drug outside of the U.S., including a list of the countries in which the drug has been marketed; a list of any countries in which the drug has been withdrawn from marketing for any reasons related to safety or effectiveness; and a list of countries in which applications for marketing are pending.

In addition to a technical review of the data submitted in the NDA, the FDA has an inspectorate that will visit selected clinical investigators to assure that the data submitted in the NDA matches the records at the investigator's site and that the patients in the study have been adequately protected through the use of written informed consent and adequate Institutional Review Board oversight of the study.

The FDA will also send inspectors to manufacturing facilities to assure compliance with cGMP regulations. These pre-approval inspections must be passed before the product can be approved for marketing.

Once an NDA is submitted but is not yet approved, an applicant may submit an amendment to the application. Such amendments may contain additional safety and or efficacy information that was not available at the time of the original filing. If the FDA determines the submitted amendment to be a "major amendment," for instance, that which contains significant new data from a previously unreported study or contains detailed new analyses of previously submitted data, they will extend the review time to account for the time necessary to complete the additional review.

Once an NDA is approved, an applicant can submit a supplement to the NDA requesting a change to the conditions of original approval. Such a change may relate to the drug substance: to delete a specification or regulatory analytical method or to change the synthesis of the drug substance or the drug product; to add or delete an ingredient, to establish a new regulatory analytical method, to use a different facility or establishment, including a different contract labeler or laboratory, or to change the labeling; to add a new indication which would need to be supported by submitted clinical studies.

2.5.11.4 Approval and Launch. Once the FDA has determined that the submitted technical information meets the statutory requirements to allow approval of the product for the intended indications and under the intended conditions of use, typically, an approveable letter will be issued which may list certain minor deficiencies that can be rapidly corrected in the application and will also ask the applicant to submit final printed labeling based on comments on the draft labeling submitted. The FDA will also usually ask for promotional material to be used in the initial advertising campaign to be assured that the product is only being promoted for the approved indications and approved conditions for use.

After the final printed labeling has been submitted, and whatever minor deficiencies were noted have been resolved, the FDA will issue an approval letter. The date of the approval letter becomes the date of approval of the application. Once the approved product is launched, the FDA will continue to monitor the promotion of the material, to assure that it is in compliance with appropriate FDA regulations, and pharmacovigilance information, to assure continued safety of the drug.

ACKNOWLEDGEMENT

We would like to thank Wendy Norris for her help in the preparation of the section on Ethics in Clinical Research and Colleen McGinley and Pat Cortesini for their assistance in the typing of this chapter.

REFERENCES

1. U. B. Sinclair, *The Jungle*, Doubleday & Co., New York, 1906.

2. E. Reis-Arndt, *Pharm. Ind.*, **49**, 136–143 (1987).

3. J. Drews, *Drug Inf. J.* **26**, 638 (1992).

4. *Pharmaceutical R & D: Costs, Risks and Rewards*, Office of Technology Assessment, Washington D.C., 1993.

5. J. A. DiMasi, R. W. Hansen, H. G. Grabowski, and L. Lasagna, *J. of Health Economics*, **10**, 107–142 (1991).

6. R. G. Halliday, A. L. Drasdo, C. E. Lumley, and S. R. Walker, *Pharmaceutical Medicine*, **6**, 281–296 (1992).

7. P. B. Crosby, *J. for Quality & Participation*, 24–27 (July/Aug. 1992).

8. D. F. Bernstein and F. J. Tiano, *J. Clin. Res. Pharmacoepidemiol.*, **5**, 1–10 (1991).

9. *Guidelines For Submitting Documentation For The Stability of Human Drugs and Biologics*, FDA Publication, 1987.

10. D. F. Bernstein and F. J. Tiano, *J. Clin. Res. Pharmacoepidemiol*, **5**, 183–193 (1992).

11. *Guidelines For Submitting Documentation For Packaging For Human Drugs and Biologics*, FDA Publication, 1987.

12. F. Douglas, "Dilemmas in Clinical Research," *Scrip Magazine*, 10–12* (June 1993).

13. R, Temple, "Trends in Pharmaceutical Development," *Drug Information J.*, **27**, 355–366 (1993).

14. C. C. Peck et al., *Clinical Pharmacology Therapeutics*, **51**, 465–473 (1992).

15. M. McDonald, "Dose Ranging Studies; The Key to Registration,"*Applied Clinical Trials*, **2**, 50–58 (1993).

16. Pharmaceutical Manufacturer's Association, Draft, pp. 1–47 (March, 1992).

17. L. B. Sheiner, *Clinical Pharmacology Therapeutics*, **50**, 4–9 (1991).

18. B. E. Rodda, C. Brooks, and G. Reynolds, *Clinical Pharmaceutical & Therepeutics*, **52**, 104–106 (1992).

19. M. S. Moran, S. Boots, N. Resnick, and C. Wallenmark, "The Measurement of Efficacy in Clinical Research and Development," *Drug Information J.*, **26**, 201–209 (1992).

20. J. Hone, "Combatting Fraud and Misconduct in Medical Research," *Scrip Magazine*, **14** (Mar. 1993).

21. D. Rennie and C. K. Gunsalus, "Scientific Misconduct: New Definition, Procedures, and Office Perhaps a New Leaf," *J. of the A.M.A.*, **269**(7), 915–917 (1993).

22. M. F. Shapiro and R. P. Charrow, "Scientific Misconduct in Investigational Drug Trials," *NEJM*, **11**, 731–734 (1985).

23. P. O'Donnell, GCP in Europe: Facing Up to Fraud, *Applied Clin. Trials*, 36–38 (199?).

24. J. N. Gibbs, "Clinical Investigations: Six Common Mistakes and How to Avoid Them," *Regulatory Affairs*, **2**, 385–386 (1990).

25. B. Spilker, *Guide to Clinical Trials*, Ra·en Press, New York, 1991, p. 814.

26. D. J. Roy, "Basic Ethical Considerations in Clinical Trials and their Rationale: the Canadian Perspective," *J. of Clin. Res. and Pharmacoepidemiol.*, **5**, 89–97 (1991).

27. R. J. Levine, "Basic Ethical Considerations in Clinical Trials and Their Rationale: The U.S. Perspective," *J. of Clin. Res. Pharmacoepidemiol.*, **5**, 99–104 (1991).

PART III

STRUCTURAL MEDICINAL CHEMISTRY

CHAPTER TEN

Three Dimensional Structure-Aided Drug Design

B. VEERAPANDIAN

La Jolla Cancer Research Foundation
La Jolla, California, USA

CONTENTS

1 Introduction, 304
2 The Structure-Aided Drug Design Process, 305
3 Methods to Derive 3-Dimensional Structures, 306
  3.1 Obtaining the target, 306
  3.2 Crystallography, 307
    3.2.1 Crystallization, 308
    3.2.2 Diffraction methods and structure
        solution, 308
    3.2.3 The electron density map, 310
    3.2.4 Model building and refinement, 310
    3.2.5 Accuracy of crystallographic
        structures, 312
  3.3 Nuclear magnetic resonance, 312
    3.3.1 The basic methodology, 313
    3.3.2 Isotope labeling, 313
    3.3.3 NMR and drug design, 314
  3.4 Homologous modeling, 315
    3.4.1 General methodology, 315
    3.4.2 Satisfaction of spatial restraints
        method, 318
    3.4.3 Construction of a 3-D structure based
        on α-carbon atoms, 318
    3.4.4 Identification of protein folding from
        distantly related sequences, 318
    3.4.5 Building loops on a framework, 318
    3.4.6 Modeling side chains, 319
    3.4.7 Modeling by a combinatorial
        approach – *ab initio* modeling, 319
    3.4.8 Model refinement, 319
    3.4.9 Simulated annealing, 320
    3.4.10 Evaluation of the structure, 320

Burger's Medicinal Chemistry and Drug Discovery,
Fifth Edition, Volume 1: Principles and Practice,
Edited by Manfred E. Wolff.
ISBN 0-471-57556-9 © 1995 John Wiley & Sons, Inc.

4 The Design Process,   320
   4.1 Identification of the site of action, 320
   4.2 Required structural accuracy in the design process, 321
   4.3 Identification of the lead compound, 321
5 Software-Aided Drug Design,   322
6 Optimization of the Identified Compounds,   323
7 Examples of Structure-Aided Drug Design,   323
   7.1 Design of drugs to treat hypertension: the renin angiotensin system, 323
   7.2 Inhibitor design for angiotensin converting enzyme, 323
   7.3 Design of renin inhibitors, 325
      7.3.1 Substrate specificity of renin and the design of peptide inhibitors, 325
      7.3.2 Inhibitor binding as revealed by crystallography, 328
      7.3.3 Structural insights based on studies with inhibitors, 328
      7.3.4 Important conclusions, 332
   7.4 Design of drugs for the treatment of AIDS, 332
      7.4.1 Crystallographic studies to design inhibitors for the HIV protease, 333
      7.4.2 Software-based inhibitor design for HIV protease, 338
      7.4.3 Typical example of SADD, 338
8 Lessons Learned,   339

1 INTRODUCTION

Molecules carry out their functional roles in biological processes by interacting with proteins, DNA, polysaccharides, lipids, or other molecules. The functional site of interaction can be an active site, in the case of an enzyme–substrate complex, or a binding epitope, in the case of a hormone–receptor complex. The topographies of the complementary surfaces of the ligand and target molecules determine the affinity and specificity of the interactions. On the basis of the conformation of the ligands and their interactions with the target molecules, new chemical compounds can be designed to act as drugs. This is made possible by understanding the 3-dimensional structure of the molecules involved and exploiting the knowledge of their molecular interactions.

The specificity of a drug depends on its selectivity to act only on its target. The factors that determine the specificity and selectivity of drug binding are the physico-chemical properties of the drug and of the target molecule. The study of drug–receptor complexation reveals that drugs exert their effects by binding to their targets through a subtle and complex interplay of intermolecular forces. Understanding these forces and predicting how a designed drug will be docked into a receptor binding site by mimicking the natural ligand is the aim of structure-aided drug design.

Technological developments in the field of structural science have considerably reduced the time and cost of structure-aided drug design. The rate limiting steps in obtaining structural information are the crystallization of the molecules and the computer manipulation of the data. Today, faster scanning processes can assess the purity of the samples and their precipitating conditions, which are essential to obtain crystals of good quality. High power radiation sources and extremely sensitive and highly automated detectors allow the rapid collection of diffraction data in a day or two, compared to several weeks before. Above all, high power computing and stereo-graphics visualization tools have paved the way for faster calculations and better molecular viewing. Sophisticated algorithms are continually being developed to calculate the intricate properties of molecules and search the ever increasing databases for specific information.

Essentially, the final purpose of all these techniques is to visualize the designed drug docked into the target molecule, in order to analyze the two molecules in detail and evaluate the forces involved in their interaction. Visualization and analysis can reveal the subtle differences in the binding between successive members of a series of drug compounds and the conformational changes induced in the target molecule as a result of their binding.

The results obtained in these studies help in designing new drugs with better binding capabilities and improved functions. Whether 3-dimensional structural information alone is sufficient to design a proper drug, is still an open question that has been addressed by many experts. The consensus opinion is that 3-dimensional structure-based approach should make the search for new drugs better and faster, if used in combination with traditional screening techniques and knowledge of molecular physicochemical properties obtained by QSAR.

The main purpose of this review is to describe the relevance of 3-dimensional structure information in designing drugs, with a brief introduction to methods like crystallography and NMR, which are instrumental in obtaining 3-dimensional structures. Approaches to structure-based homologous modeling are described. The computational and graphics approaches to the design of novel drug molecules based on the 3-dimensional structure of the target's functional site are reviewed and some examples are briefly described. We have made an effort to highlight the need and impact of structure aided methods in the process of drug design. For additional reviews the readers are referred to refs. 1–3.

2 THE STRUCTURE-AIDED DRUG DESIGN PROCESS

Structure-aided drug design is a multidisciplinary effort that fuses the ideas of traditional medicinal chemistry with the techniques of X-ray crystallography, nuclear magnetic resonance, molecular modeling, computational chemistry, small molecular 3-dimensional database search, and the *ab initio* design of ligands.

Depending on the target molecule chosen, a particular type of drug design process is selected. Current efforts are concentrated in: (1) the design of inhibitors based on the architecture of an enzyme active site, (2) the design of agonists or antagonists based on the bioactivity of proteins engineered by site directed mutagenesis, and (3) the design of small molecular agonists or antagonists based on the interfaces of hormone and receptor binding epitopes. In the "design of inhibitors based on the architecture of an enzyme active site," it is helpful to determine the 3-dimensional structure of the enzyme and of the enzyme in complex with an inhibitor at high resolution, to define precisely all the molecular interactions that are necessary for a drug to bind to its target site. Based on the architecture of the enzyme's active site and the interactions that stabilize the inhibitor, a new ligand with better binding affinity can be designed, with a shape that fits better into the active site and a charge distribution suitable for increased interaction energies. If the attempts to obtain good quality crystals of the inhibitor–enzyme complex are not successful, it is possible to resort to newer techniques based solely on the topography of the enzyme active site. These involve the computer design of novel inhibitor molecules that are complementary in "shape and electrostatics" to the active site.

The second type of drug design process is applied when proteins such as monoclonal antibodies or hormones and growth factors are to be used as drugs. The genes encoding these proteins can be cloned, mutated by site-directed mutagenesis, and expressed. The modified proteins thus obtained can be purified, kinetically characterized, and assayed to evaluate their biological functions. This cycle of mutagenesis, expression, and evaluation of the engineered protein can be repeated until a better agonist or antagonist is obtained. The knowledge of the structure of the protein drug and/or its target molecule helps this process by allowing informed decisions about which mutations to introduce in the engineered protein in order to obtain the desired functional modifications.

The third type of drug design process presents more problems than the first two, because the 3-dimensional structure of the complex between the hormone/growth factor and its membrane associated or soluble receptor has to be solved in order to identify the binding epitopes. This is a difficult task, but not insurmountable.

Structure-aided drug design has already resulted in drugs that are in clinical trial. Worth mentioning are carbonic anhydrase inhibitors to treat glaucoma; inhibitors for thymidylate synthetase as anti-cancer agents; purine nucleoside phosphorylase inhibitors as chemotherapeutic agents and as immuno-suppressants; renin inhibitors to treat hypertension; HIV protease inhibitors to treat AIDS; thrombin-based anticoagulants; rhinoviral binders as antiviral agents and few others. There are also examples of inhibitors designed on the basis of homologous protein structures: ACE inhibitors whose design studies were based on

homologous proteins such a carboxypeptidase A and thermolysin; and renin inhibitors, based on homologous aspartic proteinases. For a list of enzyme targets and their related references, see reference 4.

As mentioned above, the rate limiting steps of the crystallographic process are to obtain good quality crystals and to solve the structure *ab initio* when homologous structures are not available. Recent technological advances provide great help in obtaining accurate 3-dimensional structures. These include the application of high power synchrotron sources, data collection with the use of well-designed detectors coupled with automated data processing procedures, improved software for structure solution, and extremely powerful graphics packages to visualize molecular structures in three dimensions.

Crystallography and NMR are techniques that can elucidate the shape of unknown objects and thus allow the rational design of new drug compounds. However, they do not provide direct information regarding the *in vivo* efficacy, toxicity, pharmacokinetics and bioavailability of a drug. Therefore, structural studies have to be used in conjunction with the other existing methods of drug discovery. Once the physical shape of a drug compound is structurally defined and the modes of interaction with the target molecule are understood, then it is necessary to assess the performance of the newly designed drug by using appropriate bioassays. This cycle of drug design based on structural considerations and drug evaluation based on bioassays, have to be repeated until satisfactory results are obtained.

3 METHODS TO DERIVE THREE-DIMENSIONAL STRUCTURES

3.1 Obtaining the Target

Isolating sufficient quantities of the macromolecular target in homogeneous form is an important step, since the quality of the structure obtained by crystallography depends upon the quality of the crystals grown. Obtaining well-diffracting single crystals in turn depends upon the purity of the sample. Furthermore, tens of milligrams of protein may be needed for the initial screening of the crystallization conditions and a further supply of crystals is necessary until the drug design process is complete. It is therefore important to start by having well-standardized techniques to produce large amounts of pure protein samples.

Recombinant DNA techniques have revolutionized the process by which large quantities of biological molecules can be obtained. Once their genes have been isolated and cloned, proteins previously extractable only in trace quantities can be purified in milligram and sometimes in gram quantities, by using genetically transformed microorganisms or eukaryotic cells. The power of these techniques is demonstrated by the ability to express stable domains of complex multidomain structures, soluble receptors, and in general proteins that would otherwise be impossible to purify. Another important advantage is that the ability to express eukaryotic proteins in bacteria, without their carbohydrate moieties, which render them heterogeneous and thus unsuitable for crystallization. By using recombinant DNA techniques it is also possible to produce genetically engineered proteins suitable for *ab initio* structure solution, such as selenoenzymes for use in multiple anomalous dispersion experiments and proteins capable of binding heavy atoms through introduced cysteines, for use in multiple isomorphous replacement method.

Another advantage of recombinant DNA techniques is the ability to mutate specific amino acid residues in a protein to any other desired residues, in order to explore the structural and functional modifications that result from such mutations. Drug agonists or antagonists of a natural compound can be generated by these procedures. Site directed mutagenesis can also be used to engineer more stable proteins or proteins that can be used in place of the wild type proteins in crystallization experiments, in case the wild type proteins fail to form crystals. A new application of this technique is the "multi-termini" approach to crystallization, which involves cloning fragments of a protein with different amino- and carboxy-terminal ends and attempting to crystallize all of them. Different termini may dramatically affect the outcome of the crystallization efforts. Successful results by this method have been obtained in crystallizing and solving the structure of a fibronectin 10 type III module (5). Site-directed cysteine mutants were utilized in identifying heavy atoms sites in the Multiple Isomorphous Replacement map (6). The technique to produce recombinant proteins enriched in ^{15}N and ^{13}C for relaxation experiments is being used in the determination of structures by NMR. Apart from their use in solving structures, isotope editing methods are being used in studying the dynamic behavior of molecules in solution and in the characterization of ligand binding.

3.2 Crystallography

Because the process of structure-aided drug design is based on experimental data obtained through crystallographic and NMR techniques, a short discussion on how such data are obtained is appropriate here. For more detailed reviews on this subject refer to Blundell and Johnson (7) and Perutz (1). For a successful crystallographic laboratory, expertise in crystallization, diffraction data collection, phasing, model building, refinement and structural analysis are the basic necessities. Often the first two steps of crystallization and data collection takes about 10 to 20% of the effort, whereas the remaining steps can be accomplished entirely by utilizing computer software coupled with human skills in calculation and structure interpretation.

3.2.1 CRYSTALLIZATION. The first major obstacle one has to overcome in solving a crystal structure is to produce a well-diffracting single crystal of the protein. Producing a crystal is a trial and error process. Protein samples in micro drops are allowed to interact with a precipitating medium so that the individual protein molecules can arrange themselves onto a nucleus to form a crystalline entity. To be successful, the precipitation process should advance slowly. Because the number of parameters that can be varied is very large, automated robotic techniques and sparse matrix methods have been developed (8–10). A good quality crystal has perfect edges with regular morphology (Fig. 10.1) and exhibits good birefringence when examined through a polarizing microscope. Crystallization of proteins in zero-gravity space is expected to have a higher success

rate, due to the lack of convection and gravity. A database of previously successful crystallization conditions is also available for guidance (11, 12). Crystallographers are always striving to improve their understanding of the forces involved in the crystallization of macromolecules, in order to obtain consistently better crystals and measure diffraction data with higher resolution. Books on the "art" of crystallization have been published and can be used as a guide (13–16). Because the value of drug design studies depends on the quality of the structural information that can be obtained, which is turn depends on the quality of the crystals, expertise in crystallization is a must for a successful laboratory.

3.2.2 DIFFRACTION METHODS AND STRUCTURE SOLUTION. X-ray diffraction data from well-diffracting single crystals are used for structure solution. These data can be collected by passing powerful X-rays through the crystals and measuring the intensity of

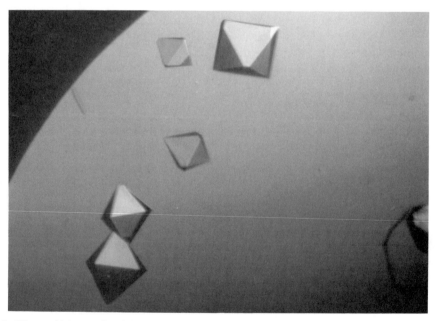

Fig. 10.1 Bipyramidal crystals of interleukin-1β, grown in a hanging drop with ammonium sulfate as the precipitant. See also color plates.

the diffracted beams with extremely sensitive computer-controlled detectors. Advances in data collection methods have been phenomenal during the past decade. An example of the diffraction data that can be collected nowadays is shown in Figure 10.2, where a synchrotron source was used on a macromolecular crystal to produce thousands of diffraction data.

The diffraction data are related to the 3-dimensional arrangement of atoms in the repeating units of the crystal by the process of Fourier transformation. The electron cloud surrounding each atom contributes to each point in the pattern. From the diffraction data only the amplitudes of the diffracted waves can be directly measured. The phases of the diffracted waves have to

be calculated separately and recombined with the experimentally obtained structural factors to reconstitute the image of the diffracting electron clouds. There is no direct way of measuring the phases of the diffracted waves and their calculation is the most formidable problem in the entire structure solution process.

At present there are two options available to solve this phase problem. The first is to solve the structure by the multiple isomorphous replacement (MIR) method, which exploits the binding of heavy atoms to proteins. The infused heavy atom scatterers allow the calculation of the initial few phases. The rest can then be generated by phase extension procedures. Structure solution by using heavy atom derivatives is

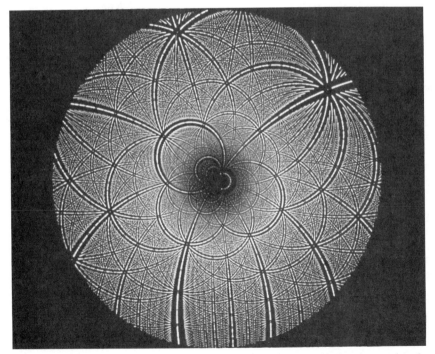

Fig. 10.2 Computer generated Laue diffraction pattern of Rubisco (ribulose bisphosphate carboxylase/oxygenase). Effective wavelength range contributing to reflections = 0.25–2.10 Å. Space group C2221, a = 157.2 Å, b = 157.2 Å, c = 201.3 Å. Crystal to film distance = 142.3 mm. Film radius = 60 mm. Number of reflections predicted in the pattern = 126,270. Each spot has been given a color code to indicate the wavelength of the contributing X-ray beam. Blue = 0.2 Å; red = 2.1 Å. Intermediate wavelengths are colored according to the colors in the visible spectrum. Courtesy of Integer A. Andersson (Uppsala, Sweden) and Janos Hajdu (Oxford, UK). See also color plates.

an art by itself (7). The second is the molecular replacement method and is applicable if a structure homologous to the protein in question has already been determined. On the basis of the known structure, the atomic positions of the unknown structure within the crystal can be determined by calculating rotational and translation matrices. The model molecule is then rotated, translated and fitted into the electron density map. Improvements in phase generation have been achieved by solvent flattening (removing the featureless map caused by water molecules occupying the spaces between the protein molecules) and by symmetry averaging (imposing restrictions on the phase values by considering the symmetrical arrangement of subunit molecules within a multisubunit complex, such as protein coat molecules within a viral particle). The initial structure solution can be obtained first to a resolution of 3–4 Å and then improved slowly by an iterative procedure of data addition, model building into the electron density map and refinement.

3.2.3 THE ELECTRON DENSITY MAP. Until a few years ago, it was difficult to construct the model of a whole protein molecule into the obtained electron density map and it took many months to complete the task. Nowadays, technologies that have been developed to visualize and manipulate electron density maps and molecular structures have facilitated this process to a great extent. Even with all these advances, the initial model building is difficult since the resolution of the electron density maps is around 3.0 Å. At such medium resolution, electron density maps are not clear: the electron clouds of the atoms appear smeared and assigning the positions of the atoms is difficult. For example, a phenyl ring appears as a lumpy donut at low resolution, but as the resolution of the data increases a distinct phenyl ring appears (Fig. 10.3), and at very high resolution

beyond 2 Å even a defined hole can be seen at the center of the ring.

3.2.4 MODEL BUILDING AND REFINEMENT. The initial attempt to build a model into an electron density map is greatly aided by the identification of: either by the heavier atoms within the molecule (such as the iron in a heme group or metal ions like Ca, Zn, Mg, etc.), or by the bigger groups (such as the tryptophane and phenylalanine aromatic rings), or by the sulfur-containing cysteines and methionines. With the positions of these groups as a starting point, the polypeptide chain can then be progressively built into the electron density map based on the amino acid sequence. The side chain conformations as observed in the map, in conjunction with the sequence information, dictate the direction of the polypeptide progression. The side chains are often recognized by looking at the size and shape of the densities branching out from the main chain. For example, arginine, lysine, and methionine are longer and continuous, whereas phenylalanine, histidine and tryptophane have flat benzyl rings. Because carbon atoms have an electron density very similar to oxygen and nitrogen atoms, the crystallographer should be knowledgeable of the rules governing the folding of polypeptide chains into a secondary structure. Such rules have been deduced by analyzing structural databases of small molecules and highly resolved macromolecules. On the basis of the electron densities alone, it is possible to fit in different but similar shaped side chains, like that of valine for threonine, aspartic acid for asparagine and glutamic acid for glutamine. Errors can be avoided by considering the possible hydrogen bonding pattern around the donor/acceptor atoms as well as the packing of surrounding atoms. The electron density fitting program FRODO (17, 18) is one of the major methodological breakthroughs in crystallography. FRODO runs on a computer-graphics workstation and allows the

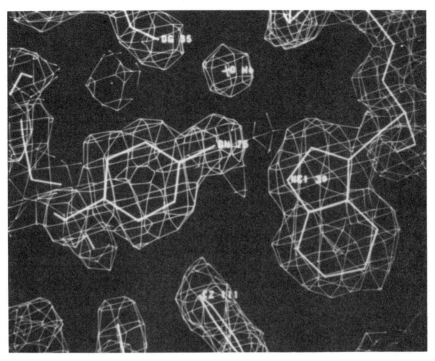

Fig. 10.3 A typical high resolution electron density picture showing the tyrosine, tryptophan and phenylalanine residue along with a water molecule. See also color plates.

crystallographer to make adjustments in order to remove incompatibilities between the model molecule and the ·calculated electron density map. The model molecule can be rotated and translated in 3-dimensions and fragments of the molecule can be locally refined by using a database of bond lengths and bond angles derived from highly refined small molecular structures. Most likely almost all the crystallographic structures are built this way. FRODO has been modified as 'O', a program that builds the molecule automatically into the electron density map with the help of a built-in database of already solved protein structures. In spite of all these automated developments, human intervention is still essential and no software can replace entirely the expertise of the crystallographer.

The initial model obtained with the procedures described above has to be refined against the restraints of the diffraction data and established structural parameters.

Many structure refining programs are available (PROLSQ, GPRLSA, RESTRAIN, TNT) to guide the crystallographer in achieving a higher resolution structure. XPLOR is another refinement program but does more than a simple refinement (19). It utilizes molecular dynamics coupled with energy minimization procedures which incorporates a pseudo-energy derived from $(F_{obs} - F_{calc})$. Due to its ability to achieve larger radius of convergence than the rest of the programs, mentioned above, XPLOR can successfully release the molecule from its trapped states of local minima, in other words can suggest correct model positions provided the errors are small. The model bias can also be checked via its free R-value procedures (20). The process of model building alternated to cycles of refinement procedures produce the desired high resolution 3-dimensional structure. This software is only a fraction of the entire list of programs used in crystallography; for a useful list see Finzel's compilation (21). Usually the coordinates of newly determined structures are submitted to the Protein Data Bank (22, 23) so that they can be used by other scientists.

3.2.5 ACCURACY OF CRYSTALLOGRAPHIC STRUCTURES. The disadvantages of crystallographic methods are that there is uncertainty in the precise positioning of atom centers while building a molecule in an experimentally obtained electron density map and that the positions of the hydrogen atoms cannot be identified, since the scattering intensity of the diffracted waves is proportional to the atomic number of the scatterer. The accuracy of the 3-dimensional structures obtained by crystallographic methods depends on several factors, like the quality of the crystals obtained (and thus the resolution with which they diffract), the types of instruments used for data acquisition, the temperature of the environment during data collection and the number of restraints introduced in the structure refinement process. Accumulation of human errors is also possible due to the time consuming process (years), but present day developments in the methodology and technology reduce the structure solution period considerably. But, it should be kept in mind that a structure obtained by crystallographic methods undergoes rigorous checking procedures against the experimentally obtained data. The accuracy of a model structure is usually measured according to statistical indicators of agreement (R-factor) between the model and the experimental data. The conformity of the model to general principles of protein stereochemistry is examined with a Ramachandran plot (24). Usually, a higher resolution of the structure (usually $2\,\text{Å}$– $1.0\,\text{Å}$) and lower R-factor ($<20\%$), indicates a better dependability of the model. On average, at $2\,\text{Å}$ resolution with a low R-factor, it is possible for the atoms to be misplaced by up to $0.3\,\text{Å}$. Ways of assessing

and minimizing errors have been reviewed by Branden and Jones (25). Well-developed algorithms are now available to assign the positions of the hydrogen atoms and they have been verified by neutron diffraction studies, with which the hydrogen atoms can be clearly identified. Clearly, the accuracy required for the design process has to be judiciously decided and experiments have to be tailored accordingly.

3.3 Nuclear Magnetic Resonance (NMR)

NMR techniques have contributed to the determination of the structures of many new proteins (26–28). The major advantage of NMR over crystallography is that the proteins need not be crystallized. In addition, it is easier to solve some structures that are difficult to be solved by crystallographic methods, such as those that contain flexible linker regions associated with globular domains. NMR is a relatively recent and still evolving technique, developed to determine the structures of macromolecules in solution. Even though solving structures greater than 75 residues by NMR is a challenge, the structures of proteins of up to about 150 amino acid residues have been successfully determined. With the development of better probes and faster computers, soon NMR procedures will be comparable to crystallographic techniques in determining many medium size molecular structures. Despite the present limitations, the structures that are solved by NMR are informative, since they reflect the nature of the molecules in aqueous media. Many small structures that have been solved by NMR in the past few years are reviewed by Hendrickson and Wuthrich (28). Examples of the larger (100–150 residues) structures that have been solved by NMR are interleukin-1β (29), hisactophilin (30), interleukin-4 (31, 32); calmodulin–peptide complex (33); and cyclophilin–cyclosporin complex (34).

In some cases the structures of the same protein solved by X-ray crystallography and NMR have been compared and analyzed. However, only in the case of interleukin-1β a single structure has been jointly refined on the basis of both crystallographic structure factors and NMR nuclear Overhauser effect measurements (35), resulting in a model that is consistent with both the experimental observations.

3.3.1 THE BASIC METHODOLOGY. The basic principle of an NMR experiment is to perturb the equilibrium of nuclear spin states with radio frequency pulses and monitor them while they relax. By analyzing the way in which the spin relaxations occur, the geometry of the molecule can be inferred.

Each atom with a nuclear spin gives rise to an individual signal (resonance), which carries information about the atom itself and its local chemical environment. For small molecules the number of resonance measurements is limited and easier to resolve. As the number of protons in the molecule increases, sophisticated techniques are needed to resolve the thousands of resonance data. To determine a molecular structure, the resonances have to be assigned to specific protons of individual amino acid residues (27, 36). Advanced techniques, such as proton-detected heteronuclear NMR, use sensitive 2-dimensional pulse sequences to perturb spin equilibrium states. Relaxation parameters like longitudinal and transverse relaxation rates and heteronuclear nuclear Overhauser effects (NOEs) can then be measured. Nuclear Overhauser effects originate from dipole–dipole interactions between protons that are closer than 5 Å and provide a mechanism for magnetization transfer between the signals corresponding to such protons in the 1 H NMR spectrum. The success of structure solution by NMR depends on obtaining a large number of NOE measurements.

Structure determination by NMR progresses by the following steps: (1) preparing the sample, (2) spectral data collection, (3) assignment of chemical shifts, (4) analysis of nuclear Overhauser effect measurements (5) assignment of secondary structural elements, (6) initial structure calculation, and (7) refinement of the structures. For reviews on the methodology of data collection and the computational aspects of structure solution by NMR (36–38).

3.3.2 ISOTOPE LABELING. The recent development of heteronuclear 3-dimensional and 4-dimensional NMR techniques, in combination with the selective or uniform enrichment of proteins with ^{15}N- and ^{13}C-labeled isotopes, allows an easier assignment of individual resonances. Atomic nuclei with odd number of protons (^{1}H, ^{13}C, ^{15}N, ^{17}O, and ^{31}P) have unpaired spins and thus give rise to large net magnetic moments, while atomic nuclei with even number of protons (^{2}H, ^{12}C, ^{14}N, ^{15}O, and ^{32}P) have paired spins that almost cancel out. Therefore, in natural proteins only hydrogen has a large magnetic moment. However, proteins expressed by using recombinant techniques can be enriched or even completely substituted with isotopically labeled amino acids. Two recent reviews discuss the preparation of isotope-labeled samples (39, 40). The 153 residues of interleukin-1β, for example, have been successfully labeled with ^{13}C and ^{15}N. As a result each proton was shifted in frequency according to the magnetic moment of the ^{13}C or ^{15}N atom to which it was attached. These shifts facilitated the assignment of resonances to particular protons and improved their resolution (41, 42). The resonance information thus obtained is used to construct a matrix. The principles of distance geometry are then applied to derive the exact fold of the protein and to refine it. Because the matrix contains a range of allowed distances for each pair of protons (between 1.4 and 5.0 Å), different structures are calculated with different sets of randomly chosen distances between neighboring protons, within the allowed range. The result is an ensemble of related structures, as shown in Figure 10.4, and the accuracy of the overall structure is expressed as the root mean square distance between the same atom in the different structures.

3.3.3. NMR AND DRUG DESIGN. NMR is also being used to identify receptor-ligand interactions (43–47). This is made possible to simplifying the NMR spectra by isotope enrichment and isotope editing, whereby the proton resonances of the bound ligand can be assigned by employing heteronuclear 3-dimensional NMR techniques. Different spectra of the receptor–ligand complex can be obtained by: (a) enriching neither the receptor nor the ligand, (b) enriching either ligand or receptor separately and (c) simultaneously enriching the ligand with ^{13}C and the receptor with ^{15}N or vice-versa. The obtained spectra can then be compared and edited to identify the resonances arising from the ligand and from the residues in the receptor binding site. From this information the residues involved in the receptor–ligand interaction can be identified.

The methods described above have been employed by complexing isotopically labeled ligands with their receptor proteins, which allowed the selective detection of the protons of the ligand (47–49). Successful results have been obtained with the solution of the structure of cyclosporin A bound to cyclophilin. In addition, a ^{13}C- and ^{15}N-enriched flavin mononucleotide was used to identify its interactions with flavodoxin. Isotope-edited NOEs were used to orient the flavodoxin ligand in the binding site of the flavin mononucleotide (50). The portions of the ligand that are exposed to the solvent were identified on the basis of the lack of ligand–receptor NOEs or paramagnetic-induced changes in the proton relaxation rates of the bound ligand. The changes in longitudinal relaxation rates of the solvent-exposed protons of a bound ligand in the presence of a paramagnetic agent can be used in defining the solvent exposed surface of a ligand when bound to the target molecules (51–54).

An alternative approach is to use an

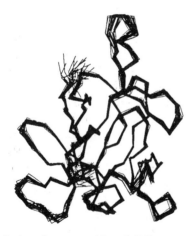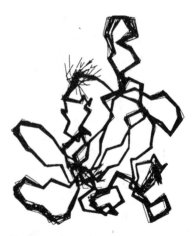

Fig. 10.4 A view of a superposition of all Cα atoms of interleukin-1β, as determined by NMR. The narrow width of the collection of Cα points along the polypeptide chain reflects the accuracy of the structure determination. The deviations on the loops indicate the dynamic mobility of the atoms. The figures were drawn using the program QUANTA, and the coordinates were extracted from PDB (7I1B.PDB, structure solved by G. M. Clore, P. T. Wingfield, and A. M. Gronenborn, see ref. 29).

isotopically labeled receptor complexed with unlabeled ligand, to identify the changes introduced by the ligand in the receptor structure (55–60). The excellent work by Arata and his colleagues is a source of encouragement for structure-based drug designers, since the receptor protein they used is a 25 kD FV fragment of an antibody, a very large protein by NMR standards. They were able to characterize the ligand binding site of this receptor and analyzed the ligand-induced conformational changes of the key residues within it.

NMR studies on the position of bound water molecules have been reported (61, 62). They are relevant for drug design efforts because desolvation is an important aspect in designing ligands that have to displace water molecules in order to bind to the receptor's binding site. Studies on metal binding proteins, such as calbindin, human factor IX, and zinc finger domains, have also been reported. For a detailed review on ligand binding studies by NMR refer to Stockman and Markley (45) and Fesik (46). Advances in NMR instrumentation coupled with recombinant techniques to produce stable isotope-labeled proteins have dramatically changed the scene of structural biology where crystallography alone reigned. The further application of NMR methods will provide even more insights into the field of molecular structures, kinetics of ligand binding, protein stability and above all in designing drugs.

3.4 Homologous Modeling

In addition to the methods based on experimental data, homologous modeling methods are being developed to derive 3-dimensional structures based on amino acid sequence information. Homologous modeling is based on existing knowledge about the structural architecture of proteins, the rules governing their folding, the essential interactions that hold proteins together and the energies involved. However, the single most important resource for the success of modeling procedures is the availability of experimentally determined structures in the Protein Data Bank (22, 23).

No definite methodology has been developed to determine the 3-dimensional folding of a protein from the amino acid sequence alone. Proteins are being purified and sequenced at an increasing pace: as of today about 103,000 sequences are available in Genbank (63). Many of these sequences can be grouped into families of proteins with common structural domains. If the 3-dimensional structure of at least one member of a family is available, then the rules governing the architecture of other members of the same family can be deciphered. The validity of these rules, and our confidence in them, increases as more and more related 3-dimensional structures are determined experimentally. These structural principles, together with the observation that certain levels of amino acid substitution can be tolerated without significantly altering the overall configuration, form the basis of homologous modeling.

3.4.1 GENERAL METHODOLOGY. As early as 1969 Sir David Phillips and his colleagues built a model of α-lactalbumin based on the structure of hen egg white lysozyme (64). Attempts by Greer to build a model structure of a member of the serine proteinases family based on the crystal structures of other homologous serine proteinases (65) and by Blundell's group to build the model of renin based on the structures of other aspartic proteinases (66), were the first few initiatives to use the existing structural knowledge for model building. Now a surge of interest and improvements in this field is seen every day.

The first step in this modeling process is to align the amino acid sequence of the protein with unknown structure against the sequence of a homologous protein whose 3-dimensional structure has already been determined. If more than one crystal structure is available, all the known structures can be superposed to a single frame of reference, to identify the structurally conserved regions (SCR) and structurally variable regions (SVR). Usually, defined secondary structural elements fall under the category of SCRs and the loops and random coils under that of SVRs. By aligning the sequences of all the known structures based on the identified SCRs, and aligning the sequence of the protein whose structure has to be identified against them, the core of the molecule can be identified (Fig. 10.5). The rest of the molecule, essentially the loops, can be later added to the core to complete the model building. The process of identifying the core has been made easier by translating the 3-dimensional model of the original structure into a structurally interpretable form of the sequence with the program JOY, which assigns specially developed structural codes to each amino acid (67). Such structure-based sequence information can be used to achieve

better alignment and core construction. Overington and Blundell built the model of bovine trypsin based on the known structures of four other serine proteinases, with an RMS difference of 0.64 Å for the 150 residues in the core of the molecule (68). By employing these modeling techniques, we built the structure of IL1-α and IL-1ra based on the crystallographic structure of IL-1β(6). Later when IL-1α's crystallographic structure was determined to a very high resolution of 1.8 Å (69), we rebuilt the model of IL-1-ra, based on the structures of IL-1α, IL1-β and the sequence alignment by JOY (Figures 10.5a and 10.5b). Even with all the sophistication in the computer algorithms, the sequence alignment had to be manually adjusted in a few regions to arrive at a sensible model. It is encouraging to note that the model of IL-1ra thus obtained has been used as a probe to solve the crystallographic structure of IL-1ra (70). Figure 10.5c shows a stereo plot of a superposition of all the three interleukin-1. The above procedures have been termed modeling by homology (66, 71, 72). An evaluation of these homology modeling

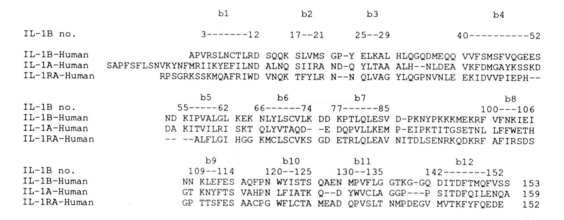

```
                       b1                b2        b3              b4
IL-1B no.              3-------12      17--21    25--29          40----------52

IL-1B-Human            APVRSLNCTLRD SQQK SLVMS GP-Y ELKAL HLQGQDMEQQ VVFSMSFVQGEES
IL-1A-Human    SAPFSFLSNVKYNFMRIIKYEFILND ALNQ SIIRA ND-Q YLTAA ALH--NLDEA VKFDMGAYKSSKD
IL-1RA-Human           RPSGRKSSKMQAFRIWD VNQK TFYLR N--N QLVAG YLQGPNVNLE EKIDVVPIEPH--

                       b5        b6          b7                          b8
IL-1B no.              55-----62  66------74  77------85                 100---106
IL-1B-Human            ND KIPVALGL KEK NLYLSCVLK DD KPTLQLESV D-PKNYPKKKMEKRF VFNKIEI
IL-1A-Human            DA KITVILRI SKT QLYVTAQD- -E DQPVLLKEM P-EIPKTITGSETNL LFFWETH
IL-1RA-Human           -- --ALFLGI HGG KMCLSCVKS GD ETRLQLEAV NITDLSENRKQDKRF AFIRSDS

                       b9         b10         b11           b12
IL-1B no.              109--114   120--125    130--135     142-------152
IL-1B-Human            NN KLEFES AQFPN WYISTS QAEN MPVFLG GTKG-GQ DITDFTMQFVSS  153
IL-1A-Human            GT KNYFTS VAHPN LFIATK Q--D YWVCLA GGP---P SITDFQILENQA  159
IL-1RA-Human           GP TTSFES AACPG WFLCTA MEAD QPVSLT NMPDEGV MVTKFYFQEDE  152
```

(a)

Fig. 10.5 (a) The amino acid sequences of IL-1α, IL-1β, and IL-1RA were aligned by the Protein Design program built within Quanta and modified based on the three dimensional structures of IL-1β and IL-1α. (b) The same sequences were aligned using the program JOY, by J. Overington. The key codes for the aminoacids are also indicated. 4i1b and 8i1b are the PDB codes for human and mouse IL-1β. il1a stands for human IL-1α. (c) Superposition of the α-carbon backbones of IL-1α, IL-1β, and IL-1RA. The model of IL-1RA was obtained as described in homology modeling.

```
                10          20          30          40          50
4i1b    v r s̄ l ñ - C T̃ L ĩ D̃ s q̄ q K̲̃ S L v m s g p ȳ e L k̲ A l h̲̃ l q g q d̃ m e q̄ q̄ v v F s M S̃
8i1b    q l h̃ - y ĩ L ĩ D̃ e q̄ q K̲̃ S L v l s̲ d p y ē L k̲̃ A l h̲ l n g q ñ i ñ̲ q Q̃ v i F S̃ M s
il1a    v k y ñ f m r I i k̃ y e F I L ñ D̃ a l ñ q̄ S̃ I i r̲ a n d q y L t̲ A a a l h - - ñ l d̃ e A v k̲ F D̃ M G
                β β   β β β β β     β β β β       β β β β        3        β β β β

                60          70          80          90          100
4i1b    f V q̄ g e - - e s n d k i P V A L G L k e k n̲ l Y L S̃ C̃ v l k d d k p t̲ L q̄ L ē s̃ V d p k n ȳ p̌ k̲̃ k
8i1b    f V q g e - - p s n̲ d k i p V A L G L k g k n̲ l Y L S̃ C̃ v m k̃ d g t p t̲ L q̄ L ē s v d p k q̄ ȳ p̌ k̲̃ k
il1a    A Y̲ k s̃ s̃ k d d̲̃ a - - k̃ i T V I L ĩ i S̲̃ k t̲ q̄ l Ỹ V t̲ A q d̃ e d - - q p V l L k e m p - - e i p k ĩ
        β                   β β β β β β β     β β β β         β β β β

                110         120         130         140         150
4i1b    - - k̲̃ M ē k ĩ F V F ñ k i e̲ i n n k l ē F ẽ S̃ a q f p n w y I S̲ T̃ s q̄ a ē n m p V f L g g t k̃ g g q
8i1b    - - k M ē k̃ ĩ F v F ñ k i e v k s̲ K̲̃ V ē F Ẽ S̃ a ē f p n w y I S̲ T̃ s q̄ a e h k p V f L g n n - s̃ g q
il1a    I t̲ g s e t n̲ l L F f w̃ ē t h̃ g t k ñ̲ y F T̃ S v a h̲ p n l f I A T k q̄ - - d y w V C̲ L A g g - - p p̌
        3 3 3       β β β β β       β β β β β       β β β         β β β

                160
4i1b    d i t d F ĩ m q̄ f v s s̃
8i1b    d̲̃ I i d̃ F t m ē s v
il1a    s i t d̃ F q i l ē n q̄ a
        β β̄ β β
```

The amino acid code is the standard one-letter code formatted using the following convention (Overington *et al.*, 1990); *italic* for positive values of ϕ; UPPER CASE for residues that are less than 7% solvent accessible; lower case for residues that are greater than 7% solvent accessible; breve ˘ for *cis*-peptide; **bold** for hydrogen bonds to main-chain NH groups; underline for hydrogen bonds to main-chain carbonyl oxygen atoms; tilde ˜ for side-chain–side-chain hydrogen bonds; cedilla ˛ for disulphide bond. The secondary structure is given below the alignment where it is present in 80% or more of the proteins: α for α-helix; β for β-strand; + for positive ϕ torsion angle.

(*b*)

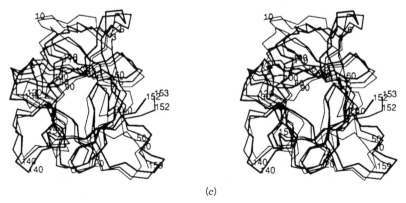

(*c*)

Fig. 10.5 (*Continued*)

procedures using the models obtained indicates that the RMS error can be as low as 1 Å (73). For a detailed review of the modeling procedures refer to refs. 74, 85, and references therein.

3.4.2 SATISFACTION OF SPATIAL RESTRAINTS METHOD. By infusing newer ideas in these modeling methodologies, sophisticated procedures are currently being developed and promising results are on the horizon. One of these novel methods is to construct models by satisfaction of spatial restraints. This method identifies the common key features of the to be modeled protein based on homology and by associating them with invariant or conserved sequences. This can be achieved more systematically by "projecting" the restraints of the three-dimensional fold onto the one dimension of the sequence (74) and then comparing the sequence templates or profiles. The 3-dimensional model is then obtained by optimally satisfying spatial restraints, which are derived from the above alignment procedure and by expressing them as probability density functions for the features restrained. For example, the probabilities for the main chain conformation of a modeled residue may be restrained by its residue type and by the main chain conformation and local similarity of an equivalent residue in a related protein (74). The method has been automated and the authors have modeled trypsin from two other serine proteinases, to show that the modelled structure deviates from the original crystallographic structure by an RMS deviation of only 0.6 Å (74).

Several other methods have been reported. In one the distance geometry approach is considered by utilizing distance constraints (76, 77). Another procedure is based on the satisfaction of main chain distance restraints (78). Neural networks and optimization in cartesian space were used to calculate a model from a Cα distance plot of a homologous protein (79).

3.4.3 CONSTRUCTION OF A 3-D STRUCTURE BASED ON α-CARBON ATOMS. Methods have been developed to estimate entire backbone coordinates based on the positions of the C-alpha atoms (80–87). These methods can be applied to modeling procedures, when homologous structures are used as the source of information to determine C-alpha positions, in combination with the loop and side chain construction algorithms (82, 88).

3.4.4 IDENTIFICATION OF PROTEIN FOLDING FROM DISTANTLY RELATED SEQUENCES. All the above modeling procedures are successful when the percentage of sequence identity of the known structures and the unknown ones is greater than 40%. The accuracy of the model decreases quickly as the sequence identity between the known and unknown structures decreases. Procedures are being developed to identify the folding of a molecule based on distantly related sequences (<30%) as a guide. This can be done by using a database of all known protein structures that are even distantly related (89, 90). Of the different approaches to determine protein folding from distantly related sequences, a significant few involve: (a) calculating amino acid substitution tables as a function of local environment (67, 91, 92); (b) optimal threading of a sequence onto a 3-dimensional structure (90); (c) topology fingerprinting (93); (d) determining the propensity of an amino acid to occur in a given local structural environment, which is defined by solvent accessibility and secondary structure (94); (e) tertiary structure recognition (95); and (f) detection of native-like models for a given sequence (96).

3.4.5 BUILDING LOOPS ON A FRAMEWORK. Loop building is a crucial part of any modeling procedure since most of the variations occur in this part of the structure. Successful results have been reported by applying interactive procedures to select loops from loop libraries and docking them into the model by visualization techniques (18, 66, 97–105). Substitutions, insertions, and deletions in loops have been modeled by regularizing a suitable fragment selected from homologous structures, by a conformation search based on minimizing the energy of a segment, or by a combination of these approaches (106–115).

3.4.6 MODELING SIDE CHAINS. Structural information derived from the Protein Data Bank has been the basis to develop side-chain building procedures. Building side-chains onto the backbone framework is based on the most similar side-chain conformations found in rotamer libraries (116, 117). In some procedures, rules that relate the side chain dihedral angle with the residue type at equivalent positions in homologous proteins have been applied (118, 119). Additional procedures have been employed, involving minimum energy conformations of selected side chains from rotamer libraries or systematic conformational searches (88, 111, 118–128). Selection of the side-chain conformation can be aided by conformationally constrained environmental amino acid substitution tables (115). Considering disulfinde bonds in the proposed model is another important aspect in constructing a model structure. The geometry of the disulfide bridges has been analyzed on the basis of observed disulfide bonds in the existing protein structures (129, 130) and this information is being incorporated in the recent modeling methods.

3.4.7 MODELING BY A COMBINATORIAL APPROACH *ab initio* MODELING. In the absence of a folding pattern to guide the model building exercise of a protein, due to the lack of experimentally determined homologous structures, combinatorial approaches can be applied (131). These depend upon the identification of secondary structural elements using conformational propensities and residue patterns. The identified secondary structural elements are then assembled based on rules governing structures. It should be remembered that at the present time there is no program available to predict accurately the secondary structure of a protein from the amino acid sequence alone. There are claims for a success rate of 63% for a single sequence prediction and 72% for multiple alignment predictions (132). Furthermore, the modeling of sections of protein backbone (cys-loop) without any homologous structural information has resulted in a general model for the binding loop of the ligand-gated ion channel (LGIC) superfamily of receptors (133).

3.4.8 MODEL REFINEMENT. After the initial model has been assembled, its stereochemistry has to be improved by adjusting intramolecular contacts and relieving steric clashes. This can be done by subjecting the model to a rigorous refinement procedure based on an available database dependent library of structural parameters. Improvements can also be made by proper energy minimization procedures (134, 135). Homologous modeling techniques have been criticized because the model ends up reflecting the taste of the modeler rather than being true to itself. There is some truth in this statement, but the lack of accuracy of a structure obtained by homologous modeling has to be weighed against the specific need for the model and its potential usefulness. In a few years it may be possible to visualize a modeled structure on a graphics screen in a matter of minutes, as long as a few homologous structures are available in the databases. This would be a great achievement in the field of 3-dimensional structure function analysis. Whether the structures based on available homologous modeling methods are sufficiently accurate to be used in drug design attempts remains to be seen, but at least they can be a source of ideas. However, one should always keep in mind that the quality of a structural model obtained by any of the *ab initio* modeling procedures available to date is not comparable to that of a structure determined by crystallography or NMR.

3.4.9 SIMULATED ANNEALING. In order to release the molecule from the trapped states of local energy minima, simulated annealing methods can be applied. These use developed force fields to calculate the atomic forces of each atoms on others. The trajectories of each part of the molecule are simulated by successive integration of the velocities. In such a simulation, the molecules are kept in a heat bath, heated by increasing the temperature such that it can randomly arrange itself in the liquid phase, and then cooled by gradually decreasing the temperature of the bath. When such a simulated annealing process is completed, the molecules arrange themselves in the lowest minimum energy ground state. The condition for such a process is that the maximum temperature is high enough and the cooling is carried out slowly. Usually the dynamics are simulated in a number of steps at short intervals (fractions of picoseconds), at every step the new trajectories are calculated for each atom and the overall energy of the system is monitored. At the final stage of the collection of the ensemble, the molecule with the lowest energy is chosen, since it presumably represents the realistic minimum energy conformation state. Solvating the system is an additional important factor, and the water molecules are kept within a box (not to be evaporated due to high trajectory values). The application of this technique has been successfully employed in structural studies by XPLOR (20) and for a detailed methodology refer to the review by Brunger and Nilges (30). This simulated annealing method has been used in homologous modeling, where the constructed molecule can be subjected to this heating and cooling procedure, preferably with harmonic restraints

on the template. In drug design studies, the designed molecule is allowed to dock into the target molecule's binding site and by simulation its dynamic behavior can be monitored.

3.4.10 EVALUATION OF THE STRUCTURE. Any one of the above mentioned methods can be employed to produce a reasonable 3-dimensional structure of the target molecule and such models are often evaluated for errors due to improper construction. Definite conformational rules for the internal parameters of a protein molecule exist and a Ramachandran Map, can be obtained by plotting ϕ and ψ values in X and Y directions. This plot can exhibit the residues that are in allowed and unallowed regions. PROCHECK (136), a program developed in Thornton's laboratory thoroughly scrutinizes the obtained structure by analyzing the distribution of its internal conformational parameters and produces valuable evaluation plots. A cleaner map with less residues in the unallowed region supports the validity of the molecular structure and increases our confidence in its accuracy.

4 THE DESIGN PROCESS

4.1 Identification of the Site of Action

The first step in the design process is to identify the site of action, where all the available tools can be used toward obtaining a compound that can bind to the target. The use of molecular graphics hardware and software is described in chapter 15. The designer has to acquire the intimate details of the target molecule by identifying the hydrogen bonds, ionic, hydrophobic and solvent interactions. Details like the domain modular structures, secondary structural arrangements, and loop architectures will guide the designer in understanding the constitution of the functional site.

Mapping such a site is the crucial task in the initial stages. In the case of an enzyme, identifying the active site is an easy task. One can visually look at it in 3-dimensions and easily draw its boundaries reasonably well. But in the case of hormones/cytokines, it is elusive. The final proof for the localization of a functional site can only be obtained when the crystal structure of the ligand, complexed with its receptor is available. An excellent example is that of human growth hormone, the hormone-receptor binding site was identified unequivocally only after the crystal structure determination of this hormone with its receptor (137).

4.2 Required Structural Accuracy in the Design Process

The accuracy required for the structure of the target protein depends upon the design process. The basic requirement is that the newly designed drug has to complement precisely the known binding site of the target molecule. This can be achieved by exploiting the structural information available in order to identify the site of drug action and the availability of space to fill. If a high resolution structure is available, the topography of the drug binding site and its environment can be accurately mapped. Only a well-defined structure will be able to reveal subtle but significant differences in the movements of atoms, binding or replacement of water molecules, localized disturbances due to charge dislocations, increase in the available space due to domain movement and flexibility of loops to close in on the ligand for better binding. These are small details, but they may heavily influence the design process. We now know in the substrate-based design of enzyme inhibitors, the presumed transition-state structure of the enzyme should be taken into account. For this purpose, the structure of the target site has to be resolved to the highest resolution possible.

4.3 Identification of the Lead Compound

Once the 3-dimensional structure of the target protein has been defined, the next step is to identify a prototype "lead compound" or a "pharmacophore". These compounds should be capable of binding to the target molecule in competition with the normally available specific biological ligands. In some cases it is not necessary to wait until the final 3-dimensional structure of the target protein has been resolved. Simultaneous experiments may yield the necessary information beforehand. A lead compound can be identified by employing the conventional screening of available libraries of compounds in parallel with the structure-based search. If multiple lead compounds are identified, then a comparison may result in the identification of the core of the pharmacophore, i.e., the parts of its chemical structure that are essential for its action as a drug. For most enzymes the substrates are known and from their chemical nature, a lead compound can be designed. However, in the case of hormone or cytokine receptors, the task of identifying a lead compound is more difficult. The functional site of interaction is usually an epitope comprising different secondary structural elements of the molecule. In this case, the knowledge of the 3-dimensional structure of the receptor functional site is a prerequisite to the structure-based search for a lead compound.

Where the 3-dimensional structure of target molecule has been determined before the lead compounds were identified, it has provided invaluable lead information. The drug design efforts to treat AIDS based on the 3-dimensional structure of HIV proteinases is one such example.

5 SOFTWARE AIDED DRUG DESIGN

The technological advances in computing and visualization methods have been a great help in developing algorithms to probe the surface of the target molecules, searching for crevices and epitopes which can act as drug binding regions. Successful attempts have been reported in docking small molecules into these binding regions by automated or investigator-aided procedures. The basic condition to be satisfied in such docking procedures is that the selected ligands should possess the appropriate geometry to fit into the binding site of the target molecule with minimal steric clashes. However, a tight fitting shape is not the only requirement. Favorable interactions between the chemical groups in the binding site and the designed compound should also be achieved. Almost all the automated docking procedures carry out systematic searches in rotational and translational space and simultaneously evaluate the electrostatic, hydrophobic or hydrogen bonding energy terms, in order to achieve the best fit of the ligand to its binding site (138, 139). The interactive docking procedures aid the investigator to optimally position a ligand into the binding site and update the energy terms as the ligand is moved (140–142).

In most of the target molecules there is a cavity-like region where the proposed drug has to bind with high specificity, in competition with other chemical groups surrounding it. The basic requirement for a compound to be an effective drug is that it has to achieve an optimal fit into the target molecule. The higher the interaction energy, the better the drug is likely to be. Thus, many programs attempt to generate structures which can be fitted into the binding sites of the target molecule as best as possible, by displacing solvent molecules and maximizing the drug-receptor interactions. For example, Kuntz and his colleagues (143, 144) developed a software called DOCK that creates a complementary image of the target site by packing within it a set of overlapping spheres of various sizes. The set of distances between the centers of the spheres (or distance matrix) is then used to create the volumetric representation of the target site. Potential ligands are also characterized in a similar fashion and their distance matrices are matched with the distance matrix of the binding site. Selected ligands are then ranked according to the match. DIRECTED DOCK is a modification of this procedure (144) in which hydrogen bonding information is used and conformational flexibility is allowed. Bacon and Moult (145) use a least squares fitting method, in which the ligand is allowed to rotate in the available space within the binding site to maximize steric contacts.

To orient the functional groups of the ligand into the binding site, energy minimization and simulated annealing procedures have been adopted in the Multiple Copy Simultaneous Search (MCSS) method (146–148). A range of small functional groups are placed inside the site and the energies of interaction are minimized using the program CHARMM and quenched by molecular dynamics procedures, resulting in the migration of the introduced groups into preferred orientations within the cavity of the binding site. The results of several of these searches are utilized in constructing a functionality map of the binding site and in identifying the preferred orientations of the functional groups of a pharmacophore in the receptor site. The program HOOK can then be used to construct new ligands by linking the bound fragments with skeletons obtained from database searches.

An extensive discussion of methods and software for fitting ligands into target sites is given in chapter 15. Searches of three-dimensional databases to obtain information for ligand design is described in chapter 13. The application of QSAR methods to these efforts is described in chapter 14.

6 OPTIMIZATION OF THE IDENTIFIED COMPOUNDS

Once the identification of the drug binding site and the selection of the lead compounds are completed, the optimization of these binding agents is carried out. Selected few compounds are synthesized and their binding constants are determined. The compounds with higher binding affinities are complexed with the target molecule and crystallized for diffraction data collection or isotope labeled to obtain NMR spectra. The structure of the bound form is determined and analyzed. Based on these results, improvements in the design can be made by optimizing the hydrogen bonds, van der Waals and electrostatic interactions. This process is repeated until a satisfactory drug is obtained.

7 EXAMPLES OF STRUCTURE-AIDED DRUG DESIGN

Having reviewed the methodologies that are essential for structure-aided drug design, some examples are now given. Numerous protein structures are being considered in the design of drugs: thymidylate synthase and dihydrofolate reductase in cancer; purine nucleoside phosphorylase in cancer and immune related diseases; carbonic anhydrase in glaucoma; thymidine phosphorylase to design better chemotherapeutic analogs and anti-HIV nucleoside analogs; aldose reductase in diabetes; neutrophil elastase in emphysema; rhino-viral coat protein in the common cold; thrombin in blood clots; HIV protease in AIDS; renin and angiotensin converting enzyme in hypertension; β-lactamases to design better antibiotics; influenza neuraminidase to design antiviral inhibitors; cytokines to mediate the immune response and so on. The list is getting longer as more and more laboratories carry out structure-based research activities.

In all cases the first step is to determine the structure of the target protein to atomic resolution. As discussed before lead compounds are identified, synthesized, and complexed with the target molecule, followed by structure solution. When the structures of the native protein molecule alone and in complex with lead compounds are known, the atomic dispositions at the protein–compound interface are analyzed, to understand the intricate network of interactions that are necessary for the complexation to occur. Based on this detailed understanding, the lead compounds are modified to optimize their complementarity with receptor subsites and to maintain key interactions. These modified compounds are assayed biologically and improved compounds are complexed again with the target molecule and the structure of the complex is determined for further improvement. The cycle is repeated until the final drug is obtained and validated by clinical studies.

Some of the structure-aided drug design studies to design inhibitors for ACE and renin and the lessons learned in designing HIV protease inhibitors to treat AIDS are discussed here.

7.1 Design of Drugs to Treat Hypertension: The Renin Angiotensin System

Renin is an enzyme that specifically cleaves human angiotensinogen at the ^{10}Leu-^{11}Val bond, thereby producing the decapeptide angiotensin I (AI) which is further cleaved by angiotensin converting enzyme (ACE) to release angiotensin II (AII). The octapeptide AII raises blood pressure.

7.2 Inhibitor Design for the Angiotensin Converting Enzyme

One of the earliest examples where 3-dimensional structural information has played a key role is the design of drugs to treat hypertension by developing inhibitors for ACE (149), an exopeptidase of 140 kD with a single polypeptide chain and a bound zinc ion. Based on the homology of this enzyme to other zinc containing proteinases like pancreatic carboxypeptidase A and thermolysin, Cushman and his colleagues designed a series of carboxyalkanoyl and mercaptoalkanoyl derivatives of proline to act as ACE inhibitors (150). The active site of carboxypeptidase A has an arginine and a cavity designed to fit an aromatic side chain. A zinc ion flanks this site by coordinating two histidines, one glutamate, and one water molecule. The C-terminal carboxylate of the substrate interacts with the arginine in the active site, and its carbonyl oxygen at the scissile bond is believed to be polarized by the positive charges of the zinc ion and of a neighboring arginine side chain (151). This polarization facilitates nucleophilic attack on the carbonyl carbon by a water molecule leading to a tetrahedral intermediate and then to proteolytic products (152).

The cleaved fragment for ACE is a dipeptide, whereas a single C-terminal residue is the substrate for carboxypeptidase A. Based on the active site configuration and the substrate sizes, the cavity of ACE was predicted to be larger than that of

carboxypeptidase A. An additional hydrogen bond donor and acceptor have to be present in the active site of ACE to interact with the peptide substrate. These structural details led to the design of the inhibitor succinylproline, which has an IC_{50} value of $3.3 \times 10^{-4}M$. Addition of a sulfur atom led to the higher affinity binder called captopril (3-mercapto-2-methylpropanol-1-proline) with an $IC_{50} = 2 \times 10^{-7}M$ (153). Modification of the cysteinyl side chain by a homophenylalanyl group led to the design of a series of inhibitors without loss of activity (154).

By modeling captopril within the active site of thermolysin, Hassall et al. identified two bonds with conformational flexibility. Designing a bicyclic derivative to abolish this and substituting the cysteyl side chain by a homophenylalanyl moiety produced an even more potent inhibitor (Cilazapril) (155, 156). Figure 10.6 shows a stereo plot of thermolysin with a compound CLT ($1 - N - (1$-carboxy-3-phenylpropyl)-L-leucyl-1-tryptophan) bound in its active site (157). These drugs obtained by structure-aided drug design, are in the market now and are used to treat hypertension. The success of these modeling studies in producing useful drugs encouraged many other scientists to take advantage of structural information in their drug discovery attempts.

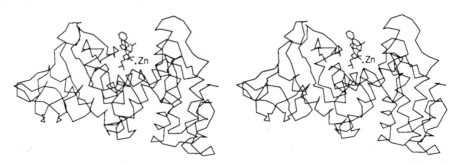

Fig. 10.6   Stereo Plot of the Cα Atoms of Thermolysin with a Compound CLT (1-*N*-(1-Carboxy-3-Phenylpropyl)-L-Leucyl-1-Tryptophan) bound in its active site. The coordinates were extracted from PDB (1TMN.PDB; Structure solved A. F. Monzingo and B. W. Matthews, 1984, see ref. 157). The active site is the deep cavity and the CLT is seen buried well within it.

7.3 Design of Renin Inhibitors

Unlike ACE, which can act on many substrates such as bradykinin, neurotensin, enkephalins, substance P and angiotensin I, renin is known to have only angiotensinogen as a substrate. Thus, it is thought that inhibitors of renin may lack the side effects associated with ACE inhibitors.

7.3.1 SUBSTRATE SPECIFICITY OF RENIN AND THE DESIGN OF PEPTIDE INHIBITORS. The N-terminal sequence of human angiotensinogen is Asp–Arg–Val–Tyr–Ile–His–Pro–Phe–His–Leu–Val–Ile–His, and renin cleaves it between the Leu–Val bond, whereas ACE cleaves the Phe–His bond. Renin is highly specific for the leucyl–valyl bond and the residues preceding and following the scissile bond. Skeggs et al. (158) defined the octapeptide –His–Pro–Phe–His–Leu–Leu–Val–Tyr– as a minimum substrate for renin. By removing the Tyr at its C-terminus this peptide was no longer a substrate, but behaved like an inhibitor. Based on this, lead compounds were designed. Pepstatine, from *Streptomyces*, is a naturally occurring inhibitor of all aspartic proteinases which contains the unusual amino acid, statine [(3S, 4S)-4-amino-3-hydroxy-6-methylheptanoic acid]. One approach is to introduce statine into the renin substrate sequence. Since renin cleaves at the scissile bond Leu–Val, modifications around this peptide bond result in nonhydrolyzable transition state isosteres. Szelke and his co-workers developed such inhibitors (Table 10.1) (159–161), the first of its kind to be used in crystallographic studies. The conformational characteristics of these inhibitors bound to the active site of aspartic proteinases provide clues that can be used to synthesize compounds of smaller in size with very high potency and specificity. Further, substrate based peptide modifications produced analogs of statine, scissile bond isosteres, like that of reduced amides, hydroxyethylenes, dihydroxyethylenes, hydroxyethylamines, ketones and difluoroketones, as well as glycol-based carboxyterminal moieties (Fig. 10.7).

Renin is a member of the aspartic proteinase family. During the period of 1983 to 1990, the 3-dimensional structures of the aspartic proteinases endothiapepsin, penicillopepsin and rhizopuspepsin were determined (162–176), whereas the structure of renin was not known. Since all these enzymes are homologous to renin and have similar active sites, the design of renin inhibitors was carried out using some of these structures. The crystal structures of various types of renin inhibitors complexed with these fungal enzymes were determined (Table 10.1). These crystals were obtained either by soaking the crystals of the enzyme in a solution of the inhibitor or by co-crystallizing the enzyme with the inhibitor. Analysis of the structures clearly revealed the conformation of the inhibitors within the enzyme active site, since most of them were solved at 2 Å resolution or better. These structural results were then combined with the IC$_{50}$ (the concentration of the inhibitor necessary to block half the activity of the enzyme) values of the inhibitors with respect to renin and a rationale was derived to synthesize even better inhibitors. Selected sets of such improved inhibitors were then complexed again and the crystal structures of the complexes were determined and analyzed. This design cycle was repeated several times to give many tighter binding renin inhibitors. Recent reports show further improvements, particularly in the design of compounds with better oral bioavailability (194). The crystallographic structures of human and mouse renin have now been solved (169–171) and the coordinates determined by Blundell's laboratory are available from PDB. Blundell and Dhanaraj have also determined the crystal structures of several additional high affinity inhibitors complexed with renin (177).

Table 10.1 Various Nonhydrolyzable Transition State Isosters as Renin Inhibitors

Name	Subsites	Inhibitor[a]	Ki/IC50[b]	Target molecule
Reduced Bond				
H-142	P6-P4'	Pro-His-Pro-Phe-His-Leu-CH2-NH-Val-Ile--His-Lys	160	Endothiapepsin
H-77	P6-P3'	DHis-Pro-Phe-His-Leu-CH2-NH-Val-Ile-His	ND	Endothiapepsin
H-256	P4-P3'	Pro-Thr-Glu-Phe-CH2-NH-Phe-Arg-GLu	60	Endothiapepsin
Hydroxyethylene				
H-261	P6-P3'	Boc-His-Pro-Phe-His-Leu-CHOH-CH2-Val-Ile-His	<1	Endothiapepsin
PD125,967	P4-P2'	Nap-Nap-His-Cha-CHOH-CH2-Leu-Ile	242	Endothiapepsin
CP-71,362	P3-P3'	Boc-Phe-His-Cha-CHOH-CH2-Leu-Lys	81	Endothiapepasin
CGP38,560	P4-P2'	Boc-Phe-His-Cha-CHOH-CH2-Val-Abu	2	Renin (human)
CH-66	P6-P4'	Boc-His-Pro-Phe-His-Leu-CHOH-CH2-Leu-Tyr-Tyr-SerNH2		Renin (mouse)
Amino Alcohol				
BW624	P1-P3'	Leu-CHOH-CH2-NH-Val-Ile-Phe	960	Endothiapepsin
BW625	P1-P3'	Leu-CHOH-CH2-NH-Val-Ile-Phe		Endothiapepsin
Statine				
Pepstatin	P4-P4'	Iva-Val-Val-Sta-CHOH-CH2-CO-NH-Ala-Sta	0.5	*Endothiapepsin
Pepstatin	P4-P4'	Iva-Val-Val-Sta-CHOH-CH2-CO-NH-Ala-Sta	17	Rhizopuspepsin
Pepstatin	P4-P4'	Iva-Val-Val-Sta-CHOH-CH2-CO-NH-Ala-Sta	1	Endothiapepsin
L-363,564	P6-P3'	Boc-His-Pro-Phe-His-Sta-CHOH-CH2-CO-NH-Leu-Phe	40	Endothiapepsin
H-189	P6-P4'	Pro-His-Pro-Phe-His-Sta-CHOH-CH2-CO-NH-Val-Ile-His-Lys	1	Endothiapepsin
L-364,099	P6-P3'	Iva-His-Pro-Phe-His-Cha-CHOH-CH2-CO-NH-Leu-Phe	420	Endothiapepsin
PD125754	P4-P3'	Boc-Phe-XGly-Cha-CHOH-CH2-CO-NH-Leu-Dmab	16180	Endothiapepsin
PD130693	P3-P1'	Dms-Pro-Bmt-CHOH-CH2-CO-NH-Mba	69	Renin (human)
CP-85,339	P4-P1'	Pro-Phe-Mcy-Cha-CHOH-CO-O-CH(CH3)2	ND	Rhizopuspepsin
Inhibitor2	P6-P3'	Iva-His-Pro-Phe-His-Sta-CHOH-CH2-CO-NH-Leu-Phe	200	Endothiapepsin
Phesta-1		Phe-Leu-Glu-Pha-Arg-Leu	ND	Endothiapepsin
Phesta-2		Thr-Phe-Asn-Ala-Pha-Arg-Glu	ND	Endothiapepsin

Statine analogues

CP-69,799	Boc-Phe-His-Cha-CHOH-CH2-N(i-Bu)-Lys-Phe	P4–P3'	270	Endothiapepsin
CP-69,799	Boc-Phe-His-Cha-CHOH-CH2-N(i-Bu)-Lys-Phe	P4–P3'		Rhizopuspepsin
PD130328	Boc-Phe-His-Pst-Mba		780	Endothiapepsin
PD135040	Smo-Phe-His-Dfs-Mor		ND	Endothiapepsin
PD133450	Smo-Phe-Scc-Gcl		6	Endothiapepsin
CP-80,794	Mor-Smc-Nor	P2–P1'	ND	Endothiapepsin
StaF2	Iva-Val-Val-Sta-CHOH-CF2-CO-NH-Me	P4–P1'	10	Penicillopepsin
Cyc-disulfide	Ibu-His-Pro-Phe-Cys-Sta-CHOH-CH2-CO-NH-Leu-Phe-Tea	P6–P3'	17	Rhizopuspepsin

Difluoroketone

CP-81,282	Mor-Phe-Nle-Cha-CH(OH)2-CF2-CO-NH-Me	P4–P1'	11	Endothiapepsin
CP-82,218	Pip-Phe-Nle-Cha-CH(OH)2-CF2-CO-NH-Me	P4–P1'		Rhizopuspepsin
StoF2	Iva-Val-Val-Sta-CH(OH)2-CF2-CO-NH-Me	P4–P1'	1	Penicillopepsin
GLYCOLS				
A63218	Etoc-Tyr-Leu-Cha-CHOH-CHOH-i-Bu	P4–P1'	10000*	Pepsin (porcine)
A66702	Etoc-Tyr-Leu-Leu-CHOH-CHOH-i-Bu	P4–P1'	10000*	Pepsin (porcine)
A62095	Etoc-Leu-Leu-Cha-CHOH-CHOH-i-Bu	P4–P1'		Pepsin (porcine)

Phosphorous-containing

Phosphinate	Iva-Val-Val-Sta-PO2H-CH2-CO-O-Et	P4–P1'	22	Penicillopepsin
Iva-Phosphonate	Iva-Val-Val-Leu-PO2H-O-Phe-OMe	P4–P1'	2.8	Penicillopepsin
Cbz-Phosphonate	Cbz-Ala-Ala-Leu-PO2H-O-Phe-OMe	P4–P1'	1600	Penicillopepsin

[a] Dhis = D-histidine, X = cyclohexylalanine, Nle = norleucine, Smo = sulfonylmorpholino Mba = methyl butylamine, Aza = azahomostatine, Pst = phosphostatine, Mor = morpholino, Ome = oxymethyl, Nor = norstatine, Boc = butyloxycarbonyl, Pha = phenylstatine, Iva = isovaleryl, Bnp = bis(1-napthyl methyl) acetyl, Chs = cyclohexyl statine, DMS = dimethylaminosulfonyl, Boc = *tert*-butyloxycarbonyl, Bmt = *N*-methyl thiourea analogue of lysine, Dfs = difluorocyclohexylstatone, Scc, Smc = analogues of cysteine, Gcl = glycol analogue of cyclohexylstatine.
[b] Values reported were either Ki or IC50.

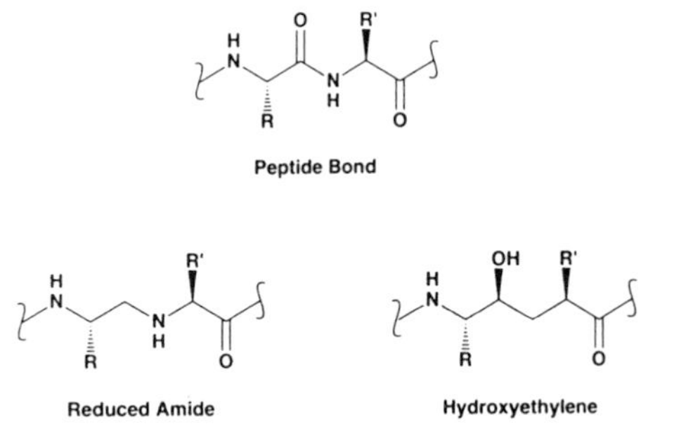

Fig. 10.7 Nonhydrolyzable transition-state isosteres as inhibitors for aspartic proteinases (for renin and as well as HIV proteases). Courtesy of Dr. Alex Wlodawer.

7.3.2 INHIBITOR BINDING AS REVEALED BY CRYSTALLOGRAPHY. The active site of all aspartic proteases is a long shallow cleft formed by the N and C terminal domains. There are two psi-type loops, each contributed by one domain, whose side chains spread across the active site. At the center of the active site there are two aspartates in close proximity, held together by a fireman grip-like hydrogen bonding pattern (164). A water molecule is found to be bound between the aspartates in all the native crystallographic structures examined. There is a hairpin loop hovering over the active site, to act as a flap that closes on top of the inhibitor after complexation. The crystallo-

graphic studies of aspartic proteinases and their complexes with many renin inhibitors have been reviewed (178, 179). Here we will not analyze such structures and complexes in detail, but will focus on their general outcome and the lessons learned in the process of discovering potent renin inhibitors to be developed into drugs.

In all these structures (Table 10.1) the inhibitors bind in an extended conformation (Fig. 10.8) and form an additional β-sheet in the active site. In almost all cases, the peptide carbonyl oxygens and the amide nitrogens of the inhibitors make hydrogen bonds with the same atoms of the enzyme, especially those in the psi loop and in the flap.

7.3.3 STRUCTURAL INSIGHTS BASED ON STUDIES WITH INHIBITORS. The H-series inhibitors, the first used in structural studies, proved to be of great value in mapping the active site and in identifying the conformation of the inhibitors and their binding interactions. These studies provided information for further modifications. Most of the renin inhibitors have been developed based on the minimal substrate sequence of angiotensinogen, by modifying the scissile Leu–Val bond to produce various nonhydrolyzable analogs (Fig. 10.7). The resulting compounds have nanomolar inhibition values (for reviews, see 180–182). The first crystallographic structure of the inhibitor (H189, in which the central amide was reduced to –CH$_2$–NH–) complexed with rhizopuspepsin and endothiapepsin, disclosed the active site of the enzyme as well as the subsites of interaction very clearly. Incorporation of the hydroxyethylene moiety –CHOH–CH$_2$– in place of –CO–NH–, was found to produce the most potent inhibitor (H261) (Table 10.1), with a nanomolar inhibition value (IC$_{50}$ = 0.7 nM) (159, 160). The crystallographic structure of H261 with endothiapepsin, resolved at the very high resolution of 1.6 Å, provided

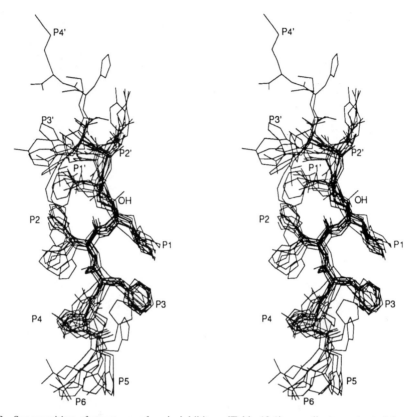

Fig. 10.8 Superposition of structures of renin inhibitors (Table 10.1), coordinates extracted from PDB.

valuable information regarding the interactions that are necessary for the side chains of the inhibitor to be fitted into the subsites of the enzyme (183). Figure 10.9a shows the active site of endothiapepsin as a surface and the H261 inhibitor as a bone model and Figure 9b shows the active site of human renin complexed with an inhibitor, CP-85339. The factors responsible for the lower binding affinity of this compound were apparent when the crystallographic structures of the statine containing inhibitors were solved and compared.

Replacement of the P1–P1' residues by statine (–CHOH–CH2–CO–NH–) into the central region of the octapeptide (in place of the residues preceding and following the scissile bond) yielded poor inhibitors (with affinities in the micro molar range), while modification of the length and side chains

of the central region yielded higher potency analogs (for a review see ref. 185). Crystallographic analysis of some of these inhibitors revealed that the statine residue occupies the two subsites of the enzyme that normally interact with the Leu and Val residues of other inhibitors, mimicking a dipeptide analogue (186). Unlike the statine containing inhibitors, the hydroxyethylene analogs do not introduce this frame shift. One common factor observed in all complexes of the enzymes with the modified peptides is that the side chains of these inhibitors occupy the enzyme subsites well and the atoms attached to the carbon-α atoms of the inhibitor adjust their positions to fit the enzyme active site. Another important aspect is that the hydroxyl group in the central region was found to be tightly bound to the active site aspartates, sug-

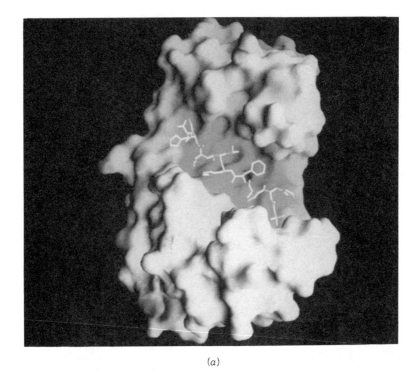

(a)

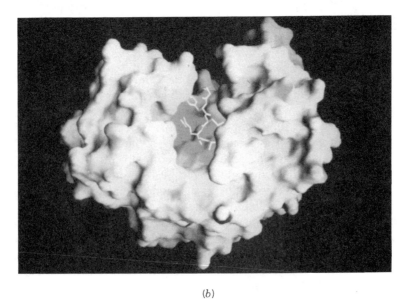

(b)

Fig. 10.9 (a) The molecular surface of endothiapepsin molecule color coded by electrostatic potential. The view is directly into the active site and the inhibitor H261, a hydroxy ethylene nanomolar binder is present in a bond representation. The intense red color portrays the highly negatively charged nature of the active site, typical of an acid proteinase. For the sake of clarity the residues of the flat region were removed. (b) Similar representation of a renin molecule complexed with a nanomolar inhibitor (CP-85339). Surface pictures were drawn by the program GRASP (184). See also color plates.

gesting that the hydroxyl group mimics the tetrahedral intermediate of natural substrates. These studies revealed that closer the analog is to the putative intermediate of hydrolysis [$-C(OH)_2NH^{2+}$], the greater its potency as an inhibitor.

In spite of its hydroxyl group in the central region, however, statine-containing compounds exhibit inferior potency, probably because statine is an atom shorter than the dipeptide and thus does not fit optimally in the enzyme active site. This leads to the conclusion that each subsite of the enzyme has to be optimally filled and that a hydroxyl moiety should be present in the inhibitor to interact with the active site aspartates and mimic the tetrahedral intermediate.

Inhibitors containing an amino alcohol ($-CHOH-CH_2-NH-$) group in the central region were designed by combining elements from the aminomethylene and hydroxyethylene isostere inhibitors. Although they have an NH group as an addition to the hydroxyethylene moiety in the central region, they were found to be less potent than H261, BW625 is an *R*-isomer with Leu–CHOH–CH2–NH–Val–Ile–Phe, and BW624 is the corresponding *S*-isomer. The IC$_{50}$ values of the *R*-form is 6 μM and that of the *S* form is 100 μM. Both of these compounds have been complexed with endothiapepsin and crystallographically analyzed (187).

An increase in potency has been obtained by substituting the side chain of the Leu preceding the scissile bond with a cyclohexylmethyl group, giving a better inhibitor than the isobutyl analog (188). Crystallographic structures containing this side chain have been determined (189–191). A comparison of their structures shows that the cyclohexylmethyl side chain makes more extensive van der Waals interactions with the enzyme subsite than the Leu side chain, and is accommodated well within the subsite. By modifying the Phe located two residues upstream of the modi-

fied Leu to naphthylalanine or bis(1-naphthylmethyl)acetyl, inhibitors with nanomolar affinities have been produced. One such inhibitor has been complexed with endothiapepsin and the structure of the complex has been solved (189). Since the modified Leu has a bulky cyclohexyl side chain and the modified Phe has a bulky naphthyl group, the subsites of the enzyme in contact with this side of the inhibitor were found to be completely filled. Significant conformational changes of the enzyme side chains forming the subsite that interacts with the modified Phe of the inhibitor have also been observed.

When orally administered, these peptide-based inhibitors are susceptible to enzymic degradation, so that the half life *in vivo* is often short. For example, the Phe-His bond is susceptible to cleavage by chymotrypsin. Modifications of the Phe or His side chains or their replacement with residues forming a nonhydrolyzable bond have been suggested. Replacing the Phe with *O*-methyl-Tyr and naphthyl derivatives was successful in making the inhibitors resistant to chymotrypsin. Another alternative is to modify the peptide bond between the Phe and His with a hydroxyethylene moiety, as in the inhibitor PD125754. The crystallographic structures of both these types of inhibitors have been determined (189). Further modifications resulted in the development of highly potent inhibitors, such as the difluorostatone-containing tripeptide inhibitor (CP81,218) which has an IC$_{50}$ of 1 nM. The crystallographic structure of CP81,218 complexed with endothiapepsin provided more information (Fig. 10.8*b*). The scissile bond surrogate, an electrophilic ketone, is hydrated in the complex. The pro-(*R*) (statinelike) hydroxyl of the tetrahedral carbonyl hydrate is hydrogen bonded to both the active site aspartates. This observation of a tetrahedral carbonyl carbon in the active site provided a basis for the model of a tetrahedral intermediate in the aspartic proteinase-mediated cleavage of the amide bond (190) and also supports the idea that the closer to the tetrahedral intermediate, better is the inhibition constant. Similar crystallographic exercises on rhizopuspepsin and penicillopepsin have been subsequently completed and confirm the above hypothesis (191, 192).

Most of the above tight binding tripeptide-like inhibitors have poor bioavailability. However, the structural data obtained revealed that the N-terminal residues are solvent accessible. By substituting polar groups at the N-termini of the inhibitors, water soluble, orally active compounds were generated. For example, amine containing N-terminal groups resulted in dramatic improvements in bioavailability. Some of these inhibitors were found to have high oral bioavailability in several animal species including primates, a significant achievement in peptide-like structures, where digestion, lack of absorption, or rapid excretion from the body often prohibit good oral characteristics (193).

7.3.4 IMPORTANT CONCLUSIONS. Regardless of the modifications in the structure of inhibitors and the consequent variations in inhibition constants, a specific set of hydrogen bonding interactions is conserved and their perturbation could lead to less potent compounds. The enzyme can accommodate a slightly lower or higher number of atoms within its active site, but such modifications may result in inhibitors with lower potency. An optimal number of atoms have to be fitted into each subsite of the enzyme active site, so that their backbone atoms are able to form the necessary set of hydrogen bonds. The potency of an inhibitor does not correlate with the hydrogen bonding interactions alone, but depends even more on the hydrophobic forces involved in its interactions with each enzyme subsite and the energy required to remove solvating

solvent (water) from portions of the inhibitor bound to the enzyme.

In many inhibitors, a hydroxyl group at the scissile bond carbonyl oxygen position is an essential factor for high potency. Analogues with even higher potency can be generated by mimicking the putative intermediate of hydrolysis. The water molecules observed in the vicinity of the aspartates that are within the active site of the unliganded enzyme have to be displaced; in other words the central region of the enzyme active site has to be desolvated to achieve better binding. To avoid hydrolysis by chymotrypsin, it is necessary to introduce additional modifications, as discussed above. In an aqueous environment the molecule is in a state of dynamic motion and it is possible that parts of its structure have to move to carry out functional aspects, as is observed in the flap and domain movements of aspartic proteinases. These flexibilities have to be taken into account in the design of inhibitor side chain modifications.

Specific interactions essential for the recognition of the substrate or the inhibitor by the enzyme and the atoms involved in such interactions should be retained. Based on crystallographic and biochemical data, a potent inhibitor is expected to have side chains resembling a Phe-His-Cyclohexylmethyl-hydroxyl group and a terminating group similar to an isobutyl group. A similar compound has been synthesized and showed nanomolar potency (182). Terminal amine-like groups have also been added, to provide better interactions with the solvent (194, 195), leading to the discovery of renin inhibitors that can be administered orally (193).

7.4 Design of Drugs for the Treatment of AIDS

Inhibiting the HIV protease (HIV PR) is one of the many strategies proposed to cure or arrest the process of AIDS. The HIV protease is essential for viral assembly and maturation (196–199). HIV reverse transcriptase and integrase are two other enzymes whose structures can be used to design drugs for antiviral therapy. The 3-dimensional structures of HIV protease and reverse transcriptase are known and efforts are underway to determine the structure of the integrase. The design of inhibitors for the HIV protease has been a major focus in many pharmaceutical and academic laboratories. Because the HIV protease has been identified as a member of the aspartic proteinase family, progress has been achieved quickly. The information derived from the design of potent, small and bioavailable renin inhibitors based on the three dimensional structures of aspartic proteases has facilitated the efforts to design inhibitors for the HIV protease.

7.4.1 CRYSTALLOGRAPHIC STUDIES TO DESIGN INHIBITORS FOR THE HIV PROTEASE.

The crystallographic structure determination of the HIV protease by Alex Wladower and his colleagues started a world wide effort to search for better HIV protease inhibitors. Even though many other groups were able to determine the crystallographic structure of HIV protease, Wladower and colleagues made their structural results available to the community. As of now there are about 175 crystallographic structures of HIV protease in complex with inhibitors (200). Excellent reviews on the structure and function of the HIV protease and its inhibitors have been published (182, 200–202) and the readers are referred to them for detailed information.

The structure of the HIV protease bear similarity to the aspartic proteinases and has the same two aspartates at the center of the active site. The major difference is that the HIV protease forms homodimers and as a consequence the active site is symmetrically structured (Fig. 10.10). Three different classes of HIV protease inhibitors are reported in the literature: (1) nonhydrolyzable transition state isosteres, similar to renin inhibitors; (2) pseudosymmetrical and C2-symmetrical compounds and (3) nonpeptidic inhibitors. Table 10.2 lists some of the inhibitors whose structures have been solved by crystallography and Figure 10.11 shows a superposition of some of them. Apart from conventional non-hydrolyzable inhibitors that mimic the transition state, symmetric inhibitors have been designed based on the C2-symmetry of the active site (Fig. 10.12). Software-aided drug design techniques have helped the identification of novel nonpeptidic lead compounds (204). Various structural features of the HIV protease were derived from the voluminous data published on inhibitor-protease complexes.

The first crystallographic structure of a reduced amide hexapeptide (MVT101) complexed to the HIV protease (205) led to the identification of the subsites of the active site. Since hydroxyethylene-containing inhibitors were observed to have nanomolar affinities for aspartic proteinases, compounds with hydroxylates at the scissile bond were designed for the HIV protease (Table 10.2). The hydroxyethylene containing octapeptide U85548e inhibits the enzyme at a concentration of less than $1\,nM$. Crystallographic results revealed that the hydroxyl group binds to the aspartates in the active site, similar to H261. This result confirmed the hypothesis that for increasing the affinity of an aspartic protease inhibitor, an hydroxyl group is the best. The next phase was to trim the inhibitor to a smaller size. This was achieved in the case of two short tripeptide mimetics, Ro-31-8588 and L-689,502 (206, 207). These are small and highly potent inhibitors, effective at less than nanomolar concentrations. The structural information derived from these studies elucidated the essential interactions of smaller peptide-mimetics with the HIV protease. Their increased potency is attrib-

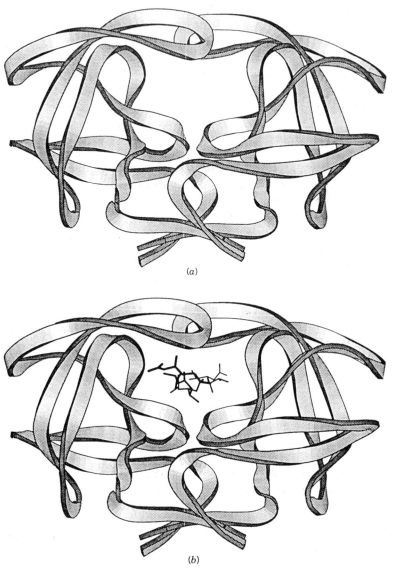

(a)

(b)

Fig. 10.10 Ribbon representation of the structure of the (a) HIV-PR enzyme and that of an (b) inhibitor complexed. The coordinates were extracted from PDB (HIV-protease complex with acetyl pepstatin, 5 HVP.PDB) (see ref. 203).

uted to the hydroxylate group in the residue preceding the scissile bond and to the bulky terminal groups. The interaction of these groups with the enzyme supports the theory that bulky termini improve the binding. The length of the peptide inhibitors can vary. For inhibitors containing an hydroxyl group on the residue preceding the scissile bond, truncation is possible to produce tetrapeptide compounds. For inhibitors other than the hydroxyethylene type, truncations that produce peptides of less than four residues lead to a reduction in potency. In general the optimum inhibitors are hydroxyethylene-based peptidomimetrics that comprise the two res-

Table 10.2 Various Nonhydrolyzable Transition State Isosters as HIV-Protease Inhibitors

Name	Subsites	Inhibitor[a]	Ki/IC50
Reduce amide			
MVT-101	P3-P3'	Ac-Thr-Ile-Nle-CH2NH-Nle-Gln-Arg	760 nM
Hydroxyethylene			
U-85548E	P5-P3'	Val-Ser-Gln-Asn-Leu-CH(OH)CH2-Val-Ile-Val	<1 nM
Ro-31-8588	P2-P3'	Boc-Cha-CH(OH)CH2-Val-Ile-Epy	0.3 nM
L-689,502	P2-P2'	Boc-Phe-CH(OH)CH2-Emt-Ahi	0.45 nM
JG-365	P4-P3'	Ac-Ser-Leu-Asn-Phe-CH(OH)CH2-NH-Pro-Ile-Val-Ome	0.24 nM
Dihydroxy			
U-75875	P3-P3'	Noa-His-Cha-CH(OH)CH(OH)-Val-Ile-Amp	<1 nM
A-77003	P3-P3'	Pyr-Val-Phe-CH(OH)CH(OH)-Phe'-Val'-Pyr'	0.15 nM
Symmetric			
A-74704	P3-P3'	Cbz-Val-Phe-CH(OH)-Phe'-Val'-Cbz'	4.5
L-700,417	P2-P2'	Ahi'-Phe'-CH(OH)-Phe-Ahi	0.65
Statine			
Pepstatin	P3-P3'	Iva-Val-Sta-CH(OH)CH2-(CO-NH)-Ala-Sta	1
Acetylpepstatin	P3-P3'	Ac-Val-Val-Sta-CHOH-CH2-Ala-Sta	1.1
PS-1	P5-P5'	Pro-Pro-Gln-Val-Psta-CH(OH)CH2-(CO-NH)-Ala-Gln-Pro-Pro	<1
AG-2	P4-P3'	Ser-Phe-Asn-Sta-CH(OH)CH2-(CO-NH)-Gln-Ile	0.5
AG-2	P4-P4'	Ser-Gln-Asn-Sta-CH(OH)CH2-(CO-NH)-Ile-Val-Gln	0.23

[a] Ac = acetyl, OMe = methoxy, Boc = *t*-butoxycarbonyl, Cbz = carbobenzyloxy, Iva = isovaleryl, Sta = statine, Psta = phenylstatine, Cha = cyclohexylalanine, Epy = ethylpyridine, Noa = 1-naphthoxyacetyl, Amp = aminomethyl-2-piridine, Pyr = (*N*-methyl-2-methylaminopyridyl)carbonyl, Ahi = 1-amino-2-hydroxyindan, Emt = *O*-ethylmorpholinyltyrosine, Prime indicates reversal of amino acid linkage.

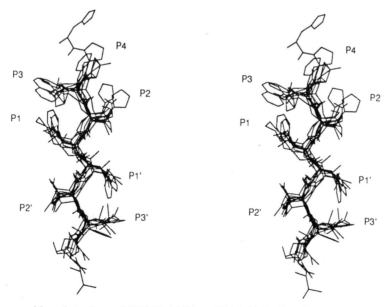

Fig. 10.11 Superposition of structures of HIV-PR inhibitors (Table 10.2). Coordinates were extracted from PDB.

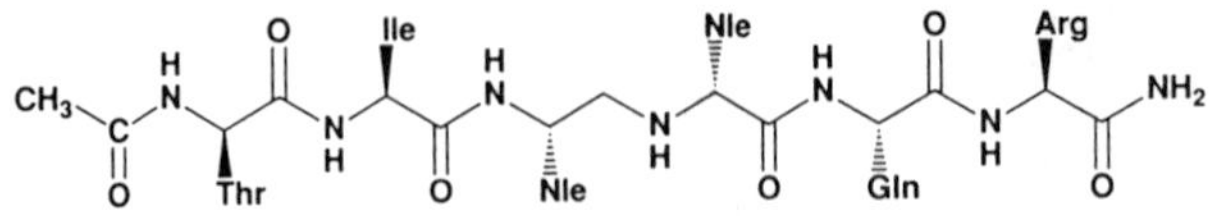

MVT-101
K_i = 780 nM

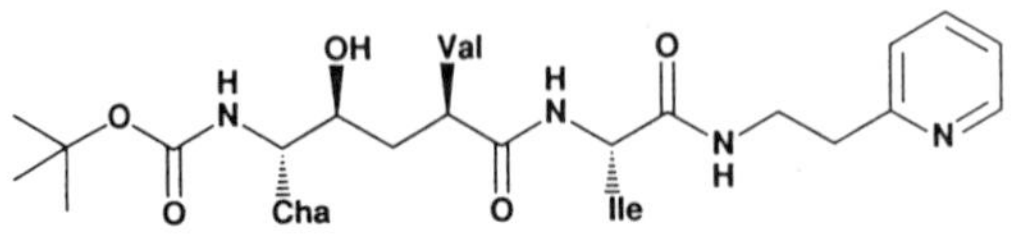

Ro-31-8588
K_i = 0.3 nM

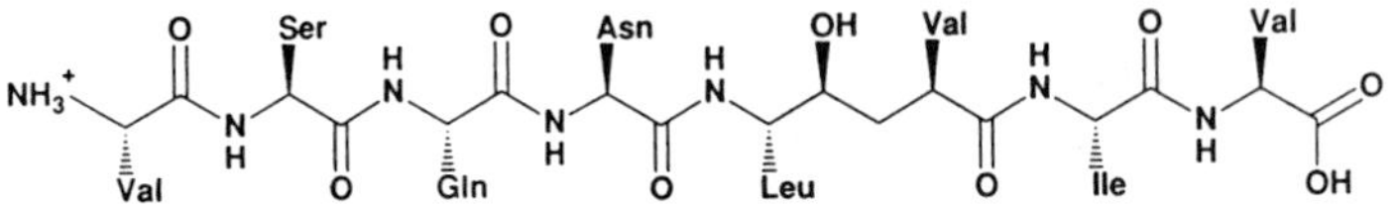

U-85548e
K_i <1 nM

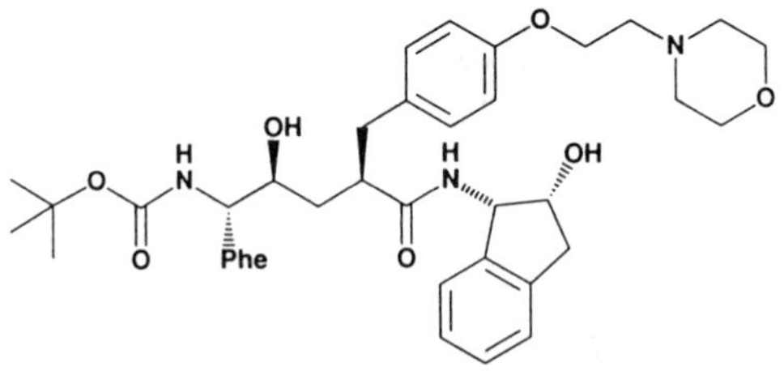

L-689,502
IC_{50} = 0.45 nM

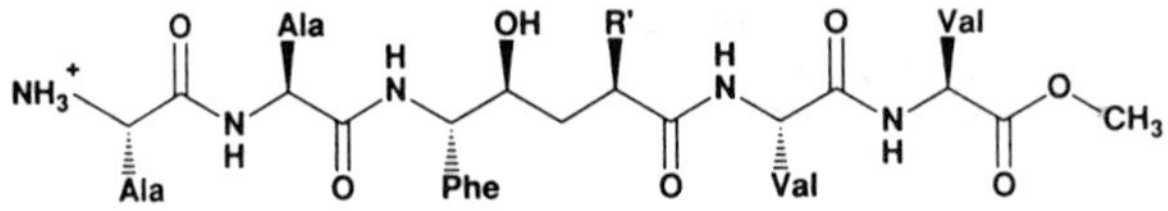

SKB-V	R	IC_{50} (nM)
a	H	4.0
b	Me	3.0
c	nPr	1.2
e	Bz	0.6

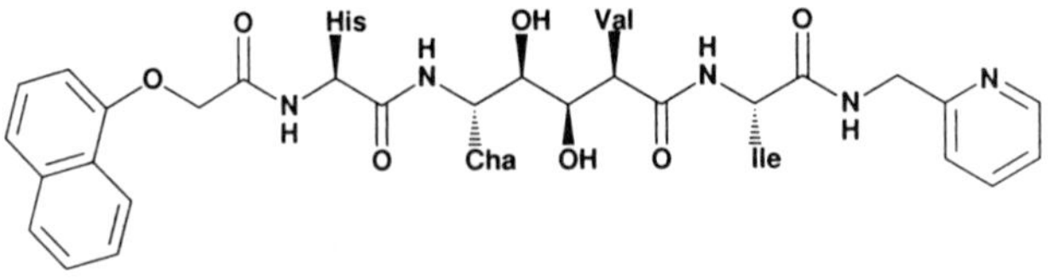

U-75875
K_i = <1.0 nM

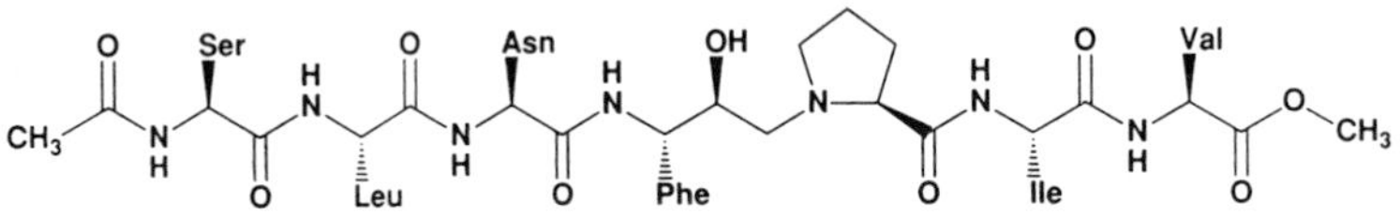

JG-365
K_i = 0.66 nM

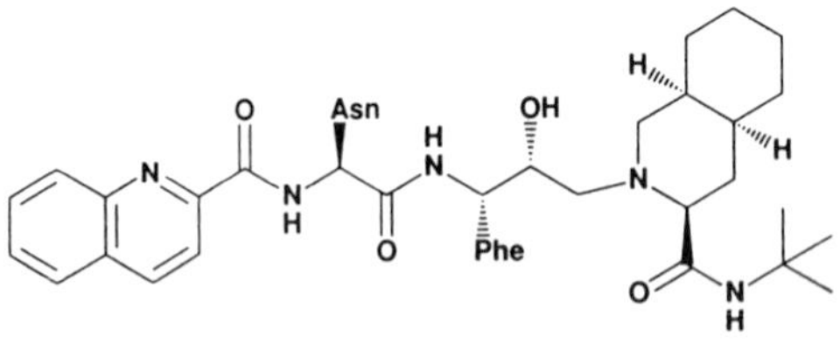

Ro-31-8959
IC_{50} < 0.4 nM

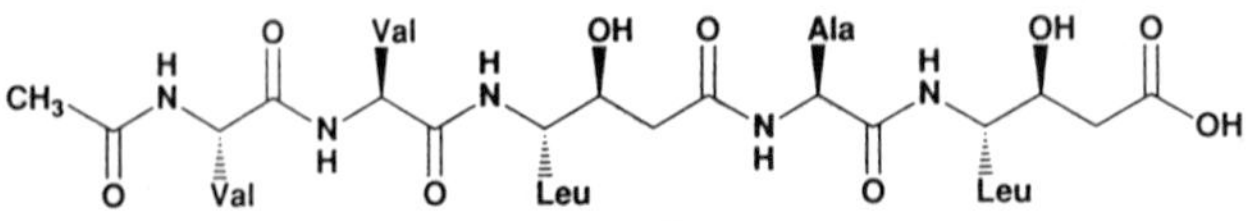

Acetylpepstatin
K_i = 20 nM

(*a*)

Fig. 10.12 (*a*) Chemical structures of nonhydrolyzable transition-state isostere inhibitors for HIV PR. Courtesy of Dr. Alex Wlodawer; (*b*) Chemical structures of symmetry based inhibitors for HIV PR. Courtesy of Dr. Alex Wlodawer.

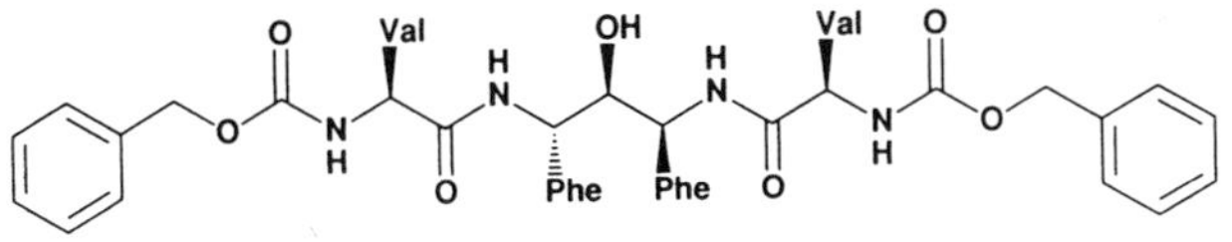

A-74704
IC_{50} = 3 nM

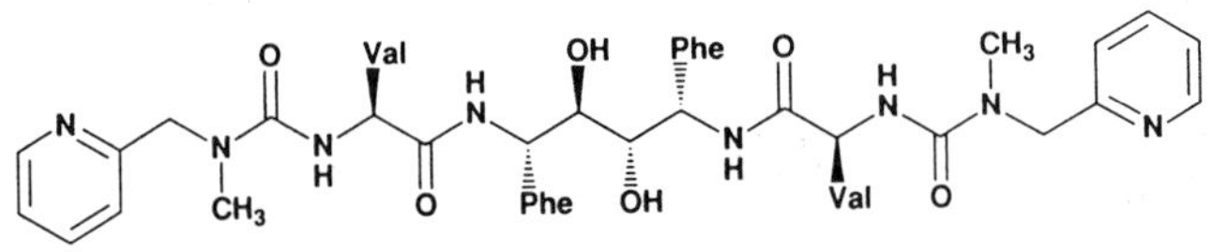

A-77003
IC_{50} = .15 nM

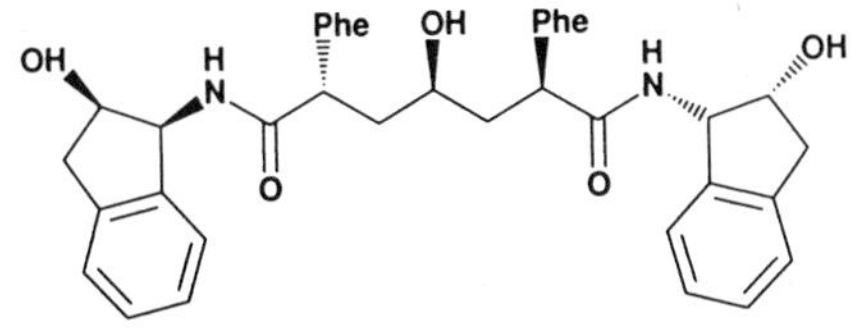

L-700,417
IC_{50} = 0.67 nM

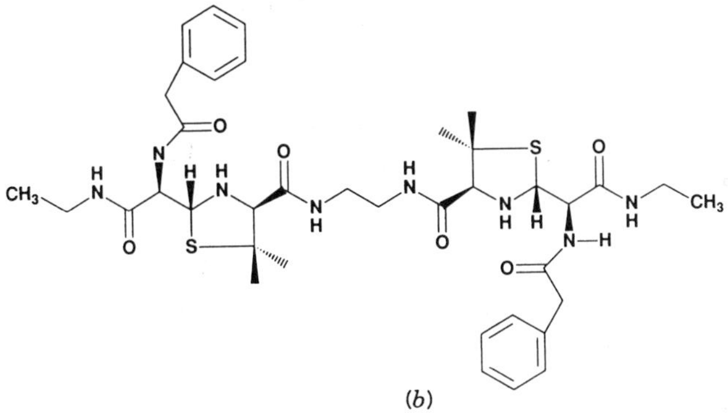

GR116624X
IC_{50} = 4.8 nM

(*b*)

Fig. 10.12 (*Continued*)

idues preceding and the two residues following the scissile bond, with large hydrophobic side chains (Phe) in the central positions and Val as terminal residues.

The crystallographic structures also indicated that a minimum number of hydrogen bonds are necessary for an inhibitor to bind to the HIV protease. A detailed analysis of hydrogen bonding in the HIV protease was reported by Appelt in his review (207). Hydrogen bond formation by a carbonyl oxygen at P2 to the amide nitrogen at P2′, is a basic condition for the binding. Increasing the number of hydrogen bonds, however, does not necessarily produce higher potency inhibitors. The design of rigid inhibitors more tightly constrained according to the subsite symmetry is preferred for entropic reasons. However, compounds with such a geometry will be difficult to synthesize. In some cases bulkier groups at the termini improve the inhibition values and in some cases they do not. Substitution of bulkier groups on the terminal residues may not produce potent inhibitors if these groups interfere with the interactions that are necessary to recognize and hold the inhibitor in the active site.

In their review article, Wlodawer and Erickson tried to determine whether symmetry is important in inhibitor design. Due to the symmetric nature of the homodimers of HIV protease and the C2 symmetry observed in its active site, a reasonable design strategy would be to synthesize symmetrical inhibitors, to provide high selectivity and potency (Table 10.2). However, crystallographic studies revealed that the atoms of the inhibitor within the active site are symmetrically positioned, even if the inhibitor is not symmetric. This has been attributed to the flexibility of the peptide-based inhibitors. Analysis of the conformations of various inhibitors revealed that their ϕ and ψ values vary widely from one another, but the side chains are always well positioned within the active site, indicating that the enzyme forces the bound inhibitor to occupy the sub sites and maximize the hydrogen bonding interactions. Even though the symmetrically related residues are found to occupy symmetrically equivalent subsites, the spanning of some of the side chains occupying many subsites lead to an apparent breakdown of subsite symmetry. So it is believed that the design for symmetric inhibitors, even though it is an exciting theme, will not prove to be of greater value than conventional design.

7.4.2 SOFTWARE-BASED INHIBITOR DESIGN FOR HIV PROTEASE.

As discussed in section 5, computer algorithms can be used in probing the active site of a molecule and can suggest lead compounds based on the structures available in small molecular databases. This idea was exploited in identifying a small molecular compound capable of binding to HIV protease (204). The program DOCK was used to identify a lead compound, bromperidol (Figure 10.13). Haloperidol, an analog of bromperidol, inhibited the HIV protease with an inhibition constant of 100 μM (204). Subsequent modifications produced a compound, UCSF8, with an improved binding constant of 15 μM. The crystallographic structure of

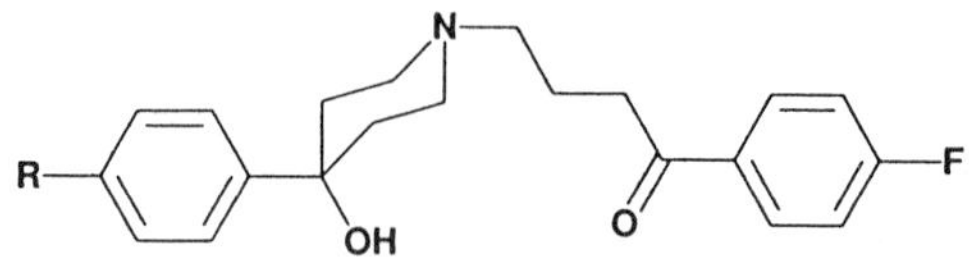

Bromperidol: R = Br
Haloperidol: R = Cl

Fig. 10.13 Non-peptide based inhibitors of HIV-protease, discovered by the program DOCK. UCSF8 is a modification of this bromperidol. Courtesy of Dr. Alex Wlodawer.

UCSF8 complexed with HIV protease has been solved (208), revealing that the flap of the enzyme, which usually folds back to cover the peptide-based inhibitors, does not do so in this case. This is an interesting observation, since the previous studies on peptide based inhibitor-enzyme complexes suggested that the movement of the flap is crucial for the inhibitor to bind. More crystallographic structures of similar complexes are necessary to elucidate the mechanism of binding of these compounds.

Traditional screening methods have also been successful in suggesting novel lead compounds. Humber et al. (209) have identified a C2-symmetric penicillin dimer. The crystallographic structure of this dimer in complex with the HIV protease has been solved (210) and reveal that even though the binding mode of this dimer inhibitor is quite different from that of conventional peptide based inhibitors, the inhibitor is still able to occupy optimally the subsites of the enzyme active site.

7.4.3 TYPICAL EXAMPLE OF STRUCTURE-AIDED DRUG DESIGN.

A typical example of a structure-aided drug design approach by applying the above said techniques has been reported recently. Lam et al. (211) from Dupont Merck have identified novel, nonpeptide inhibitors for HIV protease. On the basis of the 3-D structural information such as the active site conformation and the presence of a bound water molecule (as observed in many crystallographic studies of HIV-PR), the computational search of 3-D databases using a simplest pharmacophore provided them a clue to design novel nonpeptide cyclic ureas. Based on this basic structure, compounds that are highly selective, with relatively low molecular weight and high bioavailability were synthesized and characterized by X-ray crystallography.

Appelt, Wladower and Erickson conclude their review with a remark that is also appropriate here. By employing thermodynamic data (like that of the association constant, enthalpy, entropy, heat capacity and stoichiometry of binding) in conjunction with structural information, the factors that influence the binding of an inhibitor to an enzyme can be thoroughly understood. These data when properly utilized will lead to the design of more effective inhibitors, to be used as drugs.

8 LESSONS LEARNED

The following lessons have emerged from the studies carried out so far, to be borne in mind for a successful structure-based drug design attempt. For crystallographic studies, crystallization expertise is a must and continuous efforts to produce crystals of increasingly better quality should be maintained. Because computers and graphics play a major part in this approach, upgrading computer hardware and software dramatically improves efficiency and productivity. A combination of different strategies to reach a goal should always be considered. For example, novel enzyme inhibitors can be designed on the basis of the structure of substrates or by carrying out computational and graphic searches to identify fragments that fit into the enzyme binding site and can then be joined to form a single inhibitor molecule. Compounds that affect the activity of an enzyme by binding to sites other than the active site may also be searched for. A key element in

the success of drug design is the collaboration between structural scientists and medicinal chemists, so that the understanding of structure-based functional aspects may be complemented by intuition and imagination in designing useful chemical modifications. It is also important to continuously update the information on which the design process is based, as new information on the target molecule becomes available. Although structural information provides a rational basis in the design of smaller and better fitting compounds, the full potency of a drug has to be evaluated by designing assays to measure its metabolic stability and its efficiency in penetrating cell membranes. So far, only a few peptidominetics have been approved for clinical trials (212, 213). However, as more data are generated by structure-aided drug design, the procedures will be improved and this relatively new approach will become increasingly effective.

ACKNOWLEDGMENTS

The author wishes to thank Tom Blundell, Alex Wladower, Andrej Sali, V. N. Balaji, John Cooper, V. Dhanaraj, Peter Whittle, John Overington, Dennis Hoover, Kevin Parris, Elya Kurktchi and Alex Okun for their help in making this manuscript possible. The author wishes to extend special thanks to Elena Pasquale, for critically reading this manuscript and offering many valuable suggestions and to Jonas Hajdu for supplying the diffraction photographs. Sincere thanks also to the authors of the many reviews that were consulted: Max Perutz, C. R. Beddell, J. N. Champness, R. M. Hyde, G. R. Marshall, S. W. Fesik, M. Navia, J. Erickson, Paula Fitzgerald, Sherin Abdel-Meguid, and K. Appelt whose splendid efforts formed the foundation of this review.

REFERENCES

1. M. Perutz, *Protein Structure: New Approaches to Disease and Therapy*, W. H. Freeman & Co., New York, 1992.

2. C. R. Beddell, in The Design of Drugs to Macromolecular Targets, John Wiley & Sons, Inc., New York, 1992.

3. P. J. Whittle and T. L. Blundell, Protein-structure based drug design, in press, 1994.

4. M. A. Navia and M. A. Murcko, "Use of Structural Information in Drug Design," *Curr. Opin. Struct. Biol.*, **2**, 202–210 (1992).

5. D. Craig, D. A. Gay, J. Parello, E. Ruoslahti, and K. R. Ely, "Crystals of the Cell-binding Module of Fibronectin Obtained from a Series of Recombinant Fragments Differing in Length," *J. Mol. Biol.*, 237 (1994).

6. B. Veerapandian, G. L. Gilliland, R. Raag, A. L. Svensson, Y. Masui, Y. Hirai, and T. L. Poulos, "Functional Implications of Interleukin-1β Based on the Three-Dimensional Structure," *Proteins, Structure, Function, and Genetics*, **12**, 10–23 (1992).

7. T.L. Blundell and L. N. Johnson, *Protein Crystallography*, Academic Press, New York, 1976.

8. Crystallization Research Tools, Hampton Research, *List of Robotic Instruments*, **4-1**, 16 (1994).

9. J. Jancaric and S.H. Kim, "Sparse Matrix Sampling: A Screening Method for Crystallization of Proteins," *J. Appl. Cryst.*, **24**, 409–411 (1991).

10. R. Cudney, S. Patel, and A. McPherson, *5th ICCBM*, San Diego, Calif., 1993.

11. G. L. Gilliland, D. M. Bickham, and M. M. Tung, *NIST/CARB Biological Macromolecule Crystallization Database*, Version 2.0.

12. A. Roussel, L. Serre, M. Frey, and J. C. Fontecilla-Camps, "Rapid Access to an Updated Biological Macromolecule Crystallization Data Base through Artificial Intelligence," *J. Cryst. Growth*, **106**, 405–409 (1990).

13. A. McPherson, *Preparation and Analysis of Protein Crystals*, John Wiley & Sons, Inc., New York, 1982.

14. A. Ducruix and R. Giege, *Crystallization of Nucleic Acids and Proteins: Practical Approach*, IRL Press/Oxford University Press, New York, 1992.

15. C. W. Carter, *Protein and Nucleic Acid Crystallization Methods*, Academic Press, San Diego, Calif., 1990, p. 127.

16. H. Michel, *Crystallization of Membrane Proteins*, CRC Press, Boca Raton, Flo., 1991.

17. T. A. Jones, "A Graphics Model Building and Refinement System for Macromolecules," *J. Appl. Crystallogr.*, **1**, 268–272 (1978).

18. T. A. Jones and S. Thirup, Using Known Substructures in Protein Model Building and Crystallography, *EMBO J.*, **5**, 819–822 (1986).

19. A. T. Brunger, *X-PLOR Version 3.1. A System for X-Ray Crystallography and NMR*. Yale University Press, New Haven, Conn., 1992. A complete user's guide to X-PLOR.

20. A. T. Brunger, "Free R Value: A Novel Statistical Quantity for Assessing the Accuracy of Crystal Structures," *Nature*, 355, 472–475 (1992).

21. B. C. Finzel, "Software for Macromolecular Cystallography: A User's Overview," *Curr. Opin. Struct. Biol.*, **3**, 741–747 (1993).

22. F. C. Bernstein, T. F. Koetzle, G. J. B. Williams, E. F. Meyer, M. D. Brice, J. R. Rodgers, O. Kennard, T. Shimanouchi, and M. Tasumi, "The Protein Data Bank: A Computer-Based Archival File for Macromolecular Structures," *J. Mol. Biol.*, **112**, 535–542 (1977).

23. E. E. Abola, F. C. Bernstin, S. H. Bryant, T. F. Koetzle, and J. Weng, (1987). "Protein Data Bank," in *Crystallographic Databases, Information Content, Software Systems, Scientific Applications*, (F. H. Allen, G. Bergerhoff, and R. Sievers, Eds.), Data Commission of the International Union of Crystallography, Bonn, pp. 107–132.

24. G. N. Ramachandran and V. Sasisekaran, Representation of the Protein Main Chain Conformation, *Adv. Protein. Chem.*, **23**, 283–437 (1968).

25. C. I. Branden and T. A. Jones, "Between Subjectivity and Objectivity, *Nature*," **343**, 687–698 (1990).

26. G. M. Clore and A. M. Gronenborn, "Two, Three, and Four Dimensional NMR Methods for Obtaining Larger and More Precise Three-Dimensional Structures of Proteins in Solution," *Ann. Rev. Biophys. Chem.*, **20**, 29–63 (1991).

27. K. Wuthrich, The Development of Nuclear Magnetic Resonance Spectroscopy as a Technique for Protein Structure Determination, *Acc. Chem. Research*, **22**, 36–44 (1989).

28. W. A. Hendrickson and K. Wuthrich, *Macromolecular Structures, Atomic Structures of Biological Macromolecules Reported During 1990*, Current Biology Ltd., London, 1991.

29. G. M. Clore, P. T. Wingfield, and A. M. Gronenborn, "High-Resolution Three-dimensional Structure of Interleukin-1β in Solution by Three- and Four-dimensional Nuclear Magnetic

Resonance Spectroscopy," *Biochemistry*, **30**, 2315–2323 (1991).

30. J. Habazettl, D. Gondol, R. Wiltscheck, J. Otlweski, M. Schleicher, and T. A. Holak, "Structure of Hisactophilin is Similar to Interleukin-1β and Fibroblast Growth Factors," *J. Mol. Biol.*, **359**, 855–858 (1992).

31. L. J. Smith, C. Redfield, J. Boyd, G. M. P. Lawrence, R. G. Edwards, R. A. G. Smith, and C. M. Dobson, "The Solution Structure of a Four-Helix Bundle Protein," *J. Mol. Biol.*, **224**, 899–904 (1992).

32. R. Powers, D. S. Garrett, C. J. March, E. A. Frieden, A. M. Gronenborn, and G. M. Clore, "Three-dimensional Solution Structure of Human Interleukin-4 by Multidimensional Heteronuclear Magnetic Resonance Spectroscopy," *Science*, **256**, 1673–1677 (1992).

33. M. Ikura, G. M. Clore, A. M. Gronenborn, G. Zhu, C. B. Klee, and A. Bax, "Solution Structure of a Calmodulin-Target Peptide Complex by Multidimensional NMR," *Science*, **256**, 632–638 (1992).

34. Y. Theriault, T. M. Logan, R. Meadows, L. Yu, E. T. Olejniczak, T. E. Hoizman, R. L. Simmer, and S. W. Fesik, "Solution Structure of a Decameric Cyclosporin A-Cyclophilin Complex," *Nature*, **361**, 88–91 (1992).

35. B. Shaanan, A. M. Gronenborn, G. H. Cohen, G. L. Gilliland, B. Veerapandian, D. R. Davies, and G. M. Clore, "Combining Experimental Information from Crystal and Solution Studies: Joint X-ray and NMR Refinement," *Sciences*, **257**, 961–964 (1992).

36. K. Wuthrich, *NMR of Proteins and Nucleic Acids*, John Wiley & Sons, Inc., New York, 1986.

37. G. M. Clore and A. M. Gronenborn, "Structures of Larger Proteins in Solution: Three and Four Dimensional Heteronuclear NMR Spectroscopy," *Science*, **252**, 1390–1399.

38. A. T. Brunger and M. Nilges "Computational Challenges for Macromolecular Structure Determination by X-ray Crystallography and Solution NMR-Spectroscopy," *Quarterly Reviews of Biophysics*, **26**, 49–125 (1993).

39. G. Otting, (1992). "Experimental NMR Techniques for Studies of Protein-Ligand Interactions," *Curr. Opin. Stru. Biol.*, **3** 760–768 (1993).

40. A. Pardi, "Isotope Labelling for NMR Studies of Biomolecules," *Curr. Opin. in Str. Biol.*, **2**, 832–835 (1992).

41. L. E. Kay, G. M. Clore, A. Bax, and A. M. Gronenborn, "Four Dimensional Heteronuclear Triple-Resonance NMR Spectroscopy of Interleukin-1b in Solution," *Science*, 249, 411–414 (1990).

42. E. R. P. Zuiderweg, A. M. Petros, S. W. Fesik, and E. T. Olejniczak, "HMQC-NOE-HMQC NMR Spectroscopy: Resolving Tertiary NOE Distance Constraints in the Spectra of Larger Proteins," *J. Am. Chem. Soc.*, **113**, 370–372 1991.

43. R. H. Griffey and A. G. Redfield, "Proton-Detected "Heteronuclear Edited and Correlated Nuclear Magnetic Resonance and Nuclear Overhauser Effect in Solution," *Q. Rev. Biophys.*, **19**, 51–82 (1987).

44. G. Otting and K. Wuthrich, "Heteronuclear Filters in Two Dimensional [1H-1H]-NMR Spectroscopy: Combined Use with Isotope Labeling for Studies of Macromolecular Conformation and Intermolecular Interactions," *Q. Rev Biophys.*, **23**, 39–96 (1990).

45. S. W. Fesik, "NMR Structure-Based Drug Design," *J. Biomol. NMR*, **3**, 261–269 (1993).

46. B. J. Stockman and J. L. Markley, "NMR Analysis of Ligand Binding," *Curr. Opin. in Stru. Biol.*, **2**, 52–56 (1992).

47. S. W. Fesik, (1991a). "NMR Studies of Molecular Complexes as a Tool in Drug Design," *J. Med. Chem.*, **34**, 2937–2945 (1991).

48. A. M. Petros, G. Gemmecker, P. Neri, E. T. Olejniczak, D. Nettesheim, R. X. Xu, E. G. Gubbins, H. Smith, and S. W. Fesik, *J. Med. Chem.*, **35**, 2467–2473 (1992).

49. C. Weber, G. Wider, B. von Freyberg, R. Traber, W. Braun, H. Widmer, and K. Wuthrich, *Biochemistry*, **30**, 6563–6574 (1991).

50. B. J. Stockman, A. M. Krezel, J. L. Markley, K. G. Leonhardt, and N. A. Strauss: "Hydrogen-1, Carbon-13, and Nitrogen-15 NMR Spectroscopy of Anabaena Flavodoxin: Assignment of β-sheet and Flavin Binding Site Resonances and Analysis of Protein-Flavin Interactions," *Biochemistry*, **29**, 9600–9609 (1990).

51. E. A. M. de Jong, C. A. A. Claesen, C. J. M. Daemen, B. J. M. Harmsen, R. N. H. Konings, G. I. Tesser, and C. W. Hilbers, *J. Magn. Reson.*, **80**, 197–213 (1988).

52. A. M. Petros, L. Muller, and K. D. Kopple, *Biochemistry*, **29**, 10041–10048 (1990).

53. A. M. Petros, P. Neri, and S. W. Fesik, (1992b). *J. Biomol. NMR*, **2**, 11–18 (1992).

54. S. W. Fesik, G. Gemmecker, E. T. Olejniczak, and A. M. Petros, *J. Am. Chem. Soc.*, **113**, 7080–7081 (1991).

55. K. Kato, C. Matsunaga, T. Igarashi, H. Kim, A. Odaka, I. Shimada, and Y. Arata, "Complete

Assignment of the Methionyl Carbonyl Carbon Resonances in Switch Variant Anti-dansyl Antibodies Labeled with [13-C] Methionine," *Biochemistry*, **30**, 270–278 (1991).

56. K. Kato, C. Matsunaga, A. Odaka, S. Yamato, W. Takaha, I. Shimada, and Y. Arata (1991b). "Carbon-13 NMR Study of Switch Variant Antidansyl Antibodies, Antigen Binding and Domain-Domain Interactions," *Biochemistry*, **30**, 6604–6610 (1991).

57. H. Takahashi, T. Igarashi, I. Shimada and Y. Arata, "Preparation of the Fv Fragment from a Short-chain Mouse IgG2a Antidansyl Monoclonal Antibody and Use of Selectivity Deuterated Fv Analogues for Two-dimensional 1H-NMR Analysis of the Antigen-Antibody Interactions," *Biochemistry*, **30**, 2840–2847 (1991).

58. H. Takahashi, A. Odaka, S. Kawaminami, C. Matsunaga, K. Kato, I. Shimada, and Y. Arata, (1991b). Multinuclear NMR Study of the Structure of the Fv Fragment of the Anti-dansyl Mouse IgG2a Antibody, *Biochemistry*, **30**, 6611–6619 (1991).

59. M. Ikura, L. E. Kay, M. Krinks, and A. Bax, "Multidimensional NMR Study of Calmoldulin Complexed with the Binding Domain of Skeletal Muscle Myosin Lightchain Kinase: Indication of a Conformational Change in the Central Helix," *Biochemistry*, **30**, 5498–5504 (1991).

60. A. M. Petros, M. Kawai, J. R. Luly, and S. W. Fesik, *FEBS Lett.*, **308**, 309–314 (1992).

61. J. D. Forman-Kay, A. M. Gronenborn P. T. Wingfield, and G. M. Clore, "Determination of the Positions of Bound Water Molecules in the Solution Structure of Reduced Human Thioredoxin by Heteronuclear Three-dimensional Nuclear Magnetic Resonance Spectroscopy," *J. Mol. Biol.*, **220**, 209–216 (1991).

62. G. Otting E. Liepinsh, B.T. Farmer II, and K. Wuthrich, Protein Hydration Studied with Homonuclear 3D 1H NMR Experiments, *J. Biomol. NMR*, **1**, 209–215 (1991).

63. D. Benson, D. J. Lipman, and J. Ostell, "Genbank, An Archival for Protein Sequences," *Nucleic Acids Res.*, **21**, 2963–2965 (1993).

64. W. J. Browne, A. C. T. North, D. C. Phillips, K. Brew, T. C. Vanaman, and R. L. Hill, "A Possible Three-Dimensional Structure of Bovine Alpha-Lactalbumin Based on that of Hen egg White Lysozyme," *J. Mol. Biol.*, **42**, 65–86 (1969).

65. J. Greer, "Comparative Model-Building of the Mammalian Serine Proteases," *J. Mol. Biol.*, **153**, 1027–1042 (1981).

66. T. L. Blundell, B. L. Sibanda, M. J. E. Sternberg, and J. M. Thornton, (1987). "Knowledge-Based Prediction of Protein Structures and the Design of Novel Molecules," *Nature*, **326**, 347–352 (1987).

67. J. P. Overington, M. S. Johnson, A. Sali, and T. L. Blundell, Tertiary Structural Constraints on Protein Evolutionary Diversity: Templates, Key Residues and Structure Prediction, *Proc. R. Soc. London.*, **B241**, 132 (1990).

68. J. P. Overington, Knowledge-Based Protein Modeling, in PhD Thesis, University of London, London, 1991.

69. M. Lewis, Crystallographic Structure of IL-1α at 1.6 Å resolution, (personal communication), 1993.

70. B. Graves, 1992, personal communication.

71. A. Sali and T. L. Blundell, "Definition of General Topological Equivalence in Protein Structures: A Procedure Involving Comparison of Properties and Relationships through Simulated Annealing and Dynamic Programming," *J. Mol. Biol.*, **212**, 403–428 (1990).

72. M. B. Swindells and J. M. Thornton, "Modeling by Homology," *Curr. Opin. Struct. Biol.*, **1**, 219–223 (1991).

73. C. M. Topham, P. Thomas, J. P. Overington, M. S. Johnson, F. Eisenmenger, and T. L. Blundell, "An Assessment of COMPOSER: a Rule-based Approach to Modeling Protein Structure," *Biochem. Soc. Symp.*, **57**, 1–9 (1991).

74. A. Sali and T. L. Blundell, "Comparative Protein Modeling by Satisfaction of Spatial Restraints," *J. Mol. Biol.*, **234**, 779–815 (1993).

75. J. Bajorath, R. Stenkamp, and A. Aruffo, (1993). "Knowledge-Based Model Building of Proteins: Concepts and Examples," *Protein Science*, **2**, 1798–1810 (1993).

76. T. F. Havel and M. E. Snow, "A New Method for Building Protein Conformations from Sequence Alignments with Homologues of Known Structure," *J. Mol. Biol.*, **217**, 1–7 (1991).

77. N. Srinivasan and T. L. Blundell, An Evaluation of the Performance of an Automated Procedure for Comparative Modeling of Protein Tertiary Structure, *Protein Eng.*, **6**, 501–512 (1993).

78. T. Fujiyoshi-Yoneda, S. Yoneda, K. Kitamura, T. Amisaki, K. Ikeda, M. Inoue, and T. Ishida, (1991), "Adaptability of Restrained Molecular Dynamics for Tertiary Structure Prediction: Application to Crotalus Atrox Venom Phospholipase A2," *Prot. Eng.*, **4**, 443–450 (1991).

79. H. Bohr, J. Bohr, S. Brunak, R. M. J. Cotterill, H. Fredholm, B. Lautrup, and S. B. Petersen, A Novel Approach to Prediction of the 3-Dimen-

sional Structures of Protein Backbones by Neural Networks, *FEBS Lett.*, **261**, 43–46 (1990).

80. D. Bassolino-Klimas, and R. E. Bruccoleri, "Application of a Directed Conformational Search for Generating 3-D Coordinates for Protein Structures from α-Carbon Coordinates," *Proteins*, **14**, 465–474 (1992).

81. P. E. Correa, "The Building of Protein Structures from Cα-carbon Coordinates," *Proteins*, **7**, 366–377 (1990).

82. L. Holm, and C. Sander, "Database Algorithm for Generating Protein Backbone and Sidechain Co-ordinates from Cα trace: Application to Model Building and Detection of Co-ordinate Errors," *J. Mol. Biol.*, **218**, 183–194 (1991).

83. M. Levitt, "Accurate Modeling of Protein Conformation by Automatic Segment Matching," *J. Mol. Biol.*, **226**, 507–533 (1992).

84. Y. Luo, X. Jiang, L. Lai, C. Qu, X. Xu, and Y. Tang, "Building Protein Backbones from Cα Coordinates," *Prot. Eng.*, **5**, 147–150 (1992).

85. P. W. Payne, Reconstruction of Protein Conformations from Estimated Positions of the Cα Coordinates, *Protein Sci.*, **2**, 315–324 (1993).

86. L. S. Reid and J. M. Thornton, "Rebuilding Flavodoxin from Cα Coordinates: A Test Study," *Proteins*, **5**, 170–182 (1989).

87. A. Rey and J. Skolnick, "Efficient Algorithm for the Reconstruction of a Protein Backbone from the α-Carbon Coordinates," *J. Comp. Chem.*, **13** 443–456 (1992).

88. L. Holm and C. Sander, "Fast and Simple Monte Carlo Algorithm for Side Chain Optimization in Proteins: Application to Model Building by Homology," *Proteins Struct. Funct. Genet.*, **14**, 213–223 (1992).

89. A. V. Finkelstein and B. A. Reva, "A Search for the Most Stable Fold of Proteins," *Nature*, **351**, 497–499 (1991).

90. D. T. Jones, W. R. Taylor, and J. M. Thornton, "A New Approach to Protein Fold Recognition," *Nature*, **358**, 86–89 (1992).

91. R. Luthy, A. D. McLachlan, and D. Eisenberg, "Secondary Structure-based Profiles: Use of Structure-Conserving Scoring Tables in Searching Protein Sequence Databases for Structural Similarities, *Proteins: Struct. Funct. Genet.*, **10**, 229 (1991).

92. M. S. Johnson, J. P. Overington, and T. L. Blundell, "Alignment and Searching for Common Protein Folds Using a Data Bank of Structural Templates," *J. Mol. Biol.* **231**, 735–752 (1993).

93. A. Godzik, A. Kolinski, and J. Skolnick, "Topology Fingerprint Approach to the Inverse Protein Folding Problem," *J. Mol. Biol.*, **227**, 227–238 (1992).

94. J. U. Bowie, R. Luthy, and D. Eisenberg, "A Method to Identify Protein Sequences that Fold into a Known Three-Dimensional Structure," *Science*, **253**, 164 (1991).

95. M. S. Friedrichs, R. A. Goldstein, and P. G. Wolynes, "Generalized Protein Tertiary Structure Recognition using Associative Memory Hamiltonians," *J. Mol. Biol.*, **222**, 1013–1034 (1991).

96. M. J. Sippl and S. Weitckus, "Detection of Nativelike Models for Amino Acid Sequences of Unknown Three-Dimensional Structure in a Database of Known Protein Conformations," *Proteins*, **13**, 258–271 (1992).

97. T. L. Blundell and M. J. E. Sternberg, Computer-Aided Design in Protein Engineering, *Trends in Biotechnology*, **3**, 228–235 (1985).

98. T. L. Blundell, D. Barlow, B. L. Sibanda, J. M. Thornton, W. R. Taylor, I. J. Tickle, M. J. E. Sternberg, J. E. Pitts, I. Haneef, and A. M. Hemmings, "Three-Dimensional Structural Aspects of the Design of New Protein Molecules," *Phil. Trans. Roy. Soc.*, A **317**, 333–344 (1986).

99. B. Robson, E. Platt, R. V. Fishleigh, A. Marsden, and P. Millard, "Expert System for Protein Engineering: its Application in the Study of Chloramphenicol Acetyltransferase and Avian Pancreatic Polypeptide," *J. Mol. Graph.*, **5**, 5–17 (1987).

100. D. E. Stewart, P. K. Weiner, and J. E. Wampler, "Prediction of the Structure of Proteins using Related Structures, Energy Minimization and Computer Graphics," *J. Mol. Graph.*, **5**, 133–140 (1987).

101. M. J. Sutcliff, F. R. F. Hayes, and T. L. Blundell, "Knowledge-Based Modeling of Homologous Proteins: II. Rules for the Conformations of Substituted Side Chains," *Protein Eng.*, **1**, 385 (1987a).

102. M. J. Sutcliffe, F. R. F. Hayes, and T. L. Blundell, "Knowledge Based Modeling of Homologous Proteins, Part II: Rules for the Conformation of Substituted Sidechains," *Prot. Eng.* **1**, 385–392 (1987b).

103. M. Claessens, E. van Cutsem, I. Lasters, and S. Wodak, "Modeling the Polypeptide Backbone with Spare Parts from Known Protein Structures," *Prot. Eng.*, **2**, 335 (1989).

104. R. Unger, D. Harel, S. Wherland, and J. L. Sussman, "A 3-D Building Blocks Approach to

Analyzing and Predicting Structure of Proteins," *Proteins*, **5**, 355–373 (1989).

105. J. Greer, "Comparative Modeling Methods: Application to the Family of the Mammalian Serine Proteases," *Proteins*, **7**, 317–334 (1990).

106. R. E. Bruccoleri and M. Karplus, "Prediction of the Folding of Short Polypeptide Segments by Uniform Conformational Sampling," *Biopolymers*, **26**, 137–168 (1987).

107. P. S. Shenkin, D. L. Yarmush, R. M. Fine, H. Wang, and C. Levinthal, "Predicting antibody hypervariable loop conformation. Ensembles of random conformations for ringlike structures," *Biopolymers*, **26**, 2053–2085 (1987).

108. C. Chothia, A. M. Lesk, A. Tramontano, M. Levitt, S. J. Smith-Gill, G. Air, S. Sheriff, E. A. Padlan, D. Davies, W. R. Tulip, P. M. Colman, S. Spinelli, P. M. Alzari, and R. J. Poljak, "Conformation of immunoglobulin hypervariable regions," *Nature*, **342**, 877–883 (1989).

109. M. J. Dudek and H. A. Scheraga, "Protein Structure Prediction Using a Combination of Sequence Homology and Global Energy Minimization. I. Global Energy Minimization of Surface Loops" *J. Comp. Chem.*, **11**, 121–151 (1993).

110. A. C. R. Martin, J. C. Cheetham, and A. R. Rees, "Modeling antibody Hypervariable Loops: a Combined Algorithm," *Proc. Natl. Acad. Sci. USA*, **86**, 9268–9272 (1989).

111. M. T. Mas, K. C. Smith, D. L. Yarmush, K. Aisaka, and R. M. Fine, "Modeling the Anti-CEA Antibody Combining Site by Homology and Conformational Search," *Proteins*, **14**, 483–498 (1992).

112. J. Moult and M. N. G. James, "An Algorithm for Determining the Conformation of Polypeptide Segments in Proteins by Systematic Search." *Proteins*, **1**, 146–163 (1986).

113. B. L. Sibanda, T. L. Blundell, and J. M. Thornton, "Conformation of β-Hairpins in Protein Structures: A Systematic Classification with Applications to Modeling by Homology, Electron Density Fitting and Protein Engineering," *J. Mol. Biol.*, **206**, 759–777 (1989).

114. N. L. Summers and M. Karplus, "Modeling of Globular Proteins: a Distance-Based Search Procedure for the Construction of Insertion/Deletion Regions and Pro and Non-Pro Mutations," *J. Mol. Biol.*, **216**, 991–1016 (1990).

115. C. Topham, A. McLeod, F. Eisenmenger, J. P. Overington, M. S. Johnson, and T.L. Blundell "Fragment Ranking in Modeling of Protein Structure. Conformationally Constrained Environmental Amino Acid Substitution Tables," *J. Mol. Biol.*, **229**, 194 (1993).

116. J. W. Ponder and F. M. Richards, "Tertiary Templates for Proteins: Use of Packing Criteria in the Enumeration of Allowed Sequences for Different Structural Classes," *J. Mol. Biol.*, **193**, 775–791 (1987).

117. H. Schrauber, F. Eisenhaber, and P. Argos, "Rotamers: To Be or Not To Be? An Analysis of Amino Acid Side-Chain Conformations in Globular Proteins," *J. Mol. Biol.* **230**, 592–612 (1993).

118. N. L. Summers, W. D. Carlson, and M. Karplus, "Analysis of Side-Chain Orientations in Homologuous Proteins," *J. Mol. Biol.*, **196**, 175 (1987).

119. M. J. Sutcliff, F. R. F. Hayes, and T. L. Blundell, Knowledge-Based Modeling of Homologous Proteins: II. Rules for the Conformations of Substituted Side Chains," *Protein Eng.*, **1**, 385 (1987).

120. M. J. McGregor, S. A. Islam, and M. J. E. Sternberg, "Analysis of the Relationship Between Side-Chain Conformation and Secondary Structure in Globular Proteins," *J. Mol. Biol.*, **198**, 295–310 (1987).

121. N. L. Summers and M. Karplus, Construction of Side-chains in Homology Modeling: Application to the C-Terminal Lobe of Rhizopuspepsin," *J. Mol. Biol.*, **210**, 785–811 (1989).

122. C. A. Schiffer, J. W. Caldweml, P. A. Kollman, and R. M. Stroud, "Prediction of Homologous, Protein Structures Based on Conformational Searches and Energetics," *Proteins*, **8**, 30–43 (1990).

123. J. Singh and J. M. Thornton, "SIRIUS. An Automated Method for the Analysis of the Preferred Packing Arrangements Between Protein Groups," *J. Mol. Biol.*, **17**, 195–225 (1990).

124. C. Lee and S. Subbiah, "Prediction of Protein Side-Chain Conformation by Packing Optimization," *J. Mol. Biol.*, **217**, 373–388 (1991).

125. P. Tuffery, C. Etchebest, S. Hazout, and R. A. Lavery, "A New Approach to the Rapid Determination of Protein Side Chain Conformations," *J. Biomol. Str. Dynam.*, **8**, 1267–1289 (1991).

126. J. Desmet, M. De Maeyer, B. Hazes, and I. Lasters, "The Dead-End Elimination Theorem and Its Use in Protein Side-Chain Positioning," *Nature*, **356**, 539–542 (1992).

127. R. L. Dunbrack and M. Karplus, "Prediction of Protein Sidechain Conformations from a Backbone Conformation Dependent Rotamer Library," *J. Mol. Biol.*, **230**, 543–571 (1993).

128. C. Wilson, L. M. Gregoret, and D. A. Agard, Modeling Side-Chain Conformation for Homologous Proteins Using an Energy-Based Rotamer Search," *J. Mol. Biol.*, **229**, 996–1006 (1993).

129. J. M. Thornton, "Disulfide Bridges in Globular Proteins," *J. Mol. Biol.*, **151**, 261–287 (1981).

130. R. Sowdhamini, N. Srinivasan, B. Shoichet, D. V. Santi, C. Ramakrishnan, and P. Balaram, "Stereochemical Modeling of Disulfide Bridges. Criteria for Introduction into Proteins by Site-Directed Mutagenesis," *Prot. Eng.*, **3**, 95–103 (1989).

131. S. R. Presnell, B. I. Cohen, and F. E. Cohen, "A Segment-Based Approach to Protein Secondary Structure Prediction," *Biochemistry*, **31**, 983 (1992).

132. B. Rost, R. Schneider, and C. Sander, "Progress in Protein Structure Prediction," *Trends Biochem. Sci.*, **18**, 120–123 (1993).

133. V. B. Cockcroft, D. I. Osguthorpe, E. A. Barnard, and G. G. Lunt," *Prot. Strucr. Funct. Genet.*, **8**, 386–397 (1990).

134. C. L. Brooks III, M. Karplus, and B. M. Pettit, *Proteins: A Theoretical Perspective of Dynamics, Structure and Thermodynamics*, John Wiley & Sons, Inc., New York (1988).

135. S. J. Weiner, P. A. Kollman, D. A. Case, V. C. Singh, C. Ghio, G. Alagona, S. Profeta, and P. A. Weiner, "AMBER: Assisted Model Building with Energy Refinement. A General Program for Modeling Molecules and their Interactions," *J. Comput. Chem.*, **2**, 287–303 (1981).

136. R. A. Laskowski, M. W. MacArthur, D. S. Moss, and J. M. Thornton, "PROCHECK – A Program to Check the Stereochemical Quality of Protein Structures," *J. Appl. Cryst.*, **26**, 283–291 (1993).

137. A. M. De Vos, M. Ultsch, and A. A. Kossiakoff, Human Growth Hormone and Extracellular Domain of its Receptor: Crystal Structure of the Complex, *Science*, **255**, 306–312 (1992).

138. I. D. Kuntz, J. M. Blaney, S. J. Oatley, R. Langridge, and T. E. Ferrin, "A Geometric Approach to Macromolecule-Ligand Interactions," *J. Mol. Biol.*, **161**, 269 (1982).

139. S. J. Wodak and J. Janin "Computer Analysis of Protein-Protein Interactions," *J. Mol. Biol.*, **124**, 323 (1978).

140. B. Busetta, I. J. Tickle, and T. L. Blundell, "Docker, an Interactive Program for Simulating Protein-Receptor and Substrate Interactions," *J. Appl. Cryst.*, **16**, 432 (1983).

141. N. Pattabiraman, M. Levitt, T. E. Ferrin, and R. Langridge "Computer Graphics in Real-Time Docking with Energy Calculation and Minimization," *J. Comput. Chem.*, **6**, 432 (1985).

142. N. Tomioka, A. Itai, and Y. Iitaka, "A Method for Fast Energy Estimation and Visualization of Protein-Ligand Interaction," *J. Comput. Aided Mol. Des.*, **1**, 197 (1987).

143. I. D. Kuntz," *Science*, **257**, 1078–1082 (1992).

144. A. R. Leach and I. D. Kuntz, "Conformational Analysis of Flexible Ligands in Macromolecular Receptor Sites," *J. Comput. Chem.*, **13**, 730 (1992).

145. D. J. Bacon and J. Moult, "Docking by Least-Squares Fitting of Molecular Surface Patterns," *J. Mol. Biol.*, 225, 849 (1992).

146. P. D. J. Grootenhuis, V. J. van Geerestein, C. A. G. Haasnoot, and M. Karplus, "Molecular Modelling of Protein–Ligand Interactions," *Bull. Soc. Chim. Belg.*, **101**, 661 (1992).

147. A. Miranker and M. Karplus, "Functionality Maps of Binding Sites: a Multiple Copy Simultaneous Search Method," *Proteins: Struct. Funct. Genet.*, **11**, 29–34 (1991).

148. A. Caflisch, A. Miranker, and M. Karplus," *J. Med. Chem.*, **36**, 2142–2167 (1993).

149. M. A. Ondetti and D. W. Cushman," *Ann. Rev. Biochem.* **51**, 283–308 (1980).

150. D. W. Cushman, H. S. Cheung, E. F. Sabo, B. Rubin, and M. A. Ondetti," *Fed. Proc.*, **38**, 2778–2782 (1979).

151. W. N. Lipscomb, "Structure and Mechanism in the Enzymatic Activity of Carboxypeptidase A and Relations to Chemical Sequence," *Acc. Chem. Res.*, **3**, 81–89 (1970).

152. B. W. Matthews, "Structural Basis of the Action of Thermolysin and Related Zinc Peptidases," *Acc. Chem. Res.*, **21**, 333–339 (1988).

153. D. W. Cushman, H. S. Cheung, E. F. Sabo, and M. A. Ondetti, "Design of Potent Inhibitors of ACE," *Biochemistry*, **16**, 5484–5491 (1977).

154. A. A. Patchett, E. Harris, E. W. Tristram, M. J. Wyvratt, M. T. Wu, D. Taub, E. R. Peterson, T. J. Ikeler, J. ten Broeke, L. G. Payne, D. L. Ondeyka, E. D. Thorsett, W. J. Greenlee, N. S. Lohr, R. D. Hoffsomer, H. Joshua, W. V. Ruyle, J. W. Rothrock, S. D. Aster, A. L. Maycock, F. M. Robinson, and R. Hirschmann, "A New Class of Antiotension-Converting Enzyme Inhibitors," *Nature*, **288**, 280–283 (1980).

155. C. H. Hassell, A. Krohn, C. H. Moody, and W. A. Thomas, "The Design of New Group of ACE Inhibitors," *FEBS Lett.*, **147**, 175–179 (1982).

156. M. R. Attwood, C. H. Hassall, A. Krohn, G. Lawton and S. Redshaw, "The Design and Synthesis of the ACE Inhibitor Cilazapril and Related Bicyclic Compounds," *J. Chem. Soc. Perkins, Trans.*, **1**, 1011–1019 (1986).

157. A. F. Monzingo and B. W. Matthews, "Binding of *N*-Carboxymethyl Dipeptide Inhibitors to Thermolysin Determined by X-Ray Crystallography. A Novel Class of Transition State Analogues for Zinc Peptidases," *Biochemistry*, **23**, 5724 (1989).

158. L. T. Skeggs, K. E. Lentz, J. R. Kahn, and H. Hochstrasser," *J. Exp. Med.*, 13 (1968).

159. M. Szelke, in *Aspartic Proteinases and Their Inhibitors*, V. Kostka, Ed., de Gruyter, New York, 1985, pp. 421–441.

160. M. Szelke, M. Tree, B. J. Leckie, D. M. Jones, B. Atrash, S. Beattie, B. Donovan, A. Hallett, M. Hughes, A. F. Lever, et al.," *J. Hypertens.*, 3, 13 (1985).

161. B. J. Leckie, M. Szelke, B. Atrash, S. R. Beattie, A. Hallett, D. M. Jones, G. D. McIntyre, J. Suerias, and D. J. Webb," *Biochem. Soc. Trans.* 13, 1029 (1985).

162. M. N. G. James and A. R. Sielecki, "Structure and Refinement of Penicillopepsin at 1.8 A Resolution," *J. Mol. Biol.*, 163, 299–361 (1983).

163. K. Suguna, R. R. Bott, E. A. Padlan, E. Subramanian, S. Sheriff, G. H. Cohen, and D. Davies, "Structure and Refinement at 1.8 A Resolution of the Aspartic Proteinase from Rhizopuschinensis," *J. Mol. Biol.*, 196, 877–900 (1987).

164. T. L. Blundell, J. A. Jenkins, B. T. Sewell, L. H. Pearl, J. B. Cooper, I. J. Tickle, B. Veerapandian, and S. P. Wood, "X-ray Analyses of Aspartic Proteinases. The Three-Dimensional Structure at 2.1 A Resolution of Endothiapepsin," *J. Mol. Biol.*, 211, 919–941 (1990).

165. A. R. Sielecki, M. Fujinaga, R. J. Read, and M. N. G. James, "Refined Structure of Porcine Pepsinogen at 1.8 A Resolution," *J.M.B.*, 219, 671–692 (1991).

166. J. A. Hartsuck, G. Koelsch, and S. J. Remington, "The High Resolution Crystal Structure of Porcine Pepsinogen," *Proteins: Structure, Function and Genetics* 13, 1–25 (1992).

167. A. R. Sielecki, A. A. Fedorov, A. Boodhoo, N. S. Andreeva, and M.N.G. James, "Molecular and Crystal Structures of Monoclinic Porcine Pepsin Refined at 1.8 A Resolution," *J. Mol. Biol.*, 214, 143–170 (1990).

168. J. B. Cooper, G. Khan, G. Taylor, I. Tickle, and T. L. Blundell, "Three Dimensional Structure of the Hexagonal Crystal Form of Porcine Pepsin at 2.3 Å Resolution," *J. Mol. Biol.*, 214, 199–222 (1990).

169. V. Dhanaraj, C. G. Dealwis, C. Frazao, M. Badasso, D. L. Sibanda, I. J. Tickle, J. M. Cooper, H. P. C. Driessen, M. Newman, C. Aguilar, S. P. Wood, T. L. Blundell, P. M. Hobart, K. F. Geoghegan, M. J. Ammirati, D. E. Danley, B. A. O'Connor, and D. J. Hoover, "X-Ray Analyses of Peptide-Inhibitor Complexes Define the Structural Basis of Specificity for

Human and Mouse Renins," *Nature (London)* 357, 466–472 (1992).

170. A. R. Sielecki, K. Hayakawa, M. Fujinaga, M. E. P. Murphy, M. Fraser, A. K. Muir, C. T. Carilli, J. A. Lewicki, J. D. Baxter, and M. N. G. James, Structure of Recombinant Human Renin, a Target for Cardiovascular-Active Drugs, at 2.5 Å Resolution," *Science*, 243, 1346–1350 (1989).

171. J. Rahuel, J. P. Priestle, and M. G. Grutter, "The Crystal Structures of Recombinant Glycosylated Human Renin Alone and in Complex with a Transition State Analog Inhibitor," *J. Str. Biol.*, 107, 227–236 (1991).

172. M. Newman, F. Watson, P. Roychowdhury, H. Jones, M. Badasso, A. Cleasby, S. P. Wood, I. Tickle, and T. L. Blundell, "Structure and Refinement at 2.0 Å Resolution of the Aspartic Proteinase from Mucor Pusillus," *J. Mol. Biol.* 260–283 (1992).

173. G. L. Gilliland, E. L. Winborne, J. Nachman, and A. Wlodawer, "The Three-Dimensional Structure of Recombinant Bovine Chymosin at 2.3 A Resolution," *Proteins: Structure, Function and Genetics*, 8, 82–101 (1990).

174. M. Newman, M. Safro, C. Frazao, G. Khan, A. Zdanov, I.J. Tickle, T.L. Blundell, and N. Andreeva, "X-Ray Analyses of Aspartic Proteinases IV. Structure and Refinement at 2.2 A Resolution of Bovine Chymosin," *J. Mol. Biol.*, 221, 1295–1309 (1991).

175. E. T. Baldwin, T. N. Bhat, S. Gulnik, M. V. Hosur, R. C. Sowder, C. Cachau, J. Collins, A. M. Silva, and J Erickson, "Crystal Structures of Native and Inhibited Forms of Human Cathepsin D: Implications for Lysosomal Targeting and Drug Design," *Proc. Natl. Acad. Sci. USA*, 90, 6796–6800 (1993).

176. P. Metcalf and M. Fusek, "Two Crystal Structures for Cathepsin D: the Lysosomal Targeting Signal and Active Site," *EMBO J.*, 12, 1293–1302 (1993).

177. V. Dhanaraj and T. L. Blundell, Personal communication. Renin Inhibitors Complexed to Aspartic Proteinases are Referenced in Abdel-Meguid, 1993. References from 25 to 47, pp 772–773.

178. D. R. Davies, "The Structure and Function of Aspartic Proteinases," *Annu. Rev. Biophys. Biophys. Chem.*, 19, 189–215 (1990).

179. M. N. G. James and A. R. Sielecki," *Biological Macromolecule and Assemblies*, J. Jurnak, A. McPherson, Eds. Vol. 3, John Wiley & Sons, Inc., New York, pp. 413–482 (1987).

180. T. L. Blundell, J. Cooper, S. I. Foundling, D. M. Jones, B. Atrash, and M. Szelke, "On the Rational Design of Renin Inhibitors: X-Ray Studies of Aspartic Proteinases Complexed with Transition State Analogues," *Biochemistry*, **26**, 5585–5590 (1987).

181. J. B. Cooper and C. J. Harris, "Current Directions in Renin Inhibition," *Current Trends in Cardiovascular Patents*, **1**, 143–157 (1988).

182. S. Abdel-Meguid, "Inhibitors of Aspartic Proteinases," *Medicinal Research Reviews*, **13–6**, 731–778 (1993).

183. B. Veerapandian, J. B. Cooper, A. Sali, and T. L. Blundell, "X-Ray Analyses of Aspartic Proteinases III: Three Dimensional Structure of Endothiapepsin Complexed with a Transition-State Isostere Inhibitor of Renin at 1.6 Å Resolution." *J. Mol. Biol.*, **216**, 1017–1029 (1990).

184. A. Nicholls and B. Honig, GRASP, 1993. A molecule visualizing software.

185. W. Greenlee," *J. Med. Res. Rev.*, **10**, 173 (1990).

186. J. B. Cooper, S. I. Foundling, T. L. Blundell, J. Boger, R. A. Jupp, and J. Kay, "X-Ray Studies of Aspartic Proteinase-Statine Inhibitor Complexes," *Biochemistry*, **28**, 8596–8602 (1989).

187. J. B. Cooper, S. L. Foundling, T. Blundell, R. J. Arrowsmith, C. J. Harris, and J. N. Chapness, in *Topics in Medicinal Chemistry*, *Fourth SCI-RSC Medicinal Chemistry Symposium*, P. R. Leening, Ed., Special Publication No. 65, The Royal Society of Chemistry, London, 1988, p. 309.

188. J. Boger, L. S. Payne, D. S. Perlow, N. S. Lohr, M. Poe, E. H. Blaine, E. H. Ulm, T. W. Schorn, B. I. LaMont, T.-Y. Lin, M. Kawai, D. H. Veber, and D. Rich, "Renin Inhibitors: Syntheses of Subnanomolar, Competitive, Transition-State Analogue Inhibitors Containng a Novel Analogue of Statine," *J. Med. Chem.* **28**, 1779–1790 (1985).

189. J. Cooper, W. Quail, C. Frazao, S. I. Foundling, T. L. Blundell, C. Humblet, E. A. Lunney, W. T. Lowther, and B. M. Dunn, "X-Ray Crystallographic Analysis of Inhibition of Endothiapepsin by Cyclohexyl Renin Inhibitors," *Biochemistry* **31**, 8142–8150 (1992).

190. B. Veerapandian, J. B. Cooper, A. Sali, T. L. Blundell, R. L. Rosati, B. W. Dominy, D. B. Damon, and D. J. Hoover, "Direct Observation by X-Ray Analysis of a Tetrahedral Intermediate of Aspartic Proteinases," *Protein Science*, **1**, 322–328 (1992).

191. K. D. Parris, D. J. Hoover, D. B. Damon, and D. R. Davies, "Synthesis and Crystallographic Analysis of Two Rhizopuspepsin Inhibitor Complexes," *Biochemistry*, **31**, 8125–8141 (1992).

192. M. N. James, A. R. Sielecki, K. Hayakawa, and M. H. Gelb, "Crystallographic Analysis of Transition State Mimics Bound to Penicilopepsin: Difluorostatine- and Difluorostatone-Containing Peptides," *Biochemistry*, **31**, 3872–3886 (1992).

193. B. A. Lefker, D. J. Hoover, R. L. Rosati, W. F. Holt, W. R. Murphy, M. L. Mangiapane, M. R. Nocerini, M. J. Gumkowski, W. A. Hada, M. P. Carta, M. L. Gillaspy, S. S. Ellery, J. T. MacAndrew, K. A. Simpson, and J. Wentland," *Presented at the 206th National Meeting of the American Chemical Society*, August 22–27, 1993, ACS Abstract MEDI#4.

194. G. J. Hanson, J. S. Baran, H. S. Lowrie, S. J. Sarussi, P. C. Yang, M. Babler, S. E. Bittner, S. E. Papaioannou, and G. M. Walsh," *Biochem. Biophys. Res. Commun.*, **146**, 959 (1987).

195. H. D. Kleinert, S. H. Rosenberg, W. R. Baker, H. H. Stein, V. Klinghofer, J. Barlow, K. Spina, J. Polakowski, P. Kovar, J. Cohen, and J. Denissen," *Science* **257**, 1940 (1992).

196. N. E. Kohl, E. A. Emini, W. A. Schleif, L. J. Davis, J. C. Heimbach, et al.," *Proc. Natl. Acad. Sci. USA*, **85**, 4186–4190 (1988).

197. S. Seelmeier, H. Schmidt, V. Turk, K. von der Helm," *Proc. Natl. Acad. Sci. USA*, **85**, 6612–6616 (1988).

198. T. J. McQuade, A. G. Tomaselli, L. Liu, V. Karacostas, B. Moss et al. *Science*, **249**, 1533–1544 (1990).

199. H. Mitsuya, R. Yarchoan, S. Kageyama, and S. Broder," *FASEB J.* 5, 2369 (1991).

200. A. Wlodawer and J. Erickson, "Structure Based Inhibitors of HIV-1 Protease," *Annu. Rev. Biochem.* **62**, 543–585 (1993).

201. K. Appelt, "Crystal Structures of HIV-1 Protease-Inhibitor Complexes," *Perspectives in Drug Discovery and Design*, **1**, 23–48 (1993).

202. P. M. D. Fitzgerald, "HIV Protease-Ligand Complexes," *Curr. Opin. In Struc. Biol.*, **3**, 868–874 (1993).

203. P. M. D. Fitzgerald, B. M. McKeever, J. F. Van Middlesworth, J. P. Springer, J. C. Heimbach, C.-T. Leu, W. K. Herber, R. A. F. Dixon, and P. L. Darke, "Crystallographic Analysis of a Complex Between Human Immunodeficiency Virus Type 1 Protease and Acetyl-Pepstatin at 2.0 Å Resolution," *J. Biol. Chem.* **265**, 14209 (1990); Ribbon diagram drawn by the program MOLSCRIPT); P. Kraulis, "A Program to Produce Both Detailed and Schematic Plots of

Protein Structure," *J. Appl. Cryst.*, **24**, 946–950 (1991).

204. R. L. DesJarlais, G. L. Seibel, L. D. Kuntz, P. S. Furth, J. C. Alvarez, P. R. Ortiz de Montellano, D. L. DeCamp, L. M. Babe, and C. S. Craik," *Proc. Natl. Acad. Sci. USA*, **87**, 6644 (1990).

205. M. Miller, J. Schneider, B. K. Sathyanarayana, M. V. Toth, G. R. Marshall, L. Clawson, L. Selk, S. B. Kent, and A. Wlodawer," *Science*, **246**, 1149 (1989).

206. B. J. Graves, M. H. Hatada, J. K. Miller, M. C. Graves, S. Roy, C. M. Cook, A. Krohn, J. A. Martin, and N. A. Roberts, "The Three-Dimensional X-Ray Crystal Structure of HIV-1 Protease Complexed with a Hydroxyethylene Inhibitor," in *Structure and Function of the Aspartic Proteinases*. B. M. Dunn, Ed., Plenum Press, New York, pp. 455–560 (1992).

207. W. J. Thompson, P. M. D. Fitzgerald, M. K. Holloway, E. A. Emini, P. L. Darke, B. M. McKeever, W. A. Schleif, J. C. Quintero, J. A. Zugay, T. J. Tucker, J. E. Schwering, C. F. Homnick, J. Nunberg, J. P. Springer, and J. R. Huff, "Synthesis and Antiviral Activity of a Series of HIV-1 Protease Inhibitors with Functionality Tethered to the P1 or P1' Phenyl Substituents: X-Ray Crystal Structure Assisted Design," *J. Med. Chem.* 1685–1701 (1992).

208. E. Rutenber, E. B. Fauman, R. J. Keenan, S. Fong, P. S. Furth, P. R. Ortiz de Montellano, D. L. DeCamp, L. M. Babe, and C. S. Craik, "Structure-Based Design of Nonpeptide Inhibitors Specific for the Human Immunodeficiency Virus 1 Protease," *Proc. Natl. Acad. Sci., USA*, **87**, 6644–6648 (1990).

209. D. C. Humber, N. Cammack, J. Coates, K. N. Cobley, D. C. Orr, R. Storer, G. G. Weingarten, and M. P. Weir, "Penicillin Derived C2 Symmetric Dimers as Novel Inhibitors of HIV-1 Proteinase," *J. Med Chem.*, **35**, 3080–3081 (1992).

210. A. Wonacott, R. Cook, F. R. Hayes, M. M. Hann, H. Jhoti, P. McMeekin, A. Mistry, P. Murray-Rust, O. M. P. Singh, and M. P. Weir, "A Series of Penicillin-Derived C2-Symmetric Inhibitors of HIV-1 Proteinase: Structural and Modeling Studies," *J. Med. Chem.*, **36**, 3113–3119 (1993).

211. P. Y. S. Lam, P. K. Jadhav, C. J. Eyermann, C. N. Hodge, Y. Ru, L. T. Bacheler, J. L. Meek, M. J. Otto, M M. Rayner, Y. N. Wong, C. Chang, P. C. Weber, D. Jackson, T. R. Sharpe, and S. Erickson-Viitanen," *Science*, **263**, 380–384 (1994).

212. Dorsey et al., *206th National Meeting of the American Chemical Society*, Chicago, 1993.

213. J. S. Mills, Discovery of the HIV Proteinase Inhibitor Ro 31-8959: "A Paradigm for Drug Discovery," *Interim Antiviral News*, **1**, 18–19 (1993).

CHAPTER ELEVEN

Drug Receptors

MICHAEL WILLIAMS,
DARLENE C. DEECHER and
JAMES P. SULLIVAN

Pharmaceutical Products Division
Abbott Laboratories
Abbott Park, Illinois, USA

CONTENTS

1 Introduction,   350

2 Receptor and Enzyme Concepts,   352

3 Receptor Theory,   353
   3.1 Base ligand concepts, 353
   3.2 Historical perspectives and receptor
       theories, 355
       3.2.1 Occupancy theory, 356
       3.2.2 Rate theory, 358
       3.2.3 Inactivation theory, 358

4 Receptor Complexes and Allosteric
   Modulators,   359

5 Second and Third Messenger Systems,   361

6 Receptor Interactions and Integration,   362

7 Receptor Dynamics,   362

8 Molecular Biology of Receptors,   363
   8.1 Receptor cloning, 364
   8.2 Receptor cloning strategies, 365
   8.3 Sequence analysis of cloned receptors, 369
   8.4 Expression of cloned receptors, 370
   8.5 Structural analysis of cloned receptors, 373
   8.6 G-Protein cloned receptors, 373
       8.6.1 Structural features involved in ligand
             binding, 373
       8.6.2 Regions involved in receptor
             activation, 374
       8.6.3 Regions involved with coupling to G
             proteins, 374
   8.7 Ion channel linked receptors, 375
       8.7.1 Regions involved in ion
             permeation, 376

Burger's Medicinal Chemistry and Drug Discovery,
Fifth Edition, Volume 1: Principles and Practice,
Edited by Manfred E. Wolff.
ISBN 0-471-57556-9   © 1995 John Wiley & Sons, Inc.

8.7.2 Regions involved in ion selectivity, 376

9 Receptor Models, 377

10 Receptor Nomenclature, 377

11 Receptor Binding Assays, 378
    11.1 Practical considerations of the binding
         assay, 379
         11.1.1 Binding definitions, 379
         11.1.2 The membrane receptor assay, 381
         11.1.3 Radioligand issues, 383
         11.1.4 Receptor source, 383
         11.1.5 Separation techniques, 384
         11.1.6 Data analysis, 385

12 Receptor autoradiography, 385

13 Receptor Clones in Compound Evaluation, 386

14 Lead Compound Discovery, 387
    14.1 Compound sources, 388
         14.1.1 Natural product sources, 388
         14.1.2 Pharmacophore-based ligand
                libraries, 388
         14.1.3 Diversity-based ligand libraries, 389
         14.1.4 High-throughput screening, 390

15 Future Directions, 391

1 INTRODUCTION

The phenomenon of cell to cell communication represents the basic physiological mechanism regulating cellular homeostasis and tissue viability. At the cellular level the process can be mediated by the release of a neurotransmitter or neuromodulator from a presynaptic storage site and its subsequent interaction with a cell surface receptor, the latter interaction resulting in a functional change in the target cell. Alterations in this process of chemical neurotransmission, either an overstimulation or understimulation of the target receptor (occurring either by changes in the availability of the neurotransmitter or an alteration in the responsiveness of the signal transduction processes in the target cell), are thought to represent the molecular lesions involved in many disease states.

The concept that therapeutic agents produce their selective actions in modifying disease symptomatology by acting as "magic bullets" at discrete molecular targets within the body, is generally attributed to Paul Ehrlich at the turn of the century as part of the now seminal "lock and key" hypothesis (1). This hypothesis has described drugs as receptor ligands or enzyme substrates that selectively modulated the function of, as then unknown molecular targets to produce beneficial effects. Receptors and enzyme active sites are thus classified as drug recognition sites.

Despite quantal advances in technology over the past 100 years, the seminal receptor–ligand (RL) concept developed by Ehrlich remains the foundation of understanding receptor function, disease pathophysiology and the drug discovery process. Even though the concepts of both receptors and ligands have broadened considerably as technological advances, they have allowed a refinement of potential drug targets (Table 11.1).

From a conceptual viewpoint, the focus on the nature of the RL interaction has made the structure activity relationship (SAR) the key element in compound evaluation whether the activity is defined as biological efficacy, selectivity or bioavailability. Glennon (2) has pointedly refined the general term, SAR, into two compo-

Table 11.1 Drug Recognition Sites Classifiable as Receptors

Drug Recognition Site	Location	Example
Receptor	Cell surface	β-Adrenoceptor
	Intracellular	Peripheral benzodiazepine Receptor (mitochondrial)
Enzyme	Cell surface/ intracellular	Angiotensin-converting enzyme
Hormone responsive element	Nucleic acid	Retinoid receptors
Sense oligonucleotide	Cytoplasm	NPY-Y1[a]
Orphan receptor	Cytoplasm	COUP-TF

[a] See Reference 257.

nents—the structure affinity relationship, SAFIR, limited to the assessment of ligand interactions with their molecular targets at the affinity/recognition level and the SAR proper where the functional activity of a ligand can be determined. The SAR can also be extended to encompass the activity relationship related to the pharmacokinetics and potential toxicity of receptor ligands. For the purposes of the present overview however, the term SAR will be used in its more generic sense.

The characterization of the SAR for newly synthesised compounds, the documentation of changes in the activity of a compound associated with alterations in the various substituents on a given pharmacophore, has allowed the chemist to theoretically model the way in which a ligand interacts with its target and thus derive a putative two or three dimensional model of the receptor (or enzyme). This model can then permit the use of computer assisted molecular design (CAMD) techniques (3–5) to facilitate the design of new pharmacophores and the choice of appropriate substituents that can selectively interact with regions of the receptor or enzyme that appear crucial in defining the molecular forces involved in binding. Currently this modeling is a trial and error, iterative process consistent with CAMD being an "emerging technology" (6). When

coupled with the X-ray crystallographic information (7) related to the purified ligand target and NMR data of the RL (enzyme–substrate) interaction (8), CAMD technology can, however, be a very powerful tool limited currently only by data availability, real time computational power and necessary physiochemical assumptions to facilitate programming.

More recently, with the advent of recombinant DNA (rDNA) technology and the ability to clone and express individual receptors and enzymes in copious amounts, knowledge of the primary structure of receptors and enzymes has been relatively easy to obtain. Also, it has become evident that there are considerable similarities in structure between different classes of receptor.

Receptors can thus be divided into two major classes; G-protein coupled receptors (GPCRs) and ligand gated ion channels (LGICs). Additional receptor classes include the voltage sensitive ion channels including the various classes of calcium (9) and potassium channels (10). Using rDNA technology it has also been possible to change the amino acid composition of the target protein by altering the genetic code and introducing point mutations. This process, known as site-directed mutagenesis, permits the identification of those amino acid residues involved in aspects of ligand recognition as well as the signal transduction process (11). Similarly, chimeric receptor constructs, where large regions of different receptors are genetically combined, can be used to derive information on those regions of the receptor involved in recognition and transductional processes (12).

2 RECEPTOR AND ENZYME CONCEPTS

The major focus of this review will be on cell surface drug receptors, although the concepts involved can be extrapolated to both enzymes and intracellular drug recognition sites (Table 11.1). Thus the term receptor will be used in a generic sense to describe the various recognition sites at which drugs act. A semantic point of interest in this context relates to receptors versus drug receptors. Most known drugs produce their effects by interacting with receptors (or enzymes) for which the ligand is known. There are, however, drug receptors per se, identified by newer molecular techniques that were characterized by the ability of a drug to interact with a specific molecular site and for which the endogenous ligand is unknown. One example of this ability is the GABA/benzodiazepine (BZ) receptor complex that was initially identified through the use of radiolabeled diazepam (13). The endogenous ligand for this receptor, its own neuromodulator, has yet to be identified although various peptides and gut bacterial products have been suggested to subserve this role.

Receptor theory involves, to a very major extent, the classical enzyme kinetic model based on the Law of Mass Action, that was derived by Michaelis and Menten in 1913 (14). As with many of the more recently developed in vitro techniques for the study of the receptor–ligand (RL) interactions, the RL concept can be taken as illustrative of the ES interaction; for instance, radioligand binding can also be used to study the enzyme substrate (ES) response.

However, the use of classical enzyme theory to the study of receptors is not always directly applicable. For an enzyme, the substrate, S, undergoes a catalytic conversion to a product or products. The product is then utilized in other cellular events and is thus removed from the equilibrium situation, or alternatively can act as a feedback modulator (15) to alter the ES reaction either positively or negatively and can thus be described by the equation:

$$\text{Enzyme} + \text{substrate} \rightleftharpoons \text{ES} \rightleftharpoons \text{E}$$
$$+ \text{ product} \qquad (11.1)$$

The equilibrium nature of the ES reaction is such that the products formed can directly drive the reaction in reverse.

For the RL interaction, however, the ligand, L, binds to the receptor and alters the nature of the receptor interaction with its associated membrane components to effect a change in cellular and ultimately, tissue function. While the ligand is known to undergo a conformational change as the result of the RL interaction (16) as is the receptor, there is no chemical change in the ligand resulting from the RL interaction such that the product of the RL interaction is not directly derived from the ligand producing the effect. Thus L is chemically unchanged as a result of the RL interaction according to the equation:

$$\text{Receptor} + \text{Ligand} \rightleftharpoons \text{RL} \rightarrow \text{R}$$
$$+ \text{ cellular effect} \qquad (11.2)$$

and is not directly involved in the consequences of receptor activation, although the latter process, via changes in the activity of intracellular messenger systems, can lead to desensitization of the receptor-mediated response and thus act functionally as a feedback inhibitor of the RL interaction. These phenomena represent important distinctions in using classical enzyme theory to describe the kinetic aspects of the RL interaction, especially when using the various extrapolations of Michaelis–Menten kinetic treatments to derive theoretical treatments for such commonly used concepts of spare receptors (17), allosterically regulated receptor complexes (18), and, more recently, chaos theory (19).

3 RECEPTOR THEORY

3.1 Basic Ligand Concepts

Compounds interacting with receptors, the ligands, have two intrinsic properties: the ability to recognize and bind to the receptor—a property referred to as the *activity* or *potency* of the ligand; and the ability of the ligand to effect a change in cellular processes via activation of transmembrane transductional mechanisms, involving G-protein complexes or ion channels, the latter a measure of *efficacy*. Activity is defined in terms of the affinity of the ligand expressed as the K_i (inhibition constant) or K_d, the reciprocal of the association constant, K_a. Typically, ligands have nanomolar (10^{-9} M) to micromolar (10^{-6} M) K_i values, with agonists having lesser affinity than selective antagonists.

In addition to the affinity of a receptor for its ligand, the response to the ligand is also dependent on the number of receptors on a given tissue. This number can be measured, by radioligand binding, in terms of the B_{max}, a value expressed in terms of receptor concentration per mg protein. In peripheral tissues where nerve innervation is much more limited, the B_{max} can be in the order of femtomoles (10^{-15} M). In tissues like the brain, B_{max} values are typically in the range of femtomoles to picomoles (10^{-12} M). The number of re-

ceptors present on a tissue is not always reflective of the ability of a tissue to respond. Receptors are not always coupled to a functional transduction system and as such there has been considerable discussion on the topic of what are known as spare receptors (17). Using alkylating agents that can inactivate a good portion of the receptor population on a given tissue, as much as 90%, the receptor-inactivation technique developed by Furchgott (20), it has been possible to still elicit a full response with a given agonist in a defined system. The reasons for this response are unknown and certainly confound the process of drug targeting. One possible reason for spare receptors is to maintain tissue sensitivity when receptors that have formed RL complexes are unavailable to interact with further molecules of ligand. This disposition may relate to the phenomenon known as receptor desensitization which is discussed further below.

These recognition properties are complemented at the receptor level by structural elements determining recognition and transduction. An additional ligand property is that of *selectivity*, the degree to which the ligand interacts with the target of choice as compared to related structural targets. The degree of selectivity typically determines the side effect profile of a new compound, given that the targeted mechanism itself does not produce untoward effects when stimulated beyond the therapeutic range.

Receptor ligands consist of two major classes, agonists and antagonists, that can both bind to the receptor. Agonists by definition have intrinsic efficacy, that is their binding to the receptor leads to activation of the intracellular components involved in the physiological or pharmacological responsiveness of the cell or tissue. This efficacy may be manifest by changes in the activity of an enzyme like adenylate cyclase or by an alteration in the contractile response of an isolated, intact tissue preparation. Those properties present in a ligand that define efficacy remain largely theoretical at this point in time.

The maximal response elicited by a known agonist is, by definition, 100% of the response attainable (Fig. 11.1) and this response is reflected as an intrinsic efficacy of 1.0 (17). Antagonists, on the other hand, bind to the receptor and block the interaction of the agonist while producing no effect on the tissue on their own. This inherent lack of activity reflects an intrinsic activity of zero (0).

Antagonism can be of several types: competitive, noncompetitive and uncompetitive and irreversible (21). Competitive antagonism is usually associated with ligands that interact directly with the agonist binding site, e.g., the recognition element of the receptor. This type of antagonism can be surmounted by the addition of increasing concentrations of agonist. The resultant functional dose–response curve then undergoes a rightward shift with approximately the same shape and maximal effect, the degree of which is dependent on the concentration of antagonist used (Fig. 11.1).

The situation is more complex in the case of noncompetitive or uncompetitive antagonists. Such ligands are thought to interact at sites distinct from the agonist recognition site and can modulate agonist binding either by proximal interactions with this site from a site adjacent to the recognition site or by allosterically altering the receptor protein from a distinct site to modulate agonist activity. The latter can theoretically occur by an alteration in the affinity of the receptor for the ligand or by a change in the transductional process through which the agonist produces its response. In some circumstances this change would result in an "uncoupling" of the receptor from the G-protein, in others an increase in efficiency via the disinhibition of the actions of a facilitatory modulator. The effects of noncompetitive antagonists are usually not reversible by the addition of excess agonist.

The discussion related to antagonism so far has focused at the molecular level with the assumption that antagonist ligands produce their actions at a defined molecular target, namely the receptor. Such antagonism is known as *pharmacological antagonism* and involves the interactions between ligands and the receptor site (Fig. 11.2). *Functional antagonism* refers to the

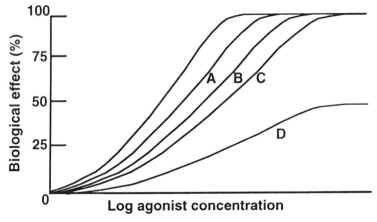

Fig. 11.1 Dose response curve. The addition of increasing concentrations of an agonist ligand causes an increase in the biological response to a maximum of 100%. When plotted on a logarithmic scale, a sigmoidal curve is attained. Addition of increasing concentrations (A < B < C) of a competitive antagonist results in a progressive rightward shift in the dose response (DR) curve. The same maximum is attained with increasing concentrations of agonist. Curve D shows a partial agonist which is unable to elicit a maximal response.

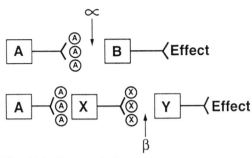

Fig. 11.2 Pharmacological and functional antagonism. In the top figure, neurotransmitter A is released and interacts with receptor A on postsynaptic cell B. Activation of cell B results in a physiological effect. Antagonist α blocks the agonist actions of neurotransmitter A by blocking its actions at receptor A, a direct pharmacological antagonism of the effects of neurotransmitter A. In the lower panel, the same neurotransmitter A is released but interacts with receptors on cell X. Activation of cell X results in the release of neurotransmitter X that in turn activates cell Y to produce a physiological effect. Antagonist β blocks the effects of neurotransmitter A by antagonizing the effects of neurotransmitter X. It thus acts as a functional antagonist of neurotransmitter A. Functional antagonism is a major caveat of intact tissue or *in vivo* studies.

situation in which an antagonist that does not interact with a given receptor can still block the actions of an agonist of that receptor and is typically reflected in the responses observed in intact tissue preparations of whole animal models.

In the hypothetical example shown in Figure 11.2, neurotransmitter A released from neuron A interacts with A-type receptors on neuron B. Antagonist α, can block the effects of A on cell B by interacting with A receptors. Antagonist α is thus a pharmacological antagonist of A receptors. In the second example in Figure 11.2, neuron A releases neurotransmitter A which interacts with A receptors located on neuron X. In turn, neuron X releases neurotransmitter X which interacts with receptors for X on neuron Y. Antagonist β is a competitive antagonist that interacts with X receptors to block the effects of X and in doing so indirectly blocks the actions of neurotransmitter A. Antagonist β is a

pharmacological antagonist of receptors for the neurotransmitter X, but a functional antagonist for neurotransmitter A. In interpreting functional data in complex systems, it is always important to remain open to the possibility that a ligand has more than one effect mediated through a single class of receptor.

Another example of functional antagonism is in the basal ganglia where receptors for the dopamine D_2 receptor and the adenosine A_{2a} receptor are colocalized in a subpopulation of neurons innervating the striatopallidal pathway (22, 23). The effects of dopamine in this pathway have been traditionally blocked using classical dopamine antagonists like haloperidol. However, adenosine can also inhibit dopamine effects in the basal ganglia by interacting with A_{2a} receptors that can in turn, by altering intracellular events, block the effects of dopamine D_2 receptor activation. Adenosine thus has the potential to act as a functional dopamine antagonist (24).

A third class of ligand is that of the inverse agonist (25, 26). Ligands of this class interact with a defined recognition site on a receptor and are not only able to block the effects of an agonist at the receptor but, to varying degrees are able to produce effects opposite to that of the agonist. Mention has already been made of the zero (0) to unity (1.0) scale to define antagonists and full agonists. By definition, inverse agonists occupy an efficacy scale of zero (0) to minus unity (−1). Examples of inverse agonists have, to date, been associated with ligand gated ion channels most notably the $GABA_A/BZ$ receptor complex (13, 25).

3.2 Historical Perspectives and Receptor Theories

Theoretical concepts of the RL interaction have typically been derived on the basis of experimental data. The earliest theory related to the nature of the RL interaction was the occupancy theory developed by Clark in 1926 (27) on the basis of the dose-response relationship (Fig. 11.1). Modifications of the seminal occupancy theory include Paton's rate theory (28) and Gosselin's inactivation theory (29). To these theories may be added the various theories involving allosteric regulation of the receptor ligand interaction (18, 30), typically associated with the receptor complexes associated with LGICs. Recent data also suggests that GPCRs, specifically the adenosine A_1 receptor, may also undergo allosteric modulation (31, 32), via the effects of the benzothiazolines (31) and the natural frog peptide, adenoregulin (32).

3.2.1 OCCUPANCY THEORY.

In 1926, Clark developed the dose–response (DR) curve to describe the interaction of acetylcholine (ACh) with muscle preparations (27). Using a logarithmic plot, antagonists like atropine were found to cause a rightward shift in the DR curve. The basic premise of occupancy theory was that the effect produced by an agonist is dependent on the number of receptors occupied by the agonist. Using the Michaelis–Menten derivation (14) of the Law of Mass Action, occupancy theory was defined by the following parameters: (i) the RL complex is reversible; (ii) the association of the receptor with the ligand to form the RL complex is a bimolecular process while the dissociation is a monomolecular process; (iii) all receptors of a given class are equivalent and bind ligand independently of one another; (iv) formation of the RL complex does not alter the free (*F*) concentration of the ligand or the affinity of the receptor for the ligand; (v) the response elicited by receptor occupancy is directly proportional to the number of receptors occupied; and (vi) the biological response is dependent on the attainment of equilibrium between R and L according to equation 11.2. Although it is

not always possible to determine the concentrations of free ligand or that of the RL complex, rearranging the latter, the equilibrium dissociation constant, K_d which equals k_{-1}/k_{+1}, can be derived from the equation:

$$K_d = ([R][L]/[RL]) \qquad (11.3)$$

and is equal to the concentration of *L* that occupies 50% of the available receptors.

The interaction of antagonist ligands with the receptor had been proposed by Gaddum (33) to result in occupancy without the elicitation of a functional response. In this way, antagonists have blocked the actions of agonist ligands. Increasing the concentration of an agonist can overcome the effects of a competitive antagonist (Fig. 11.1). Titration of the agonist dose response curve in the presence of increasing concentrations of a competitive antagonist, can generate a series of parallel curves with an increasing progression to the right (Fig. 11.1, A–C). These curves can be analyzed to yield a Schild regression plot (34) from which a pA_2 value for the antagonist can be derived. The pA_2 value represents the affinity of an antagonist for a given receptor and can be derived from a plot of log (DR-1) versus the log concentration of antagonist (Fig. 11.3) to yield the pA_2 at the intercept of the abcissa. The pA_2 value is equal to $-\log_{10} K_B$ where the K_B represents the dissociation constant for a competitive antagonist which has a slope of near unity. Non- or un-competitive antagonists which bind to sites distinct from the agonist recognition site have slopes that are significantly less than unity. The Schild plot is a frequently used method to determine the mechanism by which an antagonist produces its effects.

Another modification to Clark's occupancy theory was introduced by Ariens (35) who observed that not all cholinergic agonists were able to produce a maximal response in skeletal muscle even at sup-

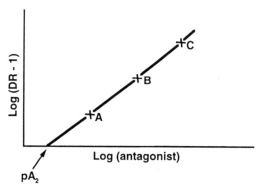

Fig. 11.3 Schild plot regression. Data from Figure 11.1 for antagonist concentrations A, B, and C were plotted by the method of Schild (35) to yield a pA2, a measure of antagonist activity. The slope of the Schild regression indicates the nature of the antagonism, a slope of unity indicating a competitive antagonist.

ramaximal concentrations. This discovery led to the introduction of the concept of *intrinsic activity* which has already been discussed. Many ligands have intrinsic efficacies that lie between zero and one and are defined as partial agonists (Fig. 11.1). These agents bind to the receptor and produce a portion of the response seen with the full agonist. Since the intrinsic efficacy spectrum reflects a combination of antagonist actions (zero) through full agonist (1.0), partial agonists are also, by definition, partial antagonists.

Another class of agonist is loosely referred to as "super agonist" where the intrinsic efficacy in a defined system is greater than the unity response elicited by the most potent agonist identified to that time. The system in which intrinsic efficacy is defined thus relies on the activity of a defined agonist being equal to 100%. Other ligands may, however, have greater effects within the system of choice because of greater intrinsic efficacy. An example is that of the muscarinic cholinergic receptor agonist, L 670,207 (36), a bioisostere of arecoline which was 70% greater efficacy than arecoline in the test system and thus has an intrinsic efficacy of 1.7. The activity associated with L 670,207 would indicate

that the reference agonist, arecoline is only able to elicit a portion of the maximal response that the issue is capable of and as such should be redefined as a partial agonist. It is critical to the practical interpretation of receptor theory that the system in which the response is defined can be stimulated to its maximum in order to set a baseline for the comparison of other compounds within it.

There is no consistent relationship between the K_i value of a ligand and its ability to elicit a full response. Thus a ligand with relatively poor affinity (10^{-7} M or greater), may still be a full agonist when a sufficient concentration interacts with the receptor. The concept of partial agonists was introduced by Stephenson (37) in introducing the concept of *efficacy*, the situation where a maximal response to an agonist could occur when only a small proportion of the total number of receptors on a tissue were occupied. This, by definition, resulted in an occupancy relationship that was nonlinear, the response occurring being defined as the stimulus S, which was the product of the fraction of receptors occupied and the ligand efficacy. The nonlinearity of the functional response can complicate data interpretation, especially when spare receptor or receptor reserve concepts are introduced (17, 38, 39) to rationalize data.

Whereas efficacy differs from intrinsic activity in that the latter is defined as a proportion of the maximal response (effect = α [RL]), Ariens modified intrinsic activity theory to bring it in line with efficacy (40). Intrinsic efficacy has been further modified to include the concentration of receptors in a tissue (20) thus making efficacy a parameter that was ligand rather than ligand and tissue dependent.

From these considerations, Kenakin (17) has defined ligand related responses in a given tissue in terms of four parameters: (i) the receptor density; (ii) the efficiency of the transductional process; (iii) the equilibrium dissociation constant of the RL complex; and (iv) the intrinsic efficacy of the ligand at the receptor.

In considering agonist effects at GPCRs, Keen (41) has noted that classical receptor theory assumes that affinity and efficacy are two separate, independent parameters. This concept may not be the case in practical terms and may be colored by many of responses being measured in classical intact tissue preparations being far removed from the receptor activation event. More recently, Tallarida has proposed (19) that receptor occupancy for exogenous ligands is primarily dependent on pharmacokinetic parameters whereas occupancy for endogenous ligands is most probably under intrinsic control. Accordingly he has introduced a feedback function defined as Φ that implies a control of RL complex stability that is dependent on the relative concentrations of free and bound ligand. Using the principles of chaos theory, Tallarida has defined the stable RL complex as an "attractor" with situations leading to loss of control for a given RL interaction as unstable points or "repellors". In addition to being both provocative and intellectually challenging, chaos theory as related to classical receptor occupancy theory may provide possible models for disease states related to receptor imbalances within a tissue.

With each new decade, the basic model of occupancy theory has been "tweaked", yet remains the seminal basis for understanding receptor function. There is still much to be learned, however, regarding the concepts of efficacy and receptor reserve (especially with the advent of newer molecular data as data related to what represents a maximal response within a tissue), the latter a moving target as newer bioisosteres of known agonists are designed (36).

3.2.2 RATE THEORY. Experimental data showing the persistence of antagonist-mediated responses and agonist "fade" where maximal responses occur transiently to be followed by lesser responses of longer duration and agonist-mediated blockade of agonist effects, led Paton to modify the concept of occupancy to include a chemically based rate term (28). Thus according to rate theory, it is not only the number of receptors occupied by a ligand that determines the response, but also the rate of RL formation. The effect, E, produced by a ligand, was considered equal to a proportionality factor, φ that included an efficacy component and the velocity, V. Thus:

$$E = \varphi Veq \qquad (11.4)$$

The rate or RL formation, like that of neurotransmitter release, is measured in quantal terms with discrete "all or none" changes in receptor-mediated events. Pharmacokinetic considerations will play a major role in determining the rate of RL formation from exogenously applied ligands (41), which most drugs are, again invoking some consideration of aspects of Tallarida's modeling of the RL complex based on chaos theory (19). The primary factor delineating occupancy and rate theory appears to be the dissociation rate constant (42). Thus if this factor is large, the ligand will be an agonist. If the factor is small, reducing the quantal response to receptor occupancy, the ligand will be an antagonist. The kinetic aspects of rate theory do not however, take into account the efficiency of transductional coupling. Rate theory has accordingly been described by Limbird (42) as "a provocative conceptualization . . . . with limited applicability."

3.2.3 INACTIVATION THEORY. The receptor inactivation theory proposed by Gosselin in 1977 (29), is a synthesis of both occupancy and rate theories. It has not been widely appreciated (17) but nonetheless provides an alternate consideration for the active study of the RL interaction.

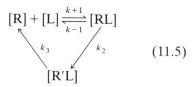

$$[R] + [L] \underset{k-1}{\overset{k+1}{\rightleftharpoons}} [RL]$$

$$k_3 \quad k_2 \qquad (11.5)$$

$$[R'L]$$

Inactivation theory assumes that the RL complex is an intermediate "active" state that gives rise to an inactive form of the receptor, R' that is part of an RL complex termed $R'L$. k_{+1} is the rate of association and k_{-1} the rate of dissociation of the RL complex (Eq. 11.5). k_2 is the rate constant for the transition from RL to $R'L$, the rate constant for the regeneration of the active form of the receptor, R is k_3. The response elicited then is proportional to the rate of R' formation which is equal to $K_3[R'L]$, a variable dependent on both the number of receptors occupied and the rate of R' formation. Unequivocal experimental data to support receptor inactivation theory has been difficult to obtain as has data to distinguish between occupancy, rate and inactivation theories of the RL interaction (17, 42). Nonetheless, the inclusion of an additional step in terms of the active receptor generation inherent in receptor inactivation theory provides a further nuance related to the potential mechanisms by which antagonists and allosteric modulatory ligands may elicit their effects on the RL interaction and the signal transduction process.

4 RECEPTOR COMPLEXES AND ALLOSTERIC MODULATORS

The various receptor theories discussed to this point have involved a simple biomolecular reaction under pseudo-first order reaction kinetics for a single ligand acting at a receptor. It appears highly unlikely that even for the relatively simple GPCRs, that the activation of a single receptor results in an interaction with only one G protein (39, 41). There is considerable evidence, however, for nonlinear concentration–response curves that provide evidence for the existence of oligomeric receptor complexes with multiple ligand binding sites similar to the enzymic complexes that have led to the concept of allosterism or cooperativity (Table 11.2).

The interactions of ligands with identical receptor sites on oligomers can result in a gradation in the interaction of sequentially bound ligand molecules. The first ligand can facilitate the binding of a second, identical ligand and so on such that the saturation curve describing the interaction of ligand with receptor is steeper than that which would be predicted from mass action kinetics. The process of one ligand, homologous or heterologous, interacting with the binding of another is thought to occur by the induction of a cooperative, conformational change in the binding protein for the second ligand from a site adjacent to the ligand recognition site. Based on the classical studies of Hill with hemoglobin (43), various models of allosterism have been developed, the best known of which are the concerted model of Monod, Wyman and Changeux (18) and the sequential, or induced fit model of Koshland, Nemethy and Filmer (30). The major criteria for these models are summarized in Table 11.2. As indicated, the two models are assumed to be comprised of oligomeric protein units with identical subunits that exist in two states that are in equilibrium with one another in the absence of ligand. The binding of a ligand induces a conformational change moving the equilibrium of the two states to favor that with the higher affinity for the ligand which in turn alters the functional properties of the receptor complex.

Not all receptor complexes are comprised of identical subunits, however. Neither are the ligands involved in producing

Table 11.2   Cooperativity Criteria—Allosteric Receptor Models

---

Concerted Model[a]

The receptor is a multicomponent oligomer comprised of a finite number of identical subunits.
The subunits are arranged symmetrically and each has a single binding site for the ligand.
The receptor complex exists in two conformational states one of which has a preference for ligand binding.
The conformational transition state involves a simultaneous shift in the state of all the subunits.
No hybrids exist—implying cooperativity.

Sequential Model[b]

The receptor complex is a multicomponent oligomer with symmetrically arranged protomers, each with a single binding site for the ligand.
The protomers exist in 2 conformational states—transition is induced by ligand binding.
Receptor symmetry is lost when the ligand is bound.
Hybrid states of the oligomer can be stabilized by protomers.
Stabilization is equivalent to negative cooperativity.

---

[a]Monod et al. (18).
[b]Koshland et al. (30).

allosteric effects identical. The $GABA_A$/ BZ(benzodiazepine) receptor (13, 44) is a ligand-gated ion channel (LGIC) that is a target site for numerous anxiolytic, anticonvulsant, muscle relaxant and hypnotic drugs that produce their effects by enhancing inhibitory neurotransmission in the CNS. The basic entities of the $GABA_A$/BZ receptor complex are a $GABA_A$ receptor, a BZ recognition site and a chloride channel. The $GABA_A$/BZ is a pentameric LGIC comprised of distinct molecular subunits. Six α, four β, three γ, a single δ, and two ρ subunits have been identified which have a distinct regional distribution in mammalian brain (45). It has been postulated, based on the number of subunits, that the $GABA_A$/ BZ LGIC receptor may exist in several thousand combinations (46). The presence of α, β, and γ subunits appears necessary for BZ sensitivity in recombinant $GABA_A$ receptors expressed in oocytes. In addition to the primary recognition sites, the $GABA_A$/BZ receptor complex has recognition sites for a number of functional allosteric modulators including: ethanol, zinc, the avermectins, barbiturates, picrotox-

inin, the neurosteroids, e.g., alfazalone (47), Ro 5-4864, the classical peripheral BZ ligand (48). The pharmacology of these allosteric sites is dependent on the subunit composition of the $GABA_A$/BZ receptor complex (45).

The *N*-methyl-D-aspartate (NMDA) receptor (49) is another LGIC that mediates certain of the effects of the principal excitatory neurotransmitter in the mammalian CNS, L-glutamate. The NMDA receptor is an oligomeric receptor complex comprised of a recognition site for NMDA, an ion channel site that binds magnesium, the dissociative anesthetics, ketamine, and phencyclidine (PCP) and the uncompetitive NMDA receptor antagonist, MK 801, and a glycine modulatory site (50). A zinc binding site, activation of which elicits a selective blockade of NMDA–evoked responses has been described (51). A polyamine binding site (52) at which spermine and possibly the anti-ischemic agent, ifenprodil (53) bind have also been described. Ligands interacting with the various recognition sites on the NMDA receptor complex offer the potential for highly complex yet subtle nuances in receptor function that while reflecting the pivotal role of this receptor in the CNS significantly complicate data interpretation within the context of classical receptor theory.

The nicotinic cholinergic receptor, nAChR (54) is another LGIC comprised of distinct α, β, γ, and δ subunits in pentameric $\alpha 2\beta\gamma\delta$ combinations (55, 56). The nAChRs found at the neuromuscular junction and at neurons differ in their subunit composition and this difference is thought to impart different functionality to the receptor oligomer (57). Although there are four different receptor subunits, recombinant studies show that combinations of α and β alone are able to form functional receptors. $\alpha_2\beta_2$, $\alpha_3\beta_2$, and $\alpha_4\beta_2$ form functional receptors with each having a different pharmacological profile (58). In contrast, the β_3 subunit in combination with the α_2, α_3, or α_4 subunits is unable to form a functional receptor. The functional contribution of the γ and δ subunits remains unknown. It is of interest that a pentamer comprised of $\alpha 7$ subunits is able to function as a functional LGIC (59). The binding of ligands to the nAChR can be modulated in an allosteric manner by the ligand, 2-methylpiperidine (2-MP) (60, 61). The uncompetitive NMDA receptor antagonist, MK 801 can also bind to the channel of the torpedo nAChR (62).

The ligands that bind to recognition sites on the oligomer and alter the functional properties of the receptor complex, are known as allosteric modulators. The central BZs, including diazepam, enhance the inhibitory responses to the central neurotransmitter, GABA (44). The nAChR allosteric modulator, 2-MP, increases ligand binding (60) and receptor function (61) whereas a number of glycine site modulators, e.g., HA 966, influence the function of the NMDA receptor complex (50). As already noted, there is also emerging evidence for allosteric modulators of the adenosine A_1-GPCR (31, 32). Cation

and anion binding sites on GPCRs also reflect the potential for allosteric modulation of receptor function.

Allosteric modulators have become popular as potential drug targets based on the hypothesis that agents that influence the effects of a neurotransmitter indirectly have a reduced side effect liability. This reduction has proven to be the case for the BZ receptor complex where the BZs have proven to be effective potentiators of GABAergic transmission (47). In contrast, directly acting $GABA_A$ agonists have proven to be ineffective clinical agents due to the magnitude of their side effects (63).

The application of classical receptor theory to situations where allosteric modulators influence primary receptor responses, considerably complicates data interpretation. This complication may be accentuated by the existence of endogenous allosteric modulators, many of which have still to be identified.

5 SECOND AND THIRD MESSENGER SYSTEMS

Historically, the signal transduction systems associated with receptors have involved the production of the cyclic nucleotides, cAMP and cGMP, from ATP and GTP, respectively, via the action of the enzymes adenylate and guanylate cyclase (64). The interaction between the classical GPCR, the G protein and effector enzyme is represented by a ternary complex that is allosterically regulated (65). The cyclic nucleotides in turn can influence the activity of other enzyme systems, the protein kinases (66), including PKA and PKC and the *trk* and tyrosine kinases (67, 68). Increased activity of these enzymes results in the phosphorylation and alteration in functional activity of various intracellular proteins that can lead to changes in the cell signalling pathways involved in receptor sensitivity (69), gene activation (70), and cell proliferation (71).

Calcium (9) and the various products of the phosphatidylinositol phosphate hydrolysis (72), (e.g., IP_3 and arachidonic acid pathways (73) are other second messengers as are the diffusable second messengers, (74) nitric oxide (NO) and (CO) carbon monoxide (75).

Receptors for ligands that produce their physiological effects via intracellular receptors present on DNA like the sex steroids (76) and the thyroid hormone/steroid receptor superfamily (77) operate independently of these classical second messenger systems. Sex steroids bind to receptors on the target cell surface and are then transported to the nucleus as an RL complex to modulator promotor regions on DNA. Ligands for the thyroid hormone/steroid receptor superfamily, many of them analogs of retinoic acid, bind to intracellular receptors or ligand-dependent transcription factors that can then bind to specific DNA sequences, the hormone responsive elements, or HREs to modulate gene expression (78). Interestingly, members of the thyroid hormone/steroid receptor superfamily can be activated independently of ligand activation. One such "orphan" receptor, COUP-TF, can be activated by phosphorylation via a dopamine D-1 receptor mechanism (79).

An additional level of complexity in the events subsequent to ligand-dependent receptor activation, involves neurotransmitter induction of gene expression (80) involving immediate-early genes like *c-fos* (81) which can lead to more long term changes in postsynaptic responsiveness.

6 RECEPTOR INTERACTIONS AND INTEGRATION

The integration of the data input into a cell has been typically thought of as a summation of the postsynaptic or postjunctional responses resulting from a variety of heterosynaptic neuronal inputs to the cell (82). This disposition may involve interreceptor interactions as in the case of the dopamine D_1 and D_2 receptors (83) with the D_2 receptor subserving a permissive role on D_1-mediated responses. There are also integrative responses to incoming signals that occur at the intracellular level and involve cross-talk between different cell signal transduction pathways as in the case of the dioxin receptor (84). The level of complexity inherent in signal transduction pathway cross-talk is staggering given the various kinases, kinase substrates, calcium-modulated events, and transcriptional and translational processes that are under the control of receptor mediated processes as well as transmitters (glutamate) that release diffusable second messengers (NO) (74) or become a part, rather than a trigger, of the second messenger (71, 78). As more becomes known about cell function at the molecular level, the greater is the complexity, especially when approaching drug targets within the cell as potential sites for selective drug actions.

7 RECEPTOR DYNAMICS

Receptors are not static entities present in the cell membrane throughout the life of the target cell but rather undergo both ligand and gene related control (39). Receptor turnover occurs as a normal consequence of cell growth with half lives that vary between hours and days (85, 86). Ligand occupancy can also alter receptor density. Given what is known about the processes of neurotransmission and neuromodulation, it is reasonable to assume that the target cells for endogenous effector agents, neurotransmitters, neuromodulators and neurohormones are under tonic control, an implicit assumption for chaos theory (19). The molecular basis of many disease states may thus reflect an over-stimulation or decrease in stimulation of a given receptor system. This inequity in turn may reflect over or underproduction of the endogenous ligand, a decrease in receptor density or function, a persistance in activation due to a maladaptation of the transduction system and so on. In Parkinson's disease, for instance, the presynaptic nerve cells in the substantia nigra that produce dopamine die as the result of an as yet unknown disease etiology. This defect results in a decrease in dopamine levels and a consequent hypersensitivity of postsynaptic responses as the homeostatic processes attempt to compensate for a lack of endogenous ligand.

An overstimulation of a given receptor system can result in receptor desensitization, a decrease in receptor number (down regulation) or function, that results in a blunted response. Because exogenously administered receptor agonists are not under normal homeostatic control (19) their effects frequently become blunted upon repeated administration. It should consequently come as no surprise that the majority of effective therapeutic agents are antagonists of receptor function.

Receptor desensitization can occur by alterations in kinase activity that alter the phosphorylation state of enzymes like NO synthase and by receptor internalization or sequestering (39, 86). Receptor downregulation can occur as the result of various drug treatments (86) and can be measured by changes in receptor tissue obtained by biopsy and autopsy. The accumulation of evidence for the association of specific receptor density changes with specific disease states, has been a major goal of biomedical research over the past 2 decades. With the unequivocal identification of such receptor losses, the molecular mechanisms involved in the disease process can be identified and used for drug targeting and disease diagnosis. Unfortunately,

many changes in receptor density prove to be difficult to replicate from one patient sample to another and frequently reflect generalized cell loss rather than specific disease-related changes. For example, in Alzheimer's Disease, the basal forebrain cholinergic system is firmly established as primary focus of the neurodegenerative process associated with the disease state. This focus is reflected in decreases in both muscarinic and cholinergic receptor densities (87). There are however well-documented changes in central dopamine, serotonin and noradrenergic systems and their receptors (87) as well as a variety of neuropeptide receptors. These findings confuse the cause and effect relationship of the disease and may reflect a generic effect on neuronal survival where cell loss is a general cause of receptor rather than a targeted loss of any one receptor system.

8 MOLECULAR BIOLOGY OF RECEPTORS

In the past ten years, the powerful tools of recombinant DNA (rDNA) technology (88–90) have permitted the isolation and sequence analysis of numerous receptors from various mammalian complimentary DNA (cDNA) libraries using the polymerase chain reaction (PCR) technique (91) to clone receptors which can then be expressed in various pro- and eukaryotic cell lines and the frog (Xenopus) oocyte.

As already discussed, structural and functional data have revealed conserved regions in receptors that are involved in ligand binding, coupling to transductional systems and ion channel formation. As a consequence, receptor cloning, sequencing, and expression have become a major focus of receptor research and an increasingly important part of the drug discovery process.

8.1 Receptor Cloning

The cloning of a receptor gene requires the isolation of the DNA encoding the protein of interest from a library of complimentary DNA sequences. Cloning receptor genes from mammalian tissues, including human, and expressing them on the surface of surrogate microbial or mammalian cells like, for example, *E. Coli*, yeast, human embryonic kidney (HEK), and Chinese hamster ovary (CHO) cells facilitate their study as isolated entities in a defined microenvironment. Once cloned and identified, the nucleotide sequence of a receptor gene can be determined and this in turn allows the primary structure of isolated receptor to be deduced (92). Analysis of the deduced protein sequences of the receptors isolated to date, indicates that each belongs to a limited number of super-families which have sequence and structural homology (Figs. 11.4 and 11.5).

The ubiquitous GPCR family of receptors that contains seven transmembrane stretches of amino acids in helical form constitutes one receptor superfamily (Fig. 11.4). In contrast, LGICs including the nicotinic, $GABA_A$, and NMDA receptors already discussed as well as the $5HT_3$ receptor are composed of protein subunits that can assemble in an oligomer (in most cases a pentamer) surrounding a membrane pore (Fig. 11.5).

From the drug discovery standpoint, the ability to specifically alter the structure of cloned receptor through modification of a small number of nucleotides, the process known as site-directed mutagenesis (11), the removal of specific regions of the receptor gene- "deletion mutagenesis" (93) and the construction of hybrid (chimeric)

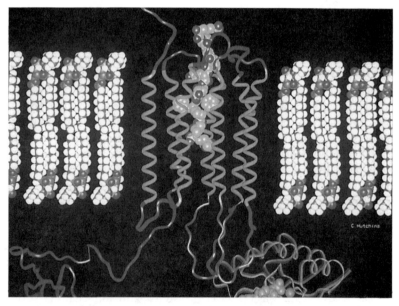

Fig. 11.4 Model of the G-protein coupled receptor (GPCR). The figure shows a stylized tertiary model for a generic GPCR. The seven α helical hydrophobic regions spanning the membrane (TM 1-7) are shown in purple. Extracellular and intracellular loops are shown in red. The *N*- and *C*-termini of the receptor are located extracellularly and intracellularly, respectively. The interaction of a ligand (yellow) with TM 2-4 and consequent coupling to an effector molecule through an appropriate G-protein (bottom right) is shown. Courtesy of Charles Hutchins, Abbott Laboratories. See also color plates.

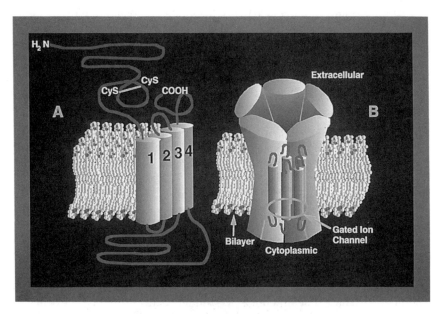

Fig. 11.5 Model of the ligand gated ion channel (LGIC). The figure shows a stylized representation for the topology in the membrane of A. A nicotinic receptor (neuronal or muscle) α-subunit and B. Arrangement of 5 subunits to form a functional LGIC. A, Four TM domains in the a-subunit are shown as cylinders (1–4). The two cysteine residues present in all members of the LGIC superfamily identified to date are also shown. B, The LGICs discussed in this section are all thought to possess pseudo-cyclic symmetry, in which the central symmetry axis delineates a gated, fluid filled pathway for ions. The walls lining the entrances are thought to reflect an excess of negatively charged groups in the case of cation selective channels. A part of the α-helical segment in TM2 from each subunit lines the narrow pore spanning the hydrophobic portion of the bilayer. See also color plates.

proteins containing, for example, the recognition site for α-adrenergic agonists and the G-protein linked region for the β-adrenergic receptor (12) or alternative loops of the dopamine D_1 and D_2 receptors (94, 95), permits a more direct analysis of the contribution that specific amino acids make to ligand recognition and functionality.

8.2 Receptor Cloning Strategies

The cloning strategy used in the isolation of receptor genes is dependent upon a number of variables including: (i) the knowledge regarding the sequence of the protein; (ii) the tissue where it is expressed; (iii) its relative abundance; and (iv) the functional properties of the protein.

These factors dictate the type of gene library to be used, and the method of cloning. A crucial decision in the isolation of a receptor gene is whether to screen a genomic or a cDNA library. A genomic DNA library contains all the genetic information of the organism from which the DNA was derived. It therefore contains structural genes as well as non-expressed sequences such as regulatory sequences. Additionally, the represented genes are structured as they occur in the genome, including introns-DNA sequences that interrupt the "message" sequences, the exons that code for a gene product, when present. A cDNA library can be derived from cellular mRNA and accordingly contain only the genetic information for the proteins expressed in a given cell or tissue. Thus, the composition of the library (types and numbers of genes represented) is highly dependent on the tissue as well as the metabolic state of the tissue from which the mRNA is isolated. The production of a cDNA or genomic library involves the insertion of cDNA or genomic sequence into an appropriate vector to create a library of sequences from which the gene of interest can be isolated. A vector is a self-replicating fragment of DNA that can be propagated in bacteria and comprises a cloning site, a series of unique restriction enzyme sites into which foreign DNA can be inserted that also allow for the selection of transfected host cells in terms of antibiotic resistance of phage lysis. Bacterial plasmids like PGEM (96) and PBr322 (97) were the vectors of choice in most early cloning experiments. These bacterial plasmids have been replaced by bacteriophages, for example, *lgt* 11 which offer the ability to clone cDNA or large (30–50 kbase) genomic fragments with significantly more colonies (1000-fold) being screened per unit time.

Hybridization of a probe to the DNA or RNA of interest is the basis of rDNA technology. All hybridization techniques depend on the ability of denatured DNA to reanneal when complimentary strands are present in an environment near, but below their melting point (Tm). In a hybridization reaction involving filter bound DNA and a single stranded DNA probe, 3 different annealing reactions can occur. First, there is the probe – DNA interaction that results in the signal indicating that the annealing has occurred. Second, there are mismatch interactions that can occur between related, but not homologous sequences. Finally, nonsequence-specific interactions can occur which result in "noise". Mismatch hybrids and nonspecific noise can be eliminated by altering the stringency of the hybridization conditions. Stringency refers to the conditions (temperature, salt concentration) that dictate the likelihood of hybridization

occurring between DNA strands that are nonhomologous. For example, as the temperature used for the hybridization reaction is increased, the stringency is increased and it becomes less likely that hybridization will occur between DNA strands that are nonhomologous, thus decreasing the background noise. Decreasing the salt concentration can also increase hybridization stringency.

Cloning methods have evolved greatly over the last decade. The cloning of the first muscarinic acetylcholine receptor serves as an example of an initial receptor cloning strategy (98). Muscarinic receptors were initially purified in quantity from porcine brain using conventional protein biochemistry techniques to permit partial amino acid sequence information to be derived. A library of cDNA clones derived from poly $(A)^+$ RNA from porcine cerebrum was then constructed (98) and screened by stringency hybridization with an oligodeoxyribonucleotide (oligo) probe containing all possible cDNA sequences predicted from the partial amino acid sequences. Initial screening yielded six clones, one of which was used as a probe to rescreen the library. Secondary screening yielded twenty seven clones. Two of these clones that apparently carried the longest cDNA inserts were analyzed for nucleotide sequence prior to subsequent expression in frog oocytes to examine the functional responses to a variety of muscarinic ligands (98). This pharmacological analysis suggested that the M_1 muscarinic receptor gene had been isolated. Sequence analysis indicated similarities to other GPCRs such as the β-adrenergic and rhodopsin receptor superfamilies. These similarities have facilitated the development of an alternative cloning strategy that was not dependent on the presence of adequate supplies of purified protein but rather assumed that when the receptor of interest is a member of a family of molecules of similar structure and function, a commonly conserved sequence could be used to design a probe for use in initial screening process.

The identification of a number of neuronal nicotinic acetylcholine receptor (nAChR) subtypes exemplifies this strategy (99). In this instance, the approach was based on the experimentally supported hypothesis (100) that although the primary structures of the nAChR from the Torpedo electric organ and vertebrate muscle are likely to be distinct from their neuronal counterparts, they are encoded by genes that have similar nucleotide sequences in regions of the receptor that share common functionality; for example, the regions modulating ion flux. Thus cDNAs encoding the subunits of the electric organ and vertebrate muscle nicotinic receptors were used as probes for low stringency screening of cDNA libraries from mRNA isolated from neural sources. These initial "fishing expeditions" yielded cDNA encoding the chick α-2 and rat α-3 subunits of the nAChR and provided the essential probes for the identification of a multigene family encoding neuronal nACRs expressed in brain and peripheral ganglia (101, 102).

While this approach has been used very successfully in the isolation of numerous GPCRs (103) and LGICs (104), it has some limitations. Because of the inherent structural similarities that exist between families of receptors, screening a cDNA library under low stringency hybridization conditions with a cross hybridizing probe may lead to the isolation of cDNA encoding subtypes of other receptors. For example, the cDNA for the 5-HT_{1A} receptor was obtained using a full length probe to the β_2-adrenoceptor using low stringency hybridization conditions (105). In addition, this strategy is unlikely to detect cDNAs corresponding to genes expressed at very low levels in tissues used in the construction of the library.

A third approach, useful in the isolation

of receptors linked to ion-channels, is cloning by functional expression in frog (*Xenopus*) oocytes. These frog eggs can efficiently express foreign receptors and ion-channels after injection of the appropriate mammalian mRNA. The expression of these proteins can be directly identified by electrophysiological measurements of the activity of an expressed receptor in response to application of an agonist. Members of the serotonin, neurokinin and glutamate receptor families have been isolated using this approach (106–108). In the case of the glutamate receptor, a cDNA library was made in an RNA expression vector, and an mRNA mixture was synthesized in vitro and assayed after injection in oocytes (108).

The application of polymerase chain reaction technology, (PCR; 91), and more recently, the ligase chain reaction (LCR, 109), to the cloning, subcloning, mutational analysis and quantification drug receptors has resulted in major advances in the isolation of novel receptors which in some cases have yet to be assigned a function. PCR was first exploited by Liebert and co-workers (110) to isolate several novel members of the GPCR family including the adenosine A_1 (111) and A_{2a} (112) receptors, and has subsequently been used to isolate cDNAs for the NK-1 (113), NK-2 (114), dopamine D_1 (115) and D_4 dopamine (116), histamine (117) and adenosine A_3 receptors (118), as well as a new subfamily of odorant receptors (119) and a novel receptor for fibroblast growth factor (120).

Using a DNA polymerase that is able to survive heating to 95°C, DNA and specific primers can be cycled through a reaction involving denaturing the DNA at 95°C, annealing at a temperature dependent upon the thermal melting point of the primers and then extending the DNA at 72°C. This cycle is typically repeated 20–40 times. PCR offers several advantages over the use

of oligonucleotide probes and low stringency screening. First, PCR-derived probes
are exactly complimentary to a single
species of receptor cDNA and they are also
longer than the oligo probes. As a result,
because conditions of high stringency can
be used, there is a marked reduction in
"false positives". Moreover, by selecting
PCR-derived partial clones with novel sequences in the highly variable regions of
G-protein linked receptors, the probability
of obtaining novel receptor sequences is
greatly enhanced.

LCR, like PCR, uses a thermostable
ligase enzyme to amplify specific sequences
of DNA a million or more times in a few
hours (109). In this type of reaction, four
oligonucleotide probes are used, two complimentary sets that are adjacent to one
another following hybridization. The DNA
ligase joins the two sets of adjacent probes
and only the neighboring oligonucleotides
are completely complimentary to the sequence of interest. Amplification is then
achieved in an identical manner to that
used for PCR.

PCR and LCR differ in the fact that
while PCR amplifies a stretch of DNA
between two primers, it yields a minimum
of information regarding the precise sequence of the amplified fragment. In contrast, LCR amplifies stretches of DNA
sequence identical to that of the probes
used. Thus LCR provides a powerful technology for the simultaneous amplification
and detection of point mutations in DNA
sequences.

From the viewpoint of receptor characterization and in designing selective ligands
for receptors, the remarkable selectivity of
the amplification process afforded by both
the PCR and LCR reactions permits their
use in the identification of receptor
subtypes present in tissues and organs even
when it is only possible to obtain small
amounts of tissue, for example, the nasal
epithelium in the case of the odorant receptors, or in cases where the target cell for

drug action is a minor tissue component.
An even greater level of sensitivity is suggested by recent reports (121, 122) that
PCR may allow the identification of the
subtype(s) of a receptor mediating a
specific physiological response in a single
cell. The chain technologies have also resulted in the identification of "orphan"
receptors that are usually members of a
defined receptor superfamily for which
there is no known ligand. These "orphan"
receptors are predominant in the thyroid
hormone/steroid receptor superfamily
(77).

The use of PCR in the identification of
dopamine receptor subtypes has resulted in
the identification of three new receptors.
Prior to the advent of molecular biological
techniques, 2 main receptor types had been
identified by classical pharmacological approaches: the D_1 and D_2 (123). Using
rDNA techniques the D_5 receptor, which is
closely related to the D_1 receptor, has been
identified (124) while the D_3 and D_4 receptors are an additional family, structurally related to the D_2 receptor (117, 125).
The identification of these additional
dopamine receptor subtypes has created
considerable excitement inasmuch as the
newly identified receptors offer the potential to develop new compounds for diseases
involving dopaminergic pathway function.

A large number of neuroleptic agents
are thought to produce their effects by
blocking the effects of D_2 receptor activation. Their marked side effects (tardive
dyskinesia, extrapyramidal symptomatology), however, limit their clinical usefulness.
The atypical neuroleptic, clozapine (126) is
a breakthrough drug that has a reduced
incidence of such side effects and represents the preferred treatment for intractable schizophrenia. The mechanism that is
responsible for this clinical profile remains
unknown despite nearly a decade of research. This unknown is problematic inasmuch as the use of clozapine is limited by a
1–2% incidence of agranulocytosis which

has in some instances proven fatal. Reports that clozapine bound to the cloned human D_4 receptor with an affinity some ten times higher than that seen at the D_2 receptor (117) as well as a preferential distribution of mRNA for the D_4 receptor in limbic regions of the brain (117) suggested, however, that this newly identified receptor might represent a target for the development of a new generation of atypical neuroleptics. However, different polymorphic forms of the human D_4 receptor have been identified (127) that display different pharmacological properties and an additional complexity to the selection of the D_4 receptor as a neuroleptic drug target.

This example of receptor cloning raises a major point of concern related to human cloning strategy. The use of limited human cDNA libraries has the potential to limit the database on which information related to receptor clones is based. It is possible that the cDNA libraries may not reflect the receptor sequence typical of the population in general. This possibility compounded with a tendency for very limited pharmacological analysis, highlights the need for caution in extrapolating data before sufficient "n values" are available from human tissues.

Receptors for thyroid hormone (T3), vitamin D3, and retinoic acid show significant sequence homology with the classical steroid hormone receptor family sensitive to glucocorticoids and sex steroids (77). In addition, there are a number of orphan receptors in this superfamily for which there are no known ligands or function (79, 128). That they have the potential to be functional is based on the fact that they are expressed as full cytoplasmic mRNAs although their expression into functional proteins has yet to be shown (79).

An additional area of caution in the use of PCR and LCR is that of contamination. Because of the magnitude of amplification process, it is possible that DNA sequences contaminating reaction vessels or in the air, can be amplified along with the clone of interest. While an obvious problem in and of itself, it assumes proportions of greater magnitude when PCR and LCR are used in the controversial forensic process of DNA "fingerprinting" (129).

8.3 Sequence Analysis of Cloned Receptors

Current models for the secondary and tertiary structure of GPCRs are based in large part on bacteriorhodopsin. This protein, which acts as a proton pump within the retinal membrane, is not linked to any G-protein (130). When analyzed by electron microscopy, bacteriorhodopsin is seen as seven α-helices, arranged in a bundle perpendicular to the plane of the lipid bilayer (131; Fig. 11.4).

Comparison of the deduced amino acid sequences of several GPCRs reveals a similar secondary structure: a single polypeptide chain containing seven hydrophobic domains of sufficient length (20–28 amino acids) to span the lipid bilayer (Fig. 11.4). These domains display a sequence similarity among most receptor classes and marked similarities among receptor subtypes. It has been noted, for example, that conserved polar residues within the transmembrane domains are always positioned on the internal side of the helices, and all but one of the conserved aromatic residues are located on the external faces of the helices (132) leading to the speculation that the highly conserved residues play an essential role in maintaining the structure of the receptor, perhaps by determining protein folding; whereas, those residues conserved only among major classes of receptors may play a role in defining their unique functional properties.

The sequences intervening the transmembrane domains, which are considerably more hydrophilic and display greater sequence diversity, form domains that are exposed intracellularly and extracellularly.

The intracellular loops and *C*-terminal fragments have been shown to be the sites of interaction with G proteins (133–135). In all members of this receptor superfamily these regions are characterized by a high content of basic amino acids. The *N*-terminal sequence of most G proteins contains putative sites for *N*-linked glycosylation and is located extracellularly (135).

LGICs which include nicotinic, GABA$_A$, glycine and 5-HT$_3$ receptors, are representative members of the second major receptor superfamily (Fig. 11.5). All of these channel proteins are characterized by highly hydrophobic stretches of 19 amino acid residues to 27 amino acid residues that span the lipid bilayer in a perpendicular or tilted helix conformation. The subunits of these receptors each contain four such transmembrane domains in the carboxy terminal region of the sequence (M1–M4); the distribution of these domains along the polypeptide is invariant for the receptors listed above (136). However, the transmembrane domains differ significantly in length even within one polypeptide, and it cannot yet be assumed that they are all α-helical.

More recently, with the application of the more advanced cloning techniques, a third superfamily of membrane bound receptors has been characterized (137) which undoubtedly will be subdivided in the near future. The subunit structure of this group of receptors has only one transmembrane domain allowing minimum exposure of the subunit to the membrane lipids which can facilitate receptor mobility and internalization. It is noteworthy that the members of this class, for example mitogenic growth factor, natriuretic peptide, neurotrophin and cytokine receptors, produce as one part of their signaling function, long–term, nuclear-based effects (137).

Sequence homology should not be used as the only criteria for the identification and assigning of a newly discovered receptor to a particular superfamily. The recently discovered receptor (138), Str16 which shows 54% homology with the dopamine receptor family, is in fact a new receptor subtype.

8.4 Expression of Cloned Receptors

The expression of a cloned receptor in a cell line, its synthesis from newly introduced cDNA, provides the opportunity to study the SAR of the RL interaction in a relatively simple environment that is usually, in its native or "wild" state, unable to synthesize the protein for the receptor targeted. Numerous receptors, for example the various dopamine receptors (117, 124, 125, 127, 139), β-2 and β-3 adrenoreceptors (140, 141) and a neuronal calcium channel (142), have been expressed in a variety of mammalian cell lines including HEK (human kidney cell line), CHO (Chinese hamster ovary), and the SHSY5Y (human neuroblastoma) cell lines, all of which are readily available from ATCC (American Type Culture Collection, Rockville, Md.). Bacterial systems are routinely used as expression systems. β-1 and β-2 adrenoceptors and 5-HT$_{1A}$ and 5-HT$_{1D}$ (143, 144) receptors have been expressed in different strains of *E. Coli* while the M$_1$ human muscarinic receptor gene has been expressed in yeast (145).

The expression of a cloned receptor is highly dependent on the vector used to transfect as well as the cell type into which the receptor is transfected. For example, the β-globin gene is expressed at a low level that cannot be induced in HeLa cells but is inducible following differentiation in MEL cells (146). Receptor expression can be stable or transient in nature. Ideally, to facilitate study of a receptor, stable expression where the receptor protein is expressed at a constant level, is the goal. Despite the best laid plans of the molecular biologist, it is not always possible to ensure stable expression where the gene for the receptor is permanently incorporated from the transfected plasmid into the genome of the target cell. In such instances, transient expression can be acceptable to demonstrate that a receptor clone has binding activity. This demonstration can be done by classical receptor binding, by the use of antibodies to the receptor or by measuring the presence of mRNA for the receptor using oligonucleotide probes. The latter method, while more sensitive, is less precise in that the presence of mRNA by no means indicates whether the protein coded for is actually expressed. There are a number of instances where mRNA changes do not correlate with changes in receptor protein (139, 147).

Stable transformants are usually selected by their ability to confer resistance to cytotoxic drugs. As only about one in 10^4 cells in a transfection will stably integrate DNA, transfection of a selectable marker linked to a non-selectable target gene permits selection of high level expression of the targeted gene by amplification of the selectable marker. The ability to co-amplify transfected DNA has permitted a 100–1000-fold increase in the expression of proteins encoded by transfected DNA (146).

While the stable expression of receptor genes is desirable for receptor characterization and ligand evaluation at the receptor, there are several critical hurdles associated with the establishment of stable cell lines. First, the gene of interest must be integrated in a functional form into the host cell chromosome. Also important is that the gene of interest not rearrange during amplification. These criteria may be difficult to achieve if the expressed gene becomes cytotoxic when overproduced. In addition, most mammalian cell expression vectors are designed to accommodate cDNAs rather than larger genomic fragments due to the size constraints imposed by the latter. As a result the efficiency of uptake of large genomic fragments and

their subsequent integration into the chromosome may be very low. Finally, the selection process leading to the stable expression of a receptor clone can take as long as 6 months and is very labor intensive.

In the case of transiently expressed receptors, the efficiency of expression depends on the number of cells that take up the transfected DNA, the gene copy number, and the expression level per gene. Most methods of DNA transfer allow 5–50% of the cells in the population to acquire DNA and express it transiently over a period of several days to several weeks. However, because the plasmid may not be incorporated into the genome, with successive cell divisions the gene of interest is lost from the cell population. A population of transiently transfected cells may also contain, in very small numbers, some stably transfected cells such that the population is heterogeneous. This heterogeneity complicates the use of the cells as the number of these cells can vary from batch to batch giving different estimates of compound activity. This variability is of special concern when a transiently expressed cell line is used to measure the functional efficacy of new chemical entities. Nonetheless, transient expression offers a convenient means by which to compare expression of a receptor gene from different vectors and to verify that any given expression plasmid is functional before initiating the more laborious procedure of isolating and characterizing stably transfected cell lines.

The relatively easy assessment of the transductional efficacy of putative ligands is a major goal in the cloning and expression of receptors. However, the association of a cloned and expressed receptor with a transduction system may not simulate the transduction process(es), for example phosphatidyl inositol (PI) turnover, cAMP accumulation, that the receptor is coupled to in its native state. While this problem is of little concern if the transduction process is only being used to demonstrate receptor activation, it presents problems when the nature of the coupling mechanism is extrapolated back to the physiological situation without the coupling process being re-examined. The magnitude of the expressed response is of further concern and requires careful examination. Depending on both the number of receptors expressed and the efficiency of their coupling to the transduction system, the maximal response will vary and give data on compounds that is a function of the passage number of the cell line rather than the receptor itself.

Such issues are of particular relevance to GPCRs. For example, three distinct molecular entities are known to be involved in the transmembrane signalling pathway for the β-adrenoceptor: the receptor itself, the G-protein- a heterotrimeric complex comprising α-, β-, and γ-subunits, and the enzyme, adenylate cyclase. When an agonist activates the receptor, the receptor binds to the G-protein and the α-subunit dissociates to stimulate formation of cAMP by adenylate cyclase. Thus, the possibility is that a transfected GPCR like the β-adrenoceptor when expressed in a cell line, could induce phosphatidyl inositol turnover or be linked to potassium conductance channels via other types of G-proteins as a result of the transfection process.

Approximately 20 different G-α and four each of the G-β and G-γ subunits have been identified (148). While the selective role of the α-subunits has been recognized for some time, recent studies indicate that the β-subunits may also contribute to receptor selectivity. The $\beta1$- and $\beta3$-subunits, for instance, have been shown to be involved specifically in the signal transduction cascades for the muscarinic M_4 and somatostatic receptors (149), respectively. The task of reconstituting the physiological signal transduction processes of a cloned receptor in a cell line may therefore be one of assessing which G-protein subunits are present in the original tissue and finding a host cell type that provides an identical mix.

The transfection and expression of ion-channel linked receptors poses a different set of challenges. As already noted, most of these receptors form a pentameric structure. With an ever increasing number of subunits of these receptors being identified by molecular biology techniques (103, 150), how is one to determine which subunits of receptors form functional receptors and, more importantly, which combination(s) of subunits are found *in vivo*?

These questions can be answered by co-expression and co-localization studies. In the case of neuronal nicotinic receptors where at least eight α and three β subunits of the receptor have been identified, functional studies of subunits encoded by cloned rat cDNAs have been performed by co-injection into oocytes of different combinations of subunit specific RNA transcribed *in vitro* (100). The expression of functional nicotinic receptors was then determined by measuring voltage or current changes across the oocyte membrane in response to acetylcholine or nicotine (151). As already discussed while $\alpha_2\beta_2$, $\alpha_3\beta_2$, and $\alpha_4\beta_2$ can form functional receptors with each having a different pharmacological profile, the β_3 in combination with α_2, α_3, or α_4 does not form a functional receptor (58). However, the possibility exists that this constraint may be due to the requirement for additional subunits to form a functional receptor or to limitations in terms of the *in vitro* assessment of functional responses. To address the issue of expression of receptors *in vivo*, *in situ* hybridization using labeled cDNA probes, and immunohistochemistry using antibodies to the different subunits can be used. Such studies for the nicotinic receptor suggest that the $\alpha_2\beta_2$ subtype is a major subtype in peripheral ganglia (151) unlike $\alpha_4\beta_2$ which is localized throughout the brain (152).

8.5 Structural Analysis of Cloned Receptors

Since all receptors bind ligands and activate an appropriate functional response as a result of the ligand binding, it is not surprising that during the course of evolution of the different superfamilies of receptors, conserved common structural features related to shared functions have occurred.

Using *in vitro* mutagenesis (11), the role of conserved domains or amino acid residues in receptor function can be studied. Within the limits of the fact that receptors in the different superfamilies bind different ligands and in one case, that of the GPCRs, are coupled to different G-proteins, it is possible to define a set of general principles that govern how ligands are bound, how agonists activate a receptor, how receptors are coupled to G-proteins and how receptor functions are regulated by post-translational modifications.

Limitations do exist in studying structure function relationships of proteins with mutagenesis. For example, changes in the activity of a receptor protein as a result of the introduction of a mutation may be observed either because the expression level of active protein is altered or because protein is modified. Therefore, determining the amount of active protein present when studying the SAR of mutated receptors is important. This measurement can often be made by determination of the stoichiometry of ligand binding, but clearly this method cannot be applied if binding affinity is beyond experimental detection (153). Immunological techniques have also been employed (154), not only to assess the quantity of protein present, but also to detect changes in subcellular localization and possibly alterations in glycosylation of the protein. Immunological techniques, however, may suffer from the limitation of being unable to distinguish between active protein and incorrectly folded or denatured protein. In spite of these limitations, mutagenesis studies have provided helpful insights into the SARs that exist among the members of the GPCR (103) and LGIC superfamilies (155).

8.6 G-Protein Coupled Receptors

The major role of the majority of GPCRs is to recognize specific hormones/regulatory molecules present in the extracellular milieu. The highly specific nature of each RL interaction would suggest that each receptor has evolved unique structural elements for ligand recognition. Only in the past 5 years however, have the techniques of *in vitro* mutagenesis have applied to the SARs for GPCRs. To date, studies have focused primarily on residues that are present in the majority of GPCRs in the hope of identifying common SAR determinants among these proteins.

8.6.1 STRUCTURAL FEATURES INVOLVED IN LIGAND BINDING. Much of the evidence obtained to date from mutagenesis studies with members of this superfamily of receptors indicates that acidic amino acids located in the membrane spanning regions are involved in ligand binding. Systematic mutagenesis of all the conserved polar residues within the hydrophobic domain of the β-adrenergic receptor did not affect the ligand binding properties of the receptor (156). However, substitution of the highly conserved Asp[79] in transmembrane region (TM)2 with uncharged amino acids resulted in a significant decrease in agonist affinity and adenylate cyclase stimulation whereas the affinity of antagonist binding was unchanged (157). In contrast, mutation of Asp[113] in TM3 adversely affected the binding of both agonists and antagonists of the receptor (158). Analysis of the amino acid sequences of other GPCRs that bind biogenic amines indicates that an acidic amino acid is conserved at the equivalent position of the β-adrenergic receptor Asp[113] in all of them, suggestive of a role for this residue as the counter ion for the amine moiety of the ligands (159).

Additionally, mutagenesis techniques have allowed identification of the receptor domains involved in determining the receptor subtype ligand binding specificity (103). For β-adrenoceptors, a chimeric receptor encompassing TM1-3 of the β_2 receptor and β_1 receptor sequence for the remainder of the protein displayed a relative agonist affinity profile similar to that of the wild type β_1 receptor (153). However, a chimera containing TM1-4 of the β_2 receptor and β_1 receptor sequence had an agonist profile typical of that observed with wild type β_2 receptors. These findings, therefore, would suggest that amino acids in TM4 confer β-adrenoceptor selectivity.

For the dopamine receptor family chimeras of the various TM regions of D_1 and D_2, receptors show that for the D_1 receptor, most changes in the TM regions to the D_2-type markedly reduce affinity for the D_1 receptor ligand, [^{3}H]SCH 23390 (95). In contrast, the D_2 receptor appears far less sensitive to replacement of TM regions with the D_1 receptor equivalent. For example, the chimera composed of D_1 TM1-5 and D_2 TM6-7 shows a 90% reduction in D_1 ligand binding as compared to the D_1 wild type. In contrast, the corresponding D_2 TM1-5 and $D_1$6-7 chimera of the D_2 receptor retains 41% of the binding of the selective D_2-receptor ligand, [^{3}H]N-0347 as that seen with the D_2 wild type receptor.

8.6.2 REGIONS INVOLVED IN RECEPTOR ACTIVATION. Disulfide bonding and thiol groups within receptors have been extensively implicated in ligand binding and agonist activation (160, 161). As a result there has been considerable effort in modifying cysteine residues using site directed mutagenic and biochemical techniques. In the case of the muscarinic acetylcholine receptor, mutagenesis of either Cys[95] in the first extracellular loop or Cys[178] in the second extracellular loop to serine generates mutant receptors that have minimal binding activity for the muscarinic antagonist, [^{3}H] QNB (160). It remains to be determined if these mutations directly affect ligand binding or alter processing of the protein and/or insertion into the plasma membrane (160). However, it appears that the role of the conserved extracellular cysteines in muscarinic and adrenoceptors may not be identical since mutant β-adrenoceptors lacking either of these residues are transported to the membrane and retain the ability to bind ligands (162).

Recent studies on the nuclear progesterone receptor that is involved in the actions of the progestin abortifacient, RU 486 (163) have shown that glycine[575] in the hormone binding domain confers binding activity for RU 486 to the chicken and hamster progesterone receptor which in their native or "wild" state cannot bind the abortifacient. Similarly, replacement of glycine[575] in the human progesterone receptor by a cysteine prevented RU 486 binding. A major finding of interest from this study was that antagonism was not an inherent property of the 11β-substituted steroids but rather that of the amino acid composition of the receptor domains.

8.6.3 REGIONS INVOLVED WITH COUPLING TO G PROTEINS. An *a priori* prediction would suggest that the cytoplasmic domains of GPCRs would be the site(s) of the receptor G-protein interaction. Similarly, since this family of receptors collectively interacts with a number of distinct G-proteins, it appears likely that the site(s) for such interactions would be located in regions that contain relatively non-similar sequences. With regard to amino acid sequence and length, the third intracellular loop is the most divergent among G-protein coupled receptors and accordingly most attention has focused on this domain of the receptor. Mutagenesis studies of the β_2-adrenoceptor (164) have shown that a small region of 8 amino acids at the N-terminal portion of the third intracellular loop was absolutely required for activation of adenylate cyclase. Further, deletion of a stretch of 12 amino acids at the C-terminal region markedly impaired the ability of the receptor to mediate stimulation of adenylate cyclase (164). Interestingly, receptors with deletions at either the N-terminal or C-terminal portion bound agonists with a single affinity that was not affected by the addition of GTP analogues. In the wild type receptor, GTP would shift agonist affinity from a low to high affinity state reflective of coupling to the receptor to G-protein. This finding, coupled with the inability of the mutant receptors to activate adenylate cyclase, indicated that the latter were not able to interact with the appropriate G-protein (164).

For the angiotensin II (A-II) type I receptor (AT1), point mutations replacing polar residues with neutral residues in the second cytosolic loop, the carboxy terminal region of the third cytosolic loop or deletional mutation of the carboxy terminal tail abolished the A-II-elicited increase in IP_3 production suggesting that the point mutated polar residues were important in receptor-G protein coupling (165).

It has been speculated that agonist binding to the receptor induces a conformational change that is responsible for the subsequent coupling to G protein subunits and the consequent transduction process (166). Secondary structure predictions indicate that regions of the N- and C-terminal portions of the third intracellular loop may form amphipathic α-helices that are extensions of TM 5 and 6. Recent theoretical, modeling and experimental data suggest that a proline residue plays a critical role in this effect (167, 168). In one study, two predicted amphiphilic helical stretches of amino acids in the third intracellular loop have been shown to align parallel to each other, in close proximity to TMs 5 and 6 (1967) suggesting that a conformational change in the helical bundles could alter the orientation of the cytoplasmic helices leading to an interaction with G-protein subunits.

However, it is important to note that other domains of the receptor – for example the second intracellular loop in the case of the β-adrenoceptor – have also been implicated in G-protein coupling (169). Thus while the N- and C-terminal regions of the third intracellular loop are the primary regions responsible for specificity in receptor G-protein interactions, these regions most likely act in concert with other cytoplasmic domains to confer full efficiency and specificity in receptor G-protein coupling process.

8.7 Ion Channel Linked Receptors

The sequence homologies that exist between neurotransmitter-gated ion channels, the LGICs, that includes the nicotinic, glycine, $GABA_A$ and $5HT_3$ receptors, suggest that the different properties of these receptors may be dependent on a limited number of amino acids within the common polypeptide backbone. The fact that invertebrates express chloride channels gated by ACh (170) and potentially by glutamate (171) demonstrates the absence of a strict relationship between neurotransmitter specificity and ion selectivity. Several chloride channels permit cations to permeate together with anions (172) suggesting that there are common structural features between anionic and cationic channels. Mutagenesis studies in combination with photoaffinity labeling and electrophysiological determinations have provided significant insight into the structural principles by which ion channels control ion permeability.

8.7.1 REGIONS INVOLVED IN ION PERMEA-
TION. Several structural models based
on amino acid sequences have been proposed that potentially explain how the subunits of the peripheral nAChR fold and
form the central pore of this ligand gated
receptor (173). Photoaffinity labeling of
two polar rings and a leucine ring in the
nAChR, spaced one α-helical turn apart,
with the channel blocker, chlorpromazine
(CPZ), suggested that M2, the second
membrane-spanning segment of each
subunit was a potential component of the
ion channel (174). Chimeric receptors constructed using bovine and electroplax δ-
subunits showed that the α-helix, M2 and
the amino acid residues connecting M2 and
M3 influence ion permeation (175).

In low divalent cation solutions, the
bovine channel has a lower conductance
than the electroplax. Interestingly, chimeras containing the M2 region of the
bovine receptor together with the electroplax sequence have shown the lower conductance property of the bovine channel
(175). Site directed mutagenesis studies
(176, 177) have shown that the charged
serine and threonine residues bracketing
the uncharged transmembrane α-helix, M2
are important in determining ion permeability.

8.7.2 REGIONS INVOLVED IN ION SELEC-
TIVITY. The anion-selective glycine and
$GABA_A$ receptors display significant
homology with cation-selective nicotinic
receptors (54, 178). Such homologies and
the finding that the glycine receptor M2
peptides can form ion channels in membranes (179) suggest that the M2 region
participates in regulating anion permeability in glycine and $GABA_A$ receptors. However, the N-terminal end of M2 in all these
anionic channels includes an additional
amino acid that has been postulated to
contribute to the difference in the ion
selectivity between ACh and glycine/
$GABA_A$ receptors (54, 179). Introduction

of three amino acids from the M2 region of
the glycine receptor into the M2 segment of
the α-7 subtype of the neuronal nAChR
converted what was a calcium permeable
channel into an anion selective channel
gated by ACh (155). The most critical
mutation for inverting the polarity of ion
selectivity was the insertion or deletion of a
neutral amino acid at position 251 in the
region linking M1 to M2 (155). On the
basis of these findings, Galzi et al. (155)
proposed that the conversion in ion selectivity is not a direct consequence of a
defined chemical alteration within the channel but rather a slight alteration in the
geometry of M2 segments which delineate
the channel. Such changes would then
modulate the accessibility of premeant ions
to putative selectivity filters located within
or outside M2.

Kinetic and electophysiological data
indicate that the nAChR can exist in interconvertible states—resting, conducting and
desensitized—that differ in the nature of
their ligand binding and channel opening
properties (180, 181). Mutation of a highly
conserved Leu^{247} located within the M2
region of α-7 subtype of the neuronal
nAChR can cause a distinct change in the
responsiveness of the receptor to agonists
and antagonists (182). Mutation of Leu^{247}
to Thr^{247} generates a mutant that, in contrast to the wild type, has two conducting
states rather than one. In addition, antagonists of the wild type receptor like
dihydro-β-erythroidine (DBE) elicit ag-
onist-type responses in the Thr^{247} mutant, a response that can be blocked by
α-bungarotoxin. Prolonged exposure to
ACh can lead to desensitization of the wild
type nAChR but leads to potentiation of
the responses to DBE in the mutant (182).
Thus changes in ionic conductance elicited
by this single mutation may represent the
conversion of a high affinity conformation
from a closed densitized state into a conducting state (182).

A role for the hydrophobic M1 segment

of amino acids in gating nicotinic and possibly other ion channels has been proposed (183). The noncompetitive antagonist, quinacrine, can only photoaffinity label the M1 helix when the channel is open. M1 is highly conserved with a central proline being found in all ligand gated ion channels. This proline produces a kink in the α-helix structure with proximal apolar residues producing nondirectional hydrophobic bonds that confer flexibility to the region. The structure of M1, its location close to the pore and the likelihood that it is the first transmembrane region after the ACh binding site, all suggest that M1 is involved in gating the channel.

Site-directed mutagenesis studies have also provided useful information on the regions of ion channel-linked receptors involved in agonist and antagonist binding. For the $GABA_A$ receptor, mutagenesis studies have identified a sequence that confers benzodiazepine (BZ) ligand binding specificity (150, 184). For the $GABA_A$ receptor channel comparison of the sequences of 3 of the α-subunits, $\alpha1$-$\alpha3$ have revealed differences in the amino terminal putative extracellular domain. The preparation of chimeric cDNAs with mixed domains of $\alpha1$ and $\alpha3$ led to the identification of Gly^{201} in $\alpha1$ as a critical determinant for high affinity BZ ligand binding to this subunit (150). Similarly, mutagenesis analysis of the $\alpha1$ and $\alpha6$ subunits resulted in the identification of a single residue (His^{102} in the $\alpha1$ and Arg^{101} in the $\alpha6$ subunit) that has conferred binding for flunitrazepam.

9 RECEPTOR MODELS

Although considerable progress has been made using receptors isolated by the standard techniques of protein biochemistry from their naturally occurring environment and, more recently, with cloned and expressed receptors, there have been various attempts to model receptor and drug recognition sites with the use of receptor antibodies and synthetic molecules (185–187).

The generation of monoclonal antibodies to receptors and the subsequent generation of antibodies to the antibodies can result in molecules with receptorlike properties. Certain of these have been studied *in vivo* to define receptor functionality with varying degrees of success. Synthetic compounds like cyclobis (paraquat-*p*-phenylene) can function as recognition sites for various aromatic ligands including dopamine and norepinephrine (187).

The contribution of these approaches may appear arcane within the context of the highly sophisticated techniques available with cloning, expression and site-directed mutagenesis. It is important to remember however, that the basic models of GPCRs that are based on bacteriorhodopsin are theoretical motifs which have yet to be unambiguously substantiated by actual data (168).

10 RECEPTOR NOMENCLATURE

The evidence used to define and characterize the existence of a new class of receptor has traditionally evolved from pharmacological studies in defined tissue preparations (188). The advent of molecular biological techniques has, however, resulted in the identification of many new receptor subtypes on the basis of cloning and sequencing of receptors and receptor subtypes which has led to considerable confusion. Indeed, Black (189) has described the identification of "receptor subtypes . . [as] . . the most flourishing branch of pharmacology." Whereas a selective ligand for a given receptor type represents one end of the spectrum of receptor characterization, an absolute assignment of the amino acid sequence of a receptor can provide the definitive molecular "fingerprint" for the receptor (or enzyme). As already noted however, sequence homology is not the only criteria for the identification of a receptor. There is also some concern regarding the use of the transmembrane sequences alone (190) to determine homology between receptors (191). Similarly, the use of classical ligand-based pharmacology to the activity of a new ligand can become an exercise in circular reasoning (189).

Many ligands are far from selective for a single receptor. Thus the integration of pharmacological and molecular data is required to advance definitively the process of receptor identification and classification. This process is a major initiative (188) of the International Union of Pharmacology (IUPHAR) for the 21st century in attempting to develop a systematic and non-redundant nomenclature.

Approaches to receptor nomenclature to date have been termed "incoherent" (192) or a "mess" (189). Since receptors have been defined on the basis of the most potent natural ligand, nomenclature can be a problem when the effector is known by different names as in the case of interleukin-1, also known as catabolin and NO, also known as EDRF (endothelium-derived relaxant factor).

The IUPHAR Committee (188) is currently involved in developing a generic system that will integrate historical precedent with a rational approach.

11 RECEPTOR BINDING ASSAYS

The development of the technique of radioligand binding has had a major impact on the way in which compounds are assayed for potential biological activity as well as in the strategies related to compound synthesis.

Radioligand binding measures the RL interaction *in vitro* using a radioactive ligand to bind with high affinity and selectivity to target receptors. The interaction of

unlabeled ("cold") ligands that have affinity for the receptor then results in a decrease in radioligand binding. This simple technique has revolutionized the compound evaluation allowing SAFIRs (3) to be determined with milligram amounts of compound in a highly cost and resource effective manner (193).

Until the early 1950s, newly synthesized compounds and compounds isolated from natural sources were assessed by a mixture of *in vivo*, whole animal screens and classical tissue assays. While many useful therapeutic agents were identified by this approach (194), the cost in terms of required amounts of compound as well as time and animal utilization were significant. *In vivo* test paradigms also suffered from the possible elimination of compounds on the basis of unknown pharmacokinetic properties. Thus test paradigms were usually rigid in terms of timing and, as a result, many potentially interesting compounds that were rapidly eliminated or had short plasma half lives were considered "inactive" because data on their actions was sought after their peak biological effect.

This type of screening approach also provided little information to the chemist regarding the discrete interaction of the drug with its target, thus limiting useful information that could be used in the design of analogues. For instance, one test procedure for antagonists of the Substance P receptor was that of reciprocal hind paw scratching in mice. Since systemic administration of Substance P induced this response, compounds that inhibited the response could potentially be classified as Substance P antagonists but could equally represent functional antagonists of the response (Fig. 11.2). The specificity of the response, ignoring caveats related to pharmacokinetics, was not ideal since the mechanism inducing the overt response and potential points of intervention to block the response were unknown. Likewise, this empirical approach would predict, in the absence of any data related to a molecular target, that since β-adrenoceptor antagonists lower blood pressure, then any compound that lowers blood pressure is by definition a β-adrenoceptor antagonist, a concept that is patently absurd. The lack of intellectual rigor in the classical screening approach compound identification generated a highly negative response from the more molecularly based sciences to this type of approach.

The 1960s saw the development of a number of *in vitro* biochemical screens that moved the measurement of the RL interaction a little closer to the molecular level. Nonetheless, the major challenge was to develop assays that measured the RL interaction independently of "downstream" events such as enzyme activation and second and third messenger systems. By such means, the ability of a compound to bind to a receptor could be determined on the basis of the SAR and thus provide the chemist with a more direct means to model the RL interaction.

It is generally accepted that pioneering work by Roth (195) and Cuatrecasas (196) led to the technology that resulted in the effective radiolabeling of ligands and the ability to measure their interaction with the receptor. Lefkowitz (197) and Hollenberg (198) made additional seminal contributions to the area, but it was Snyder's group at Johns Hopkins (199) that placed the technology of radioligand binding squarely in the forefront of modern day pharmacology and established it as a valuable tool in the drug discovery process (193).

The 1980s initiated an explosion of new receptor and receptor subtype identification using the radioligand binding approach, an explosion that has been enhanced by the melding of the tools of recombinant DNA technology to the process.

The current screening approach that involves using both receptor interactions and biologically targeted responses provide the chemist with a larger database of which to design rational compound synthesis. This screening strategy alleviates the laborious trial-and-error drug synthesis and provides the chemist with a better opportunity of designing analogs with better selectivity and specificity for a given therapeutic target.

Despite the fact that considerable research into Substance P antagonists has been conducted over the past two decades, it has only been the advent of receptor binding technology that resulted in the identification of four distinct classes of nonpeptide Substance P/neurokinin antagonist in the past 2–3 years (200).

11.1 Practical Considerations of the Binding Assay

The radioligand binding assay permits the study of the physiochemical interaction between radiolabeled ligands (radioligands) and their specific receptors *in vitro*. A radioactive form of either a neurotransmitter/hormone or biologically active compound (agonist or antagonist) is added to a membrane preparation (particulate or solubilized) and then incubated, to steady state. It is assumed that a radioligand with high affinity and specificity for a targeted receptor will bind to the receptor as part of a reversible bimolecular reaction which equilibrium obeys the Law of Mass Action. Therefore, the radioligand, L^*, has equal on and off rates for interacting with the receptor, R, at equilibrium, forming an RL^* complex. At steady state, the RL^* complex can be separated out from free radioligand using various methods described below. The ability of an unknown ligand, L to compete for the binding of the radioligand, L^*, is the basis of the radioligand approach to drug discovery.

11.1.1 BINDING DEFINITIONS. The binding of a radioligand to a membrane or protein has two components: total and non-specific binding. Total binding (T) in a radioligand binding assay represents the amount of radioactivity (L*) measured in cpm or dpm that is isolated at the end of an experiment. This measurement does not always reflect the amount of L* specifically bound to the target protein, receptor or enzyme. The radioligand can also become absorbed to nonreceptor sites in the tissue and to the reaction medium used to isolate the RL* complex. This binding does not represent a pharmacologically relevant site and this portion of radioligand binding is termed nonspecific (NS) binding. Its dimensions can be determined by the inclusion of parallel incubation tubes containing a large excess (>100-fold) of an unlabeled, or "cold" ligand that is known to specifically compete with the radioligand for the target recognition site. In the presence of excess "cold" ligand, the NS binding can be determined, and when subtracted from T (T − NS), gives the specific binding, S, of the radioligand to the receptor enzyme.

The choice of agent used to determine nonspecific binding is important. In those cases where there are a large number of different pharmacophores known to interact with the target protein, a structurally distinct entity is optimal. Using a large excess of the unlabeled form of a radioligand, which frequently occurs when there is minimal pharmacology for a target protein, can result in the phenomenon known as isotope dilution wherein there is an apparent reduction in total binding that actually reflects dilution of the isotope to a lower specific activity.

The proportion of NS binding varies depending on the assay conditions and the radioligand used. Ideally, NS should be 30% or less with S being 70% or greater. The better the signal to noise ratio (S/NS), the more accurate and reproducible the assay. Sometimes this ratio represents an ideal situation that may not be possible to achieve when developing a new assay or

radioligand. Many new assays for receptors have been developed using conditions that resulted in only 30% specific binding. While difficult to run from an experimental viewpoint, these assays usually have resulted in the iterative identification of better ligands/receptor sources/assay conditions that led to incremental improvements.

The parameters measured in a binding assay are the dissociation constant or K_d which is equal to the reciprocal of the affinity constant, K_a, and is a measure of the affinity of a radioligand for the target site; the B_{max}, which is usually measured in moles/mg protein, and is a measure of the concentration of binding sites in a given tissue source and the IC_{50} value. The K_d and B_{max} values are determined in two ways: using a saturation curve where the concentration of radioligand is increased until all the ligand recognition sites are occupied, or by measuring radioligand association and dissociation kinetics, the K_d being the ratio of the dissociation and association rate constants.

The IC_{50} value is the concentration of unlabeled radioligand required to inhibit 50% of the specific binding of the radioligand. This value is determined by running a competition curve (Fig. 11.6) with a fixed concentration of radioligand and tissue and varying concentrations of the unlabeled ligand or displacer. In order to accurately determine the IC_{50}, it is essential that sufficient data points be included. As shown in Figure 11.6, if the data used to derive the IC_{50} value are clustered over a range that reflects 40–60% of the competition curve, much useful information is lost. Ideally, the competition curve should encompass the range 10% to 90% of the competition curve. Based on Michaelis-Menten kinetics (11) when binding is the result of the interaction of the displacer with one recognition site, 10–90% of the radioligand is inhibited over an 82-fold concentration range of the displacer. The slope of the competition curve can be

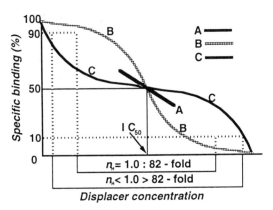

Fig. 11.6 Specific radioligand binding is indicated as 100%. Data points close to the 50% point (A) while providing a measurable IC_{50} value can limit the usefulness of the data. More complete inhibition curves (B and C) provide more useful information regarding the displacer. Displacement curve B has a Hill coefficient of unity requiring an 82-fold spread in displacer concentration to displace 10–90% of binding. Displacement curve C has a Hill coefficient of less than one, the range of displacer concentrations required to generate the 10–90% curve being greater than 82-fold reflecting more than one binding site or a noncompetitive inhibitor. If insufficient data points are generated as in A, the data obtained will not allow analysis of the type of binding or the potential existence of multiple receptor interactions.

analyzed to assess the potential cooperation of the RL interactions. When binding is complex resulting in the interaction of the displacer with more than one recognition site, a greater than 82-fold concentration of displacer is required to inhibit the same 10–90% of specific radioligand binding.

The IC_{50} value for a given compound is obviously dependent on the conditions of the assay; namely, the concentration of the radioligand used, the receptor density and the affinity of the receptor, the K_d, for the radioligand. When comparing compounds across a single assay, the T and NS control measurements usually correct for variations in receptor density from tissue batch to tissue batch as well as errors in the dilution of the radioligand. This monitoring is not the case, however, when the activity of a "cold" ligand is being compared across different radioligand binding assays. It is

then necessary to use the Cheng-Prusoff equation (201) where the K_i in a given binding assay can be derived by the relationship:

$$K_i = IC_{50}/1 + [L]/K_d \qquad (6)$$

where $[L]$ is the concentration of radioligand used and K_d is the dissociation constant for the radioligand at the receptor. This relationship corrects for inherent differences in assay conditions. If the displacing ligand has an IC_{50} value of 20 nM at an nAChR labeled by [^{3}H]-nicotine and is equally active in terms of IC_{50} value at muscarinic receptor sites labeled by [^{3}H]-QNB, a natural assumption would be that the compound is equal in activity at both sites. Feeding the information into the Cheng-Prusoff equation would, however, provide a different picture. At the nAChR (186) labeled by [^{3}H]-nicotine, the K_d value is 4 nM and the ligand concentration used was 15 nM thus the K_i value = 20/1 + [15]/4 = 4.2 nM. In contrast, at the site labeled by 0.06 nM [^{3}H]-QNB (K_d value = 0.06) this same math would yield a K_i value = 20/1 + [0.06]/0.06 = 20 nM. From being equally active in terms of IC_{50} values, the compound in question is actually 5-fold selective for the nAChR. This discrepancy underlines the need for radioligands of sufficient specific activity so that they can be used at concentrations close to or below the K_d of the receptor.

11.1.2 THE MEMBRANE RECEPTOR ASSAY. The most commonly used radioligand binding assay involves the use of membranes containing the receptor of interest under three basic experiments: (i) *competition* experiments where selected ligands or unknowns are examined with a receptor over a 100-fold concentration range to determine whether the unlabeled ligands have any affinity for the targeted receptor. For this type of assay the time of incubation and receptor concentration remain constant; (ii) *saturation* experiments where the amount of RL complex is assayed by increasing the amount of radioligand added. Again the time of incubation and receptor concentration remain constant; and (iii) association or dissociation *kinetic* experiments (ligand concentration and receptor density remain constant; time varies).

The basic technical requirements for receptor binding studies are the selection of radiolabeled ligands, agonists but more usually antagonists, because of the higher affinity of the latter, a receptor source, usually crude tissue or cell homogenate, incubation conditions that result in the formation of an RL* complex, and a method for separating bound RL* from free, unbound L*.

In order to establish that the binding of a radioligand to a tissue is a reflection of the receptor-ligand interaction rather than the simple absorption of radioligand in a nonspecific manner to the tissue, the following criteria originally developed by Cuatrecasas and Hollenberg (198) must be met:

1. Binding of radioligand to the target protein, receptor, enzyme, neurotransmitter transporter or intracellular recognition element should be saturable, indicating a finite number of specific binding sites.

2. Binding affinity should be high (K_d value $\sim 10^{-10} - 10^{-8}\,M$), consistent with a putative role as a neurohumoral agent or enzyme/transporter substrate.

3. Radioligand binding should be readily reversible, consistent with a physiological role for the ligand or enzyme/transporter substrate.

4. The distribution of binding sites, both between tissues and within the cell or tissue, or in selected or transfected cell lines, should be consistent with the proposed physiological role of the ligand recognition site.

5. The pharmacology of the binding site should have a similar agonist/antagonist rank order potency as that observed for the natural ligand and related structures in functional test procedures.

6. A simultaneous correlation of binding data with biological dose/concentration curves in identical tissue preparations should be generated.

These criteria should be additionally complemented by knowledge regarding the biological validity of the radioligand as compared to the unlabeled ligand. It is not unusual that when a compound is radiolabeled, its biological activity is diminished or even eliminated. This effect is especially true of peptide ligands (202).

The conditions for developing a binding assay are frequently determined by trial and error. Binding assays are often iterative in nature. A less than optimal assay is used to find new ligands that are then radiolabeled and used in place of the original radioligand. An example of this process is the development of a binding assay for the NMDA receptor. [³H]-Glutamate has given varying data in a number of different laboratories (203). The identification of the NMDA analog, CPP (3- (2-carboxy-piperazin-4-yl) propyl-1-phosphonic acid) (204) provided a higher affinity ligand for the NMDA receptor. The binding assay developed using [³H]-CPP (205) was a major improvement over that using [³H]-glutamate. However, the K_d value for CPP was 217 nM requiring the use of a time and labor intensive centrifugation assay. The identification of CGS 19755 using the [³H]-CPP assay and its development as a radioligand with a K_d value of 23 nM (206) resulted in a higher throughput filtration assay.

Whereas in most instances, a newly developed radioligand will work effectively under the same conditions used in its discovery, there are instances when a biologically active radiolabeled form of a new ligand shows no binding under the same conditions that resulted in its binding in unlabeled form. The reasons for this phenomenon are unknown. Nonetheless, this constraint is usually the reason when a binding assay for an "obviously better" radioligand is not feasible.

11.1.3 RADIOLIGAND ISSUES. The low concentrations of receptors found in most tissues require that the radioligands used in binding studies must have an affinity for the receptor high enough so that the dissociation constant is in the range of receptor concentration. This concentration usually requires that an antagonist rather than agonist ligand be used to define the RL interaction. For the striatal D_1 dopamine receptor, maximal receptor concentrations are in the nanomolar concentration (207). The endogenous ligand for the receptor, dopamine, has a dissociation constant in the micromolar range which precludes its use in labeling the receptor. Instead, the selective D_1 receptor antagonist, SCH 23390 with an affinity in the nanomolar range, is the current ligand of choice (208).

The choice of radioisotope used to label the ligand is a very important consideration (209). The two most common radioisotopes used in binding assays are tritium, [^{3}H] and iodine, [^{125}I]. Sulfur [^{35}S] and [^{14}C] can also be used. There are a number of advantages to using tritium. In general it is easy to introduce the isotope by reduction or methylation to a specific activity ranging between 20 and 100 Ci/mole without altering the pharmacological properties of the ligand. The half life of tritium (12.26 years) is another advantage of using tritium as the radioisotope. However, chemical stability needs to be routinely checked because of the potential for radiolysis in stored, concentrated solutions (209). [^{125}I] is used because of its high specific activity (2200 Ci/mmol) which permits the labeling of ligands that are in short supply, have affinity constants in the pM range and for which

the recognition sites are in low abundance, e.g., fmoles/mg protein. [^{125}I] however has a short-half life (~30 days) which necessitates synthesis on a monthly basis and an increased likelihood of altering the binding and biological properties of the ligand as well as an increased tendency for radiolysis.

Radiolabeled peptides represent an additional problem (202). These are more likely to bind non-specifically to the reaction vessels and various filters used in the separation of bound from free ligand. Glassware can be coated with silicates to reduce peptide binding or the assays can be conducted in polypropylene vessels (210). Radiolabeled peptides are also excellent substrates for the proteases typically present in cell homogenates. Thus assay conditions involve the use of various protease inhibitors, e.g., bacitracin, leupeptin, phenanthroline, or the inclusion of bovine serum albumin as an alternative substrate. These may interfere with binding kinetics or act as alternate binding sites for the radioligand. Care should be taken in interpreting data derived under such conditions. The kinetics of peptide ligand binding may also be problematic. Association rate constants for peptide ligands can be as much as three orders of magnitude lower than those seen for other types of radioligand. For more traditional organic radioligands, equilibrium binding occurs in the time range of 15 minutes to a maximum of 2 h. For peptide ligands, equilibrium can be taken from 5–8 h. To run a binding assay over this time period, given the caveats related to peptide stability, can lead to significant degradation of radioligand even in the presence of peptidase/protease inhibitors, pseudoirreversible binding, and receptor desensitization. As a result, many peptide binding assays are run not to equilibrium, again complicating data interpretation.

11.1.4 RECEPTOR SOURCE. The choice of a tissue or cell line as a receptor source has a significant impact on the data generated. The receptor concentration in most tissues is in the fmole to pmole range. Brain tissue has a much higher density of receptors due to the more extensive nerve innervation. The greater the concentration of receptors per unit tissue protein, the better the specific binding since the latter is usually linear with tissue concentration. Excess tissue can lead to extraneous results especially when a large proportion of the added ligand is bound. A general rule, where practicable, is to use that amount of tissue that only binds 10% of the added radioligand (210) to conform to Zone A behavior (211).

The choice of tissue species and the methods used for the preparation of tissue for the *in vitro* assay, while crucial, cannot always be done by a generic formula. For each assay, there are minor differences in the buffers and pH used to generate the receptor enriched membrane preparation. Species differences in tissue source, storage conditions and the inclusion of other factors (salts, glucose etc) also influence binding and data interpretation.

The buffer typically used is 50 mM Tris-HCl pH 7.4, hypoosmotic, when compared to the normal environment of the tissue. However, the *in vitro* assay itself is conducted under conditions that are a far cry from the situation occurring in the intact tissue. For instance, equilibrium for the association of a radioligand with the receptor is many orders of magnitude greater than the milliseconds that reflect the neurotransmission process. Thus the use of Krebs-Ringer buffers or the prehomogenization of tissues in isoosmotic sucrose solutions prior to the use of sonication of polytroning is not an entirely rational process. Both homogenization techniques result in almost complete destruction of tissue architecture, the polytron being a mechanical shear/cavitation tissue disruptor.

The development of a new binding assay proceeds largely by an oxymoronic process of logical trial and error that is dependent to a major extent on the experience of the experimenter in the area of developing such assays. There are few rules that can predict whether or not an assay will work. In many instances it is necessary to remove the endogenous ligand by washing or enzymic degradation. This elimination removes the possibility of the endogenous ligand competing with the radioligand. For instance, for binding assays targeted to adenosine receptors, unless the endogenous adenosine is removed by the action of the enzyme, adenosine deaminase, specific binding is negligible (212).

11.1.5 SEPARATION TECHNIQUES. The separation of the RL* complex from unbound (free) ligand, L* is usually accomplished by the techniques of centrifugation or filtration. While dialysis is frequently cited as a technique, its practical application to radioligand binding is minimal.

The choice of using centrifugation or filtration is dependent on the individual receptor of interest. Centrifugation is most commonly used when the K_d value for the ligand is low, e.g., greater than a 100 nM, the receptor density is low or high nonspecific binding is a problem. While effective, centrifugation is very time-consuming due to the need for 10–20 minute centrifugation runs, manual washing of the pelleted tissue and solubilization.

Filtration is the most efficient means to separate the RL* complex from free L*. At equilibrium, the assay reaction—receptor preparation, radioligand, buffer and compound—is terminated by filtration over a glass fiber or cellulose acetate filter. The RL* complex is trapped on the filter mat and the free ligand, L*, is removed by washing with ice cold buffer. Radioactivity on the filter can be directly determined by dry or scintillant counting to determine the amount of RL* complex.

With the development of the Brandel

Cell Harvester and the various microtiter plate format filtration machines, over a thousand assay tubes can be run in the same time that 180 or so tubes are run in a centrifugation assay (193). This efficiency makes filtration a higher throughput and more time and resource effective assay. The concentration of radioligand, reaction volume and amount of tissue that are used for filtration are usually less than that in centrifugation, making the assay more cost-effective.

The major criteria for the use of the filtration assay relates to the dissociation constant of the radioligand. Theoretical calculations (213) indicate that a radioligand with a K_d value of higher than 5–10 nM cannot be used in a filtration assay since the half-life of the RL* complex is in the range of 0.28–4 s. There are, however, many instances where this theoretical rule-of-thumb has no bearing and where ligands with K_d values of 20–100 nM give data that can be used to characterize both the receptor and ligands that interact with it. Some radioligands, e.g., peptides tend to bind nonspecifically in high amounts to the filters. In such cases, the filters can be pretreated with bovine serum albumin, polyethylenimine (PEI) or polyvinylpyrrolidone (PVP) to reduce such binding (214).

11.1.6 DATA ANALYSIS. The data output for a binding assay is in the form of counts per minute (cpm). Using suitable controls, cpms can be converted to pmoles of radioligand bound. Data analysis is a time-consuming and critical aspect of the binding assay. While in the past data was analyzed by pencil and graph paper or by manual downloading and reloading into inflexible, PC-based spread sheet programs, the trend towards high throughput screening has resulted in the development of LIMS, Laboratory Information Management Systems (193) together with database management systems like 4th Dimension and analysis

programs such as RS/1 (215) or EBDA (216). These are time and resource effective, objective and flexible such that the data can be analyzed and retrieved in real time.

Comments have already been made in regard to the generation of adequate numbers of data points for the derivation of accurate and informative IC_{50} value and pseudo-Hill coefficient values. When determining the K_d and B_{max} values for a new ligand, it is important that untransformed data are analyzed by a non-linear regression analysis program (217, 218). The seminal Scatchard transformation where a line to fit the data can be constructed by eye or linear regression analysis plotting B/F versus B, is mathematically flawed in that the data is transformed and the parameter, B, is present on both abcissca and ordinate. The data derived from a saturation analysis experiment where the radioligand concentration is increased with the incubation time, and the receptor concentration remains constant, can provide useful information on the number of ligand binding sites present in a tissue preparation and their relationship to one another. Are they separate sites or representing independent multiple receptors or multiple interconvertible states dependent on the assay condition and presence of ligand? The shape of a computer analyzed Scatchard plot can be used to delineate these situations using statistical evaluation of whether a dataset is best fit by a one, two or even three site model (218).

12 RECEPTOR AUTORADIOGRAPHY

Receptors can be visualized and characterized *in situ* by the technique of autoradiography (219, 220). Thin, slide-mounted tissue sections prepared on a microtome are incubated with radioligand under conditions similar to those used for regular homogenate binding. The radiolabeled slide is then juxtaposed to tritium sensitive film for a period of time dependent on the specific radioactivity of the ligand and the density of receptors in the tissue. The exposed film is then developed and the receptor density quantified by computer-assisted densitometry. While many such studies result in color enhanced images generated at a single ligand concentration reflecting the labor intensive process of reading specific areas of the film, the quantitative aspect has been approached to determine K_d and B_{max} values in different brain regions and with different drug treatments.

13 RECEPTOR CLONES IN COMPOUND EVALUATION

Considerable attention has been given in this review to the advances that are being made by rDNA technology in providing research tools to both better delineate receptor function as well as to identify new drugs. The expectation is that with time, it will be possible to rationally design new molecular entities based on knowledge of the three dimensional structure of the drug recognition site (receptor, enzyme etc.), of the SAFIR of the drug (2) and of the two together. Together with site directed mutagenesis (11), it will be theoretically possible to remove much of the "irrationality" of the present methods used to design new compounds.

rDNA technology has provided the means to produce drug recognition sites in large quantities to facilitate compound design. There are some drawbacks to this emergent technology that can be overlooked, however. Expression of the drug target in a cell line can lead to differences in the number of receptors expressed per clone, a factor dependent on the relative proportion of transient to stable expressed cells and the passage number of the transfectants (221). Thus the number of recep-

tors can vary affecting the apparent activity of unknown ligands that compete for binding with the radioligand (222).

As the drug targets of greatest interest are those in the human, the use of a human receptor or enzyme would appear ideal in defining the SAFIR/SAR of a potential drug series. A drawback however, is that nearly all the toxicology and safety studies done on a lead compound prior to clinical trials are conducted in rodents, dogs, and nonhuman primates. If there are no species differences between rat and human, this testing becomes a moot point. If on the other hand, the human target is substantially different from that in rat or dog or monkey, and there are examples of this, the safety and toxicology studies may be conducted on a compound that has limited interactions with the drug target in species other than human. Although ideal from a drug discovery viewpoint, the use of human-derived tissues should proceed with caution in conducting the laborious but equally important studies, subsequent to identification of a lead compound, that are required for clinical trials to commence.

A final point to be made, in regard to the use of transfected cell lines in receptor characterization and compound evaluation, relates to potential artifacts in the transductional readout in transfected cells. Activation of transfected receptor may result in an increase in cAMP, a second messenger effect that may already be known to be a consequence of ligand activation of the receptor in its natural state. It is also possible that the transfected receptor may activate a cell signaling pathway in the cell that is not linked to the receptor in its normal tissue environment. In this instance, the second messenger readout actually functions as a "reporter", a G-protein linked phenomenon that results from the introduction of the cDNA for a GPCR and the generic or promiscuous interaction of the receptor with the G-protein systems. The introduction of the cDNA for any

GPCR may then act to elicit a similar response. It is then advisable to use caution in extrapolating events occurring in the transfected cell to the physiological milieu of the intact tissue. A recent example of this extrapolation involves the transfection of human muscarinic receptor (mAChR) cDNA to the HEK cell line (223). Addition of muscarinic agonists to the cell line, which in its wild state does not express mAChRs, resulted in the activation of PKC and the subsequent secretion of fragments of the amyloid precursor protein (APP), the abnormal cycling of which is thought to underlie the etiology of Alzheimer's Disease. This finding was very exciting in that it potentially linked decreased cholinergic stimulation to alterations in APP processing. This phenomena can also be mimicked by stimulating the HEK cells with bradykinin or okadaic acid which also activate PKC (224), raising the distinct possibility that APP secretion from the transfected HEK cell line is a "reporter" rather than physiologically meaningful phenomenon.

14 LEAD COMPOUND DISCOVERY

As evidenced by the compound code numbers used by pharmaceutical companies, many thousands of new chemical entities have been made since the establishment of the industry in the early 20th century. A tentative hypothesis is that the major pharmaceutical companies have each made between 50,000 and 800,000 compounds during the time that they have had a dedicated compound numbering system, accessing new compounds from both fermentation and natural product sources as well as dedicated chemical efforts focused on new lead discovery. It is not unreasonable to assume therefore that somewhere in the region of 2 million to 6 million compounds have been identified in the search for new drugs to treat human disease states in the past 50 years to 70 years. One may then

pare this number down to a million in order to account for closely related structures. With this premise, it is of considerable interest to note that the *Merck Index*, a reasonable compendium of drug entities and research tools, lists only 10,100 compounds in its 1989 edition (225). Similarly, the drug compendium in the series *Comprehensive Medicinal Chemistry* lists some 5700 medicinal and pharmacological agents (226). From the hypothetical million compounds, only 1% or less therefore have proven to be of sufficient interest as either therapeutic agents or research tools.

The approach to identifying new lead structures over the past 20–30 years has focused on making the process more rational and intellectually based. Hence the ideal of computer assisted molecular modeling, NMR and x-ray crystallography being combined with the various aspects of rDNA technology is discussed above to maximize the intellectual input and minimize effort in the iteration of chemical structures that are less than optimal. Venture capital companies like Agouron and Vertex have been formed to target this approach.

Concomitantly with this evolving rational approach, the process of random screening has continued in the form of targeted screening (227). This approach minimizes the randomness of the pre 1960s screening approach discussed above by rationally choosing molecular targets thought to be involved in given disease states and screening compound sources for novel leads using the technique of radioligand binding.

While dismissed as remaining irrational, the breakthrough for this approach came in 1984 with the identification of the CCK-B antagonist, asperlicin (228) and its subsequent use as a lead structure to discover, the clinical entity, MK 329 (229). Considerable effort has been expended in the pharmaceutical industry worldwide to capitalize on this approach with significant successes that have enhanced the search for novel chemical entities as well as providing research tools to better understand receptor and enzyme function. These include the non-peptide neurokinin-antagonists, CP 96, 345 (230), RP 67580 (231) and WIN 51708 (232), the neurotensin antagonist SR 48692 (233), the arginine vasopressin antagonist, OPC 21268 (234) and the oxytocin antagonist, L-366, 509 (235).

14.1 Compound Sources

There are many potential sources for new chemicals that provide leads for new drugs including existing chemical libraries as well as natural sources that include plants, herbs, bacteria, invertebrates, and marine organisms (236, 237). A more recent strategy for compound identification is the approach termed molecular diversity (238) which has the potential to utilize the best of natural product and synthetic approaches to lead identification.

14.1.1 NATURAL PRODUCT SOURCES. As many as an estimated 70% of the drugs currently in use owe their origin to natural sources. Among these are morphine, pilocarpine, physostigmine, cocaine, digoxin, salicyclic acid, reserpine as well as a host of antibiotics (194).

Mention has already been made of the CCK-B antagonist, asperlicin (228). Screening of natural products has also led to the discovery of the immunosupressants, cyclosporin, rapamycin and FK 506 (239) which in turn have led to the identification of the immunophilins that are involved in lymphokine production.

Microbial, plant, herb, and marine sources of compounds remain viable despite the progressive loss of important ecosystems like the Amazon River Basin by deforestation (227). Drug companies are focusing on the rainforests of Costa Rica, a variety of microbial sources, plants and herbs from the Ayurvedic and Traditional Chinese Medicine Schools as well as the

emerging focus on African traditions of herbal medicine. There is considerable ongoing effort to identify the active entities present in herbal medicines as drug sources focused in entities like the Materia Medica of the Chinese University of Hong Kong (240). Marine sources are being exploited by the use of dedicated taxonomists, biologists and medicinal chemists in research centers like Harbor Branch, the University of Maryland, the University of California, San Diego, the University of Hawaii, and the Mitsubushi-Kasei and Sunbor Institutes (241).

14.1.2 PHARMACOPHORE-BASED LIGAND LIBRARIES. The majority of pharmaceutical companies have relatively large chemical libraries representing the cumulative synthetic efforts of the medicinal chemists within the company. Typically, the chemical diversity in these libraries is not extreme since the synthetic approach to drug design revolves around defined pharmacophores in lead series and the rational and systematic development of the SAR. Certain companies will thus have a large number of similar compounds based on the approaches and successes attendant to a therapeutic area.

As already noted, the radioligand binding approach to compound evaluation has provided a rapid and cost effective means to identify new lead structures. This identification can be accomplished with a minimum of compound such that intermediates of a new synthetic pathway can be screened as can the remaining supplies in samples made 50 or more years ago.

The concept of a chemical library however implies *availability*, *validity*, and *accessibility*, the latter in terms of both compounds and the data generated in the form of searchable biological databases as well as *diversity*. From a historical perspective, compound archives and databases did not always recognize the tremendous value of a chemical library. Compound storage has not been centralized, frequently residing in the chemist who had originally made the compound, such that compounds decomposed, evaporated or were lost when the chemist retired. Databases could be incomplete reflecting data only on compounds of interest with many compounds having no archival information whatsoever or incomprehensible such that the data stored had limited value.

With the recognition that chemical libraries could be evaluated in new screens using techniques like radioligand binding, their value was perceptibly increased. This was highlighted by the fact that with the continued identification of new molecular targets, for instance the immunophillins (239), the $5HT_4$ receptor (242) and the adenosine A_3 receptor (113), the chemical library would represent a completely novel resource every 3–5 years as the battery of assays in which it was used, changed. Thus compounds synthesized in the 1940s rather than being archival were potential new leads in the 1990s.

The *availability* of compounds is therefore crucial. In conducting targeted screening and a less than 1% "hit rate", the discovery of new leads was dependent on both luck (a matrix reflecting the number of assays), and the number of compounds put into these assays. With diminishing sources of compounds and their potential decomposition/evaporation and the current trend to make 10–20 mg samples of new leads for a dedicated synthetic effort, chemical libraries may not reflect the need for availability crucial to their effective use. This situation is compounded when compounds are supplied to outside investigators adding to the depletion of a valuable resource.

The issue of compound *validity* relates to the potential for the compound undergoing evaluation to have changed chemically with time. Instances have occurred where the final few milligrams of a compound of previously defined structure prove to be an exciting lead. Resynthesis of the compound

then results in a new sample of the presumed lead which then proves to be inactive reflecting the presence of an unknown and now unknowable entity in the original sample.

Accessibility to information related to a compound in the form of a database is also important even if such data is negative since it provides a base on which to judge new information. A compound that is found as a potentially novel anti-inflammatory agent may be discarded if there is data already available documenting the negative renal effects of the compound. Similarly, a compound that has been at one time a lead for a cytotoxic program may not receive much support as a potential lead in an antidepressant program.

The issue of *diversity* reflects the need to enhance the scope of the library beyond the company. This enhancement can be done by compound exchange with other companies, by acquiring compounds from university departments and commercial sources (Sigma, Bader, Mayhew, Cookson etc). Additional sources of novel synthetic compounds include the libraries of major chemical companies like Eastman Kodak and Stouffer, and more recently, chemicals made in the former Eastern Bloc countries that are now being brokered to pharmaceutical companies. In conjunction with the use of computerized cluster programs, the selection of compounds based on diverse structures can be considerably enhanced.

14.1.3 DIVERSITY-BASED LIGAND LIBRARIES. A newer aspect of compound libraries is the creation of libraries with a maximum of diversity. Some companies have generated libraries with a maximum of pharmacophore diversity of 1200–1400 compounds that is used to rapidly identify potential leads for a new drug target using the SAR generated in a binding assay. This library is constructed from compounds that are available in relatively large supply and may not necessarily be proprietary to the company. Their value is in rapidly eliminating unlikely structures in a systematic manner for each new target.

The concept of chemical diversity has received considerable attention both from a natural product perspective (237) as well as recombinant phage and synthetically produced randomized peptide libraries (238, 243). Using the latter, large numbers of peptides can be produced by phage (244), bead (245), "tea bag" (246), spatially addressable parallel chemical synthetic or microchip (247) and reaction selecting (248) methodologies. Interestingly, each of these peptide library technologies reflects the focus of venture company activities reflecting the anticipated potential of this approach. Phage is being developed Genentech, bead by Chiron, Selectide & Pharmacopeia, tea bag by Houghten, microchip by Affymax and reaction selecting by Receptor Laboratories & Darwin. Randomly generated antisense oligonucleotide (AO) and carbohydrate libraries represent other facets of this approach to chemical diversity (249).

14.1.4 HIGH-THROUGHPUT SCREENING. The first step in compound identification in the targeted screening approach is the rapid and cost effective assessment of activity in radioligand binding assays. Recent developments in hardware, a focus on microtitre plate technology and customized, user-friendly data crunching and acquisition systems have enhanced throughput in receptor binding assays. With the focus on compound flow, some targeted screening operations within the pharmaceutical industry are capable of screening 100,000 compounds or more through 10–30 dedicated assays (227, 250). The limitations to this approach are three-fold: selectivity of the RL interaction; the time taken for data generation; and the determination of whether a ligand has agonist or antagonist activity.

Selectivity of the RL interaction can readily be assessed when the compound is assayed across 10–15 assays. If a compound is active in the same concentration range across 3 or more assays, there is a good likelihood that its effects are nonselective, reflecting a potential membrane perturbation action.

The need to use scintillation counting to measure the radioactivity bound as the final readout of compound activity is time-consuming and can take up to 2 minutes per sample. With 50,000 compounds being assessed in duplicate at one concentration in 15 assays, the time required to count is 5.7 years. Obviously with the use of 10 scintillation counters the data can be made available in the same year that the assay is conducted.

Increased attention has therefore been focused on assay readouts that are not dependent on lengthy sampling of reaction products. Thus the scintillation proximity assay developed by Amersham (251) and the microphysiometer or biosensor (252) are potential approaches to reducing readout time. Another approach is that of the reporter gene where formation of the RL complex leads to the expression of a gene that produces a response that can be read immediately. One example is that of the luciferinase reporter gene assay used by Ligand Pharmaceuticals to define ligand interactions with intracellular receptors (253). The readout from the RL interaction is a quantum of light that can be measured immediately by multiple phostodiode arrays. Another approach for GPRCs involves the use of a β-galactosidase reporter gene that leads to a colorimetric readout (254).

GPCR transfected frog melanocytes represent yet another approach to determining whether a ligand is an agonist or antagonist that is independent of a reporter gene construct (255). The addition of melatonin to a transfected cell line reduces intracellular cAMP concentrations resulting in the aggregation of the pigment in the cells. Agonist stimulation of the transfected cell increases cAMP resulting in pigment dispersal, a reaction that can be immediately determined visually on a plus/minus basis but can also be quantified in terms of light transmission.

15 FUTURE DIRECTIONS

With the gradual evolution of the receptor concept over the past 100 years, the basic concepts of drugs acting at defined molecular targets has become increasingly refined. Knowledge related to receptor structure and function has increased exponentially with the advent of even more sophisticated technologies to delineate the RL interaction.

As the emergent technologies of structural biology become more amenable to real time usage, it may prove possible to reach the ultimate dream of drug discovery: the design and synthesis of new chemical entities using knowledge of the structure, conformation interactive forces defining the RL interaction at the molecular level. Indeed, it may in time be possible to design compounds on a computer screen and determine their activity by their best fit to a computerized model of the drug target. To date however, such technologies have served to dramatically improve the screening approach to compound identification.

However, drug target characterization and compound identification is a highly iterative process where both the rational and targeted screening approaches to drug discovery continue to play complimentary roles in advancing knowledge. The role of the medicinal chemist and that of the pharmacologist remain pivotal in the discovery and characterization of new therapeutic entities for diseases which today require innovative new drugs. Their role is thus to assess the usefulness of new technologies in achieving the goals of drug discovery rather than letting technology drive the goals (220, 256).

REFERENCES

1. P. Ehrlich, *Lancet*, **ii**, 445–451 (1913).
2. R. A. Glennon, *Drug Dev. Res.*, **24**, 251–274 (1992).
3. J. P. Snyder, *Med. Res. Rev.*, **11**, 641–662 (1992).
4. Y. C. Martin, *J. Med. Chem.*, **35**, 2145–2154 (1992).
5. I. D. Kuntz, *Science,* **257**, 1078–1082 (1992).
6. M. Williams, *Medications Development: Drug Discovery, Databases and Computer-Aided Drug Design*, NIDA Monograph, **134**, 1–36, 1993.
7. P. M. Dean, *Molecular Foundations of Drug-Receptor Interaction*, Cambridge University Press, Cambridge, UK, 1987, pp. 35–69.
8. S. Fesik, *J. Med. Chem.*, **34**, 2937–2945 (1991).
9. R. J. Miller, *Science*, **235**, 46–52 (1987).
10. M. Gopalakrishnan, R. A. Janis, and D. J. Triggle, *Drug Develop. Res.*, **28**, (1993).
11. M. D. Holenberg, *J. Med. Chem.*, **33**, 1275–1281 (1990).
12. B. K. Koblika, T. S. Koblika, K. W. Daniel, J. W. Regan, M. G. Caron, and R. J. Lefkowitz, *Science*, **240**, 1310–1316 (1988).
13. W. Haefely, E. Kyburz, M. Gerecke, and H. Mohler, *Adv. Drug. Res.*, **14**, 167–322, 1985.
14. L. Michaelis and M. L. Menten, *Biochem. Z.*, **49**, 333–369 (1913).
15. L. Stryer, *Biochemistry* 3rd Ed., W. H. Freeman, San Francisco, 1988, pp. 177–200.
16. R. W. Behring, T. Yamane, G. Navon, and L. W. Jelinski, *Proc. Natl. Acad. Sci. U.S.A.*, **85**, 6721–6725 (1988).
17. T. P. Kenakin, *Pharmacologic Analysis of Drug-Receptor Interaction*, Raven, New York, 1989.
18. J. Monod, J. Wyman, and J. P. Changeux, *J. Mol. Biol.*, **12**, 88–118 (1965).
19. R. J. Tallarida, *Drug Dev. Res.*, **19**, 257–274 (1990).
20. R. F. Furchgott, *Ann. Rev. Pharmacol.*, **4**, 21–38 (1964).
21. F. Wold, *Macromolecules: Structure and Function*, Prentice-Hall, Inc., Englewood Cliffs, N.J., 1971, pp. 16–40.
22. J. S. Fink, D. R. Weaver, S. A. Rivkees, R. A. Peterfreund, A. E. Pollack, E. M. Adler, and S. M. Reppert, *Mol. Brain Res.*, **14**, 186–195 (1992).
23. S. N. Schiffman, P. Halleux, R. Menu, and J.-J. Vanderhaeghen, *Drug Dev. Res.*, **28**, 381–385 (1993).
24. K. Fuxe, S. Ferre, P. Snaprud, G. von Euler, B. Johansson, and B. B. Fredholm, *Drug Dev. Res.*, **28**, 374–380 (1993).

25. C. Braestrup, in P. Krogsgaard-Larsen and H. Bundgaard, Eds. *A Textbook of Drug Design and Development*, Harwood Academic Publishers, Chur, Switzerland, 1991, pp. 335–356.

26. W. Schutz and M. Freissmith, *Trends Pharmacol. Sci.*, **13**, 376–380 (1992).

27. A. J. Clark, *The Mode of Action of Drugs on Cells*, Arnold, London, 1933.

28. W. D. M. Paton, *Proc. Roy. Soc., Ser. B.*, **154**, 21–69 (1961).

29. R. E. Gosselin, in J. M. Van Rossum, Ed., *Kinetics of Drug Action*, Springer-Verlag, Berlin, 1977, pp. 323–356.

30. D. E. Koshland, G. Nemethy, and D. Filmer, *Biochemistry*, **6**, 365–387 (1966).

31. R. F. Bruns and J. H. Fergus, *Mol. Pharmacol.*, **38**, 939–949 (1990).

32. J. W. Daly, J. Caceres, R. W. Moni, F. Gusovsky, M. Moos, Jr., K. B. Seamon, K. Milton, and C. W. Myers, *Proc. Natl. Acad. Sci. U.S.A.*, **89**, 10960–10963, 1992.

33. J. H. Gaddum, *Pharmacol. Rev.*, **9**, 211–218 (1957).

34. H. O. Schild, *Br. J. Pharmacol.*, **4**, 277–280 (1949).

35. E. J. Ariens, *Arch. Int. Pharmacodyn. Ther.*, **99**, 32–49 (1954).

36. J. Saunders and S. B. Freeman, *Trends Pharmacol. Sci.*, Suppl. 70–75 (1989).

37. R. P. Stephenson, *Br. J. Pharmacol.*, **11**, 379–393 (1956).

38. M. Nickerson, *Nature*, **178**, 697–698 (1956).

39. M. D. Hollenberg, in H. I. Yamamura, S. J. Enna, and M. J. Kuhar, Eds., *Neurotransmitter Receptor Binding*, 2nd Ed., Raven, New York, 1985, pp. 1–39.

40. J. M. Van Rossum and E. J. Ariens, *Arch. Int. Pharmacodyn. Ther.*, **136**, 385–413 (1962).

41. M. Keen, *Trends Pharmacol. Sci.*, **12**, 371–374 (1991).

42. L. Limbird, *Cell Surface Receptors*, Nijhoff, Boston, Mass., 1986.

43. A. V. Hill, *J. Physiol. (Lond.)*, **39**, 361–373 (1909).

44. W. Sieghart, *Trends Pharmacol. Sci.*, **13**, 446–450 (1992).

45. A. Doble and I. L. Martin, *Trends Pharmacol. Sci.*, **13**, 76–81 (1992).

46. D. R. Burt and G. L. Kamatchi, *FASEB J.*, **5**, 2916–3923 (1991).

47. K. W. Gee, *Mol. Neurobiol.*, **2**, 291–317 (1988).

48. A. Verma and S. H. Snyder, *Ann. Rev. Pharmacol. Toxicol.*, **39**, 307–322 (1989).

49. E. H. F. Wong and J. A. Kemp, *Ann. Rev. Pharmacol. Toxicol.*, **31**, 401–425 (1991).

50. J. W. Johnson and P. Ascher, *Nature*, **325**, 329–331 (1987).

51. C. W. Christine and D. W. Choi, *J. Neurosci.*, **10**, 108–116 (1990).

52. R. W. Ransome and N. L. Sec, *J. Neurosci.*, **10**, 830–836 (1990).

53. I. J. Reynolds and R. J. Miller, *Mol. Pharmacol.*, **36**, 738–745 (1989).

54. J.-L. Galzi, F. Revah, A. Bessis, and J.-P. Changeux, *Ann. Rev. Pharmacol. Toxicol.*, **31**, 37–72 (1991).

55. S. Numa, *Harvey Lect.*, **83**, 121–165 (1989).

56. C. W. Luetje, J. Patrick, and P. Sequela, *FASEB J.*, **4**, 2753–2760 (1990).

57. J.-P. Changeux, *Trends Pharmcol. Sci.*, **11**, 485–492 (1990).

58. R. J. Luckas and B. Bencherif, *Inter. Rev. Neurobiol.*, **34**, 25–131 (1992).

59. S. Couturier, D. Betrand, J.-M. Matter, M. C. Hernandez, S. Bertrand, N. Miller, S. Valeria, T. Barkas, and J. M. Ballivet, *Neuron*, **5**, 847–856 (1990).

60. J. Sloane, W. R. Martin, R. Hook, and J. Hernandez, *J. Med. Chem.*, **28**, 1248–1251 (1985).

61. J. L. Raszkiewicz, J. W. Turek, and S. P. Arneric, *Soc. Neurosci. Abst.*, **18**, 68.4 (1992).

62. A. Ramoa, M. Alliondon, Y. Aracaua, J. Irons, G. S. Lunt, S. Wonnacott, R. S. Aronstam, and E. X. Albuquerque, *J. Pharmacol. Exp. Ther.*, **254**, 71–81 (1990).

63. P. Krogsgaard-Larsen, H. Hjeds, E. Falch, F. S. Jorgensen, and L. Nielsen, *Adv. Drug Res.*, **17**, 381–456 (1988).

64. G. I. Drummond, *Cyclic Nucleotides in the Nervous System*, Raven, New York, 1984.

65. C. D. Mahle, H. L. Wiener, F. D. Yocca and S. Maayani, *J. Pharmacol. Exp. Ther.*, **263**, 1275–1284 (1992).

66. A. Edelman, D. Blumenthal, and E. Krebs, *Ann. Rev. Biochem.*, **56**, 567–613 (1987).

67. S. Rosenberg, *Ann. Rep. Med. Chem.*, **27**, 41–48 (1992).

68. G. Carpenter, *FASEB J.*, **6**, 3283–3289 (1992).

69. S. Kellenberger, P. Malherbe, and E. Sigel, *J. Biol. Chem.*, **267**, 25660–25663 (1992).

70. J. L. Arriza, T. M. Dawson, R. B. Simerly, L. J. Martin, M. G. Caron, S. H. Snyder, and R. J. Lefkowitz, *J. Neurosci.*, **12**, 4045–4055 (1992).

71. C. Schindler, K. Shaui, V. R. Prezioso, and J. E. Darnell, Jr., *Science*, **357**, 809–813 (1992).

72. M. J. Berridge, *Nature*, **361**, 315–325 (1993).

73. P. Needleman, J. Turk, B. Jakschik, A. R.

Morrison, and J. B. Lefkowith, *Ann. Rev. Biochem.*, **55**, 69–102 (1986).

74. G. M. Edelman and J. A. Gally, *Proc. Natl. Acad. Sci. U.S.A.*, **89**, 11651–11652 (1992).

75. A. Verma, D. J. Hirsch, C. E. Glatt, G. V. Ronnett, and S. H. Snyder, *Science*, **259**, 381–385 (1993).

76. M. Orchinik and B. S. McEwen, *Neurotransmissions*, ABI, Natick, Mass., **IX**(1), 1–6 (1993).

77. R. M. Evans, *Science*, **240**, 889–895 (1988).

78. R. Stein, in J. D. Coombes, Ed., *New Drugs from Natural Sources*, IBC, London, 1992, pp. 13–19.

79. R. F. Power, O. M. Connelly, and B. W. O'Malley, *Trends Pharmacol. Sci.*, **13**, 318–323 (1992).

80. F. O. Schmitt, in F. O. Schmitt, S. J. Bird, and F. E. Bloom, Eds., *Molecular Genetic Neuroscience*, Raven, New York, 1982, pp. 1–9.

81. T. M. Esterle and E. Sanders-Bush, *Trends Pharmacol. Sci.*, **12**, 375–379 (1991).

82. I. B. Black, *Information in the Brain. A Molecular Perspective*, MIT Press, Cambridge, Mass., 1991, pp. 77–100.

83. P. Strange, *Trends Pharmacol. Sci.*, **12**, 47–49 (1991).

84. A. Berghard, K. Gradin, I. Pongratz, M. Whitelaw, and L. Poellinger, *Mol. Cell. Biol.*, **13**, 677–689 (1993).

85. L. C. Mahan, R. M. McKernan, and P. A. Insel, *Ann. Rev. Pharmacol. Toxicol.*, **27**, 215–235 (1987).

86. I. Creese and D. R. Sibley, *Ann. Rev. Pharmacol. Toxicol.*, **21**, 357–391 (1981).

87. P. Davies, *Med. Res. Rev.*, **3**, 221–257 (1983).

88. T. Ewe, *Current Terms, Genetic Engineering*, Boehringer Ingelheim/Scriptum Redaktionsbüro, Lörrach, Germany, 1987.

89. Z. W. Hall, *An Introduction to Molecular Neurobiology*, Sinauer, Sunderland, Mass., 1992.

90. D. W. Ross, *Introduction to Molecular Medicine*, Springer-Verlag, New York, 1992.

91. K. B. Mullis and F. A. Faloona, *Methods Enzymol.*, **155**, 335–350 (1987).

92. F. Sanger, S. Nicklen, S. and A. R. Coulsen, *Proc. Natl. Acad. Sci.*, **74**, 5463–5467 (1979).

93. R. A. F. Dixon, I. S. Sigal, E. Rands, R. B. Register, M. R. Candelore, A. D. Blake, and C. D. Strader, *Nature*, **326**, 73–77 (1987).

94. L. B. Kozell, S. Starr, C. A. Machida, R. L. Neve, and K. A. Neve, *Soc. Neurosci. Abstr.*, **18**, 124.17 (1992).

95. F. Meng, A. Mansour, M. Hoversten, L. P. Taylor, and H. Akil, *Soc. Neurosci. Abstr.*, **18**, 281.13 (1992).

96. G. P. Dotto, K. Horiuchi, and N. D. Zinder, *J. Mol. Biol.*, **172**, 507–521 (1984).

97. B. Balbas, X. Soberon, E. Merino, M. Zurita, H. Lomeli, F. Valle, N. Flores, and F. Boliver, *Gene*, **50**, 3–40 (1986).

98. T. Kubo, K. Fukuda, A. Mikami, A. Maeda, H. Takahashi, M. Mishina, T. Haga, K. Haga, A. Ichiyama, K. Kangawa, M. Kojima, H. Matsuo, T. Hirose, and S. Numa, *Nature*, **323**, 411–416 (1986).

99. E. S. Deneris, J. Connolly, S. W. Rogers, and R. Duvoisin, *Trends Pharmacol. Sci.*, **12**, 34–40 (1991).

100. J. Patrick and W. B. Stallup, *Proc. Natl. Acad. Sci. U.S.A.*, **74**, 4689–4692 (1977).

101. P. Nef, C. Oneyser, T. Barkas, and M. Ballivet, in A. Maelicke, Ed., *Nicotinic Acetylcholine Receptor, Structure and Function*, Springer-Verlag, New York, 1986, pp. 417–422.

102. J. Boulter, K. Evans, D. Goldman, G. Martin, D. Treco, S. Heinemann, and J. Patrick, *Nature*, **319**, 368–374 (1986).

103. T. M. Savarese and C. M. Fraser, *Biochem. J.*, **283**, 1–19 (1992).

104. V. B. Cockcroft, D. J. Osguthorpe, E. A. Barnard, A. E. Friday, and G. G. Lunt, *Mol. Neurobiol.*, **4**, 129–169 (1990).

105. B. K. Koblika, T. Frielle, S. Collins, T. Yang-Feng, T. S. Koblika, U. Francke, R. J. Lefkowitz, and M. J. Caron, *Nature*, **329**, 75–79 (1987).

106. D. Julius, A. B. McDermott, T. Axel, and T. M. Jessell, *Science*, **241**, 558–563 (1988).

107. Y. Masu, K. Nakayama, H. Tamaki, Y. Harada, M. Kuno, and S. Nakanishi, *Nature*, **329**, 836–838 (1987).

108. K. Moriyoshi, M. Masu, T. Ishii, R. Shigemoto, N. Mizuno, and S. Nakanishi, *Nature*, **354**, 31–37 (1991).

109. T. Weiss, *Science*, **254**, 1292–1293 (1991).

110. F. Liebert, M. Parmentier, A. Lefort, C. Dinsart, J. V. Sande, C. Maenhaut, M. J. Simons, J. E. Dumont, and G. Vassart, *Science*, **244**, 569–572 (1989).

111. F. Libert, S. Schiffmann, A. Lefort, M. Parmentier, C. Gerard, J.E. Dumont, J.J. Vanderhaegen, and G. Vassart, *EMBO J.*, **10**, 1677–1682 (1991).

112. C. Maenhaut, S. J. van Sande, F. Libert, M. Abramowicz, M. Parmentier, J. J. Vanderhaegen, J. E. Dumont, G. Vassart, and S. Schiffmann, *Biochem. Biophys. Res. Comm.*, **173**, 1169–1178 (1989).

113. A. D. Hershey and J. E. Krause, *Science*, **247**, 958–962 (1990).

114. N. P. Gerard, R. L. Eddy, T. B. Shows, and C.

J. Gerard, *Biol. Chem.*, **265**, 20455–20462, (1990).

115. Q.-Y. Zhou, D. K. Grandy, L. Thambi, J. A. Kushner, H. H. M. Van Tol, R. Cone, D. Pribnow, J. Salon, J. R. Bunzow, and O. Civelli, *Nature*, **347**, 76–80 (1990).

116. H. H. M. Van-Tol, J. R. Bunzow, H. C. Guan, R. K. Sunahara, P. Seeman, H. B. Niznik, and O. Civelli, *Nature*, **350**, 610–614 (1991).

117. I. Gantz, M. Schaffer, J. DelValle, C. Logsdon, V. Campbell, M. Uhler, and T. Yamada, *Proc. Natl. Acad. Sci. U.S.A.*, **88**, 429–433 (1991).

118. F. Q.-Y Zhou, M. E. Olah, C. Li, R. A. Johnson, G. L. Stiles, G. L. Civelli, and O. Civelli, *Proc. Natl. Acad. Sci. U.S.A.*, **89**, 7432–7436 (1992).

119. L. Buck and R. Axel, *Cell*, **65**, 175–187 (1991).

120. V. Raz, Z. Kelman, A. Avivi, G. Neufeld, D. Givol, and Y. Yarden, *Oncogene*, **6**, 753–760 (1991).

121. R. N. Van Gelder, M. E. von Zastrow, A. Yool, W. C. Dement, J. D. Barchas, and J. H. Eberwine, *Proc. Natl. Acad. Sci. U.S.A.*, **87**, 1663–1667 (1990).

122. J. Eberwine, H. Yeh, K. Miyashiro, Y. Cao, S. Nair, R. Finnell, M. Zettel, and P. Coleman, *Proc. Natl. Acad. Sci. U.S.A.*, **89**, 3010–3014 (1992).

123. J. Kebabian and D. B. Calne, *Nature*, **277**, 93–96 (1979).

124. R. K. Sunahara, H. C. Guan, B. F. O'Dowd, P. Seeman, L. G. Laurier, G. Ng, S. R. George, J. Torchia, H. H. M. Van-Tol, and H. B. Niznik, *Nature*, **350**, 614–618 (1991).

125. P. Sokoloff, B. Giros, M. L. Martres, M. L. Bouthenet, and J. C. Schwartz, *Nature*, **347**, 146–151 (1990).

126. D. E. Casey, *Psychopharmacol.*, **99**, 47–53 (1989).

127. H. H. M. Van-Tol, C. M. Wu, H.-C. Guan, K. Ohara, J. R. Bunzow, O. Civelli, J. Kennedy, P. Seeman, H. B. Niznik, and V. Jovanoic, *Nature*, **358**, 149–152 (1992).

128. V. Giguere, N. Yang, P. Segui, and R. Evans, *Nature*, **331**, 91–94 (1988).

129. A. J. Jefferys, R. Wilson, R. Neumann, and J. Keyte, *J. Nuc. Acid Res.*, **16**, 10953–10959 (1988).

130. H. G. Khorana, *J. Biol. Chem.*, **263**, 7439–7442 (1988).

131. R. Henderson, J. M. Baldwin, T. A. Ceska, F. Zemlin, E. Beckmann, and K. H. J. Downing, *Mol. Biol.*, **213**, 899–929 (1990).

132. T. K. Atwood, E. E. Eliopoulos, and J. B. C. Findlay, *Gene*, **98**, 153–159 (1991).

133. J. Wess, T. I. Bonner, F. Dorje, and M. R. Brann, *Mol. Pharmacol.*, **38**, 517–523 (1990).

134. S. Wong, E. M. Parker, and E. M. Ross, *J. Biol. Chem.*, **265**, 6219–6224 (1990).

135. S. Ostrowski, M. A. Kjelsberg, M. G. Caron, and R. J. Lefkowitz, *Ann. Rev. Pharmacol. Toxicol.*, **32**, 167–183 (1992).

136. E. A. Barnard, *Trends Biochem.*, **17**, 368–374 (1992).

137. H. Thoenen, *Trends Neurosci.*, **14**, 165–170 (1991).

138. Y. Shen, D. Monsoma Jr., C. R. Gerfen, L. C. Mahan, P. A. Jose, M. M. Mouradian, and D. R. Sibley, *Mol. Pharmacol.* (1994), in press.

139. O. Civelli, J. R. Bunzow, D. K. Grandy, Q.-Y. Zhou, and H. H. M. Van-Tol, *Eur. J. Pharmacol.*, **207**, 277–286 (1991).

140. K. Koblika, R. A. F. Dixon, T. Friele, H. G. Dohlman, M. A. Bolanowski, I. S. Sigal, T. L. Yang-Feng, U. Francke, M. G. Caron, and R. W. Lefkowitz, *Proc. Natl. Acad. Sci. U.S.A.*, **84**, 46–50 (1987).

141. L. J. Emorine, S. Marullo, T. Briend, M. M. Sutron, G. Patey, K. Tate, C. Delavier-Klutchko, and A. D. Strosberg, *Science*, **245**, 1118–1121 (1989).

142. M. E. Williams, D. H. Feldman, A. F. McCue, R. Brenner, G. Velicelli, S. B. Ellis, and M. M. Harpold, *Neuron*, **8**, 71–84 (1992).

143. A. D. Strosberg and S. Marullo, *Trends Pharmacol. Sci.*, **13**, 95–98 (1992).

144. M. Freissmuth, E. Selzer, S. Marullo, W. Schutz, and A. D. Strosberg, *Proc. Natl. Acad. Sci. U.S.A.*, **88**, 8582–8586 (1991).

145. P. Payette, F. Gossard, M. Whiteway, and M. Dennis, *FEBS Lett.*, **266**, 21–25 (1990).

146. F. M. Ausbel, R. B. Brat, R. E. Kingston, D. D. Moore, J. G. Seidman, J. A. Smith, and K. Struhl, *Current Protocols in Molecular Biology*, John Wiley, & Sons, Inc., New York, 1988, 9.0.1.

147. S. G. Lee, N. Kalyan, J. Wilhelm, W.-T. Hum, S. M. Rappaport, S. Cheng, C. Dheer, C. Urbano, R. W. Hartzell, M. Ronchetti-Blume, M. Levner, and P. P. Hung, *J. Biol. Chem.*, **263**, 2917–2923 (1988).

148. R. Iyengar and L. Birnbaumer, *G Proteins*, Academic Press Inc., New York, 1990.

149. C. Kleuss, H. Scherubl, J. Hescheler, G. Schultz, and B. Wittig, *Nature*, **358**, 424–426 (1992).

150. T. M. Delorey and R. W. Olsen, *J. Biol. Chem.*, **267**, 16747–16750 (1992).

151. R. T. Boyd, M. H. Jacob, S. Couturier, M. Ballivet, and D. K. Berg, *Neuron*, **1**, 495–502 (1988).

152. P. Whiting and J. Lindstom, *Proc. Natl. Acad. Sci. U.S.A.*, **84**, 595–599 (1987).

153. S. Marullo, L. J. Emorine, A. D. Strosberg, and C. Delavier-Klutchko, *EMBO J.*, **9**, 1471–1476 (1990).

154. H.-Y. Wang, L. Lipfert, C. Malbon, and S. Bahouth, *J. Biol. Chem.*, **264**, 14424–14431 (1989).

155. J.-L. Galzi, A. Devillers-Thiery, N. Hussy, S. Bertrand, J. P. Changeux, and D. Bertrand, *Nature*, **359**, 500–505 (1992).

156. B. K. Koblika, C. McGregor, K. Daniel, T. S. Koblika, M. G. Caron, and R. J. Lefkowitz, *J. Biol. Chem.*, **262**, 15796–15802 (1987).

157. C. D. Strader, I. S. Sigal, R. B. Register, M. R. Candelore, E. Rands, and R. A. F. Dixon, *Proc. Natl. Acad. Sci. U.S.A.*, **84**, 4384–4388 (1987).

158. C. D. Strader, I. S. Sigal, M. R. Candelore, E. Rands, W. S. Hill, and R. A. F. Dixon, *J. Biol. Chem.*, **263**, 10267–10271 (1988).

159. C. D. Strader, M. R. Candelore, W. S. Hill, R. A. F. Dixon, and I. S. Sigal, *J. Biol. Chem.*, **264**, 16470–61477 (1989).

160. H. G. Dohlmann, M. G. Caron, A. DeBlasi, T. Frielle, and R. J. Lefkowitz, *Biochemistry*, **29**, 2335–2342 (1990).

161. T. M. Savarese, C.-D. Wang, J. C. Venter, and C. M. Fraser, *FASEB, J.*, **4**, A1011 (1990).

162. R. A. F. Dixon, I. S. Sigal, M. R. Candelore, R. B. Register, W. Scatterwood, W. S. Hill, E. Rands, and C. D. Strader, *EMBO J.*, **6**, 3269–3275 (1987).

163. B. Benhamou, T. Garcia, T. Lerouge, A. Vergezac, D. Goffollo, C. Bigogne, P. Chambon, and H. Gronemeyer, *Science*, **255**, 206–209 (1992).

164. C. D. Strader, R. A. F. Dixon, A. H. Cheung, M. R. Candelore, A. D. Blake, and I. S. Sigal, *J. Biol. Chem.*, **262**, 16439–16443 (1987).

165. K. Ohyama, Y. Yamano, S. Chaki, T. Kondo, and T. Inagami, *Biochem. Biophys. Res. Comm.*, **189**, 677–683 (1992).

166. A. R. Oseroff and R. H. Callender, *Biochemistry*, **13**, 4243–4248 (1974).

167. K. Maloney-Huss and T. P. Lybrand, *J. Mol. Biol.*, **40**, 8–14 (1992).

168. L. Pardo, J. A. Ballesteros, R. Osman, and H. Weinstein, *Proc. Natl. Acad. Sci. U.S.A.*, **89**, 4009–4013 (1992).

169. B. F. O'Dowd, M. Hnatowich, J. W. Regan, W. M. Leder, M. G. Caron, and R. W. Lefkowitz, *J. Biol. Chem.*, **263**, 15985–15992 (1988).

170. P. Ascher and S. Ekulkar, in B. Sakmann and E. Neher, Eds., *Single Channel Recording*, Plenum, New York, 1983, pp. 401–406.

171. J. P. Arena, K. K. Liu, P. S. Paress, and D. F. Cully, *J. Cell. Biochem.*, **16E** (suppl), 226 (1992).

172. F. Franciolini and A. Petris, *Biochem. Biophys. Acta*, **1031**, 247–259 (1990).

173. M. P. McCarthy, J. P. Earnest, E. F. Young, S. Choe, and R. M. Stroud, *Ann. Rev. Neurosci.*, **9**, 383–413 (1986).

174. J. Giraudat, J. L. Galzi, F. Revah, P. Y. Haumont, F. Lederer, and J. P. Changeux, *FEBS Lett.*, **253**, 190–198 (1989).

175. K. Imoto, C. Methfessel, B. Sakmann, M. Mishina, T. Konno, K. Fukuda, M. Kurasjki, H. Bujo, Y. Fujita, and S. Numa, *Nature*, **324**, 670–674 (1986).

176. K. Imoto, C. Busch, B. Sakmann, M. Mishina, T. Konno, J. Nakai, H. Bujo, Y. Mori, K. Fukuda, and S. Numa, *Nature*, **335**, 645–648 (1988).

177. R. J. Leonard, C. G. Labarca, P. Charnet, N. Davidson, and H. A. Lester, *Science*, **242**, 1578–1581 (1988).

178. H. Betz, *Neuron*, **5**, 383–392 (1990).

179. D. Langosch, K. Hartung, E. Grell, E. Bamberg, and H. Betz, *Biochem. Biophys. Acta.*, **1063**, 36–44 (1991).

180. T. Heidmann and J. P. Changeux, *Eur. J. Biochem.*, **94**, 281–296 (1979).

181. B. Sakmann, J. Patlak, and E. Neher, *Nature*, **286**, 71–73 (1980).

182. B. Bertrand, A. Devillers-Thiery, F. Revah, J. L. Galzi, N. Hussy, C. Mulle, S. Bertrand, M. Ballivet, and J. P. Changeux, *Proc. Natl. Acad. Sci. U.S.A.*, **89**, 1261–1265 (1992).

183. J. Dani, *Trends Neurosci.*, **12**, 125–128 (1989).

184. D. B. Pitchett and P. H. Seeburg, *Proc. Natl. Acad. Sci. U.S.A.*, **88**, 1421–1425 (1991).

185. J. C. Venter, J. A. Berzofsky, J. Lindstrom, S. Jacobs, C. M. Fraser, L. D. Kohn, W. J. Schnieder, G. L. Greene, A. D. Strosberg, and B. F. Erlanger, *Fed. Proc.*, **43**, 2532–2539 (1984).

186. P. M. Lippiello, K. G. Fernandes, J. J. Langone, and R. J. Bjercke, *J. Pharmacol. Exp. Ther.*, **257**, 1216–1224 (1991).

187. A. R. Bernado, J. F. Stoddart, and A. E. Kaifer, *J. Amer. Chem. Soc.*, **114**, 10624–10631 (1992).

188. T. P. Kenakin, R. A. Bond, and T. I. Bonner, *Pharmacol. Rev.*, **44**, 351–361 (1992).

189. J. W. Black, in J. W. Black, D. H. Jenkinson, and V. P. Gerskowitch, Eds., *Perspectives on Receptor Classification*, Liss, New York, 1987, pp. 11–15.

190. P. Hartig, T. A. Branchek, and R. L. Weinshank, *Trends Pharmacol. Sci.*, **13**, 152–159 (1992).

191. M. Williams, *Curr. Opinion Biotech.*, **4**, 85–90 (1993).

192. E. A. Ariens, *J. Receptor Res.*, **4**, 1–17 (1984).

193. M. Williams, *Med. Res. Rev.*, **11**, 147–184 (1991).

194. W. Sneader, *Comp. Med. Chem.*, **1**, 7–80 (1990).

195. J. Roth, *Metabolism*, **22**, 1059–1073 (1973).

196. P. Cuatrecasas, *Ann. Rev. Biochem.*, **43**, 169–214 (1974).

197. R. J. Lefkowitz, J. Roth, and I. Pastan, *Science*, **170**, 633–635 (1970).

198. P. Cuatrecasas and M. D. Hollenberg, *Adv. Prot. Chem.*, **30**, 251–451 (1976).

199. S. H. Snyder, *J. Med. Chem.*, **26**, 1667–1672 (1983).

200. K. J. Watling, *Trends Pharmacol. Sci.*, **13**, 226–269 (1992).

201. Y. C. Cheng and W. C. Prusoff, *Biochem. Pharmacol.*, **22**, 3099–3108 (1972).

202. R. Quirion and P. Gaudreau, *Neurosci. Biobehav. Rev.*, **9**, 413 (1985).

203. A. C. Foster and G. E. Fagg, *Brain Res. Rev.*, **7**, 103–164 (1984).

204. J. Lehman, J. Schneider, S. McPherson, D. E. Murphy, P. Bernard, C. Tsai, D. A. Bennett, G. Pastor, D. J. Steel, C. Boehm, D. L. Cheney, M. Williams, and P. L. Wood, *J. Pharmacol. Exp. Ther.*, **240**, 737–746 (1987).

205. D. E. Murphy, J. Schneider, C. Boehm, J. Lehmann, and M. Williams, *J. Pharmacol. Exp. Ther.*, **240**, 778–784 (1987).

206. D. E. Murphy, A. J. Hutchison, S. D. Hurt, M. Williams, and M. A. Sills, *Br. J. Pharmcol.*, **95**, 932–938 (1988).

207. P. Seeman, *Pharmacol. Rev.*, **32**, 279–313 (1980).

208. W. Billard, V. Ruperto, G. Crosby, L. C. Iorio, and A. Barnett, *Life Sci.*, **35**, 1885–1893 (1984).

209. C. Filer, S. Hurt, and Y. P. Wan, in M. Williams, R. A. Glennon and P. B. M. W. M. Timmermans, Eds., *Receptor Pharmacology and Function*, Dekker, New York, 1989, pp. 105–135.

210. D. B. Bylund and H. I. Yamamura, in H. I. Yamamura, S. J. Enna, and M. J. Kuhar, Eds., *Methods in Neurotransmitter Receptor Analysis*, Raven, New York, 1990, pp. 1–35.

211. O. H. Straus and A. Goldstein, *J. Gen. Physiol.*, **26**, 559–585 (1943).

212. M. Williams and E. A. Risley, *Proc. Natl. Acad. Sci. U.S.A.*, **77**, 6892–6896 (1980).

213. J. P. Bennett Jr. and H. I. Yamamura, in H. I. Yamamura, S. J. Enna, and M. J. Kuhar, Eds., *Neurotransmitter Receptor Binding*, 2nd Ed., Raven, New York, 1985, p. 69.

214. R. F. Bruns, K. Lawson-Wendling, and T.A. Pugsley, *Anal. Biochem.*, **132**, 74–81 (1983).

215. *RS/1 Release 2 Features*, Bolt, Beranek, and Newman Software Products Corp., Cambridge, Mass., 1985.

216. G. A. McPherson, in M. Williams, R. A. Glennon, and P. B. M. W. M. Timmermans, Eds., *Receptor Pharmacology and Function*, Dekker, New York, 1989, pp. 47–84.

217. P. Taylor and P. A. Insel, in W. B. Pratt and P. Taylor, Eds., *Principles of Drug Action. The Basis of Pharmacology*, Churchill-Livingstone, New York, 1990, pp. 43–97.

218. M. Williams and M. A. Sills, *Comp. Med. Chem.*, **3**, 45–80 (1991).

219. M. J. Kuhar, E. B. DeSouza, and J. Unnerstall, *Ann. Rev. Neurosci.*, **9**, 27–59 (1986).

220. M. J. Kuhar and J. R. Unnerstall, in H. I. Yamamura, S. J. Enna, and M. J. Kuhar, Eds., *Methods in Neurotransmitter Receptor Analysis*, Raven, New York, 1990, pp. 177–218.

221. M. Williams, T. Giordano, R. Elder, H. J. Reiser, and G. L. Neil, *Med. Res. Rev.*, **13**, 399–448 (1993).

222. S.-Z. Wang and E. E. El-Fakahany, *J. Pharmacol. Exp. Ther.*, **266**, 237–243 (1993).

223. R. M. Nitsch, B. E. Slack, R. J. Wurtman, and J. H. Growdon, *Science*, **258**, 304–307 (1992).

224. C. Hooper, *J. NIH Res.*, **4**, 48–54 (1992).

225. *The Merck Index*, 11th Ed., Merck Research Laboratories, Rahway, N.J., 1989.

226. P. N. Craig, *Comp. Med. Chem.*, **6**, 237–991 (1990).

227. M. Williams and M. F. Jarvis, in C. R. Clark and W. H. Moos, Eds., *Drug Discovery Technologies*, Ellis Horwood, Chichester, UK, 1990, pp. 129–166.

228. R. S. L. Chang, V. J. Lotti, R. L. Monaghan, J. Birnbaum, E. O. Stapley, M. A. Goetz, G. Albers-Schonberg, A. A. Patchett, T. M. Liesch, O. D. Hensens, and J. P. Springer, *Science*, **230**, 177–180 (1985).

229. B. E. Evans, K. E. Rittle, M. G. Bock, R. M. DiPardo, R. M. Freidinger, W. L. Whittier, N. P. Gould, G. F. Lundell, C. E. Homminick, D. F.

Veber, P. S. Anderson, R. S. L. Chang, V. J. Lotti, D. J. Cerino, T. B. Chen, P. J. King, K. A. Kunkel, J. P. Springer, and J. Hirschfield, *J. Med. Chem.*, **30**, 1229–1241 (1987).

230. R. M. Snider, J. W. Constantine, J. A. Lowe, K. P. Longo, W. S. Lebel, H. A. Woody, S. E. Drozda, M. C. Desai, F. C. Vinick, R. W. Spencer, and H.-J. Hess, *Science*, **251**, 435–437 (1991).

231. C. Garret, A. Carruette, V. Fardin, S. Moussaoui, J.-F. Peyronel, J. C. Blanchard, and P. M. Laduron, *Proc. Natl. Acad. Sci. U.S.A.*, **88**, 10208–10212 (1991).

232. B. P. Venepalli, L. D. Aimone, K. C. Appell, M. R. Bell, J. A. Dority, R. Goswani, P. L. Hall, V. Kumar, K. B. Lawrence, M. E. Logan, P. M. Scensny, J. A. Seelye, B. E. Tomczuk, and J. M. Yanni, *J. Med. Chem.*, **35**, 374–378 (1992).

233. D. Gully, M. Canton, R. Boigegrain, F. Jeanjean, J.-C. Molimared, M. Poncelet, C. Gueudet, M. Heaulme, R. Leyris, A. Brouard, D. Pelaprat, C. Labbé-Jullié, J. Mazella, P. Soubrié, J. P. Maffrand, W. Rostène, P. Kitabgi, and G. LeFur, *Proc. Natl. Acad. Sci. U.S.A.*, **90**, 65–69 (1993).

234. Y. Yamamura, H. Ogawa, T. Chihara, K. Kondo, T. Onogawa, S. Nakamura, T. Mori, M. Tominaga, and Y. Yabuuchchi, *Science*, **252**, 572–574 (1991).

235. D. J. Pettibone, B. V. Clineschmidt, M. T. Kishel, E. V. Lis, D. R. Reiss, C. J. Woyden, B. E. Evans, R. M. Freidinger, D. F. Veber, M. J. Cook, G. J. Haluska, M. J. Novy, and R. I. Lowensohn, *J. Pharmacol. Exp. Ther.*, **264**, 308–314 (1993).

236. M. F. Balandrin, J. A. Klocke, E. S. Wurtele, and W. H. Bollinger, *Science*, **228**, 1154–1160 (1985).

237. P. J. Hylands and L. J. Nisbet, *Ann. Rep. Med. Chem.*, **26**, 259–270 (1991).

238. M. A. Gallop, R. W. Barratt, W. J. Dower, S. P. A. Fodor, and E. M. Gordon, *J. Med. Chem.*, **37**, 1233–1251 (1994); E. M. Gordon, R. W. Barratt, W. J. Dower, S. P. A. Fodor, and M. A. Gallop, *J. Med. Chem.*, **37**, 1385–1401 (1994).

239. S. Schrieber, *Science*, **251**, 283–287 (1991).

240. H.-M. Chang and P. P.-H. But, *Pharmacology and Applications of Chinese Materia Medica*, World Scientific, Singapore, 1986.

241. C. W. Jefford, K. L. Rinehart, and L. S. Shield, *Pharmaceuticals and the Sea*, Technomic, Lancaster, Pa., and Basel, Switzerland, 1988.

242. A. Dumuis, R. Bouhelal, M. Sebben, R. Cory, and J. Bockhaert, *Mol. Pharmacol.*, **34**, 880–887 (1988).

243. S. Birnbaum and K. Mosbach, *Curr. Opinion Biotech.*, **3**, 49–54 (1992).

244. J. K. Scott and G. P. Smith, *Science*, **249**, 386–390 (1990).

245. K. S. Lam, S. Salamon, E. M. Hersh, V. J. Hruby, W. M. Kazmierski, and R. J. Knapp, *Nature*, **354**, 82–84 (1991).

246. R. A. Houghten, C. Pinnilla, S. E. Blondelle, J. R. Appel, C. T. Dooley, and J. H. Cuervo, *Nature*, **354**, 84–86 (1991).

247. S. P. A. Fodor, J. L. Read, M. C. Pirrung, L. Stryer, A. T. Lu, and D. Solas, *Science*, **251**, 767–773 (1991).

248. J. Vane, *Chicago Tribune*, Sunday, July 19th, 1992, Business Section, p. 1.

249. S. T. Crooke, *Ann. Rev. Pharmacol. Toxicol.*, **32**, 329–376 (1992).

250. P. M. Sweetnam, L. Caldwell, J. Lancaster, C. Bauer, Jr., B. McMillan, W. J. Kinnier, and C. H. Price, *Natural Products*, **56**, 441–455 (1993).

251. N. Cook, J. Sutton, and K. Takeuchi, *Pharma. Tech. Inter.*, Sterling Publications, London, 1992.

252. K. M. Raley-Susman, K. R. Miller, J. C. Owicki, and R. M. Sapiosky, *J. Neurosci.*, **12**, 773–780 (1992).

253. L. M. Fisher, *New York Times*, Midwest Edition, Sunday, January 24th, 1993, Business Section, p. 9.

254. K. King, H. G. Dohlman, J. Thorner, M. G. Caron, and R. J. Lefkowitz, *Science*, **250**, 121–123 (1990).

255. M. N. Potenza, G. F. Graminski, and M. R. Lerner, *Anal. Biochem.*, **206**, 315–322 (1992).

256. G. deStevens, *Prog. Drug. Res.*, **34**, 343–358 (1990).

257. C. Wahlestedt, E. M. Pich, G. F. Koob, F. Yee, and M. Helig, *Science*, **259**, 528–531 (1993).

CHAPTER TWELVE

Drug-Target Binding Forces

PETER A. KOLLMAN

Department of Pharmaceutical Chemistry
School of Pharmacy
University of California
San Francisco, California, USA

CONTENTS

1 Introduction, 399
2 Energy Components for Intermolecular
  Noncovalent Interactions in the Gas Phase, 401
    2.1 Electrostatic energy, 401
    2.2 Dispersion attraction, 402
    2.3 Exchange repulsion energy, 402
    2.4 Polarization energy, 403
    2.5 Charge transfer energy, 403
    2.6 Summary, 403
3 Thermodynamics of Association, 404
    3.1 Gas phase association, 405
    3.2 Solvation effects, 405
4 Examples of Drug-Receptor Interactions, 408
    4.1 Biotin–Avidin, 408
    4.2 DHFR–TMP, 410
    4.3 DNA–intercalator, 410
5 Summary, 411

1 INTRODUCTION

This chapter focuses mainly on the forces that hold together complexes between large and small molecules such as a "bond", which is a concept that chemists are very familiar with. A covalent bond is an attractive interaction between two atoms in which each contributes a valence electron; for example, such a bond is formed between two hydrogen atoms to make the H_2 molecule: $H + H \rightarrow H–H$. Also included is what most chemists might consider "ionic" bonds such as $Na + Cl \rightarrow Na–Cl$, even though the valence electron pair, in this case, is much closer to the chlorine atom than to the sodium atom. Examples of

Burger's Medicinal Chemistry and Drug Discovery,
Fifth Edition, Volume 1: Principles and Practice,
Edited by Manfred E. Wolff.
ISBN 0-471-57556-9 © 1995 John Wiley & Sons, Inc.

399

covalent bonds and covalent bond strengths and lengths are well described in introductory chemistry and physical chemistry textbooks (1).

However, noncovalent "bonds," where electron pairs are "conserved" in reactants and products, are the emphasis in this chapter. Examples of such interactions are "dative bonds", e.g., $H_3N: + BH_3 \rightarrow H_3N:BH_3$ and hydrogen bonds, e.g., $H_2O + H_2O \rightarrow H_2O \cdots HOH$. These noncovalent bonds provide the "force" to make drugs interact strongly with their targets.

A simple potential surface for a bonding interaction appears in Figure 12.1 which is basically the same shape for both covalent and noncovalent bonds. Most covalent bonds have a very large dissociation energy D_0, greater than 50 kcal/mol, so that at room temperature where $RT \sim 0.6$ kcal/mol (R is the universal gas constant and T is the temperature), the fraction of "broken" bonds at equilibrium $e^{-D_0/RT}$ is vanishingly small. By contrast, noncovalent bonds are much weaker, typically 1–10 kcal/mol, thus much easier to break. A significant fraction can be broken at equilibrium at room temperature. This very weakness of noncovalent bonds is what makes them so useful in biological processes because a small change in the chemical "environment" (e.g., ionic strength) can form or break such a bond. Probably the best known important noncovalent bonds are those between the strands of DNA, where hydrogen bonds hold the double helix together (2). When the cells begin to replicate, chemical signals (e.g., proteins binding to the DNA) shift the equilibrium to the single-stranded DNA, breaking these hydrogen bonds. Other important examples of noncovalent complexes include those between enzyme and substrate, "receptor" protein and hormone, antibody and antigen, and intercalator and DNA. Much of this chapter's concern is with the interaction:

$$\text{drug} + \text{receptor} \underset{k_r}{\overset{k_f}{\rightleftharpoons}} \text{complex}$$

The rate constant for association of the complex is k_f; the rate constant for dissociation of the complex is k_r; and the affinity, or association constant $K_{as} = k_f/k_r$. It is usually assumed that the biological activity of a drug is related to its affinity K_{as} for the receptor, although there are processes such as actinomycin D–DNA interactions in which the rate of dissociation k_r is more relevant to the biological activity (3).

The thermodynamic parameters of interest for the reactions above are the standard free energy (ΔG^0), enthalpy (ΔH^0), and entropy (ΔS^0) of association. These parameters are related by the equations:

$$\Delta G^0 = -RT \ln K_{as}$$

$$\Delta G^0 = \Delta H^0 - T \Delta S^0$$

This measurement of K_{as} allows one to calculate ΔG^0, the free energy of association of the complex. To find ΔH^0 and ΔS^0 separately, requires a determination of K_{as} as a function of temperature (if ΔH^0 and ΔS^0 are relatively temperature independent, a plot of $\ln K_{as}$ vs. $1/T$ can yield ΔH^0 and ΔS^0) or a calorimetric measurement of ΔH^0 directly. Since ΔH^0 and ΔS^0 themselves are often quite temperature depen-

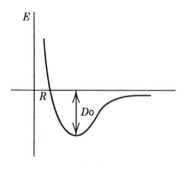

Fig. 12.1 Energy E as a function of internuclear separation R for an association reaction.

dent, the latter experiment is more definitive.

This chapter provides some background about the forces that hold molecules together, with emphasis on the noncovalent interactions of interest in biology, and attempts to relate experimental determinations of the thermodynamics of association to the forces involved in the association. The discussion in the reminder of the chapter is divided into two parts. First, the forces that hold molecules together in the gas phase and solution are discussed; the second part discusses the examples of noncovalent interactions and analyzes the binding forces in particular cases.

2 ENERGY COMPONENTS FOR INTERMOLECULAR NONCOVALENT INTERACTIONS IN THE GAS PHASE

Quantum mechanical calculations on small molecule association suggest that there are five major contributions to the energy of intermolecular interactions in the gas phase (4). The sum of these contributions is the dissociation energy of the intramolecular complex represented in Figure 12.1. Table 12.1 contains some examples of magnitudes of the different energy components for different interactions.

2.1 Electrostatic Energy

Given information on the charge distribution of two molecules A and B, the electrostatic interaction energy between them can be evaluated. Although nuclei can be treated as point positive charges, the negative charge of electrons is smeared out over space. Thus a rigorous evaluation of the electrostatic energy involves an integration over the electron clouds of the two molecules. In most cases, however, the electrons as well as the nuclei are represented by point charges, whose position and magnitude are usually chosen to reproduce known molecular properties. The strength

Table 12.1   Some Examples of Interaction Energies of Noncovalent Complexes, kcal/mol

Interaction	Interaction Energies[a]					
	$-\Delta E \equiv D_0$	ΔE_{es}	ΔE_{dis}	ΔE_{ex}	ΔE_{pol}	ΔE_{ct}
$He \cdots He$	0.02^{b}	0	-0.028	$+0.008$	0	0
$Xe \cdots Xe$	0.64^{b}	0	-0.86	0.40	0	0
$C_6H_6 \cdots C_6H_6$	$\sim 2^{c}$	$\neq 0$	$\neq 0$	$\neq 0$	$\neq 0$	$\neq 0$
$H_2O \cdots H_2O$	8.9^{d}	-9.2	(-1)	4.0	-0.5	-2.2
$TCNE \cdots OH_2$	4.1^{e}	-3.9	(-1)	2.0	-0.2	-1.0
$Li^{+} \cdots OH_2$	48.9^{f}	-51.1	(-1)	12.7	-7.8	-1.7
$F^{-} \cdots OH_2$	41.1^{f}	-37.8	(-1)	20.5	-4.9	-17.9
$NH_4^{+} \cdots F^{-}$	164.7	-181.4	(-1)	61.6	-8.3	-35.6

[a]Symbols: $-\Delta E$; calculated (or experimental) total interaction energy equal to D_0 in Figure 12.1 kcal/mole, ΔE_{es} electrostatic energy; ΔE_{dis}, dispersion energy; ΔE_{ex}, exchange repulsion energy; ΔE_{pol}, polarization energy; ΔE_{ct}, charge transfer energy (values in parentheses are estimated).
[b]See Karplus and Porter (8).
[c]See Janda et al. (13).
[d]See Umeyama and Morokuma (7); this value for ΔE is certainly too large; thus the value of Joesten and Schaad (14) in Table 12.2 has been used.
[e]See Morokuma et al. (15); TCNE, tetracyanoethylene.
[f]See Kollman (16).

and the directionality of A..B electrostatic interactions are usually dominated by
the first nonvanishing multipole moment
$\mathbf{M}_n$ of the charge distribution,

$$\mathbf{M}_n = \sum_{i=1}^{\text{\# of charges}} q_i \mathbf{r}_i^n$$

where q_i are the individual charges and $\mathbf{r}_i^n$
the vector from the origin of the coordinate
system to the ith charge (5,6). Molecules
that are charged have a nonzero zeroth
moment M_0. Ionic crystals such as Na^+Cl^-
are held together predominantly by electro-
static attraction between oppositely
charged ions. Crystals of ice I are mainly
held together by *dipolar* electrostatic forces
where $M_0 = 0$ and $\mathbf{M}_1 \neq 0$, since there are
virtually no ions in these crystals. It should
be noted here that "hydrogen bonding" is
not a separate energy component; typically
hydrogen bonds contain important energy
contributions from all five energy components, although the electrostatic component
is usually the largest contributor to this
interaction (7).

Of the intermolecular energy components, the electrostatic is the longest range
(i.e., it dies off most slowly with distance as
the two molecules separate). Ion-ion interactions die off as $1/R$; ion-dipole as $1/R^2$;
dipole–dipole as $1/R^3$, etc. In general, if
two molecules have as their first nonvanish-
ing multipole moments $\mathbf{M}_n$ and $\mathbf{M}_m$, the
electrostatic interaction energy between
them dies off as $1/R^{n+m+1}$. The electrostatic interaction energy between water, a
dipolar molecule ($n = 1$), and benzene,
whose first nonvanishing moment is a quadrupole ($m = 2$) dies off as $1/R^4$.

2.2 Dispersion Attraction

There are attractive forces existing between
all pairs of atoms, even between rare gas
atoms (He, Ar, Ne, Kr, Xe), which cause
them to condense at a sufficiently low

temperature. None of the other attractive
forces (electrostatic, polarization, charge
transfer) can explain the attraction between
rare gas atoms; it is called the dispersion
attraction (8). Even though the rare gas
atoms have no permanent dipole moments,
they are polarizable, and one has instantaneous dipole–dipole attractions in which
the presence of a locally asymmetric charge
distribution on one molecule induces an
asymmetric charge distribution on the other
molecule, e.g., $^{\delta^-}\text{He}^{\delta^+} \cdots {}^{\delta^-}\text{He}^{\delta^+}$.

The net attraction is called dispersion
attraction (often known as London or van
der Waals attraction) and is dependent on
the polarizability and the number of valence electrons of the interacting molecules.
It dies off as $1/R^6$, where R is the atom–
atom separation. The difference between
this attraction and the polarization energy
is that the latter involves the interaction of
a molecule that is already polar, with
another polar or nonpolar molecule.

2.3 Exchange Repulsion Energy

The Pauli principle keeps electrons with the
same spin spatially apart. This principle
applies whether one is dealing with electrons on the same molecule or on different
molecules and is the predominant repulsive
force (6) that keeps electrons of different
molecules from interpenetrating when noncovalent complexes are formed. Although
this repulsive term is often represented by
an analytical function of the form

$$\frac{A}{R^n} \ (n = 9 \text{ or } 12)$$

where R is the distance between molecules
or nonbonded atoms and A is a constant
which depends on the atom types, the best
available quantum mechanical calculations
suggest that this repulsion should diminish
with an exponential dependence on the
distance between the atoms (6).

2.4 Polarization Energy

When two molecules approach each other, there is charge redistribution within each molecule, leading to an additional attraction between the molecules. The energy associated with this charge redistribution is invariably attractive and is called the polarization energy. For example, if a molecule with polarizability α is placed in an electric field, E, the polarization energy is

$$E_{pol} = -\frac{1}{2}\alpha E^2$$

If the electric field is due to an ion $\mathbf{E} = q\mathbf{i}/R^2$, where q is the ionic change, i the unit vector along the ion-molecule direction, and R the ion–molecule distance, the $E_{pol} = -\frac{1}{2}\alpha q^2/R^4$ for this *ion-induced dipole* interaction. The corresponding formula for *dipole-induced dipole* interaction between two dipolar molecules is

$$E_{pol} = -\frac{1}{2}\frac{\alpha_1\mu_2^2 + \alpha_2\mu_1^2}{R^6}$$

where the μs are the dipole moments of the molecules, the αs their polarizabilities, and R the distance between molecules. The polarizability of a molecule can be broken down into atomic contributions [atomic polarizabilities are additive to a good approximation (9)], and it is roughly proportional to the number of valence electrons as well as depending on how tightly these valence electrons are bound to the nuclei. Umeyama and Morokuma (10) have calculated the ion-induced dipole contribution to the proton affinities of the simple alkyl amines. They attributed the order of *gas phase* proton affinities in the alkyl amines $[NH_3 < CH_3NH_2 < (CH_3)_2NH < (CH_3)_3N]$ to the greater polarizability of a methyl group than a hydrogen. A simple estimate using the above empirical equation for an ion-induced dipole interaction with $q = +1$, the difference in polarizabilities of a methyl and a hydrogen $(\Delta\alpha) \approx 4\,\mathrm{cm}^3$, a proton–

methyl distance of $2.0\,\text{Å}$, and a proton–proton distance of $1.6\,\text{Å}$, leads to an expected increase of $\sim 20\,\mathrm{kcal/mol}$ of proton affinity for every methyl group added to NH_3. This very qualitative estimate is of the right magnitude but about 2–3 times too large (see below).

2.5 Charge Transfer Energy

When two molecules interact, there is a small amount of electron flow from one to the other. For example, in the equilibrium geometry of the linear water dimer $HO-H\cdots OH_2$, the water molecule that is the proton acceptor has transferred about $0.05\,e^-$ to the proton donor water (10,11). The attractive energy associated with this charge transfer is the charge transfer energy and can be thought of as a mixing of an ionic resonance structure $\overset{(-)}{H-O}\cdots\overset{+}{H-OH_2}$ into the overall wave function. Although the charge transfer energy is an important contributor to the interaction energy of most noncovalent complexes, the presence of a "charge transfer" electronic transition in the visible spectrum does not mean that the charge transfer energy is the predominant force holding the complex together in its ground state. For example, the complex between benzene and I_2, earlier thought to be a prototype "charge transfer" complex, appears to be held together predominantly by electrostatic, polarization, and dispersion energies in its ground electronic state (12).

2.6 Summary

Having described the components of the interaction energies, a number of specific examples in detail need to be considered. (Table 12.1). Unlike the total interaction energy, which can be measured experimentally, the individual energy components cannot. The theoretical estimate of these quantities is often dependent on the method of calculation, but their qualitative features are usually independent of methodology.

Rare gas–rare gas interactions (He $\cdots$ He and Xe $\cdots$ Xe) have only *dispersion* attraction. The difference between the potential well depth of He $\cdots$ He and Xe $\cdots$ Xe (Fig. 12.1, D_0) at the equilibrium distance is due to the greater polarizability of the xenon atoms, thus to the greater dispersion attraction between them. A simple manifestation of this interaction is the much higher boiling point of xenon than helium, due to the greater attractive forces in xenon liquid. Miyamoto and Kollman (17) have recently shown that the single largest attractive free energy contribution to binding in the strongest known small molecule–macromolecule interaction (biotin–avidin) is the dispersion attraction.

One might intuitively expect that benzene dimer would pack together like two flat plates, but this is not the case in the gas phase (13); the crystal structure also does not have parallel alignments of benzene molecules (18). Benzene, although having no dipole moment, does have a *quadrupole* moment ($M_2 \neq 0$). A simple way to think about this quadrupole moment is to realize that a benzene C–H is somewhat electropositive and its electron cloud rather electronegative. A second benzene molecule would like to approach the first one so that its "electropositive" side approaches the other molecule's "electronegative side". The water dimer $(H_2O)_2$ and the ether ... TCNE interactions are examples of prototypal H-bonds and "charge transfer" complexes, but both are held together mainly by electrostatic forces, although the other attractive energy components contribute significantly to the total ΔE. The electrostatic component is predominant in determining all the structural parameters except the distance between molecules.

Similarly, the geometry and net attraction between Li^+ and OH_2, F^- and H_2O, and NH_4^+ and F^- are dominated by the electrostatic energy component.

Clearly, a simple molecular mechanical energy expression can represent noncovalent interactions surprisingly well (19). Such energy expressions contain only the first three terms mentioned above: electrostatic, exchange repulsion, and dispersion. By a suitable choice of parameters, charge transfer and polarization effects are implicitly included in such an expression, which is simple and easy to evaluate, along with its derivatives, for molecules with thousands of atoms. Thus, many interesting applications of such molecular mechanical methods to complex molecules have been carried out (20,21).

3 THERMODYNAMICS OF ASSOCIATION

To this point, the focus has mainly been on the energy of association between molecules; typically, in any drug-receptor interaction, what is the equilibrium constant for association K_{as} and the free energy of association ΔG^0. The difference between the free energy (ΔG^0) and energy (ΔE^0) of association is given by $\Delta G^0 = \Delta H^0 - T\Delta S^0$, and $\Delta H^0 = \Delta E^0 + (\Delta PV)$; for gas phase associations, $(\Delta PV) \cong -RT$, which is -0.6 kcal/mol at room temperature. Thus this term, when added to ΔE, favors association (the more negative ΔG, the greater tendency for association). However ΔS, the entropy of association, is typically large and negative. The reason is that one is reducing the "floppy" degrees of freedom, which have large entropies, translations, and rotations, by 6 (six translations and six rotations in the free molecules, three of each in the complex) during complex formation and replacing these with vibrations, which have lower entropies (22).

3.1 Gas Phase Association

For example, at 300 K two CH_4 molecules have a translational entropy of 69 eu and a rotational entropy of 31 eu, whereas $(CH_4)_2$ has a translational entropy of 37 eu and a rotational entropy (assuming a C . . . C distance of 4 Å) of 22 eu. Thus one can see that the translational and rotational entropy contributions to the reaction 2 $CH_4 \rightarrow (CH_4)_2$ is −41 eu. These 6 degrees of freedom become vibrations in the complex $(CH_4)_2$, and as such might contribute a vibrational entropy of about 20–30 eu. Thus for the dimerization of CH_4 in the gas phase, expected to be at 300 K $T \Delta S^0$ is about −3 to −6 kcal/mol.

As stressed in the second law of thermodynamics, the tendency for a chemical process to occur is governed both by the energy released (exothermicity) in the process and the entropy gained (the tendency of the reaction to go to a more random, disordered state). In the case of gas phase association, the energy term is invariably exothermic if the reactants approach each other in an appropriate orientation, and the entropy term is always negative, opposing association. Table 12.2 gives an example of the thermodynamics of association of water molecules in the gas phase.

Table 12.2 **Thermodynamic Functions for Gas Phase Association of Water Molecules: 2 $H_2O \rightarrow (H_2O_2)$**

Thermodynamic Function	Value for H_2O Dimerization, kcal/mol
ΔE^0 (0°K)[a]	−6.2
ΔE^0 (300°K)[a]	−4.2
ΔH^0 (300°K)[a]	−5.2
ΔS^0 (300°K)[b]	−9.0
ΔG^0 (300°K)	+3.8

[a]See Joesten and Schaad (14).
[b]Estimated, using the vibration frequencies employed by Joesten and Schaad (14).

As one can see, the entropy (ΔS^0) contribution to association of water molecules in the gas phase is substantial and negative; thus there is little tendency for water molecules to associate in the gas phase at room temperature and 1 atm pressure, even though the hydrogen bond energy is about 5 kcal/mol.

3.2 Solvation Effects

The thermodynamic cycle (Fig. 12.2) illustrates the problems faced in transferring knowledge of gas phase intermolecular interactions to solution phase phenomena. Our real interest is in ΔG_4, the solution-phase free energy of association. Until now, discussion has focused on the energy (ΔE_1), enthalpy (ΔH_1), and free energy (ΔG_1) of association in the gas phase. To be able to calculate ΔG_4, ΔG_3, the solvation free energy of the drug–receptor complex, ΔG_{2D}, the solvation free energy of the drug, and ΔG_{2R}, the solvation free energy of the receptor needs to be known. These solvation free energies are the free energies gained (or lost) by taking the molecule from a standard concentration in the gas phase to a corresponding concentration in solution. Using the thermodynamic cycle in Figure 12.2, it follows that:

$$\Delta G_4 = \Delta G_1 - \Delta G_{2D} - \Delta G_{2R} - \Delta G_3$$

$$(12.1)$$

Similar relationships hold for ΔH_4 and ΔS_4. There is no reason to expect ΔG_4 and ΔG_1

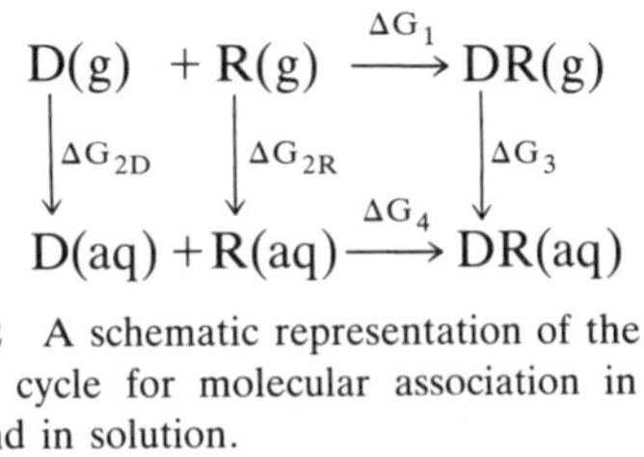

Fig. 12.2 A schematic representation of the thermodynamic cycle for molecular association in the gas phase and in solution.

to be similar, so the problem of estimating ΔG_{2D}, ΔG_{2R}, and ΔG_3 is next. ΔG_{2R} or ΔG_3, cannot be measured since this calculation would require the vaporization of a measurable amount of a receptor or drug–receptor complex. For most polar and ionic drugs, ΔG_{2D} is not measurable either. Therefore one resorts to measuring the free energy of transfer from octanol to water ΔG_{2D} (oct) rather than the free energy of transfer from the gas phase to water, ΔG_{2D}. This situation underlies the postulate of the Hansch approach (23), which suggests that the differences in ΔG_{2D}(oct) ($\Delta\Delta G_{2D}$(oct)) may be related to the biological activity of drugs, and in many cases this desolvation (water → octanol) does indeed appear to be related to drug binding and/or biological activity.

Since the individual free energies in equation 12.1 are so hard to measure, one has been led to smaller model systems to analyze the major driving force for drug-receptor association, a step taken by Kauzmann (24) in his classic paper on the forces that affect protein stability and structure. He examined the thermodynamics of association and solution of small nonpolar molecules in aqueous solution. The associations were characterized by: a large *positive* entropy term, and the solution by a large negative *entropy* with the enthalpy terms less important. Thus the well-known lack of solubility of hydrocarbons in water was not due to a net loss of hydrogen bonds; the hydrocarbons cause the water molecules to become more ordered (thus to lose entropy) so that they can still find a good hydrogen bond partner (ΔH of solution of these hydrocarbons is often negative, but much smaller in magnitude than $T\,\Delta S$ of solution). By coming together in aqueous solution, these hydrocarbons "release" some H_2Os, and this favorable $T\,\Delta S$ association has been the driving force for this association. According to many researchers, this "hydrophobic" effect of hydrocarbon groups has been a key feature in

many drug receptor associations. A lucid description of hydrophobic forces has been given by Jencks (25) and Dill (26).

Computer simulation approaches have proven very useful in enabling calculation of the association of molecules. For example, the association of two methane molecules in the gas phase would lead to a $\Delta E^0(0\,K)$ of $\sim -1\,kcal/mole$ and, by analogy with water dimer (Table 12.2), a very positive ΔG^0 (300 K) and thus no tendency for association. In aqueous solution, one can calculate, using modern statistical mechanical simulation methods, the potential of mean force for association of two molecules, which is the free energy as a function of molecular separation in solution. Although there is some controversy about whether there are both "solvent-separated" and "contact" minima for two methane molecules in aqueous solution, there is no question that methane association is quite attractive in aqueous solution compared to the gas phase (27).

One can also apply such approaches to study association of ionic and polar molecules. For example, the association of Na^+ and Cl^- has a free energy of association that is very small in magnitude, in contrast to the gas phase (28). The association of two amides through a $C{=}O\cdots H{-}N$ hydrogen bond is very favorable in vacuo, and progressively less favorable in nonpolar and aqueous solution (29). Thus, water has a significant "leveling" effect on association, making nonpolar associations more favorable and ionic and polar associations less favorable than their gas-phase counterparts.

In summary, unlike the gas phase association where ΔH_1 and ΔS_1 are invariably negative, for the corresponding thermodynamics in solution, ΔH_4 and ΔS_4 can be of either sign. The enthalpy of association ΔH_4 of two molecules in solution will be *positive* if the interactions of the solvent with the uncomplexed drug and receptor are sufficiently stronger and more exothermic $(\Delta H_3 - \Delta H_{2D} - \Delta H_{2R}$ more positive than ΔH_1 is negative) than are the interactions of the solvent with the drug-receptor complex. Similarly, the entropy of association in solution ΔS_4 can be positive if $\Delta S_3 - \Delta S_{2D} - \Delta S_{2R}$ is more positive than ΔS_1 is negative. This result can come about if the entropy gain from release of solvent from its interaction with the isolated drug and receptor is sufficiently larger than the entropy gain from release of solvent from the drug receptor complex.

An additional important point to keep in mind is that the solution phase thermodynamics may be dominated (as in the case of the hydrophobic effect, the association of nonpolar solutes in water) by changes in *solvent–solvent* interactions in the *presence* of solute. It is also important to stress that even an analysis of the relative contributions of ΔH and ΔS to ΔG may not give definitive insight into the "nature" of the drug receptor bond. For example, a large positive ΔS (and small negative ΔH) for association might come from either a hydrophobic or an ionic association (24). In either case the driving force for association is likely "release" of H_2O from "tight" binding to the solute.

One final consideration in determining either gas phase or solution phase association constants of drug-receptor complexes is conformational flexibility. Medicinal chemists have often attempted to synthesize *rigid* drugs of different stereochemistries in the hopes of finding one that fits "perfectly" into the receptor site. If, for example, the drug has three equal energy conformations and only *one* can fit the receptor site, a price must be paid of $\Delta G = +RT \ln 3$ in binding free energy relative to the drug that is "locked" in the right conformation. If the receptor has to be locked in a conformation to "accept" the drug, one must pay a similar free energy price. A nice example of the latter situation is the difference in binding free energies between "locked" and "unlocked" mac-

rocyclic crown ethers (30) that bind *t*-$BuNH_3^+$ cation.

Before turning to some examples of drug-receptor interactions, a specific example of the difference between gas phase and solution interactions will be presented. The protonation of amines has been chosen because of the large literature that has attempted to explain the irregular order of pKas of the alkyl amines ($NH_3 = 9.25$; $CH_3NH_2 = 10.66$, $(CH_3)_2NH = 10.73$ and $(CH_3)_3N = 9.81$). This reaction can be represented as:

$$R_3N + H^+ \xrightarrow{\Delta G_1} R_3N^+H$$

in the gas phase and

$$R_3N(aq) + H^+(aq) \xrightarrow{\Delta G_4} R_3NH^+(aq)$$

in aqueous solution. As has been noted in connection with Figure 12.3, the difference between the free energies of protonation in solution and the gas phase is given by:

$$\Delta G_4 - \Delta G_1 = -\Delta G_2(R_3N) - \Delta G_2(H^+)$$
$$+ \Delta G_3(R_3NH^+)$$

Recall also that the solution p$K_a = -\log K_{as} = \Delta G_4^0/2.3\,RT$. When the gas phase basicities were measured and showed a regular order, it was clear that the irregular order in solution was due to a solvation effect. In the gas phase NH_3 is a weaker base that $(CH_3)_3N$ by about 23 kcal/mol; in solution this difference is only about 1 kcal/mol.

Table 12.3 lists the free energies appropriate to the thermodynamic cycle (Fig. 12.2) for the protonation of the amines. Two points deserve strong emphasis.

1. The magnitude of ΔG_4 is much smaller than that of ΔG_1, for protonation because in aqueous solution the amines must compete with H_2O for the proton; in the gas phase there is no competition.

Table 12.3   Free Eneriges in Cycle (Fig. 12.3) for Protonation of Alkyl Amines, kcal/mol^a

R_3N	ΔG_1	$\Delta G_2(H^+)$	$\Delta G_2(R_3N)$	$\Delta G_3(R_3NH^+)$	ΔG_4
NH_3	−198.0	269.8	−2.41	−78.0	−3.79
CH_3NH_2	−210.0	269.8	−2.68	−67.7	−5.22
$(CH_3)_2NH$	−216.6	269.8	−2.41	−61.0	−5.39
$(CH_3)_3N$	−220.8	269.8	−1.34	−54.4	−4.06

^{a}See Aue (31).

2. As clearly analyzed by Aue et al. (31), the smaller the protonated amine, the more effectively solvated it is, and the better base it becomes compared to its relative rank in the gas phase.

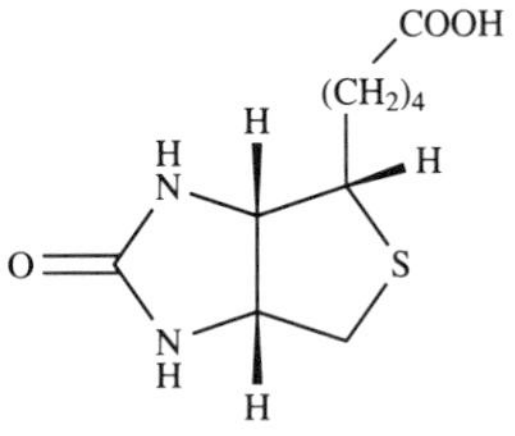

biotin

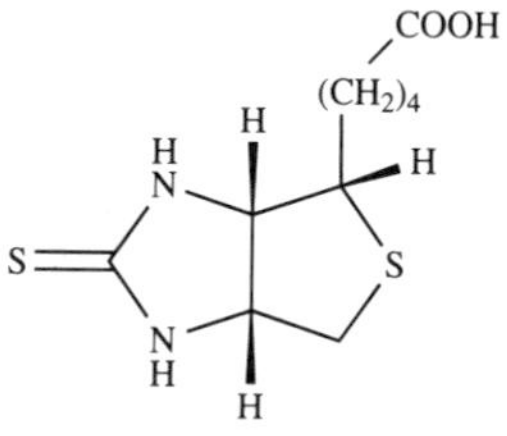

thiobiotin

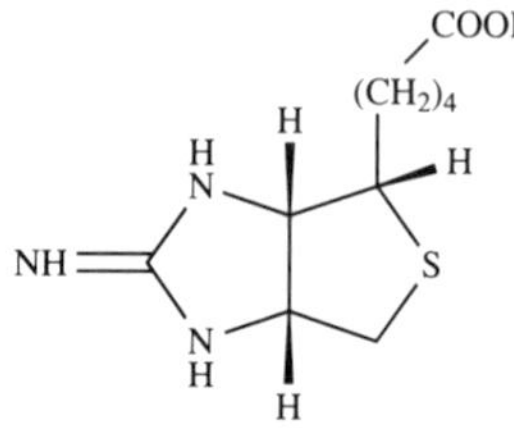

4 EXAMPLES OF DRUG–RECEPTOR INTERACTIONS

Three examples of "drug target" interactions will be discussed: (*a*) biotin–avidin (*b*) dihydrofolate reductase–trimethoprim and (*c*) DNA–intercalator. The first example is the strongest characterized protein–ligand association; the second example a prototype enzyme–inhibitor interaction; and the third example describes drugs interacting with nucleic acids.

iminobiotin

4.1 Biotin–Avidin

Biotin is the strongest known non covalent macromolecule–ligand interaction. In fact, given the small size of biotin, it is surprising to many that this association is so strong ($K_{as} \cong 10^{15}$ corresponding to a $-\Delta G$ of ~20 kcal/mole). Recently, the X-ray structure of a streptavidin (a related protein to avidin with nearly as large a biotin affinity) biotin complex was solved (32). The ureido group of biotin was thought to be the reason for the uniquely strong binding of this ligand to (strept) avidin:

Free energy calculations (17) on the relative binding of biotin, aminobiotin and thiobiotin to streptavidin, as well as absolute free energy calculations of biotin binding have been carried out. The results of these simulations are instructive in the insight they give into this association. These free energy calculations can best be understood by considering the thermodynamic cycle in Figure 12.3. The free energy calculations enable one to determine the free energies of the vertical processes by mutating one ligand into another in solution (ΔG_{solv}) and when bound in the active site (ΔG_{bind}) using molecular dynamics to create an ensemble average of the system. The difference between these calculated free energies $\Delta\Delta G_{bind}$ is equal to the difference in the observed relative free energies of ligand binding:

$$(\text{Protein})_{\text{solv}} + (\text{Ligand1})_{\text{solv}} \xrightarrow{\Delta G_{\text{bind1}}} (\text{Protein} \cdot \text{Ligand1})_{\text{solv}}$$

$$\Big\downarrow \Delta G_{\text{solv}} \qquad\qquad\qquad\qquad \Big\downarrow \Delta G_{\text{prot}}$$

$$(\text{Protein})_{\text{solv}} + (\text{Ligand2})_{\text{solv}} \xrightarrow{\Delta G_{\text{bind2}}} (\text{Protein} \cdot \text{Ligand2})_{\text{solv}}$$

$$\Delta\Delta G_{\text{bind}} = \Delta G_{\text{bind2}} - \Delta G_{\text{bind1}} = \Delta G_{\text{prot}} - \Delta G_{\text{solv}}$$

Fig. 12.3 Thermodynamic cycle for protein–ligand interactions. The experimentally measurable free energies are ΔG_{bind1} and ΔG_{bind2} (horizontal) and the calculated values (ΔG_{solv} and ΔG_{bind}) are the vertical processes.

The biotin–streptavidin system provides a "textbook case" of the relative free energies of binding biotin, aminobiotin and thiobiotin, as is illustrated in Table 12.4. First, the calculated relative free energies are in reasonable agreement with experiment; thiobiotin is calculated and observed to bind $\sim 10^3$ or $\sim 4\,\text{kcal/mole}$ more weakly to streptavidin than biotin and iminobiotin is calculated and observed to bind $\sim 10^5$ or $\sim 7\,\text{kcal/mole}$ more weakly than biotin. What is more interesting are the energy components. Thiobiotin is easier to desolvate than biotin by $\sim 9\,\text{kcal/mole}$ (ΔG_{solv}) but interacts more weakly with the protein by $\sim 13\,\text{kcal/mole}$, leading to the observed $\sim 4\,\text{kcal/mole}$ preference for biotin binding. On the other hand, iminobiotin is $\sim 5\,\text{kcal/mole}$ *harder* to desolvate than biotin, but interacts only $\sim 2\,\text{kcal/mole}$ more weakly with streptavidin, thus leading ($\Delta\Delta G_{\text{bind}} = \Delta G_{\text{bind}} - \Delta G_{\text{solv}} = 2 - (-5)$) to its $\sim 7\,\text{kcal/mole}$ weaker binding to streptavidin than biotin. The above examples illustrate the interesting tradeoff in binding and solvation effects in analysis of ligand-macromolecule interactions.

The fact that one loses only 4–$7\,\text{kcal/mole}$ out of the $\sim 20\,\text{kcal/mole}$ in free energy of binding when mutating the ureido group to its thio and imino analogue is strongly suggestive that the "ureido resonance", suggested by the crystallographers (32) who solved the structure as the reason for the unusually high K_{as}, cannot be the main reason. Calculations on the absolute free energy of biotin–streptavidin binding suggest that electrostatic effects, which might include ureido resonance (although perhaps not all of it) contribute $\sim 6\,\text{kcal/mole}$ to $\Delta\Delta G_{\text{bind}}$, whereas van der Waals effects contribute $\sim 14\,\text{kcal/mole}$.

The large contribution of van der Waals interactions (dispersion plus exchange repulsion) is surprising to many, since an individual van der Waals atom–atom dispersion attraction is very small. But there are many of them in the streptavidin active site, which, not coincidentally, contains four tryptophan residues.

Table 12.4 Results of Relative Free Energy Calculations[a] (kcal/mol)

Perturbation	ΔG_{solv}	ΔG_{prot}	$\Delta\Delta G_{\text{bind}}$	
			$\Delta G_{\text{prot}} - \Delta G_{\text{solv}}$	$\Delta G_{\text{bind2}} - \Delta G_{\text{bind1}}$
Biotin → thiobiotin	8.8 ± 0.1	12.0 ± 0.3	3.2 ± 0.3	3.6
Biotin → iminobiotin	-5.3 ± 0.1	1.2 ± 0.7	6.5 ± 0.8	6.2

[a]Errors, where listed, correspond to the half the hysteresis between forward and reverse runs.
[b]Experimental data (33).

But why do not the van der Waals interactions with water lost when one moves biotin from water to the streptavidin active site, cancel with those gained in the active site? This interaction can be understood by noting, as Sun et al. (34) and Rao and Singh (35) have, that a unique aspect of water as a solvent is its large exchange repulsion contribution to ΔG_{solv}. This exchange repulsion contribution represents the "hydrophobic effect", the fact that methane is less stable by 2 kcal/mole at a 1 M standard state in water than in the gas phase. This exchange repulsion cancels (and sometimes outweighs) the dispersion attraction which occurs for any solute when transferred from the gas phase to a condensed phase. On the other hand, in the streptavidin binding site, *preorganized* during protein synthesis, one gains dispersion attraction when biotin binds without the compensation from exchange repulsion. The magnitude of this effect is heightened by the large "atom density" both in biotin, with its bicyclic structure and in streptavidin, with its four tryptophan residues. Thus the key aspects in biotin's tight binding with (strept)avidin is the preorganization and high atom density of the protein active site (36).

4.2 DHFR–TMP

A classic example of a drug that works by species specific protein inhibition is trimethoprim (TMP). Because this drug binds to bacterial dihydrofolate reductase (DHFR) $\sim 10^4$ more tightly than to the mammalian enzyme, there is a therapeutic concentration in which the drug can be used as an antibacterial with little deleterious consequences for a mammalian host.

DHFR was the first example where the X-ray crystal structures of the enzyme protein complexes for both bacterial and mammalian enzymes have been solved. Matthews et al. (37) have suggested that a

key hydrogen bond is involved in the pyrimidine ring of TMP, which is present in the bacterial but not the mammalian enzyme complex, is responsible for the selectivity. This suggestion has not been definitively established with carbocyclic analogs, but analogs have clearly shown an important role of the three methoxy groups in TMP in causing species-selectivity. For example, the TMP analog without the three OCH_3 groups have a binding preference for the bacterial enzyme of only ~ 10.

Kuyper (38) has analyzed the structure of the bacterial and mammalian complexes and suggested that the oxygens of the $-OCH_3$ group plays a key role in species selectivity. The methoxy oxygens are significantly more solvent exposed in the bacterial complex than the mammalian. Thus, since these oxygens do not form hydrogen bonds to enzyme groups in either complex, the desolvation penalty for the oxygen is smaller in the bacterial enzyme and does not as extensively cancel the favorable hydrophobic/dispersion effects upon binding of the methoxy methyl groups. The interpretation is supported by the fact that replacing the $-OCH_3$ and CH_2CH_3 makes the molecules less species selective; such analogs bind little better to bacterial DHFR but significantly better to mammalian DHFR (39,40).

Free energy calculations/molecular dynamics have and will continue to give interesting insight into the DHFR–TMP species selectivity (39–41).

4.3 Nucleotide Intercalator

Since our first two examples have emphasized protein–small molecule interactions, our last example will be a nucleic acid–small molecule interaction.

There have been many experimental studies of the "intercalation" of flat, planar dyes into double-stranded DNA and other polynucleotides.

Table 12.5 **Thermodynamics of Binding of Drugs to DNA**

Drug[a]	ΔH^0, kcal/mol	ΔS^0, eu	ΔG^0, kcal/mol
Proflavin	−6.7	+4.7	−8.1
Ethidium bromide	−6.2	+9.4	−9.0
Actinomycin D	+2.0	+39.0	−9.6
Daunomycin	−6.5	+7.7	−8.8

[a]Conditions in all cases as follows: $T = 25°C$, 0.01 M buffer, pH = 7, 1 = 0.015 (see ref. 42).

The flexibility of the sugar–phosphate backbone allows the intercalator to be sandwiched between the nucleotides with relatively little "strain." The interaction with polynucleotides by a wide variety of intercalators has been studied by physio-chemical techniques. The driving force for association can be primarily hydrophobic, as in actinomycin D, where the driving force for association is ΔS^0 (42), or it can contain a large contribution from electrostatic effects as in ethidium bromide and adriamycin analogs, where the driving force for association is ΔH^0 (42) (Table 12.5). Both molecules have binding association constants K_{as} to DNA of about 10^6. The role of dispersion binding is not clear at this point, but it is likely to be very important as well (17). As noted above, the ability of these drugs to interfere with DNA replication is apparently related to their rate of dissociation k_r from DNA rather than to their association constant K_{as}. Muller and Crothers (3) showed that both actinomycin and actinomine had values of K_{as} similar to that of DNA, but the former had a much smaller k_r, and a much greater effect on the rate of DNA replication.

affinity. However some examples have been noted (e.g. the ureido group in biotin and the intercalation of positively charged groups into DNA) in which there might be an important polar or electrostatic driving force for binding. Again, it is difficult to ascertain whether these polar contributions come from "freeing up" water or from direct interactions, but they appear to contribute in a significant fashion to the driving force for association as well as being important in determining biological specificity. The lessons for the medicinal chemist attempting to design a drug to maximize the drug receptor association include the following:

1. Conformational flexibility can decrease the association constants in a straight-forwardly predictable way.

2. Hydrophobic effects usually contribute significantly to drug–receptor association, but one must also consider possible specific polar and ionic interactions.

3. Preorganization of the receptor or ligand is the key to optimal electrostatic or van der Waals interactions.

5 SUMMARY

The foregoing examples illustrate the likely nature of drug–receptor binding: hydrophobic and dispersion binding do contribute a substantial amount to the net binding

REFERENCES

1. P. Atkins, *Physical Chemistry*, 4th ed., W. H. Freeman, New York, 1990.

2. J. Watson, *Molecular Biology of the Gene*, 4th ed., Benjamin Cummings, Menlo Park, Calif., 1987.

3. W. Muller and D. Crothers, *J. Mol. Biol.*, **35**, 251 (1968), a discussion of actinomycin-DNA interactions.

4. K. Kitaura and K. Morokuma, *Int. J. Quant. Chem.*, **10**, 325 (1976) and J. C. G. M. van Duijnevelt-van der Rijdt and F. B. van Duijneveldt, *J. Am. Chem. Soc.*, **93**, 5644 (1971). Leading references to quantum mechanical analyses of these energy components.

5. J. Hirschfelder, C. Curtiss, and R. Bird, *Molecular Theory of Gases and Liquids*, John Wiley & Sons, New York, 1954, for an extensive discussion of the electrostatic interaction energy as a function of the multipole moments.

6. R. H. Margenau and N. Kestner, *Theory of Intermolecular Forces*, 2nd ed., Pergamon Press, Oxford, UK., 1971, contains an extensive discussion of the energy components in intermolecular interactions; see also G. Maitland, *Intermolecular Forces: Their Origin and Determination*, Oxford University Press, UK., 1987.

7. H. Umeyama and K. Morokuma, *J. Am. Chem. Soc.*, **99**, 1316 (1977).

8. M. Karplus and R. Porter, *Atoms and Molecules*, Benjamin Cummings, Menlo Park, Calif., 1971.

9. R. Lefevre, *Advan. Phys. Org. Chem.*, **3**, 1 (1965).

10. H. Umeyama and K. Morokuma, *J. Am. Chem. Soc.*, **98**, 4400 (1976).

11. P. Kollman and L. C. Allen, *Chem. Rev.*, **72**, 283 (1972), a review of charge redistribution effects in hydrogen bonds.

12. M. Hanna, *J. Am. Chem. Soc.*, **90**, 285 (1968); R. Lefevre, D. V. Radford, and P. Stiles, *J. Chem. 31 (Soc. B)*, 1297 (1968).

13. K. C. Janda, J. C. Hemminger, J. W. Winna, S. E. Novick, S. J. Harris, and W. Klemperer, *J. Chem. Phys.*, **63**, 1419 (1975).

14. M. Joesten and L. Schaad, *Hydrogen Bonding*, Dekker, New York, 1974.

15. K. Morokuma, S. Iwata, and W. Lathan, in R. Daubel and B. Pullman, Eds., *The World of Quantum Chemistry*, D. Reidel, Dordrecht, Holland, 1974, p. 277.

16. P. Kollman, *J. Am. Chem. Soc.*, **99**, 4875 (1977).

17. S. Miyamoto and P. Kollman, *Proteins*, **16**, 226 (1993).

18. G. E. Bacon, N. A. Curry, and S. A. Wilson, *Proc. Roy. Soc. Ser. A*, **279**, 98 (1964).

19. S. J. Weiner, P. A. Kollman, D. A. Case, U. C. Singh, C. Ghio, G. Alagona, S. Profeta and P. Weiner, *J. Amer. Chem. Soc.*, **106**, 765 (1984).

20. A. McCammon and S. Harvey, *Molecular Dynamics of Proteins and Nucleic Acids*, Cambridge University Press, UK., 1987.

21. P. Kollman and K. M. Merz, *Acc. Chem. Res.* **23**, 246 (1990).

22. See N. Davidson, *Statistical Mechanics*, McGraw-Hill Book Co., Inc., New York; 1962, for the explicit formulas to be used to determine the thermodynamic quantities. These relations are also discussed by M. I. Page and W. P. Jencks, *Proc. Nat. Acad. Sci. (US)*, **68**, 1678 (1971).

23. C. Hansch, in American Chemical Society Publication 30, *Biological Correlations—The Hansch Approach*, ACS, Washington, D.C., 1973.

24. W. Kauzmann, *Advan. Protein Chem.*, **14**, 1 (1975); C. Tanford, *The Hydrophobic Effect*, John Wiley & Sons, Inc., New York, 1973.

25. W. Jencks, in *Catalysis in Chemistry and Enzymology*, McGraw-Hill, New York, 1969.

26. K. Dill, *Biochem.*, **29**, 7133 (1990).

27. W. Jorgensen, J. K. Buckner, S. Boudon, and J. Tirado-Rives, *J. Chem. Phys.*, **89**, 3742 (1988).

28. L. X. Dang, J. Rice and P. Kollman, *J. Chem. Phys.*, **93**, 7528 (1990).

29. W. Jorgensen, *J. Amer. Chem. Soc.*, **111**, 3770 (1989).

30. J. Timko, S. Moore, D. Walba, P. Hiberty, and D. Cram, *J. Am. Chem. Soc.*, **99**, 4207 (1977).

31. D. Aue, H. Webb, and M. Bowers, *J. Am. Chem. Soc.*, **98**, 31, 318 (1976).

32. P. C. Weber, J. J. Ohlendorf, and F. R. Salemne, *Science*, **243**, 85 (1989).

33. N. Green, *Biochem. J.*, **101**, 774 (1966).

34. Y. Sun, D. Spellmeyer, D. Pearlman, and P. Kollman, *J. Amer. Chem. Soc.* **114**, 6798 (1992).

35. B. C. Rao and U. C. Singh, *J. Amer. Chem. Soc.* **111**, 3125 (1989); **112**, 3803 (1990).

36. S. Miyamoto and P. Kollman, *Proc. Nat. Acad. Sci.*, **90**, 8402 (1993).

37. D. Matthews, J. Bolin, J. Burridge, D. Filman, K. Volz, B. Kaufman, C. Beddell, J. Champness, D. Stammers, and J. Kraut, *J. Biol. Chem.*, **260**, 381 (1985).

38. L. Kuyper, in C. Bugg and S. Ealick, Eds., *Crystallographic and Molecular Modeling in Drug Design*, Springer-Verlag, 1989, pp. 56–79.

39. S. Fleischman and C. L. Brooks, *Proteins*, **752** (1990); C. L. Brooks and S. Fleischman, *J. Amer. Chem. Soc.*, **112**, 3307 (1990).

40. J. J. McDonald and C. L. Brooks, *J. Amer. Chem. Soc.*, **113**, 2295 (1991); **114**, 2062 (1992).

41. M. McCarrick, S. Miyamoto, P. Charifson, L. Kuyper and P. Kollman, to be submitted for publication.

42. F. Quadrifoglio and V. Crescenzi, *Biophys. Chem.*, **1**, 319 (1974); **2**, 64 (1974).

PART IV
DRUG DISCOVERY TECHNOLOGIES

Chemical Information Computing Systems in Drug Discovery

STEPHEN W. DIETRICH

Molecular Computing Systems, Inc.
Bothell, Washington, USA

CONTENTS

1 Introduction, 416
2 2D Chemical Information Management
  Software, 417
  2.1 Software function and capabilities, 419
  2.2 Specific software systems, 427
      2.2.1 DARC, 429
      2.2.2 MACCS-II, 429
      2.2.3 OSAC, 430
      2.2.4 THOR/MERLIN, 430
3 2D Chemical Information Databases, 432
  3.1 In-house 2D databases, 432
  3.2 Commercial 2D databases, 433
4 3D Chemical Information Management
  Software, 440
  4.1 Software function and capabilities, 440
  4.2 Specific software systems, 445
      4.2.1 Cambridge structural database
            system, 446
      4.2.2 ChemDBS-3D, 446
      4.2.3 MACCS-3D, 447
      4.2.4 SYBYL/3DB UNITY, 447
      4.2.5 THOR/MERLIN, 447
5 3D Chemical Information Databases, 448
  5.1 In-house 3D databases, 448
  5.2 Commercial 3D databases, 449
6 Synthetic Reaction Information Management
  Software, 452
  6.1 Software function and capabilities, 452

Burger's Medicinal Chemistry and Drug Discovery,
Fifth Edition, Volume 1: Principles and Practice,
Edited by Manfred E. Wolff.
ISBN 0-471-57556-9 © 1995 John Wiley & Sons, Inc.

6.2 Specific software systems, 457
  6.2.1 ORAC, 458
  6.2.2 REACCS, 459
  6.2.3 SYNLIB, 459
7 Synthetic Reaction Information Databases, 459
  7.1 In-house synthetic reaction databases, 459
  7.2 Commercial synthetic reaction databases, 460
8 Other Chemical Information Computing Software, 465
  8.1 Microcomputer chemical information computing software, 465
  8.2 Chemically intelligent computing software, 465
    8.2.1 SAR spreadsheets, 468
      8.2.1.1 MarkOut, 470
      8.2.1.2 Molecule spreadsheet (MDL), 470
      8.2.1.3 Molecular spreadsheet (TRIPOS), 473
    8.2.2 Log P estimation, 474
      8.2.2.1 PCMODELS (CLOGP-3), 476
      8.2.2.2 PRO-LOGP, 476
    8.2.3 PKALC, 477
    8.2.4 CHEMEST, 477
    8.2.5 TOPKAT, 478
    8.2.6 MetabolExpert, 479
    8.2.7 AUTONOM, 482
    8.2.8 SANDRA, 483
  8.3 CD-ROM Databases, 484
    8.3.1 Dictionary of natural products on CD-ROM, 484
    8.3.2 Beilstein's current facts in chemistry on CD-ROM, 486
  8.4 Integrated chemical information computing software, 486

1 INTRODUCTION

During the last two decades not only have chemical information computing software systems and databases become quite sophisticated but also reliable chemical information management tools and reliable information resources for use in research and development applications in many areas of chemistry (pharmaceutical, bioagricultural, organic synthesis, etc.) (1–9). In particular, these software tools and information resources have drastically altered how drug discovery scientists in industry and academia use and share chemical information in their research and development efforts. These software systems now allow pharmaceutical companies to manage vast amounts of proprietary chemical substance structures and information efficiently and accurately. Just as importantly, these systems now provide scientists with powerful tools for accessing, integrating, analyzing, and sharing chemical, biological and other information created in the drug discovery process. This chapter focuses on these essential roles that chemical information computing software systems and databases now play in drug discovery research and development (10, 11).

The area of chemical information computing systems encompasses a huge number of computing methodologies used in drug discovery research and development.

Therefore, for practical reasons it was necessary to limit the scope of the material covered. In particular, this chapter focuses on the current trends for application in drug discovery research in academia and industry of in-house (as opposed to on-line) chemical information computing software and databases, including:

- 2D and 3D chemical structure information management software systems and databases.
- Synthetic reaction information management software and databases.
- A widely diverse group of other chemically intelligent computing software systems (including those used for prediction of physical, chemical, and biological properties and data of specific interest to drug discovery and development scientists).

Specifically excluded from being covered are many other computing systems in chemistry, including: on-line chemical information resources; LIMS (laboratory information management systems); spectral software systems (for the collection, analysis, management, and searching of chemical spectra); "expert" software systems for synthetic reaction/route prediction; and molecular modeling, computer-assisted drug design, computational chemistry, and QSAR (quantitative structure–activity relationship) software (these last areas being covered in other chapters of this volume).

In addition, this chapter focuses, only to a limited extent, on the historical development of chemical information computing systems or the extensive theoretical research involved in developing these methodologies. Rather, the chapter primarily describes the current state-of-the-art of chemical information computing systems and databases, as applied to the drug discovery and development environment. Because of this focus, the chapter is proba-

bly unusual in that the presentation of chemical computing information systems is significantly from a view of the commercial in-house software and databases that are available and how they are used by scientists in drug discovery.

The commercial software and database vendors whose products are described in this chapter are listed in Table 13.1, together with current addresses and telephone numbers for primary U.S. and European offices. For the most current information regarding software/database product specifications, supported computer hardware, and specific software/database licensing costs, the reader should directly contact the individual vendors (especially since this information is constantly and rapidly changing). Because many of the technical capabilities of the software and database products have not been adequately described in the scientific literature, a number of the chapter references are (of necessity) to technical brochures, datasheets, manuals, and other publications obtained from the software and database vendors. Again, the reader should contact the vendor directly for copies of these items (or at least to obtain equivalent, appropriate information regarding the technical capabilities of the software and database products).

2 2D CHEMICAL INFORMATION MANAGEMENT SOFTWARE

2D chemical information management software systems provide the capability for the capture, registration, searching, retrieval, and management of 2D chemical information (1, 3, 8). In particular, this information includes both chemical structures as well as associated compound information. Because a knowledge of chemical structures and associated data is key for successful new drug discovery research and development, these 2D chemical information manage-

Table 13.1 Chemical Information Computing Software and Database Vendors

Vendor	Address and Telephone Number
ACS	ACS Software, American Chemical Society, Distribution Office, P.O. Box 57136, West End Station, Washington, DC 20037, U.S.; Telephone 1-(202) 872-4363.
Cambridge	Cambridge Crystallographic Data Centre, Dr. O. Kennard, Director, Cambridge Crystallographic Data Centre, University Chemistry Laboratory, Lensfield Road, Cambridge CB2 1EW, UK. Dr. W. L. Duax, Medical Foundation of Buffalo, Research Institute, 73 High Street, Buffalo, NY 14203-1196, U.S.
Chapman & Hall	Chapman & Hall Limited, 2–6 Boundary Row, London SE1 8HN, UK, Telephone 44-071-865-0066. Chapman & Hall, Inc., 29 West 35th Street, New York, NY, U.S.; Telephone 1-(212) 244-3336.
Chemical Design	Chemical Design Limited, Unit 12, 7 West Way, Oxford OX2 0JB, UK, Telephone 44-(0865)-251483. Chemical Design Inc., Suite 120, 200 Route 17 South, Mahwah, NJ 07430, U.S.; Telephone 1-(201) 529-3323.
CompuDrug	CompuDrug NA, Inc., P.O. Box 23196, Rochester, NY 14692, U.S., Telephone 1-(716) 292-6830. CompuDrug Chemistry Ltd., Hollan Ernoe ut., H-1136 Budapest, Hungary; Telephone 36-1-112-4874.
CSC	Cambridge Scientific Computing, Inc., 875 Massachusetts Avenue, Cambridge, MA 02139, U.S.; Telephone 1-(617) 491-6862.
Current Drugs	Current Drugs Ltd., 34–42 Cleveland Street, London W1P 5FB, UK; Telephone 44-(071)-3230323.
Daylight	Daylight Chemical Information Systems, Inc., 18500 Von Karman Ave., Suite #450, Irvine, CA 92715, U.S.; Telephone 1-(714) 476-0451.
DCG	Distributed Chemical Graphics, Inc., 1326 Carol Road, Meadowbrook, PA 19046, U.S.; Telephone 1-(215) 885-3706.
Derwent	Derwent Publications Ltd., Rochdale House, 128 Theobalds Road, London WC1X 8RP, UK, Telephone 44-(071)-2425823. Derwent Inc., 1313 Dolley Madison Boulevard, Suite 401, McLean, VA 22101, U.S.; Telephone 1(703) 790-0400.
Fraser Williams	Fraser Williams (Scientific Systems) Ltd., London House, London Road South, Poynton Cheshire SK12 1YP, UK; Telephone 44-(0625) 871126.
HDI	Health Designs, Inc., 183 Main Street, Rochester, NY 14604, U.S.; Telephone 1-(716) 546-1464.
HDS	Hampden Data Services Ltd., 167 Oxford Road, Cowley, Oxford, OX4 3ES, UK; Telephone 44-(0865) 747250.
InfoChem	InfoChem GmbH, Landsberger Strasse 408, 8000 Munich 60, Germany; Telephone 49-8958-30-02.
ISI	Institute for Scientific Information, 3501 Market Street, Philadelphia, PA 19104, U.S.; Telephone 1-(215) 386-0100. ISI European Branch, Brunel Science Park, Brunel University, Uxbridge, UB8 3PQ, UK; Telephone 44-(895)-270016.
MDL	Molecular Design Limited, 2132 Farallon Drive, San Leandro, CA 94577, U.S.; Telephone 1-(510) 895-1313. Molecular Design MDL AG, Muhlebachweg 9, CH-4123 Allschwil 2, Switzerland; Telephone 41-61-4812180.

Table 13.1 (*Continued*)

Vendor	Address and Telephone Number
ORAC	ORAC Limited: Formerly located in Leeds, UK. Following a merger with Molecular Design Limited in March, 1991, the ORAC organization was consolidated into MDL in March 1992. Research sites still using software and databases originally licensed from ORAC Limited should contact MDL for information regarding these products.
PH&M	Pool, Heller, & Milne, Inc., 9520 Linden Avenue, Bethesda, MD 20814, U.S.; Telephone 1-(301)-493-6595.
Questel	Questel, Le Capitole, 55 avenue des Champs Pierreux, 92029 NANTERRE Cedex, France; Telephone 33-(1)-4614-5555. Questel Inc., 2300 Clarendon Blvd., Suite 1111, Arlington, VA 22201, U.S.; Telephone 1-(703) 527-7501.
Springer-Verlag	Springer-Verlag Heidelberg, Marketing New Media/Handbooks, Tiergartenstrasse 17, W-6900, Heidelberg 1, FR Germany; Telephone 49-6221-487-457. Springer-Verlag New York, Inc., Electronic Media Department, 175 Fifth Avenue, New York, NY 10010, U.S.; Telephone 1-(212) 460-1682.
TDS	Technical Database Services, Inc., Suite 2300, 10 Columbus Circle, New York, NY 10019, U.S.; Telephone 1-(212) 245-0044.
TRIPOS	TRIPOS Associates Inc., 1699 South Hanley Road, Suite 303, St. Louis, Mo 63144, U.S.; Telephone 1-(314) 647-1099. TRIPOS Associates Inc., Centennial Court, Easthampstead Road, Brachnell, Berkshire RG12 1NN, UK. Telephone 44-(344)-300144.

ment software systems have become standard features at most pharmaceutical companies and now are used as integral tools for information capture, management, and access in new drug discovery research and development. The following chapter subsections describe the unique capabilities of these 2D chemical information software systems and databases and especially how they are used in the new drug discovery process.

2.1 Software Function and Capabilities

All the different chemical information management software systems (both commercial and those developed in-house by companies and academics) each differ in their specific capabilities and how their individual user interfaces have been designed. However, each of the more successful and advanced systems have a certain core base of functionality, usually including most of the capabilities described in the following paragraphs.

Most importantly, a chemical information management software system must possess chemical intelligence, that is, the software must possess a solid understanding of and an ability to handle chemical structures and chemistry. This chemical intelligence is actually an ability of the software to understand and apply rules regarding chemical structures as they are represented to the software by the user (e.g., as a chemical connection table or as a graphical drawing of a chemical structure). This chemical intelligence typically includes (but may not necessarily be limited to) a knowledge and understanding of:

- Atoms and different atom types (including isotopes).
- Bonds and different bond types (e.g., single, double, triple, aromatic).

- Chemical constitution.
- Valence and different valence states.
- Atomic charges (including radicals).
- Stereochemistry (including: stereoisomers and geometric isomers; ambiguous and even relative stereochemistry).
- Aromaticity.
- Tautomers.

Each of the 2D chemical information software systems varies slightly in its chemical intelligence and abilities to handle these areas, but the most significant areas of difference usually involve stereochemistry (e.g., ability to handle allene stereochemistry or stereochemistry other than standard tetrahedral stereo centers) and aromaticity (e.g., perception of aromatic systems other than 5- or 6-membered rings). This built-in chemical intelligence is what makes chemical information software systems unique (as compared to other information management software) in their ability to analyze, manipulate, and manage chemical structures and chemical information. This capability and software knowledge ("intelligence") is essential (and must be robust and consistent) if a chemical information computing software system is to perform its primary specialized functions of chemical structure storage, manipulation, searching, retrieval, display, drawing, etc., correctly.

Typically, each of these chemical information software systems uses several standard user menus, each with a specific function; for instance, chemical structure drawing; compound and data registration; substructure search query specification; database searching for structures and data; retrieval and review of structures and data from the chemical database; report generation and output, etc. Choosing of program options by the user is usually graphical selection of a menu button and/or typing of commands.

Chemical structures can be entered (specified) by the user in a number of ways.

The user may graphically enter ("draw") a chemical structure, usually in much the same way that a chemist would draw or sketch a chemical structure on paper (12). Although many graphic drawing devices have been used (e.g., tablet or light pen), the "mouse" is now the most common input device used for chemical structure drawing. First the atom/bond skeleton is entered, followed by addition of any stereochemistry, charges, isotope designations, etc. Templates of preconstructed structural fragments are often used to facilitate and speed the drawing process, especially for more complex compounds. Usually as a structure is being drawn, the chemical information software is continually analyzing the structure and using its chemical intelligence to insure the drawn chemical structure is consistent with its chemical intelligence ("rules") regarding chemistry (atoms, bonds, etc.). If the structure is to be a substructure search query (see below), the substructure query features are usually then added. A structure can also be retrieved (and then modified, if so desired) from a chemical database or an external user computer file. Besides storing chemical structures in their chemical databases, 2D chemical information software systems are capable of saving a chemical structure to (or retrieving the structure from) an external computer file, which is a human-readable chemical connection table. The most commonly encountered of these chemical connection file formats are Molecular Design Limited's MOLFILE (13) and the Standard Molecular Data (SMD) Format, a software-independent connection table format originally proposed by a consortium of European chemical and pharmaceutical companies (14–17). Systems for entry of chemical structures as linear text strings (representing atoms, bonds, etc.) have been and are still used with some software systems, and most significantly include WLN (Wiswesser Line Notation) (18–20) and SMILES (Daylight Chemical

Information Systems, Inc.; see Section 2.2.4). These linear notation methods for chemical structure representation and entry are not now widely used by the majority of the chemical information software user community, primarily because of the excellent software capabilities which have continued to develop and be enhanced for graphical chemical structure drawing.

Modern chemical structure database software systems gained their first extensive use (and commercial success) in the 1980s at pharmaceutical companies because of their capabilities to store and manage chemical structures (through "registration" into chemical structure databases). This trend was quite important, because it finally allowed drug companies to easily and accurately manage by computer their very often large collections of proprietary chemical entities. The registration process usually consists of a user first entering a chemical structure and then asking the software to register the compound in one of its chemical databases. The software analyzes the structure and then searches the database to see if the compound (and sometimes even stereoisomers or tautomers) has already been registered. Depending on the software or how the database have been set up, the user may or may not be allowed to register duplicates structures into the chemical database. If the user gives the OK for registration, the software then adds the structure to its database files, also incorporating substructural keys to facilitate subsequent database substructure searches (see below). The different chemical information management software systems vary in their abilities to handle (i.e., register and understand) more complex chemical structures: e.g., polymers, mixtures of compounds, and inorganics (especially involving complex stereochemistry).

In addition to their ability to register chemical structures in their chemical databases, chemical information management software systems also possess the ability to store chemical information associated with the chemical structures in these databases. At pharmaceutical companies typically this information storage would include additional text and/or numeric data that is included on the new chemical entity datasheet when it is submitted by a scientist to a central registration group for registration into the corporate proprietary chemical database. Each pharmaceutical company differs in what information is entered on these datasheets and what portion of that information is captured (registered) in the chemical database together with the structure. Such captured associated chemical data could typically include information such as: compound number, chemical name(s), chemist's name, date and amount prepared, laboratory notebook reference, sample lot/batch code, literature reference(s), reason for preparation of the compound, physical/chemical properties (form, color, MP, BP, refractive index, pK_a, solubility, etc.), analytical/spectroscopic references information, amount of sample in inventory, etc. This associated chemical information can be specific to the compound registered or even specific for individual lots/batches of the compound. Chemical information software systems excel at managing chemical structure information, but are not nearly as efficient or sophisticated in handling this associated chemical textual and numeric information. Hence, a number of pharmaceutical companies instead register much of this associated chemical data in other associated relational databases (see below) instead of in the chemical information database. Some drug companies have attempted, however, to register and manage biological and other data in 2D chemical information databases (21).

The chemical information management software systems provide a number of methods for searching for chemical structures in their chemical information databases. For a basic structure search, the user draws a chemical structure, and the software then searches to see if the compound has been registered in the chemical database. Using a unique coding algorithm for any chemical structure, such "exact" chemical structure searches are extremely rapid (22–24). These exact chemical structure searches can usually be enlarged to include searches for any stereoisomers or tautomers of the compound in the chemical database. The result of the search (or any chemical database search) is then a list of one or more "hits" which match the search query and which can be reviewed by the user as chemical structures retrieved by the software from the chemical database and then graphically displayed. In any R&D (Research and Development) chemical research environment (including drug discovery) the ability to simply draw a chemical structure, to search a large chemical database, and to retrieve that structure and data registered with it all in the matter of a minute or less is an amazingly efficient process. This fact is especially true compared to old manual chemical information management systems and even early chemical information management systems. This ability to so easily and rapidly find and access chemical compound information has, just in itself, significantly changed how drug discovery scientists access, use, and share chemical compound information in their research efforts.

Another common type of chemical database search is the chemical substructure search (12, 25). In contrast to exact structure searches (for which unfilled valences on atoms are assumed to be hydrogens), unfilled valence positions on atoms in substructure searches are assumed to be possibly substituted (unless otherwise restricted). In addition, substructure searches can be made quite specific through the addition of one or more substructure query "features" to the search query (Fig. 13.1). These searches could include query features such as:

- Requiring that a bond be a chain bond.
- Allowing a bond to be a single or a double bond.
- Allowing no substituents at an open position.
- Requiring a particular atom to be one of a list of atoms (e.g., F, Cl, or Br).
- Not allowing a particular atom to be one of a list of atoms (e.g., not O or S).
- Not allowing any other rings to be fused to a ring in the search query structure.

In addition, some chemical information software allow for the construction of even more complex and powerful generic or "markush" substructure search queries (26). For example, these could include complex structure search query features such as:

- There must be a COOH, $CONH_2$, or COOR substituent at a specific position.
- If there is an OH or OCH_3 substituent at one specific position, then there must be a halogen substituent at another specific position.

These sort of generic searches are especially of value for pharmaceutical companies when such searches are performed to identify chemical entities in large corporate proprietary chemical structure databases in support of patent applications or defenses (Fig. 13.2).

Substructure searching of chemical databases (especially for very large databases) is made quite efficient through the use of substructure keys. When each compound is originally registered in a chemical database, the software analyzes the chemical structure and sets a number of substructural keys (as many as 1000) in the database for that compound. For example, if a compound contains a carbonyl group, a key in the database could be set indicating the presence of this substructural feature in the compound. When the software later per-

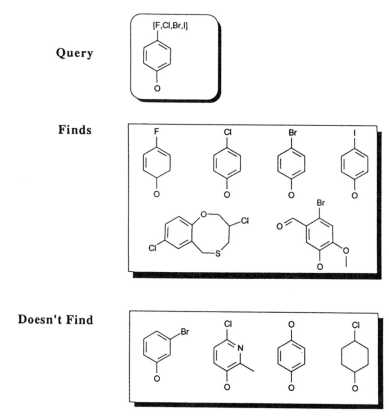

Fig. 13.1 An example of a MACCS-II substructure search query and chemical structures that would and would not be found in a subsequent substructure search of a MACCS-II 2D chemical structure database. The query is a phenyl ring substituted with an oxygen atom and a para halogen substituent (F, Cl, Br, or I). The substructure query allows (but does not require) substituents on the oxygen atom and the other phenyl ring positions.

forms a search for a compound query drawn by a user, it first analyzes the search query for the presence of any of the substructural fragments and then performs a rapid key search for any compound in the database that has all the same keys. This initial screening usually quickly reduces the number of possible matches to a fraction of the original database entries. At this point an exact final atom-by-atom, bond-by-bond, etc. comparison is made between the substructure search query and this smaller database list to provide the final list of database "hits" which match the substructure query. While slower than exact structure searches, substructure searches are still quite rapid (usually 0.5 to several minutes, depending on how many compounds were

not eliminated from consideration with the initial screening).

Substructure searches of chemical databases with 2D chemical information management software has proven to be an extremely valuable tool for drug discovery research and development scientists. For example, in developing the SAR (structure–activity relationship) for a drug class, potential appropriate bioassay candidates can quickly be located in a large corporate proprietary compound database or even from the FCD database of commercially available organic compounds (see Section 3.2). Because of the large manpower and monetary expenses associated with synthesizing each compound for bioactivity screening, this ability to possibly identify sources

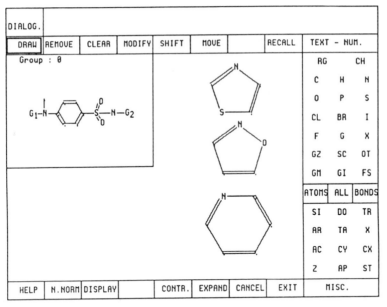

Fig. 13.2 DARC draw menu showing a generic substructure search query in the process of being defined by the user: Here the G_2 substituent in the substructure query is being defined as any one of these three heterocyclic rings.

of already synthesized and available chemical compound samples for bioactivity testing can facilitate the drug discovery process by reducing the cost and significantly accelerating the speed of the process for SAR development and investigation for a drug class.

A more recent but quite popular type of chemical structure database searching implemented in chemical information management software systems is the "similarity" search (27–29). An exact chemical structure is drawn by the user and is used as the query for the similarity search. The query is analyzed by the software for the presence of a number of molecular substructural features or properties. Each structure in the database is then compared to the query and scored as to its similarity as compared to the search query structure (e.g., how many of the substructural features/properties present in the query are also present in each database structure). The set of similarity search hits is those database structures most similar to the query structure (for example, with a % similarity greater than some value, say 70%). Although many substructural features/properties and scoring methods have been investigated for similarity searches of chemical databases, most commercial chemical information systems have implemented a large, fixed set (usually 1,000+) of simple substructural search keys for their similarity searches. The pre-determination of these keys for each compound at time of registration into the database allows the software systems to subsequently perform these similarity searches quickly and in fact essentially as fast as standard substructure searches. Similarity searching appears to provide a useful tool (complementing substructure searching) for drug discovery scientists attempting to select compounds for screening and appears to be a reliable and popular method to select compounds which are similar but still substructurally different in structure as compared to a target compound. With a new lead structure this can be an especially effective way to select structures similar to a target compound for bioactivity screening in order to broadly examine the SAR for the lead structure. (Still another approach to 2D chemical database searching is the "dissimilarity" search, which attempts to select compounds especially for random screening that are as dissimilar as possible (30). This capability generally has not yet been implemented in the commercial 2D chemical information management software systems.)

Chemical information management software systems also allow for searching of the associated compound information that is stored in their chemical databases. Depending on the type of data being searched, this can include text, numeric, or keyword searches. Because chemical information software is optimized and intended primarily for management and searching of chemical information structures, these associated chemical data searches are often comparatively inefficient and limited in their capabilities. Consequently these searches can sometimes be quite slow, especially when involving text string searches of associated chemical data in large chemical databases. Despite these shortcomings, searching and retrieval of associated compound data in chemical databases are often of great value and use for drug discovery research and development efforts. Provided that the appropriate chemical information has been registered in the chemical information database, associated data searches could be used, for example, to find:

- All compounds which have been prepared by an individual chemist.
- All compounds prepared for a specific drug discovery/development program in the last three years.
- A compound for which the scientist only knows a trivial name.

Chemical structure searches combined with associated data searches in a chemical database can effectively increase the value of the captured data for the drug discovery process. For example, having prepared a compound, a scientist might want to look at NMR spectra that had been done for other compounds with similar structures in the company's corporate compound database. A substructure search for the desired parent chemical structure followed by an associated compound data search for those substructure search hits which have references to NMR spectra, would easily yield the information that the scientist needs.

Many pharmaceutical companies have found that it is much more efficient and practical to register associated chemical data into SQL-relational databases rather than directly into chemical databases for two primary reasons. First, relational database management software systems are much more efficient and flexible (as compared to most chemical information management software) in their registration, management, searching, and retrieval of text, numeric, and keyword data. Second, by their very nature relational database software systems are able to handle much more complex associated chemical data interrelationships than chemical information management software. For example, a single compound registered into a chemical database may have been prepared several times (different batches or lots). Each batch or lot may have assays results from a number of biological and analytical assays, some assays may have been repeated any number of times, and any single assay may have generated a number of data (e.g., several doses and several biological responses). In addition, there may be detailed chemical sample inventory data for each batch/lot that was prepared. A relational database software system would have no problem handling even more complex associated chemical data interrelationships than this (such as actually are found at many drug companies), while most chemical information management software would be hard pressed to do this efficiently.

At a number of pharmaceutical companies, associated compound information for compounds in the company's proprietary chemical entity database is usually registered into relational databases by one of two methods. If the associated compound information is not readily available at the time the structure is initially registered into the chemical database, the associated compound information (once available) is later directly entered into the relational database using the relational database management software. Typically this entry would include associated data that was not included on the new chemical entity datasheet used for registration of the compound into the chemical database: e.g., biological screening data registered into a relational bioassay database or chemical sample availability data entered into a relational chemical sample inventory database. If the associated compound information is readily available at the time the structure is initially registered into the chemical database, the associated compound information is indirectly registered at the same time into the relational database using the chemical management software and an interface to the relational database system. Typically this registration would include associated data that was included on the new chemical entity datasheet used for registration of the compound into the chemical database; for example, name of the chemist who prepared the compound or date that the compound was prepared. The associated chemical information in the relational databases is usually "linked" back to the appropriate compound in the chemical database through one or more data elements that both the relational and chemical databases share in common, e.g., the company compound number assigned to the chemical entity.

The integration of chemical information management software and databases with other drug discovery research and development software systems and databases has proved to be an invaluable information

access tool and competitive advantage for many pharmaceutical companies (31–35). This approach has allowed scientists, simultaneous, linked access to and sharing of information from critical yet different computer-based R&D information resources. This linkage is best illustrated with a couple of hypothetical scenarios (which are actually quite common now at many drug companies). As a first example, a scientist performs a substructure search of the corporate proprietary chemical database with the chemical information management software in order to retrieve all structures in a particular drug class being investigated by a drug discovery program team. The compound numbers for the resulting substructure search "hits" are used (with an interface between the chemical information and relational database software systems) to search a relational database of bioassay data for results of any of these compounds in two different biological screening tests. The chemical structures from the chemical database and the biological testing data from the relational bioassay database are combined into a single graphics report in a SAR (structure-activity relationship) style table, with each row representing a single compound and the columns containing the compound chemical structure (graphically shown), the company compound number, and the results (if available) for the two bioassays. These reports could be regularly updated by the chemist and used for presentations and discussions at the regular drug discovery program team meetings. In the second example, a scientist has discovered a new drug lead compound and wants to investigate similar compounds from the large corporate proprietary chemical compound database. The scientist first performs a similarity search of the corporate chemical compound database based on the lead compound structure. The compound numbers for the resulting similarity search "hits" are used (with an interface between the chemical information and relational database software systems) to search a relational database of chemical sample inventory availability information for these compounds. The chemical structures from the chemical database and the sample availability information from the relational chemical inventory database are combined into a single graphics report in a SAR (structure-activity relationship) style table, with each row representing a single compound and the columns containing the compound chemical structure (graphically shown), the compound number, and the sample availability data. This report is used by the scientist to request samples from the chemical sample inventory and dispensing group for use in bioassay screening tests in order to further investigate the structure-activity relationship for the new drug lead compound.

The commercial chemical information management software systems all provide standard user menus that can be used without change for compound and data registration, database searching, structure and data retrieval, and generation of standard reports with structures and/or data. Also these software systems provide the software capabilities for extensive modification of the user interface with the system, allowing essentially unlimited flexibility and versatility for developing and implementing customized applications and user interfaces. This extensive approach is employed in the pharmaceutical industry for implementation of a wide variety of customized applications that best meet the chemical information management and access requirements of each individual company. For example, these requirements have included customized chemical information management software applications to facilitate:

- Registration of chemical structures and associated chemical data into chemical and relational databases.

- Searching and retrieval of chemical structures and complex associated chemical data simultaneously from both chemical and relational databases.

- Generation of customized reports (e.g., Fig. 13.3) containing chemical structures and associated chemical data from chemical and related relational databases, often in a SAR (structure-activity relationship) or molecular spreadsheet style format most useful for drug discovery scientists.

The commercial chemical information management software systems also include software capabilities to allow for development of customized applications for the analysis, comparison, and manipulation of chemical structures. This customization is probably one of the most sophisticated manifestations of the chemical intelligence inherent in chemical information management software. It provides the ability to use this software for the design and implementation of chemically intelligent "expert" software applications for a variety of drug discovery research and development uses (see Section 8.2 below).

2.2 Specific Software Systems

Since the 1960s a number of pharmaceutical companies have undertaken major software development efforts to create software systems for the management of their in-house, proprietary corporate chemical compound information. Three of the most successful and best-documented of these efforts include Upjohn's COUSIN software system (36–40), ICI's CROSSBOW software system (41–43), and Pfizer's SOCRATES system (44). Moving into the 1980s, however, there was a rapid trend for the development and marketing of commercial chemical information management software systems. During this period most

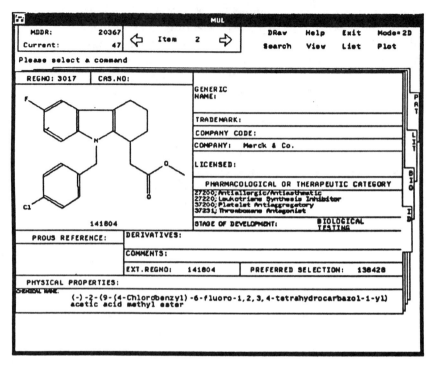

Fig. 13.3 Example of a customized MACCS-II report, generated with the customized MACCS-II interface for accessing data and structures from the MACCS-II MDDR database.

pharmaceutical companies (large and small) adopted one of these commercial software systems for management and access to their chemical compound information. This shift apparently took place because most pharmaceutical companies found that it was much more cost-effective for them to license and pay support for a commercial chemical information management software system as opposed to developing, enhancing, and maintaining their own system on an on-going basis. This shift is due in part to the complex and continual-

ly changing software for chemical information management and the need for its ability to interface with other information systems. A list of the current major commercial 2D chemical information management software systems is presented on Table 13.2, with further description of their individual characteristics included in the following chapter subsections.

Although not listed in this chapter as a 2D chemical information software system, the SYBYL/3D UNITY 3D chemical information management software (TRIPOS

Table 13.2   Major Commercial 2D Chemical Information Software Systems

Software	Vendor	Hardware Platforms	Major Markets
DARC	Questel	VAX/VMS	Europe
MACCS-II	MDL	VAX/VMS, IBM, Fujitsu	U.S., Europe, Japan
OSAC	ORAC	VAX/VMS	Europe
THOR/MERLIN	Daylight	VAX/VMS, UNIX Workstations	U.S., Europe

Associates, Inc.; Section 4.2.4) actually includes essentially all the 2D chemical information management software capabilities described earlier. SYBYL/3D UNITY was originally developed and marketed as a 3D chemical information management software system, integrated with the SYBYL molecular modeling software. As to whether this software may also become a significant player in the future for 2D chemical information management at pharmaceutical companies remains to be seen.

2.2.1 DARC. The DARC (Description, Acquisition, Retrieval, Correlation) chemical information management software (Questel) was originally developed for searching of on-line DARC chemical structure databases, but is also marketed as an in-house 2D chemical information management software system almost exclusively in Europe (45, 46). The chemical structure generic query search capabilities in the DARC software are especially powerful, reflecting the emphasis of the on-line DARC patent database searching capabilities. The DARC Communication Modules and host interface software provide the necessary software for users to develop and implement customized interfaces to other software and to associated compound data stored in relational databases (45, 47, 48). 2D chemical databases that can be licensed for use with the DARC software are described in Section 3.2.

2.2.2 MACCS-II. The MACCS (Molecular ACCess System) chemical information management software (49–52) and now the MACCS-II software have been marketed by Molecular Design Limited since 1979, with MACCS-II now the predominant commercial 2D chemical information management software system installed worldwide (especially at pharmaceutical companies) (53). The MACCS-II basic user interface (menus) are quite similar to that of Molecular Design Limited's REACCS synthetic

reaction information management software (Section 6.2.2). MACCS-II includes two internal programming languages [MACCS-II Sequence Language and MACCS-II PL (Programming Language)], which provide significant capabilities for user customization. Molecular Design Limited also offers a number of software modules for licensing as add-ons to the MACCS-II software to extend its 2D chemical information management software capabilities:

- The Customization Module (Mod C) significantly expands the functionality and capabilities of the MACCS-II Sequence Language for creating customized user applications and is required for most of the other MACCS-II modules;
- The Database Interface Module (Mod D) provides the software interface links to relational software systems (e.g., ORACLE, INGRES, etc.) for the registration, searching, and retrieval of associated chemical data from relational databases;
- The Power Search Module (Mod P) primarily extends the chemical structure search capabilities of the basic MACCS-II software to include generic/Markush substructure search queries (54); and
- The Substance Module (Mod S) primarily extends the chemical structures that the basic MACCS-II chemical information software can handle to include chemical mixtures (Fig. 13.4) and organic polymers (55).

Molecular Design Limited with the MACCS-II software and modules has made an intensive and successful effort to market to the pharmaceutical industry. It has done this emphasizing the ability to interface MACCS-II and its databases to other information software systems and databases, the capability to develop customized applications with the MACCS-II sequence language, and its dominance in the 2D chemi-

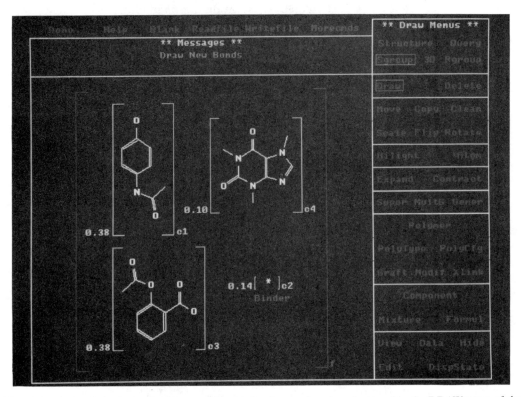

Fig. 13.4 A chemical mixture (in this case a formulation for a pain reliever) entered in the DRAW menu of the MACCS-II 2D chemical information management software with Molecular Design Limited's Substance Module: The "c(n)" bracket labels indicate the order in which the components are added to the formulation, while the fractional numbers represent the relative amounts added. The formulation even includes a nonstructural component, a nonspecified "binder".

cal information management software market. 2D chemical databases that can be licensed for use with the MACCS-II software are described in Section 3.2.

2.2.3 OSAC. The OSAC (Organic Structures Accessed by Computer) chemical information management software (ORAC Ltd.) has a limited number of installations at pharmaceutical companies and academic institutions in England and continental Europe (56). OSAC's user interface is similar to that of ORAC Ltd.'s ORAC synthetic reaction information management software (Section 6.2.1). OSAC's customized flexibility and interfaces with other software systems and databases are available through its Host Language Interface

software (57, 58). Following the merger of ORAC Ltd. with Molecular Design Limited (MDL) in 1991 and the consolidation of ORAC Ltd. into MDL in 1992, it appears that MDL will continue to support the OSAC software until sometime in 1994. MDL is attempting to facilitate the transition of previous OSAC customers to its MACCS-II or ISIS software systems in anticipation of this eventuality, but some industrial and academic drug discovery scientists may still encounter the OSAC software in the meantime. 2D chemical databases for use with the OSAC software are described in Section 3.2.

2.2.4 THOR/MERLIN. THOR (THesaurus-Oriented Retrieval) and MERLIN are two software systems marketed by Daylight Chemical Information Systems, Inc. for 2D chemical information management (24). THOR is software for the basic registration, management, and retrieval of chemical structures and data from the THOR chemical information databases. The MERLIN software performs the chemical substructure, superstructure, and similarity searches in the THOR databases (Fig. 13.5). The software permits graphical chemical structure entry, as well as entry using the SMILES (Simplified Molecular

Input Line Entry System) structure specification language, a simple linear string of connected atom, bond, and stereochemistry symbols (59–61). Chemical structures are normally displayed not from a user-supplied drawing but by automatic structure depiction using a software module called DEPICT (62). An extremely powerful set of programmer software tools are available from Daylight Chemical Information Systems, Inc. for the development of customized software, especially for expert chemical computing software (e.g., see Section

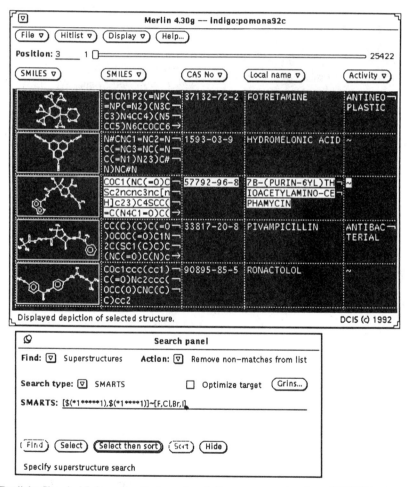

Fig. 13.5 Daylight Chemical Information Systems, Inc: Software screens showing a MERLIN substructure query panel and the results of the subsequent MERLIN substructure search of a THOR database, presented in a spreadsheet style format (chemical structure, SMILES, CAS Registry Number, chemical name, and biological activity).

8.2.2.1) and molecular modeling/drug design applications (63, 64). The original Daylight Chemical Information Software Systems, Inc. software has its origins in chemically intelligent computing software development efforts undertaken for the Pomona College Medicinal Chemistry Project (65, 66). 2D chemical databases that can be licensed for use with the THOR/MERLIN software are described in Section 3.2.

3 2D CHEMICAL INFORMATION DATABASES

3.1 In-House 2D Databases

By 1990 essentially all of the large pharmaceutical companies (and most of the smaller pharmaceutical companies) had used one of the major commercial chemical information management software systems to create chemical structure databases for their proprietary chemical compounds (31, 32). These databases can contain as many as several hundred thousand registered chemical structures (for a large drug company) or as few as just several thousand registered chemical structures (for a smaller drug company). A number of the pharmaceutical company takeovers and mergers in the 1980s and early 1990s resulted in the combining of chemical structure databases from the companies involved to create some of the larger corporate chemical structure databases. These in-house chemical structure databases of proprietary compounds were usually built by several approaches, including:

- Graphically drawing the chemical structures from original hardcopy records (usually corporate chemical compound datasheets or cards) and then registering the chemical structures into the database.
- Automated computer conversion (usual-

ly only partially successful) of the chemical structures in older chemical structure software systems into chemical connection tables that could be registered into the new database.

For the larger corporate compound databases, there database building efforts were typically very manpower intensive projects, taking several years to complete and included extensive QC efforts in order to ensure reasonably reliable database information quality and accuracy.

Corporate chemical structure databases at pharmaceutical companies are dynamic (not static) information resources. New chemical entities are usually being registered daily into these databases, as they are synthesized by the drug discovery and development scientists. At many pharmaceutical companies the responsible drug discovery scientist is required to complete some sort of hardcopy datasheet for each newly synthesized chemical entity, showing the chemical structure (including stereochemical and salt information) and including other relevant information regarding the sample (notebook reference, research program/project name, physical data, analytical data, synthesizing chemist, data synthesized, inventory data, etc.). This chemical datasheet is then usually submitted to a centralized registration group which checks the corporate database for "prior" registration, assigns a company compound number (for new chemical entities), and registers the chemical structure into the corporate proprietary chemical structure database. Often at the same time, the associated chemical compound sample data from the datasheet is also registered into the corporate compound database and/or into an associated relational software system database. Most pharmaceutical companies have their own unique (and often complex) company compound numbering system, which often may include sub-numbering or additional codes to designate different compound salts or stereoisomers. At many pharmaceutical companies there is a standard policy that any compound submitted for testing (biological, analytical, etc.) must first be assigned a company compound number (which obviously implies simultaneous registration into the corporate chemical structure database). This simple sort of policy (when rigorously followed) can be an extremely effective mechanism for a large pharmaceutical firm with hundreds (or even thousands) of drug discovery research and development scientists for creating and maintaining an up-to-date, complete, and accurate database for tracking and providing access to information for its new chemical entities. Many companies typically also register samples of any compounds that are obtained from external sources (i.e., from outside of the company) for biological testing purposes.

Some pharmaceutical companies have multiple research and development sites in the same country, in different countries, and often even on different continents. Some of these companies may have separate corporate chemical structure databases at each site, but there is, presently, a trend for many companies to maintain a single, large corporate database (and compound numbering system) for all its R&D sites at a single location. Scientists at other R&D sites either remotely access the centralized database from the other sites, or copies of the "master" corporate compound database are periodically distributed to the other R&D sites for local access there. Several companies (e.g., SmithKline Beecham and Glaxo) have taken this one step further, in that a master corporate chemical structure database for all its worldwide R&D sites is maintained at a single site in the United States (or Europe) with a second copy at a key R&D site on the other continent. Nightly automated computer programs are run which update the copy database with any changes that have been made to the master corporate

database. In essence, these companies have managed to provide immediate access for all their R&D scientists worldwide to current available proprietary chemical entity information for the entire pharmaceutical worldwide R&D organization.

These in-house databases of proprietary new chemical entities are a key information resource for most pharmaceutical companies. These databases do more than just provide a convenient means for electronically tracking a company's valuable proprietary chemical structure data. These databases are often the key link whereby drug discovery and development scientists are able to access related and essential information in other information resource databases (e.g., bioactivity data, inventory data, chemical sample tracking data, analytical data, etc.). Because of this ability, these corporate chemical structure databases at pharmaceutical companies are normally easily accessible by all drug discovery research and development scientists on centralized time-sharing computing systems (e.g., VAX, IBM).

3.2 Commercial 2D Databases

All of the chemical information management software vendors and some traditional book publishers also offer a variety of valuable 2D chemical structure databases for licensing and use in-house with the chemical information software systems described above. The chemical structures and associated data in these 2D databases are derived from a diverse range of information sources, including the scientific literature, patents, and even catalogs of fine organic chemical suppliers (67). Each database has its specific emphasis, and many of them are of particular value for drug discovery research and development scientists. A list of the commercial 2D chemical structure databases is presented in Table 13.3, with further description of their content and use

Table 13.3   Commercially Available 2D Chemical Structure Databases

Database	Vendor	Format	Description
ACD	MDL	MACCS-II	ACD = Available Chemical Directory = FCD database (see below) plus information on chemicals available in bulk quantities. Updated 2x/year.
DARC–CHCD	Questel	DARC	CHCD = Chapman & Hall Chemical Database. 250,000 organic structures with physical/chemical data, literature references, chemical names/synonyms, use, etc.
FCD	MDL	MACCS-II	FCD = Fine Chemicals Directory. Combined catalogs of 65+ commercial suppliers of fine organic chemicals. Contains chemical structures and supplier information, including catalog #'s and price/quantity information. Updated 2X/year.
FCD	Fraser Williams	DARC	FCD = Fine Chemicals Directory. See description for MDL's FCD database above and in the text.
MDDR	MDL	MACCS-II	MDDR = MACCS Drug Data Report. Database of Prous Science Publisher's journal *Drug Data Reports* since 1988. Summary of new bioactive molecules from patents and the scientific literature. Contains chemical structures, biological activity data, patent/bibliographic references, etc. Updated 2x/year.
PKFILE	MDL	MACCS-II	Experimental pK_a data for 3,400+ molecules. No longer distributed.
POMONA92	Daylight	THOR	Partition coefficients, pK_a values, and bioactivities (about 25,000 structures). Developed by the Pomona Collete Medicinal Chemistry Project.
SDF	Derwent	DARC, MACCS-II, OSAC	SDF = Standard Drug File. Information on approximately 40,750 drug molecules (1964–present).
Therapeutic Patent Fast-Alert	Current Drugs, PH&M	MACCS-II	Weekly worldwide pharmaceutical patents current awareness database.

in drug discovery included as the remainder of this chapter subsection.

The DARC-CHCD (DARC Chapman & Hall Chemical Database) database (QUESTEL) is a large, consolidated database of chemical and physical data together with key literature references and chemical structures for about 250,000 organic compounds (68, 69). The database is based on a number of Chapman & Hall compendia:

- *Dictionary of Organic Compounds*, 5th

ed., and subsequent annual supplements (70).

- *Dictionary of Organometallic Compounds* and subsequent supplements (71).
- *Dictionary of Antibiotics & Related Substances* (72).
- *Dictionary of Organophosphorous Compounds* (73).
- *Dictionary of Alkaloids* (74)
- *Dictionary of Drugs* (75).
- *Dictionary of Steroids* (76).
- *Carbohydrates* (Chapman & Hall Chemistry Sourcebook) (77).
- *Amino Acids and Peptides* (Chapman & Hall Chemistry Sourcebook) (78).

The chemical structures are stored in a DARC database, while the associated chemical, physical, and literature reference textual data are contained in a related RDB database. The associated data includes Chapman & Hall compound number, chemical name and synonyms, molecular formula and weight, Chapman & Hall reference, general comments (source, synthesis, use, etc.), physical and chemical description (state, color, recrystallization solvent, solubility data, density data, melting point, boiling point, etc.), and complete scientific literature bibliographic information. The database is provided with a number of customized DARC forms for display and plotting of retrieved chemical structures and data (Fig. 13.6). The database is planned for two updates per year.

The FCD database (Fine Chemicals Directory; Molecular Design Limited) was one of the first and certainly most successful of the commercially available 2D chemical structure databases. Basically the MAC-CS-II database is a compendium of the catalogs of more than 65 international suppliers of fine chemicals for over 90,000 compounds and more than 210,000 database entries (79, 80). Each database entry includes the chemical structure and the following associated chemical data: chemical name and synonyms (as listed by each supplier), molecular formula, molecular weight, supplier name, supplier catalog number(s), price/quantity information (for suppliers who publish price lists), CAS Registry Number, purity data (e.g., 97%),

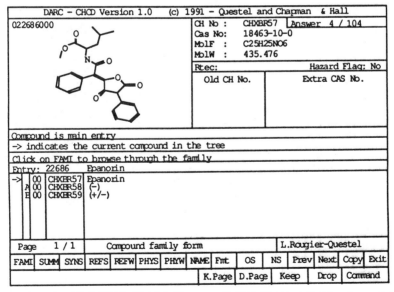

Fig. 13.6 A customized DARC-CHCD (DARC Chapman & Hall Chemical Database) report form, showing retrieval of a chemical structure and basic associated data.

and other miscellaneous supplier catalog information (e.g., salt and stereoisomer data). The database and its documentation also contain addresses and telephone numbers for each supplier's United States, European, and Japanese offices. The database can be searched by chemical structure (or substructure) and by any of the associated chemical data. For drug discovery scientists, the FCD database is used extensively at many pharmaceutical companies for two purposes. First, by performing appropriate structural and data searches, a scientist can quickly identify sources and pricing for specific organic chemicals to be used as synthetic starting materials, intermediates, or unusual reagents for the preparation of potential drug molecules or for other research needs (e.g., analytical testing,). Second, by using substructure and similarity searches, scientists can identify

commercially available compounds for biological screening. This strategy can be an especially effective (and cost-effective) means for obtaining screening samples for initially investigating structure activity-relationships for newly identified potential drug series. MDL provides an easy-to-use customized MACCS-II user interface for accessing, searching, reviewing, and producing reports from the FCD database (Fig. 13.7). (For licensees of the MDL FCD database, Fraser Williams (Scientific Systems) Ltd. can provide a DARC in-house formatted version of the database.)

The ACD database (Available Chemicals Directory; Molecular Design Limited) consists of the FCD MACCS-II database expanded with additional entries for compounds available from commercial chemical suppliers in bulk quantities (over 25 kilograms) (80, 81) (Fig. 13.7). In addition to

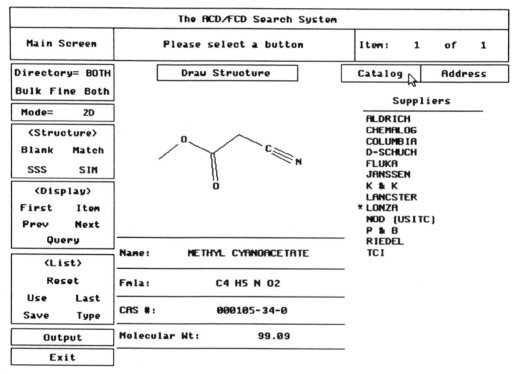

Fig. 13.7 A customized MACCS-II interface menu illustrating retrieval of a chemical structure from the Molecular Design Limited combined FCD/ACD MACCS-II databases. The Catalog menu option would subsequently show complete supplier information (catalog #'s, pricing, etc.) for this compound.

this combined catalog collection from over 70 suppliers, the ACD includes bulk chemical information derived from the United States International Trade Commission Publication, *Synthetic Organic Chemicals*. Searches can be limited to compounds available in bulk, research-scale amounts, or both. Even as a new chemical entity is identified in the later stages of drug discovery research as a potential development candidate, it becomes necessary to evaluate the costs of one or more possible scaled-up synthetic routes that may be used to produce the significant amounts of drug molecule needed for development studies (e.g., drug metabolism, pharmacokinetics, short and long term toxicity, analytical formulations, and eventually clinical trials). The specific bulk chemical availability information in the ACD database can help the development synthetic chemist (who normally is working on a combined drug discovery and development program/project team) with this process by providing ready access to this information for a large number of possible suppliers.

The MDDR database (MACCS-II Drug Data Report; Molecular Design Limited) is essentially a complete electronic version of Prous Scientific Publisher's journal, *Drug Data Reports* since July 1988 (80, 82). The journal contains current information on approximately 10,000 new bioactive compounds (and related derivatives) each year. The initial information for new molecules is abstracted by Prous from patent entries from 11 international patent offices. The MDDR MACCS-II database semi-annual updates by MDL add about 5,000 new molecules to the database, as well as updating existing database entries with additional information from various sources, including correspondence, publications, and symposia/scientific meetings. Each database entry contains the chemical structure and the associated information, including: chemical names (systematic chemical name, synonyms, trademark,

generic name, and company code), Prous Registry Number, descriptions of biological activity, patent information (inventor company, number, source, title, etc.), molecular formula, molecular weight, CAS Registry Number (if available), compound development stage, companies involved in license agreements, and full bibliographic references. With the MDDR database, MDL provides an essential user-interface for easily searching and reviewing the structures and data in the database, as well as for generating customized reports (Fig. 13.3). The interface consists of four screens (menus + display forms): (1) An identification screen for performing structure and data searches of the database and for reviewing the basic chemical structure and data retrieved for each molecule; (2) a biological information screen for displaying more extensive biological information; (3) a literature references screen for displaying detailed literature reference data; and (4) a patent information screen for displaying more detailed patent reference information. Especially in the pharmaceutical industry, drug discovery scientists must keep abreast of current developments in the patent literature for new bioactive compounds. A current knowledge of patent activity by other pharmaceutical companies assists the drug discovery scientist in evaluating the research efforts at the other companies and whether these patents may impact the patent potential of compounds being investigated in current drug discovery and development programs at his/her own company. In addition, review of pertinent patents of bioactive compounds can provide insight or creative inspiration for the drug discovery scientist in pursuing new drug discovery therapeutic strategies. There are a number of on-line patent abstract databases (which usually are complicated enough to require an experienced information specialist for searching), as well as printed patent abstracts, however, continually searching for only a few possible relevant patent abstracts can be laborious. The availability of an in-house patent abstract database for bioactive compounds (such as MDDR) potentially provides drug discovery scientists with the opportunity of easily accessing, searching, browsing, and remaining current with the relevant patent literature. Timeliness (i.e., updates only twice each year) may be a problem, but more frequent database updating would solve the problem (see the discussion below regarding the Therapeutic Patent Fast-Alert database).

The PKFILE database (Molecular Design Limited, developed in conjunction with Rhone Poulenc-Recherches) contains 10,700 acid/base dissociation constants (pK_a values) from the scientific literature for more than 3,400 molecules (mostly organics) (80). The database is no longer distributed, but scientists may encounter original copies of this database still being used at some pharmaceutical research sites, The PKFILE contains chemical structures, pK_a values, solvent system data, molecular weight, literature reference, temperature, and proton source information. The database has been distributed without a customized user interface, contributing unfortunately, perhaps, to its demise as a commercial product. pK_a values of drug molecules play an important role in almost every aspect of drug bioactivity, including absorption, distribution, excretion, metabolism, receptor binding, etc. Drug discovery and development scientists need to know pK_a values for compounds actually prepared and being tested, as well as predicted pK_a values for compounds that might be potentially synthesized, in order both to interpret and understand the effect of molecular pK_a on observed bioactivity and to help design new molecules with appropriate pK_a values to maximize desired bioactivity effects. A representative 2D chemical structure database of experimental pK_a values for organic compounds, coupled with a customized user-interface and an appropriate expert

system for theoretical pK_a prediction, may eventually serve this need.

The POMONA92 database (Daylight Chemical Information Systems, Inc.) is a THOR database containing experimental partition coefficients (Log P values) and acid/base dissociation constants (pK_a values) for about 25,000 organic compounds (83, 84). The database originally had been developed (and is still updated at least once each year) by the Pomona College Medicinal Chemistry Project (65, 66). The database has a significant representation of compounds of interest in pharmaceutical research and development. The scientific literature coverage for the Log P values is comprehensive. Partition coefficients in all solvent systems are included, but the most useful 1-octanol/water partition coefficients predominate. The most accurate and reliable experimental 1-octanol/water Log P values (as judged by the Pomona College Medicinal Chemistry Project) are additionally noted in the database (as LOGPSTAR values). The scientific literature coverage for the pK_a values is extensive, with an emphasis for inclusion only of the most reliable pK_a values in water (although other solvent systems are included). Besides the chemical structures, associated data in the POMONA92 database include pharmacological activity data (where available), WLN's, CAS Registry Numbers, molecular formula, molecular weight, literature references, and experimental conditions of measurement (solvent, temperature, pH, method, etc.). For many years (when originally distributed by the Pomona College Medicinal Chemistry Project and now as distributed by Daylight Chemical Information System, Inc.), the POMONA92 database (also called the POMONA MED CHEM database) has proven to be a successful and much-used database for pharmaceutical drug discovery and development research in both academia and industry. The Log P and pK_a values for a drug molecule often have a significant impact on the compound's bioactivity (influencing absorption, biodistribution, metabolism, excretion, receptor interactions, etc.). For a scientist to be able to examine values for a compound that are similar to ones that he or she is planning to or has already prepared, in order to assist with assessing how these properties might affect a potential drug molecule's bioactivity, can be very useful. In addition, the experimental Log P values in the database serve as a valuable adjunct to the CLOGP-3 software (for estimation of Log P values), in that the accuracy of the CLOGP-3 software in calculating Log P values can be evaluated by comparing the calculated versus experimental values in the database for similar compounds (83). The POMONA92 database is also available with estimated 1-octanol/water partition coefficients and molar refractivities, as computed by CLOGP-3 and CMR (see Section 8.2.2.1 below).

The SDF (Standard Drug File) database (Derwent Publications Ltd.) is a database of information on drug molecules (marketed and in development) worldwide and is based on non-patent technical and scientific literature sources (85–87). Associated drug molecule data in the database include CAS Registry Numbers, molecular formulae, Derwent Registry Names, synonyms (e.g., INN, USAN, and other approved names, as well as trade names by country and company), biological activity mechanism of action, and pharmacological activity. For marketed drugs, information (extracted from official compendia) is included for indications, contra-indications, interactions, precautions, and adverse effects. The database is available in DARC, MACCS-II, and OSAC formats, as well as in SMD (Standard Molecular Data) file format. Updated about two times per year, the SDF with Graphics Database Version 6.0 (September 1992) contains 40,750 drug compounds, together with 149,000 drug names and synonyms and 8,900 mechanism of action entries.

The Therapeutic Patent Fast-Alert database (Current Drugs Ltd. and Pool, Heller, & Milne, Inc.; MACCS-II format) is a current awareness type database of potential new drugs abstracted from new patents worldwide in the pharmaceutical and biotechnology fields (beginning in 1992) (88). Patent documents in the database include European, Worldwide PCT, U.S. granted, and UK applications. Areas of database emphasis include anticancer agents, drugs for hormonal and metabolic diseases, anti-inflammatories, respiratory and GI agents, antimicrobials, antivirals, vaccines, CNS active agents, cardiovascular agents, blood products, and immunological agents. Approximately 140 patents are reviewed and abstracted for the database each week. Database updates are weekly, with only a brief delay between publication and shipping of the update diskettes to the database user. Besides patent chemical structure/substructure data, the database also includes information relative to the referenced patents: title, patent assignee, inventor(s), patent number, priority application number, application date, merit rating ("3" = patents with special significance; "1" = less significant patents), informative abstract, section codes, index terms, biology, chemistry, patent page number, cross-references, and accession number. The database is also available in ChemBase format (see Section 8.1). A MACCS-II graphical forms "front-end" (supplied with the database) simplifies searching for the database user.

The Institute for Scientific Information (ISI) is also planning for marketing by 4Q93 of an electronic version (MACCS-II chemical connection table plus associated data format, ready for MACCS-II database inclusion) of its *Index Chemicus*, a weekly current awareness publication covering new chemical compounds reported in over 100 international pharmaceutical and chemical journals. Information on 200,000+ new organic compounds are covered each year, including chemical structures, bibliographic references, author literature abstracts, chemical name, molecular formula and weight, isolated intermediates, and biological activity (if available). Updates will be provided bimonthly.

4 3D CHEMICAL INFORMATION MANAGEMENT SOFTWARE

A fairly recent and significant development in chemical information computing systems (and the molecular modeling/drug design field) has been the development of sophisticated 3D chemical information management software systems (89–96), useful for the capture (registration), management, searching, and retrieval of 3D chemical structures and associated 3D chemical structure data. As described below, such software systems/databases have been the focus of extensive (and still on-going) research and application, especially in the drug discovery field. The 3D chemical information management software systems and databases can be viewed (at least in part) as extensions of the 2D chemical information management software systems and databases. That is, besides understanding and handling 2D chemical structures, the 3D software/databases also understand and handle 3D chemical structure information. The following chapter subsections describe the capabilities of these 3D chemical information management software systems and databases and how they are utilized in industry and academia in new drug discovery R&D.

4.1 Software Function and Capabilities

3D chemical information management software systems are much newer and are still much more the focus of active research investigation and development efforts, as compared to the available 2D chemical information management software systems. Therefore the various proprietary (industrial and academic) and commercial 3D chemical information management software systems currently tend to differ considerably in their specific capabilities and interfaces and in their 3D searching techniques for 3D chemical model databases (90, 92, 94). The most common software capabilities of these 3D software systems are described in the following paragraphs.

3D chemical information software systems must of necessity possess the chemical intelligence of 2D chemical information software systems regarding 2D chemical structures (as described in detail in section 2.1). In addition, the 3D software must also possess chemical intelligence and capabilities regarding 3D chemical structure models (and even 3D chemical structure model properties) and of the use of this chemical intelligence for 3D searching and other 3D software applications (as described below). This additional 3D chemical intelligence typically includes a knowledge and understanding of a number of 3D characteristics associated with 3D chemical structure 3D models, including 3D atomic coordinates as well as various geometric features associated with 3D chemical structures and 3D chemical structure searching (distances, angles, dihedral angles, etc.).

The 3D chemical information software systems typically employ a number of standard users menus, each with a specific function; for example, 3D chemical model entry and registration; registration of associated 3D chemical model data; 3D chemical structure/substructure/pharmacophore search query specification; 3D database searching for 3D models and data; retrieval of 3D structures and data from the 3D database; etc. As with the corresponding 2D software systems, choice of program options by the user is usually graphical selection of menu buttons and/or typing of commands.

Normally new 3D chemical structure

models are not directly entered interactively by the user (primarily because of the complexity and amount of data that would have to be laboriously typed in). Instead, already constructed 3D chemical structure models are usually brought directly into the 3D chemical information management software from one of several sources, including:

- External computer files, which contain a 3D structure model generated from another software system (e.g., CONCORD, see Section 5.1) or a molecular modeling/computational chemistry system.
- Directly from a 3D chemical structure model builder or calculator in a molecular modeling system.
- External computer files which contain 3D structures from experimental crystallographic studies.

3D chemical model registration, by the 3D chemical information management software systems into 3D chemical structure model databases, usually includes the 3D atomic coordinates for at least one 3D model for each 2D chemical structure. Some 3D software systems allow for and registration of multiple 3D models, all of which are associated with a single 2D chemical structure registered in the database. Depending on the specific software system, the 3D software may associate the 3D chemical structure model(s) with a 2D chemical structure already registered in the database or the 3D software may also generate the appropriate 2D structure and register the 2D structure and 3D model simultaneously in the database. The 3D software will usually analyze the 3D chemical structure at the time of registration and also generate the register the 3D substructure search keys needed for subsequent 3D chemical structure searching of the 3D chemical model database. Depending on

the specific 3D software system, registration may also include a conformational analysis of the chemical structure, with registration of a single 3D chemical structure model together with precalculated keys to allow for conformational flexibility in searching.

3D chemical structure software systems and databases also normally register and manage both simple and complex associated 3D chemical model data which might include:

- References (scientific literature or in-house laboratory notebook) to experimental crystallographic structures.
- Description of various computational methodologies used for generation of the 3D models from 2D chemical structures.
- Various parameters indicating the quality/reliability of the experimental or theoretical 3D chemical model structures.
- Specific assigned atomic, bond, molecular, or substructural physical/chemical properties (charge distribution, shape, hydrophobicity, etc.).

Associated 3D chemical model data is usually registered into the 3D databases and not in associated relational database systems.

3D chemical information management software systems offer a variety of techniques for searching 3D chemical model databases. With 2D chemical structure information also registered in the 3D databases, most of the 3D software systems permit the user to perform the same types of 2D searches of the databases as are possible with 2D chemical information management software (i.e., exact 2D structure, 2D substructure, 2D similarity, etc.). These 2D searches can be performed independently or combined with 3D model searching (described below).

The 3D chemical information management software systems (both developed in-house in academia and industry, as well as those licensed from software vendors) vary considerably in the methodologies they employ for 3D chemical model searching in 3D databases (90, 94). These 3D search capability differences reflect both the differing objectives of the 3D searching, as well as the different computational and analysis methodologies that are implemented in the different 3D software systems.

The most prevalent form of searching employed in the 3D software systems are 3D geometric searches. Such searches first consist of the user specifying (usually graphically drawing) a search query which contains intramolecular relationships between geometric features or objects that can be calculated from the 3D structures in a 3D chemical model database. These can include geometric features such as:

- Points (e.g., atomic nucleus or electron lone pair position, center of mass of several atoms, arbitrary points (dummy atoms) calculated from other geometric features).
- Lines (e.g., calculated from two or more points).
- Planes (e.g., calculated from three or more points).

The user then adds (again usually graphically) geometric constraints to these geometric objects in order to specify the pharmacophore or model that is desired in order to search for the specified model among the 3D models in the 3D database. These geometric constraints can be used to construct quite complex search queries. Typical, simple geometric constraints that could be specified include:

- A distance (actually normally a distance range) between two points (e.g., between two atoms or between an atom and a lone pair of electrons);

- An angle (normally an angle range) defined by three points (e.g., for any three atoms);
- A torsional angle (normally a torsional angle range) defined by four points (e.g., for any four atoms);
- A sphere of exclusion (i.e., a specified 3D volume which may not contain any atoms of the 3D database model structure) calculated from distances between dummy atoms and actual atom(s) in the 3D model.

Unless signed torsional angles are included in a 3D geometric search query, the search will generally not distinguish between enantiomers in the 3D database.

3D chemical model databases typically employ 3D search keys (analogous to 2D substructure search keys) that are used in a 3D geometric search to screen out 3D database models that will not meet the 3D geometric search query constraints (97, 98). This specification is usually critical in order to greatly increase the speed at which the 3D geometric searches can be performed. These 3D geometric keys usually correspond to 3D geometric features that are frequently used in 3D geometric searches (primarily distances and angles). When each 3D model is originally registered in a 3D chemical model database, the software analyzes the 3D structure and sets a large number of 3D geometric keys (often several thousand) in the 3D database for that model. For example, if a 3D model contains an oxygen to oxygen distance of 2.5–3.5 Angstroms, a key in the database could be set indicating the presence of this 3D geometric feature in the compound. A different key would be set if the 3D model contains an oxygen to oxygen distance of 3.5–4.5 Angstroms. As the first step in 3D geometric searches, this initial screening usually quickly reduces the number of possible matches to a fraction of the original database models. At this point an exact final analysis and comparison is made between the 3D geometric search query and this smaller 3D database list to provide the final list of database "hits" which match the 3D geometric search query. 3D geometric searches of 3D databases are usually slower than structure and substructure searches of 2D databases, but are often still interactive for simple 3D geometric search queries. 3D database size, the efficiency of the 3D keys in eliminating 3D models from consideration, and the complexity of the 3D geometric search query can considerably increase the time for these searches.

Most drug molecules and potential drug molecules are not rigid structures. They typically contain one or more degrees of conformation flexibility and can adopt a number of reasonable, low-energy conformations in solution and at their potential interactions sites (receptors). Also typically, the conformation responsible for a drug molecule's bioactivity is not necessarily the global minimum energy conformation. If only a single 3D model (e.g., from a crystal structure or a theoretical calculation) is registered in a 3D database for each structure, 3D searching of the database will examine only one of many possible energetically possible conformations for most of the models and those may not correspond to the conformation(s) that could impart bioactivity to those structures. One solution would be to perform extensive conformational analyses of 3D models at time of registration, and then to register all energetically reasonable conformations into the 3D database. This strategy, however would result in very large 3D databases and greatly increased 3D search times. Some of the 3D chemical information management software systems do allow for multiple model registration and 3D searching in their 3D chemical model databases. Another option would be to register a single low-energy conformation for each model in the 3D database, with appropriate information regarding the conformational flexibility of the model also

registered into the database. Appropriate chemical knowledge/intelligence and computing techniques could be used both for rapid prescreening of the models as well as for the actual analysis of the possible conformations for the models. Many of these 3D conformational search techniques certainly are perhaps better characterized as molecular modeling methodologies, considerably more complex in the expertise and time required compared to that suggested by this simplistic description of searching in 3D chemical information management software systems. 3D searching with conformational flexibility for the 3D database models is currently and will certainly continue to be the object of much intensive computer sciences, molecular modeling, and computational chemistry research in academia, at pharmaceutical companies, and by the commercial 3D software vendors.

Another more recent type of 3D searching employs 3D similarity searches of 3D chemical model databases (analogous to 2D similarity searching of 2D chemical structure databases: see Section 2.1). In this type of 3D database searching, the user specifies a single exact 3D model (e.g., of a bioactive drug molecule) to be used as the 3D similarity search query. The model is then analyzed by the 3D software for the presence of a number of 3D molecular features or properties. Each 3D model in the database is then compared to the query and scored as to its similarity as compared to the search query structure (e.g., how many of the 3D features/properties present in the query are also present in each database model). The set of 3D similarity search hits is those 3D database models most similar to the 3D query structure (for example, with a % similarity greater than some value, say 70%). Willett et al. have investigated the use of different possible 3D model features/properties which could be used to detect 3D model similarity of compounds in 3D databases (99, 100).

These studies have indicated that 3D similarity searches are most effective when based on an intra-atomic distance profile (i.e., similarity based on having specific atoms separated by similar distances in the 3D database models as compared to the 3D model query). 3D similarity searching is a reasonably rapid technique that will also, likely, continue to be the object of extensive inquiry and investigation in drug discovery research, because of the potential of this approach for identifying potential drug molecules for testing in SAR and pharmacophore model development.

Other more complex methods for 3D database have also been actively investigated and used in drug discovery research studies. These more sophisticated and complicated 3D search methodologies have been primarily implemented in in-house (academia and industrial) 3D software and molecular modeling systems and much less so in "traditional", commercial 3D chemical information management software. Such 3D database searching applications, usually for identification of possible bioactive molecules based on complex pharmacophore models and/or known receptor binding sites, include methodologies as diverse as:

- 3D searching based on search query shape, electronic distributions, and other 3D pharmacophore properties.
- 3D searching (often involving 3D model properties and conformational flexibility) to identify structures from 3D databases which could favorably dock as ligands with a known macromolecular receptor.
- 3D searching of 3D databases to identify and use 3D substructural fragments for the automated construction (i.e., "design") of new structures (i.e., potential drug molecules) based on an active drug structure and/or a 3D drug pharmacophore model.

3D searching of 3D chemical model databases have a variety of valuable applications in new drug discovery research. In particular, Martin provides a nice perspective overview of this topic, citing numerous examples of 3D database searching in drug discovery and design (90). These applications of 3D database searching for drug discovery research include:

- Identification (based on a 3D drug pharmacophore model) of available, already synthesized compounds (from commercial or in-house databases) for bioactivity testing.
- Design of new bioactive molecules for synthesis and bioactivity testing based on an established 3D pharmacophore model.
- Design of new chemical structures (including structures incorporating specific conformational constraints) for synthesis and testing in order to develop or test a 3D drug pharmacophore model.

Most certainly the area of 3D databases and searching will be the object of continued intense investigation and new software development in the coming decade, as drug discovery scientists strive to design, implement, and use ever more sophisticated software tools for the design, analysis, and suggestion of potential new drug molecules.

3D chemical information management software systems allow for searching (text and/or numeric) and retrieval of associated 3D chemical information registered in 3D chemical model databases. 2D substructure, 3D geometric, and associated 3D data searches can often be combined to provide for more complex search queries that match a complex pharmacophore model. For example, such a search might include an aliphatic nitrogen atom in a chain and an aromatic hydroxyl group (2D substructural query features), where the nitrogen atom to oxygen atom distance is 2.5–3.5 Angstroms (3D query feature) and there is a positive charge (calculated and registered in the 3D database) of at least a certain magnitude (3D associated data query).

A key and highly desirable feature for 3D chemical information management software systems is as close and as integrated an interface with a 3D molecular graphics modeling system as possible. Ideally this interface would consist of a one-step command, menu button, or graphics window to allow moving back and forth between 3D software and the molecular graphics modeling software. In particular, this command would allow for immediate and direct visualization, manipulation, and comparison (and even further analyses) in the molecular graphics modeling software of the list of "hit" models found by a 3D search of a 3D database. Without such capabilities it would be necessary to save the 3D model "hits" to an external computer file, which could be subsequently read and used later by the 3D molecular graphics modeling software. The closer the integration of the 3D search/database and molecular graphics software, the more immediately useful (and user friendly) 3D databases and searching are for drug discovery applications.

The 3D chemical information software systems also vary considerably in their ability to be customized for a variety of applications, including automating 3D structure/associated data registration and even modifying the 3D searching methodologies used by the 3D software. When such customizability is available, the 3D software usually employs a high-level internal software language for accomplishing the customization.

4.2 Specific Software Systems

As mentioned earlier, 3D chemical information management and searching software is still a very active area of research for software and methodology development. For this reason there are a number of innovative 3D software systems in use and still under continuing development in drug discovery research organizations in both academia and industry (90, 101–103). Most of these innovative systems are proprietary systems that most drug discovery scientists will not encounter in their own research. Many of these are also actually fairly complex computer assisted drug design software systems and so will not be described here.

Even now many drug discovery scientists (especially in industry) are more likely to encounter one of the commercial 3D chemical information management software systems. A list of the current major commercial 3D chemical information management software systems is presented in Table 13.4, with further description of their individual characteristics included in the

Table 13.4 Major Commercial 3D Chemical Information Software Systems

Software	Vendor	Hardware Platforms	Major Markets
Cambridge Structural Database System	Cambridge	VAX/VMS, IBM, UNIX Workstations	Worldwide
ChemDBS-3D	Chemical Design	VAX/VMS, UNIX Workstations	U.S., Europe
MACCS-3D	MDL	VAX/VMS, IBM, Fujitsu	U.S., Europe, Japan
SYBYL/3D UNITY	TRIPOS	VAX/VMS, IBM PC, Macintosh, UNIX Workstations	U.S., Europe, Japan
THOR/MERLIN	Daylight	VAX/VMS, UNIX Workstations	U.S., Europe, Japan

following chapter subsections. This list is not comprehensive, as other molecular modeling software vendors may also offer software for creating and searching 3D chemical structure databases (usually as integrated software totally within their molecular modeling systems), but the major 3D chemical information management software vendors are described.

4.2.1 CAMBRIDGE STRUCTURAL DATABASE SYSTEM. The Cambridge Structural Database System (Cambridge Crystallographic Data Centre) is software specifically for searching and retrieving experimental 3D crystallographic structures and associated data from the Cambridge Structural Database (See Section 5.2) (104, 105). Software components of Version 4 of the system provide for 2D searching (structure/substructure/similarity) and 3D searching (primarily geometric) of this database, as well as complete searching of the associated

textual and numeric data for the 3D crystallographic structures. Development of a menu-driven user interface still continues with this system, with additional enhancements and integration planned for Version 5 of the software.

4.2.2 CHEMDBS-3D. The ChemDBS-3D software (Chemical Design Limited) is directly interfaced as a module associated with the Chem-X computer graphics molecular modeling software system (Fig. 13.8) (106, 107). (Chemical Design Limited does not market a similar 2D-only chemical information management software system.). ChemDBS-3D performs a conformational analysis of each 3D model at the time it is being registered into a 3D database. The low energy conformations are used to set a number of 3D conformation search keys, and these keys and the first low energy conformation are registered into the 3D database. When performing 3D

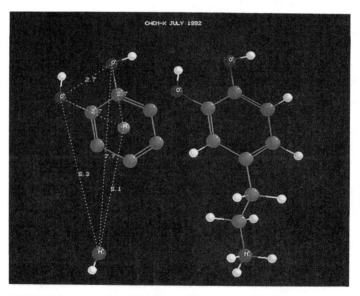

Fig. 13.8 A ChemDBS-3D 3D search query (shown on the left) for compounds which match a pharmacophore model for dopamine (shown on the right): The pharmacophore model search query includes a hydrogen bond donor, a hydrogen bond acceptor, a positive charge, and aromatic ring center atoms (connected with yellow dashed lines). The numbers on the dashed lines indicate the distance in Angstroms between the search center atoms. This query would be used for 3D searches by Chem-X with ChemDBS-3D for compounds which match this dopamine pharmacophore model. See also color plates.

searches with conformational flexibility, the ChemDBS-3D software regenerates and then thoroughly searches all the appropriate 3D conformations for a model, if the model passes the conformational search key prescreening. This approach for 3D searching with conformation flexibility has been critically investigated as to whether this approach significantly increases the number of 3D search hits as compared to searching only a single low energy model in 3D databases (108). 3D chemical structure model databases that can be licensed for use with the ChemDBS-3D software are described in Section 5.2.

4.2.3 MACCS-3D. The MACCS-3D software (Molecular Design Limited) is the direct result of an extension of the Molecular Design Limited's MACCS-II 2D chemical information management software to 3D chemical information management and searching (109–111). Initially developed by Molecular Design Limited with a consortium of industrial partners (primarily pharmaceutical companies), MACCS-3D is actually an add-on module to the MACCS-II software. 2D structures and associated 2D data are registered into a 2D chemical structure database. The 3D models are associated with the structures in the 2D database, but are in essence registered into a separate 3D model database, together with associated 3D model data. Thus, MACCS-3D possesses the full functionality of the underlying MACCS-II 2D software, as well as the added 3D model/data registration and searching capabilities of the 3D software. 3D searches are primarily geometric, although Molecular Design Limited is actively investigating implementation and alternative methods of 3D searching with conformational flexibility (112, 113). The MACCS-3D software provides for direct visualization and manipulation of 3D database models (e.g., hits from a 3D search), but these capabilities are much less sophisticated than those found in computer graphics molecular modeling systems. There are as yet, no direct interfaces of MACCS-3D to molecular graphics modeling systems, although the 3D models can be written to external files for subsequent use by a molecular graphics modeling system for additional 3D model manipulation, comparison, analysis, etc. 3D chemical structure model databases that can be licensed for use with the MACCS-3D software are described in Section 5.2.

4.2.4 SYBYL/3DB UNITY. The SYBYL/3DB UNITY software (TRIPOS Associates, Inc.) is directly interfaced as a module associated with the SYBYL computer graphics molecular modeling software system (Fig. 13.9) (114, 115). The complete 2D and 3D chemical information management software capabilities (registration, management, searching, interfaces to relational databases, etc.) are combined in SYBYL/3DB UNITY. TRIPOS at this point does not yet market a similar 2D-only chemical information management software system. TRIPOS is also implementing 3D conformational flexibility searching into the SYBYL/3DB UNITY software. The ability to create customized SYBYL/3DB UNITY applications is provided through an extended version of the SYBYL Programming language (the internal high-level programming language of the SYBYL software), as well as with a planned customizable report writer. At this time there are no 3D chemical structure model databases that can be licensed for use with the SYBYL/3DB UNITY software.

4.2.5 THOR/MERLIN. Daylight Chemical Information Software Systems, Inc. does not license separate software systems for handling 2D and 3D chemical structures and data. Rather, Daylight's THOR and MERLIN software (see Section 2.2.4) are capable of managing both 2D chemical structures and any number of 3D structure models with each 2D structure (83). The

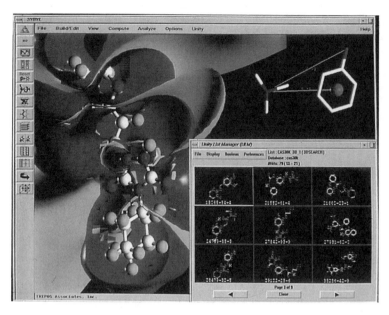

Fig. 13.9 Graphics screens showing the overall integration of SYBYL/3DB UNITY with the SYBYL molecular modeling software system. A 3D search query defined with SYBYL/3DB UNITY (in the upper right hand corner) specifies two distances which describe the pharmacophore or biologically active region of a dopamine agonist. This 3D geometric pharmacophore search definition was then used for a search of a 30K model subset 3D database of the *Chemical Abstracts Registry*. UNITY's List Manager (in the lower right hand corner) displays the search results for review and further analysis. The SYBYL molecular modeling software (on the left) depicts one of the resultant 3D search hits, displayed with an isopotential surface. See also color plates.

Daylight software is also capable of displaying 2D structures as well as the 3D chemical structure models (Fig. 13.10). The Daylight software does not explicitly provide extensive 3D searching software tools/interfaces. Rather it is assumed that the software users will implement customized 3D searching methodologies and applications best suited to their 3D search needs using the Daylight high-level, chemically intelligent programming and query specification languages. This approach has been taken for the 3D database structure implemented in MENTHOR (116), for the 3D geometric searching and new drug molecule design software capabilities implemented in ALADDIN (63, 64), and for generation of 3D conformers in Daylight's RUBICON software. 3D chemical structure model databases that can be licensed

for use with the THOR/MERLIN software are described in Section 5.2.

5 3D CHEMICAL INFORMATION DATABASES

5.1 In-House 3D Databases

One of the primary uses of 3D chemical information management software systems in the pharmaceutical industry has been for companies to build 3D chemical model databases based on the chemical structures registered in their corporate proprietary 2D chemical structure databases. As these corporate 2D databases can be quite large (typically 50,000 to 200,000 compounds), the CONCORD software (distributed by

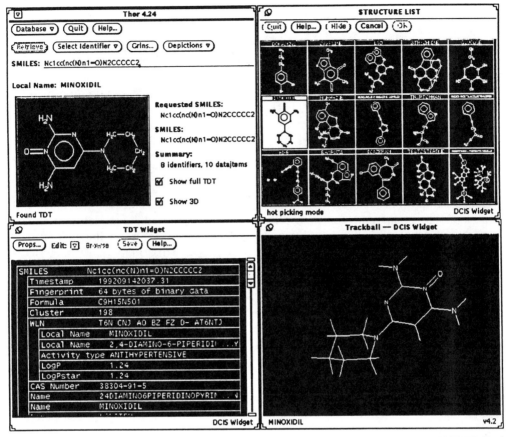

Fig. 13.10 The Daylight Chemical Information Software, Inc., software was used to read a SMILES file (an external computer file containing a number of SMILES chemical structures) and then to create a Structure List Screen compound list. Graphical selection of the Minoxidil structure from the Structure List Screen permits automatic presentation of the basic THOR database screen for this compound. Additional graphical selections permit display of the TDT (THOR Data Tree) Screen, showing associated chemical data for this compound in the THOR database (e.g., SMILES, molecular formula, WLN, chemical names, biological activity, experimental Log P values, CAS Registry Number, etc.). Finally selection of a 3D view screen allows the user to see a 3D depiction of the compound.

TRIPOS Associates, Inc.) (117, 118) has most often been used to generate the needed 3D models from the 2D chemical database structures rapidly (119). 3D chemical databases also provide an appropriate mechanism for academic and industrial drug discovery research groups for the capture of 3D chemical structures solved in-house with crystallographic studies. A number of companies have also converted the 3D crystallographic structures from the Cambridge Structural Database into 3D

databases to take advantage of the 3D search capabilities of the commercial 3D chemical information management software systems (e.g., MACCS-3D and THOR/MERLIN) (120).

5.2 Commercial 3D Databases

Most of the 2D chemical information management software vendors offer a number of 3D chemical structure databases for licensing and use in-house with their 3D chemical information software systems described above. Most typically, these 3D database have been constructed by the software vendors directly from the 2D versions of their databases using the CONCORD software program (117, 118). (Whenever CONCORD is used to generate 3D structures from the 2D structures in a large database, inevitably CONCORD is unable to construct 3D models for some of the compounds. Therefore these "derived" 3D databases inevitably contain most (but not all) of the compounds in their 2D counterparts). All of the 2D chemical structures and associated data from the 2D databases are usually included in the 3D databases, together with the 3D structures. As with the 2D databases, each 3D database has its own specific emphasis, and

many of them are of particular interest for pharmaceutical research and development. A list of the commercial 3D chemical structure databases available for licensing is presented in Table 13.5, with some description of their content and use in drug discovery included as the remainder of this section.

The CMC-3D (Comprehensive Medicinal Chemistry-3D; Molecular Design Limited) is a 3D database of Pergamon Press' *Comprehensive Medicinal Chemistry* (121, 122). The database contains CONCORD-generated 3D models of 5,800 compounds from the drug compendium in this six-volume work which have been actively investigated or marketed as drugs. Besides the 2D structures and 3D models, the database includes the following associated compound data: generic name, CAS Re-

Table 13.5   Commercially Available 3D Chemical Structure Databases

Database	Vendor	Format	Description
CMC-3D	MDL	MACCS-3D	3D database of Pergamon Press's *Comprehensive Medicinal Chemistry*
CSD	Cambridge	Cambridge	CSD = Cambridge Structural Database. 86,000+ experimental crystallographic 3D structures
FCD-3D	MDL	MACCS-3D	3D version of MDL's FCD 2D database
MDDR-3D	MDL	MACCS-3D	3D version of MDL's MDDR 2D database
POMONA92-3D	Daylight	THOR	3D version of Daylight's POMONA92 2D database
SDF-3D	Chemical Design	ChemDBS-3D	3D database of Derwent's Standard Drug File
3D Dictionary of Drugs	Chemical Design	ChemDBS-3D	3D database of the Chapman & Hall's *Dictionary of Drugs*
3D Dictionary of Fine Chemicals	Chemical Design	ChemDBS-3D	3D database of Chapman & Hall's *Dictionary of Organic Compounds*
3D Dictionary of Natural Products	Chemical Design	ChemDBS-3D	3D database of Chapman & Hall's *Dictionary of Alkaloids*, *Dictionary of Antibiotics & Related Substances*, and *Dictionary of Terpenoids*, 50,000 compounds

gistry Number, drug class, originating company, original references, reference to the *Comprehensive Medicinal Chemistry* page location, molecular weight and formula, Log *P* data, and pK_a values. Molecular Design Limited does not offer a 2D-only version of this database for licensing.

The CSD (Cambridge Structural Database; Cambridge Crystallographic Data Centre) is a 3D database of 86,000+ experimental crystallographic structures derived from scientific literature X-ray and neutron diffraction studies of organocarbon compounds (104, 105). The database contains 2D chemical structures, 3D models in the form of complete numerical crystallographic results, and associated text/ numeric data (bibliographic references, comments, etc.)

The FCD-3D database (Fine Chemicals Directory-3D; Molecular Design Limited) is a 3D version of Molecular Design Limited's 2D FCD database (123, 124). This version contains more than 60,000 CONCORD-generated 3D models, as well as the 2D structures and associated chemical and supplier information found in the 2D version of the database. The database is supplied with a menu-driven FCD-3D Search System front-end (written in MAC-CS-II sequence language) to facilitate searching and retrieval of 3D models, 2D structures, and associated database data. The database is updated two times each year. Similarly, the MDDR-3D database (MACCS-II Drug Data Report-3D; Molecular Design Limited) is a 3D version of Molecular Design Limited's 2D MDDR database (123, 125). It contains more than 16,000 CONCORD-generated 3D models, as well as the 2D structures and associated chemical and patent/company information found in the 2D version of the database. The database is updated two times each year. The POMONA92-3D database (Daylight Chemical Information Systems, Inc.) is a 3D version of Daylight's POMONA92 2D database (84). It contains CONCORD-

generated 3D coordinates for most of the structures in the POMONA92 2D database, as well as the 2D structures and associated chemical/physical/bioactivity information found in the 2D version of the database. The database is updated whenever the POMONA92 2D database is updated.

The SDF-3D database (Standard Drug File-3D; Chemical Design Ltd.) is a 3D version of Derwent's SDF 2D database (126, 127). The database contains 3D models (built with Chemical Design Ltd.'s Chem-X software) for over 31,000 compounds, together with the associated compound data found in the 2D version of the database. Chemical Design Ltd. also offers three 3D databases based on "Dictionaries" from Chapman & Hall and build from 2D structures using Chemical Design Ltd.'s Chem-X software (128). (These databases appear to be essentially a 3D version of Questel's 2D DARC-CHCD database). The 3D Dictionary of Drugs database is a 3D database based on Chapman & Hall's *Dictionary of Drugs* (75, 129–131) and contains 3D models for about 13,000 compounds. The 3D Dictionary of Fine Chemicals database is a 3D database based on Chapman & Hall's *Dictionary of Organic Compounds* (70, 131) and contains 3D models for about 120,000 compounds. The 3D Dictionary of Natural Products database (131) is a 3D database based on Chapman & Hall's *Dictionary of Alkaloids* (74), *Dictionary of Antibiotics & Related Substances* (72), and *Dictionary of Terpenoids* (132) and contains 3D models for about 120,000 compounds. Each of these Chemical Design Ltd. Chapman & Hall databases contains for each compound a 3D coordinate set for a low energy conformation; conformational keys for searching; Chapman & Hall printed book cross reference; and (when available) the following associated compound data: CAS Registry Number, compound names, systematic names, activity type (for the 3D

Dictionary of Drugs database), and use/importance statement and/or source (for the 3D Dictionary of Fine Chemicals and Natural Products databases).

6 SYNTHETIC REACTION INFORMATION MANAGEMENT SOFTWARE

Synthetic reaction information management software systems are concerned with the capture, management, searching, and retrieval of synthetic reaction information (133, 134). This information includes the chemical structures of both reactants and products, information regarding the actual synthetic transformation, and associated reaction information. Over the last decade use of synthetic reaction information management software for searching and retrieving information from synthetic reaction databases has become a common information resource tool for synthesis planning in drug discovery research. The following chapter subsections describe the software capabilities of synthetic reaction information management software, synthetic reaction databases available for searching, and how these databases are used by synthetic chemists in drug discovery research and development.

6.1 Software Function and Capabilities

Just as with 2D chemical information management software, all of the different synthetic reaction information management software systems differ in their specific capabilities and in their end user interfaces. However, each of the commercial systems possesses most of the same software capabilities for synthetic reaction registration, management, searching, and retrieval, as described below.

Synthetic reaction information management software must handle more complex information concerning chemical compounds than 2D chemical information management software in that the former must deal with both reactant and product chemical structures, as well as specific molecular information regarding the synthetic transformation (e.g., which atoms and bonds are involved in the reaction). Because of this complexity, synthetic reaction software systems usually possess all of the chemical intelligence capabilities described earlier for 2D chemical information management software. In addition, the synthetic reaction information management software must also have the chemical intelligence to understand, manage, and search chemical information regarding the actual synthetic transformation for each reaction. This understanding usually entails chemical information which corresponds to one-to-one "mapping" of reactants and products. For each reaction the software is able to establish and track a one-to-one correspondence for each atom and bond in the reactants with the corresponding atoms and bonds in the products, also resulting in a consequential knowledge of which specific bonds are being broken or formed in the synthetic transformation (135).

Each of the synthetic reaction information management software systems uses several standard user menus as its primary user interface for specific functions: reactant and product drawing; compound and synthetic reaction data registration; search query specification (Fig. 13.11), database searching for structures and/or data, retrieval and review of reactions from synthetic reaction databases (e.g., Fig. 13.12–13.14), report generation and output, etc. The user chooses program options either graphically using menu buttons and/or by typing commands.

Chemical structures (reactant and product molecules) are entered using essentially the same methods described in detail above for chemical structure entry in 2D chemical information management systems: the

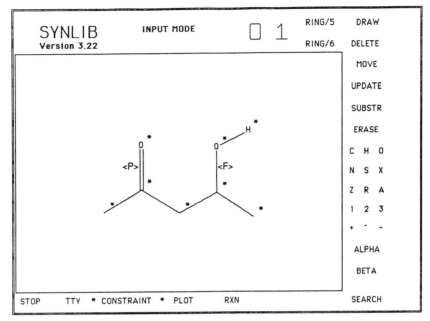

Fig. 13.11 A SYNLIB INPUT MODE screen showing a search query for the preparation of betahydroxyketones. The * symbols mark atoms that must be present in the reaction product. The added search constraints indicate that C=O bond must be present in the reactants and is preserved in the synthesis and that the C–OH bond is formed in the synthesis.

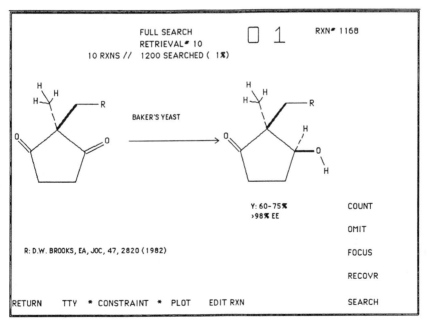

Fig. 13.12 A SYNLIB SEARCH MODE screen showing a reaction retrieved from the SYNLIB Master Chemical Reaction Library database using the reaction search query shown in Figure 13.11. R = Scientific Literature Reference; Y = Reaction Yield; %EE = Enantiomeric Excess (optical purity).

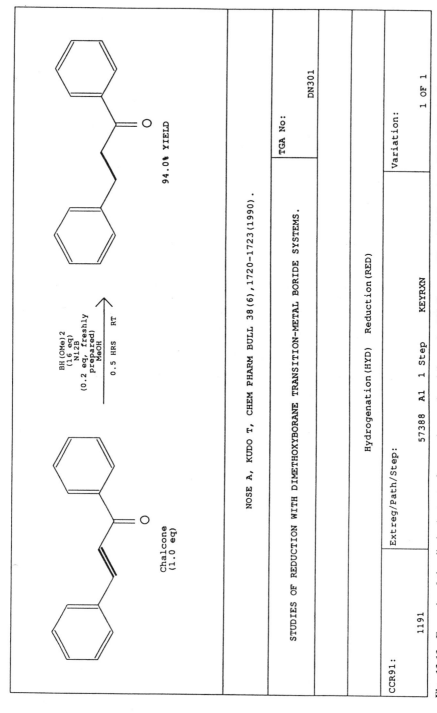

Chalcone
(1.0 eq)

BH(OMe)2
(16 eq)
Ni2B
(0.2 eq, freshly
prepared)
MeOH

0.5 HRS   RT

94.0% YIELD

NOSE A, KUDO T, CHEM PHARM BULL 38(6),1720-1723(1990).

STUDIES OF REDUCTION WITH DIMETHOXYBORANE TRANSITION-METAL BORIDE SYSTEMS.

	TGA No:			
				DN301

Hydrogenation(HYD)   Reduction(RED)

Extreg/Path/Step:				Variation:

CCR91:		57388 A1 1 Step KEYRXN		1 OF 1
1191				

Fig. 13.13 Example of the display/output of a reaction retrieved from the ISI Current Chemical Reactions REACCS database: a one-step reduction of an olefinic bond in the presence of a keto group.

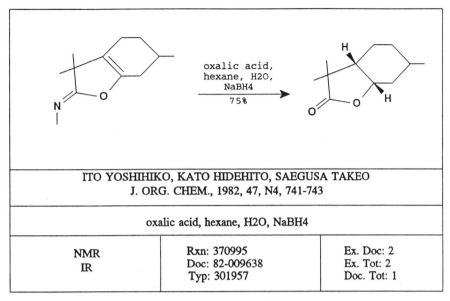

ITO YOSHIHIKO, KATO HIDEHITO, SAEGUSA TAKEO J. ORG. CHEM., 1982, 47, N4, 741-743		
oxalic acid, hexane, H2O, NaBH4		
NMR IR	Rxn: 370995 Doc: 82-009638 Typ: 301957	Ex. Doc: 2 Ex. Tot: 2 Doc. Tot: 1

Fig. 13.14 A typical reaction record retrieved from the ChemReact REACCS database showing a stereoselective synthetic method for gamma-lactones.

structures can be graphically drawn or can be retrieved from external computer chemical structure connection table files. Synthetic reaction software systems are also capable of saving or retrieving entire reactions (reactant and product structures, as well as information regarding the synthetic transformation) to/from external computer files.

Registration of a reaction into a synthetic reaction database with a synthetic reaction information management software system is similar to, but more complicated than, compound registration into chemical databases with 2D chemical information management software. First, the user draws the reactant and product structures (and there may be more than one of each of these). When asked to register the reaction into a synthetic reaction database, the software analyzes the structures and then usually attempts to perform an automatic "mapping" of the reactant and product molecule atoms and bonds. The user is given the option of correcting the mapping and is usually asked to input some other

information regarding the reaction: e.g., reagent(s), temperature, yield. After the software searches the synthetic reaction database for duplicate reactions, the software, if given the OK by the user, registers the reaction into the synthetic reaction database. Substructure search keys and similarity keys are also determined and registered into the reaction database by the software at this point for the reaction.

Besides registering the actual reactant and product molecules, synthetic reaction information management software systems also possess the ability to store other information associated with the synthetic reactions in these databases. Typically this associated synthetic reaction information (text and/or numeric) might include: reaction type (e.g., oxidation, Diels Alder, etc.); scientific literature reference(s) from which the reaction information was abstracted; information regarding reaction limitations and variations; general comments regarding the synthetic procedure; information regarding product purification and purity; etc. In contrast to many 2D chemical databases, synthetic reaction databases tend to be completely self-contained in their data; for instance, all of the associated synthetic reaction information is registered in the synthetic reaction database and not in relational databases. Reaction type associated synthetic reaction information is often keyword data (i.e., the reaction type entered must be taken from a pre-defined list of reaction types). Some synthetic reaction software is actually capable of automatically analyzing a synthetic transformation and to suggest appropriate keyword(s) to be used to describe the reaction.

The synthetic reaction information management software systems provide a number of methods for searching the reactions in synthetic reaction databases. The results of any synthetic reaction database search is a list of "hits", which match the reaction search query. Review of these hits by the user usually involves display of reactants, products, and associated synthetic reaction data graphically in a standard report form format. Typically most synthetic reaction information management software permit simultaneous searching of more than one synthetic reaction database, using a single synthetic reaction search query.

For a basic reaction search, the user draws and specifies one or more exact product and/or reactant chemical structures. The software analyzes these structures and uses this information to perform the reaction database search for matches. In much the same manner as used for 2D chemical database substructure searches, the user can also add substructure search query features to any of the reactant or product chemical structures. A search of a synthetic reaction database with such a query by the synthetic reaction software is then essentially a synthetic reaction substructure search. In addition, most of the synthetic reaction information software systems also allow the user to specify required one-to-one mapping of any atoms and/or bonds for the reactant and product structures (135). The user is usually also allowed to specify which bonds are required to have been broken in the reactants in the synthetic transformation, which bonds must have formed in the products in the synthetic transformation, and/or even specific bonds that must be resent in both reactants and products (Fig. 13.11). Generally most synthetic reaction information management software systems do not provide for the specification of generic/markush substructure search queries.

In one form or another each of the synthetic reaction information management software systems also provide for the ability to perform "similarity" searches of synthetic reaction databases (136, 137). In such a case, the user can often specify that the similarity search to be performed is based on similarity to the reactant and/or product structures specified in the search query or is based on similarity to the actual synthetic transformation in the search query. In the latter case this basis usually involves searching the synthetic reaction database for reactions ranked as to their similarity for the atoms/bonds and their immediate environment involved in the synthetic transformation specified in the search query.

Synthetic reaction information management software systems also provide the ability to perform searches of the associated synthetic reaction information stored in synthetic reaction databases. These are similar to associated compound data searches in 2D chemical databases, and can include text, numeric, or keyword searches. Typical searches might include searching for all articles by a specific author or for all reactions with a specific keyword reaction type.

Synthetic reaction information software systems vary considerably in their capabilities to be customized by the user. Despite this, in most cases users of the commercial synthetic software systems do little, if any, customization of the users interfaces to this software, preferring instead to use the standard user interface menus as provided by the software vendors. Customization has been limited primarily to modifying the format of the forms that are used for review and report generation of the reaction structures and associated data from the synthetic reaction databases. This limitation is likely to change in the near future, as efforts are made to integrate and interface synthetic chemical information management software and databases with predictive synthetic reaction software systems (computer-aided synthesis, reaction generators, reaction analysis and prediction, etc.) (138–140).

Synthetic reaction information management software systems and their use for searching and retrieval of synthetic method information from reaction databases have become a well-accepted and valuable information resource for drug discovery research and development, both at pharmaceutical companies and in academia. There are several reasons and drug discovery R&D applications that can account for this wide-spread acceptance. For the research synthetic chemist attempting to synthesize new chemical entities in a drug class for bioactivity testing, searches of available reaction databases of synthetic methods abstracted from the scientific synthetic literature can help with identification of possible synthetic routes for the preparation of the new compounds, facilitating and hopefully accelerating SAR (structure–activity relationship) development for the drug class. The development synthetic chemist is concerned with fewer synthetic routes for synthesis of a few drug development candidates, but efficient synthetic route identification is crucial for preparation of considerable amounts of these compounds. Rapid identification of even a single key, efficient synthetic transformation through searches of synthetic reaction databases can cut days/weeks (and huge development costs) from the drug develop-

ment process. Synthetic reaction information management software and synthetic reaction databases abstracted from the scientific synthetic literature have also proven to be an effective means for many drug discovery synthetic chemists to keep up with the current synthetic literature. This process is accomplished by regular browsing of available synthetic reaction databases and their periodic updates by the synthetic chemist. All of these valuable drug discovery uses of the synthetic reaction information management software and databases are in part the result of several key factors, including:

- Careful abstracting and inclusion of representative (rather than comprehensive) synthetic reactions from the current scientific synthetic literature in synthetic reaction databases available for licensing.
- Unlimited access to the software and databases in-house for searching and browsing by the synthetic chemists themselves, without having to worry about the costs of extensive on-line literature searches that in many cases are performed by an on-line search specialist (rather than by the synthetic chemist) (141).

6.2 Specific Software Systems

Very few companies have attempted to develop and still maintain their own synthetic reaction information management software. Most pharmaceutical companies and academic drug discovery groups that use synthetic reaction information software have relied instead on licensing one of the commercial systems. This licensing is apparently because of the manpower costs that would be needed to develop, maintain, and enhance such a system in-house, and the desire to use the valuable synthetic reaction databases that are licensed for use with the commercial software systems. A list of the current major commercial synthetic reaction information management software systems is presented on Table 13.6, with further description of their individual characteristics included in the following chapter sub-sections. (Questel did develop a DARC-like synthetic reaction information management software system, RMS-DARC (142), but it was discontinued in favor of an interface between the DARC chemical information management software

and the ORAC synthetic reaction information management software).

6.2.1 ORAC. The ORAC (Organic Structures Accessed by Computer) synthetic reaction information management software (ORAC Ltd.) was developed at the University of Leeds (Fig. 13.15) and has a limited number of installations at pharmaceutical companies and academic institutions in England, continental Europe, and Japan (143–145). ORAC's user interface is similar to that of ORAC Ltd.'s OSAC 2D

Table 13.6 Major Commercial Synthetic Reaction Software Vendors

Software	Vendor	Hardware Platforms	Major Markets
ORAC	ORAC	VAX/VMS, Macintosh	U.S., Europe, Japan
REACCS	MDL	VAX/VMS, IBM, Fujitsu	U.S., Europe, Japan
SYNLIB	DCG	VAX/VMS, Macintosh	U.S., Europe, Japan

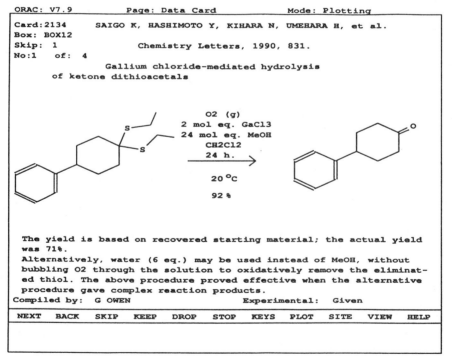

Fig. 13.15 Typical ORAC chemical reaction database management software screen displaying retrieval of a reaction and associated data.

chemical information management software (Section 2.2.3). ORAC makes extensive use of keyword associated synthetic reaction data in its synthetic reaction databases, including reaction types, intermediates, reagents, solvents, etc. (146). With the consolidation of ORAC Ltd. into MDL in 1992, it appears that MDL will continue to support the ORAC software until sometime in 1994. MDL is attempting to facilitate the transition of previous ORAC customers to its REACCS or ISIS software systems in anticipation of this eventuality, but some industrial and academic drug discovery scientists may still encounter the ORAC software/databases in the meantime. Synthetic reaction databases for use with the ORAC software are described in Section 7.2.

6.2.2 REACCS.. The REACCS synthetic reaction information management software (Molecular Design Limited) is easily the most widely licensed software of this type worldwide, including at pharmaceutical companies but with few academic installations (53, 147–152). The REACCS basic user interface (menus) is quite similar to that of Molecular Design Limited's MAC-CS-II chemical information management software (Section 2.2.2). REACCS provides for only limited keyword associated synthetic reaction data for reaction types in its synthetic reaction databases. The large number of synthetic reaction databases that can be licensed for use with the REACCS software are described in Section 7.2.

6.2.3 SYNLIB. The SYNLIB (SYNthesis LIBrary) synthetic reaction information management software (Distributed Chemical Graphics, Inc.) was originally developed at Columbia University and Smith-Kline & French Laboratories (Fig. 13.11 and Fig. 13.12) (153–159). SYNLIB has had a significant number of both industrial and academic installations worldwide. The software has not used keyword data, but does make extensive use of textual and numeric associated synthetic reaction data in its synthetic reaction databases. Synthetic reaction databases that can be licensed for use with the SYNLIB software are described in Section 7.2.

7 SYNTHETIC REACTION INFORMATION DATABASES

7.1 In-House Synthetic Reaction Databases

As described earlier in this chapter, most pharmaceutical companies have developed comprehensive chemical structure information databases for tracking their proprietary new chemical entities (i.e., potential drug molecules) and associated chemical, biological testing, and inventory data. In sharp contrast, only a few pharmaceutical companies have made an effort to develop "in-house" synthetic reaction databases as a means for tracking the synthetic methods for preparations of those proprietary new chemical entities (151). This precedent has happened despite the fact that the software (current commercial synthetic reaction information software systems) is available for registration and capture of such synthetic data. In addition, the logical timing exists for such synthetic information capture, (for example, at the time of registration of the basic new chemical entity information, either from hardcopy corporate new compound datasheets or through electronic submission by the chemists. Apparently, most pharmaceutical companies have deemed not to undertake synthetic reaction information capture for several reasons: Only a certain part of the synthetic chemistry performed at pharmaceutical companies is viewed as truly novel and worth the effort to capture. Also, even with concurrent capture of the synthetic information at time of new compound registration, the manpower to do this information capture would probably be nearly equal to that needed to register the compounds alone. Most companies apparently have decided so far that complete "in-house" synthetic reaction capture cannot be cost justified. For those cases when specific synthetic route information is needed, synthetic chemists at most drug companies have relied on several alternative routes for obtaining that information: from original hardcopy new compound datasheets; from notebooks references in the corporate chemical compound database for chemical samples; from the patent and scientific literature (when this information has been published); and (probably most often) from another chemist at the company who was actually involved with the original synthetic work (if he or she is still around). It is reasonable to anticipate that more pharmaceutical companies may eventually begin to selectively capture certain key synthetic reactions in "in-house" synthetic reaction databases. This procedure could logically include compounds which have moved from the research stage into development, synthetic reactions which truly demonstrate novel proprietary synthetic methods, and representative synthetic pathways for the preparation of analogous series of compounds.

Development of "in-house" synthetic reaction databases is apparently just as rare in academia, even though this decision might at first thought appear to be a reasonable mechanism for capture of such information for an individual academic drug discovery research laboratory or group (160). Most academic groups that have undertaken any such synthetic information capture (especially with the SYNLIB synthetic reaction information software), have tended to turn that information over to the software supplier for inclusion instead in a general current synthetic literature database that the vendor distributes. This strategy relieves the academic research group from maintaining a comprehensive synthetic reaction database,

while allowing those key synthetic methods deemed worthy of capture to be included in a commercially distributed database that all drug discovery scientists can have access to.

7.2 Commercial Synthetic Reaction Databases

The predominant use of synthetic reaction information management software and databases in drug discovery research at pharmaceutical companies and in academia has been the licensing and searching of commercially available synthetic reaction databases (67, 134, 161). These synthetic reaction databases are licensed by the commercial software vendors for use with their synthetic reaction software systems. Some of these databases have a specific synthetic emphasis such as chiral transformations or metal catalyzed reactions; but many databases have been constructed from well-established published synthetic information resources (e.g., specific books, compendia, or published abstracts from the synthetic literature).

The on-line synthetic reaction information resource CASREACT (162) attempts to provide a comprehensive database of synthetic reaction transformations abstracted from the current scientific literature. In contrast, the commercially available synthetic reaction databases available for in-house licensing and searching have focused primarily on creating synthetic reaction databases that are representative (rather than comprehensive) in their coverage and inclusion of synthetic reactions (163). For example, one of these databases may contain only a single (but hopefully representative) example of a specific synthetic transformation, even though there may be dozens of essentially identical reactions described in one or more scientific articles. This selection is usually based on an abstractor's own objective (subjective?) criteria as to what reactions to include, but this approach appears to be accepted and popular with most synthetic chemists who want a representative view of the current synthetic scientific literature.

Published articles have attempted to evaluate the coverage of the different commercially available synthetic reaction databases available for REACCS, ORAC, and SYNLIB. In one of these articles (164), the authors have concluded that databases available for these three synthetic reaction software systems do not excessively duplicate each other (in fact, they probably compliment each other), as far as cited scientific journal references for specific synthetic transformations. So far, however, no objective study has been done comparing how well these commercially available synthetic reaction databases each provide comprehensive coverage of representative examples of all possible synthetic methods from the scientific literature for one or more specific types of synthetic transformations. Each synthetic reaction database has its specific emphasis, and many of them are of potential value for drug discovery research and development scientists. A list of the commercially available synthetic reaction databases is presented in Table 13., with further description of their content included as the remainder of this chapter subsection.

The CCR (Current Chemical Reactions) database (Institute for Scientific Information) reflects about 25,000–30,000 new synthetic methodology reactions abstracted by the staff at ISI each year from the scientific literature for the ISI monthly publication *Current Chemical Reactions* (Fig. 13.13). Each year's database update coverage includes about 14,000 new synthetic methods (single- and multi-step syntheses) from over 350 journals. Since 1988, coverage has also included the U.S. Patent literature (about 1,000 each year). Author journal abstracts were included beginning in 1991 (165).

The CHC (Comprehensive Heterocyclic Chemistry) database (Molecular Design Limited; ORAC Limited) is an electronic version of the heterocyclic chemistry (38,000 reactions) from Pergamon Press' eight-volume compendium *Comprehensive Heterocyclic Chemistry* (Fig. 13.16) (166). The compendium and the database encompass the scientific literature from the early 1830s through 1983, including the old German literature. The database covers important synthetic methodologies pertaining to heterocyclic compounds, focusing on three areas: synthesis of heterocyclic compounds, reactions of heterocyclic systems, and the use of heterocycles for synthesizing other molecules. The database bibliographic references include the original reaction literature references, as well as specific references to the bound volumes of *Comprehensive Heterocyclic Chemistry* (167, 168).

The ChemReact database (Springer-Verlag; InfoChem GmbH; Pool, Heller, & Milne: REACCS format) is an abstraction of 370,00 different reactions from the VINITI database (built 1975–1988 by the All-Union Institute of Scientific and Technical Information [VINITI] of the USSR Academy of Sciences and the German Zentrale Informationsverarbeitung [ZIC] from articles abstracted from over 1,000 journals) (Fig. 13.14). The entire 1,800,000 reactions in the original VINITI database can be viewed for any reaction types found in the ChemReact database. The ChemReact database reactions are drawn from 137 key scientific journals (169).

The ChemSynth database (Springer-Verlag; InfoChem GmbH; Pool, Heller & Milne: REACCS format) is an 8,000 reaction subset of the ChemReact database including only those reactions which had been reported more than once in leading journals and whose yield was at least 50% (169).

The CHIRAS database (Molecular Design Limited) is a collection of asymmetric synthesis reactions abstracted from the scientific literature by synthetic chemists in

Table 13.7   Commercially Available Synthetic Reaction Databases

Database	Vendor	Format	Description
CCR	ISI	REACCS	CCR = Current Chemical Reactions. Synthetic reactions abstracted by ISI from the current scientific and U.S. Patent literature for *Current Chemical Reactions* (1986–present).
CHC	MDL	REACCS	CHC = Comprehensive Heterocyclic Chemistry. Reactions involving heterocyclic compounds based on Pergamon Press's compendium *Comprehensive Heterocyclic Chemistry*
CHC	ORAC	ORAC	CHC = Comprehensive Heterocyclic Chemistry. See description for MDL's CHC database above and in the text.
ChemReact	Springer-Verlag, InfoChem, PH&M	REACCS	370,000 reactions abstracted from the synthetic literature by Russian and German Scientists (1975–1988).
ChemSynth	Springer-Verlag, InfoChem PH&M	REACCS	80,000 reaction subset of the ChemReact database.
CHIRAS	MDL	REACCS	Database of asymmetric syntheses abstracted from the scientific literature (1975–present).
CIRX	MDL	REACCS	CIRX = ChemInform RX. 60,000 reactions/year abstracted from the current synthetic literature and published in the journal *ChemInform* (1991–present).
CLF	MDL	REACCS	CLF = Current Literature File. Significant new and improved synthetic methods abstracted from the current literature by academic chemists for MDL.
CSM	MDL	REACCS	CSM = Current Synthetic Methods. A representative subset of MDL's CIRX database, 8,000 reactions/year.
METALYSIS	MDL	REACCS	Database of transition-metal-mediated reactions abstracted from the scientific literature (1974–present).
ORAC CORE DATABASE	ORAC	ORAC	70,000 reactions abstracted from the current and past synthetic literature by ORAC Ltd. staff and academic collaborators.
ORGSYN	MDL	REACCS	Database of *Organic Syntheses*. Verified and exceptionally reproducible synthetic reactions (1921–present).
REACCS-JSM	MDL	REACCS	Database of Derwent's *Journal of Synthetic Methods* (JSM), Reactions abstracted from the literature since 1980, using Theilheimer's selection criteria.

Table 13.7   (Continued)

Database	Vendor	Format	Description
SYNLIB Master Chemical Reaction Library	DCG	SYNLIB	69,000 reactions abstracted from the current and retrospective synthetic literature by an international consortium of academic and industrial chemists.
THEILHEIMER	MDL	REACCS	Database of W. Theilheimer's *Synthetic Methods of Organic Chemistry*; Covers the synthetic chemical literature from 1946–1980, emphasizing high-yield functional group transformations.
THEILHEIMER	ORAC	ORAC	See description for MDL's THEILHEIMER database above and in the text.

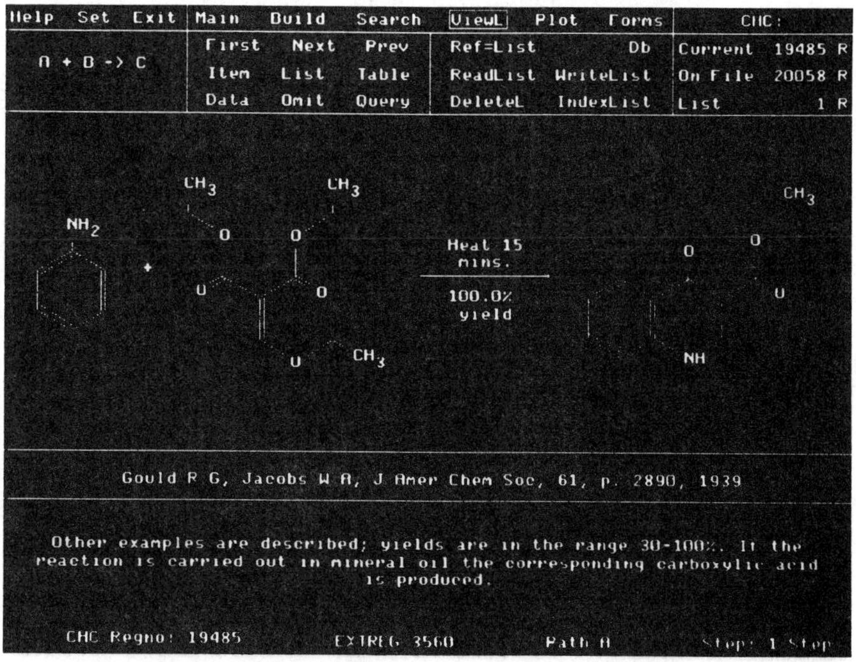

Fig. 13.16 Example of a synthetic reaction retrieved from the Molecular Design Limited REACCS CHC (Comprehensive Heterocyclic Chemistry) database.

industry and academia for Molecular Design Limited. The original database covered the asymmetric synthesis literature from 1975–1988, yielding approximately 11,000 reactions, with subsequent annual database updates. Besides the usual reaction information (reactants, products, reagents, yield, literature reference, etc.), the CHIRAS database also includes information specific to asymmetric syntheses, including method of stereochemical analysis and quantitative stereochemical information (enantiomeric excess, diastereomeric excess, optical purity, etc.). The database includes reactions with controlled absolute and relative sterochemistry (170).

The CIRX (ChemInform RX) database (Molecular Design Limited) is derived from the journal *ChemInform*, which is published weekly by the German organization Fachinformationszentrum Chemie GmbH (FIZ Chemie), Bayer AG, and the German Chemical Society. Chemists from Bayer AG and FIZ Chemie, abstract 20,000 articles each year from over 250 international journals, including 11,000 abstracts with synthetic reaction information. *ChemInform* emphasizes novel syntheses and preparative methods in organic chemistry, including: new reactions and syntheses, including enzymatic and microbial processes; application of known reactions for synthesizing new compounds or classes of compounds; improved synthetic methods and new reagents; syntheses of natural products of general importance; and syntheses of novel organo-element compounds and new catalysts. Beginning with 1991, the ChemInform RX database will include approximately 60,000 reactions per year taken from *ChemInform*, with yearly updates each covering the previous year (171).

The CLF (Current Literature File) database (Molecular Design Limited) includes novel and significantly improved synthetic methods, including multifunctional reactions, and topics of current interest to synthetic chemists. The reactions are abstracted from the current scientific literature by academic chemists for Molecular Design Limited. The CLF database covers the synthetic literature from 1983 to the present. The database is updated semi-annually with approximately 4,000 new reaction/year. Current database size is 33,000+ reactions (172, 173).

The CSM (Current Synthetic Methodology) database (Molecular Design Limited) is a representative subset of the much larger CIRX database (see above). The selection of reactions for the CSM database will focus on reactions which describe new synthetic methodologies, reactions involving use of new reagents, regio, chemo, and stereo-selective reactions carried out on

multifunctional substrates, and single step reactions. Starting with 1991, twice a year database updates will expand the CSM database by about 8,000 reactions/year (174).

The METALYSIS database (Molecular Design Limited) includes transition-metal-mediated reactions abstracted from the scientific literature. The database covers over 30 journals from 1974 to the present, providing a database of approximately 10,000 reactions that is updated yearly. The reactions emphasize the chemical activation and transformation of organic compounds by organotransition metal complexes, both catalytically and stoichiometrically (175).

The ORAC Core database (ORAC Limited) consists of over 70,000 reactions covering all areas of organic chemistry and abstracted from the current and past synthetic literature by ORAC Limited staff and a group of academic collaborators worldwide (168). Before the integration of ORAC Limitation into Molecular Design Limited, this database was updated once each year. Apparently Molecular Design Limited will be converting this database into a REACCS version in the near future.

The ORGSYN database (Molecular Design Limited) is an electronic version of the synthetic reactions in the series *Organic Syntheses* (176), Volumes 1–72, 1921–1992. The ORGSYN database is a small collection (5000 + reactions) of experimentally verified and therefore easily reproduced synthetic preparations. The database is updated annually (177).

The REACCS-JSM database (Molecular Design Limited) is an electronic version of the synthetic reactions in the *Journal of Synthetic Methods* (JSM: published by the Chemical Reaction Documentation Service, Derwent Publications Limited) (178). Beginning with Volume 6 in 1980, the REACCS-JSM database takes up where the Theilheimer database (see below) leaves off. Reactions are included using the selection criteria established by Theilheimer for new synthetic procedures, high-yield functional group transformations, and improvements to existing synthetic methods. In addition, the REACCS-JSM database includes the worldwide patent literature information found in JSM. The database is updated yearly with approximately 3000 new reactions abstracted from the patent literature and 150 international journals. Current database size is about 36,000 reactions (179).

The SYNLIB Master Chemical Reaction Library database (Distributed Chemical Graphics, Inc.) consists of over 69,000 reactions (as of January 1991) abstracted from the current and retrospective synthetic literature by an international consortium of academic and industrial chemists. The emphasis for this database is the building of a high quality collection of important and useful reactions representative of advances in synthetic chemistry. Updated once each year, the database continues to grow by approximately 5000 new entries each year (about 3000 reactions from the retrospective literature and about 2000 reaction from the current literature (180, 181).

The Theilheimer database (Molecular Design Limited; ORAC Limited) is an electronic version of the synthetic reactions in W. Theilheimer's compendium *Synthetic Methods of Organic Chemistry* (182). The database covers volumes 1–35 (1946–1981): 46,818 reactions for the REACCS database and 41,873 reactions for the ORAC database (168, 183). Theilheimer's annual synthetic literature abstracts has emphasized novel and improved synthetic methods, including high-yield functional group transformations.

8 OTHER CHEMICAL INFORMATION COMPUTING SOFTWARE

8.1 Microcomputer Chemical Information Computing Software

All of the major 2D chemical, 3D chemical, and synthetic reaction information management software systems described in the preceding sections are extensively used in drug discovery research at most large- and medium-sized pharmaceutical companies worldwide. This usage is often not the case (especially for the 2D chemical information management software systems) at many smaller pharmaceutical companies and in academic laboratories for a number of reasons. First, the software and database licensing costs can be prohibitive and not cost-justifiable for the relatively small drug discovery research and development organizations at a small company or at an academic institution. The relatively small chemical information management needs of these smaller drug discovery organizations often do not require the more complex and sophisticated chemical information handling capabilities of such software nor are these smaller organizations able to justify the manpower needed to administer such systems and create complex customized applications. Fortunately there are a number of relatively inexpensive yet capable microcomputer-based (IBM-compatible PC and/or Macintosh) chemical information management systems that are more suitable for use by small companies or academic research laboratories (or even for an individual chemist) (184–188).

The different microcomputer-based 2D chemical information management software packages vary considerably in their capabilities but most incorporate the basic chemical intelligence and most crucial capabilities of the large 2D commercial systems. This capability usually includes:

- Interactive chemical structure drawing for compound entry
- Registration of chemical structures and associated compound data into chemical databases
- Exact structure, substructure, and associated compound data searching of the chemical databases
- Generation of combined structure and

associated data reports for output to laser printers.

These capabilities are usually sufficient for the chemical information management of most smaller drug discovery research organizations, laboratories, or individual chemists. The microcomputer-based systems usually lack many of the more complex software capabilities of the larger commercial systems, such as seamless interfaces to relational software systems and internal high-level software languages for development of customized applications.

In the area of 2D chemical information management, these microcomputer-based software systems include:

- ChemBase (Molecular Design Limited) is probably the most sophisticated of these microcomputer-based packages (53, 189–191). ChemBase is unique in that it includes capabilities for both 2D chemical information and synthetic reaction information management/databases/searching. It runs on IBM-compatible PC under MS DOS. ChemBase provides the user considerable capabilities for the creation of customized chemical structure/data screens and reports. Not surprisingly, ChemBase can read and write standard Molecular Design Limited MACCS-II and REACCS compound/reaction chemical connection table files (13). ChemBase can be linked with MACCS-II running on minicomputer/mainframe CPU's. A few pharmaceutical companies actually do their initial new proprietary chemical entity registration in ChemBase. Then (usually each night) chemical structure/data files are moved from ChemBase on the PC to MACCS-II on a minicomputer/mainframe CPU for registration into the complete MACCS-II corporate proprietary chemical database.
- PSIDOM/PsiBase/PsiGen (Hampden

Data Services Ltd.) (186, 187) software runs on IBM-compatible PCs under MS DOS or Microsoft Windows. The PsiGen module of PSIDOM is used for structure input and display. The PsiBase Module of PSIDOM permits chemical structure and substructure searching of PSIDOM databases.

- HTSS/TREE (IBM-compatible PC's; Technical Database Services, Inc.) (187, 192).
- ChemFinder (Cambridge Scientific Computing, Inc. (193–195) runs on Macintoshs, with availability planned for IBM-compatible PCs under Microsoft Windows and for UNIX workstations. This software allows for searching of chemical structure files by chemical structure or substructure. ChemFinder is part of ChemOffice, a series of microcomputer-based products marketed by Cambridge Scientific Computing, Inc. and includes the quite popular software packages ChemDraw and Chem3D (with which ChemFinder is totally compatible (Fig. 13.17).

A number of these microcomputer chemical information computing software packages (and a number of other microcomputer software packages of interest to chemists) are available from ACS software at significant discounts for ACS members and academics. Also of interest in this area of microcomputer-based chemical information computing software are the CD-ROM chemical information databases with associated search software (see Section 8.3), as well as the microcomputer-based chemically intelligent computing software packages described in Section 8.2.

8.2 Chemically Intelligent Computing Software

In this chapter the phrase "chemically intelligent computing software" is used to

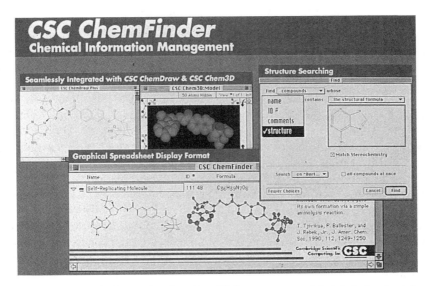

Fig. 13.17 Cambridge Scientific Computing, Inc. ChemFinder screens on a Macintosh showing integration with ChemDraw and Chem 3D.

describe software systems which contain a knowledge or understanding not just of chemical structures but also their graphical display. This chapter has been extended to include the manipulation, analysis, comparison, and searching of such chemical structure information. This knowledge certainly would describe the 2D and 3D chemical information computing software systems and synthetic reaction software systems covered in earlier sections of this chapter. Without trying to venture into the areas of molecular modeling, computational drug design, and quantitative structure-activity relationships (QSAR), topics adequately covered in other chapters there are also a number of other chemically intelligent computing systems which are useful for predicting molecular physical, chemical, or bioactivity properties of interest to medicinal chemists and other scientists involved in the drug discovery process.

Most of these chemically intelligent software systems utilize a standard 2D molecular structure, for example, information on atoms, bonds, stereochemistry, charges, etc.) as their primary data input. 2D struc-

tures are usually provided by the user either by graphically drawing the structure, by textual input of a linear string representation for the molecule, or from a computer file containing a chemical structure connection table. Once the specific predictive task is defined, the software then usually performs a number of complex analyses of the chemical structure (based on the software's "chemical intelligence"), identifying (as needed) specific molecular structure characteristics. For example, this process could include identification of specific substructural fragments (e.g., presence or absence of an aliphatic nitro group), as well as identification of chemical substructure inter-relationships (e.g., are there strong electron attracting substituents on the same aromatic ring as a carboxyl group). Most of these chemically intelligent software systems at this point then attempt to employ well-established computational algorithms or methodologies for their predictions or estimations. These predictive models or methodologies tend to be fairly simple in their actual computations, but are often quite complex in their logic and rationale for molecular physical, chemical, or bioactivity prediction based on chemical structure. These chemically intelligent computing systems range all the way from true expert systems based on artificial intelligence software to computational implementation of simple predictive models.

This area of chemically intelligent computing software systems includes a broad diversity of applications that are of interest for scientists involved in the drug discovery and development process. This is also an area of very active research (academic and industrial) for developing new chemical computing methodologies and approaches. In addition, both large and small information and software vendors have been rapidly developing and introducing a wide variety of such chemically intelligent computing systems as software products. While it is impossible to exhaustively describe all of these new software products, a list of the more established and successful of these predictive software systems is provided in Table 13.8. This list is meant to provide an overview of the amazing broad diversity of chemically intelligent computing systems that have been introduced in the last few years, and which may be of specific interest and relevance to scientists involved in drug discovery and development research (both in academia and the pharmaceutical industry). Each of these software systems is described in some detail in the chapter sub-sections below.

8.2.1 SAR SPREADSHEETS. The structure–activity relationship (SAR) table is a primary mechanism whereby drug discovery scientists (especially medicinal chemists) are able to organize, analyze, and interpret relationships between variations in chemical structure, biological activity, and molecular physical/chemical properties for a series of compounds. (For example, see any current issue of *J. Med. Chem.* or *Eur. J. Med. Chem.*). This table is usually applied to an analog series of structures for an active set of compounds. The SAR table

has also proven to be an extremely effective means for medicinal chemists and biologists (in particular with typical interdisciplinary drug discovery R&D teams in the pharmaceutical industry) to share SAR data for series of potentially new drug molecules. The increasing sophistication in chemically intelligent computing software in the last several years has made possible the introduction of software systems capable of automatically analyzing a series of chemical structures and (with input of additional chemical or biological data) to generate such SAR tables. Although an almost unlimited variety of formats is possible for such SAR tables, typically they display the following features:

- Each row represents one compound
- Each column represents one compound feature (structure, substituents, compound data such as compound # or notebook references, bioactivity data, physical/chemical property data, etc.).
- The chemical structure can consist of a 2D graphical presentation of each complete chemical structure. More typically, a parent substructure (with indicated substituent positions and/or linking groups) is presented graphically at the top of the SAR table. In this case, one or more columns of the SAR table indicate the variations in the chemical structures, each handling a single substituent position or linking group.

In terms of software for generating SAR tables, the term "SAR spreadsheet" should probably be reserved for software that incorporates appropriate "hot-wired" interfaces to 2D chemical structure databases (which typically are used for storage of chemical structures and chemical compound data) and to relational software databases (which typically are used for storage of other information; for example, bioactivity data, sample inventory data,

Table 13.8 Some Chemically Intelligent Computing Software Systems

Software	Vendor	Description
MarkOut	Fraser Williams	Generation of chemical structure/chemical property/biological activity SAR (structure–activity relationship) tables; VAX/VMS or IBM mainframe-based.
Molecule Spreadsheet	MDL	Generation of chemical structure/chemical property/biological activity SAR (structure–activity relationship) tables; VAX/VMS or IBM mainframe-based.
Molecular Spreadsheet	TRIPOS	Generation of chemical structure/chemical property/biological activity SAR (structure-activity relationship) tables; VAX/VMS, PC, Macintosh, and UNIX workstation-based.
PCMODELS	Daylight	CLOGP-3 = Estimation of n-octanol-water partition coefficients for organic compounds (Log P values). CMR = molar refractivity prediction for organic compounds MR values; VAX/VMS or UNIX workstation-based.
PRO-LOGP	CompuDrug	Estimation of n-octanol/water partition coefficients (Log P values). PC or VAX/VMS-based.
PKALC	CompuDrug	Estimation of pK_a values for organic compounds. PC-based.
CHEMEST	TDS	Estimation of a wide variety of physical and chemical properties for organic comounds; PC or VAX/VMS-based.
TOPKAT	HDI	Application of QSAR models for prediction/estimation of toxicity for organic compounds; PC or VAX/VMS-based.
MetabolExpert	CompuDrug	Expert system for drug metabolism prediction; PC or VAX/VMS-based.
AUTONOM	Springer-Verlag	Generation of IUPAC systematic nomenclature of organic compounds based on chemical structure; PC-based.
SANDRA	Springer-Verlag	Determination of location of compounds in *The Beilstein Handbook of Organic Chemistry*, based on input chemical structure; PC-based.

etc.). (The term "hot-wired" interfaces is taken here to mean that the software is able to directly extract the desired structures and data from the databases, without the user needing to generate intermediate computer files containing the desired structures and data). An ideal SAR spreadsheet might also contain "hot-wired" connections to software for estimating molecular physical-chemical properties. The continuing developments in current SAR table and spreadsheet generating software are a significant step in the complex integration of diverse information sources and resources in the drug discovery and development process. The software capabilities of the commercial 2D chemical information management software systems for allowing creation of customized interfaces, reports, and applications are often used at drug companies to generate such SAR spreadsheets. In addition, several examples of currently available software systems specifically for generating molecular SAR Tables or spreadsheets are described in the following chapter subsections.

8.2.1.1 *MarkOut*. MarkOut (Fraser Williams Ltd.) was one of the first chemically intelligent commercial software systems (PC or VAX/VMS based) for the generation of structure activity relationship (SAR) tables (196, 197). Typically MarkOut has been for use with a list of chemical structures from an in-house 2D chemical structure database (e.g., MACCS-II, OSAC, or DARC: greater MarkOut software customization is required for extraction of structures from MACCS-II and OSAC databases than from DARC databases, for which there is a simpler and more integrated MarkOut chemical structure interface). Given a list of structures from an in-house 2D chemical structure database (or a computer file of chemical structure connection tables), MarkOut first reads in the complete set of chemical structures. This software then employs there specific steps in its analysis of these structures for subsequent generation of the SAR table: (A) the complete set of structures is analyzed in order to identify the maximum common substructure; (B) the appropriate and smallest number of substituent positions for the common substructure are identified; and (C) the specific substituents for each substituent position for each structure are identified based on a pre-defined substituent library, which may be supplemented with additional user-defined substituents. (Within the context of MarkOut software, substituent positions and substituent include both substituent groups attached to a common substructure as well as substructural linking groups with-

in a common substructure such as $-O-$, $-CH_2-$, $-NH-$.

The MarkOut software user may select from 3 different strategies for deriving the chemical structure analyses for the SAR table: (1) the MarkOut software is allowed to perform a completely automated analysis of the structures, performing all of steps A to C above, identifying the common substructure, substituent positions, and substituents for each compound; (2) the user provides the common substructure and MarkOut then automatically performs steps B and C above, identifying substituent positions and the specific substituents for each compound; or (3) the user provides a common substructure and identification of the substituent positions and MarkOut then automatically performs step C above, identifying the specific substituents for each compound. MarkOut then presents to the user a basic structure analysis table, which the user may manipulate (sorting, deleting entries, etc.) and to which the user may specify the addition of additional columns (i.e., compound, bioactivity, and physical/chemical data for each structure). Additional data is typically imported from formatted computer files which the user has created from other information sources chemical database, relational database, chemical property prediction software, etc.). This process basically completes the MarkOut SAR Table generation, which can be viewed on-line at a graphics computer terminal or which may output to a computer file for hardcopy laser printer reports (Fig. 13.18) or inclusion in external PC WP documents. MarkOut also provides the capability for the user to modify/specify the exact formatting of its SAR table reports.

8.2.1.2 *Molecule Spreadsheet (MDL)*. Molecule Spreadsheet (Molecular Design Limited) is a true SAR spreadsheet (as described above), allowing direct incorporation of chemical structures and data

| MARKOUT Version 2.10; (C) Copyright 1990 Fraser Williams. | 28-OCT-1992 18:01 |

HSV1 Thymidine Kinase Inhibition

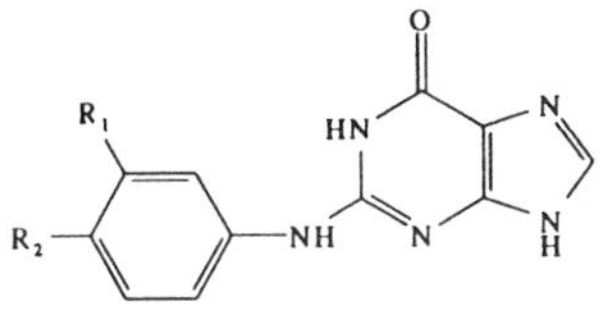

Compd #	R 1	R 2	Pi-R1	Pi-R2	Log(1/IC50)
01	CF3	H	0.88	0.00	6.82
03	H	Br	0.00	0.86	6.00
04	CH2Br	H	0.79	0.00	6.00
07	Cl	H	0.71	0.00	5.82
08	Br	H	0.86	0.00	5.82
10	Br	Br	0.86	0.86	5.52
12	CN	H	-0.57	0.00	5.30
13	Et	Me	1.02	0.56	5.16
15	H	H	0.00	0.00	5.10
16	Cl	Me	0.71	0.56	4.92
18	H	Et	0.00	1.02	4.70
22	H	CF3	0.00	0.88	4.52
26	H	I	0.00	1.12	4.40
32	H	OH	0.00	-0.67	3.85

Fig. 13.18 A MarkOut-generated SAR (structure–activity relationship) table for the inhibition of herpes simplex virus type 11 (HSV1) thymidine kinase by a series of substituted N^2-phenylguanines: Pi–R1 and Pi–R2 values are Hansch π hydrophobic substituent parameters (198) for the R_1 and R_2 substituent groups. Log (1/IC50) values refer to concentrations of inhibitor necessary to inhibit the enzyme 50% under standard conditions. Chemical structures, π substituent parameters, and log (1/IC_{50}) data were taken from Tables II and III of ref. 199.

from chemical databases and from relational databases (200–202). The Molecule Spreadsheet software is actually a MACCS-II sequence language applications program, including use of the MACCS-II sequence language capabilities for analysis of the chemical structures (and their substructures) for the SAR tables it produces (Fig. 13.19). The program uses three menus that correspond to three basic tasks that the user must perform in order to generate the SAR spreadsheets (204, 205). The first menu permits definition of the spreadsheet organization, including specification of:

- The MACCS-II and relational databases to be accessed.
- The specific fields (including chemical structure) from the databases to be included in the datasheet.
- Definition of new fields (i.e. additional datasheet columns) that are mathematical, string manipulation, or relational functions of other data fields.

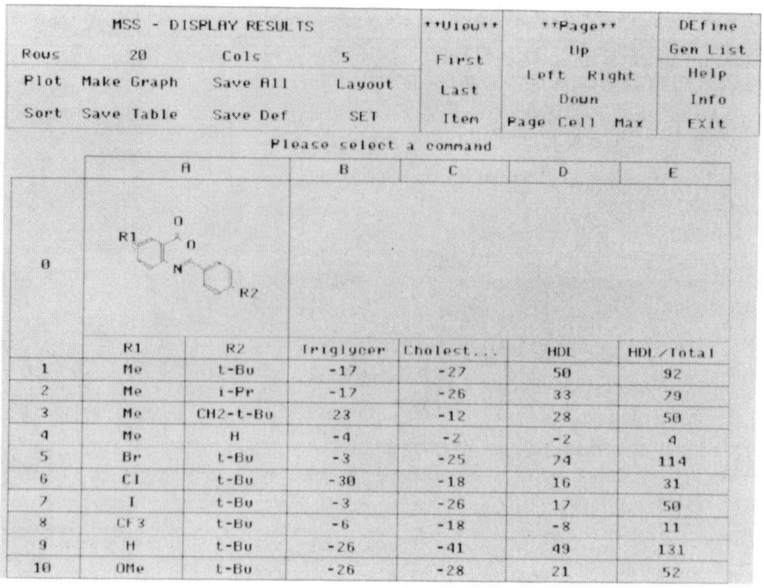

MSS - DISPLAY RESULTS					**View**	**Page**	DEfine
Rows	20	Cols		5	First	Up	Gen List
Plot	Make Graph	Save All		Layout	Last	Left Right	Help
						Down	Info
Sort	Save Table	Save Def		SET	Item	Page Cell Max	Exit

Please select a command

	A	B	C	D	E
0	R1 ⬡ O N R2				

	R1	R2	Triglycer	Cholest...	HDL	HDL/Total
1	Me	t-Bu	-17	-27	50	92
2	Me	i-Pr	-17	-26	33	79
3	Me	CH2-t-Bu	23	-12	28	50
4	Me	H	-4	-2	-2	4
5	Br	t-Bu	-3	-25	74	114
6	Cl	t-Bu	-30	-18	16	31
7	I	t-Bu	-3	-26	17	50
8	CF3	t-Bu	-6	-18	-8	11
9	H	t-Bu	-26	-41	49	131
10	OMe	t-Bu	-26	-28	21	52

Fig. 13.19 Molecular Design Limited Molecule Spreadsheet (MSS) screen showing a chemical structure–biological activity SAR (structure–activity relationship): In this example (data from ref. 203), a group of high density lipoprotein (HDL) elevators is compared for their effect on the plasma levels (by percentage change) of triglycerides, total cholesterol, HDL, and HDL/total cholesterol.

- Saving the spreadsheet definition to a computer file.

The second menu allows the user to generate a list of compounds from the MACCS-II database that will be used for the SAR table, including:

- Drawing a chemical structure search query and then searching the MACCS-II database for compounds which match the query.
- Searching the MACCS-II database or the relational database textual and numeric data fields.
- Reviewing the list of MACCS-II database compounds resulting from the search(es), with the user allowed to deleted unwanted compounds from the list.

The third menu allows viewing, modifying, and saving of the completed SAR spreadsheet, including:

- Graphically browsing through the SAR spreadsheet.
- Saving the SAR datasheet to a computer file.
- Sending a plot of the SAR spreadsheet to a laser printer.

For each chemical structure on the compound list, one of the following (from the MACCS-II database) can be included in the SAR spreadsheet:

- The compound chemical name.
- The complete chemical structure.
- Specific substituents in individual columns. (In this case, the user is required to provide a common substructure and to identify the substituent positions. The software is then able to automatically identify the substituents, based on a library of substituent translation files).

When actually searching a MACCS-II database from within Molecule Spreadsheet for a list of chemical structures, the user is allowed to perform all the substructure search types normally allowed in MACCS-II, including substructure searches, similarity searches, and substructure searches employing the additional query specification capabilities available with the MACCS-II Power Search and Substance Modules. Additionally, the Molecule Spreadsheet software allows the user a fair amount of flexibility for arranging the data fields on the spreadsheet, sorting the datasheet entries based on data in one or more of the data fields, and modifying the column widths and row heights. The Molecule Spreadsheet software even allows the user to select either a horizontal orientation (each row represents a compound and each column represents a chemical structure, a substitution, or a data field) or a vertical orientation (row and column definitions now reversed). Note that (unlike Mark-Out) for a list of compounds from a MACCS-II database, Molecule Spreadsheet does not itself automatically perform a complete structure/substructure analysis in order to define the largest common substructure and to identify the substituent positions. The common substructure and substituent position definitions are left to the user. The Molecule Spreadsheet does not readily permit incorporation or additional compound data from computer files or from physical/chemical property prediction software (although this inclusion can be accomplished with some in-house customization).

8.2.1.3 *Molecular Spreadsheet* (*TRIPOS*).
Molecular Spreadsheet (TRIPOS Associates, Inc.; VAX, PC, Macintosh, or UNIX workstation based) is the most complex and sophisticated of the SAR spreadsheet software systems (206). Molecular Spreadsheet has been made an integrated part of the SYBYL molecular modeling system (TRIPOS Associates, Inc.) (207). In addition, Molecular Spreadsheet is closely integrated with the SYBYL/2DB UNITY software and 2D/3D chemical structure databases. The basic and more advanced features and capabilities of Molecular Spreadsheet include the following:

- Definition of a list of compounds to be included from SYBYL/3DB Unity 2D/3D chemical structure databases (with full access to the SYBYL/3DB UNITY chemical structure search capabilities for generating such a list).

- Inclusion of complete compound structures and/or automatically identified substituents for a common substructure.

- Direct inclusion of numeric and textual data fields from SYBYL/3DB UNITY 2D/3D chemical structure databases and from relational databases to which the Molecular Spreadsheet is interfaced.

- Full capabilities for modification of the spread sheet definition (e.g. addition or deletion of columns) and addition/deletion of compounds (rows) from the datasheet.

- Inclusion as spreadsheet columns of approximately 40 predefined and automatically generated molecular metrics, based on properties such as geometry, charge distributions, substituent properties, etc.

- A variety of statistical methodologies for analysis of spreadsheet data.

- Interactive generation of several sophisticated graphic presentations of spreadsheet data.

- Inclusion of user defined data fields, as well as import of data from external software (e.g. for prediction of molecular physical/chemical properties), using the SYBYL programming language (SPL).

- Interactive browsing of a spreadsheet filled with chemical structures and data.

- Availability of a sophisticated report

generator for creating customized SAR reports from the spreadsheet.

- Direct interfacing to all the molecular visualization, manipulation, and computational techniques of the SYBYL molecular modeling software.

Inclusion of all this functionality into Molecular Spreadsheet makes it an extremely powerful and flexible drug discovery research tool. Much of the value of Molecular Spreadsheet lies in its essentially seamless integration with SYBYL and the other TRIPOS molecular modeling software. It remains to be seen whether Molecular Spreadsheet will be primarily a sophisticated integrated research tool used by scientists experienced with molecular modeling, drug design, and the SYBYL software, or whether it will also be accepted as a more general, integrated research tool used by a much broader group of R&D scientists involved in the drug discovery process (especially at pharmaceutical companies).

8.2.2 LOG *P* ESTIMATION. The *n*-octanol/water partition coefficient (Log *P*) of organic compounds has proven to be one of the most significant and successful molecular physical/properties used in drug design, discovery, and development (198). Initially, estimation of Log *P* values were made (usually manually) using the Hansch additivity approach:

$$\text{Log } P(\text{Compound}) = \text{Log } P(\text{Unsubstituted}$$

$$\text{Parent Compound}) + \sum \pi \text{ (Substituents)}$$

where π is a substituent constant measuring the hydrophobicity of a substituent. Subsequently a variety of different approaches have been evaluated for estimating Log *P* values, but the most successful of

these has been using the substructural fragment methodology (65):

$$\text{Log } P(\text{Compound}) = \sum \text{ (Substructural}$$

$$\text{Fragment Contributions)} + \sum \text{ (Correction}$$

$$\text{Factors)}$$

Several chemically intelligent computer software implementations for automated Log *P* estimation for organic compounds have been developed and are used frequently in drug discovery and development research, as described in the following chapter subsections.

8.2.2.1 *PCMODELS (CLOGP*-3). CLOGP-3, one of the physical–chemical property prediction models of the PCMODELS software (Daylight Chemical Information Systems, Inc.; VAX/VMS based), estimates *n*-octanol-water Log *P* values, based on algorithms developed by the Pomona College Medicinal Chemistry Project (65, 66, 83). The software program, CLOGP, for the prediction of Log *P* values was actually originally implemented in a fairly simple, hard-wired, but successful version of the fragment method estimation algorithm (208). Subsequently the very popular CLOGP-3 software program for *n*-octanol/water Log *P* estimation by the fragment methodology of Leo (65) was implemented by the Pomona College Medicinal Chemistry Project (66). The success of this approach lies not only in the fragment method for Log *P* calculation, but also in the flexible and powerful chemically intelligent computing software tools developed at the Pomona Medicinal Chemistry Project (24). Daylight Chemical Information Systems, Inc. has subsequently taken over continued development and commercial distribution of the CLOGP-3 software and the chemically intelligent computing software tools. The continued development and enhancement of the

CLOGP-3 Log P prediction algorithm and knowledge base still resides with the Pomona College Medicinal Chemistry Project.

The rule base for CLOGP-3 consists of the substructural analysis of a chemical structure, which identification of the substructural fragments and correction factors needed for the Log P calculation. The knowledge base for CLOGP-3 consists of the substructural fragment values and the correction factor values. These values may be supplemented with new values by the user (i.e., new substructural fragment values and correction factor values may be added to the CLOGP-3 knowledge base).

The CLOGP-3 software provides an unusual, but extremely fast and friendly user software interface for its n-octanol/water Log P estimations. Chemical structures may be entered using the SMILES linear string chemical structure notation (59–61), can be graphically drawn, or can be read in from chemical structure connection table computer files. The CLOGP-3 software is unusual (compared to most other chemically intelligent computing software) in that it utilizes its own depiction algorithm to generate and display a 2D chemical structure based solely on the chemical connection table of the compound (62). The chemical structure is automatically substructurally analyzed by the CLOGP-3 software, and the Log P value is calculated using the appropriate substructural fragment values and correction factors. CLOGP-3 then generates a report, displaying the structure, the calculated Log P estimate, and information regarding the various substructural fragments and correction values used in the estimation (Fig. 13.20). The THOR POMONA92 database

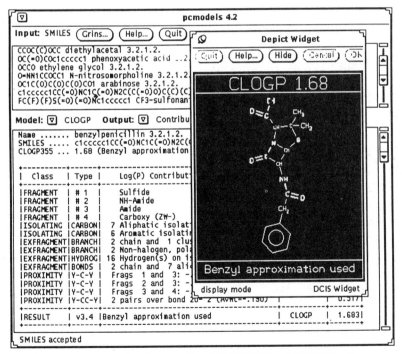

Fig. 13.20 Daylight Chemical Information Systems, Inc. PCMODELS and DEPICT software screens showing a CLOGP-3 estimation of the Log P (1-octanol/water partition coefficient) value for benzylpenicillin: Note that the PCMODELS software also provides a detailed description of the software's analysis of the chemical structure and the substructural fragment contributions and correction terms used to calculate the Log P estimate.

(see Section 3.2 above) is also searched by CLOGP-3 to determine if it contains any reliable *n*-octanol/water Log *P* values from the scientific literature for the structure. If available, that experimental Log *P* value is also included in the CLOGP-3 report. The CLOGP-3 reports can also be output to computer files for subsequent laser printer hardcopy output, if the user so desires.

The *n*-octanol-water partition coefficient has consistently proven to be a valuable physical/chemical molecular parameter for drug discovery scientists when used both for interpreting and predicting drug bioactivity (209, 210). This capability includes not only quantitative modeling applications (e.g., quantitative structure-activity relationship studies), but also qualitative SAR analyses of drug bioactivity/physical property relationships. Drug bioactivity effects often influenced by molecular hydrophobicity (as modeled by Log *P*) include absorption, biodistribution, receptor binding, excretion, etc. The importance of Log *P* in influencing so many facets of drug bioactivity makes a knowledge of its quantitative value and variation within an active analog set of compounds of obvious importance to scientists throughout the drug discovery, design, and development process. Although experimental methodologies are well established for the direct measurement of Log *P* values, the usual factors of time and cost require that the majority of Log *P* values analyzed by drug discovery scientists must be theoretically estimated (with chemically intelligent software such as CLOGP-3) (211).

The PCMODELS software (Daylight Chemical Information Software Systems, Inc.) also incorporates the CMR software. CMR, using substructural analysis and summation of fragment terms (much like the CLOGP-3 software), calculates estimates of molar refractivity for organic compounds. Also, this molar refractivity estimation methodology has been developed and implemented at The Pomona College Medicinal Chemistry Project using the chemically intelligent computing software tools developed there. Molecular and substituent molar refractivity (MR) parameter values are used primarily in QSAR studies as a model for combined molecular bulk and polarizability interactions of drug molecules with biological macromolecules (i.e., as an estimator of polar, as opposed to hydrophobic, interactions) (198).

8.2.2.2 *PRO-LOGP.* PRO-LOGP (CompuDrug NA, Inc.) is an artificial intelligence (AI) rule-based expert software system (PC or VAX/VMS based and developed in the PROLOG AI language) for the estimation of partition coefficients (Log *P* values) of organic molecules (212). This software package uses Rekker's fragment method (213–215) to provide *n*-octanol-water partition coefficient predictions for organic compounds. Like the Leo CLOGP-3 Log *P* estimation methodology (65, 198), Rekker's original fragment method for Log *P* prediction utilizes the summation of the contributions of specified substructural fragments in a chemical structure to provide its Log *P* estimation. It is a simpler algorithm, however, without a number of the more complex features of the Leo method (e.g., contributions for bonds, branching, electronic effects). Rekker has introduced the use of correction terms in his Log *P* estimation methodology, including corrections for proximity of effects of polar groups, conjugated double bonds, aryl–aryl conjugation, aromatic cross conjugation, and aromatic unit condensation (216). These additional features have been incorporated into another PC based PROLOG AI expert system for Log *P* estimation using Rekker's methodology (217).

Chemical structures can be entered into the PRO-LOGP software by the user either graphically or as chemical connection table file. The program then automatically analyzes the chemical structure and its substructures and then calculates the estimated partition coefficient value. PRO-LOGP finally generates a report which graphically depicts the structure and summarizes the estimated $\text{Log} P$ calculation. The knowledge base of PRO-LOGP (its substructural fragment values and correction factor values) can be added to by the user. Obviously, the same comments made above regarding the use and value of the GLOGP-3 software for partition coefficient estimation and use in drug discovery and development apply for the PRO-LOGP expert software system.

8.2.3 PKALC.

PKALC (CompuDrug NA, Inc.) is an expert PC-based software program which predicts acid-base dissociation constants (pK_a values) for organic compounds using Hammett and Taft linear free energy relationship equations (218), by the methodologies described by Perrin et al. (219). This software allows the user to graphically draw a molecule or to read in an MDL-formatted MOLFILE chemical structure connection table (13). After analyzing the chemical structure and comparing it with available models, the software attempts to predict the compound pK_a:

$$pK_a = pK_a^0 - \rho \sum \sigma$$

where $pK_a^0 =$ the acid/base dissociation constant for the unsubstituted parent structure, $\rho =$ the linear free energy relationship constant indicating the sensitivity of the parent molecule dissociation constant to the electronic effects of substituents, and $\sum \sigma =$ the sum of Hammett or Taft substituents constants, which reflect the electronic effects of the substituents. The software allows some extension beyond the basic Hammett and Taft linear free energy relationships models by applying simple "rules of thumb" (e.g. σ estimation in some cases if the experimentally derived σ constant is not available for a substituent,

extension of simple Hammett equations for some polyaromatic acids/bases by the method of Dewar and Grisdale (220–223)). The program is capable of handling structures with multiple acidic/basic centers, and a statistical factor is applied to correct pK_a values for compounds with multiple equivalent acidic/basic sites. Despite the chemical intelligence and predictive capabilities of the software, the user must still be careful and aware that PKALC may fail or give erroneous results in a number of more complex acid/base situations: e.g., cis and trans isomer differences, covalent hydration, keto–enol tautomerism, lack of an appropriate Taft/Hammett equation or missing σ value(s). The software is also capable of producing hardcopy graphics reports. The more sophisticated user can also modify the program's knowledge base, which includes parent structures and data needed for the Hammett and Taft linear free energy equation definitions, as well as substituent substructures and data needed for the Hammett and Taft σ constant definitions.

8.2.4 CHEMEST.

CHEMEST (Technical Database Services, Inc.) is a PC or VAX/VMS software package that calculates 11 different physical, chemical, and environmental properties for a wide variety of classes of organic compounds (224). The software, developed by Arthur D. Little, Inc., in part is under contract with the U.S. Environmental Protection Agency and the U.S. Army (225). The software is a basic implementation of 36 property estimations methods based on the compilation of Lyman et al. (226). Of particular interest to drug discovery and development scientists, the software incorporates a number of well-established computational models for prediction of water solubility, boiling point, melting point, vapor pressure, and pK_a for organic compounds. Unlike the other chemically intelligent computing software described in this chapter, CHEMEST does not utilize 2D chemical structures (i.e., chemical connection table data) and their analysis for its implementation of the physical/chemical property estimation methods. Instead CHEMEST relies on a textual dialogue with the user to obtain sufficient physical, chemical, and substructural information and analysis regarding the compound so that the software can apply the appropriate parameters and the correct property prediction model. Lastly, CHEMEST generates a textual terminal or computer file report, including the predicted value for the physical/chemical property, information on how the software calculated the predicted value, and some estimate of error for the prediction.

Many of the CHEMEST physical/chemical property prediction models actually require significant knowledge by the user of the models, if the software is to be adequately and correctly used. For this reason, availability and consultation by the user to the CHEMEST User's Guide (224) and ideally also to Lyman's book (226) are practically essential. Based on current trends in the development of chemically intelligent software for physical/chemical property prediction (e.g., CLOGP-3), it can be anticipated that more sophisticated software will be developed in the future which can predict these properties in a more automated manner (i.e. with 2D chemical structure input and automated substructure/substructure analysis for the prediction models, relying only minimally on user input).

8.2.5 TOPKAT. TOPKAT (Health Designs, Inc.) is a PC or VAX/VMS software package for the estimation of toxic, environmental, biological, and other effects of chemicals, based on compound structure and statistically-derived QSAR (quantitative structure-activity relationship) models. Of particular interest for drug discovery and development, separate models have been developed and incorporated into

TOPKAT to estimate carcinogenicity (227–232), mutagenicity (Ames test) (231, 233, 234), teratogenicity (228, 235), rat oral LD50 (236, 237), and rabbit eye and skin irritancy (Draize) (338, 239) for organic compounds. Each of the TOPKAT models has been developed through a series of similar steps (228, 232, 240). First a series of compounds is selected which have well-documented experimental data (usually from public sources; for example, the EPA) for a specific biological effect. A number of parameters (based on chemical structure) are then derived for each compound as molecular properties or characteristics which may correlate with the specific biological effect. These parameters include keys to indicate the presence of specific substructural fragments, molecular connectivity indices (241), topological shape-descriptive indices (242, 243), and some electronic/atomic charge parameters (233, 243–245). Appropriate statistical correlation procedures (including stepwise discriminant analysis, multiple regression analysis, and cross-validation) are then used to generate a final predictive model which contains those parameters which statistically best correlate with specific observed biological effect for the set of compounds.

Chemical structures can be entered into the TOPKAT software by the user either graphically, as a linear SMILES string with automatic graphical structure depiction (based on the Daylight Chemical Information Systems SMILES interpreter and DEPICT software) (24, 60–62), or as a chemical connection table file. The program then automatically analyzes the chemical structure, generates the appropriate parameter values, and calculates the estimated biological activity for the selected TOPKAT predictive model. TOPKAT finally generates a report (Fig. 13.21), which graphically depicts the structure and summarizes the estimated biological activity (including information on the reliability of

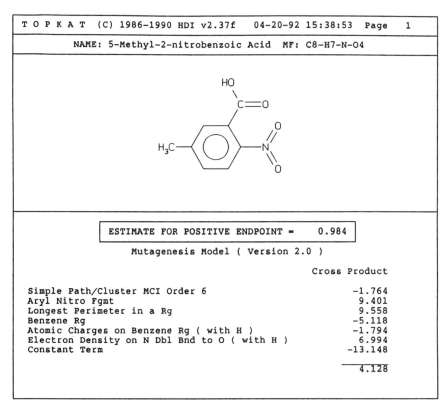

```
T O P K A T  (C) 1986-1990 HDI v2.37f    04-20-92 15:38:53  Page   1

         NAME: 5-Methyl-2-nitrobenzoic Acid  MF: C8-H7-N-O4
```

```
              ┌──────────────────────────────────────────────┐
              │  ESTIMATE FOR POSITIVE ENDPOINT =   0.984      │
              └──────────────────────────────────────────────┘
                   Mutagenesis Model ( Version 2.0 )

                                                    Cross Product

        Simple Path/Cluster MCI Order 6                  -1.764
        Aryl Nitro Fgmt                                   9.401
        Longest Perimeter in a Rg                         9.558
        Benzene Rg                                       -5.118
        Atomic Charges on Benzene Rg ( with H )          -1.794
        Electron Density on N Dbl Bnd to O ( with H )     6.994
        Constant Term                                   -13.148
                                                    ─────────────
                                                         4.128
```

Fig. 13.21 The first page of a typical TOPKAT toxicity report, in this case predicting a 98.4% probability that 5-methyl-2-nitrobenzoic acid is a mutagen. Also listed are the various substructural fragments and molecular property parameters found in the structure and in the TOPKAT mutagenicity model and their contributions which were used for the mutagenicity prediction. Subsequent to this TOPKAT mutagenicity prediction prediction, this compound was indeed found to be mutagenic (Ames test).

the estimate and the parameters used for the estimate). Additional report data with graphical structures define in more extensive detail the exact molecular features used (or excluded) for the bioactivity prediction (Fig. 13.22).

Chemically intelligent software (such as TOPKAT) for the prediction or estimation of biotoxicity for compounds based on chemical structure could prove extremely valuable for medicinal chemists in several ways: The results from the predictive models could be used to prioritize testing schedules for novel compounds; to suggest or recommend substructural features to avoid during development of a new drug class; to assess possible toxicity when testing is too expensive or unavailable, or possibly even to eliminate some whole animal testing (e.g. for eye and skin irritation). The long term success of such an approach to estimate bio-toxicity effects for compounds based on chemical structure will ultimately depend on demonstrated examples of correct predictions in its application in the drug research and development environment.

8.2.6 METABOLEXPERT. MetabolExpert (ComputDrug NA, Inc.) is an artificial intelligence (AI) rule-based expert software system for the prediction of possible (and probable) metabolic transformations of organic molecules (246–248). This software

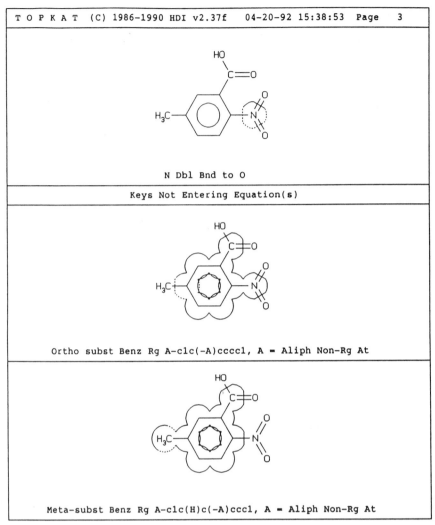

T O P K A T   (C) 1986–1990 HDI v2.37f   04-20-92 15:38:53   Page   3

N Dbl Bnd to O

Keys Not Entering Equation(s)

Ortho subst Benz Rg A-c1c(-A)cccc1, A ▬ Aliph Non-Rg At

Meta-subst Benz Rg A-c1c(H)c(-A)ccc1, A ▬ Aliph Non-Rg At

Fig. 13.22 The third page of the TOPKAT toxicity report predicting the mutagenicity of 5-methyl-2-nitrobenzoic acid (see Fig. 13.21): The upper box displays a substructural feature (nitrogen double bond to oxygen) that was used for one of the electronic parameters employed in the TOPKAT mutagenicity prediction. The bottom two boxes display two substructural fragments found in the compound but which are not present in the TOPKAT mutagenicity model (and hence did not contribute to the mutagenicity prediction). TOPKAT verifies that substructural molecular features and properties found in a compound but not in its toxicity models are adequately represented in the original set of compounds used for derivation of the model (i.e., that these substructural features and properties truly do not contribute to the toxicity model, rather than being omitted merely because they were inadequately represented in the original set of compounds).

has been developed in the PROLOG AI language and is available both for PCs and in a more sophisticated version for DEC VAX/VMS computers. MetabolExpert employs two different methods for predicting metabolites, with rules based on well-docu-mented metabolic transformations of xeno-biotics. The knowledge base for these rules was originally based on the classic drug metabolism references of Jenner and Testa (249, 250) but has been expanded to in-clude additional metabolic transformations from the scientific literature. MetabolExpert is an open expert software system, providing the option for the user to supplement the MetabolExpert knowledge base with additional metabolic transformation trees (e.g. from new scientific research or proprietary industrial information on metabolism of chemical compounds).

The first and more general algorithm employed by MetabolExpert for predicting metabolic transformations is not species specific, uses a general knowledge (rule) base of approximately 250 common metabolic transformations, and employs a general rule search for prediction of probable metabolic transformations. Once the software has analyzed an input structure, the rules are applied to the structure by the expert software system to predict possible metabolism of the compound.

The second algorithm employed by MetabolExpert for predicting metabolic transformations is species specific. The VAX/VMS version of MetabolExpert uses about 900 complete species specific metabolic trees, while the PC version uses about 250. This second algorithm usually generates a smaller (but more probable) number of potential metabolites (as compared to the first, more general algorithm) by considering the compounds in the metabolic trees as potential analogs of the compound being investigated. Once MetabolExpert has analyzed the submitted structure, analogue from the metabolic trees are selected either on the basis of "metabolic similarity' or on the basis of shared substructures. Potential metabolites of the submitted compound are then generated, employing (if possible) the metabolic transformations observed in the metabolic trees of the analogs for the selected species.

As with other successful chemically intelligent computing systems, structures can be submitted by the user to MetabolExpert for analysis either by direct graphical entry or from a chemical connection table file for the structure. Having analyzed the structure and employing one of two algorithms described above, MetabolExpert then generates a report, which contains schematic, graphic presentations of the potential metabolic trees for the submitted compound (Fig. 13.23). Detailed information can also be output for the user, describing the rationale and steps employed by the program in its analyses and generation of potential metabolites.

An expert metabolite prediction software system (such as MetabolExpert) has enormous potential in the drug discovery process, both during the initial stages of research and especially as a new chemical entity reaches the later stages of research and becomes a potential candidate for development. For the medicinal chemist the ability to predict probable metabolites a the potential drug molecule could be of value in the design of prodrugs which would be metabolically activated *in vivo*. Similarly, knowledge of likely metabolites could help explain the metabolic inactivation of a compound *in vivo* and obviously help with the structural modification so as

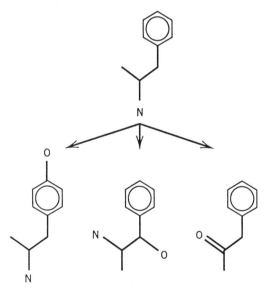

Fig. 13.23 A MetabolExpert output/report of a partial metabolic tree predicted for amphetamine in humans.

to avoid such metabolic inactivation. In addition, metabolism prediction for a series of compounds could assist with design of analogues whose metabolites possess more desirable physical properties for activity (e.g., changes in hydrophobicity, solubility, pK_a which significantly affect biodistribution, excretion, serum half-life, etc.). As a potential drug becomes a candidate for developing (or even moves into development), a knowledge of likely drug metabolites (especially unusual metabolic transformations) could be of great value for the drug metabolism and pharmacokinetics scientists in anticipating probable metabolites in their research studies. (This knowledge could be of particular value when coupled with other software systems for estimating molecular physical/chemical properties, in that a knowledge of the anticipated physical/chemical properties of drug metabolites can greatly assist with experimental design/conditions for identifying and quantitating such species).

The weakest link in the MetabolExpert type of approach for prediction of drug metabolites is not in the underlying concepts or its implementation as an expert software system but rather lies in the knowledge base upon which software is dependent. Probably several million new chemical entities have been synthesized and tested for bioactivity as potential drug molecules. Unfortunately, only a small fraction of these compounds have had complete metabolic trees determined, and often only in one species. Also, the relative importance of competing metabolic transformations, further complicated by species metabolic, biodistribution, and excretion differences, is often not known, even for established metabolic trees for individual compounds. This disclosure should be viewed not as a criticism of the MetabolExpert type of approach for predicting probable drug metabolites, but rather as an indication that this methodology will likely increase in accuracy and value for the drug

discovery process as the metabolic knowledge base expands in depth, breadth, and complexity in the future.

8.2.7 AUTONOM. AUTONOM (AUTOmatic NOMenclature; developed by the Beilstein Institute; marketed by Springer-Verlag) is a PC-based software program for the generation of IUPAC systematic chemical nomenclature of organic compounds (251–254). The user graphically draws and edits the structure within AUTONOM (or the program can read a chemical connection table computer file). Using its chemical knowledge and its understanding of chemical nomenclature, AUTONOM then automatically analyzes the structure, identifying the parent fragment, ring systems, chains, and functional groups. If the software detects no problems or unknown areas in its structural analysis, it then constructs a unique IUPAC-compatible chemical name (Fig. 13.24). Otherwise, AUTONOM generates a diagnostic message, explaining why it could not construct a name. Tests at the Beilstein Institute show that AUTONOM Version 1.0 will generate a name for about 71% of typical organic compounds submitted. Virtually 100% of these names will be correct IUPAC systematic nomenclature. For the other 29% of organic compounds, AUTONOM generates no name, because of extremely complex nomenclature situations or if the compound contains structural characteristics that are outside of AUTONOM's knowledge or capabilities to handle.

AUTONOM's primary short-coming is that Version 1.0 ignores all stereochemistry, although it will still generate an IUPAC systematic name. Other limitations of AUTONOM Version 1.0 include:

- Non-hydrogen atom limit = 100 atoms.
- Ring and chain size limit = 44 atoms.
- Isotopes, charged species, salts, radicals, multi-component mixtures, and inorganic compounds are not handled.

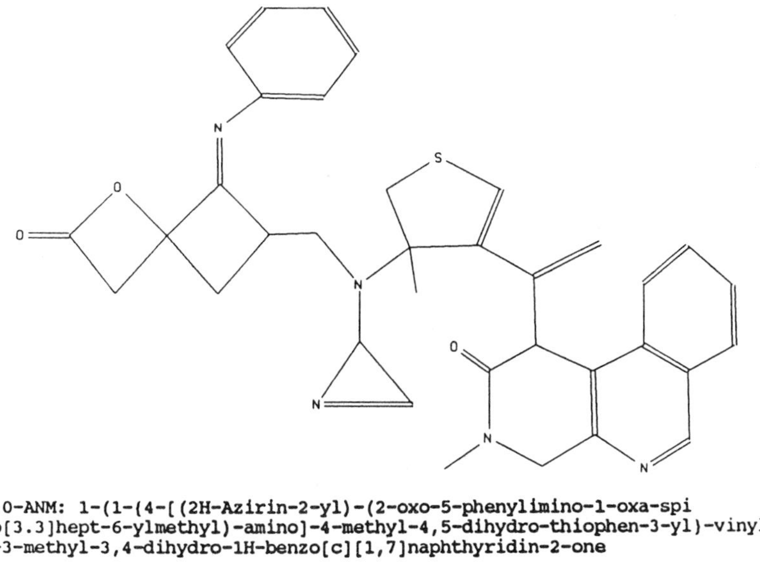

1.0-ANM: 1-(1-(4-[(2H-Azirin-2-yl)-(2-oxo-5-phenylimino-1-oxa-spi
ro[3.3]hept-6-ylmethyl)-amino]-4-methyl-4,5-dihydro-thiophen-3-yl)-vinyl
)-3-methyl-3,4-dihydro-1H-benzo[c][1,7]naphthyridin-2-one

Fig. 13.24 An output report from AUTONOM showing the IUPAC systematic chemical nomenclature generated for a complex organic compound from the chemical structure which was submitted to the software.

Correct and accurate chemical nomenclature is important for drug discovery research and development scientists (and for pharmaceutical companies themselves) for several reasons:

- For patent filings.
- For clinical trial and new drug applications and documentation.
- For research documentation (whether in a single research laboratory in academia or for an entire pharmaceutical company).
- For clear scientific communication (at meetings/symposia, in journal articles, in research and grant proposals, and internally for a research group, department, or even company).

However, IUPAC nomenclature rules can be quite complex, making manual naming of many complicated compounds (as drug discovery scientists are prone to synthesize) quite difficult. Obviously a software tool such as AUTONOM (with its chemical and nomenclature intelligence)

which can facilitate and hopefully even automate the naming process will save the scientist (or the information specialist for the scientist) considerable time and effort that can be directed to higher priority tasks in the drug discovery process. The basic concept of AUTONOM (i.e., complete systematic IUPAC naming of a compound based solely on chemical structure input) is a reasonable and needed capability. It is reasonable (hopeful) to anticipate that subsequent versions of AUTONOM will include handling of stereochemistry and other structural features not presently handled now by this software.

8.2.8 SANDRA. SANDRA (Structure AND Reference Analyser; developed by Beilstein Institute; marketed by Springer-Verlag) is a PC-based software package (255–259) to assist users in locating information for specific compounds in *The Beilstein Handbook of Organic Chemistry* (260). At present the Beilstein Handbook contains relevant and critically evaluated data published in the scientific literature on the preparation and properties of all organic compounds. The complete work consists of a number of series of volumes, each covering a specific period of time. The location of information from the Beilstein Handbook for any specific compound requires a selective search technique and some knowledge of the complex Beilstein system of compound ordering. Using SANDRA, however, a user merely graphically inputs the target structure. The software then analyzes the chemical structure and (based on its knowledge of *The Beilstein Handbook of Organic Chemistry* system of compound ordering) provides the user with a location (series, volume, sub-volume, section) to almost precisely where information regarding the compound can be found. SANDRA is an unusual but good example of a chemically intelligent computing software package that (because of its chemical structure knowledge and analysis expertise) can facilitate the access by scientists to chemical information and data for specific compounds from a large and complex data resource.

8.3 CD-ROM Databases

Another interesting recent development in chemical information computing software systems and databases has been the commercial introduction of chemical information databases on CD-ROM, packaged together with chemically intelligent chemical structure/substructure searching software on PCs (261). As described below for two of these CD-ROM databases, this development has proven to be an economical means for providing convenient in-house access for scientists (either in the laboratory or in a company/institution library) to large specialized chemical information databases which otherwise had been available only in books or on-line. The chemical intelligence incorporated in the search software is what clearly distinguishes these chemical information systems/data-

bases from other simpler CD-ROM databases, which typically provide only for text or numeric searching. The more sophisticated chemical search and display software supplied with these CD-ROM databases allow the user to input a chemical structure or substructure graphically, to perform the desired search, to review the hits graphically, and to save the results to a computer file. The usual text and numeric searches can also be performed on the associated chemical and other data in the CD-ROM database. These CD-ROM chemical databases plus search software systems are so far only stand-alone PC systems, as yet with no direct interfaces to other chemical information software systems.

8.3.1 DICTIONARY OF NATURAL PRODUCTS ON CD-ROM. The CHCD Dictionary of Natural Products on CD-ROM (Chapman & Hall) database consists of over 80,000 natural products, including chemical structures, chemical and physical data, and key literature references (262). The database was constructed from all the natural products contained in the Chapman & Hall books *Dictionary of Organic Compounds* (70), *Dictionary of Antibiotics & Related Substances* (72), *Dictionary of Alkaloids* (74), *Dictionary of Steroids* (76), and *Dictionary of Terpenoids* (132). Chemical classes covered (in descending order of representation) include terpenoids, alkaloids, miscellaneous compounds, antibiotics, amino acids and peptides, steroids, flavinoids, carbohydrates, and lipids. The entire system runs under Microsoft Windows on a PC. The complete software/database package incorporates the Psi-Base PC software (Hampden Data Services) for its chemical structure/substructure drawing, searching, and display and the Headfast software (Head Software International) for its text searches and display. The 80,000 natural products are grouped together according to chemical and biosynthetic similarity, yielding a database with 33,000 actual entries. For example, stereo-isomers and derivatives of parent compounds are listed within the same entry. Associated data included in the CD-ROM database are as extensive as in the original Chapman & Hall books and include chemical name(s) (entry name, CAS name, synonyms, trivial and archaic names), molecular formula and weight, hazardous and toxic properties, CAS Registry Number, physical description (state, color, indication of stability), melting/boiling point, relative density, refractive index, optical rotation, solubility, pK_a values, compound type, use or importance, biological source with extensive taxonomic listings, biological activity including pharmacological actions, etc. The included references concentrate on natural occurrence and isolation, structural characterization, synthesis, and uses. The chemical structure and data display (Fig. 13.25) mimic very closely the format used

in the Chapman & Hall books from which the database was derived.

These Chapman & Hall books have proven to be invaluable scientific information resources for scientists involved with drug discovery research involving natural products and derivatives. Simple and ready access to the wealth of natural products chemical structures and associated data contained in the CHCD Dictionary of Natural Products on CD-ROM, represents a significant step in truly making this information available for drug discovery scientists for use in their research. Hopefully this availability is an indicator of a trend for other important scientific chemical information resources (which previously had only been available in book format). While this would appear to be a standard information resource that should be available in scientific libraries, this particular CD-ROM database is appropriately priced and valuable enough so that one would expect

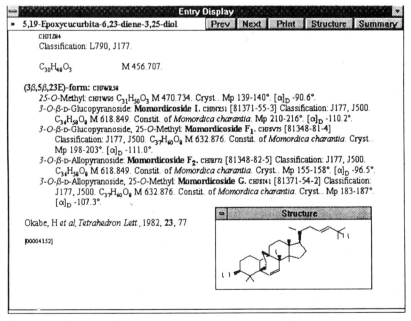

Fig. 13.25 PC screens (Microsoft Windows) showing retrieval of a chemical structure and associated chemical data from the Chapman & Hall CHCD Dictionary of Natural Products on CD-ROM.

that it would also be common in laboratory research groups involved with natural products in the drug discovery environment.

8.3.2 BEILSTEIN'S CURRENT FACTS IN CHEMISTRY ON CD-ROM.

Beilstein's Current Facts in Chemistry on CD-ROM database (developed by the Beilstein Institute; marketed by Springer-Verlag) is a PC-based CD-ROM database of organic chemical structures, data, and references abstracted from the scientific literature by the Beilstein Institute (263, 264). The CD-ROM disks are updated quarterly (beginning in 1990), with each covering approximately 300,000 compounds from the previous 12 months' scientific literature. The chemical data are abstracted from 82 key scientific journals and include structures, reactions, preparations, physical properties, toxicological and environmental data, keywords, citations, authors, etc. The coverage of the Beilstein's Current Facts in Chemistry on CD-ROM database is apparently a distillation of the more extensive current chemical data contained in *The Beilstein Handbook of Organic Chemistry* (260) and in the Beilstein On-Line Database (STN, DIALOG, or Maxwell/Online-ORBIT). Specific references are given in the CD-ROM database to these other two Beilstein information sources, allowing the user to go to these for more extensive data, if desired. The Beilstein's Current Facts in Chemistry on CD-ROM database is provided with an integrated PC software system (developed by Fraser Williams Ltd.) for chemical structure drawing, structure and substructure searching, and display of chemical structures and associated data from the CD-ROM database.

Depending on the quality and key-wording of the data covered in the Beilstein's Current Facts in Chemistry on CD-ROM database, this could prove to be an additional valuable information resource for drug discovery scientists in maintaining their current awareness of the chemical literature. The generic coverage of this database makes it most likely to be an information resource available in scientific libraries, rather than in individual research labs.

8.4 Integrated Chemical Information Computing Software

Most commercial chemical information computing software systems were originally developed to be used on large interactive time-sharing minicomputers/mainframes (e.g. DEC VAX/VMS or IBM mainframes), accessed by users from graphics terminals (or PCs running graphics emulation software). Also, the individual chemical computing software systems operated fairly independently of each other, with only moderately effective interfaces to other R&D information sources. A current and strong continuing trend in the pharmaceutical industry is an emphasis on the development of software systems with as complete and as seamless (i.e., transparent to the user) as possible integration and interfacing of chemical information computing systems (2D, 3D, reaction, and expert) to other drug discovery information systems and databases and on a variety of computing platforms using different operating systems (265). Also, the recent development of relatively inexpensive, extremely powerful microcomputers and workstations has prompted many pharmaceutical companies to exploit these hardware capabilities to distribute computing loads from large interactive, time-sharing computers to these powerful "personal" platforms. Key corporate databases (e.g., 2D chemical, 3D chemical, and reaction information databases, relational databases of bioactivity data; etc.) usually still need to be centralized, for example, located on a single CPU, for access by scientists throughout the industrial R&D organization.

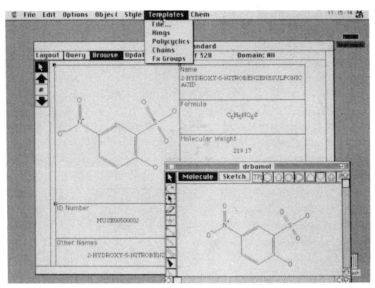

Fig. 13.26 Simultaneous display of Molecular Design Limited's ISIS/Draw (smaller window) and ISIS/Base (larger window) on a Macintosh.

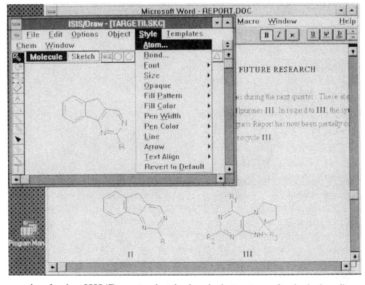

Fig. 13.27 An example of using ISIS/Draw to sketch chemical structures for inclusion (by cut-and-paste on a microcomputer) in a word processing document (in this case, Microsoft Word). See also color plates.

The ISIS software (Molecular Design Limited) has been developed and has been marketed with exactly this intent in mind (and as a successor to MDL's MACCS-II, REACCS, and MACCS-3D software systems). The software consists of three basic components (Fig. 13.26):

- ISIS/Draw (installed on the local workstation/microcomputer) for drawing of chemical structures and search queries (2D, 3D, and reaction) (266); cut-and-paste capabilities are also available for direct import of chemical structure drawings into various word-processing packages (e.g., Microsoft Word: see Fig. 13.27) for report generation.

- ISIS/Base (installed on the local workstation/microcomputer) for local analysis and manipulation of chemical structures and data; creation of local chemical databases; customized report generation;

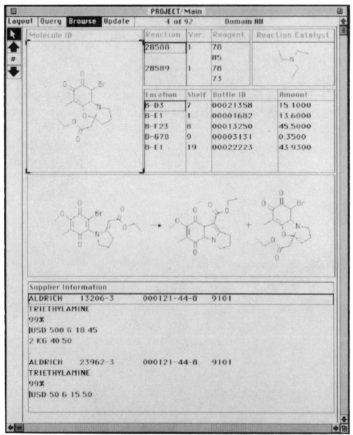

Fig. 13.28 An ISIS/Base customized screen demonstrating integrated and coordinated retrieval of chemical structures, reactions, and associated data from MACCS-II 2D chemical structure databases, a REACCS synthetic reaction database, and a relational database. A search of a MACCS-II database (e.g., a proprietary corporate database) first retrieves the structure in the upper left corner. This structure is used to automatically search a REACCS database for its preparation, yielding the reaction in the center of the screen and the reaction information (including catalyst structure) in the boxes in the upper right corner. The catalyst information automatically triggers a search of a relational chemical inventory database (yielding the in-house chemical sample availability information in the boxes just below the reaction information), as well as a search of the FCD MACCS-II database (yielding the chemical supplier information for the catalyst in the bottom box).

submission of search queries to and retrieval of search results from centralized chemical and relational databases.

- ISIS/Host: software installed on a centralized CPU for centralized database registrations, performing the actual chemical and relational database searches submitted by users from ISIS/Base on workstations/microcomputers, and handling communications between itself and ISIS/Base.

The ISIS software is intended to permit simultaneous access (registration, searching, information retrieval, etc.) by a user to multiple MACCS, REACCS, MACCS-3D, and relational databases, while off-loading some of the computing load from the centralized CPU to the workstation/microcomputer (Fig. 13.28). ISIS/Draw and ISIS-Base are also distributed by ACS software with discounts for ACS members.

The SYBYL/3DB UNITY software possesses most of the capabilities for such a comprehensive, distributed chemical information computing system. It remains to be seen whether this software will also become a viable player in this distributed chemical and scientific information computing systems market. The Daylight Chemical Information Systems software (although also potentially capable of this comprehensive, distributed approach to pharmaceutical drug discovery computing) is apparently presently viewed by most large pharmaceutical companies primarily as a powerful chemical information computing research system (as opposed to a "production" chemical information management software system).

REFERENCES

1. J. E. Ash, P. A. Chubb, S. E. Ward, S. M. Welford, and P. Willett, *Communication, Storage and Retrieval of Chemical Information*, Ellis Horwood Limited, Chichester, England, 1985.

2. F. H. Allen and M. F. Lynch, *Chem. Brit.*, **25**, 1101–1104, 1108 (1989).

3. W. A. Warr, Ed., *Chemical Structures: The International Language of Chemistry*, Springer-Verlag, Berlin, 1988.

4. T. R. Hagadone in ref. 3, pp. 23–41.

5. J. E. Ash and E. Hyde, Eds., *Chemical Information Systems*, Ellis Horwood Limited, Chichester, England, 1975.

6. H. R. Collier, Ed., "Chemical Information: Information in Chemistry, Pharmacology and Patents," *Proceedings of the Montreux 1989, International Chemical Information Conference*, Montreux, September 26–28, 1989, Springer-Verlag, Berlin, 1989.

7. P. Willett, *J. Chemom.*, **1**, 139–155 (1987).

8. J. E. Ash, W. A. Warr, and P. Willett, *Chemical Structure Systems: Computational Techniques for Representation, Searching, and Processing of Structural Information*, Ellis Horwood Limited, Chichester, England, 1991.

9. W. T. Wipke, S. R. Heller, R. J. Feldmann, and E. Hyde, Eds., *Computer Representation and Manipulation of Chemical Information*, John Wiley & Sons, Inc., New York, 1974.

10. S. W. Dietrich, *Med. Chem. Res.*, **2**, 127–147 (1992).

11. F. Choplin in C. Hansch, P. G. Sammes, and J. B. Taylor, Eds., *Comprehensive Medicinal Chemistry: The Rational Design, Mechanistic Study & Therapeutic Applications of Chemical Compounds*, Vol. 4, Pergamon Press, Oxford, England, 1990, Chapter 17.2, pp. 33–58.

12. S. Anderson, *J. Mol. Graphics*, **2**, 83–90 (1984).

13. A. Dalby, J. G. Nourse, W. D. Hounshell, A. K. I. Gushurst, D. L. Grier, B. A. Leland, and J. Laufer, *J. Chem. Inf. Comput. Sci.*, **32**, 244–255 (1992).

14. H. Bebak, C. Buse, W. T. Donner, P. Hoever, H. Jacob, H. Klaus, J. Pesch, J. Roemelt, P. Schilling, B. Woost, and C. Zirz, *J. Chem. Inf. Comput. Sci.*, **29**, 1–5 (1989).

15. J. M. Barnard, *J. Chem. Inf. Comput. Sci.*, **30**, 81–96 (1990).

16. H. Bebak, C. Buse, W. T. Donner, P. Hoever, H. Jacob, H. Klaus, J. Pesch, J. Roemelt, P. Schilling, B. Woost, and C. Zirz in W. A. Warr, Ed., *Chemical Structure Information Systems: Interfaces, Communication, and Standards*, ACS Symposium Series No. 400, American Chemical Society, Washington, D.C., 1989, Chap. 11, pp. 105–117.

17. J. S. Garavelli in ref. 16, Chapt. 12, pp. 118–124.

18. J. J. Vollmer, *J. Chem. Ed.*, **60**, 192–196 (1983).

19. W. A. Warr, *J. Chem. Inf. Comput. Sci.*, **22**, 98–101 (1982).

20. E. G. Smith, *The Wiswesser Line-Formula Chemical Notation*, McGraw-Hill Book Company, New York, 1968.

21. S. Barcza, L. A. Kelly, S. S. Wahrman, and R. E. Kirschenbaum, *J. Chem. Inf. Comput. Sci.*, **25**, 55–59 (1985).

22. H. L. Morgan, *J. Chem. Doc.*, **5**, 107–113 (1965).

23. W. T. Wipke and T. M. Dyott, *J. Amer. Chem. Soc.*, **96**, 4834–4842 (1974).

24. D. Weininger and J. L. Weininger in C. Hansch, P. G. Sammes, and J. B. Taylor, Eds., *Comprehensive Medicinal Chemistry: The Rational Design, Mechanistic Study & Therapeutic Applications of Chemical Compounds*, Vol. 4, Pergamon Press, Oxford, England, 1990, Chapter 17.3, pp. 59–82.

25. M. G. Hicks and C. Jochum, *J. Chem. Inf. Comput. Sci.*, **30**, 191–199 (1990).

26. J. M. Barnard, Ed., *Computer Handling of Generic Chemical Structures*, Gower Publishing Company Limited, Aldershot, England, 1984.

27. P. Willett, *Similarity and Clustering in Chemical Information Systems*, Research Studies Press Ltd., Letchworth, England, 1987.

28. P. Gund, *J. Med. Chem.*, **34**, 3408 (1991).

29. M. A. Johnson and G. M. Maggiora, *Concepts and Applications of Molecular Similarity*, Wiley-Interscience, New York, 1990.

30. M. S. Lajiness in C. Silipo and A. Vittoria, Eds., "QSAR: Rational Approaches to the Design of Bioactive Compounds," *Proceedings of the VIII European Symposium on Quantitative Structure-Activity Relationships*, Sorrento, Italy, September 9–13, 1988, Elsevier Scientific Publishers B. V., Amsterdam, 1991, pp. 201–204.

31. H. H. Shlevin, M. M. Graham, D. F. Pennington, and W. von Wartburg in ref. 3, pp. 79–90.

32. W. L. Henckler, D. L. Allison, P. L. Combs, G. S. Franklin, W. B. Gall, and S. J. Sallamack in ref. 3, pp. 91–95.

33. E. K. F. Ahrens in ref. 3, pp. 97–111.

34. S. Barcza, H. W. Mah, M. H. Myers, and S. S. Wahrman, *J. Chem. Inf. Comput. Sci.*, **26**, 198–204 (1986).

35. S. Barcza, L. A. Kelly, and C. D. Lenz, *J. Chem. Inf. Comput. Sci.*, **30**, 243–251 (1990).

36. T. R. Hagadone, *J. Chem. Inf. Comput. Sci.*, **32**, 515–521 (1992).

37. W. J. Howe and T. R. Hagadone, *J. Chem. Inf. Comput. Sci.*, **22**, 8–15 (1982).

38. T. R. Hagadone and W. J. Howe, *J. Chem. Inf. Comput. Sci.*, **22**, 182–186 (1982).

39. T. R. Hagadone and M. S. Lajiness, *Tetrahedron Comput. Methodol.*, **1**, 219–230 (1988).

40. W. J. Howe and T. R. Hagadone in W. J. Howe, M. M. Milne, and A. F. Pennell, Eds., *Retrieval of Medicinal Chemical Information*, ACS Symposium Series No. 84, American Chemical Society, Washington, D.C., 1978, Chapt. 8, pp. 107–131.

41. D. R. Eakin, E. Hyde, and G. Palmer, *Pestic. Sci.*, **5**, 319–326 (1974).

42. D. R. Eakin in J. E. Ash and E. Hyde, Eds., *Chemical Information Systems*, Ellis Horwood Limited, Chichester, England, 1975, Chap. 14, pp. 227–242.

43. E. E. Townsley and W. A. Warr in W. J. Howe, M. M. Milne, and A. F. Pennell, Eds., *Retrieval of Medicinal Chemical Information*, ACS Symposium Series No. 84, American Chemical Society, Washington, D.C., 1978, Chap. 6, pp. 73–84.

44. D. Bawden, T. K. Devon, D. T. Faulkner, J. D. Fisher, J. M. Leach, R. J. Reeves, and F. E. Woodward in ref. 3, pp. 63–75.

45. J.-P. Gay, G. Auneveux, and F. Chabernaud in ref. 16, Chapt. 10, pp. 89–104.

46. P. Attias, *J. Chem. Inf. Comput. Sci.*, **23**, 102–108 (1983).

47. A. J. C. M. de Jong and A. M. C. Deibel in ref. 3, pp. 45–51.

48. J. P. Gay and H. Alardo in H. R. Collier, Ed., "Chemical Information: Information in Chemistry, Pharmacology and Patents," *Proceedings of the Montreux 1989 International Chemical Information Conference*, Montreux, Switzerland, September 26–28, 1989, pp. 221–236.

49. G. W. Adamson, J. M. Bird, G. Palmer, and W. A. Warr, *J. Chem. Inf. Comput. Sci.*, **25**, 90–92 (1985).

50. J. D. Dill, W. D. Hounshell, S. Marson, S. Peacock, and W. T. Wipke, *182nd American Chemical Society National Meeting*, New York, August 23–28, 1981.

51. D. J. Polton, *Online Review*, **6**, 235–242 (1982).

52. W. A. Warr in *Proceedings of the 7th International Online Information Meeting*, London, December 6–8, 1983, Learned Information Ltd., Oxford, England, 1983, pp. 91–93.

53. S. V. Kasparek, *Computer Graphics and Chemical Structures: Database Management Systems: CAS Registry, ChemBase, REACCS, MACCS-*

II, Chem Talk, John Wiley & Sons Inc., New York, 1990.

54. W. T. Wipke, J. G. Nourse, and T. Moock in J. M. Barnard, Ed., *Computer Handling of Generic Chemical Structures*, Gower Publishing Company Limited, Aldershot, England, 1984, Chapter 15, pp. 167–178.

55. A. J. Gushurst, J. G. Nourse, W. G. Hounshell, B. A. Leland, and D. G. Raich, *J. Chem. Inf. Comput. Sci.*, **31**, 447–454 (1991).

56. D. S. Magrill in ref. 3, pp. 53–62.

57. A. P. Johnson, K. Burt, A. P. F. Cook, K. M. Higgins, G. A. Hopkinson, and G. Singh in ref. 16, Chapt. 5, pp. 50–58.

58. *HLI: Host Language Interface*, technical datasheet, ORAC Ltd., Leeds, England, 1991.

59. J. L. Weininger, *Chemical Design Automation News*, **1**(8), 2, 12–15 (1986).

60. D. Weininger, *J. Chem. Inf. Comput. Sci.*, **28**, 31–36 (1988).

61. D. Weininger, A. Weininger, and J. L. Weininger, *J. Chem. Inf. Comput. Sci.*, **29**, 97–101 (1989).

62. D. Weininger, *J. Chem. Inf. Comput. Sci.*, **30**, 237–243 (1990).

63. Y. C. Martin, *Tetrahedron Comput. Methodol.*, **3**, 15–25 (1990).

64. J. H. Van Drie, D. Weininger, and Y. C. Martin, *J. Comput.-Aided Mol. Des.*, **3**, 225–251 (1989).

65. A. J. Leo in C. Hansch, P. G. Sammes, and J. B. Taylor, Eds., *Comprehensive Medicinal Chemistry: The Rational Design, Mechanistic Study & Therapeutic Applications of Chemical Compounds*, Vol. 4, Pergamon Press, Oxford, England, 1990, Chapter 18.7, pp. 295–319.

66. Pomona College Medicinal Chemistry Project, Chemistry Department, Pomona College, Claremont, Calif.

67. L. M. Dumont, *Can. Chem. News*, **40**(6) 17–20 (June 1988).

68. *The Inhouse DARC Newsletter*, No. 1 Questel, Paris, Jan. 1992.

69. *DARC-CHCD: Chapman & Hall Chemical Database*, technical manual, Questel, Paris, April 1992.

70. *Dictionary of Organic Compounds*, 5th Edition and Supplements, Chapman & Hall, New York, 1982–1991.

71. *Dictionary of Organometallic Compounds*, and Supplements, Chapman & Hall, New York, 1984–1990.

72. B. W. Bycroft, Ed., *Dictionary of Antibiotics & Related Substances*, Chapman & Hall, New York, 1987.

73. R. S. Edmundson, Ed., *Dictionary of Or-ganophosphorous Compounds*, Chapman & Hall, New York, 1987.

74. I. Southon and J. Buckingham, Eds., *Dictionary of Alkaloids*, Chapman & Hall, New York, 1989.

75. J. Elks and C. R. Ganellin, *Dictionary of Drugs*, Chapman & Hall, New York, 1990.

76. R. A. Hill, D. N. Kirk, H. L. J. Makin, and G. M. Murphy, Eds., *Dictionary of Steroids*, Chapman & Hall, New York, 1991.

77. P. M. Collins, *Carbohydrates*, Chapman & Hall Chemistry Sourcebooks, Chapman & Hall, New York, 1986.

78. J. S. Davies, Ed., *Amino Acids and Peptides*, Chapman & Hall Chemistry Sourcebooks, Chapman & Hall, New York, 1985.

79. *FCD: The Fine Chemicals Directory*, technical datasheet, Molecular Design Limited, San Leandro, Calif., Aug. 1990.

80. *Guide To Molecular Databases Manual*, Molecular Design Limited, San Leandro, Calif., Oct. 1989.

81. *ACD: The Available Chemicals Directory*, technical datasheet, Molecular Design Limited, San Leandro, Calif., Jan. 1991.

82. *MDDR: The MACCS-II Drug Data Report*, technical datasheet, Molecular Design Limited, San Leandro, Calif., Dec. 1991.

83. *Daylight Software Manual Version 4.2*, Daylight Chemical Information Systems, Inc., Irvine, Calif., March 20, 1992.

84. *Daylight Version 4.2 Software: Databases*, product description datasheet, Daylight Chemical Information Systems, Inc., Irvine, Calif., Feb. 1992.

85. *Standard Drug File with Graphics: Version 4.0*, technical brochure, Derwent Publications Ltd., London, Oct. 1990.

86. *SDF with Graphics: Version 5.0*, technical datasheet, Derwent Publications Ltd., London, April 1992.

87. *SDF with Graphics: Version 6.0*, technical datasheet, Derwent Publications Ltd., London, Sept. 1992.

88. *What Drugs Are in Development?*, Therapeutic Patent Fast-Alert Database technical brochure, Current Drugs Ltd., London, 1992.

89. D. R. Henry in P. S. Magee, D. R. Henry, and J. H. Block, Eds., *Probing Bioactive Mechanisms*, *ACS Symposium Series No. 413*, American Chemical Society, Washington, D. C., 1989, Chapt. 2, pp. 26–36.

90. Y. C. Martin, *J. Med. Chem.*, **35**, 2145–2154 (1992).

91. S. Borman, *Chem. Eng. News.* **70**(32) 18–26, (Aug. 10, 1992).

92. Y. C. Martin and P. Willett, *Tetrahedron Comput. Methodol.*, **3**, 527–530 (1990).

93. P. Willett in D. I. Raitt, Ed., "Online Information 90," *Proceedings of the 14th International Online Information Meeting*, London, December 11–13, 1990, Learned Information Ltd., Oxford, England, 1990, pp. 115–136.

94. Y. C. Martin, M. G. Bures, and P. Willett in K. B. Lipkowitz and D. B. Boyd, Eds., *Reviews in Computational Chemistry*, VCH Publishers, Inc., New York, 1990, Chapt. 6, pp. 213–263.

95. P. Willett, *Chemical Design Automation News*, **6**(7) 1, 24–28, 31 (July 1991).

96. P. Willett, *Three-Dimensional Chemical Structure Handling*, Research Studies Press Ltd., Taunton, Somerset, England (1991).

97. A. T. Brint, E. Mitchell, and P. Willett in ref. 3, pp. 131–144.

98. J. K. Cringean, C. A. Pepperrell, A. R. Poirrette, and P. Willett, *Tetrahedron Comput. Methodol.*, **3**, 37–46 (1990).

99. C. A. Pepperrell, R. Taylor, and P. Willett, *Tetrahedron Comput. Methodol.*, **3**, 575–593 (1990).

100. C. A. Pepperrell and P. Willett, *J. Comput.-Aided Mol. Des.*, **5**, 455–474 (1991).

101. R. P. Sheridan, A. Rusinko III, R. Nilakantan, and R. Venkataraghavan, *Proc. Natl. Acad. Sci. U.S.A.*, **86**, 8165–8169 (1989).

102. R. P. Sheridan, R. Nilakantan, A. Rusinko III, N. Bauman, K. S. Haraki, and R. Venkataraghavan, *J. Chem. Inf. Comput. Sci.*, **29**, 255–260 (1989).

103. P. A. Bartlet, G. T. Shea, S. J. Telfer, and S. Waterman in S. M. Roberts, S. V. Ley, and M. M. Campbell, Eds., *Chemical and Biological Problems in Molecular Recognition*, Royal Society of Chemistry, London, 1989, pp. 182–196.

104. F. H. Allen, J. E. Davies, J. J. Galloy, O. Johnson, O. Kennard, C. F. Macrae, E. M. Mitchell, G. F. Mitchell, J. M. Smith, and D. G. Watson, *J. Chem. Inf. Comput. Sci.*, **31**, 187–204 (1991).

105. F. H. Allen and O. Kennard, *Chemical Design Automation News*, **8**(1) 1, 31–37 (Jan. 1993).

106. N. W. Murrall and E. K. Davies, *J. Chem. Inf. Comput. Sci.*, **30**, 312–316 (1990).

107. *Chem-X Reference Guide*, Chemical Design Ltd., Oxford, England, July 1992.

108. K. S. Haraki, R. P. Sheridan, R. Venkataraghavan, D. A. Dunn, and R. McCulloch, *Tetrahedron Comput. Methodol.*, **3**, 565–573 (1990).

109. O. F. Guner, D. W. Hughes, and L. M. Dumont, *J. Chem. Inf. Comput. Sci.*, **31**, 408–414 (1991).

110. B. D. Christie, D. R. Henry, W. T. Wipke, and T. E. Moock, *Tetrahedron Comput. Methodol.*, **3**, 653–664 (1990).

111. B. D. Christie, D. R. Henry, O. F. Guner, and T. E. Moock in D. I. Raitt, Ed., "Online Information 90," *Proceedings of the 14th International Online Information Meeting*, London, December 11–13, 1990, Learned Information Ltd., Oxford, England, 1990, pp. 137–161.

112. O. F. Guner, D. R. Henry, and R. S. Pearlman, *J. Chem. Inf. Comput. Sci.*, **32**, 101–109 (1992).

113. O. F. Guner, D. R. Henry, T. E. Moock, and R. S. Pearlman, *Tetrahedron Comput. Methodol.*, **3**, 557–563 (1990).

114. *SYBYL/3DB UNITY: Chemical Information Software: Version 1.0, System Manuals 1 & 2*, TRIPOS Associates, Inc., St. Louis, Mo., June 1992.

115. *SYBYL/3DB UNITY: Chemical Information Software: Version 1.0, User's Manual*, TRIPOS Associates, Inc., St. Louis, Mo., June 1992.

116. Y. C. Martin, E. B. Danaher, C. S. May, and D. Weininger, *J. Comput.-Aided Mol. Des.*, **2**, 15–29 (1988).

117. A. Rusinko III, J. M. Skell, R. Balducci, and R. S. Pearlman, *192nd American Chemical Society National Meeting*, Anaheim, Calif., Sept. 7–12, 1986.

118. R. S. Pearlman, *Chemical Design Automation News*, **2**(1), 1, 5–7 (Jan. 1987).

119. A. Rusinko III, R. P. Sheridan, R. Nilakantan, K. S. Haraki, N. Bauman, and R. Venkataraghavan, *J. Chem. Inf. Comput. Sci.*, **29**, 251–255 (1989).

120. M. A. Pleiss, *Tetrahedron Comput. Methodol.*, **3**, 549–556 (1990).

121. C. Hansch, P. G. Sammes, and J. B. Taylor, Eds., *Comprehensive Medicinal Chemistry: The Rational Design, Mechanistic Study & Therapeutic Applications of Chemical Compounds*, Pergamon Press, Oxford, England, 1990.

122. *CMC-3D: Comprehensive Medicinal Chemistry-3D*, technical datasheet, Molecular Design Limited, San Leandro, Calif., Aug. 1990.

123. D. R. Henry, P. J. McHale, B. D. Christie, and D. Hillman, *Tetrahedron Comput. Methodol.*, **3**, 531–536 (1990).

124. *FCD-3D: The Three-Dimensional Version of the Fine Chemicals Directory*, technical datasheet,

Molecular Design Limited, San Leandro, Calif., Sept. 1990.

125. *MDDR-3D: The Three-Dimensional Version of the MACCS-II Drug Data Report*, technical datasheet, Molecular Design Limited, San Leandro, Calif., 1990.

126. *Derwent Publications Standard Drug File 3D Database from Chemical Design*, technical datasheet, Chemical Design Inc., Mahwah, N.J., Oct. 1992.

127. "Database News", *Chemical Design News*, Chemical Design Ltd., Oxford, England, Summer 1992.

128. *Chapman & Hall 3-D Databases from Chemical Design*, technical datasheet, Chemical Design Inc., Mahwah, N.J., Oct. 1992.

129. K. Davies and R. Upton, *Tetrahedron Comput. Methodol.*, **3**, 665–671 (1990).

130. "Chem-X Builds Dictionary of Drugs", Chemical Design News, Chemical Design Ltd., Oxford, UK, Winter 1990/1991.

131. "3D Databases Grow", *Chemical Design News*, Chemical Design Ltd., Oxford, England, Spring 1992.

132. J. D. Connolly and R. A. Hill, Eds., *Dictionary of Terpenoids*, Chapman & Hall, New York, 1992.

133. P. Willett, Ed., *Modern Approaches to Chemical Reaction Searching*, Gower Publishing Company Limited, Aldershot, England, 1986.

134. E. Zass, *J. Chem. Inf. Comput. Sci.*, **30**, 360–372 (1990).

135. T. E. Moock, J. G. Nourse, D. Grier, and W. D. Hounshell in ref. 3, pp. 303–313.

136. G. Grethe and T. E. Moock, *J. Chem. Inf. Comput. Sci.*, **30**, 511–520 (1990).

137. T. E. Moock, D. L. Grier, W. Hounshell, G. Grethe, K. Cronin, J. G. Nourse, and J. Theodosiou, *Tetrahedron Comput. Methodol.*, **1**, 117–128 (1988).

138. D. W. Elrod in ref. 3, pp. 331–341.

139. W. Sieber in ref. 3, 361–366.

140. "Synthesis Design Interface," *The Newsletter of ORAC Limited*, Spring 1990, ORAC Ltd., Leeds, England.

141. C. Jochum in H. Collier, Ed., "Recent Advances in Chemical Information," *Proceedings of the Montreux 1991 International Chemical Information Conference*, Annecy, France, September 23–25, 1991, The Royal Society of Chemistry, Cambridge, England, 1992, pp. 1–6.

142. J. P. Gay in P. Willett, Ed., *Modern Approaches*

to *Chemical Reaction Searching*, Gower Publishing Company Limited, Aldershot, England, 1986, Chapt. 8, pp. 87–91.

143. A. P. Johnson, *Chem. Brit.*, **26**, 28–32 (Jan. 1985).

144. A. P. Johnson and A. P. Cook in P. Willett, Ed., *Modern Approaches to Chemical Reaction Searching*, Gower Publishing Company Limited, Aldershot, England, 1986, Chapt. 14, pp. 184–201.

145. A. P. Johnson, C. Marshall, A. P. F. Cook, K. M. Higgins, and G. A. Hopkinson, *192nd American Chemical Society National Meeting*, Anaheim, Calif., Sept. 7–12, 1986.

146. A. P. Johnson in ref. 3, pp. 297–301.

147. W. T. Wipke, J. Dill, D. Hounshell, T. Moock, and D. Grier in P. Willett, Ed., *Modern Approaches to Chemical Reaction Searching*, Gower Publishing Company Limited, Aldershot, England, 1986, Chapt. 9, pp. 92–117.

148. G. Grethe, D. del Rey, J. G. Jacobson, and M. VanDuyne in ref. 3, pp. 315–329.

149. S. E. French, *Chemtech*, **17**, 106–111 (1987).

150. J. E. Mills, C. A. Maryanoff, K. L. Sorgi, L. Scott, and R. Stanzione, *J. Chem. Inf. Comput. Sci.*, **28**, 153–155 (1988).

151. J. E. Mills, C. A. Maryanoff, K. L. Sorgi, R. Stanzione, L. Scott, L. Herring, J Spink, B. Baughman, and W. Bullock, *J. Chem. Inf. Comput. Sci.*, **28**, 155–159 (1988).

152. J. E. Mills and B. Baughman, *J. Chem. Inf. Comput. Sci.*, **30**, 431–435 (1990).

153. J. Boother, *Chem. Brit.*, 36–37 (Jan. 1985).

154. D. F. Chodosh in P. Willett, Ed., *Modern Approaches to Chemical Reaction Searching*, Gower Publishing Company Limited, Aldershot, England, 1986, Chapt. 10, pp. 118–145.

155. D. F. Chodosh, J. Hill, L. Shpilsky, and W. L. Mendelson, *Recl. Trav. Chim. Pays-Bas*, **111**, 247–254 (1992).

156. D. F. Chodosh and W. L. Mendelson, *Pharm. Tech.*, **7**(3), 90–92 (March 1983).

157. D. Chodosh and W. L. Mendelson, *Drug Info. J.*, **17**, 231–238 (1983).

158. *SYNLIB User Manual*, Distributed Chemical Graphics, Inc., Meadowbrook, Penn., 1991.

160. M. Bersohn, *192nd American Chemical Society National Meeting*, Anaheim, Calif., Sept. 7–12, 1986.

160. D. Chodosh, Distributed Chemical Graphics, Inc., Meadowbrook, Penn., Dec. 1992, personal communication.

161. A. Barth, *J. Chem. Inf. Comput. Sci.*, **30**, 384–393 (1990).

162. J. E. Blake and R. C. Dana, *J. Chem. Inf. Comput. Sci.*, **30**, 394–399 (1990).

163. R. E. Buntrock, *Database*, **11**(6) 124–127 (Dec. 1988).

164. J. H. Borkent, F. Oukes, and J. H. Noordik, *J. Chem. Inf. Comput. Sci.*, **28**, 148–150 (1988).

165. *The Current Chemical Reactions Database*, technical brochure, Institute for Scientific Information, Philadelphia, Penn., 1992.

166. A. R. Katritzky and C. W. Rees, Eds., *Comprehensive Heterocyclic Chemistry: The Structure, Reactions, Synthesis and Uses of Heterocyclic Compounds*, Pergamon Press, Oxford, England, 1984.

167. *CHC: Comprehensive Heterocyclic Chemistry*, technical datasheet, Molecular Design Limited, San Leandro, Calif., June 1991.

168. *ORAC Reaction Databases*, technical datasheet, ORAC Ltd., Leeds, England, 1991.

169. *Reaction Databases*, technical brochure, Springer-Verlag, New York, 1992.

170. *CHIRAS: The Database of Asymmetric Synthesis*, technical datasheet, Molecular Design Limited, San Leandro, Calif., March 1992.

171. *ChemInform RX: The Reaction Database from MDL and FIZ Chemie*, technical datasheet, Molecular Design Limited, San Leandro, Calif., 1992.

172. M. Gall, W. Thaisrivongs, J. Torrado, and M. Weinshelbaum, *192nd American Chemical Society National Meeting*, Anaheim, Calif., Sept. 7–12, 1986.

173. *CLF: The Current Literature File*, technical datasheet, Molecular Design Limited, San Leandro, Calif., September 1990.

174. *Current Synthetic Methodology (CSM)*, technical datasheet, Molecular Design Limited, San Leandro, Calif., April 1992.

175. *METALYSIS: A Reaction Database of Transition-Metal-Mediated Chemistry*, technical datasheet, Molecular Design Limited, San Leandro, Calif., Aug. 1991.

176. *Organic Syntheses*, John Wiley & Sons, New York, Vol. 1–72, 1921–1992.

177. *ORGSYN: The Organic Syntheses Database*, technical datasheet, Molecular Design Limited, San Leandro, Calif., Nov. 1988.

178. *Journal of Synthetic Methods*, **6–18**, (1980–1992).

179. *REACCS-JSM: The Journal of Synthetic Methods Database for REACCS*, technical datasheet, Molecular Design Limited, San Leandro, Calif., Aug. 1990.

180. *SYNthesis LIBrary*, technical datasheet, Distributed Chemical Graphics, Inc., Meadowbrook, Penn., June 1991.

181. *SYNLIB for Synthesis Ideas*, technical datasheet, Distributed Chemical Graphics, Inc., Meadowbrook, Penn., June 1991.

182. W. Theilheimer, Ed., *Synthetic Methods of Organic Chemistry*, S. Karger, Basel and New York, Vol. 1–35, 1946–1981.

183. *Theilheimer: The Synthetic Methods of Organic Chemistry Reaction Database*, technical datasheet, Molecular Design limited, San Leandro, Calif., Nov. 1991.

184. W. G. Town, *Chem. Brit.*, **25**, 1118–1120 (1989).

185. S. R. Heller and D. E. Meyer, *Chem. Int.*, **12**, 89–94 (1990).

186. D. E. Meyer in ref. 3, pp. 251–259.

187. D. E. Meyer and W. A. Warr, Eds., *Chemical Structure Software for Personal Computers*, American Chemical Society, Washington, D.C., 1988.

188. D. E. Meyer in W. A. Warr, Ed., *Graphics for Chemical Structures: Integration with Text and Data*, ACS Symposium Series No. 341, American Chemical Society, Washington, D.C., 1987, Chapt. 4, pp. 29–36.

189. B. Curry-Koenig and C. Seiter, *American Laboratory*, **18**, 70, 72, 74, 76, 78 (May 1986).

190. C. Seiter and P. Cohan, *American Laboratory*, **18**, 40, 42, 44, 46–47 (Sept. 1986).

191. J. C. Marshall, *J. Chem. Inf. Comput. Sci.*, **27**, 47–49 (1987).

192. M. Z. Nagy, S. Kozics, T. Veszpremi, and P. Bruck in ref. 3, pp. 127–130.

193. R. Cohen, *MacWeek* (Jan. 27, 1992).

194. *CSC ChemFinder: Desktop Chemical Information Management*, technical datasheet, Cambridge Scientific Computing, Inc., Cambridge, Mass., 1992.

195. *The CSC ChemOffice: Drawing, Modeling, and Information Management*, technical datasheet, Cambridge Scientific Computing, Inc., Cambridge, Mass., 1992.

196. *MarkOut Version 2.1 User Guide*, Fraser Williams (Scientific Systems) Ltd., Poynton, Cheshire, England, August 1990.

197. *MarkOut*, technical brochure, Fraser Williams (Scientific Systems) Limited, Poynton, Cheshire, England, November 1991.

198. C. Hansch and A. Leo, *Substituent Constants for Correlation Analysis in Chemistry and Biology*, John Wiley & Sons, Inc., New York, 1979.

199. J. Gambino, F. Focher, C. Hildebrand, G. Maga, T. Noonan, S. Spadari, and G. Wright, *J. Med. Chem.*, **35**, 2979–2983 (1992).

200. O. Guner, *Molecular Connection*, **10**(6) (Dec. 1991).

201. L. M. Dumont, *Molecular Connection*, **10**(2), 6–7, (April 1991).

202. "MACCS-II Spreadsheet Excels," *Molecular Connection*, **9**(6) 4, (Dec. 1990).

203. G. Fenton, C. G. Newton, B. M. Wyman, P. Bagge. D. I. Iron, D. Riddell, and G. D. Jones, *J. Med. Chem.* **32**, 265–272 (1989).

204. *Molecule Spreadsheet User Guide*, Molecular Design Limited, San Leandro, Calif., Dec. 1990.

205. *Molecule Spreadsheet User Guide: Addendum for Revision 1.2*, Molecular Design Limited, San Leandro, Calif., Dec. 1991.

206. "TRIPOS' Molecular Spreadsheet: Expanding the Reach of Computational Chemistry", *Product Viewpoint*, **5**(14) (Aug. 19, 1992).

207. *SYBYL Molecular Spreadsheet*, technical brochure, TRIPOS Associates, Inc., St. Louis, Mo., 1991.

208. J. T. Chou and P. C. Jurs, *J. Chem. Inf. Comput. Sci.*, **19**, 172–178 (1979).

209. Y. C. Martin, *Quantitative Drug Design: A Critical Introduction*, Marcel Dekker, Inc., New York, 1978.

210. T. Fujita in C. Hansch, P. G. Sammes, and J. B. Taylor, Eds., *Comprehensive Medicinal Chemistry: The Rational Design, Mechanistic Study & Therapeutic Applications of Chemical Compounds*, Vol. 4, Pergamon Press, Oxford, England, 1990, Chapt. 21.1, pp. 497–560.

211. K. H. Kim and Y. C. Martin, *J. Pharm. Sci.*, **75**, 637–638 (1986).

212. F. Darvas, I. Erdos, and G. Teglas in D. Hadzi and B. Jerman-Blazic, Eds., *QSAR in Drug Design and Toxicology*, Elsevier Publishers B. V., Amsterdam, 1987, pp. 70–73.

213. R. F. Rekker in J. A. K. Buisman, Ed., *Biological Activity and Chemical Structure*, Elsevier Scientific Publishing Company, Amsterdam, 1977, pp. 231–238.

214. R. F. Rekker, *The Hydrophobic Fragmental Constant: Its Derivation and Application: A Means of Characterizing Membrane Systems*, Elsevier Scientific Publishing Company, Amsterdam, 1977.

215. G. G. Nys and R. F. Rekker, *Chim. Therap.*, **8**, 521–535 (1973).

216. R. F. Rekker and H. M. de Kort, *Eur. J. Med. Chem.*, **14**, 479–488 (1979).

217. K. Takeuchi, C. Kuroda, and M. Ishida, *J. Chem. Inf. Comput. Sci.*, **30**, 22–26 (1990).

218. *PKALC: Version 1.0: Calculation of pK_a Values from Structure*, user manual, CompuDrug NA, Inc., Rochester, N.Y., 1992.

219. D. D. Perrin, B. Dempsey, and E. P. Serjeant, *pK_a Prediction for Organic Acids and Bases*, Chapman & Hall Ltd., London, 1981.

220. M. J. S. Dewar and P. J. Grisdale, *J. Amer. Chem. Soc.*, **84**, 3539–3541 (1962).

221. *Ibid.*, 3541–3546 (1962).

222. *Ibid.*, 3546–3548 (1962).

223. *Ibid.*, 3548–3553 (1962).

224. *CHEMEST: A Program for Chemical Property Estimation: User's Guide*, Technical Database Services, Inc. and Arthur D. Little, Inc., New York, 1987.

225. W. Lyman, W. Reehl, and D. Rosenblatt, Eds., *Research and Development of Methods for Estimating Physicochemical Properties of Organic Compounds of Environmental Concern*, Final Report (in 2 Parts), Phase II, prepared for the U.S. Army Medical Bioengineering Research and Development Laboratory, Fort Detrick, Frederick, Md, June 1981.

226. W. J. Lyman, W. F. Reehl, and D. H Rosenblatt, *Handbook of Chemical Property Estimation Methods: Environmental Behavior of Organic Compounds*, McGraw-Hill Book Company, New York, 1982; reprinted by American Chemical Society, Washington, D.C., 1990.

227. K. Enslein and H. H. Borgstedt, *Toxicol. Letters*, **49**, 107–121 (1989).

228. K. Enslein, *Pharmacol. Rev.*, **36**, 131S–135S (1984).

229. V. K. Gombar, K. Enslein, J. B. Hart, B. W. Blake, and H. H. Borgstedt, *Risk Analysis*, **11**, 509–517 (1991).

230. K. Enslein, B. W. Blake, and H. H. Borgstedt, *Mutagenesis*, **5**, 305–306 (1990).

231. B. W. Blake, K. Enslein, V. K. Gombar, and H. H. Borgstedt, *Mut. Res.*, **241**, 261–271 (1990).

232. K. Enslein, H. H Borgstedt, M. E. Tomb, B. W. Blake, and J. B. Hart, *Toxicol. Ind. Health*, **3**, 267–287 (1987).

233. V. K. Gombar and K. Enslein, *Quant. Struct.-Act. Relat.*, **9**, 321–325 (1990).

234. K. Enslein, B. W. Blake, M. E. Tomb, and H. H. Borgstedt, *In Vitro Toxicol.*, **1**, 33–44 (1986).

235. V. K. Gombar, H. H. Borgstedt, K. Enslein, J. B. Hart, and B. W. Blake, *Quant. Struct.-Act. Relat.*, **10**, 306–332 (1991).

236. K. Enslein and P. N. Craig, *J. Envir. Path. Toxicol.*, **2**, 115–121 (1978).

237. K. Enslein, T. M. Tuzzeo, H. H. Borgstedt, B.

W. Blake, and J. B. Hart in K. L. E. Kaiser, Ed., *QSAR in Environmental Toxicology-II: Proceedings of the 2nd International Workshop*, D. Reidel Publishing Company, Dordrecht, Holland, 1987, pp. 91–106.

238. K. Enslein, B. W. Blake, T. M. Tuzzeo, H. H. Borgstedt, J. B. Hart, and H. Salem, *In Vitro Toxicol.*, **2**, 1–14 (1988).

239. K. Enslein, H. H. Borgstedt, B. W. Blake, and J. B. Hart, *In Vitro Toxicol.*, **1**, 129–147 (1987).

240. *TOPKAT*, technical brochure, Health Designs, Inc., Rochester, N.Y., August 1990.

241. L. B. Kier and L. H. Hall, *Molecular Connectivity in Structure-Activity Analysis*, Research Studies Press Ltd., Letchworth, England, 1986.

242. V. K. Gombar and D. V. S. Jain, *Ind. J. Chem.*, **26A**, 554–555 (1987).

243. V. K. Gombar and K. Enslein, *In Vitro Toxicol.*, **2**, 117–127 (1989).

244. J. Gasteiger and M. Marsili, *Tetrahedron*, **36**, 3219–3228 (1980).

245. J. Mullay, *J. Comp. Chem.*, **9**, 399–405 (1988).

246. F. Darvas, *J. Mol. Graphics*, **6**, 80–86 (1988).

247. F. Darvas in K. L. E. Kaiser, Ed., *QSAR in Environmental Toxicology*, Vol. II, D. Reidel Publishing Co., Dordrecht, Holland, 1987, p. 71.

248. P. Zurer, *Chem. Eng. News*, **66**(38), 27, (Sept. 19, 1988).

249. B. Testa and P. Jenner, *Drug Metabolism: Clinical and Biochemical Aspects*, Marcel Dekker, Inc., New York, 1976.

250. P. Jenner and B. Testa, Eds., *Concepts in Drug Metabolism*, Marcel Dekker, Inc., New York and Basel, 1981.

251. J. L. Wisniewski, *J. Chem. Inf. Comput. Sci.*, **30**, 324–332 (1990).

252. L. Goebels, A. J. Lawson, and J. L. Wisniewski, *J. Chem. Inf. Comput. Sci.*, **31**, 216–225 (1991).

253. *AUTONOM Version 1.0 User Guide*, Springer-Verlag, Berlin, 1991.

254. R. A. Glennon, *J. Med. Chem.*, **35**, 4918 (1992).

255. Y. Wolman, *J. Chem. Inf. Comput. Sci.*, **27**, 144–145 (1987).

256. SANDRA: *Your Window to Beilstein:* Version *2.0*, technical datasheet, Springer-Verlag, Berlin, 1992.

257. S. R. Heller, *Database*, **10**(4), 47–52 (Aug. 1987).

258. A. Lawson, *192nd American Chemical Society National Meeting*, Anaheim, Calif., Sept. 7–12, 1986.

259. A. J. Lawson in W. A. Warr, Ed., *Graphics for Chemical Structures: Integration with Text and Data*, ACS Symposium Series No. *341*, American Chemical Society, Washington, D.C., 1987, Chapt. 8, pp. 80–87.

260. *The Beilstein Handbook of Organic Chemistry*, Basic and Supplementary Series, Beilstein Institute, Frankfurt and Springer-Verlag, Berlin, 1918–1992.

261. L. Domokos, C. Jochum, and H. Maier in H. R. Collier, Ed., "Chemical Information: Information in Chemistry, Pharmacology and Patents," Proceedings of the Montreux 1989 International Chemical Information Conference, Montreux, Switzerland, September 26–28, 1989, Springer-Verlag, Berlin, 1989, pp. 191–199.

262. *CHCD Dictionary of Natural Products on CD-ROM*, technical brochure, Chapman & Hall Limited, London, England, 1992.

263. S. R. Heller, *J. Chem. Inf. Comput. Sci.*, **31**, 430–432 (1991).

264. *Beilstein Current Facts in Chemistry: The Bench Tool for Chemists*, technical brochure, Springer-Verlag, New York, 1991.

265. D. H. Smith in ref. 16, Chap. 3, pp. 18–40.

266. W. G. Town, *J. Chem. Inf. Comput. Sci.*, **32**, 393–394 (1992).

CHAPTER FOURTEEN

The Quantitative Analysis of Structure–Activity Relationships

HUGO KUBINYI

BASF, Hauptlaboratorium
Ludwigshafen, Germany

CONTENTS

1 Introduction, 498
  1.1 History and development of QSAR, 498
  1.2 Drug-receptor interactions, 500
  1.3 Biological data. The additivity of group
     contributions, 503

2 Parameters, 505
  2.1 Lipophilicity parameters, 509
  2.2 The measurement of partition coefficients and
     related lipophilicity parameters, 511
  2.3 Lipophilicity contributions and the calculation
     of partition coefficients, 512
  2.4 Polarizability parameters, 513
  2.5 Electronic parameters, 513
  2.6 Steric parameters, 515
  2.7 Other parameters, 515
  2.8 Indicator variables, 516

3 Quantitative Models, 517
  3.1 The extrathermodynamic approach (Hansch
     analysis), 517
  3.2 The additivity model (Free Wilson
     analysis), 520
  3.3 The relationships between Hansch and Free
     Wilson analysis (the mixed approach), 522
  3.4 Nonlinear relationships, 523
  3.5 Dissociation and ionization of acids and
     bases, 526
  3.6 Other QSAR approaches, 527

4 Statistical Methods, 528

Burger's Medicinal Chemistry and Drug Discovery,
Fifth Edition, Volume 1: Principles and Practice,
Edited by Manfred E. Wolff.
ISBN 0-471-57556-9 © 1995 John Wiley & Sons, Inc.

4.1 Regression analysis, 528
4.2 Partial least squares (PLS) analysis and other multivariate statistical methods, 530
5 Design of Test Series in QSAR, 532
6 Applications of Hansch Analysis, 533
6.1 Enzyme inhibition, 534
6.2 Other *in vitro* data, 536
6.3 Pharmacokinetic data, 538
6.4 Other biological data, 539
6.5 Activity-activity relationships, 540
7 Applications of Free Wilson Analysis and Related Models, 541
8 3D-QSAR Approaches, 543
8.1 Stereochemistry and drug action, 543
8.2 Active site interaction models, 544
8.3 Comparative molecular field analysis (CoMFA), 546
9 Summary and Conclusions, 550

1 INTRODUCTION

1.1 History and Development of QSAR

The concept of quantitative structure–activity relationships (QSAR) dates back to the nineteenth century. Crum-Brown and Fraser (1) published equation 14.1 in 1868, which is considered to be the first formulation of a quantitative structure–activity relationship: the "physiological activity" Φ was expressed as a function of the chemical structure C.

$$\Phi = f(C) \qquad (14.1)$$

A few decades later Richet (2), Meyer (3), and Overton (4) independently found linear relationships between lipophilicity, expressed as solubility or oil–water partition coefficients, and biological effects, like toxicity and narcotic activity (5). Fühner realized that within homologous series narcotic activities increase in a geometric progression, i.e., $1:3:3^2:3^3$, etc. (6).

Many other studies confirmed these relationships, using different lipophilicity parameters to describe various nonspecific biological activities. Ferguson (7) observed a "cut-off" of biological activities beyond a certain range of lipophilicity and gave a thermodynamic interpretation for such nonlinear structure–activity relationships.

Bruice, Kharasch, and Winzler (8) formulated group contributions to biological activity values in a series of thyroid hormone analogs, which may be considered as a first Free Wilson-type analysis. On the other hand, Zahradnik (9–11) tried to apply the concept of the Hammett equation (eq. 14.2) (12), which describes the reactivities of aromatic organic compounds in a quantitative manner, to biological data (eq. 14.3; τ_i is the biological activity value of the *i*th member of a series, τ_{Et} is the activity value of the ethyl compound within the same series, β is a substituent constant, which corresponds to the electronic σ parameter in the Hammett equation, and α is a constant characterizing the biological system, which corresponds to the Hammett reaction constant ρ).

$$\log k_{R-X} - \log k_{R-H} = \rho\sigma \qquad (14.2)$$

$$\log \tau_i - \log \tau_{Et} = \alpha\beta \qquad (14.3)$$

Equation 14.3 applies only to nonspecific biological activities, most often within homologous series. At about the same time Hansen derived a Hammett-type relationship between the toxicities of substituted benzoic acids and the electronic σ constants of their substituents (13).

In the early sixties two different quantitative approaches were developed, one by Hansch and Fujita (14, 15), the other by Free and Wilson (16), later called Hansch analysis (linear free energy-related approach or extrathermodynamic approach) and Free Wilson analysis, respectively. The concept of Hansch and Fujita was to combine different physicochemical parameters in a linear additive manner (eq. 14.4; log $1/C$ = logarithm of the inverse molar dose that produces a certain biological response; log P = logarithm of the n-octanol/water partition coefficient P), to define a calculated lipophilicity parameter π (eq. 14.5), to be used instead of measured lipophilicity values, and to formulate a parabolic model for the nonlinear dependence of biological activities on lipophilicity (eq. 14.6) (17–19).

$$\log 1/C = a \log P + b\sigma$$
$$+ \cdots + \text{const.} \quad (14.4)$$

$$\pi_{X} = \log P_{R-X} - \log P_{R-H} \quad (14.5)$$

$$\log 1/C = a(\log P)^2 + b \log P + c\sigma$$
$$+ \cdots + \text{const.} \quad (14.6)$$

The Free Wilson model in its currently used version (20) can be expressed by equation 14.7, where a_{ij} is the group contribution of a substituent X_i in the position j and μ is the biological activity value of a reference compound.

$$\log 1/C = \sum a_{ij} + \mu \quad (14.7)$$

Improvements resulted from the combination of Hansch equations with indicator variables (21) to a mixed Hansch/Free Wilson model (22) and from the formulation of nonlinear models other than the parabolic model, e.g., the bilinear model (eq. 14.8) (23).

$$\log 1/C = a \log P$$
$$- b \log(\beta P + 1) + c \quad (14.8)$$

Pattern recognition methods (24, 25) have been applied in QSAR studies; new statistical techniques, e.g. the partial least squares (PLS) method (26, 27), now offer better opportunities to correlate large numbers of variables with biological activity values of a limited number of objects.

Three-dimensional quantitative structure–activity relationships (3D-QSAR) were developed from the first attempts to map a receptor surface from the results of Hansch analyses (e.g. 28). Höltje (29, 30) postulated certain amino acid side chains as binding partners, calculated interaction energies in standard geometries, and correlated these energies with biological activity values. Other approaches of mapping a receptor surface are the distance geometry method (31, 32) and the program GRID for the calculation of interaction energies between different probe atoms and the surface of a protein whose 3D structure is known from crystallographic analysis (33).

Comparative molecular field analysis (CoMFA) correlates different fields of ligands with their biological activities (34–38). The molecules of a chemically related series are superimposed according to a pharmacophore hypothesis and a grid is laid over the molecules. The values of the steric and electrostatic fields (and optionally other fields) are calculated in every grid point for each molecule of the series. An appropriate multivariate statistical method, e.g. PLS analysis, correlates thousands of such energy values with biological activities.

The book *Quantitative Drug Design*, volume IV of the six-volume set *Comprehensive Medicinal Chemistry* (39), covers the whole field of QSAR. Numerous other monographs on QSAR methodology and applications (40–47), on physicochemical parameters (48–56), and on related topics (57–64) have been published. In addition, there are several monograph series (65–67), proceedings of QSAR and QSAR-related symposia (68–84), the journal *Quantitative Structure–Activity Relationships*, especially the abstracts section of this journal (85) which year by year contains about 400–500 excellently prepared abstracts of QSAR-related publications, other abstracts services (86–88), as well as some other journals (89) which contain QSAR publications as their regular content.

The history of QSAR has been reviewed in books (e.g. 40) and in dedicated articles (5, 90–93).

1.2 Drug-Receptor Interactions

The interactions of drugs with their biological counterparts are determined by intermolecular forces. QSAR studies derive models for the correlation of biological activities with physicochemical parameters (Hansch analysis) or with indicator variables encoding different structural features (Free Wilson analysis). Drugs, which exert their biological effects by interaction with a specific target, be it an enzyme, a receptor, an ion channel, a nucleic acid, or any other biological macromolecule, must have a three-dimensional structure which in its surface properties is more or less complementary to the binding site. The better the fit of the drug and the complementarity of the surface properties are, the higher is the affinity of the drug to its binding site and the higher may be its biological activity.

In addition to the complementarity of the 3D structures and the surface properties, the drug has to reach the binding site. Even in simple *in vitro* experiments, e.g., in enzyme inhibition, the surrounding water molecules compete to form hydrogen bonds to the binding site and to the functional groups of the ligand. In complex biological systems, like in cells, isolated organs, or whole animal experiments, a certain range of lipophilicity enables the drug to cross lipid membranes as well as aqueous phases.

QSAR methods are used to prove hypotheses regarding the dependence of biological activities on physicochemical interactions. The different interactions between a ligand and its binding site can be "seen" in three dimensions if protein crystallography-derived 3D structures are available. However, structure-based drug design only concerns ligand design and does not consider transport and distribution properties or metabolic degradation. These areas still remain in the field of classical QSAR studies.

In nonspecific biological activities caused by membrane perturbation, only the distribution of the drug and its local concentration in a certain membrane compartment is responsible for its biological activity.

The concept of specific receptors (94, 95) functioning as binding sites of drugs goes back to investigations by Langley (96), Fischer (97), and Ehrlich (98). In the following the term "receptor" is sometimes used as a synonym for any biological target, e.g., a specific binding site at a macromolecule; in a strict sense receptors are soluble or membrane-bound proteins that are able to produce a certain biological response by a series of mostly unknown events. As receptors are reviewed in chapter 11, only a few aspects relevant to quantitative structure–activity relationships will be discussed here.

In the meantime the originally static lock and key model was modified to a more realistic picture, with flexible drug molecules and dynamic receptors (99, 100). Whenever a ligand approaches its binding site, both partners may change their shape (induced fit, flexible fit). The three-dimensional structures of some membrane-bound proteins and receptor-type protein complexes are known at atomic resolution, e.g., the photosynthetic reaction center (101), the light-driven proton pump bacteriorhodopsin (102), and the bacterial membrane-channel porin (103). Some attempts have been made to model G protein-coupled receptors (104–106) because of their similarity in the number of trans-membrane domains to bacteriorhodopsin. Most of our knowledge regarding the geometry of ligand-binding site interactions results from 3D structures of soluble proteins, especially of enzymes and their inhibitor complexes (107–110).

Herbette (111, 112) investigated the partitioning into and the distribution of drugs in biological membranes; the correct spatial arrangement of the drug and its correct orientation in the membrane with respect to the surface of the membrane-embedded receptor is considered to be of utmost importance for the drug–receptor interaction.

The affinity of a drug D to its binding site at the receptor R is determined by the energy difference ΔG between the free states of both partners and the drug-receptor complex $[DR]$, which is made up from the enthalpy change ΔH and the entropy change ΔS (eq. 14.9). ΔG is related to the equilibrium constant K for the reaction $D + R = [DR]$ by equation 14.10.

$$\Delta G = \Delta H - T \, \Delta S \qquad (14.9)$$

$$\Delta G = -2.303RT \log K \qquad (14.10)$$

Covalent bonds have energy ranges of about 170–$600 \, \text{kJ} \cdot \text{mol}^{-1}$. As they are irreversible, they are not relevant to drug-receptor interactions; only alkylating agents (e.g., antitumor drugs) and suicide enzyme inhibitors (e.g., the penicillins and cephalosporins) form covalent bonds.

Electrostatic interactions are important attractive forces (59, 113–115), due to their relative strength. The molecular electrostatic fields of the drug and its binding site are considered to be responsible for the relative orientation of the ligand and for the first contact to the binding site (59).

Most interactions between charged groups include hydrogen bonds. Their energy values depend on the distance, the interaction geometry (59, 114, 116), and the solvation-desolvation energy balance. Different energy values are given in literature; from the investigation of muteins the values of charged hydrogen bonds were estimated to be mainly in the range of 15–$19 \, \text{kJ} \cdot \text{mol}^{-1}$, while those of neutral hydrogen bonds were estimated to be 2–$6 \, \text{kJ} \cdot \text{mol}^{-1}$ (117–119).

Correspondingly the introduction of a neutral hydrogen bond increases affinity by a factor of about 2–20, whereas the introduction of a charged hydrogen bond increases it by a factor of 400–2000 (119). Differences in free-energy values, being derived from ligands containing a hydroxy group and ligands having a hydrogen atom instead, have been compiled for different enzymes (120). From a recent comparison of the binding energies of amide–amide hydrogen bonds in aqueous solution and in nonpolar solvents it was concluded that earlier values of neutral hydrogen bond energies may be too small (121).

Dispersion forces are attractive forces between atoms at close distances; local dipole moments, which result from the movement of the electrons in a molecule, induce dipoles in the opposite molecule, leading to electrostatic attractions. Repulsive forces are obtained at closer distances, due to an unfavorable overlap of the van der Waals spheres of both molecules. Dipole–dipole interactions and dispersion forces are much weaker than other electrostatic interactions; however, if there is a close contact between both molecules over a relatively large surface area, they may sum up to higher values.

Hydrophobic interactions are most important for noncovalent interactions in aqueous solution. Loosely associated water molecules at hydrophobic surfaces have a degree of order and are thus in an unfavorable entropic state. The association of the hydrophobic areas of a ligand and its binding site releases the ordered water molecules, which leads to a gain in entropy; however, the actual strength of the hydrophobic effect still is under discussion (115, 122).

Negative contributions result from the loss of translational and rotational energies of the ligand in the bound state, from the loss of internal rotational degrees of freedom (conformational entropy), and from the desolvation enthalpy of polar groups of both partners. Rigid analogs containing the correct conformation of the pharmacophore are often much more active and show a higher degree of selectivity than the more flexible ones.

The contribution of electrostatic interactions is often overemphasized because the negative influence of desolvation is neglected. But hydrophobic interactions also have negative consequences: decreasing solubility renders transport and distribution in the biological system more difficult or even impossible if a drug molecule becomes too lipophilic.

The different contributions to the overall free energy of ligand binding to a biological macromolecule (113, 115, 123, 124) and the role of the surrounding water molecules (59, 125) have been reviewed; the most important favorable and unfavorable enthalpic and entropic contributions are summarized in Figure 14.1.

No general conclusions can be drawn whether the binding of agonists and antagonists is stabilized either by enthalpic or by entropic contributions (126). The dispute, whether QSAR really helps to find the optimum within a series of biologically active molecules, cannot generally be decided. The QSAR results depend on the validity of the underlying hypotheses and on the precision of the biological data. Most often QSAR analyses are retrospective studies. For new compounds within a

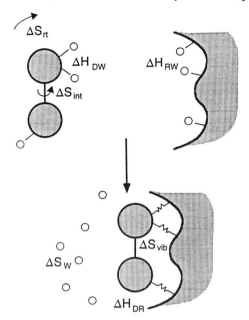

Fig. 14.1 Drug-receptor interactions. ΔH_{dw} and ΔH_{rw} are the enthalpies of hydration of the drug and the receptor, respectively, ΔH_{dr} is the enthalpic contribution of the drug–receptor interaction, ΔS_{rt} is the overall rotational and translational entropy, and ΔS_{int} is the internal entropy of the free drug. ΔS_w is the increase in entropy due to the release of bound water molecules (small circles) and ΔS_{vib} is the entropy gain due to new low-frequency vibrational modes associated with the drug receptor noncovalent interaction. Reproduced from Figure 1 of ref. 123 with permission from the American Chemical Society, Washington, D.C.

congeneric series the quality of prediction of the biological activity values depends on the spanned parameter space, on the distance of the new analogs to the other compounds, on the conformational flexibility of the ligand and its binding site, on multiple binding modes, and on differences in transport and metabolism.

Prediction is not the primary goal of QSAR analyses. QSAR helps to analyze the structure–activity relationships and to find e.g., the optimum of lipophilicity or size of a certain group. QSAR also enables medicinal chemists to look at their structures in terms of physicochemical properties instead of only considering certain pharmacophoric groups in it.

Rational drug design did not start with

QSAR. Chemists and biologists always followed rational guidelines, depending on the state of knowledge at their time. However, our knowledge about the influence of lipophilicity on drug transport and distribution in a biological system (i.e., the concept of optimum lipophilicity) and on the relative importance of the different physicochemical properties being responsible for receptor affinity mainly evolved from QSAR studies.

1.3 Biological Data—The Additivity of Group Contributions

All kinds of biological data (41, 127, 128) can be described by quantitative structure–activity relationships, provided they are in the right scale:

- Affinity data, such as substrate or receptor binding constants.
- Rate constants, such as association, dissociation, and Michealis-Menten constants.
- Inhibition constants, especially IC_{50} and K_i values of different enzymes.
- Pharmacokinetic parameters.
- *In vitro* biological activity values.
- *In vivo* biological activity values, i.e. various pharmacodynamic and toxic activities of drugs.

Each single step of drug distribution and binding corresponds to partitioning between an aqueous and a nonaqueous phase, the latter being a membrane or another lipid phase, a serum protein, the active site of an enzyme, or the binding site of a receptor. In the case of biological data which result from a sequence of several independent processes (e.g., whole animal data), sometimes one effect predominates, e.g., the bioavailability, the penetration of the blood–brain barrier, or the affinity to the receptor site. The relationships and the resulting QSAR equations may become much more complex if several of these effects overlap. Equilibrium constants are related to free energy values ΔG by equation 14.10. Thus rate constants (not % absorption or % concentration in a certain compartment) or equilibrium constants (e.g., K_i values, not % inhibition at a certain concentration) must be used in QSAR studies. All biological response values have to be transformed to equieffective molar doses, i.e., to molar dose levels which produce or prevent a certain pharmacodynamic effect. Corresponding to equation 14.10, the data have to be expressed in a logarithmic scale. Inverse logarithms, i.e. logarithms of reciprocal molar concentrations (e.g., $\log 1/C$ or pC), are preferred to obtain higher values for more active compounds (values in this scale are directly comparable to pH and pK_a values). There is another reason to use the logarithmic scale for biological activity values. A precondition for the application of regression analysis is a normal distribution of the experimental error; for biological experiments this only holds true in the logarithmic scale.

Thus, $\log 1/C$ (C being a molar concentration producing a certain effect, e.g., an ED_{50} value), $\log 1/K_i$, pI_{50}, $\log k$ values, etc., are correct biological parameters for QSAR studies. Other data, such as mg/kg values, sometimes give satisfactory results as they are, at least within a small molecular weight range, correlated to molar doses; the same holds true for some % effect or % concentration data. However, in good QSAR practice the use of such scales should be avoided. Linear values (instead of logarithmic values) are sometimes found in the QSAR literature; if they only cover a small range, they are correlated to logarithmic values. Any conclusions drawn from a comparison of the results, as to whether one or the other scale might be "better," are meaningless; the results only reflect an excessively narrow range of data and fortuitous errors may lead to wrong interpretations.

A medicinal chemist, whether familiar with the principles of quantitative structure–activity relationships or not, implicitly applies the additivity concept of group contributions to biological activity values. In general, the assumption of a more or less strict additivity of group contributions has been proven to be correct by thousands of QSAR equations and by a few dedicated investigations which will be discussed below.

Andrews (113, 123) showed that certain functional groups contribute to receptor affinity in a more or less constant range. He used equation 14.11 (ΔS_{rt} = overall translational and rotational entropy of the drug in solution; n_{DOF} and E_{DOF} = numbers and energies of internal degrees of freedom; n_X and E_X = numbers and energies of interaction of different functional groups) to calculate "mean binding energies" *AVERAGE* ΔG and derived equation 14.12 (all energy values in $kJ \cdot mol^{-1}$) from the affinity constants of 200 different ligands; the term $T \Delta S_{rt}$ (first term at the right side of eq. 14.12) was fixed at $-59 \, kJ \cdot mol^{-1}$.

$$AVERAGE \; \Delta G = T \, \Delta S_{rt} + n_{DOF} \cdot E_{DOF}$$

$$+ \sum n_X \cdot E_X \quad (14.11)$$

$$AVERAGE \; \Delta G = -59 - 3.0 n_{DOF}$$

$$+ 3.0 n_{C(sp^2)} + 3.4 n_{C(sp^3)} + 48 n_{N^+}$$

$$+ 5.0 n_N + 34 n_{CO_2^-} + 42 n_{PO_4^{2-}} + 10.5 n_{OH}$$

$$+ 14.2 n_{C=O} + 4.6 n_{O,S} + 5.4 n_{Hal} \quad (14.12)$$

Equation 14.12 is not predictive; the intrinsic binding energy contributions cover a wide range, if being calculated from different subsets. *AVERAGE* ΔG means that there are "poor fit compounds," binding much worse than predicted by equation 14.12, and "exceptional fit compounds," binding much better. Thus the values of

equation 14.12 should be interpreted as the lower limits of interaction energies in a geometrically favorable arrangement of the interacting groups.

General rules of bioisosterism (129–131) are reflected by equation 14.12. However, significant exceptions may be obtained, dependent on the biological system. Bartlett (132, 133) described thermolysin inhibitors, where the exchange of the –NH– group of phosphonamidate analogs against oxygen (phosphonates) reduces affinities to the enzyme by a factor of about 1000, while in the case of the –CH_2– analogs (phosphinates) affinities are retained. The –NH– group interacts as a hydrogen bond donor with an acceptor atom at the binding site. The phosphonamidate and the phosphonate groups are hydrated in solution, which is unfavorable for binding; only in the phosphonamidates is this negative effect counterbalanced by a hydrogen bond to the binding site. Therefore the situation is balanced for the phosphonamidates as well as for the phosphinates (no hydrogen bonds at all); it is highly unfavorable for the phosphonates, explaining the large differences in their affinities.

Another limitation of the concept of bioisosterism arises from different conformational preferences of closely related analogs. Even small structural variations of X in Phe-X-Phe (e.g., in going from $X =$ –O– to $X = $ –NH–) drastically change the conformation maps (134); the results of semiempirical calculations (134) are identical to the experimental data for the corresponding structures, as contained in the Cambridge database of crystal structures (135).

Evidence for additivity of binding energies has been derived in cases where a small molecule A and a larger molecule B interact with different parts of a binding site. If such molecules are combined to A–B, the group A may be considered as a substituent of the larger molecule B (the "anchor principle") (136, 137). As most of the loss of entropy upon binding can be attributed to the binding of B, the difference of free energy values between B and AB reflects the true binding energy of A. Additivity in this sense has elegantly been proven by a series of single and double/ multiple point mutation experiments in proteins (119, 138), demonstrating a strict additivity of multiple exchanges as compared to single exchanges.

In only a few investigations has the number of various kinds of interactions of ligands with their binding sites been correlated with affinities or with some other type of biological activity. The shift of the oxygen binding curves of hemoglobins is a function of the different interactions of the allosteric effector molecules with the protein (eq. 14.13; n_I and n_C are the numbers of ionic and covalent interactions) (139). In equation 14.13 and in all the following QSAR equations the values given in parentheses after the regression coefficients are the 95% confidence intervals, n is the number of compounds, r is the multiple correlation coefficient, s is the standard deviation, and F is the Fisher significance ratio (Section 4.1).

$$\Delta G = -3.14(\pm 0.62)n_I - 6.78(\pm 1.39)n_C$$
$$- 8.29(\pm 2.87) \quad (14.13)$$
$$(n = 29; \ r = 0.928; \ s = 3.34; \ F = 81.15)$$

Equation 14.13 shows that the binding energies of the ligands to the various hemoglobins can be explained by the numbers of ionic and covalent interactions; a reversible covalent bond contributes about twice as much as an ionic interaction.

The different contacts of thermolysin inhibitors to their binding site were correlated with inhibitory potencies (eq. 14.14, recalculated; $NPHO$ = total complementary nonpolar carbon contacts, i.e., hydrophobic interactions; $NHBOND$ = buried hydrogen bonds) (140).

$$\log 1/K_i = 0.624(\pm 0.10)NPHO$$
$$+ 0.217(\pm 0.08)NHBOND$$
$$- 3.623(\pm 0.59) \quad (14.14)$$
$$(n = 9; \ r = 0.993; \ s = 0.228; \ F = 202.51)$$

There is sufficient evidence that the additivity of group contributions to biological data is an intrinsic feature resulting from the thermodynamic relationships between the free energies of binding and biological activity values. Deviations arise from the nonlinear dependences of transport and distribution on lipophilicity, from steric crowding of ligand groups, leading to conformational distortions, from multiple binding modes, from changes in the mechanism of action, and from different metabolic pathways.

2 PARAMETERS

Parameters are needed to describe the intermolecular forces of the drug–receptor interaction and the transport and distribution of drugs in a quantitative manner and to correlate them with biological activities. The most important physicochemical and other parameters in this respect are

- Lipophilicity parameters, e.g., partition coefficients and chromatographic parameters.
- Polarizability parameters, e.g., molar refractivity.
- Electronic parameters, e.g., Hammett σ constants, field and resonance parameters, charge transfer constants, dipole moments, and quantum chemical parameters.
- Steric parameters, derived from linear free energy relationships or from geometric considerations.
- Parameters such as molecular weight,

geometric parameters, conformational entropies, connectivity indices, and other topological parameters.

- Indicator variables.

Although hundreds of different parameters have been used in QSAR studies in the past 30 years, there is a lack of adequate parameters to describe some important interactions such as the membrane partitioning of drugs, the strength of hydrogen bonds, the influence of desolvation energies on drug-receptor affinities, and steric interactions with a (most often unknown) binding site.

Early parameter collections included π, π^-, σ_m, σ_p, $\mathscr{F}$, $\mathscr{R}$, and MR values (141–143) of aromatic substituents. In 1979 all known π, MR, σ, and E_s values of about 2000 different substituents were compiled in a book (50); in addition, π, MR, $\mathscr{F}$, $\mathscr{R}$, σ_m, σ_p, and indicator variables for hydrogen bond acceptor and donor properties of the most important aromatic substituents as well as hydrophobic fragmental constants, hydrogen bond acceptor and donor properties, MR, and $\mathscr{F}$ values of selected aliphatic substituents were included. By cluster analysis the substituents were separated into different groups to allow a rational selection of substituents in the design of new analogs (50, 144). Physicochemical parameters, the underlying theories, and their use in QSAR studies have been reviewed in several other monographs (39–43, 48, 49, 51, 52, 54–56) and in dedicated articles (e.g., 145–148).

The most comprehensive review on physicochemical parameters mentions more than 220 different parameters and contains a table of 58 parameters of 59 different substituents, groups, and fragments, together with a correlation matrix of all 58 parameters (148). Later 16 parameters were added to this compilation (149, 150); all parameters are included in a commercially available database DESBASE (151). An in-house compilation of Eli Lilly contains more than 17,000 physicochemical parameters of 3,000 different substituents (152).

Principal component analysis (PCA, compare Section 4.2) reduces the multidimensional data matrices of physicochemical properties to fewer, orthogonal dimensions (149, 150, 153–158). Six properties (aqueous solvation energy, partition coefficient, boiling point, molar refractivity, volume, and vaporization enthalpy) of 114 liquid compounds are nearly quantitatively correlated with two principal components, termed B (bulk) and C (cohesiveness); some other properties can be explained by B and C and additional minor components D, E, and F (154, 155).

Principal component analysis of electronic parameters shows that more than 90% of the information is contained in their first principal component (156). A principal component analysis of seven different chemical descriptors of aromatic substituents leads to a clear grouping of substituents in a plot of the first two components according to hydrogen bond acceptors, hydrogen bond donors, alkyl groups, and halogens (157). Nine descriptor variables, i.e., π, MR, σ_m, σ_p, and the STERIMOL parameters of 100 aromatic substituents (Table 14.1) were investigated by PCA (158). The first component is mainly related to steric bulk and hydrophobicity, the second one to electronic parameters, and the third one again to hydrophobicity and shape.

Principal component analysis was also used to investigate 74 parameters of 59 different substituents (149, 150). Five significant components contain about 84% of the total variance; lipophilic, steric, and electronic parameters are nicely separated in a plot of the first two components, whereas several less well-defined properties are close to the origin of this diagram.

Amino acids have been characterized by a principal component analysis of their side-chain properties (159, 160). These

Table 14.1 Representative Parameters of Aromatic Substituents[a]

Substituents	π	MR^b	σ_m	σ_p	L	$B_i{}^c$	$B_{ii}{}^c$	$B_{iii}{}^c$	$B_{iv}{}^c$
Br	0.86	0.888	0.39	0.23	3.83	1.95	1.95	1.95	1.95
Cl	0.71	0.603	0.37	0.23	3.52	1.80	1.80	1.80	1.80
F	0.14	0.092	0.34	0.06	2.65	1.35	1.35	1.35	1.35
SO$_2$F	0.05	0.865	0.80	0.91	3.50	2.03	2.70	2.45	2.51
SF$_5$	1.23	0.989	0.61	0.68	4.65	2.49	2.49	2.49	2.49
I	1.12	1.394	0.35	0.18	4.23	2.15	2.15	2.15	2.15
NO	−1.20	0.520	0.62	0.91	3.44	1.70	2.44	1.70	1.70
NO$_2$	−0.28	0.736	0.71	0.78	3.44	1.70	1.70	2.44	2.44
N$_3$	0.46	1.020	0.27	0.15	4.62	1.50	4.18	2.34	2.57
H	0.00	0.103	0.00	0.00	2.06	1.00	1.00	1.00	1.00
OH	−0.67	0.285	0.12	−0.37	2.74	1.35	1.93	1.35	1.35
SH	0.39	0.922	0.25	0.15	3.47	1.70	2.33	1.70	1.70
NH$_2$	−1.23	0.542	−0.16	−0.66	2.93	1.50	1.50	1.84	1.84
SO$_2$NH$_2$	−1.82	1.228	0.46	0.57	3.82	2.11	3.07	2.67	2.67
NHNH$_2$	−0.88	0.844	−0.02	−0.55	3.40	1.50	2.82	1.84	1.84
N=CCl$_2$	0.41	1.835	0.21	0.13	5.65	1.70	1.80	1.84	4.54
CF$_3$	0.88	0.502	0.43	0.54	3.30	1.98	2.61	2.44	2.44
OCF$_3$	1.04	0.786	0.38	0.35	4.57	1.35	3.33	2.44	2.44
SCF$_3$	1.44	1.381	0.40	0.50	4.89	1.70	3.69	2.44	2.44
CN	−0.57	0.633	0.56	0.66	4.23	1.60	1.60	1.60	1.60
NCS	1.15	1.724	0.48	0.38	4.29	1.50	2.24	1.64	1.76
SCN	0.41	1.340	0.41	0.52	4.08	1.70	4.45	1.70	1.70
SO$_2$CF$_3$	0.55	1.286	0.79	0.93	4.11	2.11	3.64	2.67	2.67
NHCN	−0.26	1.014	0.21	0.06	3.53	1.50	3.08	1.90	1.90
CHO	−0.65	0.688	0.35	0.42	3.53	1.60	1.60	2.00	2.36
CO$_2$H	−0.32	0.693	0.37	0.45	3.91	1.60	1.60	2.36	2.66
CH$_2$Br	0.79	1.339	0.12	0.14	4.09	1.52	3.75	1.95	1.95
CH$_2$Cl	0.17	1.049	0.11	0.12	3.89	1.52	3.46	1.90	1.90
CH$_2$I	1.50	1.886	0.10	0.11	4.36	1.52	4.15	2.15	2.15
NHCHO	−0.98	1.031	0.19	0.00	4.22	1.50	1.50	1.94	3.61
CONH$_2$	−1.49	0.981	0.28	0.36	4.06	1.60	1.60	2.42	3.07
CH=NOH	−0.38	1.028	0.22	0.10	4.88	1.60	1.60	1.92	3.11
CH$_3$	0.56	0.565	−0.07	−0.17	3.00	1.52	2.04	1.90	1.90
NHCONH$_2$	−1.30	1.372	−0.03	−0.24	5.09	1.84	1.84	1.94	3.61
NHCSNH$_2$	−1.40	2.219	0.22	0.16	4.62	1.50	4.18	2.34	2.57
OCH$_3$	−0.02	0.787	0.12	−0.27	3.98	1.35	2.87	1.90	1.90
CH$_2$OH	−1.03	0.719	0.00	0.00	3.97	1.52	2.70	1.90	1.90
SOCH$_3$	−1.58	1.370	0.52	0.49	4.03	1.60	2.93	2.49	3.36
OSO$_2$CH$_3$	−0.88	1.699	0.39	0.36	4.03	1.35	3.86	1.90	3.57
SO$_2$CH$_3$	−1.63	1.349	0.60	0.72	4.37	2.11	3.15	2.67	2.67
SCH$_3$	0.61	1.382	0.15	0.00	4.30	1.70	3.26	1.90	1.90
NHCH$_3$	−0.47	1.033	−0.30	−0.84	3.53	1.50	3.08	1.90	1.90
NHSO$_2$CH$_3$	−1.18	1.817	0.20	0.03	4.06	1.50	1.90	3.59	3.88
CF$_2$CF$_3$	1.68	0.923	0.47	0.52	4.11	1.98	3.64	2.44	2.44
C≡CH	0.40	0.955	0.21	0.23	4.66	1.60	1.60	1.60	1.60
NHCOCF$_3$	0.08	1.430	0.30	0.12					
CH$_2$CN	−0.57	1.011	0.16	0.01	3.99	1.52	4.12	1.90	1.90
CH=CHNO$_2$	0.11	1.642	0.32	0.26	4.29	1.60	3.24	1.83	4.21

Table 14.1 *(Continued)*

Substituents	π	MR^b	σ_m	σ_p	L	$B_i{}^c$	$B_{ii}{}^c$	$B_{iii}{}^c$	$B_{iv}{}^c$
CH=CH$_2$	0.82	1.099	0.05	−0.02	4.29	1.60	1.60	2.00	3.09
COCH$_3$	−0.55	1.118	0.38	0.50	4.06	1.90	1.90	2.36	2.93
SCOCH$_3$	0.10	1.842	0.39	0.44	5.19	1.70	4.01	1.90	1.90
OCOCH$_3$	−0.64	1.247	0.39	0.31	4.87	1.35	3.68	1.90	1.90
CO$_2$CH$_3$	−0.01	1.289	0.37	0.45	4.85	1.90	1.90	2.36	3.36
NHCOCH$_3$	−0.97	1.493	0.21	0.00	5.15	1.50	3.61	1.90	1.94
CONHCH$_3$	−1.27	1.457	0.35	0.36	5.00	1.60	2.23	2.42	3.07
CH$_2$CH$_3$	1.02	1.030	−0.07	−0.15	4.11	1.52	2.97	1.90	1.90
OCH$_2$CH$_3$	0.38	1.247	0.10	−0.24	4.92	1.35	3.36	1.35	1.90
CH$_2$OCH$_3$	−0.78	1.207	0.02	0.03	4.91	1.52	2.88	1.90	1.90
SC$_2$H$_5$	1.07	1.842	0.18	0.03	5.24	1.70	3.97	1.90	1.90
NHC$_2$H$_5$	0.08	1.498	−0.24	−0.61	4.96	1.50	3.42	1.90	1.90
SO$_2$C$_2$H$_5$	−1.09	1.814	0.60	0.72	5.31	2.11	3.67	2.67	2.67
NMe$_2$	0.18	1.555	−0.15	−0.83	3.53	1.50	2.56	2.80	2.80
PMe$_2$	0.44	2.119	0.03	0.31	3.88	2.00	2.97	2.84	3.29
cyclo-Propyl	1.14	1.353	−0.07	−0.21	4.14	1.98	2.24	2.29	2.88
CO$_2$C$_2$H$_5$	0.51	1.747	0.37	0.45	5.96	1.90	1.90	2.36	4.29
(CH$_2$)$_2$CO$_2$H	−0.29	1.652	−0.03	−0.07	5.96	1.52	3.05	2.35	2.67
NHCO$_2$C$_2$H$_5$	0.17	2.118	0.07	−0.15	4.45	1.50	4.97	1.90	5.57
CHMe$_2$	1.53	1.496	−0.07	−0.15	4.11	2.04	2.76	3.16	3.16
n-C$_3$H$_7$	1.55	1.496	−0.07	−0.13	5.05	1.52	3.49	1.90	1.90
OCHMe$_2$	0.85	1.706	0.10	−0.45	4.59	1.35	3.61	1.90	3.16
OC$_3$H$_7$	0.85	1.706	0.10	−0.25	6.05	1.35	4.30	1.90	1.90
SC$_3$H$_7$	1.61	2.307	0.15	0.00	6.21	1.70	4.90	1.90	1.90
NHC$_3$H$_7$	0.62	1.963	−0.24	−0.61	6.07	1.50	4.36	1.90	1.90
2-Thienyl	1.61	2.404	0.09	0.05	5.97	1.65	1.77	3.13	3.16
CH=CHCOCH$_3$	−0.06	2.110	0.21	−0.01	5.80	1.60	3.24	1.83	3.73
COC$_3$H$_7$	0.53	2.048	0.38	0.50	4.67	2.36	3.69	3.16	3.16
CO$_2$C$_3$H$_7$	1.07	2.217	0.37	0.45	6.90	1.90	1.90	2.36	4.83
sec-C$_4$H$_9$	2.04	1.959		−0.12	5.02	1.90	3.16	2.76	3.49
iso-C$_4$H$_9$		1.959		−0.12	5.05	1.52	4.21	1.90	3.16
n-C$_4$H$_9$	2.13	1.969	−0.08	−0.16	6.17	1.52	4.42	1.90	1.90
tert-C$_4$H$_9$	1.98	1.962	−0.10	−0.20	4.11	2.59	2.97	2.86	2.86
OC$_4$H$_9$	1.55	2.166	0.10	−0.32	6.99	1.35	4.79	1.90	1.90
NHC$_4$H$_9$	1.16	2.426	−0.34	−0.51	7.01	1.50	4.97	1.90	1.90
C$_5$H$_{11}$	2.67	2.426	−0.08	−0.16	7.11	1.52	4.94	1.90	1.90
C$_6$H$_5$	1.96	2.536	0.06	−0.01	6.28	1.70	1.70	3.11	3.11
N=NC$_6$H$_5$	1.69	3.131	0.32	0.39	8.43	1.70	1.70	1.92	4.31
OC$_6$H$_5$	2.08	2.768	0.25	−0.03	4.51	1.35	5.89	3.11	3.11
SO$_2$C$_6$H$_5$	0.27	3.320	0.61	0.70	5.82	2.11	6.01	2.67	2.67
OSO$_2$C$_6$H$_5$	0.93	3.670	0.36	0.33	8.20	1.61	3.64	1.80	3.57
NHC$_6$H$_5$	1.37	3.004	−0.12	−0.40	4.53	1.50	5.95	3.11	3.11
NHSO$_2$C$_6$H$_5$	0.45	3.788	0.16	0.01					
cyclo-Hexyl	2.51	2.669	−0.15	−0.22	6.17	2.04	3.49	3.16	3.16
COC$_6$H$_5$	1.05	3.033	0.34	0.43	4.57	2.36	5.98	3.11	3.11
OCOC$_6$H$_5$	1.46	3.233	0.21	0.13	8.15	1.70	4.40	1.70	1.84
N=CHC$_6$H$_5$	−0.29	3.301	−0.08	−0.55	8.40	1.70	3.55	1.80	3.66
CN=NC$_6$H$_5$	−0.29	3.301	0.35	0.42	8.50	1.70	1.70	2.36	4.07

Table 14.1   (*Continued*)

Substituents	π	MR^b	σ_m	σ_p	L	$B_i{}^c$	$B_{ii}{}^c$	$B_{iii}{}^c$	$B_{iv}{}^c$
$CH_2C_6H_5$	2.01	3.001	-0.08	-0.09	3.63	1.52	6.02	3.11	3.11
$CH_2OC_6H_5$	1.66	3.219	0.03	0.04	8.19	1.52	3.09	3.11	3.11
$C\equiv CC_6H_5$	2.65	3.321	0.14	0.16	8.88	1.70	1.70	3.11	3.11
$NHCOC_6H_5$	0.49	3.464	0.02	-0.19	8.40	1.94	3.61	3.11	3.11

[a]Reproduced from Table 1 of ref. 158 with permission from VCH Verlagsgesellschaft mbH, Weinheim, Germany.

[b]MR is scaled by a factor of 0.1, as usual.

[c]$B_i - B_{iv}$ are defined as in ref. 158; B_i is the smallest value orthogonal to L, B_{ii} is opposite to B_i; B_{iii} and B_{iv} are orthogonal to B_i and B_{ii} and arranged in such a manner that $B_{iii} < B_{iv}$.

scales (instead of the original variables) were recommended for structure–activity analyses.

Principal component scores have several advantages: the individual error of a single parameter value is usually not contained in the principal components; the problem of missing values is greatly reduced; correlation of biological activities with the first few components (which can be interpreted in terms of lipophilicity, bulk, and electronic properties) gives a clear picture which property might be responsible for the variation in biological activity values. However, higher components can no longer be interpreted in physicochemical terms.

2.1 Lipophilicity Parameters

No other physicochemical property has attracted as much interest in QSAR studies as lipophilicity (161, 162), due to its direct relationship to solubility in aqueous phases, to membrane permeation, and to its entropic contribution to binding. Several monographs (49, 50, 54, 56) and numerous reviews (e.g., 148, 162–168) have been published, a recent article by Taylor (162) providing the most comprehensive overview.

Lipophilicity (hydrophobicity) is defined by the partitioning of a compound between an aqueous and a nonaqueous phase (eq.

14.15; $P = n$-octanol/water partition coefficient).

$$P = c_{org}/c_{aq} \qquad (14.15)$$

n-Octanol is the organic solvent of choice since the pioneering work of Hansch on partition coefficients and lipophilicity parameters derived from these partition coefficients (14, 15, 17, 18) because it has many important advantages as compared to other systems (162, 163, 169). It is a good model of the lipid constituents of biological membranes, due to its long alkyl chain and the polar hydroxy group. Its hydroxy group is a hydrogen bond donor and a hydrogen bond acceptor, interacting with a large variety of polar groups of different solutes. It dissolves many more organic compounds than alkanes, cycloalkanes, or aromatic solvents. Although the aqueous phase of the n-octanol/water system contains nearly no octanol at equilibrium, the octanol phase dissolves an appreciable amount of water (thus polar groups need not be dehydrated on their transfer from the aqueous phase to the organic phase). n-Octanol has a low vapor pressure, allowing reproducible measurements, but its vapor pressure is high enough to allow its removal under mild conditions. n-Octanol is UV-transparent over a large range, making the quantitative determination of many compounds relatively easy. By far the most partition coefficients have been measured in n-octanol/water (50, 170); also calculated partition coefficients refer to this system. Last but not least, many lipophilicity-activity relationships, using n-octanol/water partition coefficients or lipophilicity parameters derived therefrom, prove the relevance of this system (e.g., 18, 19, 171).

The use of a standard system for drug partitioning is justified by the Collander equation (eq. 14.16) (172), which correlates partition coefficients from different solvent systems.

$$\log P_2 = a \log P_1 + c \qquad (14.16)$$

Numerous examples (163, 173–175) confirm the validity of Collander-type relationships; for some solvents different equations have been obtained for hydrogen bond donor and acceptor solutes (163).

Equation 14.17 relates the partitioning of some alcohols between human erythrocyte membranes and aqueous buffer to n-octanol/water partition coefficients (176).

$$\log P_{\mathrm{membrane}} = 1.003(\pm 0.13) \log P_{\mathrm{oct}}$$
$$- 0.883(\pm 0.39) \quad (14.17)$$
$$(n = 5; \; r = 0.998; \; s = 0.082)$$

Several hundreds of linear relationships between various (mostly nonspecific) biological data and n-octanol/water partition coefficients have been published (e.g., 18, 171).

However, the choice of n-octanol/water as the standard system for drug partitioning must be reconsidered. Principal component analysis of partition coefficients from different solvent systems (177–179) shows that lipophilicity depends on solute bulk, polar, and hydrogen bonding effects (178, 179).

Hydrogen bonding ability values I_{H} of different functional groups were first defined by Seiler (180) as the differences between cyclohexane/water and n-octanol/

water partition coefficients (eq. 14.18).

$$\Delta \log P = \log P_{\mathrm{oct}} - \log P_{\mathrm{cyclohexane}}$$
$$= \sum I_{\mathrm{H}} - 0.16 \qquad (14.18)$$
$$(n = 195; \; r = 0.967; \; s = 0.333; \; F = 107)$$

Corresponding scales can be derived e.g., from $\log P$ values measured in n-octanol/water, heptane/water, and other systems (181), from the "water dragging effect" (the ability of a solute to carry water molecules from the aqueous phase into an organic solvent, e.g., dibutyl ether) (182, 183), and from water/gas-phase equilibrium constants of different solutes (184). The significance of hydrogen bonding parameters in QSAR studies has been discussed (185, 186) and examples for their application have been given (185, 187–191), the most interesting ones being relationships between the blood–brain barrier penetration of H_2-antihistaminic drugs and $\Delta \log P$ (187, 188), the difference between n-octanol/water and cyclohexane/water partition coefficients ($\log C_{\mathrm{brain}}/C_{\mathrm{blood}}$ vs. $\Delta \log P$: $n = 6$; $r = 0.980$; $s = 0.249$; and $n = 20$; $r = 0.831$; $s = 0.439$).

The solvents alkane (inert), n-octanol (amphiprotic), chloroform (hydrogen bond donor), and propylene glycol dipelargonate (PGDP; hydrogen bond acceptor) were proposed to model different membranes and tissues (192, 193). While n-octanol seems to be relevant for amphiprotic regions of a membrane, PGDP resembles more its lipid part and should be considered as a supplementary solvent.

Systematic investigations by Herbette (111, 112, 194–198), based on membrane/water partition coefficient measurements and neutron diffraction experiments, show that an isotropic two-phase solvent system cannot be a good model for the lipid bilayer of membranes, with their inner hydrophobic part and the outer, polar and negatively charged surface of the phospholipids. Indeed, biological membrane/buffer partition coefficients of drugs significantly differ from those measured in *n*-octanol/water systems.

The important role of membranes in drug action was also recognized by Seydel (199–201). In the drug/membrane interaction, the action of the membrane on the drug molecules and *vice versa* the action of the drug on the membrane properties (201), exert an important, hitherto mostly neglected effect on drug activity.

The role of biomembranes in mediating the receptor subtype selectivities of peptides was investigated by Schwyzer (202, 203).

2.2 The Measurement of Partition Coefficients and Related Lipophilicity Parameters

The measurement of partition coefficients (40, 41, 49, 146, 162, 163, 204, 205) is not as easy as one would expect from their simple definition (eq. 14.15). Practical problems arise for polar and highly lipophilic ($\log P > 4$) compounds; even small impurities may distort the experimental values drastically. Phases must be equilibrated in advance; after adding the solute and having attained equilibrium, centrifugation is necessary to separate phases quantitatively. Partition coefficients should be determined with as small amounts of solute as possible to avoid association phenomena in either phase; aqueous buffers should not contain extractable ions. Solute concentrations should be determined in both phases; at least two independent measurements should be made.

Alternatives to the classical shake flask method are e.g., filter probe methods (206, 207), the AKUFVE method (208), and different centrifugal partition chromatographic techniques (209–212). Most techniques have been reviewed (162, 204, 205, 212).

Chromatographic parameters from reversed phase thin-layer chromatography are occasionally used as substitutes for partition coefficients (213–216). Silica gel plates, being coated with hydrophobic phases, are eluated with aqueous/organic solvent systems. Equation 14.19 converts the resulting R_f values to R_M values, which are true measures of lipophilicity (214) and closely correlated with $\log P$ values (215, 216).

$$R_M = \log(1/R_f - 1) \qquad (14.19)$$

Chromatographic R_M values are useful as rough estimates of lipophilicity. Compounds need not be pure; only traces of material are needed. A wide range of hydrophilic and lipophilic congeners can be investigated. The measurement of practically insoluble analogs poses no problems. No quantitative method for concentration determination is needed. Several compounds can be investigated simultaneously. The main disadvantage is a certain lack of reproducibility. Nowadays high performance liquid chromatography (HPLC) (217–222) is the method of choice in many (especially industrial) laboratories. Log k' values, which are calculated from equation 14.20 (t_r is the retention time of the compound and t_0 the retention time of the solvent front), are closely correlated to *n*-octanol/water partition coefficients, e.g., by equation 14.21 (218).

$$k' = (t_r - t_0)/t_0 \qquad (14.20)$$

$$\log P = 1.025(\pm 0.06) \log k'$$
$$+ 0.797 \qquad (14.21)$$

$$(n = 33; \ r = 0.987; \ s = 0.127)$$

Technical details, including solid support, coating and column filling techniques, eluents, and factors affecting reproducibility have been reviewed (162, 222, 223). Lipophilicity values from HPLC measurements are not on a unique scale. But with the help of standard compounds, for which classical shake flask partition coefficients are known, the log k' values can be converted to n-octanol/water partition coefficients.

2.3 Lipophilicity Contributions and the Calculation of Partition Coefficients

Partition coefficients are, like some other molecular properties, additive constitutive parameters. Hansch defined a lipophilicity parameter π (eq. 14.5, Section 1.1) (15, 17, 18, 163, 205, 224, 225), in the manner that Hammett σ constants (eq. 14.2, Section 1.1) are defined.

The only difference between equation 14.5 and the Hammett equation is the absence of a term like ρ, because π values refer to aromatic substituents and, if not stated otherwise, to n-octanol/water partition coefficients. Slightly different π values are obtained for meta- and para-substituents. Although even more π scales exist in the literature, nowadays the π values which were derived from monosubstituted benzenes are used most often.

A new lipophilicity parameter was defined by Rekker. The hydrophobic fragmental constant f (eq. 14.22) (49, 56, 226–228) is the lipophilicity contribution of a substituent or fragment and is no longer based on the exchange of H against X, as π values are.

$$\log P = \sum a_i f_i \qquad (14.22)$$

f Scales were not only derived for n-octanol/water but also for other solvent systems, e.g., alkane/water, chloroform/water, and PGDP/water systems (162, 192, 193). Methylene group fragment values are known for 24 different organic solvent/water systems (229, 230); they reg-

ularly decrease with increasing water content of the organic phase, i.e., with increasing polarity of the solvent.

The new f system, later modified by Leo and Hansch (50, 231, 232) and others (233, 234), allowed the *de novo* calculation of partition coefficients. The computer program CLOGP (166, 235), developed from the hydrophobic fragmental constant approach of Leo and Hansch, was later largely extended and fully computerized (e.g., 168, 205, 236–238) to its current version (239). The input of structures is being done in SMILES notation (239–242), an easy and powerful language for converting chemical structures into a computer-readable form (e.g., n-butanol = CCCCO; benzoic acid = c1ccccc1C(=O)O).

Calculations based on the two different f scales, the one by Rekker, derived from a set of a thousand compounds by statistical methods (228), and the other by Leo and Hansch, derived from a few highly accurate measurements of appropriate standard compounds (231), have been compared in their predictive ability (56, 148, 243, 244). Although partially computerized versions of the Rekker method have been developed (245, 246), CLOGP is by far the most convenient, advanced, and reliable computer program for the calculation of n-octanol/water partition coefficients.

Some other atom-, bond-, and group-based calculation procedures (e.g., refs. 247–254) have been reviewed and critically commented (162).

From a theoretical point of view it might be better to explain lipophilicity by other molecular properties, e.g., the BC(DEF) parameters (154, 155), solubility, solvent accessible surface, or charge distributions calculated from semiempirical methods (e.g., refs. 179, 255–267, and references cited therein); however, although some of the results allow a better understanding of the intrinsic nature of lipophilicity, none of these alternative approaches led to a reliable log P prediction system so far.

2.4 Polarizability Parameters

Molar volume MV, molar refractivity MR, and parachor PA are closely interrelated (268) (eqs. 14.23–14.25; MW = molecular weight, ρ = density, n = refractive index; γ = surface tension). Although molar refractivity has attracted much attention (50, 269–271); molar volume (55, 272) and parachor (50, 273) have only rarely been used.

$$MV = MW/\rho \qquad (14.23)$$

$$MR = MV \cdot \frac{n^2 - 1}{n^2 + 2} \qquad (14.24)$$

$$PA = MV \cdot \gamma^{1/4} \qquad (14.25)$$

MR still is the chameleon among the physicochemical parameters, despite its broad application in QSAR studies; it has been correlated with lipophilicity, with molar volume, and with steric bulk (41, 91, 274). The refractive index-related correction term in MR accounts for polarizability and thus for the size and the polarity of a certain group (148, 162). For hydrophobic substituents there is a close interrelation between volume, surface, lipophilicity, and MR, which breaks when polar substituents are included.

Many QSAR studies of ligand–enzyme interactions show that substituents modeled by MR bind in polar areas and substituents modeled by π bind in hydrophobic space (271, 275).

The different nature of MR, as compared to hydrophobic and steric properties, can only be detected in cases where a proper selection of substituents allows this. One such example is the inhibition of malate dehydrogenase by 4-hydroxyquinoline-3-carboxylic acids, where the interaction of the ligands with the enzyme is described better by MR (pI_{50} vs. MR: $n = 13$; $r = 0.939$; $s = 0.315$) than by π (pI_{50} vs. π: $n = 13$; $r = 0.604$; $s = 0.716$), and the

respiration inhibition of ascites tumor cells by the same set of compounds, where the transport into or the accumulation in the cells is described better by π (pI_{50} vs. π: $n = 14$; $r = 0.933$; $s = 0.280$) than by MR (pI_{50} vs. MR: $n = 14$; $r = 0.699$; $s = 0.554$) (276). Atomic molar polarizability contributions have been defined (250–252). The CLOGP program also contains a routine for the calculation of MR values (239).

2.5 Electronic Parameters

Electronic properties of molecules (12, 40–43, 53, 57, 148, 277–280) can be described by a wide variety of different parameters: Hammett σ constants, field and resonance parameters $\mathscr{F}$ and $\mathscr{R}$, pK_a values, parameters derived from molecular spectroscopy, charge-transfer constants, dipole moments, hydrogen bonding parameters, and parameters derived from quantum chemical calculations. In contrast to global molecular properties, such as lipophilicity and molar refractivity, they normally refer to a certain atom or group.

Considering electronic effects, one has to differentiate between inductive (field) effects and resonance effects. Due to the characteristic features of a benzene ring, σ_m mainly describes the inductive effect while σ_p stands for a combination of both effects, with the resonance effect predominating. Over the decades many different σ scales have developed in organic chemistry, besides σ_m and σ_p also σ^+ (to account for substituents which donate electrons to the aromatic ring system by direct resonance interaction), σ^- (for corresponding acceptor substituents), σ^0 and σ^n (normal or unexalted σ constants), σ_I and σ_R (inductive and resonance contributions), etc.

In 1968, Swain and Lupton (281) defined field and resonance components $\mathscr{F}$ and $\mathscr{R}$ and correlated 43 different electronic parameters with linear combinations of these two parameters, e.g. equations 14.26 and 14.27.

$$\sigma_m = 0.60(\pm 0.00)\mathscr{F} + 0.27(\pm 0.00)\mathscr{R}$$
$$+ 0.00(\pm 0.00) \quad (14.26)$$
$$(n = 42; \, r = 1.00; \, s = 0.00)$$

$$\sigma_p = 0.56(\pm 0.00)\mathscr{F} + 1.00(\pm 0.00)\mathscr{R}$$
$$+ 0.00(\pm 0.00) \quad (14.27)$$
$$(n = 42; \, r = 1.00; \, s = 0.00)$$

Despite considerable discussion *pro* (282, 283) and *contra* (284–288) the validity of the underlying assumptions, the separation of σ values into inductive and resonance effects seems to be justified, at least from a practical point of view.

A recent compilation (289) contains σ_m, σ_p, and redefined $\mathscr{F}$ and $\mathscr{R}$ values (50, 141) of 530 substituents, together with σ_p^+, σ_p^-, $\mathscr{R}^+$, and $\mathscr{R}^-$ values of 223 substituents as well as other electronic parameters, derived from spectroscopic data; factoring σ values into different field and resonance contributions is reviewed. In addition, optimized and normalized S (field-inductive σ bond perturbation) and P (resonance π bond perturbation; orthogonal to S) values have been used in QSAR studies (290).

Aliphatic σ constants (σ^* values) are defined by equation 14.28, where $\log k$ and $\log k_0$ are the rate constants of acid- and base-catalyzed hydrolysis of RCOOR′ and $CH_3COOR′$, respectively (279, 291).

$$\sigma^* = [\log(k/k_0)_B - \log(k/k_0)_A]/2.48$$
$$(14.28)$$

pK_a Values (53, 278) may be used as substitutes for σ values. However, if they are taken to describe the relative amounts of the unionized form of drugs, their use is inadequate (see Section 3.5); one of the rare exceptions is e.g., eq. 14.29 (antibac-

terial activities of sulfonamides vs. *Escherichia coli*) (292).

$$\log 1/C = 1.044(\pm 0.13)pK_a$$
$$- 1.640(\pm 0.18) \log(\beta.10^{pK_a} + 1)$$
$$+ 0.275$$
$$(14.29)$$
$$\log \beta = -5.96 \quad pK_a \text{ optimum} = 6.2$$
$$(n = 39; \, r = 0.956; \, s = 0.275)$$

Parameters derived from molecular spectroscopy, e.g., from infrared or NMR data, have been used in QSAR studies (e.g., refs. 148, 293–295). They can be extremely helpful in describing the electronic influence of substituents for which no σ values are known, which applies to most heterocyclic systems. Charge-transfer constants C_T (296) and κ (297, 298) have been derived but have not attracted much attention in QSAR studies. The use of dipole moments μ (279, 299) in QSAR studies was proposed by Lien (299–301); group dipole moments are published for 311 aromatic (300) and 214 aliphatic substituents (301).

Hydrogen bonding parameters have, in part, been discussed earlier in this chapter (Section 2.1). In addition to Seiler's I_H values (180) several other scales were derived, e.g., by Hansch and Leo (discriminating donor, acceptor, and neutral substituents) (50, 302) and by Taft (pK_{HB} values) (303); the subject has been reviewed (279).

Quantum chemical parameters (280) were frequently abused in early QSAR studies; the uncritical combination of many different values, e.g., net atomic charges, charge densities, superdelocalizabilities, electrostatic potentials, values for inductive, resonance, and polarizability effects, HOMO and LUMO energies, etc., often ended in chance correlations. Currently some proper applications demonstrate their usefulness in QSAR studies (304–308).

Rapid calculation procedures for electronic effects in organic molecules were proposed by Gasteiger and Marsili (309–311) as an alternative to *ab initio* and semiempirical quantum chemical calculations, which are relatively time-consuming procedures.

2.6 Steric Parameters

Steric effects are difficult to describe, due to the most often unknown 3D structures of the binding sites of drugs. Several reviews on steric effects and steric descriptors (50, 52, 270, 291, 312–315) contribute to this problem but a general solution seems to be inherently impossible.

E_s constants, defined by equation 14.30 (acid-catalyzed hydrolysis of RCOOR' vs. CH_3COOR') (291), were the first parameters which were used to describe steric effects in QSAR studies.

$$E_s = \log(k/k_0)_A \qquad (14.30)$$

Charton (316) defined a steric substituent parameter v (r_v = minimum van der Waals radius of a substituent) (eq. 14.31), which is highly correlated with E_s values (eq. 14.32) (50).

$$v_X = r_{vX} - r_{vH} = r_{vX} - 1.20 \qquad (14.31)$$

$$E_s = -2.062(\pm0.86)v - 0.194(\pm0.10)$$
$$(14.32)$$
$$(n = 104; \ r = 0.978; \ s = 0.250)$$

Hancock (317) modified E_s to E_s^c values by correcting them for the number of α-hydrogen atoms, n_H. A simple steric parameter S_b was formulated on the basis of substituent branching (318). Fujita expressed E_s^c values of substituents of the type $CR^1R^2R^3$ as a weighted sum of the individual E_s^c values of R^1, R^2, and R^3 (319) to overcome problems with steric parameters of unsymmetrical substituents. Other

parameters related to size, e.g., van der Waals volumes, molar volumes, solvent accessible surface, molar refractivity, etc., have been used to describe steric effects in QSAR equations (148, 270).

A real progress resulted from the definition of the STERIMOL parameters L, B_1, B_2, B_3, and B_4 (314, 315). L is defined as the length of the substituent along the axis of its substitution to the parent skeleton; the width parameters B are all orthogonal to L and have angles of 90 degrees to each other; they are arranged in such a manner that B_1 has the smallest and B_4 the largest value. A slightly different definition was used by Skagerberg et al. (Table 14.1, Section 2) (158). Later the width parameters were reduced to B_1, being the smallest, and B_5, now being the largest width orthogonal to L, but independent of the angle between B_1 and B_5 (315, 320). Applications of the STERIMOL parameters in QSAR studies have been reviewed (270, 314, 315, 320).

Compilations of different steric parameters are given in refs. 148, 270, 314, and 315.

2.7 Other Parameters

Molecular weight was used by Lien (321) to improve the fit of parabolic Hansch equations. However, in this case the MW term only accounted for systematic deviations between the parabolic model and the experimental data (322).

A more appropriate use of MW was demonstrated in a QSAR study of the multidrug resistance of tumor cells, where the MW term stands for the dependence of biological activities on diffusion rate constants. The relationship between MW and volume implies that $\sqrt[3]{MW}$, corresponding to a linear dimension of size, should be better suited than $\log MW$ ($n = 29$; $r = 0.871$; $s = 0.394$) (323), which is indeed the case ($n = 40$; $r = 0.891$; $s = 0.344$) (324).

Geometric parameters are derived from known or hypothetical pharmacophores; thus they only apply to certain sets of compounds. The use of conformational entropy values as parameters in QSAR studies has been proposed (325–327).

A large (unfortunately much too large) group of parameters in QSAR studies are topological indices, e.g., different connectivity values χ, based on the characterization of chemical structures by graph theory. Since the first papers on molecular connectivity values and their use in correlation analysis and QSAR studies appeared (328–331), a large number of publications followed, most of them by Kier and Hall (for reviews see 48, 52, 148, 270, 332–335).

Molecular connectivity indices χ are calculated from molecular formulas in a unique manner and, due to their mathematical definition, some physicochemical properties of branched and unbranched isomers can be described with high accuracy (48, 333). It is this relationship to physicochemical properties such as partition coefficient, molar refractivity, and steric properties, which allows a quantitative description of (most often nonspecific) biological activities within closely related series.

In addition to normal and valence connectivity (336, 337) values, many other topological indices, e.g., shape descriptors and electrotopological indices, have been defined (for reviews see refs. 52, 148, 270, 333, 335). The use of topological indices in QSAR has been criticized (e.g., 148, 162, 164, 270, 338). In contrast to general recommendations on the selection of biologically meaningful parameters (290), the physicochemical meaning of the topological parameters is never clear. Chance correlations may arise from the uncritical combination of a large number of closely interrelated connectivity terms. In many cases standard deviations of regression coefficients are given instead of confidence intervals, suggesting that terms are significant which in reality are not significant.

Although Taylor's comments on topological indices are generally favorable, with respect to QSAR studies he considers their use as unsuitable (162).

2.8 Indicator Variables

Indicator variables (sometimes called dummy variables or *de novo* constants) are used in linear multiple regression analysis (339, 340) to account for certain features which cannot be described by continuous variables (21, 22, 41, 341, 342). In QSAR equations they normally stand for a certain structural element, be it a substituent or another molecular fragment; thus, Free Wilson analysis may be interpreted as a regression analysis approach using only indicator variables (21, 22, 341, 342).

Indicator variables have also been used to account for other structural features, e.g., intramolecular hydrogen bonding, hydrogen donor and acceptor properties, ortho effects, cis/trans isomerism, different parent skeletons, different test models, etc. (22, 341).

The proper use of an indicator variable is demonstrated with two subsets of papain ligands; equation 14.33 was derived for a series of N-mesyl-glycine phenyl esters and equation 14.34 for a corresponding series of N-benzoyl-glycine phenyl esters (343).

$$\log 1/K_m = 0.529(\pm 0.23)MR$$
$$+ 0.370(\pm 0.20)\sigma$$
$$+ 1.877(\pm 0.13) \qquad (14.33)$$
$$(n = 13; \; r = 0.935; \; s = 0.105; \; F = 34.51)$$

$$\log 1/K_m = 0.771(\pm 0.67)MR$$
$$+ 0.728(\pm 0.37)\sigma$$
$$+ 3.623(\pm 0.34) \qquad (14.34)$$
$$(n = 7; \; r = 0.971; \; s = 0.148; \; F = 32.85)$$

The coefficients of the MR and σ terms are not significantly different, but the constant terms are. The combination of equations 14.33 and 14.34 with the help of an indicator variable I ($I = 1$ for mesylamides; $I = 0$ for benzamides) leads to equation 14.35 (343) (recalculated).

$$\log 1/K_m = 0.569(\pm 0.26)MR$$
$$+ 0.561(\pm 0.19)\sigma$$
$$- 1.922(\pm 0.15)I$$
$$+ 3.743(\pm 0.17) \qquad (14.35)$$
$$(n = 20; \; r = 0.990; \; s = 0.148; \; F = 272.04)$$

Indicator variables are especially useful in the early phases of a QSAR analysis and for large, complex data sets. Different subsets can be combined with their help, until the real dependence of biological activity values on some physicochemical parameters can be derived from a more extensive structural variation.

3 QUANTITATIVE MODELS

3.1 The Extrathermodynamic Approach (Hansch Analysis)

Hansch analysis (14, 15, 17, 18, 40–44, 344) correlates biological activity values with physicochemical properties; thus, Hansch analysis is indeed a property–property relationship model. As practically all parameters used in Hansch analysis are linear free energy-related values (i.e., derived from rate or equilibrium constants), the terms "linear free energy-related approach" or "extrathermodynamic approach" (344) are used as synonyms for Hansch analysis.

Early attempts to correlate biological activity values with lipophilicity explained only nonspecific structure–activity relationships; the concept of a general biological Hammett equation (eq. 14.3, Section 1.1) failed. A methodological breakthrough resulted from the combination of different physicochemical parameters in one equa-

tion, e.g., equation 14.36 ($k_1, k_2, k_3 =$ coefficients determined by linear multiple regression analysis to fit the biological data).

$$\log 1/C = k_1 \log P + k_2 \sigma + k_3 \quad (14.36)$$

For *in vivo* data equation 14.36 was extended to equation 14.37 by including a parabolic lipophilicity term. The idea behind equation 14.37 was that molecules which are too hydrophilic or too lipophilic will not be able to cross lipophilic and hydrophilic barriers, respectively. Therefore they will have a lower probability to arrive at the receptor site than molecules with intermediate lipophilicity, being readily soluble in aqueous phases as well as in lipid phases.

$$\log 1/C = -k_1(\log P)^2 + k_2 \log P$$
$$+ k_3 \sigma + k_4 \quad (14.37)$$

Complex dependences of biological activities on physicochemical properties can be described by such multiparameter equations. In the last two decades nearly all conceivable combinations of lipophilic, polarizability, electronic, and steric parameters have been used and correlated with biological activity values in linear, parabolic, and bilinear equations.

Only one example is given here to describe and explain the application of Hansch analysis (for further examples see Section 6). Hansch and Lien (345) derived equation 14.38 for the antiadrenergic activities of a series of α-bromo-phenethylamines (Table 14.2; only some selected physicochemical parameters are included; slightly different results are obtained if different scales, e.g., π values from the phenoxyacetic acid system, $\pi_{benzene}$ values, or any other π values are used).

$$\log 1/C = 1.22\pi - 1.59\sigma + 7.89$$
$$(14.38)$$
$$(n = 22; \; r = 0.918; \; s = 0.238)$$

Table 14.2 Antiadrenergic Activities of *meta-* and *para*-substituted *N,N*-Dimethyl-α-bromophenethylamines[a]

meta (X)	para (Y)	π	σ^+	E_s^{meta}	log 1/C obsd.	log 1/C calc.[b]	log 1/C calc.[c]
H	H	0.00	0.00	1.24	7.46	7.82	7.88
H	F	0.15	−0.07	1.24	8.16	8.09	8.17
H	Cl	0.70	0.11	1.24	8.68	8.46	8.60
H	Br	1.02	0.15	1.24	8.89	8.77	8.94
H	I	1.26	0.14	1.24	9.25	9.06	9.26
H	Me	0.52	−0.31	1.24	9.30	8.87	8.98
F	H	0.13	0.35	0.78	7.52	7.45	7.43
Cl	H	0.76	0.40	0.27	8.16	8.11	8.05
Br	H	0.94	0.41	0.08	8.30	8.30	8.22
I	H	1.15	0.36	−0.16	8.40	8.61	8.51
Me	H	0.51	−0.07	0.00	8.46	8.51	8.36
Cl	F	0.91	0.33	0.27	8.19	8.38	8.34
Br	F	1.09	0.34	0.08	8.57	8.57	8.51
Me	F	0.66	−0.14	0.00	8.82	8.78	8.65
Cl	Cl	1.46	0.51	0.27	8.89	8.75	8.77
Br	Cl	1.64	0.52	0.08	8.92	8.94	8.94
Me	Cl	1.21	0.04	0.00	8.96	9.15	9.08
Cl	Br	1.78	0.55	0.27	9.00	9.06	9.11
Br	Br	1.96	0.56	0.08	9.35	9.25	9.29
Me	Br	1.53	0.08	0.00	9.22	9.46	9.43
Me	Me	1.03	−0.38	0.00	9.30	9.56	9.47
Br	Me	1.46	0.10	0.08	9.52	9.35	9.33

[a]Refs. 290, 347.
[b]eq. 14.40.
[c]eq. 14.41.

Cammarata (346) presented equation 14.39 (recalculated) which describes meta-substituents by their π and σ values and para-substituents by a steric parameter r_v^{para}.

$$\log 1/C = 0.747(\pm 0.26)\pi_m$$
$$- 0.911(\pm 0.52)\sigma_m$$
$$+ 1.666(\pm 0.26)r_v^{para}$$
$$+ 5.769(\pm 0.45) \qquad (14.39)$$
$$(n = 22; \; r = 0.962; \; s = 0.168; \; F = 74.01)$$

Equation 14.39 was criticized by Unger and Hansch (290) in a noteworthy paper, which constitutes a milestone in the development of Hansch analysis. They formulated rules for the derivation of extrathermodynamic equations which are summarized below because of their general validity:

- A wide range of different parameters, i.e., $\log P$ or π, σ, *MR*, and steric parameters, should be tried. The parameters selected for the "best equation" should be essentially independent.
- All "reasonable" parameters must be validated by an appropriate statistical

procedure, e.g., by stepwise regression. The "best equation" is normally the one with the lowest standard deviation, all terms being significant.

- All things being equal, one should accept the simplest model.
- One should have at least five to six data points per variable to avoid chance correlations.
- It is important to have a model which is consistent with the known physical-organic and biomedicinal chemistry of the process under consideration.

Following these recommendations, Unger and Hansch reconsidered the mechanism of action of the α-bromo-phenethylamines and argued that σ^+ instead of σ might be a better electronic descriptor, because the compounds are supposed to interact with the receptor site via the formation of an ethyleneiminium and subsequently a benzyl cation. They derived equation 14.40 (290) (recalculated), which gave a much better description of the data than equation 14.38.

$$\log 1/C = 1.151(\pm 0.19)\pi$$

$$- 1.464(\pm 0.38)\sigma^+$$

$$+ 7.817(\pm 0.19) \quad (14.40)$$

$$(n = 22; \ r = 0.945; \ s = 0.196; \ F = 78.63)$$

Several other equations were derived, separating hydrophobic and electronic effects in different positions and splitting electronic parameters into field and resonance effects (290). Later equation 14.41 was derived from the assumption that hydrophobic and electronic influences are identical in the meta- and para-positions, but that there might be a steric hindrance for meta-substituents (347).

$$\log 1/C = 1.259(\pm 0.19)\pi$$

$$- 1.460(\pm 0.34)\sigma^+$$

$$+ 0.208(\pm 0.17)E_s^{meta}$$

$$+ 7.619(\pm 0.24) \quad (14.41)$$

$$(n = 22; \ r = 0.959; \ s = 0.173; \ F = 69.24)$$

Equations 14.38–14.41 reveal a typical dilemma in Hansch analysis: although equations 14.40 and 14.41 are significantly better than equation 14.38 and are based on more reasonable assumptions than equation 14.39, which one is the "best" equation? The differences in the correlation coefficients r and in the standard deviations s of eqs. 14.40 and 14.41 are rather small. The confidence interval of the E_s term in equation 14.41 is relatively large and the F value of equation 14.41 is smaller than the one of equation 14.40, indicating that there may be too few degrees of freedom to favor equation 14.41; on the other hand, the additional E_s term in equation 14.41 is justified by a sequential F test (see Section 4.1). The equations are derived from a less well-designed group of compounds (the importance of a proper selection of substituents is discussed in Section 5). With the evidence on hand it is impossible to differentiate between both equations and to prefer either one.

In addition to the ambiguity of the results, there is another serious problem in Hansch analysis. One compound of the original series, the *para*-phenyl analog, has been omitted in equations 14.38–14.41 because of its bad fit. This procedure is the only choice if a single compound represents a largely different substituent which could only be described by a separate parameter. But most often the exclusion of data points is an arbitrary and dangerous procedure. An important effect may be overlooked or a false hypothesis may be incorrectly justified if one starts from a wrong selection of so-called "outliers".

Topliss investigated the risk of chance correlations in Hansch analyses in a systematic manner; for a given number of compounds the chance of obtaining correlation coefficients larger than 0.9 not only increases with the number of variables included in the equation, but also with the number of variables from which the different variable combinations are selected (348, 349).

The biological activity values of new analogs can be predicted from Hansch equations. Of course, different predictions result from different equations. If a point to be predicted is far outside the included parameter range there is not only a risk, but certainly a guarantee for failure.

Predictive ability is often considered to be a criterion in quantitative structure–activity analyses. However, it should be realized that the main purpose of Hansch analysis is not prediction, but a better understanding. Hypotheses can be established which are proven or disproven by synthesis and testing of new analogs. If the predicted values are close to the experimental ones, the model can be accepted. Otherwise the hypothesis was wrong or limited to a certain parameter range; new conclusions and a new model must be derived.

The factors which influence significance and validity of QSAR relationships have been reviewed (350–356).

3.2 The Additivity Model (Free Wilson Analysis)

The Free Wilson approach (16, 20, 341, 342) is a true structure–activity relationship model. An indicator variable is generated for each structural feature which deviates from an arbitrarily chosen reference compound. Values 1, indicating the presence of a certain substituent or structural feature, and 0, indicating its absence, are correlated with the biological activity values by linear multiple-regression analysis. The resulting regression coefficients of the indicator variables are the biological activity contributions of the corresponding structural elements. "Mathematical model", "additivity

model", or "*de novo* approach" are synonyms for the Free Wilson method.

Free Wilson analysis was not as simple in its original formulation (16). No reference compound was selected and so-called symmetry equations were generated to avoid the problem of linear dependences between the variables.

As nowadays only the modification described by Fujita and Ban (eq. 14.7, Section 1.1) (20, 341, 342) is used, no details of the original Free Wilson model are discussed here. In comparison to the classical version, the Fujita Ban variant offers some important advantages. The table for regression analysis can be easily generated. Addition and elimination of compounds is simple and does not significantly change the values of other regression coefficients. Any compound may be chosen as the reference compound; singularity problems are avoided. The values of the group contributions are directly related to Hansch analysis-derived group contributions (Section 3.3); Fujita Ban-type indicator variables can be combined with Hansch analysis to a mixed approach (see Sections 2.8 and 3.3) (22, 341, 342).

Table 14.3 results if the Free Wilson method is applied to the compounds of Table 14.2 and if the unsubstituted parent compound is selected as the reference compound; regression analysis of these data gives equation 14.42 (341, 342, 347).

$$\log 1/C = -0.301(\pm0.50)[m\text{-F}]$$
$$+ 0.207(\pm0.29)[m\text{-Cl}]$$
$$+ 0.434(\pm0.27)[m\text{-Br}]$$
$$+ 0.579(\pm0.50)[m\text{-I}]$$
$$+ 0.454(\pm0.27)[m\text{-Me}]$$
$$+ 0.340(\pm0.30)[p\text{-F}]$$
$$+ 0.768(\pm0.30)[p\text{-Cl}]$$
$$+ 1.020(\pm0.30)[p\text{-Br}]$$

Table 14.3 Antiadrenergic Activities of *meta*- and *para*-substituted *N,N*-Dimethyl-α-bromo-phenethylamines[a]

$$X$$
$$Y-\underset{Br}{C_6H_3}-CHCH_2NMe_2\cdot HCl$$

meta (X)	para (Y)	meta- F	Cl	Br	I	Me	para- F	Cl	Br	I	Me	log 1/C obsd.	log 1/C calc.[b]
H	H											7.46	7.82
H	F						1					8.16	8.16
H	Cl							1				8.68	8.59
H	Br								1			8.89	8.84
H	I									1		9.25	9.25
H	Me										1	9.30	9.08
F	H	1										7.52	7.52
Cl	H		1									8.16	8.03
Br	H			1								8.30	8.26
I	H				1							8.40	8.40
Me	H					1						8.46	8.28
Cl	F		1				1					8.19	8.37
Br	F			1			1					8.57	8.60
Me	F					1	1					8.82	8.62
Cl	Cl		1					1				8.89	8.80
Br	Cl			1				1				8.92	9.02
Me	Cl					1		1				8.96	9.04
Cl	Br		1						1			9.00	9.05
Br	Br			1					1			9.35	9.28
Me	Br					1			1			9.22	9.30
Me	Me					1					1	9.30	9.53
Br	Me			1							1	9.52	9.51

[a]Matrix for Free Wilson analysis (342, 347).
[b]Eq. 14.42.

$$+ 1.429(\pm 0.50)[p\text{-I}]$$
$$+ 1.256(\pm 0.33)[p\text{-Me}]$$
$$+ 7.821(\pm 0.27) \qquad (14.42)$$
$$(n = 22; \ r = 0.969; \ s = 0.194; \ F = 16.99)$$

Different regression coefficients are obtained if any other compound is chosen as the reference compound or if the classical Free Wilson model is applied. However, these values are only linearly shifted to the values of equation 14.42; all statistical parameters are identical, with the only exception of the 95% confidence intervals (341, 342, 357).

Free Wilson analysis is easy to apply. Especially in the early phases of structure–activity analyses it offers a simple way to derive substituent contributions and to have a first look on their possible dependence on physicochemical properties. However, Free Wilson analysis also has some shortcomings. Structural variation is necessary in at least two different positions of substitution. A substituent which occurs only once in the data set leads to a single point determination; the corresponding group contribution contains the whole experimental error of this one activity value. Only a common activity contribution can be derived for substituents which always occur together in two different positions of the molecule. In most cases a large number of parameters is needed to describe relatively few compounds, sometimes leading to equations being statistically not significant. Predictions for substituents which are not included in the analysis are generally impossible.

Free Wilson analysis is limited to linear additive relationships (its application to nonlinear relationships and the combination with Hansch analysis is described in Section 3.3). A detailed discussion of scope and limitations of Free Wilson analysis is given in refs. 341 and 342.

Modifications including only significant variables (e.g., 358, 359), like the "reduced Free Wilson model" (360–362) and the BEL-FREE method (363), have not generally been accepted.

The DARC-PELCO approach (364–367) is a simple application of a hyperstructure concept in Free Wilson analysis; it is useless for structure–activity analyses, due to the much too large number of variables (341, 342). The results from Hansch, Free Wilson, and DARC-PELCO analyses have been compared (366–368); no advantages of the latter approach can be seen.

3.3 The Relationships between Hansch and Free Wilson Analysis (The Mixed Approach)

Hansch analysis and the Free Wilson model differ in their application, but they are nevertheless closely related (341, 342, 369). From the general formulation of a linear Hansch equation (eq. 14.43; Φ_i is any physicochemical property) group contributions a_i can be derived for each substituent under consideration (eq. 14.44; Φ_{ij} is the

physicochemical property j of the substituent X_i).

$$\log 1/C = k_1\Phi_1 + k_2\Phi_2 + \cdots + k_n\Phi_n + c$$

$$= \sum k_j\Phi_j + c \qquad (14.43)$$

$$a_i = \sum k_j\Phi_{ij} \qquad (14.44)$$

This theoretical relationship was first recognized by Singer and Purcell (370); although it was questioned by Cammarata (346, 371), later investigations confirmed it theoretically and by practical examples (341, 342, 347, 369). If all physicochemical properties are normalized to $\Phi_j = 0$ for hydrogen and if the corresponding Free Wilson group contributions also refer to hydrogen, the values of the group contributions are, within experimental error, numerically equivalent (341, 342, 347).

According to equation 14.44, the Free Wilson group contributions contain all possible physicochemical contributions of a substituent; correspondingly a Free Wilson analysis always gives the upper limit of correlation which can be achieved by a linear Hansch analysis. Free Wilson analysis of a data set shows whether a linear additive model is suited for the analysis; only in some cases a good fit is obtained for nonlinear data, especially if there are only few degrees of freedom (22, 341, 342, 369).

Bocek and Kopecky proposed an additive model with additional interaction terms (eq. 14.45, reformulated; $e_X e_Y$ = interaction term) (372, 373), which is related to nonlinear Hansch analysis (22, 347, 370). However, due to the large number of variables, this modification has never been used.

$$\log 1/C = \sum a_i + \sum e_X e_Y + c \qquad (14.45)$$

Due to the relationships between Hansch

and Free Wilson analysis, indicator variables (Section 2.8) can be included in Hansch analyses (e.g., 21, 374, 375). Both models can be combined to a mixed approach, in a linear (eq. 14.46) and a nonlinear form (eq. 14.47), which offers the advantages of both, Hansch and Free Wilson analysis, and widens their applicability (22).

$$\log 1/C = k_1\Phi_1 + k_2\Phi_2 + \cdots + k_n\Phi_n$$
$$+ \sum a_i + c$$
$$= \sum k_j\Phi_j + \sum a_i + c \quad (14.46)$$

$$\log 1/C = b_1\Phi_1^2 + b_2\Phi_2^2 + \cdots + k_1\Phi_1 + k_2\Phi_2$$
$$+ \cdots + k_n\Phi_n + \sum a_i + c$$
$$= \sum b_j\Phi_j^2 + \sum k_j\Phi_j + \sum a_i + c$$
$$(14.47)$$

The mixed approach allows the description of data sets, where structural variation is sufficient to derive a Hansch-type relationship for one or several sites of substitution, while for others indicator variables are appropriate because structural variation is too narrow. For a successful application of the mixed approach it is highly recommended to derive Hansch equations for each subset and to compare whether they correspond to each other or not, before combining them into one equation with the help of indicator variables (e.g., eqs. 14.33–14.35, Section 2.8).

Today the mixed approach is the most powerful tool for the quantitative description of large and structurally diverse data sets. Numerous Hansch analyses including Free Wilson-type variables have been published (examples are discussed in Section 6).

3.4 Nonlinear Relationships

Nonlinear relationships between biological activities and lipophilicity are very common. Although biological activities most often linearly increase with increasing lipophilicity (171), such an increase is no longer obtained if a certain range of lipophilicity is surpassed; biological activities remain constant or decrease more or less rapidly with further increase of lipophilicity (7, 19). Many reviews deal with nonlinear lipophilicity–activity relationships (19, 164, 167, 322, 376).

Different explanations have been given for this effect, the kinetics of drug transport in biological systems and the distribution of drugs in different compartments of a biological system being the most common. In addition, limited space for hydrophobic groups at the binding site, allosteric effects, increased metabolism of higher, lipophilic analogs, end product inhibition by lipophilic products of an enzymatic reaction, micelle formation or limited solubility of higher analogs, and, last but not least, the principle of minimum receptor occupation have been discussed as alternative reasons (19).

Hansch formulated a parabolic model (eq. 14.6, Section 1.1) (15, 17–19) for the mathematical description of nonlinear relationships. A computer simulation of the transport of drugs in a biological system, using hypothetical rate constants of drug transfer, supported the parabolic model (377), although the computer simulation showed some systematic deviations at the sides of the parabola.

Franke developed another empirical model to bridge the gap between so many linear relationships and a nonlinear model. He formulated two different equations, one (eq. 14.48) for the left linear part and another (eq. 14.49; $\log P_x$ = critical $\log P$ value, where the linear relationship changes into a nonlinear one) for the right side, the nonlinear part (378). In many practical cases the Franke model gives a better fit than the parabolic model.

$$\log 1/C = a \log P + c$$

$$\text{(if } \log P < \log P_x \text{)} \quad (14.48)$$

$$\log 1/C = \alpha (\log P)^2 + \beta \log P + \gamma$$

$$\text{(if } \log P > \log P_x \text{)} \quad (14.49)$$

McFarland considered the probability of a molecule to enter a lipid phase (eq. 14.50) or an aqueous phase (eq. 14.51) from the aqueous/lipid interface ($p_{i,j}$ = probabilities) (379).

$$p_{0,1} = \frac{P}{P+1} \quad (14.50)$$

$$p_{1,0} = \frac{1}{P+1} \quad (14.51)$$

From these equations he derived the probability of a molecule to cross different aqueous and lipid barriers and to arrive at the receptor by multiplying the different probabilities (eq. 14.52; $p_{1,2} = p_{1,0}$, $p_{2,3} = p_{0,1}$, etc.); equation 14.53 (c_r = concentration in the receptor phase) is obtained after appropriate transformation of equation 14.52 (164, 322, 379).

$$p_{0,n} = p_{0,1} \cdot p_{1,2} \cdot p_{2,3} \cdots p_{n-1,n}$$

$$= \frac{P^{n/2}}{(P+1)^n} \quad (14.52)$$

$$\log c_r = a \log P - 2a \log(P+1) + c \quad (14.53)$$

Symmetrical curves with linear ascending and descending sides, having their optimum at $\log P = 0$, result from equation 14.53.

Hyde followed the equilibrium approach of Higuchi and Davis (380), but considered much simpler model systems (381, 382). Equation 14.54 (slope = 1) and equation 14.55 (different slopes of the ascending left side) describe nonlinear relationships with linear left sides, leveling off to a plateau

(381, 382); only such lipophilicity–activity relationships can be described by this model (164, 322).

$$\log 1/C = \log P - \log(aP + 1) + c \quad (14.54)$$

$$\log 1/C = b \log P - \log(aP^b + 1) + c \quad (14.55)$$

The bilinear model (eq. 14.56) was derived from a reconsideration of the McFarland model, taking into account the different volumes of aqueous and organic phases of a biological system (23, 164, 322, 383–385).

$$\log 1/C = a \log P - b \log(\beta P + 1) + c \quad (14.56)$$

A different form of the bilinear model (e.g., eq. 14.57) has to be used in the case of physicochemical parameters which already are in the logarithmic scale.

$$\log 1/C = a\pi - b \log(\beta \cdot 10^\pi + 1) + c \quad (14.57)$$

Equations 14.56 and 14.57 may be considered as extensions of equations 14.53–14.55. In contrast to these equations, the bilinear model is generally applicable for the quantitative description of a wide variety of nonlinear lipophilicity–activity relationships. In addition to the parameters that are calculated by linear regression analysis it contains a nonlinear parameter β, which is estimated by stepwise iteration (383, 384). The term a in equation 14.56 is the slope of the left linear part of the lipophilicity–activity relationship, the value $(a - b)$ corresponds to the slope on the right side. In the case of unsymmetrical curves the site of the lipophilicity optimum is described much better by the bilinear model than by the parabolic model.

The bilinear model is confirmed by simulations, using rate constants of drug transport that were determined in a three-component system water/n-octanol/water (386). Equations 14.58 and 14.59 could be derived for the rate constants k_1 (from the aqueous phase into the organic phase) and k_2 (from the organic phase into the aqueous phase) (387).

$$\log k_1 = \log P - \log(\beta P + 1) + c \qquad (14.58)$$

$$\log k_2 = -\log(\beta P + 1) + c \qquad (14.59)$$

Both equations were confirmed by independent investigations of larger series of structurally different substances, including neutral compounds, ionized compounds, and quaternary ion pairs, with molecular weights in the range <100 to >500 dalton (388–390).

Equation 14.56 can be derived from diffusion theory as well as from equilibrium models, indicating that the bilinear model is valid under kinetic control as well as under equilibrium or pseudo-equilibrium conditions (164, 322, 383, 391, 392).

The parabolic model still has its place in structure–activity analyses; it is the simpler model, easier to calculate, and most often a sufficient approximation of the true structure–activity relationship. The calculation of bilinear equations is relatively time-consuming, as compared to the parabolic model; strange results may be obtained in ill-conditioned data sets. On the other hand, the bilinear model explains many data sets much better than the parabolic model (e.g. Fig. 14.2) (23, 164, 322).

Other models, closely related to the bilinear model, have been derived for the quantitative description of nonlinear structure–activity relationships (41, 146, 393–398); none of these models combines general applicability and ease of calculation to

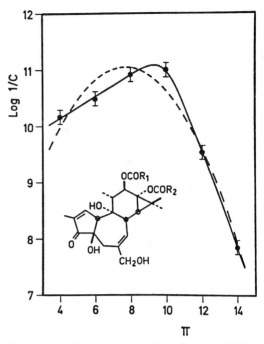

Fig. 14.2 Inflammatory activities of phorbol-12,13-diesters; comparison of the bilinear model ($r = 1.000$; solid line) and the parabolic model ($r = 0.978$; dashed line). Reproduced from Figure 3 of ref. 383 with permission from Editio Cantor Verlag, Aulendorf, Germany.

the same extent as the parabolic and the bilinear models do.

Other nonlinear relationships are known in addition to nonlinear lipophilicity–activity relationships. Most common are nonlinear dependences on molar refractivity, e.g., resulting from a limited binding site at the receptor (for examples see Section 6.1), but also other kinds of nonlinear relationships, e.g., on steric parameters, are frequently obtained. Even electronic parameters (eq. 14.29, Section 2.5) or molecular weight have been used in nonlinear equations. Cross product terms, e.g., $MR_1 \cdot MR_2 \cdot MR_3$ (399), should be avoided because they are highly interrelated to squared terms ($MR_1 \cdot MR_2 \cdot MR_3$ vs. a combination of ΣMR^2, MR_1, MR_2, and MR_3: $n = 71$; $r = 0.993$) (164).

3.5 Dissociation and Ionization of Acids and Bases

Ions are, due to their charge, much more polar than neutral compounds. The dependence of the apparent partition coefficients P_{app} on pH values, pK_a values, P_u (partition coefficient of the neutral, unionized form) and P_i (partition coefficient of the ionized form) values is described by equations 14.60 (acids) (Fig. 14.3) and 14.61 (bases) (for reviews see refs. 41, 146, 162, 164, 400).

$$\log P_{app} = \log(P_u \cdot 10^{pK_a} + P_i \cdot 10^{pH})$$
$$- \log(10^{pK_a} + 10^{pH}) \quad (14.60)$$

$$\log P_{app} = \log(P_u \cdot 10^{pH} + P_i \cdot 10^{pK_a})$$
$$- \log(10^{pK_a} + 10^{pH}) \quad (14.61)$$

Sigmoidal curves are obtained for the pH dependence of $\log P_{app}$ values (173, 401–404). At pH values where the neutral form predominates ($pH < pK_a$ for acids; $pH > pK_a$ for bases), P_{app} values are identical with P_u values. With increasing ionization, the $\log P_{app}$ values decrease linearly with increasing (acids) or decreasing (bases) pH values, till again a constant P_{app} value is obtained, because now only the ionic form contributes to partitioning ($P_{app} = P_i$).

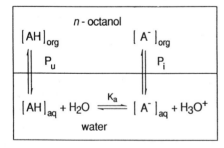

Fig. 14.3 Dissociation and partitioning equilibria of an acid AH in a two-compartment system n-octanol/aqueous buffer. Redrawn from Figure 2 of ref. 164 with permission from Birkhäuser Verlag AG, Basel, Switzerland.

Complex pH dependences are obtained in the case of compounds having more than one ionizable group (e.g., 162, 404, 405).

P_i values are about 3 to 5 decades smaller than the corresponding P_u values; the distance can be larger, e.g., for salicyclic acid, which contains two acidic groups (404), but also much smaller, e.g., for chenodesoxycholic acid, which forms micelles (403), or in the presence of lipophilic counter ions (404). Lipophilicity and polarizability of the counterion have a significant influence on the partitioning of ion pairs (e.g. refs. 406–409).

The concentrations of A^- and BH^+ in the organic phase may be neglected for compounds which are not too lipophilic; much simpler equations than equations 14.60 and 14.61 can be used to estimate the $\log P_{app}$ values of most acids (eq. 14.62) and bases (eq. 14.63) at a given pH value.

$$\log P_{app} = \log P_u - \log(1 + 10^{pH - pK_a})$$
$$(14.62)$$

$$\log P_{app} = \log P_u - \log(1 + 10^{pK_a - pH})$$
$$(14.63)$$

Scherrer (410–412) calculated $\log D$ ($= \log P_{app}$) values by equations 14.62 and 14.63, respectively, and used them instead of the most often inappropriate ($pK_a - pH$) terms; the ($pK_a - pH$) approximation (413) only holds true for pH ranges where the compounds predominantly exist in their ionized forms.

Equation 14.64 (322) correlates the buccal absorption rate constants of an acid (p-hexylphenylacetic acid, $pK_a = 4.36$) and a base (propranolol, $pK_a = 9.45$) at different pH values (411) with $\log P_{app}$ values.

$$\log k_{abs} = 0.448(\pm 0.05) \log P_{app}$$
$$- 0.448(\pm 0.05) \log(\beta P_{app} + 1)$$
$$- 1.689 \quad (14.64)$$

$$\log \beta = -2.792$$

$$(n = 12; \, r = 0.988; \, s = 0.102)$$

Log P_{app} values are appropriate in all cases where rate constants are involved, but not for binding or other equilibrium systems (162). The correct approach for equilibrium systems is demonstrated by equation 14.65 (K_i = inhibition of monoamine oxidase by amines and alcohols; $I = 0$ for amines, $I = 1$ for alcohols), where the biological data have been corrected for the concentration of the unionized form (164).

$$\log 1/K_i + \log(1 + 10^{pK_a - pH})$$

$$= 3.130(\pm 0.17) \log P$$

$$- 3.797(\pm 0.32) \log(\beta P + 1)$$

$$- 3.507(\pm 0.12)I + 3.379 \qquad (14.65)$$

$$\log \beta = -1.781 \quad \text{optimum} \log P = 2.45$$

$$(n = 21; \, r = 0.999; \, s = 0.118)$$

Deviations from simple pH partition hypothesis (i.e., the pH absorption profiles should be parallel to the pH partition profiles) (e.g., 414, 415), called pH shift, are obtained for highly lipophilic compounds; their absorption profiles are shifted to higher (acids) or lower (bases) pH values. The higher the lipophilicity of the neutral species is, the higher is the observed pH shift, which can easily be explained by the assumption of an aqueous diffusion layer at the aqueous/organic interface (162, 416, 417).

Much more complex models were derived for the quantitative description of biological data of ionizable compounds; applications to practical examples are discussed in Section 6.3 and in refs. 41, 146, 164, 400, and 418–420.

Several methods have been described for the simultaneous determination of n-octanol/water $\log P$ values and pK_a values (404, 405, 421–427).

3.6 Other QSAR Approaches

Pattern recognition techniques have attracted much attention in the past two decades (24, 25, 58, 428–434). In principle there is no difference between the classical QSAR methods and pattern recognition, only the number of variables in a pattern recognition study is much higher than in Hansch analysis. A training set (usually 50–70% of the data) is chosen to derive a quantitative model for the prediction of the rest of the data (the test set). Many problems are associated with the proper selection of the training set (e.g., ref. 435) and the limitations coming from stepwise regression analysis (too few degrees of freedom, interrelated variables). More consistent results are obtained using other multivariate methods, like principal component analysis or soft modeling techniques, e.g., SIMCA or PLS analysis (Section 4.2), instead of regression analysis.

The application of pattern recognition methods, at least in combination with a reasonable preselection of variables and use of the PLS method, seems to be justified for groups of congeneric drugs which have the same mechanism of action. However, its abuse to correlate and predict "toxic, mutagenic, teratogenic, carcinogenic" and other global biological properties (436, 437) must be criticized. A more reliable approach seems to be a rule-based expert system which compares and categorizes structures of new compounds with respect to the information extracted from a large database, e.g., the CASE (computer automated structure evaluation) programs (438–440). CASE and MULTICASE (including a hierarchical selection of descriptors) (441) are artificial intelligence programs which automatically identify molecular features that contribute to (biophores) or reduce (biophobe fragments) biological activity.

A machine learning program GOLEM from the field of inductive logic programming was applied to model the structure–activity relationships of dihydrofolate reductase inhibitors (442).

Many different but inherently related QSAR approaches start from a hyperstructure, which is a hypothetical molecule including all structural features of the molecules under investigation. The presence and absence of certain hyperstructure atoms or groups in the individual molecules are correlated with biological activities in a stepwise optimization procedure. In the topological pharmacophore methods (443–447), e.g., LOCON (443, 444, 446), LOGANA (444–446), and EVAL (447), Free Wilson-type indicator variables are (in a stepwise procedure) connected by logical operators to correlate structures and activities. Also the minimal steric difference (MSD) (52, 448–450), MCD (Monte Carlo version of MSD) (52, 451), minimal topological difference (MTD) (52, 450, 452–456), and SIBIS (457) methods (for reviews see 52, 270, 450) define hypothetical hypermolecules; values of +1, 0, and −1 are assigned to different positions of the hypermolecule and the distance of each molecule to the optimum selection of these values is correlated with biological activities.

Magee (458, 459) combined the hyperstructure concept with the strategies of Hansch analysis and the mixed approach (Section 3.3). As only several atoms or groups of a molecule modulate biological activity, each position of the hypermolecule can be characterized as being favorable, unfavorable, or indifferent for biological activity. Positional effects for lipophilic interactions, polarizability, electronegativity, steric interactions, and hydrogen bonding can be assigned to certain positions.

All these methods regard hypermolecules as rigid frames but molecular shape analysis (MSA) (270, 460–469) considers conformational flexibility. Minimum energy conformations are calculated for all molecules within a series and their volumes are compared to a reference structure; the resulting volume differences are then correlated with biological activities.

A recent development in QSAR is the application of neural networks (470–478); further investigations, comparing classical approaches and neural networks (e.g., ref. 478), are required to evaluate the scope and limitations of neural nets. Some problems, e.g., the design of the network, lack of convergence, chance correlations, or overtraining of the network, have been critically discussed (473, 477, 478).

4 STATISTICAL METHODS

4.1 Regression Analysis

Regression analysis (339, 340, 479) correlates independent X variables (e.g., physicochemical parameters, indicator variables) and dependent Y variables (e.g., biological data). The dependent variables contain an error term ε, while the independent variables are supposed to contain no error. In reality, the physicochemical parameters of a QSAR equation also contain experimental error, but in most cases this error is much smaller than the error in the biological data.

Equations 14.66 and 14.67 describe a regression model containing two X variables, which is the simplest case of linear multiple regression analysis.

$$y_{obs} = ax_1 + bx_2 + c + \varepsilon \quad (14.66)$$

$$y_{calc} = ax_1 + bx_2 + c \quad (14.67)$$

Since $\Sigma \varepsilon^2 = \Sigma \Delta^2 = \Sigma(y_{obs} - y_{calc})^2$ shall be a minimum, the function $f = \Sigma(y_{obs} - ax_1 - bx_2 - c)^2$ is differentiated according to $df/da = df/db = df/dc = 0$. The coefficients a, b, and c of equation 14.67 are calculated from the resulting equations, the so-called "normal equations".

The correlation coefficient r (eq. 14.68) is a relative measure of the quality of fit of the model. Its value depends on the overall variance of the data; r^2 is a measure of the explained variance, most often given as a percentage value. The overall (total) variance S_{yy} is defined by equation 14.69, the unexplained variance (SSQ = sum of squared error; residual variance; variance not explained by the model) by equation 14.70.

$$r^2 = 1 - \Sigma \Delta^2 / S_{yy} \qquad (14.68)$$

$$S_{yy} = \Sigma(y_{obs} - y_{mean})^2 = \Sigma y^2 - (\Sigma y)^2/n \qquad (14.69)$$

$$\Sigma \Delta^2 = SSQ = \Sigma(y_{obs} - y_{calc})^2 \qquad (14.70)$$

The standard deviation s (eq. 14.71) is an absolute measure of the quality of fit. Its value considers the number of objects n and the number of variables k. Thus s does not only depend on the goodness of fit, but also on the number of degrees of freedom, $DF = n - k - 1$; the larger the number of objects and the smaller the number of variables is, the smaller will be its value for a certain value of $\Sigma \Delta^2$.

$$s^2 = \frac{\Sigma \Delta^2}{n - k - 1} = \frac{(1 - r^2) \cdot S_{yy}}{n - k - 1} \qquad (14.71)$$

The F value (eq. 14.72) is a measure of the statistical significance of the regression model; the influence of the number of variables included in the model is even larger than for the standard deviation s.

$$F = \frac{r^2(n - k - 1)}{k(1 - r^2)} \qquad (14.72)$$

The confidence intervals of the coefficients a, b, and c in equation 14.67 indicate the significance of each individual regression term.

Two different regression models, containing different numbers of variables k_1 (smaller number) and k_2 (larger number), can be compared by a sequential (partial) F-Test (eq. 14.73). The model containing the larger number of variables is justified if the resulting F value proves a 95% significance for the introduction of the additional $(k_2 - k_1)$ variables.

$$F = \frac{(r_2^2 - r_1^2)(n - k_2 - 1)}{(k_2 - k_1)(1 - r_2^2)} \qquad (14.73)$$

Equation 14.73 is used in automated algorithms to derive a regression model in a stepwise manner (e.g., by a forward selection procedure with intermediate proof whether already included variables become insignificant at a later step) (340). Whereas such procedures avoid the testing of hundreds or even thousands of different variable combinations, in the case of a large number of (partially interrelated) variables often a local optimum results and the global optimum is missed.

A better procedure in QSAR studies is first to derive a physicochemical model from the biological mechanism of action for a small subset of compounds. In the next steps, more and more compounds are added by introducing new variables for new positions of structural variation or by combining different subsets with the help of indicator variables (e.g., eqs. 14.33–14.35, Section 2.8).

A QSAR equation can be accepted if the correlation coefficient is around or better than 0.9, if the standard deviation is not much larger than the standard deviation of the biological data (corresponding to their mean error, normally around 0.3; smaller for *in vitro* data), if its F value indicates that the overall significance level is better than 95%, and if all the individual regression coefficients are justified at the 95% significance level (i.e., if their confidence intervals are smaller than the values of the regression coefficients). The equation has to be rejected if the number of variables is unreasonably large or if the standard deviation s is smaller than the error in the biological data (overprediction by the model).

Outliers constitute a serious problem in QSAR studies. Most often they are omitted from the data set without further comments, which is not a good practice. A lot of information might be derived from the careful inspection and consideration of the residuals of a multiple regression analysis (e.g., refs. 480) and of so-called outliers (e.g., refs. 481, 482).

The proper application of regression analysis (as well as of other multivariate statistical methods) in QSAR studies and the validity of the obtained results have been reviewed (354–356).

4.2 Partial Least Squares (PLS) Analysis and Other Multivariate Statistical Methods

Discriminant analysis (41, 428, 483–487) separates objects with different properties, e.g., active and inactive compounds, by deriving a function of other features (e.g., different physicochemical properties) which gives the best separation of the individual classes. A training set is used and the quality of fit is checked with the help of a test set. COMPACT (computer optimized molecular parametric analysis of chemical toxicity) (488, 489) is a discriminant analysis approach to predict carcinogenicity and other forms of toxicity.

The ALS (Adaptive least squares) method (344, 490–492), a modification of discriminant analysis, separates several activity classes (e.g., data ordered by a rating score) by a discriminant function. OR-MUCS (ordered multicategorial classification using simplex technique) (493) is an ALS-related approach which uses a simplex technique for the derivation of the discriminant function. A fuzzy ALS version

was recently applied to QSAR studies (494).

Regression analysis and discriminant analysis are extremely sensitive to interrelated X variables; multivariate statistical methods which reduce the dimensionality of the X block are robust in this respect. Factor analysis (FA) and principal component analysis (PCA) (495–498) derive vectors which are orthogonal and contain, in decreasing order, the maximum amount of information that can stepwise be extracted from the X block. These principal components are then correlated with biological activity data. Applications of FA and PCA in QSAR are illustrated by several studies (e.g., refs. 499–503).

The SIMCA method (354, 428, 504–507) is a class modeling technique which places objects from p-dimensional space into lower dimension boxes (e.g., a line, plane, or hyperplane); the size of the box is determined by the scatter of the data. Separate principal component models are derived to discriminate objects of different classes.

The most promising new approach in multivariate statistics is the partial least squares (PLS) method (26, 27, 428, 508–511). Hundreds or even thousands of independent variables (the X block) can be correlated with one or several dependent variables (the Y block). PLS analysis is a principal component-like method in which the vectors are not independently extracted for the X and the Y block. As in the SIMCA method, the NIPALS (nonlinear iterative partial least squares) algorithm (512) is applied to derive a certain number of vectors for each block which, in contrast to the principal components derived by PCA, are slightly shifted to their exact positions. The vectors are still located in their corresponding boxes, but the correlation of corresponding X block- and Y block-derived vectors is optimized (Fig. 14.4) (27, 428, 508, 509).

Often perfect correlations are obtained

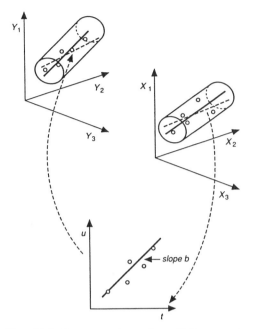

Fig. 14.4 Representation of a PLS regression through the inner relation u = b.t. The solid lines in X- and Y-space are the principal components and the dashed lines are the PLS vectors. These are slightly skewed to account for the correlation between the two data blocks. Redrawn from Figure 9, p. 698, of ref. 428 with permission from Pergamon Press Ltd., Oxford, UK.

in PLS analyses, due to the usually large numbers of X variables. A cross-validation procedure (356, 513) must be used to select the model having the highest predictive value; several PLS runs are performed in which one (leave one out-technique) or several objects are eliminated from the data set. Only the excluded objects are predicted by the corresponding model. The standard deviation s_{PRESS} (derived from PRESS, the sum of the squared errors of these predictions, divided by the number of degrees of freedom) (513) is taken as the criterion for the optimum number of components. If too many components are extracted, overprediction results and PRESS and s_{PRESS} increase. SDEP (standard deviation of the error of predictions) (514, 515) corresponds to s_{PRESS}, the only difference

being that the number of degrees of freedom is not considered in the calculation of the SDEP value.

The squared correlation coefficient r^2 is defined as in regression analysis. A r^2_{PRESS} value can be formulated for cross-validation runs using PRESS instead of the unexplained variance (513). Cross-validated r^2 values always are more or less smaller than the r^2 values including all objects (r^2_{FIT}), depending on the quality of the model. In severe cases of overprediction, negative r^2_{PRESS} values are obtained, indicating that the predictions from the model are even worse than the y_{mean} value. Bootstrapping (356, 513) is a procedure in which n random selections out of the original set of n objects are performed several times to simulate different samplings from a larger set of objects. Confidence intervals for each term can be estimated from such a procedure, giving an independent measure of the stability of the PLS model.

Although the PLS method is claimed to be a robust modeling technique, experience shows that variables not contributing to prediction obscure the result. A procedure for variable elimination from large X blocks, called GOLPE (generating optimal linear PLS estimations), was developed (516, 517) to solve this problem.

PLS analysis is the method of choice in 3D-QSAR methods like comparative molecular field analysis (CoMFA) (Section 8.3).

Cluster analysis separates and groups objects according to their distances in multidimensional space; different algorithms are described to agglomerate related objects, most often in a hierarchical manner. Its application for the rational selection of substituents in drug design (50, 144) and for QSAR studies (e.g., refs. 518–521) has been discussed. The results from cluster analysis and from nonlinear mapping, a method which projects data from multidimensional space to fewer, e.g., two dimensions (the nonlinear map) by a principal componentlike iterative procedure, have been compared (519).

Cluster significance analysis (CSA) (483, 522–524) is a graphical method to look at the clustering of active compounds in a space that is made up of various physicochemical parameters. Qualitative or rank ordered biological data can be used; a significance probability value is calculated to judge whether any cluster must be considered as a chance occurrence or not.

5 DESIGN OF TEST SERIES IN QSAR

A prerequisite for a QSAR study is a congeneric series of compounds, all having the same mechanism of action. While congenericity is not easy to define, it is clear from common experience that all compounds of a set should have the same molecular frame, i.e., an identical parent compound with structural variation in one or several positions.

Parameter intercorrelation in less well designed data sets was recognized as a problem in QSAR from the very beginning. The first contribution to solve this problem in a proper manner was made by Craig (525); he proposed to look at 2D plots of physicochemical properties and to choose substituents from all different quadrants. This graphical method is easy to apply and different physicochemical properties can be plotted against each other. Substituents are selected by the chemist by the relative ease of synthesis. The disadvantage of Craig diagrams is that they are restricted to at most three dimensions (526) while it is *a priori* unknown which physicochemical properties will be responsible for the biological activities.

Parameter focusing is a related technique (527). Different 2D plots of physicochemical properties are drawn to find out which parameter combination separates active and inactive compounds to the largest extent.

A sequential simplex technique was proposed by Darvas (528) to find the most active analog within a series in a stepwise procedure. Despite some successful applications (528, 529) the method has limitations: only two physicochemical parameters are considered simultaneously and the method is only suited for retrospective analyses or for cases where synthesis is not the rate-limiting step, as compared to biological testing.

A real advance in design strategy resulted from the Topliss operational schemes (530, 531). The Topliss scheme starts from two analogs, e.g. a compound bearing hydrogen at a phenyl ring and the corresponding *p*-Cl analog. In relation to the parent compound the *p*-Cl analog may have higher, equal, or lower biological activity. Correspondingly, in the next step more lipophilic analogs (in the case of higher activity of the *p*-Cl analog) or more hydrophilic analogs, e.g., *p*-OMe (lower activity of *p*-Cl) are proposed by the operational scheme. If the activity of the H and Cl analogs is about the same, either the lipophilicity or the electron acceptor properties of the chlorine substituent are unfavorable, while the other property might increase biological activity. Thus a lipophilic donor substituent, e.g., Me, and a not too lipophilic acceptor substituent, e.g., the NO_2 group, are the next proposals. If activity is increased in any direction, this guides further syntheses; if not, it has to be considered that large substituents in the para-position may be unfavorable and the same procedure as above is applied to the meta-position. For aliphatic substitution a corresponding scheme was developed. A manual method was proposed by Topliss (532) as a modification of his operational schemes: a larger number of substituents is selected in the first step to derive the dependence of biological activities on π (linear and nonlinear) and σ with a minimum number of analogs. This latter approach has been criticized because of collinearity and unbalanced spanning of the parameter space (533).

The different approaches proposed by Topliss should not be understood as rigid schemes; they are strategies which have to be adjusted to each problem. A recent review (350) lists more than 50 references where the Topliss methods have been applied, mostly in medicinal chemistry. It was shown that optimum activity would have rapidly been reached in many series of compounds (534), following the Topliss scheme; on the other hand, there are at least some examples where the Topliss method failed (350, 526).

2^n-Factorial design techniques are quite common in experimental design (535–537). They have successfully been applied to series design in lead structure optimization, using $+$ and $-$ or $+$, 0, and $-$ as descriptors for each physicochemical property of the different substituents (538–541). Several physicochemical properties can simultaneously be considered in a factorial design.

More objective procedures for series design are clustering methods in multidimensional parameter space (50, 144, 350; Section 2); substituents from different clusters are selected for synthesis. As this approach cannot automatically avoid collinearity or multicollinearity, different standard sets of aromatic substituents have been proposed (e.g., refs. 542, 543). A distance mapping technique selects further substituents on the criterion of a maximum distance to the substituents which already are included (542). A modification (544) of this approach uses the determinant of the parameter correlation matrix for substituent selection.

D-optimal design methods (340, 350, 545) calculate the determinant of the variance–covariance matrix; its value is largest for substituent sets with maximum variance and minimum covariance in their physicochemical properties. In some other approaches synthetic accessability has been

included as an additional selection feature (545–547).

Other design methods, such as principal component methods, combined with multidimensional mapping (153), and a two-dimensional mapping of intraclass correlation matrices (548) have been reviewed (350). Principal components of properties were also used in fractional design methods (549, 550) and in D-optimal design (550).

Other design strategies are applied in Free Wilson analysis (341, 551). While in Hansch analysis structural modification is sometimes restricted to one position of substitution, including a relatively large number of different substituents, in Free Wilson analysis at least two different positions of substitution must be modified. Each substituent in every position should be included several times, otherwise the corresponding group contribution will include the experimental error of this one biological activity value. Also for Free Wilson analyses a factorial design technique (551) and a quantitative procedure to extract an optimal set out of all possible analogs have been proposed (552).

Experimental design strategies for QSAR studies have been reviewed (350, 540) and compared by more than 20 different criteria (350); some of their practical limitations have been discussed (350, 533, 545).

6 APPLICATIONS OF HANSCH ANALYSIS

In the original definition of the extrathermodynamic approach a linear combination of lipophilic and electronic terms accounted for drug receptor interaction, and a nonlinear lipophilicity relationship was included to model transport and distribution of the drugs (15, 17, 18). Only in special cases, e.g., in enzyme inhibition, is an isolated process measured and described. In other biological systems much more complex relationships are to be expected, an exception being pharmacokinetic data, where only rate constants or concentrations of different drugs in certain compartments are described in a quantitative manner.

Thousands of Hansch equations have been published in the past 30 years. A database already contains about 3000 QSAR equations of biological data as well as 3000 linear free energy relationships in organic chemistry (553), allowing systematic comparisons of different biological effects and of the effects of a certain group of compounds on different biological systems; comparative structure–activity relationships (554) will provide further insight on the intrinsic nature of drug-receptor interactions.

Only a few typical examples are discussed below to demonstrate the proper application of Hansch analysis and its value in medicinal chemistry and in rational drug design. More examples are given in refs. 39–44; QSAR publications are regularly reviewed in the abstracts section of the journal *Quantitative Structure–Activity Relationships* (85) and by some other abstracts services (86–88).

6.1 Enzyme Inhibition

Significant progress in QSAR came from Hansch analyses of enzyme inhibitors (399, 555–558), especially in combination with protein 3D structures and molecular graphics (271, 559–564). Most of our knowledge on the quantitative aspects of ligand–protein interactions has been derived from protein crystallography and from QSAR studies, especially from the systematic work of Hansch and his group on dihydrofolate reductase and on cysteine and serine proteases.

Dihydrofolate reductase (DHFR) is by far the best investigated enzyme. 3D structures of binary and ternary DHFR complexes from different bacteria and verte-

brates have been published and an extremely large number of QSAR equations, both for the isolated enzyme and for growth inhibition of whole cells, has been derived (271, 344, 555, 559, 565–580). DHFR was also the target of early attempts of a structure-based drug design using crystallographic information (581, 582).

Some QSAR equations derived for 5-(X-benzyl)-2,4-diamino-pyrimidines as inhibitors of DHFR from different species are given below (eqs. 14.74–14.78) (559).

For *Escherichia coli* DHFR:

$$\log 1/K_{i\,\text{app}} = 0.75(\pm 0.26)\pi_{3,4,5}$$

$$- 1.07(\pm 0.34)\log(\beta \cdot 10^{\pi_{3,4,5}} + 1)$$

$$+ 1.36(\pm 0.24)MR'_{3,5}$$

$$+ 0.88(\pm 0.29)MR'_4 + 6.20 \qquad (14.74)$$

$$\log \beta = 0.12 \quad \text{optimum } \pi = 0.25$$

$$(n = 43; r = 0.903; s = 0.290)$$

For *Lactobacillus casei* DHFR:

$$\log 1/K_{i\,\text{app}} = 0.31(\pm 0.11)\pi_{3,4}$$

$$- 0.88(\pm 0.24)\log(\beta \cdot 10^{\pi_{3,4}} + 1)$$

$$+ 0.95(\pm 0.21)MR'_{3,4} + 5.32 \qquad (14.75)$$

$$\log \beta = -1.33 \quad \text{optimum } \pi = 1.05$$

$$(n = 42; r = 0.876; s = 0.222)$$

For chicken liver DHFR:

$$\log 1/K_{i\,\text{app}} = 0.55(\pm 0.19)\pi_{3,4,5}$$

$$- 0.43(\pm 0.35)\log(\beta \cdot 10^{\pi_{3,4,5}} + 1)$$

$$+ 0.20(\pm 0.10)MR_3$$

$$+ 0.32(\pm 0.26)\, \Sigma\, \sigma + 4.46 \qquad (14.76)$$

$$\log \beta = -0.222 \quad \text{no optimum } (b < a)$$

$$(n = 39; r = 0.900; s = 0.241)$$

For bovine liver DHFR:

$$\log 1/K_{i\ app} = 0.48(\pm0.11)\pi_{3,5}$$

$$-1.25(\pm0.40)\log(\beta \cdot 10^{\pi_{3,5}} + 1)$$

$$+0.13(\pm0.10)MR_3$$

$$+0.24(\pm0.24)\sum \sigma + 5.43 \qquad (14.77)$$

$$\log \beta = -1.98 \quad \text{optimum } \pi = 1.52$$

$$(n = 42; r = 0.875; s = 0.227)$$

For human lymphoblastoid DHFR:

$$\log 1/K_{i\ app} = 0.59(\pm0.20)\pi_{3,5}$$

$$-0.63(\pm0.59)\log(\beta \cdot 10^{\pi_{3,5}} + 1)$$

$$+0.19(\pm0.14)\pi_4$$

$$+0.19(\pm0.15)MR_3$$

$$+0.30(\pm0.28)\sum \sigma + 4.03 \qquad (14.78)$$

$$\log \beta = -0.82 \quad \text{optimum } \pi = 1.94$$

$$(n = 38; r = 0.879; s = 0.266)$$

Although the equations in general look the same, some striking differences can be seen on a closer inspection. First, the vertebrate, but not the bacterial DHFR equations contain an electronic parameter in addition to lipophilicity and molar refractivity terms. Secondly, in the case of *L. casei* (eq. 14.75) the 5-position of the benzyl group does not contribute to biological activity at all. An explanation could be derived from the 3D structure of *L. casei* DHFR, in comparison to the *E. coli* DHFR structure. The active sites of both enzymes are more or less identical in the geometries of the protein backbone and the amino acid side chains, yet there is one striking difference. The *E. coli* DHFR contains a methionine side chain in the area where the 5-substituents bind. In the *L. casei* DHFR there is a relatively rigid leucine side chain which obviously interferes with the 5-substituents; positive contributions from lipophilicity and

polarizability are counterbalanced by their steric bulk.

Another well-investigated enzyme is the cysteine protease papain (eqs. 14.33–14.35, Section 2.8; eqs. 14.79–14.81) (271, 343, 561, 583–589).

N-(X-Benzoyl)-glycine methyl esters (583):

$$\log 1/K_m = 1.01(\pm0.11)\pi + 1.46$$

$$(14.79)$$

$$(n = 16; r = 0.981; s = 0.165)$$

N-Benzoyl-glycine X-phenyl esters (584):

$$\log 1/K_m = 1.03(\pm0.25)\pi_3'$$

$$+0.57(\pm0.20)\sigma$$

$$+0.61(\pm0.29)MR_4$$

$$+3.80(\pm0.17) \qquad (14.80)$$

$$(n = 25; r = 0.907; s = 0.208)$$

N-Mesyl-glycine X-phenyl esters (561):

$$\log 1/K_m = 0.61(\pm0.09)\pi_3'$$

$$+0.55(\pm0.20)\sigma$$

$$+0.46(\pm0.11)MR_4$$

$$+2.00(\pm0.12) \qquad (14.81)$$

$$(n = 32; r = 0.945; s = 0.178)$$

A comparison of equations 14.79–14.81 and an inspection of the 3D structure of papain show that the substituents of the *N*-benzoyl group (eq. 14.79) are located in hydrophobic space, while the phenyl ester group binds in a polar environment. Similar equations were derived for the closely related cysteine hydrolases actinidin (271, 585–587), bromelain (583, 586, 587), and ficin (586, 587).

N-Benzoyl-glycine X-phenyl esters (eq. 14.80) were also investigated as inhibitors of the serine proteases chymotrypsin ($n = 28$; $r = 0.945$; $s = 0.081$) (271, 563) and trypsin $(n = 10; \quad r = 0.961; \quad s = 0.100)$ (271, 590).

The inhibition of trypsin by benz-amidines and naphth-2-yl-amidines is described by equations 14.82 and 14.83, respectively (271, 591).

$$\log 1/K_i = -0.59(\pm 0.49)MR_4$$
$$+ 0.88(\pm 0.52)\log(\beta \cdot 10^{MR_4} + 1)$$
$$+ 0.23(\pm 0.07)\pi'_3$$
$$- 0.74(\pm 0.20)\sigma$$
$$+ 0.20(\pm 0.30)I\text{-}M$$
$$+ 0.65(\pm 0.22)I\text{-}1$$
$$+ 0.43(\pm 0.19)I\text{-}2$$
$$+ 0.51(\pm 0.15)I\text{-}3$$
$$+ 1.38(\pm 0.28) \qquad (14.82)$$

optimum $MR_4 = 1.03$

$(n = 104; r = 0.924; s = 0.222)$

$$\log 1/K_i = 0.47(\pm 0.19)MR_4$$
$$- 1.40(\pm 0.40)\sigma$$
$$+ 2.59(\pm 0.24) \qquad (14.83)$$

$(n = 21; r = 0.915; s = 0.322)$

Out of many other Hansch analyses derived for different enzymes, only investigations on alcohol dehydrogenase (271, 592–594), butyrylcholinesterase (595), carbonic anhydrase (271, 596, 597), chymotrypsin (271, 399, 557, 598, 599), DNA polymerase (600), β-glucosidase (601), glycolic acid oxidase (602), guanine deaminase (556, 603), monoamine oxidase (164, 604), HSV-thymidine kinase (605), and xanthine oxidase (556, 606) shall be mentioned here.

A recent compilation of QSAR studies on enzyme inhibitors (558) reviews more than 400 Hansch equations.

6.2 Other *in vitro* Data

Specific and nonspecific binding of drugs to proteins (other than enzymes) show significant differences. The serum albumin binding of miscellaneous neutral compounds can be explained by their lipophilicity ($\log 1/C$ vs. π: $n = 42$; $r = 0.960$; $s = 0.159$) but not by their polarizability ($\log 1/C$ vs. MR: $r = 0.307$) (18, 607). The highly specific, polar binding of phenyl-β-D-glucosides to concanavalin A is described much better by a polarizability term MR ($\log M_{50}$ vs. MR: $n = 19$; $r = 0.954$; $s = 0.038$) than by lipophilicity ($\log M_{50}$ vs. π: $r = 0.664$) (608).

Structure–activity relationships in immunochemistry (21, 314, 344, 609–612) reveal the importance of steric interactions in the QSAR of hapten–antibody interactions (314, 344, 612).

Systematic investigations have been performed over more than one decade on the QSAR of muscarinic receptor ligands (613, 614). An equation for the acetylcholine receptor affinity of quaternary ammonium compounds was used to predict the potency of a new, structurally different analogue (615). The compound was synthesized and tested; however, the prediction turned out to be completely wrong (616); observed and predicted affinities differed by 6 log units (!), once again showing the risk of predictions for structurally dissimilar compounds which are too far outside the included parameter range. A reanalysis of the data gave an equation which led to a better prediction for the affinity of this compound (error: 1.4 log units) (350).

QSAR studies of H_1-receptor antagonists (617), serotonin antagonists and uptake inhibitors (618), and receptor binding and thyroxine binding protein affinity of thyroid hormone analogs (619) have been reviewed. In addition, Hansch analyses for binding to the β-adrenergic receptor (620, 621), the benzodiazepin receptor (622), the tetrachlorodibenzodioxin (TCDD) receptor

(623, 624), the dopamine receptor (625), the estrogen receptor (626), and dopamine-, norepinephrine-, and serotonin-uptake inhibition (627) shall be mentioned here. Some QSAR studies of receptor agonists and antagonists are discussed in ref. 95.

Another well-investigated class of compounds are calcium antagonists (344, 628–635). Multiparameter equations have been derived for verapamil-type compounds ($n = 75$; $r = 0.89$; $s = 0.33$) (635), while a chemically closely related series of compounds turned out to be potent α-adrenergic antagonists ($n = 59$; $r = 0.92$; $s = 0.37$) (636).

Nonspecific hemolytic, antibacterial, and antifungal *in vitro* activities generally follow linear (18, 171), parabolic (18, 19), and bilinear (23, 322) lipophilicity–activity relationships. Many bilinear equations have correlation coefficients r close to 1.00 (322); it seems that at least in some cases the biological activity depends on the critical micelle concentration of the compounds (637). QSAR studies of antibacterial sulfa drugs (e.g., eq. 14.29, Section 2.5) (344, 638) and some other examples of specific antibacterial activities (41, 42, 344) have been reviewed.

Much work has been done to elucidate the molecular mechanisms of drug resistance. Comparative QSAR equations were derived for bacterial DHFR and bacterial cell cultures (200, 201, 271, 555, 566, 574) and for different tumor cell lines (271, 555, 559, 567, 568, 570, 573, 576), all being sensitive and resistant to methotrexate (MTX). Much higher lipophilicity optima are obtained for resistant cells (566, 568, 570, 573); from this evidence Hansch concluded that a change in the membrane properties should be responsible for the MTX resistance. Seydel (200, 201) found differences in the dose response curves of *Escherichia coli* strains that are sensitive and resistant to trimethoprim (TMP), to be responsible for TMP resistance. Lipophilic analogs still bind to the enzyme, but they are no longer antagonists; the higher, amphiphilic analogs are nonspecific membrane-perturbing agents. Chloroquine resistance and multidrug resistance were explained in the same manner (200).

Multidrug resistance (MDR) is the acquired resistance of tumor cells against a wide variety of structurally diverse, polar and lipophilic, small and large antitumor drugs, caused by a single antitumor agent. The QSAR of MDR shows linear and nonlinear dependences on lipophilicity and on the size of the molecules (307, 323, 324). A nonlinear dependence on size can be explained with the inability of medium-sized molecules to reenter the cells after they are eliminated *via* an active transport by the over-expressed glycoprotein GP-170, either by passive diffusion (pathway of the small molecules) or by endocytosis (pathway of the large molecules) (323).

Another well-investigated field in QSAR are mutagenic agents (305–308, 639–642). The QSAR equations of a series of 1-(X-phenyl)-3,3-dialkyltriazenes show that mutagenic activity (and presumably carcinogenicity) can be minimized with relatively little loss in antitumor potency.

Quantum chemical indices were used to describe such activities (305–308); much more heterogeneous sets can be combined in a QSAR equation, e.g. aromatic analogs and heteroaromatic compounds, for which no σ values are available (eq. 14.84; TA98 = mutagenic activity in *Salmonella typhimurium*, strain TA98; ε_{LUMO} = energy of the lowest unoccupied molecular orbital) (308).

$$\log TA98 = 0.65(\pm0.16)\log P$$
$$- 2.90(\pm0.59)\log(\beta P + 1)$$
$$- 1.38(\pm0.25)\varepsilon_{LUMO}$$
$$+ 1.88(\pm0.39)I_1$$
$$- 2.89(\pm0.81)I_a$$
$$- 4.15(\pm0.58) \qquad (14.84)$$
$$\log \beta = -5.48 \quad \text{optimum} \log P = 4.93$$
$$(n = 188; r = 0.900; s = 0.886)$$

6.3 Pharmacokinetic Data

Pharmacokinetics describes the time dependence of transport and distribution of a drug in the different compartments of a biological system, e.g., rate constants of absorption, blood and tissue levels, and metabolism and elimination rate constants (415). Quantitative structure–pharmacokinetics relationships (376, 385, 394, 395, 413, 643–646) investigate the structural dependence of such parameters in chemically related groups of compounds.

Model simulations (see Section 3.4) substantiate that the lipophilicity dependence of the rate constants of drug transport should follow bilinear relationships (41, 146, 164, 322, 383, 385). Indeed bilinear equations have been derived for the transport rate constants of various barbiturates in an absorption simulator, from an aqueous phase (pH = 3) through an organic membrane into another aqueous phase (pH 7.5), simulating the gastric absorption of these compounds ($n = 23$; $r = 0.992$; $s = 0.081$) (385), and for the buccal absorption of homologous alkanoic acids (385). Much more complex models correlate the buccal absorption rate constants of these acids at different pH values (420).

Gastric and intestinal absorption rates of neutral carbamates are described by equations 14.85 and 14.86 (385), respectively.

$$\log k_{abs} = 0.138(\pm 0.06) \log P$$
$$- 0.228(\pm 0.16) \log(\beta P + 1)$$
$$- 2.244 \qquad (14.85)$$

$$\log \beta = -1.678 \quad \text{optimum} \log P = 1.87$$

$$(n = 8; r = 0.971; s = 0.030; F = 22.14)$$

$$\log k_{abs} = 0.234(\pm 0.10) \log P$$
$$- 0.502(\pm 0.15) \log(\beta P + 1)$$
$$- 0.786 \qquad (14.86)$$

$$\log \beta = -0.621 \quad \text{optimum} \log P = 0.56$$

$$(n = 8; r = 0.989; s = 0.031; F = 61.10)$$

The blood–brain barrier inhibits the passage of hydrophilic compounds from the blood into the central nervous system (CNS). For various groups of CNS-active drugs lipophilicity optima for blood-brain barrier penetration at $\log P$ values around 2.1 (647), 1.8–2.0 (648, 649), 1.4–2.7 (413, 650), and 0.9–2.5 (651) have been reported (376, 652). The rat brain capillary permeability coefficients P_c of a wide variety of compounds, ranging from water (MW = 18) to bleomycin (MW = 1400), can be described by equation 14.87 (652), giving evidence for the importance of the size of the molecules (approximated by $\log MW$) for diffusion and pore transport.

$$\log P_c = 0.50(\pm 0.10) \log P$$
$$- 1.43(\pm 0.58) \log MW - 1.84 \qquad (14.87)$$
$$(n = 23; r = 0.927; s = 0.461)$$

The blood–brain barrier penetration of H_2-receptor antihistaminics has been correlated with $\Delta \log P$, the difference between n-octanol/water and cyclohexane/water partition coefficients (Section 2.1) (187, 188). Using Λ_{alk}, a hydrogen bonding capability parameter, and V_M, the van der Waals volume, an even better correlation could be obtained ($n = 20$; $r = 0.934$; $s = 0.290$) (653).

Hansch emphasized the importance of lipophilicity for nonspecific side effects of drugs (652). Hydrophobic drugs do not only pass the blood–brain barrier (e.g., sedative side effects of most antihistaminics), they are also slowly eliminated from the biological system, are more inhibitory to biochemical systems than hydrophilic compounds, induce cytochrome P-450 (654), and reactive species may be formed in their metabolism. Thus, without convincing evidence to the contrary, drugs should be made as hydrophilic as possible (652).

Also the placenta has a barrier for hydrophilic and very lipophilic compounds; correspondingly quantitative relationships could be derived for the placental transfer ratios TR of various drugs (eq. 14.88, recalculated) (655).

$$\log TR = 0.354(\pm 0.06) \log P$$

$$- 0.469(\pm 0.13) \log(\beta P + 1)$$

$$- 0.116(\pm 0.07) \qquad (14.88)$$

$$\log \beta = -0.658 \quad \text{optimum} \log P = 1.15$$

$$(n = 21; r = 0.949; s = 0.106; F = 51.17)$$

The diffusion of drugs into milk and prostatic fluid has been reviewed (413, 643). A comprehensive review on quantitative structure–pharmacokinetics relationships (395) tabulates about 100 equations, including absorption, distribution, protein binding, elimination, and metabolism of drugs.

6.4 Other Biological Data

Numerous kinds of biological activities have been correlated with physicochemical properties; only a few selected examples from different indications will be discussed here.

The local anesthetic activities of lidocaine analogs have been compared to their acute toxicities (656). Possible reasons for the differences between both activities have been discussed, but no structural proposals were derived for local anesthetics with lower toxicity.

The antiadrenergic activities of α-bromo-phenethylamines are described by equations 14.38–14.41 (Section 3.1). The β_1- and β_2-antagonistic activities of a series of 4-imidazol-2'-yl-phenoxy-propanolamines were compared (657); MR must be about 2 for maximum β_1-antagonism, while electron-acceptor substituents increase β_2-antagonistic potency.

Structure–activity relationships of antimalarials attracted much attention (658, 659) because of an extensive program of the Walter Reed Army Institute for Medical Research during the Vietnam war. Equation 14.89 correlates the antimalarial activities of phenanthrenecarbinols and related analogs in mice (659).

$$\log 1/C = 0.576(\pm 0.09) \sum \sigma$$

$$+ 0.168(\pm 0.05) \sum \pi$$

$$+ 0.105(\pm 0.05) \log P$$

$$- 0.167(\pm 0.07) \log(\beta P + 1)$$

$$- 0.169(\pm 0.10)c\text{-side}$$

$$+ 0.319(\pm 0.136)CNR_2$$

$$- 0.139(\pm 0.06)AB$$

$$- 0.795(\pm 0.06) < 3\text{-cures}$$

$$+ 0.278(\pm 0.11)MR\text{-}4'\text{-}Q$$

$$+ 0.252(\pm 0.18)\text{Me-6,8-}Q$$

$$+ 0.084(\pm 0.10)2\text{-Pip}$$

$$+ 0.151(\pm 0.19)NBrPy$$

$$- 0.683(\pm 0.22)Q2P378$$

$$+ 0.267(\pm 0.11)Py$$

$$+ 2.726(\pm 0.15) \qquad (14.89)$$

$$\log \beta = -3.959 \quad \text{optimum} \log P = 4.19$$

$$(n = 646; s = 0.898; s = 0.309)$$

Inflammatory (Fig. 14.2, Section 3.4) (23, 383) and tumor promoting activities (660) of phorbol esters show a nonlinear dependence on lipophilicity, giving evidence that skin permeation after topical application of the compounds is responsible for biological activity.

Quantitative structure–activity relationships of antitumor drugs have been reviewed (661–663). Out of many studies performed by Hansch et al. (e.g., 664–669) some are discussed here to demonstrate how QSAR results can be used to decide on the probability of success of further research.

The antitumor activities of aniline mustards are correlated to the hydrolysis rate constants of these compounds; also acute toxicity parallels antitumor efficacy (664). The antileukemic activity of $1-$(X-aryl)-3,3-dialkyltriazenes is increased by electron donor substituents X. Chemical instability (the 4-OCH_3 analog has a half-life of only 12 min) precludes the introduction of donor substituents (665). In addition, the acute toxicities of these compounds are correlated with their antitumor activities; thus, no more syntheses and testing of new analogs were recommended on the basis of this comparative QSAR study (666).

Equation 14.90 was derived for the antitumor activities of 9-anilinoacridines (669). The coefficients of the $\Sigma \pi$ terms indicate that activity falls off more rapidly for the hydrophilic analogs; as the parent compound has a $\log P$ value of about 4.8, the lipophilicity optimum can be estimated to be close to $\log P = 0$.

$$\log 1/D_{50} = 0.63(\pm 0.27) \sum \pi$$
$$- 0.75(\pm 0.23) \log(\beta_1 \cdot 10^{\Sigma \pi} + 1)$$
$$- 1.01(\pm 0.09) \sum \sigma$$
$$- 1.21(\pm 0.36) R_{BS}$$
$$- 0.26(\pm 0.16) MR_2$$
$$+ 4.95(\pm 0.75) MR_3$$
$$- 5.13(\pm 0.86) \log(\beta_2 \cdot 10^{MR_3} + 1)$$
$$- 0.67(\pm 0.12) I_{3,6}$$
$$- 1.67(\pm 0.20) E_s\text{-}3'$$
$$- 1.57(\pm 0.21)(E_s - 3')^2$$
$$+ 0.58(\pm 0.13) I\text{-}NO_2$$
$$+ 0.87(\pm 0.31) I_{DAT}$$
$$+ 0.52(\pm 0.17) I_{BS}$$

$$+ 9.24(\pm 1.33) \qquad\qquad (14.90)$$

$$\log \beta_1 = 5.64 \quad \text{optimum} \sum \pi = -4.93$$
$$\log \beta_2 = 0.01 \quad \text{optimum } MR_3 = 1.44$$
$$\text{optimum } E_s\text{-}3' = -0.53$$
$$(n = 509; s = 0.893; s = 0.305)$$

QSAR studies on hallucinogens (670) and on drugs acting at the central nervous system (671) have been reviewed; together both reviews contain about 260 QSAR equations. Also the QSAR of steroids, having a wide variety of different biological activities, has been reviewed (672).

6.5 Activity–Activity Relationships

Activity–activity relationships, i.e. the comparison of biological activities of a group of compounds in different biological test models, were originally not the domain of QSAR analyses. However, in industrial practice such relationships and their quantitative description are of utmost importance. Instead of thousands of animals, nowadays enzyme inhibition, receptor binding, and cell culture data are used to derive activity profiles of classes of compounds and to predict the pharmacodynamic effects of new drugs from simple and efficient *in vitro* test models.

Most often linear relationships are obtained between different kinds of biological activities for the same group of compounds, provided both activities are caused by the same mechanism of action and no drug transport or distribution processes are involved (e.g., refs. 128, 344).

For α_2-adrenergic clonidine analogs Timmermans determined $\log P_{app}$ values (n-octanol/buffer, pH = 7.4), binding affinities to α_1-adrenoceptors, $IC_{50}\alpha_1$ (displacement of the α_1-antagonist prazosin), binding affinities to α_2-adrenoceptors, $IC_{50}\alpha_2$ (displacement of the α_2-agonist clonidine), antihypertensive activities (mediated by a central mechanism) in anesthetized normotensive rats ($ED_{25\%}$, i.v. application), and hypertensive activities (mediated by peripheral α-stimulation, which in the absence of central nervous system regulation causes blood vessel contraction) in pithed rats ($ED_{60\,mm}$, i.v. application) (673, 674). The pC_{60} values are directly related to $IC_{50}\alpha_2$ values (eq. 14.91), because the site of application of the drugs and the site of action are identical. On the other hand, a parabolic lipophilicity relationship had to be included to correlate antihypertensive activities (pC_{25} values) and $IC_{50}\alpha_2$ values (673, 674), because after i.v. application the drugs have to cross the blood–brain barrier to be able to achieve their central effect. A slightly better description of the data is obtained if the bilinear model is used instead (eq. 14.92) (675, 676).

$$pC_{60} = 1.16(\pm 0.21) \log 1/IC_{50}\alpha_2 - 0.96$$

$$(14.91)$$

$$(n = 21; r = 0.936; s = 0.317)$$

$$pC_{25} = 0.81(\pm 0.22) \log P$$
$$- 3.37(\pm 1.02) \log(\beta P + 1)$$
$$+ 1.07(\pm 0.20) \log 1/IC_{50}\alpha_2 - 1.16$$

$$(14.92)$$

$$\log \beta = -1.99 \quad \text{optimum} \log P = 1.48$$

$$(n = 21; r = 0.971; s = 0.284)$$

Compounds with $\log P$ values around 1.5 have the highest antihypertensive selectivity, because they easily penetrate the blood–brain barrier. Much more important is the result that both biological effects can be predicted from the simple binding assay (eq. 14.91) together with lipophilicity measurements (eq. 14.92). The determination of pC_{25} and pC_{60} values of a single compound needs about twenty to fifty rats; the

brain homogenate of only one rat is sufficient to measure the *in vitro* binding affinities of a large number of analogs.

A spectral mapping technique, based on principal component analysis, has been developed for the two-dimensional interpretation of multidimensional activity data (677–679); it was successfully applied to characterize the activity profiles of drugs according to their pharmacological effects in different test models.

Principal component analysis and QSAR have been used to analyze various biological test systems for the quantification of ecotoxic compounds (680). The QSAR of *in vitro* approaches for developing non-animal methods to substitute the *in vivo* LD_{50} test has been reviewed (681).

7 APPLICATIONS OF FREE WILSON ANALYSIS AND RELATED MODELS

Free Wilson analysis never became as popular as the Hansch model. Only a few hundred applications (341, 342) have been published since 1964.

From the results of a Free Wilson analysis of antimalarial 2-phenylquinolinylmethanols (34 variables; $n = 69$; $r = 0.905$; $s = 0.359$) Hansch equations could be derived for the activity contributions in different positions of the molecules (682). This analysis helped in the stepwise derivation of Hansch equations for structurally related phenanthreneaminoalkylcarbinols (658) and finally led to equation 14.89 (Section 6.4) for a much larger group of analogs (659).

Some other examples of stepwise derivation of Hansch equations from Free Wilson analyses and for the improvement of Hansch equations from the results of Free Wilson analyses have been published (22, 341, 347).

Different sets of compounds were used in a Free Wilson analysis of analgesic benzomorphans; the first one included all compounds (38 variables; $n = 99$; $r = 0.893$; $s = 0.466$), a second one only contained the racemic compounds (36 variables; $n = 86$; $r = 0.909$; $s = 0.457$) and a last one excluded all single point determinations (20 variables, $n = 70$; $r = 0.879$; $s = 0.457$) (683). Two extra variables accounted for (+)-enantiomers ($a_i = -0.97$) and (−)-enantiomers ($a_i = 0.17$) in the first set. The group contributions of the benzomorphans could be used to predict the biological activity values of a group of morphinanes, which are some orders of magnitude more active than the benzomorphanes ($\log 1/C_{obs}$ vs. $\log 1/C_{calc}$: $n = 6$; $r = 0.950$; $s = 0.254$) (683).

Different group contributions were calculated for the R- and S-substituents in a Free Wilson analysis of norepinephrine-uptake inhibiting phenethylamines, including achiral analogs, racemates, pure enantiomers, but also diastereomeric mixtures (nine variables; $n = 30$; $r = 0.963$; $s = 0.276$) (684). The assignment of 0.5 to R- and S-positions (1 to either position in the case of pure enantiomers) is correct for the racemates; a ratio of 0.5:0.5:0.5:0.5 was assigned to the two independent chiral centers of the diastereomeric mixtures, which is an arbitrary and most often wrong assumption.

A comparative study of the inhibitory activities of benzamidines (37 variables) against the serine proteases thrombin ($n = 83$; $r = 0.90$; $s = 0.39$), plasmin ($n = 82$; $r = 0.96$; $s = 0.24$), and trypsin ($n = 84$; $r = 0.91$; $s = 0.35$) (685) shows differences between the group contributions of different substituents, giving some hints for analogs having higher selectivities against the different enzymes. Free Wilson analyses which include too many single-point determinations suggest a much better fit of the biological data than is obtained without these values. For the hallucinogenic properties of phenylalkylamines excellent

statistical parameters are obtained if all members are included in the analysis (15 variables; $n = 23$; $r = 0.985$; $s = 0.182$; $F = 15.28$; recalculated F value) (341, 686). The correlation coefficient is much lower and the overall significance decreases considerably if the single point determinations are eliminated (7 variables; $n = 15$; $r = 0.896$; $s = 0.182$; $F = 4.08$) (341); the standard deviation s remains constant (same number of degrees of freedom), indicating that it is the only reliable statistical parameter in such cases.

Sometimes Free Wilson analyses are presented in graphical form (e.g., 359, 687), which allows an easier interpretation of the results if many variables in different positions are involved.

Nonadditivity in Free Wilson analyses due to nonlinear lipophilicity–activity relationships has been discussed in Section 3.3 (22, 341, 342, 369, 370). Another type of nonadditivity is observed (341, 676) in a Free Wilson analysis of the affinities of quaternary ammonium compounds to the postganglionic acetylcholine receptor (688). While the whole set of compounds can be described by only 15 variables ($n = 128$; $r = 0.991$; $s = 0.231$), a closer inspection of the group contributions shows that they do not behave in an additive manner; certain substituents, e.g., a phenyl group, have significantly different effects if they are introduced into different residues (changing e.g., R = H to R = C_6H_5), e.g., into R-CH_2COO- (+1.30), into $C_6H_5CH(R)$-COO- (+2.10), or into $C_6H_{11}CH(R)$-COO- (+3.07) (341, 676).

Free Wilson analyses may include far fewer variables than substituents, if nonsignificant group contributions are eliminated. 28 Indicator variables and 15 interaction terms were investigated to describe the inhibition of dihydrofolate reductase by 2,4-diaminopyrimidines; 9 indicator variables and 2 interaction terms were selected and equation 14.93 was derived, out of

2047 possible linear combinations of any numbers of these variables (358).

$$\log 1/C = 0.365(\pm 0.12)I\text{-}1$$

$$+ 1.013(\pm 0.12)I\text{-}8$$

$$- 0.784(\pm 0.19)I\text{-}9$$

$$+ 0.419(\pm 0.20)I\text{-}13$$

$$- 0.220(\pm 0.09)I\text{-}15$$

$$+ 0.513(\pm 0.18)I\text{-}20$$

$$+ 0.674(\pm 0.23)I\text{-}4.I\text{-}8$$

$$+ 7.174(\pm 0.07) \qquad (14.93)$$

$$(n = 105; r = 0.903; s = 0.229)$$

In a series of ACTH-derived peptides the same quality of fit was obtained if only 11 group contributions ($n = 52$; $r = 0.984$; $s = 0.406$; $F = 112$) were used instead of the original set of 24 variables ($n = 52$; $r = 0.986$; $s = 0.464$; $F = 40$) (359); the standard deviation s is even smaller, because a slight increase in the sum of squared errors is counterbalanced by the larger number of degrees of freedom.

More applications of Free Wilson analysis are reviewed in textbooks (e.g., 40–43) and in dedicated articles (341, 342). Some statistical problems in Free Wilson analysis are discussed in ref. 689.

The computer-automated structure evaluation (CASE) (Section 3.6) of 9-anilinoacridines is illustrated by equation 14.94 (439); several biophores and biophobes (fragments differentiating active and inactive analogs) were automatically selected (out of nearly 200 descriptors) by the CASE program and correlated to anti-tumor activities.

$$\log 1/D_{50} = 0.63n_1F_1 + 0.31n_2F_2$$

$$+ 0.20n_3F_3 - 1.85n_4F_4$$

$$+ 0.16n_5F_5 + 0.51n_6F_6$$

$$- 0.34n_7F_7 - 0.21n_8F_8$$

$$+ 0.41n_9F_9 + 0.40n_{10}F_{10}$$

$$+ 0.37n_{11}F_{11} - 0.40n_{12}F_{12}$$

$$- 0.35n_{13}F_{13} - 0.26n_{14}F_{14}$$

$$- 0.08 \log P + 4.11 \qquad (14.94)$$

$$(n = 461; r = 0.805; s = 0.46; F = 54.52)$$

The minimal topological difference (MTD) method (Section 3.6) has been applied to a series of progesterone analogs. A hypermolecule was constructed and the different atomic positions were characterized in a stepwise procedure as being beneficial ($\varepsilon = -1$), irrelevant ($\varepsilon = 0$), or detrimental ($\varepsilon = +1$) to biological activities. Afterwards the MTD values of each member of the series against this optimized map were calculated; together with a side chain-corrected lipophilicity parameter f they are correlated to the relative binding affinities (RBA) to the progesterone receptor (eq. 14.95) (456).

$$\log RBA = 0.696(\pm 0.09)f$$

$$- 0.744(\pm 0.13)MTD$$

$$+ 3.917(\pm 0.66) \qquad (14.95)$$

$$(n = 55; r = 0.935; s = 0.331)$$

8 3D-QSAR APPROACHES

8.1 Stereochemistry and Drug Action

Stereochemistry plays an important role for the biological activity of drugs. Optical enantiomers have identical chemical and physicochemical properties, except their different influence on the rotation of polarized light. However, a binding site is a chiral environment that discriminates between the different enantiomers of an optically active drug as if they were different molecules. Several contributions by Ariëns and Lehmann (690–697) stress the important influence of chirality on biological activity. The situation is even worse in diastereomeric mixtures, for two reasons: first, 2^n species (n being the number of asymmetric centers) are involved and secondly, the relative amounts of the different racemates in the mixture vary largely. Labetalol, a β-antiadrenergic drug having two different centers of optical asymmetry, shows different pharmacological characteristics for its enantiomers (691). Whenever possible, pure enantiomers are nowadays developed and introduced into the pharmaceutical market; the only exceptions are compounds, where identical pharmacological profiles are found for both enantiomers, or compounds where the much higher price of one enantiomer, as compared to the racemate, precludes such a selection.

Different QSAR equations have been derived for different enantiomers of phenoxypropionic acids (698), giving evidence for the validity of Pfeiffer's rule (690, 699) that the activity ratio (the eudismic index) of the active (eutomer) vs. the less active enantiomer (distomer) increases with increasing activity of the more active one. There has been some dispute whether Pfeiffer's rule indeed is generally valid or not (700–704).

Schaper derived quantitative models for the dependence of the biological activity of a racemate on the activities of the pure enantiomers (705); not only quantitative, but also qualitative differences were observed for the different enantiomers (706). On the other hand, different enantiomers of chymotrypsin ligands could be combined in one equation under the assumption that the group with the largest MR value binds in a hydrophobic cleft (the so-called ρ_2 area), while the smaller groups bind in ρ_1 space (707).

The proper parametrization of optically active compounds in Free Wilson analysis has been discussed in Section 7.

8.2 Active Site Interaction Models

Early attempts to map the properties of an unknown receptor (binding site) started from qualitative structure–activity relationships (708), from MO calculations of preferred conformations of ligands (709) and from the interpretation of multiparameter Hansch equations (e.g., eq. 14.28). Pharmacophoric pattern searching and receptor mapping (41, 128, 271, 710–712) use information from the QSAR's in the different positions of the ligands and also from ligands with restricted internal rotations (rigid analogs) to derive the structural elements being necessary for receptor affinity (the pharmacophore) and to conclude on the properties at the different sites of the receptor surface (the receptor map) (e.g., refs. 28, 619, 713–719).

Systematic investigations on the interaction energies of ligands to hypothetical receptor sites have been performed by Höltje for chloramphenicol binding to ribosomes (29, 30, 720, 721), pyrimidinone H_2-antihistaminics (721, 722), acetylcholinesterase substrates (720, 723), cyclopropylamine inhibitors of monoamine oxidase (724, 725), antihypertensive benzothiadiazine-1,1-dioxides (726), norepinephrine-uptake inhibition by phenethylamines (727), sulfonamide binding to serum albumin (728), calcium antagonism of verapamil analogs (729, 730), binding, calcium agonism, and calcium antagonism of 1,4-dihydropyridines (731–734), and 5-HT_2 agonism of 2,5-dimethoxy-phenethylamines (735). Simple organic molecules are models of the different amino acid side chains, e.g., n-propane for aliphatic amino acids, acetamide for amide side chains, toluene, p-cresole, and 3-methylindole for aromatic amino acids, n-propylguanidine (positively charged) for basic amino acids, acetate (negatively charged) for acidic amino acids, and methanol for serine. Next, the interaction energies of each molecule are calculated using several of these probes; all analogs of a series are placed in standard geometries and in certain distances to the hypothetical amino acid side chains. The resulting energies are then correlated to receptor affinities or to biological activities. 3D coordinates from protein crystallography were used to calculate the interaction energies of sulfonamide inhibitors to erythrocytic carboanhydrase (736) and of methotrexate analogs to dihydrofolate reductase (737).

In general, good to excellent correlations are obtained for certain amino acid side chains, while others fail to explain the structure–activity relationship. The concept of pharmacophore identification based on molecular electrostatic potentials has been reviewed (738).

A corresponding strategy was followed by Goodford and largely extended to the computer program GRID (33, 125, 739). GRID calculates interaction energies of probe atoms around a protein surface of known three-dimensional structure, giving contour maps of energy values. Negative contour values can be interpreted as regions of attraction between the probe atom and the protein. Methyl (CH_3), amino groups (NH_2), charged amino groups (NH_3^+), carbonyl oxygens (O), carboxy oxygen (O^-), hydroxyl (OH), and water (H_2O) are used as probe atoms and groups; empirical hydrogen-bond potentials were derived for the determination of energetically favorable binding sites of proteins and of small molecules (739). Thus GRID is suited for the design of new ligands, to calculate fields for CoMFA-related 3D-QSAR approaches (Section 8.3), and to model a receptor map for series of active analogs (739).

Audry et al. defined molecular lipophilicity potentials (740–742) for the determination of the lipophilic and hydrophilic regions of a molecule. Abraham and Leo (743) proposed the conversion of hydrophobic fragmental constants to atomic contributions for the evaluation of hydrophobic interactions between molecules. The program HINT (744–746) maps such hydrophobic fields of molecules for 3D-QSAR studies; hydrophobic atom constants were estimated from published hydrophobic fragmental constants f (50, 743) and applied to calculate the hydrophobic field in a grid around the molecule (744). HINT can also be used to estimate $\log P$ values of molecules (746).

Distance geometry, originally introduced by Crippen (747), is an approach to calculate 3D coordinates from a set of distances; nowadays it is routinely used for the calculation of 3D structures of organic compounds, peptides, and small proteins from 2D-NMR measurements. The distance geometry approach was extended for receptor modeling (31, 748–750) and Crippen demonstrated its application to the QSAR of DHFR inhibitors (31, 32, 555, 750–754). Approximate 3D structures of the ligands are constructed and low energy conformations are selected. Each ligand is characterized by ligand points, i.e., by positions of atoms or groups, and by defining upper and lower boundaries of the distances between these points. Also the binding site is defined by points, which can be either empty (a ligand point may be there) or filled (no ligand allowed); allowed binding modes result from conformations where all ligand points occupy empty space. The smallest set of site points is determined and interaction parameters are calculated by a least squares procedure. Scope and limitations of the distance geometry approach have been discussed (750).

Voronoi binding site models (755–757) are an approach to correlate binding affinities of ligands to proposed site geometries which are projected to the surface of polyhedra. Without further hypotheses concerning how the ligands bind and which parts of the ligands interact, the allowed conformational space of each ligand is searched for the conformations and binding modes which are the energetically most favorable ones.

REMOTEDISC (receptor modeling from the three-dimensional structure and physicochemical properties of the ligand molecules) (758–761) starts from the low-energy conformation of a reference compound. Low-energy conformations of all other analogs are automatically superimposed to achieve a maximum overlap of atom-based physicochemical properties and the relative importance of the different properties at different regions of the active site is determined.

Doweyko developed the so-called hypothetical active site lattice (HASL) model (762). Minimum energy conformations are calculated for similar or dissimilar ligands and all molecules are placed in a three-dimensional grid. A user-selected physicochemical property, e.g., lipophilicity or electron density, is added to it as the fourth dimension. The resulting multidimensional lattices are automatically superimposed by an iterative fitting. In this manner a hypothetical active site lattice is formed to predict the relative orientations and affinities of the ligands. Wiese and Coats (763) modified the HASL approach by using PLS analysis instead of the iterative fitting and obtained better results, especially in the predictive ability of the models.

A logico-structural approach to computer-assisted drug design (764) was further developed to a three-dimensional structure-activity expert system Apex-3D (765, 766), which recognizes pharmacophores in biologically active molecules. Various descriptors are used, e.g., aromatic ring centers, lipophilic regions, electronic and hydrogen bond donor and acceptor properties, quantum chemical indices, as well as atomic contributions to hydrophobicity and molar refractivity. The program compares the descriptors and their distances for active

and inactive analogs and stores the results as rules in a knowledge base, which can be used to predict the activities of new compounds. Apex-3D is claimed to be more robust than classical QSAR methods.

8.3 Comparative Molecular Field Analysis (CoMFA)

Comparative molecular field analysis (CoMFA) slowly developed from the first attempts to place molecules in a grid and to correlate field properties of the molecules with biological activities (34–38, 767–769).

There are several important and critical steps in a CoMFA study (Fig. 14.5) (36, 770–772). First, a group of compounds having a common pharmacophore is selected. Then three-dimensional structures of

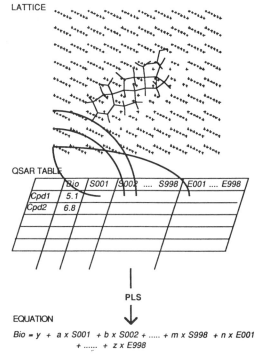

Fig. 14.5 The CoMFA method: Alignment, field calculation in a grid, and QSAR table for PLS analysis. Reproduced from Figure 1 of ref. 36 with permission from the American Chemical Society, Washington, D.C.

reasonable conformations must be generated from the two-dimensional structures. Several 2D/3D conversion procedures are in use or have been described in literature, e.g., CONCORD (773, 774), AIMB (775), WIZARD and COBRA (776–780), CORINA (781), and MIMUMBA (782). Methods for searching the conformational space of small and medium-sized molecules have been reviewed (783). As an alternative, 3D structures derived from crystallographic analyses can be used.

The (optionally) energy-minimized structures are fitted to each other, using a pharmacophore hypothesis and postulating orientation rules. While chemical similarity (784, 785) is not easy to define on an objective basis, every medicinal chemist has some hypothesis or intuition how a pharmacophore can be extracted from a series of molecules. Rational methods for the alignment of congeneric molecules are the active analog approach (712, 786–789) and the distance geometry method (31, 750). Several other attempts have been made to develop and use computer-assisted or computer-automated procedures (e.g., 765, 766, 790–799) for the superposition.

In the alignment of molecules it must be considered that multiple binding modes of chemically closely related analogs seem to be relatively common. As more and more 3D structures of ligand–protein complexes have become known, more and more examples of multiple binding modes have been identified, e.g., for the binding of α- and β-N-acetyl-glucosamines to lysozyme (800), for thermolysin inhibitors (801), binding of dihydrofolate and methotrexate to DHFR (802, 803), viral coat protein ligands (804), binding of isomeric phenylimidazole inhibitors to cytochrome P-450 (805), trimethoprim analogs (806), carbonic anhydrase inhibitors (807), purine nucleoside phosphorylase inhibitors (Fig. 14.6) (808), thrombin inhibitors (809, 810), and thyroid hormone analogs (811). In some of these cases only smaller changes

are observed, nevertheless having a drastic influence on the structure–activity relationships (e.g., Fig. 14.6) (808). In other cases the binding of some analogs is just in the reverse direction (801, 804), ring systems turn around by 180 degrees (e.g., 802, 803), or totally new, unexpected binding modes are observed (e.g., 800, 805).

On the other hand, there is at least one example of an identical binding mode of chemically different analogs: thiorphan and *retro*-thiorphan bind in the same manner (despite of the reverse direction of the amide bonds in both molecules), due to a slight modification of their interaction geometries (812).

Once the molecules are aligned, a grid or lattice is established which surrounds the set of analogs in potential receptor space. Steric and electrostatic fields are calculated for each molecule in every grid point, leading to thousands of columns in the X block. For the steric field a $(a/r^{12} - b/r^{6})$ Lennard-Jones potential is calculated, the electrostatic field is a $1/r$ Coulomb potential. Large positive energy values, i.e., grid points "inside" the molecules, are set constant at certain cut-off values. Normally the steric and electrostatic fields are kept separate for ease of interpretation of the results. Grid points without variance (e.g., inside all molecules) or with small variance (e.g., in the corners of the grid box, far away from the molecules) are eliminated before the PLS analysis is performed.

Other fields than those implemented in the CoMFA program have been proposed for 3D-QSAR analyses, e.g. different interaction fields calculated by the program GRID (33, 739) or hydrophobic fields derived from HINT (744–746) (Section 8.2). In addition, any other parameters, e.g., physicochemical properties, such as log P or quantum chemical indices, may be added to the X block if they are properly weighted; due to the large number of variables included, PLS analysis will not find an unweighted single variable, even if

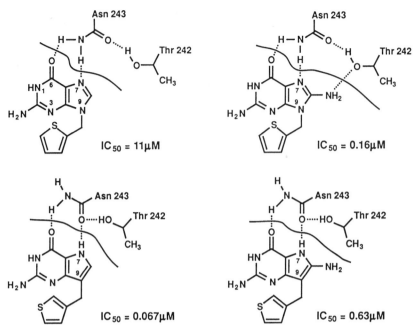

Fig. 14.6 Binding of unsubstituted (left) and 8-amino-substituted (right) purines (upper formulas) and 9-deazapurines (lower formulas), with R = 2-thienylmethyl (purines) and R = 3-thienylmethyl (9-deazapurines) to purine nucleoside phosphorylase. When N7 has an attached hydrogen (9-deazapurines), Asn-243 undergoes a shift to form a highly favorable N(7)-H···O hydrogen bond, increasing the affinity of the unsubstituted analog by a factor of 170 (left formulas). Introduction of an 8-amino group leads to a new hydrogen bond to Thr-242, thereby increasing inhibitory potency of the purine by a factor of 70 (upper formulas). No such hydrogen bond can be formed to the 8-amino group of the 9-deazapurine; on the contrary, the methyl group of Thr-242 approaches the 8-amino group, generating a hydrophobic environment which decreases binding by a factor of 10. Proposed hydrogen bonds, derived from X-ray structure analyses of the inhibitor complexes, are shown as dotted lines. Redrawn from ref. 808 with permission from the copyright owner.

the contribution of this variable to fit and prediction is significant.

The molecular alignment, i.e., the selection and relative orientation of a certain 3D structure out of (most often) several conformers of each molecule, is the most important determinant in a CoMFA study. Recently a field fit procedure (813, 814) has been proposed to improve the alignment. No better results could be obtained in comparative studies if 3D coordinates from X-ray structures were used instead of the user-defined alignment of the ligands (815).

The next step in a CoMFA study is a partial least squares (PLS) analysis (Section 4.2) to determine a minimal set of grid points necessary to explain the measured biological activities of the compounds.

Most often a good to excellent fit is obtained; the predictive value of the model must be checked by cross-validation. If necessary, the model is refined and the analysis is repeated until a model with high predictive ability is obtained. The PLS variant GOLPE (516, 517) seems to be better suited than ordinary PLS analysis because it eliminates variables not contributing to prediction in a stepwise procedure.

The risk of chance correlations in CoMFA studies seems to be low if arbitrary orientations of the molecules are chosen instead of a reasonable alignment (813, 814) or if series of random numbers are correlated to biological activities (816). On the other hand, CoMFA offers many different options; while this flexibility of CoMFA makes it a powerful tool to perform a QSAR study, the risk of user-generated chance correlations becomes relatively high. Even cross-validation offers no guarantee to avoid such fortuitous (but subjective) results.

CoMFA results are most often presented in graphical form, with contours for favorable and unfavorable regions of the different fields. Difference maps were proposed as tools to analyze and identify areas of interest with respect to activity and selectivity, if two different biological activities are compared (817). Biological activities of new compounds can be predicted by transforming the PLS result into a multiple regression equation (e.g., 509, 818).

CoMFA and related 3D-QSAR approaches have been applied to correlate various physicochemical properties with molecular fields. Equilibrium constants of the hydration of carbonyl groups could be explained by a combination of C=O bond order, steric, and electrostatic fields (813). 3D-QSAR studies which correlate σ, inductive, and resonance parameters of benzoic acids (819, 820) as well as pK_a values of clonidine analogs (821), show that a H^+ field precisely describes such electronic parameters, e.g., $\sigma_{m,p}$ of benzoic acids ($n = 49$; $r_{FIT} = 0.976$; $s_{FIT} = 0.082$; $s_{PRESS} = 0.093$). Some steric parameters of benzoic acids could be described by a steric field, while E_s values of acetic acid methyl esters need a combination of steric and electrostatic fields ($n = 21$; $r_{FIT} = 0.984$; $s_{FIT} = 0.133$; $s_{PRESS} = 0.209$) (820). New steric and electronic parameters for classical QSAR analyses have been derived from CoMFA fields (822).

Results from CoMFA studies were compared to classical QSAR equations (823–827) and to results from the minimal topological difference (MTD) method (828). Examples for the comparison of Hansch equations with CoMFA studies are e.g., the papain hydrolysis of N-benzoylglycine

pyridyl esters (823, 824), the emulsin-catalyzed hydrolysis of phenyl-β-D-glucosides (824), the mutagenicity of substituted (o-phenylenediamine)platinum dichlorides (824), dihydrofolate reductase inhibition (824), and some other biological activities (825–827).

The CoMFA methodology has also been applied to describe nonlinear lipophilicity–activity relationships (829, 830). However, despite the simplicity of the analyses and the good correlations obtained in these studies, a ligand interaction-based model like the CoMFA method should not be used to model nonlinear effects arising from transport and distribution; no reasonable results can be expected for sets of compounds which are no homologous series.

Due to the definition of the method, many CoMFA studies and related 3D-QSAR studies deal with the quantitative description of ligand protein interactions, such as

- Enzyme inhibition, e.g., angiotensin converting enzyme inhibition (35, 772, 831, 832), prostaglandin synthase inhibition (772), renin inhibition (815), thermolysin inhibition (815), and tyrosine kinase inhibition (833);

- Substrate properties of enzyme ligands, e.g., the toxic activation of MPTP analogs by monoamine oxidase (834, 835);

- Receptor binding, e.g., benzodiazepine receptor binding (836–838), binding of tetrahydrocannabinol analogs to the cannabinoid receptor (839), binding of CCK-A antagonists (840), affinity of phenyltropane carboxylic acids to the cocaine binding site (841), D_2-receptor affinity of clozapine analogs (842) and salicylamides (843), muscarinic receptor binding (844), binding of non-NMDA antagonists (845), σ-receptor ligands (846), 5-HT$_{1A}$-serotonin receptor ligands (847), and the affinity of halogenated dibenzofurans, dibenzodioxins, and biphenyls to the tetrachlorodibenzodioxin receptor (517, 848);

- Other ligand–protein interactions, e.g., the binding of steroids to various carrier proteins (35, 36, 745, 772, 817, 818, 828), GABA-uptake inhibition (35), ligand binding to viral coat proteins (815, 849), and antigenic complexes between peptides and a histocompatibility glycoprotein (850).

CoMFA was also applied to correlate various other biological activities, e.g., the diuretic activities of sulfonamides in the isolated perfused tubulus of rabbit kidney (851) and bone resorption regulation by biphosphonate esters (852). However, the more distant the biological activities from a pure ligand-receptor interaction are, e.g., the toxicities of alkanes in mice (830) or the anticoccidial activities of triazines in chicken (853), the more unrealistic becomes the application of 3D-QSAR methods.

The important influence of different CoMFA options on the obtained results has been demonstrated (851). More objective alignment procedures, different fields (e.g., a better consideration of polarizability), and better variable selection procedures are needed; in addition, systematic investigations are necessary to find out which of the different CoMFA options should be selected to obtain stable results. Methodology and applications, theoretical and practical aspects, as well as some limitations of CoMFA and other 3D-QSAR approaches have been reviewed (38).

9 SUMMARY AND CONCLUSIONS

Classical QSAR methods still play an important role in drug design, despite the progress in protein crystallography and molecular modeling. They are cheap and easy tools to derive and to prove hypotheses on structure–activity relationships in a quantitative manner, especially in those cases where the 3D structure of the biological target is unknown. In addition, 3D structure-based drug design is only applicable to ligand design; the quantitative description of transport, distribution, and metabolism of drugs is still the domain of classical QSAR methods.

Predictions from QSAR studies (e.g., refs. 43, 344, 350, 545, 854–859) and success stories of QSAR-guided drug design have been reviewed (344, 860, 861). Although in most cases QSAR does not directly contribute to the development of a new drug, with the increasing evidence of the importance of lipophilicity, dissociation, polarizability, electronic and hydrogen bonding interactions, and steric fit on drug action, our ability and performance in drug development increases. QSAR neither brings the solution of all our problems, nor can it only be considered as an academic game; *"the great advantage of the QSAR paradigm lies not in the extrapolations which can be made from known QSAR to fantastically potent new drugs, but in the less spectacular slow development of science in medicinal chemistry"* (855).

As stated earlier, prediction is not the main goal of a QSAR analysis. General conclusions on the reduction of toxic properties, on selectivity, on optimum lipophilicity to pass the blood–brain barrier or, on the other hand, to avoid CNS side effects, are more important for the optimization of a lead structure. QSAR also helps to decide when to stop a synthetic program (666, 856). Another example of a proper QSAR application is given in equations 14.91 and 14.92 (Section 6.5), describing the antihypertensive and hypertensive activities of clonidine analogs. While no predictions for more active analogs can be derived, three most important conclusions can be drawn from these equations: first, further analogs can be tested in simple *in vitro* systems instead of whole animal models, secondly, log P values around 1.5 are optimal for the CNS-mediated antihypertensive activity, and thirdly, one cannot expect to separate the antihypertensive activity from the peripheral hypertensive side effect.

In speculating about the future of QSAR, Hansch (862) stated that the situation may be compared to the development of the Hammett σ constant till 1968, when 43 variations of σ existed. Today, there is rather broad agreement that only four of them, σ, σ^0, σ^-, and σ^+, are needed; however, still no agreement exists how σ can be factored into field and resonance effects. In deriving a single QSAR equation, one can never be sure that the relationship is a causal one; neither statistical tools nor any other criteria can help in this respect. Only the comparison of QSAR equations from different but related sources (553, 554, 862) can assure the relevance of certain parameters, e.g., lipophilicity for cytochrome P-450 induction by different series of compounds and in different systems (654, 862) or the importance of a σ term in the description of the hydrolysis rate constants of glycine ester amides by different proteases (554, 862). Understanding of true structure–activity relationships will depend on lateral validation of QSAR, i.e., relating a new QSAR to a matrix of self-consistent structure-activity relationships (862).

The problem of validation of QSAR studies has also been approached from a statistical point of view (863). Since the biological activity of a compound is most often a combination of several known and unknown subeffects, it is important to measure a fairly large number of different biological effects in different test systems. To aggregate these several effects to one magic number, "the biological activity", reduces the information content; with certain exceptions, e.g., nonspecific, lipophilicity-related biological activities, separate QSAR's must be derived for each structural class of chemicals to distinguish between compounds with different mechanisms of biological action. Multiparameter tables should be used together with a multivariate characterization approach. The training set should be selected by a statistical design method. An appropriate data modeling and data analysis system should be used, e.g., PLS analysis or, in the case of a single activity variable, multiple regression. A validation procedure must be performed. The real criterion for the validity of a model is always synthesis and testing of new analogs. Biological hypotheses can only be tested on a quantitative basis. We have to live with the fact that only few QSAR studies fulfill these (by no means exaggerated) demands.

The state of the art and some other aspects of the future development of QSAR (564, 862, 864) and computer-aided drug design (825, 864–866) have recently been reviewed.

With the largely increasing number of 3D structures of enzymes and enzyme inhibitor complexes also our understanding of the corresponding QSAR equations will increase (271, 562, 564). CoMFA and CoMFA-related 3D-QSAR approaches (38) are powerful new tools but they will not displace classical QSAR studies. New and hopefully better parameters may be derived from comparative molecular field analyses (822). On the other hand, CoMFA cannot describe biological activities other than ligand-protein interactions, if no global physicochemical parameters are included in the data tables; if they are, then CoMFA imitates classical Hansch analysis. From the current limitations of both methodologies it seems that they may approach each other and may even grow together in the future.

It is the combination of so many different effects which contribute to biological activity that makes the formulation of a sound QSAR model so difficult. To repeat only the most important factors:

- Lipophilicity and ionization are responsible for the transport and the distribution in a biological system.
- The drug receptor interaction is a highly specialized hydrophobic, polar, electronic, and steric interaction; the lipophilicity pattern, the electron density distribution, and the polarizability pattern at the surface of the drug and its binding site contribute to the interaction energy.
- Neither the drug nor its binding site are completely rigid systems; a flexible fit occurs during the binding of the drug.
- The drug molecule must be considered in three dimensions, with restricted rotations or at least conformational barriers around certain bonds.
- It is evident that a drug cannot bind in a conformation which is energetically highly unfavorable; however, this does not imply that only minimum energy conformations of a drug are able to interact with the receptor.
- The change of a favorable conformation to a less favorable one has to be taken into account in those cases, where a higher net free energy results from the new conformation of the ligand.
- Even structurally closely related analogs may bind in a completely different manner.
- The solvation-desolvation balance may be favorable or unfavorable for binding.
- The insertion of water molecules between the ligand and its binding site has to be considered.
- Entropy effects play an important, but much too often neglected role.

We have the ability to intuitively extract high-level information from facts at different levels, without being programmed like a computer. QSAR cannot and will never substitute the creativity and intuition of an experienced medicinal chemist or biologist.

But our logical reasoning is limited to one or two, at most three dimensions; QSAR aims in the objective interpretation of multidimensional results in medicinal chemistry to an extent which is far beyond the intellectual capacity of the human mind.

NOTE

A greatly expanded version of this chapter has been published as a book (867).

REFERENCES

1. A. Crum-Brown and T. R. Fraser, *Trans. Roy. Soc. Edinburgh*, **25**, 151–203, 693–739 (1868–1869).
2. M. C. Richet, *Compt. Rend. Soc. Biol.* (*Paris*) **45**, 775–776 (1893).
3. H. Meyer, *Arch. Exp. Path. Pharm.*, **42**, 109–118 (1899).
4. E. Overton, *Studien über die Narkose, zugleich ein Beitrag zur allgemeinen Pharmakologie*, G. Fischer, Jena, 1901; English translation by R. L. Lipnick, Ed., *Studies on Narcosis, Charles Ernest Overton*, Chapman and Hall, London, 1991.
5. R. L. Lipnick, *Trends Pharmacol. Sci.*, **7**, 161–164 (1986); **10**, 265–269 (1989).
6. H. Fühner and E. Neubauer, *Arch. Exp. Path. Pharm.*, **56**, 333–345 (1907).
7. J. Ferguson, *Proc. Roy. Soc., Ser.* **B 127**, 387–404 (1939).
8. T. C. Bruice, N. Kharasch, and R. J. Winzler, *Arch. Biochem. Biophys.* **62**, 305–317 (1956).
9. R. Zahradnik and M. Chvapil, *Experientia*, **16**, 511–512 (1960).
10. R. Zahradnik, *Arch. Int. Pharmacodyn. Ther.*, **135**, 311–329 (1962).
11. R. Zahradnik, *Experientia*, **18**, 534–536 (1962).
12. L. P. Hammett, *Physical Organic Chemistry. Reaction Rates, Equilibria and Mechanism*, 2nd ed., McGraw-Hill, New York, 1970.
13. O. R. Hansen, *Acta Chem. Scand.*, **16**, 1593–1600 (1962).
14. C. Hansch, P. P. Maloney, T. Fujita, and R. M. Muir, *Nature*, **194**, 178–180 (1962).
15. C. Hansch and T. Fujita, *J. Am. Chem. Soc.*, **86**, 1616–1626 (1964).

16. S. M. Free Jr. and J. W. Wilson, *J. Med. Chem.*, **7**, 395–399 (1964).

17. C. Hansch, *Acc. Chem. Res.*, **2**, 232–239 (1969).

18. C. Hansch, *Drug Design*, Vol. I, E. J. Ariëns, Ed., Academic Press, New York, 1971, pp. 271–342.

19. C. Hansch and J. M. Clayton, *J. Pharm. Sci.*, **62**, 1–21 (1973).

20. T. Fujita and T. Ban, *J. Med. Chem.*, **14**, 148–152 (1971).

21. C. Hansch and M. Yoshimoto, *J. Med. Chem.*, **17**, 1160–1167 (1974).

22. H. Kubinyi, *J. Med. Chem.*, **19**, 587–600 (1976).

23. H. Kubinyi, *J. Med. Chem.*, **20**, 625–629 (1977).

24. W. E. Brugger, A. J. Stuper, and P. C. Jurs, *J. Chem. Inf. Comput. Sci.*, **16**, 105–110 (1976).

25. G. L. Kirschner and B. R. Kowalski, *Drug Design*, Vol. VIII, E. J. Ariëns, Ed., Academic Press, New York, 1979, pp. 73–131.

26. S. Wold, A. Ruhe, H. Wold, and W. J. Dunn III, *SIAM J. Sci. Stat. Comput.*, **5**, 735–743 (1984).

27. W. J. Dunn III, S. Wold, U. Edlund, S. Hellberg, and J. Gasteiger, *Quant. Struct.-Act. Relat.*, **3**, 131–137 (1984); *erratum* **4**, 82 (1985).

28. J. Y. Fukunaga, C. Hansch, and E. E. Steller, *J. Med. Chem.*, **19**, 605–611 (1976).

29. H.-D. Höltje and L. B. Kier, *J. Med. Chem.*, **17**, 814–819 (1974).

30. H.-D. Höltje and M. Tintelnot, *Quant. Struct.-Act. Relat.*, **3**, 6–9 (1984).

31. G. M. Crippen, *J. Med. Chem.*, **22**, 988–997 (1979).

32. A. K. Ghose and G. M. Crippen, *J. Med. Chem.*, **25**, 892–899 (1982).

33. P. J. Goodford, *J. Med. Chem.*, **28**, 849–857 (1985).

34. M. Wise, *QSAR and Strategies in the Design of Bioactive Compounds, Proceedings of the 5th European QSAR Symposium, Bad Segeberg, 1984*, J. K. Seydel, Ed., VCH, Weinheim, 1985, pp. 19–29.

35. R. D. Cramer III and J. D. Bunce, *QSAR in Drug Design and Toxicology, Proceedings of the 6th European QSAR Symposium, Portoroz, 1986*, D. Hadzi and B. Jerman-Blazic, Eds., *Pharmacochem. Libr.*, Vol. 10, Elsevier, Amsterdam, 1987, pp. 3–12.

36. R. D. Cramer III, D. E. Patterson, and J. D. Bunce, *J. Am. Chem. Soc.*, **110**, 5959–5967 (1988).

37. U.S. Pat. 5,025,388 (June 18, 1991), R.D. Cramer and S. B. Wold.

38. H. Kubinyi, Ed., *3D QSAR in Drug Design, Theory, Methods, and Applications*, ESCOM Science Publishers, Lieden, 1993.

39. C. A. Ramsden, Ed., *Quantitative Drug Design*, Vol. 4 of *Comprehensive Medicinal Chemistry. The Rational Design, Mechanistic Study & Therapeutic Application of Chemical Compounds*, C. Hansch, P. G. Sammes, and J. B. Taylor, Eds., Pergamon Press, Oxford, 1990.

40. W. P. Purcell, G. E. Bass, and J. M. Clayton, *Strategy of Drug Design. A Molecular Guide to Biological Activity*, Wiley, New York, 1973.

41. Y. C. Martin, *Quantitative Drug Design, A Critical Introduction*, Medicinal Research Series, Vol. 8, Marcel Dekker, New York, 1978.

42. J. K. Seydel and K.-J. Schaper, *Chemische Struktur und biologische Aktivität von Wirkstoffen, Methoden der Quantitativen Struktur-Wirkung-Analyse*, Verlag Chemie, Weinheim, 1979.

43. R. Franke, *Optimierungsmethoden in der Wirkstoff-Forschung. Quantitative Struktur-Wirkungs-Analyse*, Akademie-Verlag, Berlin, 1980; revised English translation: R. Franke, *Theoretical Drug Design Methods*, *Pharmacochem. Libr.*, Vol. 7, Elsevier, Amsterdam, 1984.

44. J. G. Topliss, Ed., *Quantitative Structure-Activity Relationships of Drugs*, Academic Press, New York, 1983.

45. L. Goldberg, Ed., *Structure-Activity Correlation as a Predictive Tool in Toxicology, Fundamentals, Methods, and Applications*, Hemisphere, Washington, 1983.

46. G. Jolles and K. R. H. Woolridge, Eds., *Drug Design: Fact or Fantasy?*, Academic Press, London, 1984.

47. W. Karcher and J. Devilers, Eds., *Practical Application of Quantitative Structure-Activity Relationships (QSAR) in Environmental Chemistry and Toxicology*, Chemical and Environmental Sciences, Vol. I, Kluwer Academic Publishers for the European Communities, Dordrecht, 1990.

48. L. B. Kier and L. H. Hall, *Molecular Connectivity in Chemistry and Drug Research*, Academic Press, New York, 1976.

49. R. F. Rekker, *The Hydrophobic Fragmental Constant. Its Derivation and Application, A Means of Characterizing Membrane Systems*, *Pharmacochem. Libr.* Vol. 1, Elsevier, Amsterdam, 1977.

50. C. Hansch and A. Leo, *Substituent Constants for Correlation Analysis in Chemistry and Biology*, Wiley, New York, 1979.

51. S. H. Yalkowsky, A. A. Sinkula, and S. C.

Valvani, Eds., *Physical Chemical Properties of Drugs, Medicinal Research Series*, Vol. 10, Marcel Dekker, New York, 1980.

52. A. T. Balaban, A. Chiriac, I. Motoc, and Z. Simon, *Steric Fit in Quantitative Structure-Activity Relations, Lecture Notes in Chemistry*, Vol. 15, Springer-Verlag, Berlin, 1980.

53. D. D. Perrin, B. Dempsey, and E. P. Serjeant, *pK$_a$ Prediction for Organic Acids and Bases*, Chapman and Hall, London, 1981.

54. W. J. Dunn III, J. H. Block, and R. S. Pearlman, Eds., *Partition Coefficient: Determination and Estimation*, Pergamon, New York, 1986.

55. J. C. McGowan and A. Mellors, *Molecular Volumes in Chemistry and Biology: Applications Including Partitioning and Toxicity*, Ellis Horwood Ltd., Chichester, 1986.

56. R. F. Rekker and R. Mannhold, *Calculation of Drug Lipophilicity. The Hydrophobic Fragmental Constant Approach*, VCH, Weinheim, 1992.

57. N. B. Chapman and J. Shorter, Eds., *Correlation Analysis in Chemistry: Recent Advances*, Plenum Press, New York, 1978.

58. A. J. Stuper, W. E. Brugger, and P. C. Jurs, *Computer Assisted Studies of Chemical Structure and Biological Function*, Wiley, New York, 1979.

59. P. M. Dean, *Molecular Foundations of Drug-Receptor Interaction*, Cambridge University Press, Cambridge, 1987.

60. Y. C. Martin, E. Kutter, and V. Austel, *Modern Drug Research, Paths to Better and Safety Drugs, Medicinal Research Series*, Vol. 12, Marcel Dekker, New York, 1989.

61. W. G. Richards, Ed., *Computer-Aided Molecular Design*, IBC Technical Services, London, 1989.

62. T. J. Perun and C. L. Propst, *Computer-Aided Drug Design, Methods and Applications*, Marcel Dekker, New York, 1989.

63. M. A. Johnson and G. M. Maggiora, Eds., *Concepts and Applications of Molecular Similarity*, Wiley, New York, 1990.

64. C. G. Wermuth, N. Koga, H. König, and B. W. Metcalf, Eds., *Medicinal Chemistry for the 21st Century*, Blackwell Scientific Publications, Oxford, 1992.

65. E. J. Ariëns, Ed., *Drug Design*, Vol. I (1971)–Vol. X (1980), Academic Press, New York.

66. E. Jucker, Ed., *Fortschr. Arzneimittelforsch.* (*Prog. Drug Res.*), **1**, ff (1959).

67. *Pharmacochem. Libr.*, Vol. 1, ff (1977) ff.

68. R. F. Gould, Ed., *Biological Correlations—The Hansch Approach, Advan. Chem. Ser.*, **114** (1972).

69. M. Tichy, Ed., *Quantitative Structure-Activity Relationships* (*Proceedings of the Conference on Chemical Structure-Biological Activity Relationships: Quantitative Approaches, Prague, 1973*), *Experientia Suppl.*, **23**, Birkhäuser Verlag, Basel, 1976.

70. J. A. Keverling Buisman, Ed., *Biological Activity and Chemical Structure, Proceedings of the IUPAC-IUPHAR Symposium, Noordwijkerhout, 1977*), *Pharmocochem. Libr.*, Vol. 2, Elsevier, Amsterdam, 1977.

71. R. Franke and P. Oehme, Eds., *Quantitative Structure-Activity Analysis, Proceedings of the Second Symposium on Chemical Structure-Biological Activity Relationships: Quantitative Approaches, Suhl, 1976*, Akademie-Verlag, Berlin, 1978.

72. E. C. Olsen and P. E. Christofferson, Eds., *Computer-Assisted Drug Design, ACS Symp. Series* 112, American Chemical Society, Washington, D.C., 1979.

73. J. Knoll and F. Darvas, Eds., *Chemical Structure-Biological Activity Relationships. Quantitative Approaches, Proceedings of the 3rd European QSAR Symposium, Budapest, 1979*, Akadémiai Kiadó, Budapest, 1980.

74. J. A. Keverling Buisman, Ed., *Strategy in Drug Research, Proceedings of the Second IUPAC-IUPHAR Symposium, Noordwijkerhout, 1981*, *Pharmacochem. Libr.*, Vol. 4, Elsevier, Amsterdam, 1982.

75. J. C. Dearden, Ed., *Quantitative Approaches to Drug Design, Proceedings of the 4th European Symposium on Chemical Structure-Biological Activity: Quantitative Approaches, Bath, 1982*), *Pharmacochem. Libr.*, Vol. 6, Elsevier, Amsterdam, 1983.

76. M. Kuchar, Ed., *QSAR in Design of Bioactive Compounds, Proceedings of the 1st Telesymposium on Medicinal Chemistry, 1984*), Prous Science Publishers, Barcelona, 1984.

77. M. Tichy, Ed., *QSAR in Toxicology and Xenobiochemistry, Proceedings of a Symposium, Prague, 1984, Pharmacochem. Libr.*, Vol. 8, Elsevier, Amsterdam, 1985.

78. J. K. Seydel, Ed., *QSAR and Strategies in the Design of Bioactive Compounds, Proceedings of the 5th European Symposium on QSAR, Bad Segeberg, 1984*, VCH, Weinheim, 1985.

79. A. F. Harms, Ed., *Innovative Approaches in Drug Research, Proceedings of the Third Noordwijkerhout Symposium on Medicinal Chemistry, Noordwijkerhout, 1985*), *Pharmacochem. Libr.*, Vol. 9, Elsevier, 1986.

80. D. Hadzi and B. Jerman-Blazic, Eds., *QSAR in*

Drug Design and Toxicology, Proceedings of the 6th European Symposium on QSAR, Portoroz, 1986), *Pharmacochem. Libr.*, Vol. 10, Elsevier, Amsterdam, 1987.

81. K. L. E. Kaiser, Ed., *QSAR in Environmental Toxicology*, Reidel, Dordrecht, 1987.

82. J. L. Fauchère, Ed., *QSAR: Quantitative Structure-Activity Relationships in Drug Design* (*Proceedings of the 7th European Symposium on QSAR, Interlaken, 1988*), *Progr. Clin. Biol. Research*, **291** (1989).

83. C. Silipo and A. Vittoria, Eds., *QSAR: Rational Approaches to the Design of Bioactive Compounds, Proceedings of the 8th European Symposium on QSAR, Sorrento, 1990, Pharmacochem. Libr.*, Vol. 16, Elsevier, Amsterdam, 1991.

84. C. G. Wermuth, Ed., *Trends in QSAR and Molecular Modelling 1992, Proceedings of the 9th European Symposium on Structure-Activity Relationships: QSAR and Molecular Modelling, Strasbourg, 1992, ESCOM Science Publishers, Leiden*, 1993.

85. F. Darvas, Ed., "Abstracts of Publications Related to QSAR", *Quant. Struct.-Act. Relat.*, **1** (1982) ff.

86. CAS Selects "Structure-Activity Relationships", *Chemical Abstracts Service* (service code 04S), Columbus, Ohio, U.S.

87. *Ringdoc Drug Information, Profile 38, Structure Activity*, Derwent Publications Ltd., London, England.

88. *Molecular Modelling & Computational Chemistry Results*, **1** (1992) ff.

89. (a) *J. Med. Chem.*; (b) *Eur. J. Med. Chem.*; (c) *Med. Chem. Res.*; (d) *J. Comput.-Aided Mol. Des.*

90. P. N. Craig, *Drug. Inf. J.*, **18**, 123–30 (1984).

91. M. S. Tute in ref. 39, pp. 1–31.

92. R. F. Rekker, *Quant. Struct.-Act. Relat.*, **11**, 195–199 (1992).

93. H. van de Waterbeemd, *Quant. Struct.-Act. Relat.*, **11**, 200–204 (1992).

94. E. J. Ariëns, *Drug Design*, Vol. I, E. J. Ariëns, Ed., Academic Press, New York, 1971, pp. 1–270.

95. J. C. Emmett, Ed., *Membranes & Receptors*, Vol. 3 of *Comprehensive Medicinal Chemistry. The Rational Design, Mechanistic Study & Therapeutic Application of Chemical Compounds*, C. Hansch, P. G. Sammes, and J. B. Taylor, Eds., Pergamon Press, Oxford, 1990.

96. J. N. Langley, *J. Physiol.* (*London*), **1**, 339–369 (1878).

97. E. Fischer, *Ber. Dtsch. Chem. Ges.*, **27**, 2985–2993 (1894).

98. P. Ehrlich, *Lancet II*, 445–451 (1913).

99. R. J. P. Williams, *Angew. Chem. Int. Ed. Engl.*, **16**, 766–777 (1977).

100. G. C. K. Roberts in ref. 75, pp. 91–98.

101. J. Deisenhofer and H. Michel, *Science*, **245**, 1463–1480 (1989).

102. R. Henderson, J. M. Baldwin, T. A. Ceska, F. Zemlin, E. Beckmann, and K. H. Downing, *J. Mol. Biol.*, **213**, 899–929 (1990).

103. M. S. Weiss, U. Abele, J. Weckesser, W. Welte, E. Schiltz, and G. E. Schulz, *Science*, **254**, 1627–1630 (1991).

104. J. Findlay and E. Eliopoulos, *Trends Pharmacol. Sci.*, **11**, 492–499 (1990).

105. S. Trumpp-Kallmeyer, J. Hoflack, A. Bruinvels, and M. Hibert, *J. Med. Chem.*, **35**, 3448–3462 (1992).

106. C. Humblet and T. Mirzadegan, *Ann. Rep. Med. Chem.*, **27**, 291–300 (1992).

107. F. C. Bernstein, T. F. Koetzle, G. J. B. Williams, E. F. Meyer Jr., M. D. Brice, J. R. Rodgers, O. Kennard, T. Shimanouchi, and M. Tasumi, *J. Mol. Biol.*, **112**, 535–542 (1977).

108. T. L. Blundell and L. N. Johnson, *Protein Crystallography*, Academic Press, London, 1976.

109. C. Branden and J. Tooze, *Introduction to Protein Structure*, Garland Publishing Company, New York, 1991.

110. W. Bode and R. Huber, *Eur. J. Biochem.*, **204**, 433–451 (1992).

111. L. G. Herbette, D. W. Chester, and D. G. Rhodes, *Biophys. J.*, **49**, 91–94 (1986).

112. R. P. Mason, D. G. Rhodes, and L. G. Herbette, *J. Med. Chem.*, **34**, 869–877 (1991).

113. P. R. Andrews and M. Tintelnot in ref. 39, pp. 321–347.

114. M. Tintelnot and P. R. Andrews, *J. Comput.-Aided Mol. Des.*, **3**, 67–84 (1989).

115. D. H. Williams, *Aldrichimica Acta*, **24**, 71–80 (1991); **25**, 9 (1992).

116. P. Murray-Rust and J. P. Glusker, *J. Am. Chem. Soc.*, **106**, 1018–1025 (1984).

117. A. R. Fersht, J.-P. Shi, J. Knill-Jones, D. M. Lowe, A. J. Wilkinson, D. M. Blow, P. Brick, P. Carter, M. M. Y. Waye, and G. Winter, *Nature*, **314**, 235–238 (1985).

118. A. R. Fersht, *Trends Biochem. Sci.*, **12**, 301–304 (1987).

119. W. H. J. Ward, D. Timms, and A. R. Fersht, *Trends Pharmacol. Sci.*, **11**, 280–284 (1990).

120. R. Wolfenden and W. M. Kati, *Acc. Chem. Res.*, **24**, 209–215 (1991).

121. A. J. Doig and D. H. Williams, *J. Am. Chem. Soc.*, **114**, 338–343 (1992).

122. K. A. Sharp, A. Nicholls, R. Friedman, and B. Honig, *Biochemistry*, **30**, 9686–9697 (1991).

123. P. R. Andrews, D. J. Craik, and J. L. Martin, *J. Med. Chem.*, **27**, 1648–1657 (1984).

124. P. Andrews, *Trends Pharmacol. Sci.*, **7**, 148–151 (1986).

125. P. J. Goodford in ref. 83, pp. 49–55.

126. R. Hitzemann, *Trends Pharmacol. Sci.*, **9**, 408–411 (1988).

127. M. Williams and M. A. Sills in ref. 95, pp. 45–80.

128. Y. C. Martin, E. N. Bush, and J. J. Kyncl in ref. 39, pp. 349–373.

129. C. Hansch, *Intra-Science Chem. Rept.*, **8**, 17–25 (1974).

130. C. W. Thornber, *Chem. Soc. Rev.*, **8**, 563–580 (1979).

131. A. Burger, *Fortschr. Arzneimittelforsch.* (*Prog. Drug. Res.*), **37**, 287–371 (1991).

132. P. A. Bartlett and C. K. Marlowe, *Science*, **235**, 569–571 (1987).

133. B. P. Morgan, J. M. Scholtz, M. D. Ballinger, I. D. Zipkin, and P. A. Bartlett, *J. Am. Chem. Soc.*, **113**, 297–307 (1991).

134. G. Klebe, *Struct. Chem.*, **1**, 597–616 (1990).

135. F. H. Allen, J. E. Davies, J. J. Galloy, O. Johnson, O. Kennard, C. F. Macrae, E. M. Mitchell, G. F. Mitchell, J. M. Smith, and D. G. Watson, *J. Chem. Inf. Comput. Sci.*, **31**, 187–204 (1991).

136. M. I. Page, *Angew. Chem. Int. Ed. Engl.*, **16**, 449–459 (1977).

137. W. P. Jencks, *Proc. Natl. Acad. Sci. USA*, **78**, 4046–4050 (1981).

138. J. A. Wells, *Biochemistry*, **29**, 8509–8517 (1990).

139. C. R. Beddell, P. J. Goodford, D. K. Stammers, and R. Wootton, *Br. J. Pharmac.* **65**, 535–543 (1979).

140. R. Bohacek and C. McMartin, *J. Med. Chem.*, **35**, 1671–1684 (1992).

141. C. Hansch, A. Leo, S. H. Unger, K. H. Kim, D. Nikaitani, and E. J. Lien, *J. Med. Chem.*, **16**, 1207–1216 (1973).

142. C. Hansch, S. D. Rockwell, P. Y. C. Jow, A. Leo, and E. E. Steller, *J. Med. Chem.*, **20**, 304–306 (1977).

143. F. E. Norrington, R. M. Hyde, S. G. Williams, and R. Wootton, *J. Med. Chem.*, **18**, 604–607 (1975).

144. C. Hansch, S. H. Unger, and A. B. Forsythe, *J. Med. Chem.*, **16**, 1217–1222 (1973).

145. A. Verloop, *Drug Design*, Vol. III, E. J. Ariëns, Ed., Academic Press, New York, 1972, pp. 133–187.

146. Y. C. Martin, *Drug Design*, Vol. VIII, E. J. Ariëns, Ed., Academic Press, New York, 1979, pp. 1–72.

147. R. Franke in ref. 78, pp. 59–78.

148. H. van de Waterbeemd and B. Testa, *Adv. Drug. Res.*, **16**, 85–225 (1987).

149. H. van de Waterbeemd, B. Testa, P.-A. Carrupt, and N. El Tayar in ref. 82, pp. 123–126.

150. H. van de Waterbeemd, N. El Tayar, P.-A. Carrupt, and B. Testa, *J. Comput.-Aided Mol. Des.*, **3**, 111–132 (1989).

151. H. van de Waterbeemd, P.-A. Carrupt, and N. El Tayar in ref. 82, pp. 101–103.

152. D. B. Boyd and C. M. Seward in ref. 83, pp. 167–170.

153. W. J. Streich, S. Dove, and R. Franke, *J. Med. Chem.*, **23**, 1452–1456 (1980).

154. R. D. Cramer III, *J. Am. Chem. Soc.*, **102**, 1837–1849, 1849–1859 (1980).

155. R. D. Cramer III, *Quant. Struct.-Act. Relat.*, **2**, 7–12, 13–19 (1983).

156. R. Hyde in ref. 82, pp. 91–95.

157. S. Alunni, S. Clementi, U. Edlund, D. Johnels, S. Hellberg, M. Sjöström, and S. World, *Acta Chem. Scand.*, **B 37**, 47–53 (1983).

158. B. Skagerberg, D. Bonelli, S. Clementi, G. Cruciani, and C. Ebert, *Quant. Struct.-Act. Relat.*, **8**, 32–38 (1989).

159. M. Sjöstrom and S. Wold, *J. Mol. Evol.*, **22**, 272–277 (1985).

160. J. Jonsson, L. Eriksson, S. Hellberg, M. Sjöström, and S. Wold, *Quant. Struct.-Act. Relat.*, **8**, 204–209 (1989).

161. K. A. Dill, *Science*, **250**, 297 (1990).

162. P. J. Taylor in ref. 39, pp. 241–294.

163. A. Leo, C. Hansch, and D. Elkins, *Chem. Rev.*, **71**, 525–616 (1971).

164. H. Kubinyi, *Fortschr. Arzneimittelforsch.* (*Prog. Drug Res.*), **23**, 97–198 (1979).

165. E. A. Coats in ref. 51, pp. 111–139.

166. J. T. Chou and P. C. Jurs in ref. 51, pp. 163–199.

167. J. C. Dearden, *Environ. Health Perspect.*, **61**, 203–228 (1985).

168. A. J. Leo in ref. 39, pp. 295–319.

169. R. N. Smith, C. Hansch, and M. M. Ames, *J. Pharm. Sci.*, **64**, 599–606 (1975).

170. C. Hansch and A. Leo, *Partition Coefficient Data Bank*, MEDCHEM Project, Pomona College, Claremont, Calif.

171. C. Hansch and W. J. Dunn III, *J. Pharm. Sci.*, **61**, 1–19 (1972).

172. R. Collander, *Acta Chem. Scand.*, **5**, 774–780 (1951).

173. K. C. Yeh and W. I. Higuchi, *J. Pharm. Sci.*, **65**, 80–86 (1976).

174. A. Leo and C. Hansch, *J. Org. Chem.*, **36**, 1539–1544 (1971).

175. A. Leo in ref. 68, pp. 51–60.

176. P. Seeman, S. Roth, and H. Schneider, *Biochim. Biophys. Acta*, **225**, 171–184 (1971).

177. W. J. Dunn III and S. Wold, *Acta Chem. Scand.*, **B 32**, 536–542 (1978).

178. R. Franke, R. Kühne and S. Dove in ref. 75, pp. 15–32.

179. M. G. Koehler, S. Grigoras, and W. J. Dunn III, *Quant. Struct.-Act. Relat.*, **7**, 150–159 (1988).

180. P. Seiler, *Eur. J. Med. Chem.*, **9**, 473–479 (1974).

181. N. El Tayar, R.-S. Tsai, B. Testa, P.-A. Carrupt, and A. Leo, *J. Pharm. Sci.*, **80**, 590–598 (1991).

182. W. Fan, N. El Tayar, B. Testa, and L. B. Kier, *J. Phys. Chem.*, **94**, 4764–4766 (1990).

183. W. Fan, N. El Tayar, B. Testa, P.-A. Carrupt, and L. B. Kier in ref. 83, pp. 67–70.

184. R. Wolfenden, *Science*, **222**, 1087–1093 (1983).

185. T. Fujita, T. Nishioka and M. Nakajima, *J. Med. Chem.*, **20**, 1071–1081 (1977).

186. D. Hadzi, J. Kidric, J. Koller, and J. Mavri, *J. Mol. Struct. (Theochem)* **237**, 137–150 (1990).

187. R. C. Young, R. C. Mitchell, T. H. Brown, C. R. Ganellin, R. Griffiths, M. Jones, K. K. Rana, D. Saunders, I. R. Smith, N. E. Sore, and T. J. Wilks, *J. Med. Chem.*, **31**, 656–671 (1988).

188. C. R. Ganellin, T. H. Brown, R. Griffiths, M. Jones, R. C. Mitchell, K. Rana, D. Saunders, I. R. Smith, N. E. Sore, T. J. Wilks, and R. C. Young in ref. 83, pp. 103–110.

189. P. D. Leeson, R. W. Carling, K. James, J. D. Smith, K. W. Moore, E. H. F. Wong, and R. Baker, *J. Med. Chem.*, **33**, 1296–1305 (1990).

190. M. H. Abraham, G. S. Whiting, Y. Alarie, J. J. Morris, P. J. Taylor, R. M. Doherty, R. W. Taft, and G. D. Nielsen, *Quant. Struct.-Act. Relat.*, **9**, 6–10 (1990).

191. C. Altomare, R.-S. Tsai, N. El Tayar, B. Testa, P.-A. Carrupt, A. Carotti, and P. G. De Benedetti in ref. 83, pp. 139–142.

192. D. E. Leahy, P. J. Taylor, and A. R. Wait, *Quant. Struct.-Act. Relat.*, **8**, 17–31 (1989).

193. D. E. Leahy, J. J. Morris, P. J. Taylor, and A. R. Wait, *J. Chem. Soc. Perkin Trans.*, **2**, 705–722, 723–731 (1992).

194. D. G. Rhodes, J. G. Sarmiento, and L. G. Herbette, *Mol. Pharmacol.*, **27**, 612–623 (1985).

195. L. G. Herbette and S. M. Gruner, *Dev. Cardiovasc.*, **68**, 353–365 (1987).

196. L. G. Herbette, Y. M. H. Vant Erve, and D. G. Rhodes, *J. Mol. Cell. Cardiol.*, **21**, 187–201 (1989).

197. R. P. Mason, G. E. Gonye, D. W. Chester, and L. G. Herbette, *Biophys. J.*, **55**, 769–778 (1989).

198. L. G. Herbette, D. G. Rhodes, and R. P. Mason, *Drug Des. Delivery*, **7**, 75–118 (1991).

199. J. K. Seydel, H.-P. Cordes, M. Wiese, H. Chi, N. Croes, R. Hanpft, H. Lüllmann, K. Mohr, M. Patten, Y. Padberg, R. Lüllmann-Rauch, S. Vellguth, W. R. Meindl, and H. Schönenberger, *Quant. Struct.-Act. Relat.*, **8**, 266–278 (1989).

200. J. K. Seydel, M. Wiese, H. P. Cordes, H. L. Chi, K.-J. Schaper, E. A. Coats, B. Kutscher, and H. Emig in ref. 83, pp. 367–376.

201. J. K. Seydel, M. Albores Velasco, E. A. Coats, H. P. Cordes, B. Kunz, and M. Wiese, *Quant. Struct.-Act. Relat.*, **11**, 205–210 (1992).

202. R. Schwyzer, *J. Receptor Res.*, **11**, 45–57 (1991).

203. R. Schwyzer, *Biopolymers*, **31**, 785–792 (1991).

204. J. C. Dearden and G. M. Bresnen, *Quant. Struct.-Act. Relat.*, **7**, 133–144 (1988).

205. A. J. Leo, *Methods Enzymol.*, **202**, 544–591 (1991).

206. E. Tomlinson, S. S. Davis, G. D. Parr, M. James, N. Farraj, J. F. M. Kinkel, D. Gaisser, and H. J. Wynne in ref. 54, pp. 83–99.

207. A. Hersey, A. P. Hill, R. M. Hyde, and D. J. Livingstone, *Quant. Struct.-Act. Relat.*, **8**, 288–296 (1989).

208. S. S. Davis, G. Elson, E. Tomlinson, G. Harrison, and J. C. Dearden, *Chem. Ind. (London)*, 677–683 (1976).

209. R. A. Menges, G. L. Bertrand, and D. W. Armstrong, *J. Liquid Chromatogr.*, **13**, 3061–3077 (1990).

210. P. Vallat, N. El Tayar, B. Testa, I. Slacanin, A. Marston, and K. Hostettmann, *J. Chromatogr.*, **504**, 411–419 (1990).

211. R.-S. Tsai, N. El Tayar, B. Testa, and Y. Ito, *J. Chromatogr.*, **538**, 119–123 (1991).

212. N. El Tayar, R.-S. Tsai, P. Vallat, C. Altomare, and B. Testa, *J. Chromatogr.*, **556**, 181–194 (1991).

213. C. B. C. Boyce and B. V. Milborrow, *Nature*, **208**, 537–539 (1965).

214. E. Tomlinson, *J. Chromatogr.*, **113**, 1–45 (1975).

215. G. L. Biagi, M. Recanatini, A. M. Barbaro, M. C. Guerra, A. Sapone, P. A. Borea, and M. C. Pietrogrande in ref. 83, pp. 83–90.

216. K. P. Dross, R. Mannhold, and R. F. Rekker, *Quant. Struct.-Act. Relat.* **11**, 36–44 (1992).

217. M. S. Mirrlees, S. J. Moulton, C. T. Murphy, and P. J. Taylor, *J. Med. Chem.*, **19**, 615–619 (1976).

218. S. H. Unger, J. R. Cook, and J. S. Hollenberg, *J. Pharm. Sci.*, **67**, 1364–1367 (1978).

219. S. H. Unger and G. H. Chiang, *J. Med. Chem.*, **24**, 262–270 (1981).

220. S. J. Lewis, M. S. Mirrlees, and P. J. Taylor, *Quant. Struct.-Act. Relat.*, **2**, 1–6, 100–111 (1983).

221. J. E. Haky and A. M. Young, *J. Liquid Chromatogr.*, **7**, 675–689 (1984).

222. R. M. Smith and C. M. Burr, *J. Chromatogr.*, **475**, 75–83 (1989).

223. R. Kaliszan, *Quant. Struct.-Act. Relat.*, **9**, 83–87 (1990).

224. T. Fujita, J. Iwasa, and C. Hansch, *J. Am. Chem. Soc.*, **86**, 5175–5180 (1964).

225. C. Hansch, A. Leo, and D. Nikaitani, *J. Org. Chem.*, **37**, 3090–3092 (1972).

226. G. G. Nys and R. F. Rekker, *Chim. Ther.*, **8**, 521–535 (1973).

227. G. G. Nys and R. F. Rekker, *Eur. J. Med. Chem.*, **9**, 361–375 (1974).

228. R. F. Rekker and H. M. De Kort, *Eur. J. Med. Chem.*, **14**, 479–488 (1979).

229. S. S. Davis, T. Higuchi, and J. H. Rytting, *Adv. Pharm. Sci.* **4**, 73–261 (1974).

230. P. J. Taylor in ref. 83, pp. 123–126.

231. A. Leo, P. Y. C. Jow, C. Silipo, and C. Hansch, *J. Med. Chem.*, **18**, 865–868 (1975).

232. A. J. Leo, *Eur. J. Med. Chem.*, **15**, 484 (1980).

233. M. A. Pleiss and G. L. Grunewald, *J. Med. Chem.*, **26**, 1760–1764 (1983).

234. H. van de Waterbeemd and B. Testa, *Int. J. Pharm.*, **14**, 29–41 (1983).

235. J. T. Chou and P. C. Jurs, *J. Chem. Inf. Comput. Sci.*, **19**, 172–178 (1979).

236. A. J. Leo, *J. Pharm. Sci.*, **76**, 166–168 (1987).

237. A. J. Leo in ref. 82, pp. 53–58.

238. A. J. Leo in ref. 83, pp. 349–352.

239. *MEDCHEM Software Manual, Releases 3.54* (VMS version), 1989, and 4.2 (UNIX version), 1992, Daylight Chemical Information Systems, Irvine, Calif.

240. D. Weininger, *J. Chem. Inf. Comput. Sci.*, **28**, 31–36 (1988).

241. D. Weininger, A. Weininger, and J. L. Weininger, *J. Chem. Inf. Comput. Sci.*, **29**, 97–101 (1989).

242. D. Weininger and J. L. Weininger in ref. 39, pp. 59–82.

243. J. M. Mayer, H. van de Waterbeemd, and B. Testa, *Eur. J. Med. Chem.* **17**, 17–25 (1982).

244. R. Mannhold, K. P. Dross, and R. F. Rekker, *Quant. Struct.-Act. Relat.* **9**, 21–28 (1990).

245. H. van de Waterbeemd, *Hydrophobicity of Organic Compounds. How to Calculate it by PC's*, Booksoft, Vol. 1, F. Darvas, Ed., CompuDrug, Vienna, 1986.

246. K. Takeuchi, C. Kuroda, and M. Ishida, *J. Chem. Inf. Comput. Sci.*, **30**, 22–26 (1990).

247. J. Hine and P. D. Mookerjee, *J. Org. Chem.*, **40**, 292–298 (1975).

248. P. Broto, G. Moreau, and C. Vandycke, *Eur. J. Med. Chem.*, **19**, 71–78 (1984).

249. A. K. Ghose and G. M. Crippen, *J. Comput. Chem.*, **7**, 565–577 (1986).

250. A. K. Ghose and G. M. Crippen, *J. Chem. Inf. Comput. Sci.*, **27**, 21–35 (1987).

251. A. K. Ghose, A. Pritchett, and G. M. Crippen, *J. Comput. Chem.*, **9**, 80–90 (1988).

252. V. N. Viswanadhan, A. K. Ghose, G. R. Revankar, and R. K. Robins, *J. Chem. Inf. Comput. Sci.*, **29**, 163–172 (1989).

253. T. Suzuki and Y. Kudo, *J. Comput.-Aided Mol. Des.*, **4**, 155–198 (1990).

254. T. Suzuki, *J. Comput.-Aided Mol. Des.*, **5**, 149–166 (1991).

255. A. Leo, C. Hansch, and P. Y. C. Jow, *J. Med. Chem.*, **19**, 611–615 (1976).

256. T. Bultsma, *Eur. J. Med. Chem.*, **15**, 371–374 (1980).

257. S. C. Valvani and S. H. Yalkowsky in ref. 51, pp. 201–229.

258. R. S. Pearlman in ref. 51, pp. 321–347.

259. K. Iwase, K. Komatsu, S. Hirono, S. Nakagawa, and I. Moriguchi, *Chem. Pharm. Bull.*, **33**, 2114–2121 (1985).

260. W. J. Dunn III, M. G. Koehler, and S. Grigoras, *J. Med. Chem.*, **30**, 1121–1126 (1987).

261. K. Kasai, H. Umeyama, and A. Tomonaga, *Bull. Chem. Soc. Jpn.*, **61**, 2701–2706 (1988).

262. W. J. Dunn III in ref. 82, pp. 47–51.

263. N. Bodor, Z. Gabanyi, and C.-K. Wong, *J. Am. Chem. Soc.*, **111**, 3783–3786 (1989).

264. J. de Bruijn and J. Hermens, *Quant. Struct.-Act. Relat.*, **9**, 11–21 (1990).

265. W. J. Dunn III, P. I. Nagy, E. R. Collantes, W.

G. Glen, G. Alagona, and C. Ghio in ref. 83, pp. 59–65.

266. Y. Sasaki, H. Kubodera, T. Matuszaki, and H. Umeyama, *J. Pharmacobio-Dyn.*, **14**, 207–214 (1991).

267. N. Bodor and M.-J. Huang, *J. Pharm. Sci.*, **81**, 272–281 (1992).

268. I. Moriguchi, *Chem. Pharm. Bull.*, **23**, 247–257 (1975).

269. W. J. Dunn III, *Eur. J. Med. Chem.*, **12**, 109–112 (1977).

270. C. Silipo and A. Vittoria in ref. 39, pp. 153–204.

271. J. M. Blaney and C. Hansch in ref. 39, pp. 459–496.

272. M. Gryllaki, H. van de Waterbeemd, and B. Testa in ref. 78, pp. 273–276.

273. P. Ahmad, C. A. Fyfe, and A. Mellors, *Biochem. Pharmacol.*, **24**, 1103–1109 (1975).

274. J. C. Dearden, S. J. A. Bradburne, and M. H. Abraham in ref. 83, pp. 143–150.

275. C. Hansch and J. M. Blaney in ref. 46, pp. 185–208.

276. K. J. Shah and E. A. Coats, *J. Med. Chem.*, **20**, 1001–1006 (1977).

277. N. B. Chapman and J. Shorter, Eds., *Advances in Linear Free Energy Relationships*, Plenum Press, London, 1972.

278. D. D. Perrin in ref. 51, pp. 1–48.

279. K. Bowden in ref. 39, pp. 205–239.

280. G. H. Loew and S. K. Burt in ref. 39, pp. 105–123.

281. C. G. Swain and E. C. Lupton Jr., *J. Am. Chem. Soc.*, **90**, 4328–4337 (1968).

282. C. G. Swain, S. H. Unger, N. R. Rosenquist, and M. S. Swain, *J. Am. Chem. Soc.*, **105**, 492–502 (1983).

283. C. G. Swain, *J. Org. Chem.*, **49**, 2005–2010 (1984).

284. O. Exner in ref. 277, pp. 1–69.

285. J. Shorter in ref. 57, pp. 119–173.

286. W. F. Reynolds and R. D. Topsom, *J. Org. Chem.*, **49**, 1989–1992 (1984).

287. A. J. Hoefnagel, W. Oosterbeek, and B. M. Wepster, *J. Org. Chem.*, **49**, 1993–1997 (1984).

288. M. Charton, *J. Org. Chem.*, **49**, 1997–2001 (1984).

289. C. Hansch, A. Leo, and R. W. Taft, *Chem. Rev.*, **91**, 165–195 (1991).

290. S. H. Unger and C. Hansch, *J. Med. Chem.*, **16**, 745–749 (1973).

291. R. W. Taft Jr., *Steric Effects in Organic Chemistry*, M. S. Newman, Ed., Wiley, New York, 1956, pp. 556–675.

292. C. Silipo and A. Vittoria, *Farmaco Ed. Sci.*, **34**, 858–868 (1979).

293. J. K. Seydel, *Drug Design*, Vol. I, E. J. Ariëns, Ed., Academic Press, New York, 1971, pp. 343–379.

294. J.-L. Fauchère and J. Lauterwein, *Quant. Struct.-Act. Relat.*, **4**, 11–13 (1985).

295. P. G. De Benedetti, *Adv. Drug. Res.*, **16**, 227–279 (1987).

296. B. Hetnarski and R. D. O'Brien, *J. Med. Chem.*, **18**, 29–33 (1975).

297. R. Foster, R. M. Hyde, and D. J. Livingstone, *J. Pharm. Sci.*, **67**, 1310–1313 (1978).

298. D. J. Livingstone, R. M. Hyde, and R. Foster, *Eur. J. Med. Chem.*, **14**, 393–397 (1979).

299. E. J. Lien, R. C. H. Liao, and H. G. Shinouda, *J. Pharm. Sci.*, **68**, 463–465 (1979).

300. E. J. Lien, Z.-R. Guo, R.-L. Li, and C.-T. Su, *J. Pharm. Sci.*, **71**, 641–655 (1982).

301. W.-Y. Li, Z.-R. Guo, and E. J. Lien, *J. Pharm. Sci.*, **73**, 553–558 (1984).

302. C. Hansch, A. Vittoria, C. Silipo, and P. Y. C. Jow, *J. Med. Chem.*, **18**, 546–548 (1975).

303. J. Mitsky, L. Joris, and R. W. Taft, *J. Am. Chem. Soc.*, **94**, 3442–3445 (1972).

304. J. C. Dearden and R. M. Nicholson, *Pestic. Sci.*, **17**, 305–310 (1986).

305. A. J. Shusterman, A. K. Debnath, C. Hansch, G. W. Horn, F. R. Fronczek, A. C. Greene, and S. F. Watkins, *Mol. Pharmacol.*, **36**, 939–944 (1989).

306. R. L. Lopez de Compadre, A. K. Debnath, A. J. Shustermann, and C. Hansch, *Environ. Mol. Mutagen.*, **15**, 44–55 (1990).

307. C. Hansch in ref. 83, pp. 3–10.

308. A. K. Debnath, R. L. Lopez de Compadre, G. Debnath, A. J. Shusterman, and C. Hansch, *J. Med. Chem.*, **34**, 786–797 (1991).

309. J. Gasteiger and M. Marsili, *Tetrahedron*, **36**, 3219–3288 (1980).

310. J. Gasteiger, M. G. Hutchings, M. Marsili, and H. Saller in ref. 78, pp. 90–97.

311. J. Gasteiger, M. G. Hutchings, B. Christoph, L. Gann, C. Hiller, P. Löw, M. Marsili, H. Saller, and K. Yuki, *Topics Curr. Chem.*, **137**, 19–73 (1987).

312. S. H. Unger and C. Hansch, *Prog. Phys. Org. Chem.*, **12**, 91–118 (1976).

313. T. Fujita, *Pure & Appl. Chem.*, **50**, 987–994 (1978).

314. A. Verloop, W. Hoogenstraaten, and J. Tipker,

Drug Design, Vol. VII, E. J. Ariëns, Ed., Academic Press, New York, 1976, pp. 165–207.

315. A. Verloop, *The STERIMOL Approach to Drug Design*, Marcel Dekker, New York, 1987.

316. M. Charton, *Topics Curr. Chem.*, **114**, 57–91 (1983).

317. C. K. Hancock, E. A. Meyers, and B. J. Yager, *J. Am. Chem. Soc.*, **83**, 4211–4213 (1961).

318. V. Austel, E. Kutter, and W. Kalbfleisch, *Arzneim.-Forsch.* (*Drug Res.*) **29**, 585–587 (1979).

319. T. Fujita and H. Iwamura, *Topics Curr. Chem.*, **114**, 119–157 (1983).

320. A. Verloop in ref. 78, pp. 98–104.

321. E. J. Lien and P. H. Wang, *J. Pharm. Sci.*, **69**, 648–650 (1980).

322. H. Kubinyi in ref. 76, pp. 321–346.

323. C. D. Selassie, C. Hansch, and T. A. Khwaja, *J. Med. Chem.*, **33**, 1914–1919 (1990).

324. C. D. Selassie, personal communication.

325. F. Avbelj and D. Hadzi, *Mol. Pharmacol.*, **27**, 466–470 (1985).

326. R. L. Lopez de Compadre, R. A. Pearlstein, A. J. Hopfinger, and J. K. Seydel, *J. Med. Chem.*, **30**, 900–906 (1987); erratum **31**, 2315 (1988).

327. A. J. Hopfinger, R. L. Lopez de Compadre, M. G. Koehler, and S. Emery, *Quant. Struct.-Act. Relat.*, **6**, 111–117 (1987).

328. L. B. Kier, L. H. Hall, W. J. Murray, and M. Randic, *J. Pharm. Sci.*, **64**, 1971–1974 (1975).

329. L. H. Hall, L. B. Kier, and W. J. Murray, *J. Pharm. Sci.*, **64**, 1974–1977 (1975).

330. W. J. Murray, L. H. Hall, and L. B. Kier, *J. Pharm. Sci.*, **64**, 1978–1981 (1975).

331. L. B. Kier, W. J. Murray, and L. H. Hall, *J. Med. Chem.*, **18**, 1272–1274 (1975).

332. L. B. Kier in ref. 51, pp. 277–319.

333. L. B. Kier and L. H. Hall, *Molecular Connectivity in Structure-Activity Analysis*, Research Studies Press, Letchworth, 1986.

334. K. Osmialowski and R. Kaliszan, *Quant. Struct.-Act. Relat.*, **10**, 125–134 (1991).

335. L. H. Hall and L. B. Kier, *Reviews in Computational Chemistry II*, K. B. Lipkowitz and D. B. Boyd, Eds., VCH Publishers, New York, 1991, pp. 367–422.

336. L. B. Kier and L. H. Hall, *J. Pharm. Sci.*, **70**, 583–589 (1981).

337. L. B. Kier and L. H. Hall, *J. Pharm. Sci.*, **72**, 1170–1173 (1983).

338. R. L. Lopez de Compadre, C. M. Compadre, R. Castillo, and W. J. Dunn III, *Eur. J. Med. Chem.*, **18**, 569–571 (1983).

339. C. Daniels and F. S. Wood, *Fitting Equations to Data*, Wiley, New York, 1980.

340. N. R. Draper and H. Smith, *Applied Regression Analysis*, 2nd ed., Wiley, New York, 1981.

341. H. Kubinyi in ref. 39, pp. 589–643.

342. H. Kubinyi, *Quant. Struct.-Act. Relat.*, **7**, 121–133 (1988).

343. C. Hansch and D. F. Calef, *J. Org. Chem.*, **41**, 1240–1243 (1976).

344. T. Fujita in ref. 39, pp. 497–560.

345. C. Hansch and E. J. Lien, *Biochem. Pharmacol.*, **17**, 709–720 (1968).

346. A. Cammarata, *J. Med. Chem.*, **15**, 573–577 (1972).

347. H. Kubinyi and O.-H. Kehrhahn, *J. Med. Chem.*, **19**, 578–586 (1976).

348. J. G. Topliss and R. J. Costello, *J. Med. Chem.*, **15**, 1066–1068 (1972).

349. J. G. Topliss and R. P. Edwards, *J. Med. Chem.*, **22**, 1238–1244 (1979).

350. M. A. Pleiss and S. H. Unger in ref. 39, pp. 561–587.

351. A. Cammarata, R. C. Allen, J. K. Seydel, and E. Wempe, *J. Pharm. Sci.* **59**, 1496–1499 (1970).

352. P. N. Craig, C. H. Hansch, J. W. McFarland, Y. C. Martin, W. P. Purcell, and R. Zahradnik, *J. Med. Chem.*, **14**, 447 (1971).

353. W. P. Purcell, *Eur. J. Med. Chem.*, **10**, 335–339 (1975).

354. S. Wold and W. J. Dunn III, *J. Chem. Inf. Comput. Sci.*, **23**, 6–13 (1983).

355. R. Benigni and A. Giuliani, *Quant. Struct.-Act. Relat.*, **10**, 99–100 (1991).

356. S. Wold, *Quant. Struct.-Act. Relat.*, **10**, 191–193 (1991).

357. H. Kubinyi and O.-H. Kehrhahn, *J. Med. Chem.*, **19**, 1040–1049 (1976).

358. C. Hansch, C. Silipo and E. E. Steller, *J. Pharm. Sci.*, **64**, 1186–1191 (1975).

359. J. Kelder and H. M. Greven, *Rev. Chim. Pays-Bas*, **98**, 168–172 (1979).

360. P. P. Mager, H. Mager, and A. Barth, *Sci. Pharm.*, **47**, 265–297 (1979).

361. P. P. Mager, *Med. Res. Rev.*, **3**, 435–498 (1983).

362. P. P. Mager, *Pharmazie*, **45**, 359–360 (1990).

363. F. Darvas, J. Röhricht, Z. Budai, and B. Bordás, *Advances in Pharmacological Research and Practice, Proceedings of the 3rd Congress of the Hungarian Pharmacological Society, Budapest, 1979*, Vol. 3, J. Knoll, Ed., Pergamon Press, 1980, pp. 25–38.

364. J.-E. Dubois, D. Laurent, and A. Aranda, *J. Chim. Phys.*, **70**, 1608–1615, 1616–1624 (1973).

365. J.-E. Dubois, D. Laurent, P. Bost, S. Chambaud, and C. Mercier, *Eur. J. Med. Chem.*, **11**, 225–236 (1976).

366. B. Duperray, M. Chastrette, M. Cohen Makabeh, and H. Pacheco, *Eur. J. Med. Chem.*, **11**, 323–336, 433–437 (1976).

367. C. Mercier and J. E. Dubois, *Eur. J. Med. Chem.*, **14**, 415–423 (1979).

368. L. H. Hall and L. B. Kier, *Eur. J. Med. Chem.*, **13**, 89–92 (1978).

369. L. J. Schaad, B. A. Hess Jr., W. P. Purcell, A. Cammarata, R. Franke, and H. Kubinyi, *J. Med. Chem.*, **24**, 900–901 (1981).

370. J. A. Singer and W. P. Purcell, *J. Med. Chem.*, **10**, 1000–1002 (1967).

371. A. Cammarata and T. M. Bustard, *J. Med. Chem.*, **17**, 981–985 (1974).

372. K. Bocek, J. Kopecky, M. Krivucova, and D. Vlachova, *Experientia*, **20**, 667–668 (1964).

373. J. Kopecky, K. Bocek, and D. Vlachova, *Nature*, **207**, 981 (1965).

374. C. Hansch, *J. Org. Chem.*, **35**, 620–621 (1970).

375. Y. C. Martin and K. R. Lynn, *J. Med. Chem.*, **14**, 1162–1166 (1971).

376. J. C. Dearden in ref. 39, pp. 375–411.

377. J. T. Penniston, L. Beckett, D. L. Bentley, and C. Hansch, *Mol. Pharmacol.*, **5**, 333–341 (1969).

378. R. Franke and W. Schmidt, *Acta. Biol. Med. Germ.*, **31**, 273–287 (1973).

379. J. W. McFarland, *J. Med. Chem.*, **13**, 1192–1196 (1970).

380. T. Higuchi and S. S. Davis, *J. Pharm. Sci.*, **59**, 1376–1383 (1970).

381. R. M. Hyde, *J. Med. Chem.*, **18**, 231–233 (1975).

382. R. M. Hyde, *Chem. Ind.* (*London*), 859–862 (1977).

383. H. Kubinyi, *Arzneim.-Forsch.* (*Drug Res.*), **26**, 1991–1997 (1976).

384. H. Kubinyi and O.-H. Kehrhahn, *Arzneim.-Forsch.* (*Drug Res.*), **28**, 598–601 (1978).

385. H. Kubinyi, *Arzneim.-Forsch.* (*Drug Res.*), **29**, 1067–1080 (1979).

386. B. C. Lippold and G. F. Schneider, *Arzneim.-Forsch.* (*Drug Res.*), **25**, 843–852, 1683–1686 (1975).

387. H. Kubinyi, *J. Pharm. Sci.*, **67**, 262–263 (1978).

388. H. van de Waterbeemd, S. van Boeckel, A. Jansen, and K. Geeritsma, *Eur. J. Med. Chem.*, **15**, 279–282 (1980).

389. H, van de Waterbeemd, P. van Bakel, and A. Jansen, *J. Pharm. Sci.*, **70**, 1081–1082 (1981).

390. F. H. N. de Haan, T. de Vringer, J. T. M. van de Waterbeemd, and A. C. A. Jansen, *Int. J. Pharm.*, **13**, 75–87 (1982).

391. E. R. Cooper, B. Berner, and R. D. Bruce, *J. Pharm. Sci.*, **70**, 57–59 (1981).

392. B. Berner and E. R. Cooper, *J. Pharm. Sci.*, **73**, 102–106 (1984).

393. S. H. Yalkowski and G. L. Flynn, *J. Pharm. Sci.*, **62**, 210–217 (1973).

394. J. K. Seydel in ref. 74, pp. 179–201.

395. J. K. Seydel and K.-J. Schaper, *Pharmac. Ther.*, **15**, 131–182 (1982).

396. S. Baláz, E. Sturdík, M. Hrmová, M. Breza, and T. Liptaj, *Eur. J. Med. Chem.*, **19**, 167–171 (1984).

397. S. Baláz, M. Wiese, H.-L. Chi, and J. K. Seydel, *Anal. Chim. Acta*, **235**, 195–207 (1990).

398. S. Baláz, M. Wiese, and J. K. Seydel, *Quant. Struct.-Act. Relat.*, **11**, 45–49 (1992).

399. C. Hansch, C. Grieco, C. Silipo, and A. Vittoria, *J. Med. Chem.*, **20**, 1420–1435 (1977).

400. Y. C. Martin in ref. 51, pp. 49–110.

401. G. le Petit, *Pharmazie*, **32**, 289–291 (1977).

402. G. le Petit, *Pharmazie*, **35**, 696–698 (1980).

403. K. Klemm and U. Krüger, *Arzneim.-Forsch.* (*Drug. Res.*), **29**, 2–11 (1979).

404. F. H. Clarke and N. M. Cahoon, *J. Pharm. Sci.*, **76**, 611–620 (1987).

405. K.-J. Schaper, *J. Chem. Research* (**S**), 357 (1979).

406. K. S. Murthy and G. Zografi, *J. Pharm. Sci.*, **59**, 1281–1285 (1970).

407. B. C. Lippold and G. F. Schneider, *Pharmazie*, **31**, 237–239 (1976).

408. B. C. Lippold and W. A. Lettenbauer, *Pharmazie*, **33**, 221–225 (1978).

409. P.-H. Wang and E. J. Lien, *J. Pharm. Sci.*, **69**, 662–668 (1980).

410. R. A. Scherrer and S. M. Howard, *J. Med. Chem.*, **20**, 53–58 (1977).

411. R. A. Scherrer and S. M. Howard in ref. 72, pp. 507–526.

412. R. A. Scherrer, *Pesticide Synthesis Through Rational Approaches*, P. S. Magee, G. K. Kohn, and J. J. Menn, Eds., *ACS Symp. Series*, **255**, 225–246 (1984).

413. E. J. Lien, *Drug Design*, Vol. V, E. J. Ariëns, Ed., Academic Press, 1975, pp. 81–132.

414. P. A. Shore, B. B. Brodie, and C. A. M. Hogben, *J. Pharmac. Exptl. Therap.*, **119**, 361–369 (1957).

415. J. G. Wagner, *Fundamentals of Clinical Pharmacokinetics*, Drug Intelligence Publications, Inc., Hamilton, 1975.

416. D. Winne, *J. Pharmacokin. Biopharm.*, **5**, 53–94 (1977).

417. A. Tsuji, E. Miyamoto, N. Hashimoto, and T. Yamana, *J. Pharm. Sci.* **67**, 1705–1711 (1978).

418. Y. C. Martin and J. J. Hackbarth, *J. Med. Chem.*, **19**, 1033–1039 (1976).

419. Y. C. Martin in ref. 71, pp. 351–358.

420. K.-J. Schaper, *Quant. Struct.-Act. Relat.*, **1**, 13–27 (1982).

421. S. S. Davis and G. Elson, *J. Pharm. Pharmacol.*, **26 S**, 90 P (1974).

422. P. Seiler, *Eur. J. Med. Chem.*, **9**, 663–665 (1974).

423. J. J. Kaufman, N. M. Semo, and W. S. Koski, *J. Med. Chem.*, **18**, 647–655 (1975).

424. K. Ezumi and T. Kubota, *Chem. Pharm. Bull.*, **28**, 85–91 (1980).

425. F. H. Clarke, *J. Pharm. Sci.*, **73**, 226–230 (1984).

426. F. H. Clarke in ref. 78, pp. 264–267.

427. A. Avdeef in ref. 83, pp. 119–122.

428. W. J. Dunn III and S. Wold in ref. 39, pp. 691–714.

429. K. Fukunaga, *Introduction to Statistical Pattern Recognition*, Academic Press, New York, 1972.

430. K. Varmuza, *Pattern Recognition in Chemistry*, *Lecture Notes in Chemistry* 21, Springer-Verlag, Berlin, 1980.

431. B. R. Kowalski and C. F. Bender, *J. Am. Chem. Soc.*, **94**, 5632–5639 (1972).

432. H. J. Wijnne in ref. 70, pp. 211–229.

433. P. C. Jurs, J. T. Chou, and M. Yuan in ref. 72, pp. 103–129.

434. D. J. Livingstone, *Methods Enzymol*, **203**, 613–638 (1991).

435. R. J. Mathews, *J. Am. Chem. Soc.*, **97**, 935–936 (1975).

436. P. N. Craig in ref. 39, pp. 645–666.

437. V. K. Gombar, H. H. Borgstedt, K. Enslein, J. B. Hart, and B. W. Blake, *Quant. Struct.-Act. Relat.*, **10**, 306–332 (1991).

438. G. Klopman, *J. Am. Chem. Soc.*, **106**, 7315–7321 (1984).

439. G. Klopman and O. T. Macina, *Mol. Pharmacol.*, **31**, 457–476 (1987).

440. G. Klopman and M. L. Dimayuga, *J. Comput.-Aided Mol. Des.*, **4**, 117–130 (1990).

441. G. Klopman, *Quant. Struct.-Act. Relat*, **11**, 176–184 (1992).

442. R. D. King, S. Muggleton, R. A. Lewis, and M. J. E. Sternberg, *Proc. Natl. Acad. Sci. USA*, **89**, 11322–11326 (1992).

443. S. Hübel, T. Rösner, and R. Franke, *Pharmazie*, **35**, 424–433 (1980).

444. R. Franke, S. Huebel, and W. J. Streich, *Environ. Health Perspect*, **61**, 239–255 (1985).

445. W. J. Streich and R. Franke, *Quant. Struct.-Act. Relat.*, **4**, 13–18 (1985).

446. R. Franke and W. J. Streich, *Quant. Struct.-Act. Relat.*, **4**, 51–63, 63–69 (1985).

447. S. Hübel and R. Franke in ref. 83, pp. 177–180.

448. Z. Simon and Z. Szabadai, *Stud. Biophys.*, **39**, 123–132 (1973).

449. Z. Simon, *Angew. Chem. Int. Ed. Engl.*, **13**, 719–727 (1974).

450. Z. Simon, A. Chiriac, S. Holban, D. Ciubotariu, and G. I. Mihalas, *Minimum Steric Difference—The MTD Method for QSAR Studies*, Research Studies Press, Letchworth, 1984.

451. I. Motoc, *Topics Curr. Chem.*, **114**, 93–105 (1983).

452. Z. Simon, A. Chiriac, I. Motoc, S. Holban, D. Ciubotariu, and Z. Szabadai, *Stud. Biophys.*, **55**, 217–226 (1976).

453. Z. Simon, S. Holban, I. Motoc, M. Mracec, C. Chiriac, F. Kerek, D. Ciubotariu, Z. Szabadai, R. D. Pop, and I. Schwartz, *Stud. Biophys.*, **59**, 181–197 (1976).

454. Z. Simon, I. I. Badilescu, and T. Racovitan, *J. Theor. Biol.*, **66**, 485–495 (1977).

455. V. Popoviciu, S. Holban, I. I. Badilescu, and Z. Simon, *Stud. Biophys.* **69**, 75–76 (1978).

456. Z. Simon and M. Bohl, *Quant. Struct.-Act. Relat.*, **11**, 23–28 (1992).

457. I. Motoc, *Quant. Struct.-Act. Relat.*, **3**, 43–47, 47–51 (1984).

458. P. S. Magee in ref. 83, pp. 549–552.

459. P. S. Magee, *Quant. Struct.-Act. Relat.*, **9**, 202–215 (1990).

460. A. J. Hopfinger, *J. Am. Chem. Soc.*, **102**, 7196–7206 (1980).

461. C. Battershell, D. Malhotra, and A. J. Hopfinger, *J. Med. Chem.*, **24**, 812–818 (1981).

462. A. J. Hopfinger, *J. Med. Chem.*, **24**, 818–822 (1981).

463. A. J. Hopfinger, *Arch. Biochem. Biophys.*, **206**, 153–163 (1981).

464. A. J. Hopfinger and R. Potenzone Jr., *Mol. Pharmacol.*, **21**, 187–195 (1982).

465. A. J. Hopfinger, *J. Med. Chem.*, **26**, 990–996 (1983).

466. A. J. Hopfinger, *Quant. Struct.-Act. Relat.*, **3**, 1–5 (1984).

467. M. Mabilia, R. A. Pearlstein, and A. J. Hopfinger, *Eur. J. Med. Chem.*, **20**, 163–174 (1985).

468. D. E. Walters and A. J. Hopfinger, *J. Mol. Struct. (Theochem)*, **134**, 317–323 (1986).

469. A. J. Hopfinger and B. J. Burke in ref. 63, pp. 173–209.

470. T. Aoyama, Y. Suzuki, and H. Ichikawa, *J. Med. Chem.*, **33**, 905–908, 2583–2590 (1990).

471. V. S. Rose, I. F. Croall, and H. J. MacFie, *Quant. Struct.-Act. Relat.* **10**, 6–15 (1991); erratum **10**, 141 (1991).

472. M. Wiese, *Quant. Struct.-Act. Relat.*, **10**, 369–371 (1991).

473. T. A. Andrea and H. Kalayeh, *J. Med. Chem.*, **34**, 2824–2836 (1991).

474. T. Aoyama and H. Ichikawa, *Chem. Pharm. Bull.*, **39**, 358–366, 372–378 (1991).

475. M. Chastrette and J. Y. de Saint Laumer, *Eur. J. Med. Chem.*, **26**, 829–833 (1991).

476. D. J. Livingstone, G. Hesketh, D. Clayworth, *J. Mol. Graphics*, **9**, 115–118 (1991).

477. D. T. Manallack and D. J. Livingstone, *Med. Chem. Res.*, **2**, 181–190 (1992).

478. S.-S. So and W. G. Richards, *J. Med. Chem.*, **35**, 3201–3207 (1992).

479. G. W. Snedecor and W. G. Cochran, *Statistical Methods*, The Iowa State University Press, Ames, 1973.

480. Y. J. Jeng and A. Martin, *J. Pharm. Sci.*, **74**, 1053–1057 (1985).

481. J. K. Seydel and K.-J. Schaper in ref. 74, pp. 337–354.

482. R. L. Lipnick, *Sci. Total Environ.*, **109–110**, 131–153 (1991).

483. J. W. McFarland and D. J. Gans in ref. 39, pp. 667–689.

484. Y. C. Martin, J. B. Holland, C. H. Jarboe, and N. Plotnikoff, *J. Med. Chem.*, **17**, 409–413 (1974).

485. G. Prakash and E. M. Hodnett, *J. Med. Chem.*, **21**, 369–374 (1978).

486. D. R. Henry and J. H. Block, *J. Med. Chem.*, **22**, 465–472 (1979).

487. C. C. Smith, C. S. Genther and E. A. Coats, *Eur. J. Med. Chem.*, **14**, 271–276 (1979).

488. D. F. V. Lewis, C. Ioannides, and D. V. Parke, *Mutagenesis*, **5**, 433–435 (1990).

489. D. F. V. Lewis, C. Ioannides, and D. V. Parke in ref. 83, pp. 525–527.

490. I. Moriguchi and K. Komatsu, *Chem. Pharm. Bull.*, **25**, 2800–2802 (1977).

491. I. Moriguchi, K. Komatsu, and Y. Matsushita, *J. Med. Chem.*, **23**, 20–26 (1980).

492. I. Moriguchi, K. Komatsu, and Y. Matsushita, *Anal. Chim. Acta*, **133**, 625–636 (1981).

493. Y. Takahashi, Y. Miyashita, H. Abe, and S. Sasaki, *Bunseki Kagaku*, **33**, E487–E494 (1984); *Chem. Abstracts*, **102**, 105 720 n (1985).

494. I. Moriguchi, S. Hirono, Q. Liu, and I. Nakagome, *Quant. Struct.-Act. Relat.*, **11**, 325–331 (1992).

495. E. R. Malinowski and D. G. Howery, *Factor Analysis in Chemistry*, Wiley, New York, 1980.

496. W. R. Dillon and M. Goldstein, *Multivariate Analysis: Methods and Applications*, Wiley, New York, 1984.

497. I. T. Joliffe, *Principal Component Analysis*, Springer-Verlag, New York, 1986.

498. S. Wold, K. Esbensen, and P. Geladi, *Chemom. Intell. Lab. Syst.*, **2**, 37–52 (1987).

499. E. A. Coats, H.-P. Cordes, V. M. Kulkarni, M. Richter, K.-J. Schaper, M. Wiese, and J. K. Seydel, *Quant. Struct.-Act. Relat.*, **4**, 99–109 (1985).

500. K.-J. Schaper and J. K. Seydel in ref. 78, pp. 173–189.

501. T. Kubota, J. Hanamura, K. Kano, and B. Uno, *Chem. Pharm. Bull.*, **33**, 1488–1495 (1985).

502. M. Wiese, J. K. Seydel, H. Pieper, G. Krüger, K. R. Noll and J. Keck, *Quant. Struct.-Act. Relat.*, **6**, 164–172 (1987).

503. V. S. Rose, J. Wood, and H. J. H. MacFie, *Quant. Struct.-Act. Relat.*, **10**, 359–368 (1991).

504. W. J. Dunn III, S. Wold, and Y. C. Martin, *J. Med. Chem.*, **21**, 922–930 (1978).

505. W. J. Dunn III and S. Wold, *J. Med. Chem.*, **21**, 1001–1007 (1978).

506. W. J. Dunn III and S. Wold, *Bioorg. Chem.*, **9**, 505–523 (1980).

507. S. Wold, W. J. Dunn III, and S. Hellberg in ref. 46, pp. 95–117.

508. S. Wold, H. Martens, and H. Wold, *Matrix Pencils*, Lecture Notes in Mathematics, A. Ruhe and B. Kagström, Eds., Springer-Verlag Heidelberg, 1983, pp. 286–293.

509. B. Nordén, U. Edlund, D. Johnels, and S. Wold, *Quant. Struct.-Act. Relat.*, **2**, 73–76 (1983).

510. S. Wold, C. Albano, W. J. Dunn III, K. Esbensen, S. Hellberg, E. Johansson, and M. Sjöström, *Food Research and Data Analysis*, H. Martens and H. Russwurm Jr., Eds., Applied Science Publishers, London, 1983, pp. 147–188.

511. S. Wold, C. Albano, W. J. Dunn III, U. Edlund, K. Esbenson, P. Geladi, S. Hellberg, E. Johansson, W. Lindberg, and M. Sjöström, *Chemometrics, Mathematics and Statistics in Chemistry*, B. R. Kowalski, Ed., Reidel Publishing Company, Dordrecht, 1984, pp. 17–95.

512. H. Wold, *Perspectives in Probability and Statistics, Papers in Honour of M. S. Bartlett*, J. Gani, Ed., Academic Press, London, 1975.

513. R. D. Cramer III, J. D. Bunce, D. E. Patterson, and I. E. Frank, *Quant. Struct.-Act. Relat.*, **7**, 18–25 (1988); *erratum* **7**, 91 (1988).

514. G. Cruciani, M. Baroni, D. Bonelli, S. Clementi, C. Ebert, and B. Skagerberg, *Quant. Struct.-Act. Relat.*, **9**, 101–107 (1990).

515. G. Cruciani, M. Baroni, S. Clementi, G. Costantino, D. Riganelli, and B. Skagerberg, *J. Chemometrics*, **6**, 335–346 (1992).

516. M. Baroni, S. Clementi, G. Cruciani, G. Costantino, D. Riganelli, and E. Oberrauch, *J. Chemometrics*, **6**, 347–356 (1992).

517. M. Baroni, G. Costantino, G. Cruciani, D. Riganelli, R. Valigi, and S. Clementi, *Quant. Struct.-Act. Relat.*, **12**, 9–20 (1993).

518. W. J. Dunn III, M. J. Greenberg, and S. S. Callejas, *J. Med. Chem.*, **19**, 1299–1301 (1976).

519. Y. Takahashi, Y. Miyashita, H. Abe, and S.-I. Sasaki, *Anal. Chem. Acta*, **122**, 241–247 (1980).

520. P. Wilett, *Anal. Chim. Acta*, **136**, 29–37 (1982).

521. P. C. Jurs and R. G. Lawson, *Chemom. Intell. Lab. Syst.*, **10**, 81–83 (1991).

522. J. W. McFarland and D. J. Gans, *J. Med. Chem.*, **29**, 505–514 (1986).

523. *Ibid.*, **30**, 46–49 (1987).

524. J. W. McFarland and D. J. Gans, *Drug. Information J.*, **24**, 705–711 (1990).

525. P. N. Craig, *J. Med. Chem.*, **14**, 680–684 (1971).

526. R. D. Cramer III, K. M. Snader, C. R. Willis, L. W. Chakrin, J. Thomas, and B. M. Sutton, *J. Med. Chem.*, **22**, 714–725 (1979).

527. P. S. Magee, *IUPAC Pesticide Chemistry: Human Welfare and the Environment*, Vol. 1, J. Miyamoto and P. C. Kearney, Eds., Pergamon Press, Oxford, 1983, pp. 251–260.

528. F. Darvas, *J. Med. Chem.*, **17**, 799–804 (1974).

529. R. D. Gilliom, W. P. Purcell, and T. R. Bosin, *Eur. J. Med. Chem.*, **12**, 187–192 (1977).

530. J. G. Topliss, *J. Med. Chem.*, **15**, 1006–1011 (1972).

531. J. G. Topliss and Y. C. Martin, *Drug Design*, Vol. V, E. J. Ariëns, Ed., Academic Press, New York, 1975, pp. 1–21.

532. J. G. Topliss, *J. Med. Chem.*, **20**, 463–469 (1977).

533. Y. C. Martin and H. N. Panas, *J. Med. Chem.*, **22**, 784–791 (1979).

534. Y. C. Martin and W. J. Dunn III, *J. Med. Chem.*, **16**, 578–579 (1973).

535. W. G. Cochran and B. M. Cox, *Experimental Designs*, 2nd Ed., Wiley, New York, 1957.

536. R. G. Petersen, *Design and Analysis of Experiments*, Marcel Dekker, New York, 1985.

537. S. N. Deming and S. L. Morgan, *Experimental Design: A Chemometric Approach*, Elsevier, Amsterdam, 1987.

538. V. Austel, *Eur. J. Med. Chem.*, **17**, 9–16, 339–347 (1982).

539. V. Austel, *Quant. Struct.-Act. Relat.*, **2**, 59–65 (1983).

540. V. Austel, *Drugs of the Future*, **9**, 349–365 (1984).

541. V. Austel, *Topics Curr. Chem.*, **114**, 7–19 (1983).

542. R. Wootton, R. Cranfield, G. C. Sheppey, and P. J. Goodford, *J. Med. Chem.*, **18**, 607–613 (1975).

543. K. R. H. Woolridge, *Eur. J. Med. Chem.*, **15**, 63–66 (1980).

544. R. Wootton, *J. Med. Chem.*, **26**, 275–277 (1983).

545. S. H. Unger, *Drug Design*, Vol. IX, E. J. Ariëns, Ed., Academic Press, New York, 1980, pp. 47–119.

546. K.-J. Schaper in ref. 75, pp. 235–236.

547. D. M. Borth, R. J. McKay, and J. R. Elliott, *Technometrics*, **27**, 25–35 (1985).

548. S. Dove, W. J. Streich, and R. Franke, *J. Med. Chem.*, **23**, 1456–1459 (1980).

549. B. Skagerberg, S. Clementi, M. Sjöström, M.-L. Tosato, and S. Wold in ref. 82, pp. 127–130.

550. S. Clementi, G. Cruciani, M. Baroni, and B. Skagerberg in ref. 83, pp. 217–222.

551. V. Austel in ref. 78, pp. 247–250.

552. C. Cativiela, J. Elguero, D. Mathieu, E. Melendez, and R. Phan Tan Luu, *Eur. J. Med. Chem.*, **18**, 359–363 (1983).

553. C. Hansch, A. Leo, and L. Zhang, eds., *Comprehensive Quantitative Structure-Activity Relationships: C-QSAR*, Pomona College, Claremont, Calif., 1992.

554. C. Hansch in ref. 82, pp. 23–30.

555. J. M. Blaney, C. Hansch, C. Silipo, and A. Vittoria, *Chem. Rev.*, **84**, 333–407 (1984).

556. C. Silipo and C. Hansch, *J. Med. Chem.*, **19**, 62–71 (1976).

557. M. Yoshimoto and C. Hansch, *J. Med. Chem.*, **19**, 71–98 (1976).

558. S. P. Gupta, *Chem. Rev.*, **87**, 1183–1253 (1987).

559. R.-L. Li, C. Hansch, D. Matthews, J. M. Blaney, R. Langridge, T. J. Delcamp, S. S. Susten, and J. H. Freisheim, *Quant. Struct.-Act. Relat.*, **1**, 1–7 (1982).

560. C. Hansch, *Drug Intell. Clin. Pharm.*, **16**, 391–396 (1982).

561. A. Carotti, R. N. Smith, S. Wong, C. Hansch, J. M. Blaney, and R. Langridge, *Arch. Biochem. Biophys.*, **229**, 112–125 (1984).

562. C. Hansch and T. E. Klein, *Acc. Chem. Res.*, **19**, 392–400 (1986).

563. L. Morgenstern, M. Recanatini, T. E. Klein, W.

Steinmetz, C.-Z. Yang, R. Langridge, and C. Hansch, *J. Biol. Chem.*, **262**, 10767–10772 (1987).

564. C. Hansch and T. E. Klein, *Methods Enzymol.*, **202**, 512–543 (1991).

565. C. Silipo and C. Hansch, *J. Am. Chem. Soc.*, **97**, 6849–6861 (1975).

566. E. A. Coats, C. S. Genther, S. W. Dietrich, Z.-R. Guo, and C. Hansch, *J. Med. Chem.*, **24**, 1422–1429 (1981).

567. T. A. Khwaja, S. Pentecost, C. D. Selassie, Z.-R. Guo, and C. Hansch, *J. Med. Chem.*, **25**, 153–156 (1982).

568. C. D. Selassie, Z.-R. Guo, C. Hansch, T. A. Khwaja, and S. Pentecost, *J. Med. Chem.*, **25**, 157–161 (1982).

569. R.-L. Li, C. Hansch, and B. T. Kaufman, *J. Med. Chem.*, **25**, 435–440 (1982).

570. C. D. Selassie, R.-L. Li, C. Hansch, T. A. Hansch, T. A. Khwaja, and C. B. Dias, *J. Med. Chem.*, **25**, 518–522 (1982).

571. C. Hansch, R.-L. Li, J. M. Blaney, and R. Langridge, *J. Med. Chem.*, **25**, 777–784 (1982).

572. C. Hansch, B. A. Hathaway, Z.-R. Guo, C. D. Selassie, S. W. Dietrich, J. M. Blaney, R. Langridge, K. W. Volz, and B. T. Kaufman, *J. Med. Chem.*, **27**, 129–143 (1984).

573. C. D. Selassie, C. Hansch, T. A. Khwaja, C. B. Dias, and S. Pentecost, *J. Med. Chem.*, **27**, 347–357 (1984).

574. E. A. Coats, C. S. Genther, C. D. Selassie, C. D. Strong, and C. Hansch, *J. Med. Chem.*, **28**, 1910–1916 (1985).

575. C. D. Selassie, Z.-X. Fang, R.-L. Li, C. Hansch, T. Klein, R. Langridge, and B. T. Kaufman, *J. Med. Chem.*, **29**, 621–626 (1986).

576. C. D. Selassie, C. D. Strong, C. Hansch, T. J. Delcamp, J. H. Freisheim, and T. A. Khwaja, *Cancer Res.*, **46**, 744–756 (1986).

577. R. G. Booth, C. D. Selassie, C. Hansch, and D. V. Santi, *J. Med. Chem.*, **30**, 1218–1224 (1987).

578. R.-L. Li and M. Poe, *J. Med. Chem.*, **31**, 366–370 (1988).

579. C. D. Selassie, R. L. Li, C. H. Hansch, T. Klein, R. Langridge, B. T. Kaufman, J. Freisheim, and T. Khwaja in ref. 82, pp. 341–344.

580. C. D. Selassie, R.-L. Li, M. Poe, and C. Hansch, *J. Med. Chem.*, **34**, 46–54 (1991).

581. L. F. Kuyper, B. Roth, D. P. Baccanari, R. Ferone, C. R. Beddell, J. N. Champness, D. K. Stammers, J. G. Dann, F. E. Norrington, D. J. Baker, and P. J. Goodford, *J. Med. Chem.*, **28**, 303–311 (1985).

582. K.-H. Czaplinsky, M. Kansy, J. K. Seydel, and R. Haller, *Quant. Struct.-Act. Relat.*, **6**, 70–72 (1987).

583. C. Hansch, R. N. Smith, A. Rockoff, D. F. Calef, P. Y. C. Jow, and J. Y. Fukunaga, *Arch. Biochem. Biophys.*, **183**, 383–392 (1977).

584. R. N. Smith, C. Hansch, K. H. Kim, B. Omiya, G. Fukumura, C. D. Selassie, P. Y. C. Jow, J. M. Blaney, and R. Langridge, *Arch. Biochem. Biophys.*, **215**, 319–328 (1982).

585. A. Carotti, C. Hansch, M. M. Mueller, and J. M. Blaney, *J. Med. Chem.*, **27**, 1401–1405 (1984); erratum **28**, 261 (1985).

586. A. Carotti, G. Casini, and C. Hansch, *J. Med. Chem.*, **27**, 1427–1431 (1984).

587. A. Carotti, C. Raguseo, and C. Hansch, *Chem.-Biol. Interactions*, **52**, 279–288 (1985).

588. C. M. Compadre, C. Hansch, T. E. Klein, and R. Langridge, *Biochim. Biophys. Acta*, **1038**, 158–163 (1990).

589. C. M. Compadre, C. Hansch, T. E. Klein, J. Petridou-Fischer, C. D. Selassie, R. N. Smith, W. Steinmetz, C.-Z. Yang, and G.-Z. Yang, *Biochim. Biophys. Acta*, **1079**, 43–52 (1991).

590. C. D. Selassie, M. Chow, and C. Hansch, *Chem.-Biol. Interactions*, **68**, 13–25 (1988).

591. M. Recanatini, T. Klein, C.-Z. Yang, J. McClarin, R. Langridge, and C. Hansch, *Mol. Pharmacol.*, **29**, 436–446 (1986).

592. N. W. Cornell, C. Hansch, K. H. Kim, and K. Henegar, *Arch. Biochem. Biophys.*, **227**, 81–90 (1983).

593. C. Hansch, T. Klein, J. McClarin, R. Langridge, and N. W. Cornell, *J. Med. Chem.*, **29**, 615–620 (1986).

594. C. Hansch and J.-P. Bjorkroth, *J. Org. Chem.*, **51**, 5461–5462 (1986).

595. F. Barbato, B. Cappello, C. Silipo, and A. Vittoria, *Farmaco Ed. Sci.*, **37**, 519–536 (1982).

596. C. Hansch, J. McClarin, T. Klein, and R. Langridge, *Mol. Pharmacol.* **27**, 493–498 (1985).

597. A. Carotti, C. Raguseo, F. Campagna, R. Langridge, and T. E. Klein, *Quant. Struct.-Act. Relat.*, **8**, 1–10 (1989).

598. C. Grieco, C. Hansch, C. Silipo, R. N. Smith, A. Vittoria, and K. Yamada, *Arch. Biochem. Biophys.*, **194**, 542–551 (1979).

599. C. Silipo, C. Hansch, C. Grieco, and A. Vittoria, *Arch. Biochem. Biophys.*, **194**, 552–557 (1979).

600. G. E. Wright and J. J. Gambino, *J. Med. Chem.*, **27**, 181–185 (1984).

601. M. P. Dale, H. E. Ensley, K. Kern, K. A. R. Sastry, and L. D. Byers, *Biochemistry*, **24**, 3530–3539 (1985).

602. C. S. Rooney, W. C. Randall, K. B. Streeter, C.

Ziegler, E. J. Cragoe Jr., H. Schwam, S. R. Michelson, H. W. R. Williams, E. Eichler, D. E. Duggan, E. H. Ulm, and R. M. Noll, *J. Med. Chem.*, **26**, 700–714 (1983).

603. C. Silipo and C. Hansch, *Mol. Pharmacol.*, **10**, 954–962 (1974).

604. Y. Martin, W. B. Martin, and J. D. Taylor, *J. Med. Chem.*, **18**, 883–888 (1975).

605. J. Gambino, F. Focher, C. Hildebrand, G. Maga, T. Noonan, S. Spadari, and G. Wright, *J. Med. Chem.*, **35**, 2979–2983 (1992).

606. C. Silipo and C. Hansch, *Farmaco Ed. Sci.*, **30**, 35–46 (1975).

607. A. Leo, C. Hansch, and C. Church, *J. Med. Chem.*, **12**, 766–771 (1969).

608. C. Hansch, *Adv. Pharmac. Chemother.*, **13**, 45–81 (1975).

609. E. Kutter and C. Hansch, *Arch. Biochem. Biophys.*, **135**, 126–135 (1969).

610. M. Yoshimoto, C. Hansch and P. Y. C. Jow, *Chem. Pharm. Bull.*, **23**, 437–444 (1975).

611. C. Hansch, M. Yoshimoto, and M. H. Doll, *J. Med. Chem.*, **19**, 1089–1093 (1976).

612. C. Hansch and P. Moser, *Immunochemistry*, **15**, 535–540 (1978).

613. P. Pratesi, G. Caliendo, C. Silipo, and A. Vittoria, *Quant. Struct.-Act. Relat.*, **11**, 1–17 (1992).

614. P. Pratesi, G. Caliendo, C. Silipo, and A. Vittoria, *Quant. Struct.-Act. Relat.*, **11**, 151–161 (1992).

615. E. J. Lien, E. J. Ariëns, and A. J. Beld, *Eur. J. Pharmacol.*, **35**, 245–252 (1976).

616. G. Lambrecht, U. Moser, and E. Mutschler, *Eur. J. Med. Chem.*, **15**, 305–310 (1980).

617. A. M. ter Laak, M. J. van Drooge, H. Timmerman, and G. M. Donné-op den Kelder, *Quant. Struct.-Act. Relat.*, **11**, 348–363 (1992).

618. C. Hansch and J. Caldwell, *J. Comput.-Aided Mol. Des.*, **5**, 441–453 (1991).

619. S. W. Dietrich, M. B. Bolger, P. A. Kollman, and E. C. Jorgensen, *J. Med. Chem.*, **20**, 863–880 (1977).

620. A. P. IJzerman, G. H. J. Aué, T. Bultsma, M. R. Linschoten, and H. Timmerman, *J. Med. Chem.*, **28**, 1328–1334 (1985).

621. A. P. IJzerman, T. Bultsma, and H. Timmerman, *J. Med. Chem.*, **29**, 549–554 (1986).

622. P. A. Borea, M. C. Pietrogrande, and G. L. Biagi, *Biochem. Pharmacol.* **37**, 3953–3957 (1988).

623. S. Bandiera, T. W. Sawyer, M. A. Campbell, T. Fujita, and S. Safe, *Biochem. Pharmacol.*, **32**, 3803–3813 (1983).

624. S. Safe, S. Bandiera, T. Sawyer, B. Zmudzka, G. Mason, M. Romkes, M. A. Denomme, J. Sparling, A. B. Okey, and T. Fujita, *Environ. Health Perspect.*, **61**, 21–33 (1985).

625. N. El Tayar, G. J. Kilpatrick, H. van de Waterbeemd, B. Testa, P. Jenner, and C. D. Marsden, *Eur. J. Med. Chem.*, **23**, 173–182 (1988).

626. S. P. Gupta and A. Handa, *Res. Commun. Chem. Pathol. Pharmacol.*, **55**, 357–366 (1987).

627. P. Singh and A. Goyal, *Arzneim.-Forsch. (Drug Res.)*, **37**, 51–54 (1987).

628. W. Seidel, H. Meyer, L. Born, S. Kazda, and W. Dompert in ref. 78, pp. 366–369.

629. R. Mannhold, *Drugs of Today*, **20**, 69–90 (1984).

630. M. Mahmoudian and W. G. Richards, *J. Pharm. Pharmacol.*, **38**, 272–276 (1986).

631. A. Goll, H. Glossmann, and R. Mannhold, *Arch. Pharmacol.*, **334**, 303–312 (1986).

632. R. Mannhold, R. Bayer, M. Ronsdorf, and L. Martens, *Arzneim.-Forsch. (Drug Res.)*, **37**, 419–424 (1987).

633. R. A. Coburn, M. Wierzba, M. J. Suto, A. J. Solo, A. M. Triggle, and D. J. Triggle, *J. Med. Chem.*, **31**, 2103–2107 (1988).

634. K. Mitani, T. Yoshida, E. Koshinaka, H. Kato, Y. Ito, and T. Fujita, *Chem. Pharm. Bull.*, **36**, 776–783 (1988).

635. K. Mitani, S. Sakurai, T. Suzuki, K. Morikawa, E. Koshinaka, H. Kato, Y. Ito, and T. Fujita, *Chem. Pharm. Bull.*, **36**, 4103–4120 (1988).

636. K. Mitani, S. Sakurai, T. Suzuki, K. Morikawa, E. Koshinaka, H. Kato, Y. Ito, and T. Fujita, *Chem. Pharm. Bull.*, **36**, 4121–4135 (1988).

637. G. E. Bass, L. J. Powers, and E. O. Dillingham, *J. Pharm. Sci.*, **65**, 1525–1527 (1976).

638. P. G. De Benedetti, *Fortschr. Arzneimittelforsch. (Prog. Drug Res.)*, **36**, 361–417 (1991).

639. B. H. Venger, C. Hansch, G. J. Hatheway, and Y. U. Amrein, *J. Med. Chem.*, **22**, 473–476 (1979).

640. C. Hansch, B. H. Venger, and A. Panthananickal, *J. Med. Chem.*, **23**, 459–461 (1980).

641. A. Leo, A. Panthananickal, C. Hansch, J. Theiss, M. Shimkin, and A. W. Andrews, *J. Med. Chem.*, **24**, 859–864 (1981).

642. C. Hansch, *Sci. Total Environ.*, **109–110**, 17–30 (1991).

643. E. J. Lien, *Ann. Rev. Pharmacol. Toxicol.*, **21**, 31–61 (1981).

644. V. Austel and E. Kutter in ref. 44, pp. 437–496.

645. E. J. Lien, *Fortschr. Arzneimittelforsch. (Prog. Drug Res.)*, **29**, 67–95 (1985).

646. J. M. Mayer and H. van de Waterbeemd, *Environ. Health Perspect.*, **61**, 295–306 (1985).

647. C. Hansch, A. R. Steward, S. M. Anderson, and D. Bentley, *J. Med. Chem.*, **11**, 1–11 (1968).

648. C. Hansch, *Farmaco Ed. Sci.*, **23**, 293–320 (1968).

649. C. Hansch, A. R. Steward, and J. Iwasa, *Mol. Pharmacol.*, **1**, 87–92 (1965).

650. E. J. Lien, G. L. Tong, J. T. Chou, and L. L. Lien, *J. Pharm. Sci.*, **62**, 246–250 (1973).

651. D. D. Dischino, M. J. Welch, M. R. Kilbourn, and M. E. Raichle, *J. Nucl. Med.*, **24**, 1030–1038 (1983).

652. C. Hansch, J. P. Björkroth, and A. Leo, *J. Pharm. Sci.*, **76**, 663–687 (1987).

653. H. van de Waterbeemd and M. Kansy, *Chimia*, **46**, 299–303 (1992).

654. C. Hansch, J. F. Sinclair, and P. R. Sinclair, *Quant. Struct.-Act. Relat.*, **9**, 223–226 (1990).

655. J. P. Akbaraly, J. J. Leng, G. Bozler, and J. K. Seydel in ref. 78, pp. 313–317.

656. M. Recanatini, P. Valenti, and P. Da Re, *Quant. Struct.-Act. Relat.*, **7**, 12–18 (1988).

657. S. Dove, A. Koch, and R. Franke, *Acta Pharm. Jugosl.*, **36**, 119–134 (1986).

658. P. N. Craig and C. H. Hansch, *J. Med. Chem.*, **16**, 661–667 (1973).

659. K. H. Kim, C. Hansch, J. Y. Fukunaga, E. E. Steller, P. Y. C. Jow, P. N. Craig, and J. Page, *J. Med. Chem.*, **22**, 366–391 (1979).

660. F. Rippmann, *Quant. Struct.-Act. Relat.*, **9**, 1–5 (1990).

661. C. Hansch, *Farmaco Ed. Sci.*, **34**, 89–104 (1979).

662. R. F. Rekker, *Dev. Pharmacol.*, **3**, 23–46 (1983).

663. H. Kubinyi, *J. Cancer Res. Clin. Oncol.*, **116**, 529–537 (1990).

664. A. Panthananickal, C. Hansch, A. Leo, and F. R. Quinn, *J. Med. Chem.*, **21**, 16–26 (1978).

665. G. J. Hatheway, C. Hansch, K. H. Kim, S. R. Milstein, C. L. Schmidt, R. N. Smith, and F. R. Quinn, *J. Med. Chem.*, **21**, 563–574 (1978).

666. C. Hansch, G. J. Hatheway, F. R. Quinn, and N. Greenberg, *J. Med. Chem.*, **21**, 574–577 (1978).

667. A. Panthananickal, C. Hansch, and A. Leo, *J. Med. Chem.*, **22**, 1267–1269 (1979).

668. C. Hansch, A. Leo, C. Schmidt, P. Y. C. Low, and J. A. Montgomery, *J. Med. Chem.*, **23**, 1095–1101 (1980).

669. W. A. Denny, B. F. Cain, G. J. Atwell, C. Hansch, A. Panthananickal, and A. Leo, *J. Med. Chem.*, **25**, 276–315 (1982).

670. S. P. Gupta, P. Singh, and M. C. Bindal, *Chem. Rev.*, **83**, 633–649 (1983).

671. S. P. Gupta, *Chem. Rev.*, **89**, 1765–1800 (1989).

672. F. J. Zeelen, *Quant. Struct.-Act. Relat.*, **5**, 131–137 (1986).

673. P. B. M. W. M. Timmermans, A. de Jonge, J. C. A. van Meel, F. P. Slothorst-Grisdijk, E. Lam, and P. A. van Zwieten, *J. Med. Chem.*, **24**, 502–507 (1981).

674. P. B. M. W. M. Timmermans, A. de Jonge, M. J. M. C. Thoolen, B. Wilffert, H. Batink, and P. A. van Zwieten, *J. Med. Chem.*, **27**, 495–503 (1984).

675. H. Kubinyi, *Chemie in unserer Zeit*, **20**, 191–202 (1986).

676. H. Kubinyi, *Physical Property Prediction in Organic Chemistry*, C. Jochum, M. G. Hicks, and J. Sunkel, Eds., Springer-Verlag, Berlin, 1988, pp. 235–247.

677. P. J. Lewi, *Arzneim.-Forsch. (Drug Res.)*, **26**, 1295–1300 (1976).

678. P. J. Lewi, *Drug Design*, Vol. VII, E. J. Ariëns, Ed., Academic Press, New York, 1976, pp. 209–278.

679. P. J. Lewi, *Chemom. Intell. Lab. Syst.*, **5**, 105–116 (1989).

680. M. Nendza and J. K. Seydel, *Quant. Struct.-Act. Relat.*, **7**, 165–174 (1988); erratum **7**, 250 (1988).

681. J. C. Phillips, W. B. Gibson, J. Yam, C. L. Alden, and G. C. Hard, *Food Chem. Toxicol.*, **28**, 375–394 (1990).

682. P. N. Craig, *J. Med. Chem.*, **15**, 144–149 (1972).

683. R. Katz, S. F. Osborne, and F. Ionescu, *J. Med. Chem.*, **20**, 1413–1419 (1977).

684. T. Ban and T. Fujita, *J. Med. Chem.*, **12**, 353–356 (1969).

685. D. Labes and V. Hagen, *Pharmazie*, **34**, 554–556 (1979).

686. M. C. Bindal, P. Singh, and S. P. Gupta, *Arzneim.-Forsch. (Drug Res.)* **32**, 719–721 (1982).

687. J. Kelder, T. de Boer, J. S. de Graaf, and J. H. Wieringa in ref. 78, pp. 162–169.

688. F. B. Abramson, R. B. Barlow, M. G. Mustafa, and R. P. Stephenson, *Br. J. Pharmac.*, **37**, 207–233 (1969).

689. D. L. Duewer, *J. Chemometrics*, **4**, 299–321 (1990).

690. P. A. Lehmann, J. F. Rodrigues de Miranda, and E. J. Ariëns, *Fortschr. Arzneimittelforsch. (Prog. Drug Res.)*, **20**, 101–142 (1976).

691. E. J. Ariëns, *Eur. J. Clin. Pharmacol.*, **26**, 663–668 (1984).

692. E. J. Ariëns, *Trends Pharmacol. Sci.*, **7**, 200–205 (1986).

693. P. A. Lehmann F., *Trends Pharmacol. Sci.*, **7**, 281–285 (1986).

694. E. J. Ariëns, *Med. Res. Rev.*, **7**, 367–387 (1987).

695. E. J. Ariëns in ref. 82, pp. 3–6.

696. E. J. Ariëns, *Chirality in Drug Design and Synthesis*, C. Brown, Ed., Academic Press, New York, 1990, pp. 29–43.

697. E. J. Ariëns, *Quant. Struct.-Act. Relat.*, **11**, 190–194 (1992).

698. E. J. Lien, J. F. Rodrigues de Miranda, and E. J. Ariëns, *Mol. Pharmacol.* **12**, 598–604 (1976).

699. C. C. Pfeiffer, *Science*, **124**, 29–30 (1956).

700. R. B. Barlow, *Trends Pharmacol. Sci.*, **11**, 148–150 (1990).

701. F. Gualtieri, *Trends Pharmacol. Sci.*, **11**, 315–316 (199).

702. F. Gualtieri, M. N. Romanelli, and E. Teodori, *Chirality*, **2**, 79–84 (1990).

703. E. Teodori, M. N. Romanelli, and F. Gualtieri in ref. 83, pp. 451–456.

704. P. A. Lehmann F. in ref. 83, pp. 457–460.

705. K.-J. Schaper in ref. 82, pp. 41–44.

706. K.-J. Schaper in ref. 83, pp. 25–32.

707. M. Yoshimoto and C. Hansch, *J. Org. Chem.*, **41**, 2269–2273 (1976).

708. A. H. Beckett and A. F. Casy, *J. Pharm. Pharmacol.*, **6**, 986–999 (1954).

709. L. B. Kier, *Fundamental Concepts in Drug-Receptor Interactions*, J. F. Danielli, J. F. Moran, and D. J. Triggle, Eds., Academic Press, New York, 1968, pp. 15–45.

710. P. Gund, *Ann. Rep. Med. Chem.*, **14**, 299–308 (1979).

711. C. Humblet and G. R. Marshall, *Ann. Rep. Med. Chem.*, **15**, 267–276 (1980).

712. G. R. Marshall and C. B. Naylor in ref. 39, pp. 431–458.

713. P. Gund and T. Y. Shen, *J. Med. Chem.*, **20**, 1146–1152 (1977).

714. T. A. Andrea, E. C. Jorgensen, and P. A. Kollman, *Int. J. Quantum. Chem.*, *Quantum Biol. Symp.*, **5**, 191–200 (1978).

715. G. L. Olson, H.-C. Cheung, K. D. Morgan, J. F. Blount, L. Todaro, L. Berger, A. B. Davidson, and E. Boff, *J. Med. Chem.*, **24**, 1026–1034 (1981).

716. J. R. Sufrin, D. A. Dunn, and G. R. Marshall, *Mol. Pharmacol.*, **19**, 307–313 (1981).

717. L. G. Humber, F. T. Bruderlein, A. H. Philipp, M. Götz, and K. Voith, *J. Med. Chem.*, **22**, 761–767 (1986).

718. M. F. Hibert, M. W. Gittos, D. N. Middlemiss, A. K. Mir, and J. R. Fozard, *J. Med. Chem.*, **31**, 1087–1093 (1988).

719. M. Ohta and H. Koga, *J. Med. Chem.*, **34**, 131–139 (1991).

720. H.-D. Höltje, *Pharmazie in unserer Zeit*, **4**, 109–117 (1975).

721. H.-D. Höltje, M. Tintelnot, and P. Baranowski, *Proceedings of the 9th International Congress of Pharmacology*, Vol. 2, W. Paton, J. Mitchell, and P. Turner, Eds., The Macmillan Press, London, 1984, pp. 75–79.

722. H.-D. Höltje, P. Baranowski, J.-P. Spengler, and W. Schunack, *Arch. Pharm.*, **318**, 542–548 (1985).

723. H.-D. Höltje and L. B. Kier, *J. Pharm. Sci.*, **64**, 418–420 (1975).

724. H.-D. Höltje, *Pharm. Acta Helv.*, **54**, 125–134 (1979).

725. H.-D. Höltje, *Arch. Pharm.*, **308**, 438–444 (1975).

726. H.-D. Höltje, *Arch. Pharm.*, **309**, 480–485 (1976).

727. H.-D. Höltje and L. Vogelgesang, *Arch. Pharm.*, **312**, 578–586 (1979).

728. H.-D. Höltje and P. Adler, *Arch. Pharm.*, **320**, 234–240 (1987).

729. H.-D. Höltje, *Arch. Pharm.*, **315**, 317–323 (1982).

730. H.-D. Höltje and P. Baranowski, *Arch. Pharm.*, **316**, 154–160 (1983).

731. H.-D. Höltje and S. Marrer, *J. Comput.-Aided Mol. Des.*, **1**, 23–30 (1987).

732. H.-D. Höltje and S. Marrer, *Quant. Struct.-Act. Relat.*, **7**, 174–178 (1988).

733. H.-D. Höltje in ref. 82, pp. 237–241.

734. H.-D. Höltje, *Quant. Struct.-Act. Relat.*, **11**, 224–227 (1992).

735. H.-D. Höltje and H. Briem in ref. 83, pp. 245–252.

736. H.-D. Höltje and H. Simon, *Arch. Pharm.*, **317**, 506–516 (1984).

737. H.-D. Höltje and P. Zunker, *J. Mol. Struct. (Theochem)*, **134**, 429–436 (1986).

738. H.-D. Höltje in ref. 64, pp. 181–189.

739. D. N. A. Boobbyer, P. J. Goodford, P. M. McWhinnie, and R. C. Wade, *J. Med. Chem.*, **32**, 1083–1094 (1989).

740. E. Audry, J. P. Dubost, J. C. Colleter, and P. Dallet, *Eur. J. Med. Chem.*, **21**, 71–72 (1986).

741. F. Croizet, M. H. Langlois, J. P. Dubost, P. Braquet, E. Audry, P. Dallet, and J. C. Colleter, *J. Mol. Graphics*, **8**, 153–155 (1990).

742. F. Croizet, J. P. Dubost, M. H. Langlois, and E. Audry, *Quant. Struct.-Act. Relat.*, **10**, 211–215 (1991).

743. D. J. Abraham and A. J. Leo, *Proteins: Struct. Funct. Genetics*, **2**, 130–152 (1987).

744. F. C. Wireko, G. E. Kellog, and D. J. Abraham, *J. Med. Chem.*, **34**, 758–767 (1991).

745. G. E. Kellog, S. F. Semus, and D. J. Abraham, *J. Comput.-Aided Mol. Des.*, **5**, 545–552 (1991).

746. G. E. Kellog, G. S. Joshi, and D. J. Abraham, *Med. Chem. Res.*, **1**, 444–453 (1992).

747. G. M. Crippen, *J. Comput. Phys.*, **24**, 96–107 (1977).

748. G. M. Donné-Op den Kelder, *J. Comput.-Aided Mol. Des.*, **1**, 257–264 (1987).

749. G. M. Donné-Op den Kelder, *Trends Pharmacol. Sci.*, **9**, 391–393 (1988).

750. A. K. Ghose and G. M. Crippen in ref. 39, pp. 715–733.

751. G. M. Crippen, *J. Med. Chem.*, **23**, 599–606 (1980).

752. A. K. Ghose and G. M. Crippen, *J. Med. Chem.*, **26**, 996–1010 (1983).

753. *Ibid.*, **27**, 901–914 (1984).

754. *Ibid.*, **28**, 333–346 (1985).

755. G. M. Crippen, *J. Comput. Chem.*, **8**, 943–955 (1987).

756. L. G. Boulu and G. M. Crippen, *J. Comput. Chem.*, **10**, 673–682 (1989).

757. L. G. Boulu, G. M. Crippen, H. A. Barton, H. Kwon, and M. A. Marletta, *J. Med. Chem.*, **33**, 771–775 (1990).

758. A. K. Ghose, G. M. Crippen, G. Revankar, P. A. McKernan, D. F. Smee, and R. K. Robins, *J. Med. Chem.*, **32**, 746–756 (1989).

759. A. K. Ghose and G. M. Crippen, *Mol. Pharmacol.*, **37**, 725–734 (1990).

760. V. N. Viswanadhan, A. K. Ghose, and J. N. Weinstein, *Biochem. Biophys. Acta*, **1039**, 356–366 (1990).

761. V. N. Viswanadhan, A. K. Ghose, N. B. Hanna, S. S. Matsumoto, T. L. Avery, G. R. Revankar, and R. K. Robins, *J. Med. Chem.*, **34**, 526–532 (1991).

762. A. M. Doweyko, *J. Med. Chem.*, **41**, 1396–1406 (1988).

763. M. Wiese and E. A. Coats in ref. 83, pp. 343–346.

764. V. E. Golender and A. B. Rozenblit, *Drug Design*, Vol. IX, E. J. Ariëns, Eds., Academic Press, New York, 1980, pp. 299–337.

765. E. Vorpagel, C. Herd, and V. Golender, personal communication.

766. Apex-3D, BIOSYM Technologies, Inc., San Diego, Calif.

767. R. D. Cramer III and M. Milne, *Abstracts of Papers, Am. Chem. Soc.*, April 1979, Computer Chemistry Section, no. 44.

768. M. Wise, R. D. Cramer, D. Smith, and I. Exman in ref. 75, pp. 145–146.

769. M. Wise, *Molecular Graphics and Drug Design*, *Top. Mol. Pharmacol.*, **3**, A. S. V. Burgen, G. C. K. Roberts, and M. S. Tute, eds., Elsevier, New York, 1986, pp. 183–194.

770. SYBYL/QSAR, Version 5.5, February 1992; TRIPOS Associates, Inc., St. Louis, Missouri.

771. G. R. Marshall and R. D. Cramer III, *Trends Pharmacol. Sci.*, **9**, 285–289 (1988).

772. R. D. Cramer III, D. E. Patterson, and J. D. Bunce in ref. 82, pp. 161–165.

773. R. S. Pearlman, *Chem. Design Automation News*, **2**(1), 1–7 (1987); **8**(8), 3–15 (1993).

774. A. Rusinko III, J. M. Skell, R. Balcucci, C. M. McGarity, and R. S. Pearlman, CONCORD, Tripos Associates, Inc., St. Louis, Missouri.

775. W. T. Wipke and M. A. Hahn, *Tetrahedron Comp. Methodology*, **1**, 141–167 (1988).

776. D. P. Dolata and R. E. Carter, *J. Chem. Inf. Comput. Sci.*, **27**, 36–47 (1987).

777. D. P. Dolata, A. R. Leach, and K. Prout, *J. Comput.-Aided Mol. Des.*, **1**, 73–85 (1987).

778. A. R. Leach, K. Prout, and D. P. Dolata, *J. Comput.-Aided Mol. Des.*, **2**, 107–123 (1988); **4**, 271–282 (1990).

779. A. R. Leach, K. Prout, and D. P. Dolata, *J. Comput. Chem.*, **11**, 680–693 (1990).

780. A. R. Leach and K. Prout, *J. Comput. Chem.*, **11**, 1193–1205 (1990).

781. J. Gasteiger, C. Rudolph, and J. Sadowski, *Tetrahedron Comp. Methodology*, **3**, 537–547 (1990).

782. G. Klebe and T. Mietzner, *Organic Crystal Chemistry*, D. W. Jones, Ed., Oxford University Press, Oxford, in press.

783. A. R. Leach, *Reviews in Computational Chemistry*, Vol. II, K. B. Lipkowitz and D. B. Boyd, Eds., VCH Publishers, New York, 1991, pp. 1–55.

784. P. M. Dean in ref. 63, pp. 211–238.

785. Y. C. Martin, M. G. Bures, and P. Willett, *Reviews in Computational Chemistry*, K. B. Lipkowitz and D. B. Boyd, Eds., VCH Publishers, New York, 1990, pp. 213–263.

786. G. R. Marshall, C. D. Barry, A. E. Bosshard, R. A. Dammkoehler, and D. A. Dunn in ref. 72, pp. 205–226.

787. C. Humblet and G. R. Marshall, *Drug. Dev. Res.*, **1**, 409–434 (1981).

788. D. Mayer, C. B. Naylor, I. Motoc, and G. R. Marshall, *J. Comput.-Aided Mol. Des.*, **1**, 3–16 (1987).

789. R. A. Dammkoehler, S. F. Karasek, E. F. B. Shands, and G. R. Marshall, *J. Comput.-Aided Mol. Des.*, **3**, 3–21 (1989).

790. A. T. Brint and P. Willett, *J. Chem. Inf. Comput. Sci.*, **27**, 152–158 (1987).

791. S. Namasivayam and P. M. Dean, *J. Mol. Graphics*, **4**, 46–50 (1986).

792. P. M. Dean and P.-L. Chau, *J. Mol. Graphics*, **5**, 152–158 (1987).

793. P. M. Dean, P. Callow, and P.-L. Chau, *J. Mol. Graphics* **6**, 28–34 (1988).

794. Y. Kato, A. Itai, and Y. Iitaka, *Tetrahedron*, **43**, 5229–5236 (1987).

795. A. Itai, N. Tomioka, Y. Kato, Y. Nishibata, and S. Saito in ref. 64, pp. 191–212.

796. F. Manaut, E. Lozoya, and F. Sanz in ref. 83, pp. 339–342.

797. R. B. Hermann and D. K. Herron, *J. Comput.-Aided Mol. Des.*, **5**, 511–524 (1991).

798. J. H. Van Drie, D. Weininger, and Y. C. Martin, *J. Comput.-Aided Mol. Des.*, **3**, 225–251 (1989).

799. Y. C. Martin, M. G. Bures, E. A. Danaher, J. DeLazzer, I. Lico, and P. A. Pavlik, *J. Comput.-Aided Mol. Des.*, **7**, 83–102 (1993).

800. T. Imoto, L. N. Johnson, A. C. T. North, D. C. Phillips, and J. A. Rupley, *The Enzymes*, 3rd Ed., Vol. VII, P. D. Boyer, ed., Academic Press, New York, 1972, pp. 665–868.

801. W. R. Kester and B. W. Matthews, *Biochemistry*, **16**, 2506–2516 (1977).

802. J. T. Bolin, D. J. Filman, D. A. Matthews, R. C. Hamlin, and J. Kraut, *J. Biol. Chem.*, **257**, 13650–13662 (1982).

803. C. Bystroff, S. J. Oatley, and J. Kraut, *Biochemistry*, **29**, 3263–3277 (1990).

804. G. D. Diana, A. M. Treasurywala, T. T. Bailey, R. C. Oglesby, D. C. Pevear, and F. J. Dutko, *J. Med. Chem.*, **33**, 1306–1311 (1990).

805. T. L. Poulos and A. J. Howard, *Biochemistry*, **26**, 8165–8174 (1987).

806. V. Cody and P. A. Sutton in ref. 82, pp. 247–250.

807. J. J. Baldwin, G. S. Ponticello, P. S. Anderson, M. E. Christy, M. A. Murcko, W. C. Randall, H. Schwam, M. F. Sugrue, J. P. Springer, P. Gautheron, J. Grove, P. Mallorga, M.-P. Viader, B. M. McKeever, and M. A. Navia, *J. Med. Chem.*, **32**, 2510–2513 (1989).

808. (a) S. E. Ealick, Y. S. Babu, C. E. Bugg, M. D. Erion, W. C. Guida, J. A. Montgomery, and J. A. Secrist III, *Proc. Natl. Acad. Sci. U.S.A.*, **88**, 11540–11544 (1991); (b) J. A. Montgomery, S. Niwas, J. D. Rose, J. A. Secrist III, Y. S. Babu,

C. E. Bugg, M. D. Erion, W. C. Guide, and S. E. Ealick, *J. Med. Chem.*, **36**, 55–69 (1993).

809. D. W. Banner and P. Hadváry, *J. Biol. Chem.*, **266**, 20085–20093 (1991).

810. H. Brandstetter, D. Turk, H. W. Hoeffken, D. Grosse, J. Stürzebecher, P. D. Martin, B. F. P. Edwards, and W. Bode, *J. Mol. Biol.*, **226**, 1085–1099 (1992).

811. A. Wojtczak, J. Luft, and V. Cody, *J. Biol. Chem.*, **267**, 353–357 (1992).

812. S. L. Roderick, M. C. Fournie-Zaluski, B. P. Roques, and B. W. Matthews, *Biochemistry*, **28**, 1493–1497 (1989).

813. M. Clark, R. D. Cramer III, D. M. Jones, D. E. Patterson, and P. E. Simeroth, *Tetrahedron Comp. Methodology*, **3**, 47–59 (1990).

814. R. D. Cramer III, M. Clark, P. Simeroth, and D. E. Patterson in ref. 83, pp. 239–242.

815. G. Klebe and U. Abraham, *J. Med. Chem.*, **36**, 70–80 (1993).

816. M. Clark and R. D. Cramer III, *Quant. Struct.-Act. Relat.*, **12**, 137–145 (1993).

817. U. Norinder, *J. Comput.-Aided Mol. Des.*, **5**, 419–426 (1991).

818. *Ibid.*, **4**, 381–389 (1990).

819. K. H. Kim and Y. C. Martin, *J. Org. Chem.*, **56**, 2723–2729 (1991).

820. K. H. Kim and Y. C. Martin in ref. 83, pp. 151–154.

821. K. H. Kim and Y. C. Martin, *J. Med. Chem.*, **34**, 2056–2060 (1991).

822. H. van de Waterbeemd, P. A. Carrupt, N. El Tayar, B. Testa, and L. B. Kier, ref. 84, pp. 69–75.

823. K. H. Kim, *Med. Chem. Res.*, **1**, 259–264 (1991).

824. K. H. Kim, *Quant. Struct.-Act. Relat.*, **11**, 127–134 (1992).

825. Y. C. Martin, K.-H. Kim, and M. G. Bures in ref. 64, pp. 295–317.

826. K. H. Kim, *Quant. Struct.-Act. Relat.*, **11**, 453–460 (1992).

827. K. H. Kim in ref. 84, pp. 245–251.

828. T. I. Oprea, D. Ciubotariu, T. I. Sulea, and Z. Simon, *Quant. Struct.-Act. Relat.*, **12**, 21–26 (1993).

829. K. H. Kim, *Med. Chem. Res.*, **2**, 22–27 (1992).

830. K. H. Kim, *Quant. Struct.-Act. Relat.*, **11**, 309–317 (1992).

831. G. R. Marshall, D. Mayer, C. B. Naylor, E. E. Hodgkin, and R. D. Cramer III in ref. 82, pp. 287–295.

832. S. A. DePriest, E. F. B. Shands, R. A. Dammkoehler, and G. R. Marshall in ref. 83, pp. 405–414.

833. M. C. Nicklaus, G. W. A. Milne, and T. R. Burke Jr., *J. Comput.-Aided Mol. Des.*, **6**, 487–504 (1992).

834. G. Maret, N. El Tayar, P.-A. Carrupt, B. Testa, P. Jenner, and M. Baird, *Biochem. Pharmacol.*, **40**, 783–792 (1990).

835. C. Altomare, P. A. Carrupt, P. Gaillard, N. El Tayar, B. Testa, and A. Carotti, *Chem. Res. Toxicol.*, **5**, 366–375 (1992).

836. M. S. Allen, Y.-C. Tan, M. L. Trudell, K. Narayanan, L. R. Schindler, M. J. Martin, C. Schultz, T. J. Hagen, K. F. Koehler, P. W. Codding, P. Skolnick, and J. M. Cook, *J. Med. Chem.*, **33**, 2343–2357 (1990).

837. M. S. Allen, A. J. LaLoggia, L. J. Dorn, M. J. Martin, G. Costantino, T. J. Hagen, K. F. Koehler, P. Skolnick, and J. M. Cook, *J. Med. Chem.*, **35**, 4001–4010 (1992).

838. G. Greco, E. Novellino, C. Silipo, and A. Vittoria, *Quant. Struct.-Act. Relat.*, **11**, 461–477 (1992).

839. B. F. Thomas, D. R. Compton, B. R. Martin, and S. F. Semus, *Mol. Pharmacol.*, **40**, 656–665 (1991).

840. S. Rault, R. Bureau, J. C. Pilo, and M. Robba, *J. Comput.-Aided Mol. Des.*, **6**, 553–568 (1992).

841. F. I. Carroll, Y. Gao, M. A. Rahman, P. Abraham, K. Parham, A. H. Lewin, J. W. Boja, and M. J. Kuhar, *J. Med. Chem.*, **34**, 2719–2725 (1991).

842. J. F. Liegeois, L. Dupont, and J. Delarge, *J. Pharm. Belg.*, **47**, 100–108 (1992).

843. U. Norinder and T. Högberg, *Quant. Struct.-Act. Relat.*, **10**, 1–5 (1991); erratum **10**, 141 (1991).

844. G. Greco, E. Novellino, C. Silipo, and A. Vittoria, *Quant. Struct.-Act. Relat.*, **10**, 289–299 (1991).

845. L. Naerum and J. S. Jensen in ref. 83, pp. 489–492.

846. S. Y. Ablordeppey, M. B. El-Ashmawy, and R. A. Glennon, *Med. Chem. Res.*, **1**, 425–438 (1991).

847. M. A. El-Bermawy, H. Lotter, and R. A. Glennon, *Med. Chem. Res.*, **2**, 290–297 (1992).

848. C. L. Waller and J. D. McKinney, *J. Med. Chem.*, **35**, 3660–3666 (1992).

849. G. D. Diana, P. Kowalczyk, A. M. Treasurywala, R. C. Oglesby, D. C. Pevear, and F. J. Dutko, *J. Med. Chem.*, **35**, 1002–1008 (1992).

850. D. Rognan, M. J. Reddehase, U. H. Koszinowski, and G. Folkers, *Proteins*, **13**, 70–85 (1992).

851. U. Thibaut, G. Folkers, and H. J. Roth in ref. 83, pp. 431–434.

852. J.-P. Björkroth, T. A. Pakkanen, J. Lindroos, E. Pohjala, H. Hanhijärvi, L. Laurén, R. Hannuniemi, A. Juhakoski, K. Kippo, and T. Kleimola, *J. Med. Chem.*, **34**, 2338–2343 (1991).

853. J. W. McFarland, *J. Med. Chem.*, **35**, 2543–2550 (1992).

854. C. Hansch, *J. Med. Chem.*, **19**, 1–6 (1976).

855. C. Hansch in ref. 70, pp. 47–61.

856. C. Hansch, *Drug Rev. Res.*, **1**, 267–309 (1981).

857. Y. C. Martin, *J. Med. Chem.*, **24**, 229–237 (1981).

858. T. Fujita in ref. 46, pp. 19–33.

859. A. J. Hopfinger, *J. Med. Chem.*, **28**, 1133–1139 (1985).

860. D. B. Boyd, *Reviews in Computational Chemistry*, K. B. Lipkowitz and D. B. Boyd, Eds., VCH Publishers, New York, 1990, pp. 355–371.

861. T. Fujita, *QSAR in Design of Bioactive Compounds*, M. Kuchar, Ed., Prous Science Publishers, Barcelona, 1992, pp. 3–22.

862. C. Hansch in ref. 64, pp. 281–293.

863. S. Wold, P. Berntsson, L. Eriksson, G. Geladi, S. Hellberg, E. Johansson, J. Jonsson, M. Kettaneh-Wold, F. Lindgren, S. Rännar, M. Sandberg, and M. Sjöström in ref. 83, pp. 15–24.

864. Y. C. Martin, *Methods Enzymol*, **203**, 587–613 (1991).

865. G. R. Marshall in ref. 64, pp. 163–178.

866. R. Mannhold, *Quant. Struct.-Act. Relat.*, **11**, 232–236 (1992).

867. H. Kubinyi, *QSAR. Hansch Analysis and Related Approaches*, *Methods and Principles in Medicinal Chemistry*, R. Mannhold, P. Krogsgaard-Larsen, and H. Timmerman, Eds., Vol. 1, VCH, Weinheim, 1993.

CHAPTER FIFTEEN

Molecular Modeling in Drug Design

GARLAND R. MARSHALL

Center for Molecular Design
Washington University
St. Louis, Missouri, USA

CONTENTS

1 Introduction, 574

2 Background and Methods, 575
  2.1 Molecular mechanics, 575
    2.1.1 Force fields, 575
    2.1.2 Electrostatics, 578
    2.1.3 The potential surface, 582
    2.1.4 Systematic search and conformational analysis, 583
    2.1.5 Statistical mechanics, 589
    2.1.6 Molecular dynamics, 590
    2.1.7 Monte Carlo simulations, 592
    2.1.8 Thermodynamic cycle integration, 594
    2.1.9 Non-Boltzmann sampling, 595
  2.2 Quantum mechanics: applications in molecular mechanics, 596
    2.2.1 Charge and electrostatics, 596
    2.2.2 Parameter development for force fields, 598
    2.2.3 Modeling chemical reactions and design of transition-state inhibitors, 599

3 Known Receptors, 599
  3.1 Definition of site, 600
  3.2 Characterization of site, 604
    3.2.1 Hydrogen bonding and other group binding sites, 604
    3.2.2 Electrostatic and hydrophobic fields, 605
  3.3 Design of ligands, 607
    3.3.1 Visually assisted design, 607
    3.3.2 Three-dimensional databases, 607
    3.3.3 *De Novo* design, 610
  3.4 Calculation of affinity, 613

Burger's Medicinal Chemistry and Drug Discovery,
Fifth Edition, Volume 1: Principles and Practice,
Edited by Manfred E. Wolff.
ISBN 0-471-57556-9   © 1995 John Wiley & Sons, Inc.

    3.4.1 Components of binding affinity, 613
    3.4.2 Binding energetics and comparisons, 614
    3.4.3 Simulations and the thermodynamic
          cycle, 615
    3.4.4 Multiple binding modes, 617
  3.5 Homology modeling, 617
4 Unknown Receptors, 618
  4.1 Pharmacophore versus binding-site
      models, 619
    4.1.1 Pharmacophore models, 619
    4.1.2 Binding-site models, 621
    4.1.3 Molecular extensions, 622
    4.1.4 Activity versus affinity, 623
  4.2 Searching for similarity, 627
    4.2.1 Simple comparisons, 627
    4.2.2 Visualization of molecular
          properties, 628
  4.3 Molecular comparisons, 631
    4.3.1 Volume mapping, 631
    4.3.2 Field effects, 632
    4.3.3 Directionality, 633
    4.3.4 Locus maps, 633
    4.3.5 Vector maps and conformational
          mimicry, 633
  4.4 Finding the common pattern, 635
    4.4.1 Constrained minimization, 636
    4.4.2 Systematic search and the active analog
          approach, 637
    4.4.3 Strategic reductions of computational
          complexity, 638
    4.4.4 Alternative approaches, 640
    4.4.5 Receptor mapping, 642
    4.4.6 Model receptor sites, 644
    4.4.7 Assessment of model predictability, 645
5 Conclusion, 649

1 INTRODUCTION

By historical imperative, the role of molecular modeling in drug design has been divided into two separate paradigms: one centered on the structure–activity problem, which attempts to rationalize biological activity in the absence of detailed, three-dimensional structural information about the receptor, and the other focused on understanding the interactions seen in receptor–ligand complexes, which uses the known three-dimensional structure of the therapeutic target to design novel drugs. The rapid increase in relevant structural information, as a result of advances in molecular biology that is used to generate the target proteins in adequate quantities for study, and the equally impressive gains in NMR (1–3) and crystallography that provide three-dimensional structures have stimulated the need for design tools, and the molecular modeling community is rapidly evolving useful approaches. The more common problem, however, is one in which the receptor can only be inferred from pharmacological studies and little, if any, structural information is available to guide modeling. Nevertheless, useful information that can guide the design and synthesis of potential novel therapeutics can be developed from an analysis of structure–activity data in the three-dimensional framework provided by current molecular modeling techniques. While most of the techniques and approaches described here have broader application than shown, the examples chosen should be sufficient to illustrate their use. A number of reviews (4–8) of computer-aided drug design have relevant sections covering portions of this chapter and are recommended for a more complete overview.

2 BACKGROUND AND METHODS

2.1 Molecular Mechanics

Molecular mechanics treats a molecule as a collection of atoms whose interactions can be described by Newtonian mechanics (9). Because the mass of the nuclei is much greater than the mass of the electrons, one can separate (the Born-Oppenheimer approximation) the Schrödinger equation into a product of two functions: one for electrons and one for nuclei. For the purposes of molecular mechanics, which was initially developed to interpret spectroscopic data, the electronic function is ignored, i.e., the charge distribution is assumed to remain constant during changes in the position of the nuclei. Because molecular mechanics is based on classical physics, it cannot provide information about the electronic properties of molecules under study that are generally assumed fixed during the parameterization of the force field with experimental data.

A few words about the basics of molecular mechanics (9, 10) may provide the elements of understanding for what follows. This is not meant to be comprehensive, but rather a simple overview to remind the reader of a few crucial points. The interactions between atoms are divided into bonded and nonbonded classes. Nonbonded forces between atoms are based on

an attractive interaction that has a firm theoretical basis and varies as the inverse of the 6th power of the distance between the atoms. It is balanced by a repulsion between the electronic clouds as the atoms come close, and this interaction has been represented empirically by a variety of functional forms, exponential, 12th power or 9th power of the distance between the atoms. The coefficients for these two interactions are parameterized for atom types, usually by element, so that the minimum of the combined functions corresponds to the sum of the experimental van der Waals radii for the two atoms.

In addition, bonded atoms are considered a special case with a "spring constant" determining the energy of deformation from experimental bond lengths. Atoms directly bonded to the same atom (one–three interactions) are eliminated from the van der Waals list and have a special energetic term relating the deviation from an ideal bond angle. Atoms having a one–four interaction define a torsional relation that is usually parameterized based on the types of the four connected atoms defining the torsion angle. The numerous combinations of atom types require an enormous number of parameters to be determined from either theoretical (quantum mechanics) and/or experimental data. Simplified force fields in which the torsional parameters depend only on the atoms at the end of a bond have been developed to give approximate geometries for further refinement by quantum mechanics.

2.1.1 FORCE FIELDS. The basic assumption underlying molecular mechanics is that classical physical concepts can be used to represent the forces between atoms. In other words, one can approximate the potential energy surface by the summation of a set of equations representing pairwise and multibody interactions. These equations represent forces between atoms related to bonded and nonbonded interactions. Pairwise interactions are often represented by a harmonic potential ($1/2K_b[b - b_0]^2$) and obeying Hooke's law (derived for a spring) for bonded atoms restores the bond distance to an equilibrium value b_0 and for nonbonded atoms, to a van der Waals potential ($C_{12}(i, j)/r_{ij}^{12} - C_6(i, j)/r_{ij}^6$). Similarly, distortion from an equilibrium valence angle (θ_0) that describes the angle between three bonded atoms sharing a common atom is also penalized ($1/2K_\theta[\theta - \theta_0]^2$). A third class of interaction, which depends on the dihedral angle ϕ between four bonded atoms, is the torsional potential ($K_\phi[1 + \cos(\phi - \delta)]$) used to account for orbital delocalization and to compensate for other deficiencies in the force field. A harmonic term ($1/2K_\xi[\xi - \xi_0]^2$) is often introduced for dihedral angles ξ that are relatively fixed, such as those in aromatic rings. Coulomb's law ($q_i q_j/(4\pi\varepsilon_0\varepsilon_r r_{ij})$) is the simplest approach to the contribution of electrostatics to the potential V:

$$V = \sum 1/2K_b[b - b_0]^2 + \sum 1/2K_\theta[\theta - \theta_0]^2$$
$$+ \sum 1/2K_\xi[\xi - \xi_0]^2$$
$$+ \sum K_\phi[1 + \cos(\phi - \delta)]$$
$$+ \sum [C_{12}(i, j)/r_{ij}^{12} - C_6(i, j)/r_{ij}^6]$$
$$+ \sum q_i q_j/(4\pi\varepsilon_0\varepsilon_r r_{ij})$$

A central issue is the number of different atom types that are used in a particular force field. There is always a compromise between increasing the number to allow for the inclusion of more environmental effects versus the increase in the number of parameters to be determined to represent adequately a new atom type. In general, the more subtypes of atoms (how many different kinds of nitrogens, for example), the less likely that the parameters for a particular application will be available in the force field. The extreme, of course,

would be a special atom type for each kind of atomic environment in which the parameters were chosen so that the calculated properties of each molecule would simply reproduce the experimental observations. One major assumption, therefore, is that the force constants (parameters) and equilibrium values of the equations are functions of a limited number of atom types and can be transferred from one molecular environment to another. This assumption holds reasonably well when one is primarily interested in geometric issues, but is not as valid in molecular spectroscopy. This has led to the introduction of additional equations, the so-called cross-terms, that allow more parameters to account for correlations between bond lengths and bond angles ($K_{b\theta}[b - b_0][\theta - \theta_0]$), dihedral angles and bond angles, etc. Because of the lack of adequate parameterization of the more complex force fields, which are usually specialized to one kind of molecule (e.g., proteins or nucleic acids), more simplified force fields have gained some popularity because of their general applicability. Examples are the Tripos force field (11), the COSMIC force field (12), and the White and Bovill (13) force field that uses only two atom types (those at the end of the bond to parameterize the torsional potential rather than the four types of the atoms used to define the torsional angle). One only has to consider the number of combinations of 20 atom subtypes taken 4 at time (16,000) versus 2 at a time (400) to understand the explosion of parameters that occurs with increased atom subtypes. The simplifying assumption in parameterization of the torsional potential reduces to some extent the quality of the results (14) but allows the use of the simplified force fields (11) in many situations in which other force fields would lack appropriate parameters. The situation can become complicated, however. For example, the amide bond is normally represented by one set of parameters whether the configuration is *cis* or *trans*. Recent experimental data are quite compelling that the electronic states for the two configurations are different and different parameter sets should be used for accurate results (Fig. 15.1). Only AMBER/OPLS currently distinguishes between these two conformational states (15). Certainly, the limited parameterization of simplified force fields would not allow accurate prediction of spectra, which are more reflective of the dynamic behavior of the molecule. Accurate estimates of energy may require accurate representation of the dynamics of molecules and may justify the derivation of the larger number of parameters. The new version of the Allinger force field, MM3, has the objective of reproducing spectral data more accurately than MM2 (16). Much of chemistry remains to be incorporated into appropriate force fields. Only recently have adequate modi-

fications been made to the force fields developed for organic molecules so that they can include some metals (17–20).

Because different force fields may use different mathematical representations of the forces between atoms and the details of their parameterization also will generally differ, it is unwise to use parameters derived for one force field to replace missing parameters in another. One often hears of a "balanced" parameter set that reproduces well the phenomena under consideration but that is often inadequate for other applications. A comparison by Burkert and Allinger (9) showed the different van der Waals (VDW) potentials used in several of the popular force fields, and the situation has not improved in the intervening years. Because of other differences in parameters and functional forms of the equations used in the rest of the individual force fields,

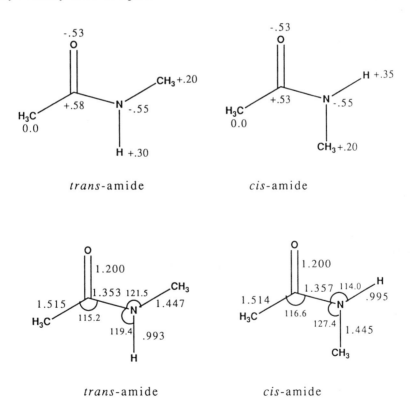

Fig. 15.1 Differences in OPLS charge distribution (*top*) between cis and trans isomers of amide bond and geometries calculated by *ab initio* and adapted for the figure (15).

these quite different approaches to the VDW potential give excellent results when used in the correct combination. Indiscriminant combination of one part of a force field with another derived independently would lead to considerable divergence in the calculated results from experimental observation.

The most extreme difference between force fields arises in the method by which the hydrogen bond is included. Because atoms involved in a hydrogen bond are often closer than the sum of their VDW radii, they must be handled in a special manner. Several force fields have special functional forms with angular dependence that have special VDW parameters to ensure that not only the correct close approach of the atoms involved is calculated correctly but the correct angular distribution observed for hydrogen bonds is also reproduced. Hagler et al. (21) use an amide hydrogen with a zero VDW radius for hydrogen bonding and a slightly greater nitrogen radius to give a correct amide hydrogen bond distance. The charges on the atoms involved (including the amide hydrogen) are adjusted to give an appropriate balance of VDW repulsion and dipole attraction. Clearly, the method for handling the electrostatic interaction is an integral part of each force field and cannot be modified independently.

2.1.2 ELECTROSTATICS. The most difficult aspect of molecular mechanics is electrostatics (22–25). In most force fields, the electronic distribution surrounding each atom is treated as a monopole with a simple Coulombic term for the interaction. The effect of the surrounding medium is generally treated with a continuum model by use of a dielectric constant. More detailed approaches with distributed multipole representations of the electron distribution (26) and/or efforts to deal with dielectric inhomogeneity through solution of the Poisson equation are clear improve-

ments but have yet to be routinely used. Other difficulties arise in dealing with macromolecular systems as the electrostatic interaction is long ranged ($1/r$) and the interactions cannot be arbitrarily terminated with distance. Electrostatic interactions range from those operating only at very short distances that are nonspecific (dispersive interactions, r^{-6} dependence) to those operating at very long distances with a high degree of specificity (charge–charge interactions, r^{-1} dependence).

Dispersive interactions, r^{-6}, are caused by the interaction of induced dipoles within the electron clouds as molecules come in proximity. They are responsible for the attractive part of the nonbonded van der Waals interaction.

Dipole–dipole interactions, r^{-3}, occur because of the nonsymmetric distribution of electrons between atoms of different size and electronegativity; bonds have associated permanent dipoles. The interaction energy between two of these dipoles depends on their relative orientation. This is basically the interaction underlying the phenomenon of the hydrogen bond. While some force field authors use a special hydrogen bonding potential with an orientation dependence, simple partial charge representations combined with appropriate VDW parameters can reproduce the effect as well (21).

Charge-dipole interactions, r^{-2}, are explained as a charge interacting with a permanent dipole which can be handled simply by considering the charge interacting with the two charges at the poles of the dipole. Alternatively, if the distance between the poles of the dipole is small compared with that between the centers of the ion and the dipole, then the potential energy, Φ, can be approximated as

$$\Phi = e\mu \cos \Theta / r^2$$

where e = charge of ion
μ = dipole moment

Θ = angle between the vector connecting the center of dipole with the charge and dipole orientation

r = distance between the center of the ion and the center of the dipole

Charge-charge interactions, r^{-1}, are explained as the energy of interaction between two charges q_1 and q_2 and is given by Coulomb's law:

$$E = \frac{q_1 q_2}{4\pi\varepsilon r_{12}}$$

where r_{12} = distance separating the charges

ε = dielectric constant of the medium

To evaluate atom–atom interactions using Coulomb's law, the concept of net atomic charge is invoked. This amounts to representing charge as a point (a monopole), and is an artificial construct. Nevertheless, this is the common method. Recent improvements in calculating an appropriate set of point charges to reproduce accurately the molecular electrostatic potential derived by accurate quantum calculations have been reported (27).

In an effort to increase the quality of electrostatic representations, dipole and higher multipole moments have been used. There are advantages in these more accurate representations with a relatively small computational increase due to the reductions in distances over which the higher moments must be summed, but they do require additional effort in the derivation of the parameters for the higher moments themselves. A good example is the distributed multipole model of electrostatics derived for peptides. A recent review (28) discussed the problems of deriving a distributed multipole expansion of charge representation that accurately reproduces the molecular electrostatic potential derived from quantum calculations. Comparisons were made between atomic multipole,

bond dipole, and restricted bond dipole models. It was found that a model for the electrostatic potential based on bond dipoles supplemented with monopoles (for ions) and atomic dipoles (for lone pairs) is most useful. Dipole–dipole energy converges much faster than monopole–monopole energy. Molecular charge at any desired position in a molecule is not a physically measurable quantity; one can only calculate a delocalized electron probability distribution from quantum theory. Clearly, the more complex the representation, the more accurately one can approximate the quantum mechanical results, and the more realistic should be the results obtained. One complexity of electrostatics is the long distances over which interactions occur. Appropriate means of truncating the long-range forces to maintain the accuracy of simulations are necessary (29–31), and progress in better approximations has been reported (32). The difficulties with cutoff schemes were demonstrated (33, 34) by significant variations in the behavior of a 17-residue helical peptide, simulated with explicit waters as various electrostatic schemes were employed, and by studies (35) of a pentapeptide in aqueous ionic solution (36). In both cases, the Ewald approximation, for which periodicity is assumed and which allows summation over much longer distances, gave superior results (33–35).

2.1.2.1 *The Dielectric Problem and Solvation* While methods of localizing charge just described may give reasonable results, the use of Coulomb's law with a dielectric constant, a scaling factor related to the polarizability of the medium between the charges, is clearly of concern. The dielectric at the molecular level is neither homogeneous nor continuous, nor even well defined, and thus it violates the basic assumption of Coulomb's law. While the use of a low, uniform dielectric is more correct in dynamical simulations where all solute and solvent atoms are explicitly included, a variety of comparisons of experimental data with the results of calculation using a simplified solvent model have led to the realization that much better approaches are needed. Initial efforts led to the proposal of a variable dielectric ($1/R$ or $1/4R$) (37). More recently, use of approaches that model the inhomogeneity of the dielectric at the interface between the solute and solvent by use of the Poisson-Boltzman equation have shown considerable promise (38, 39). An alternative approach using the mirror charge approximation has been described (40). Excellent reviews of the electrostatic problem have appeared, to which the reader is referred (22–25).

Much effort has been given to simple continuum models of solvation to explain the origin of solvent effects on conformational equilibria and reaction rates. The current status of such efforts, as well as simulations to rationalize solvation effects, has been reviewed (41). There are two general approaches to the continuum models. The first is reaction field theory (Bell, Kirkwood, Onsager) that follows the classical treatment of Debye-Huckel. The solvent is considered in terms of charge distribution, polarizability, and dielectric constant. The solvation energy is determined simply by considering the solute as a point dipole that interacts with the induced charge distribution in the solvent (Onsager reaction field). An extension by Sinangolou in the 1960s partitioned solvation energy into cavity formation, solvent–solute interaction, and the "free volume" of the solute. The logical extension of this approach is the scaled-particle theory by which the free energy of formation of a hard-sphere cavity for a hard-sphere solute of diameter σ_2 in a hard-sphere solvent of diameter σ_1 and number density ρ is scaled to the exact solution for small cavity sizes (42). Alternatively, the virtual charge approach uses a system of effective and virtual charges

interacting in the gas phase. The Hamiltonian of the system is modified to include an imaginary particle, a "solvaton," with an opposite charge for each of the solute atoms; it is solved by a SCF procedure. These continuum models have met with limited success (trends and relative effects of solvation can be predicted), but highly specific molecular interaction, such as those involving hydrogen bonding groups, cannot be accommodated.

In the equation for calculating affinity of a drug for a receptor, the ligand is solvated either by the receptor or by the solvent. This competition means that the accurate determination of the free energy of solvation is important in understanding differences in affinities. Solvation free energy (G_{sol}) can be approximated by three terms: G_{cav}, the formation of a cavity in the solvent to hold the solute, and G_{vdw} and G_{pol}, the interaction between solute and solvent divided between the VDW and electrostatic forces:

$$G_{sol} = G_{cav} + G_{vdw} + G_{pol}$$

There are four theoretical approaches to the problem.

Scaled Particle Theory. The essence of the scaled particle theory (42) is that formation of a cavity in a fluid requires work. The theory for hard spheres has been well developed from statistical mechanics, and the work $W(R, \rho)$ can be calculated as follows:

$$
\begin{aligned}
W(R, \rho)/kT = {} & -\ln(1 - y) + (3y/1 - y)R \\
& + [(3y/1 - y) \\
& + 9/2 \cdot (y/1 - y)^2]R^2 \\
& + yPR^3/rkT
\end{aligned}
$$

where $y = \pi\rho\sigma_1^3/6$, $R = \sigma_2/\sigma_1$, σ_2 is the diameter of the hard-sphere solute, σ_1 is the diameter of the solvent, and ρ is the number density of the fluid (N/V). Because this theory includes no interaction between solvent and solute, i.e., only G_{cav} is calculated, effective volumes for nonspherical compounds with interactive groups are normally calibrated from experiment. This is one way to deal with the energy of interaction between solvent and solute (43).

Charge Image (or Virtual Charge) Method (Method for G_{pol} Calculation). The charge image method replaces the solute-continuum model with one in which a system of charges derived from the solute and virtual charges in the adjacent space interact in the gas phase (40). A set of mirror charges reflected at the dielectric boundary are created and used in the calculation of the electrostatics.

Boundary Element Method (Method for G_{pol} Calculation). For the boundary element method, the system is modeled by calculating the appropriate surface charges at the dielectric boundary (44). This is similar to fitting charges at atomic centers to reproduce the molecular electrostatic potential. For a quantum mechanical equivalent, Tomasi and co-workers (45) introduced a charge distribution on the surface of a cavity of realistic shape to introduce the solvation term in the Hamiltonian of the solute. The charge distribution on the surface of the cavity depends on the solute's electric field, which is affected in turn by polarization from the cavity's surface. An iterative QM procedure is used to obtain the perturbation term.

Poisson-Boltzmann Equation (Method for G_{pol} Calculation). Generalization of Debye-Huckel theory leads directly to the Poisson-Boltzmann equation, which describes the electrostatic potential of a field of charges with dielectric discontinuities (39). This equation has been solved analytically for spherical and elliptical cavities but must be solved by finite difference methods on a grid for more complicated systems. One exciting advance in this area is the development of an approximate equation for the reaction field acting on a macromolecular solute due to the surrounding water and ions (46). By combining these equations with conventional molecular dynamics, solvation-free energies were obtained similar to those with explicit solvent molecules at little computational cost over vacuum simulations. This implies that a more correct solution to the electrostatics problem might minimize the solvation problem. Other approaches to evaluations of G_{sol} have recently appeared in the literature. Still and co-workers (47) estimated $G_{cav} + G_{vdw}$ by the solvent-accessible surface area times 7.2 cal/mol/Å^2. G_{pol} is estimated from the generalized Born equation. Effective solvation terms have been added to molecular mechanics force fields to improve molecular dynamics simulations without the cost of modeling explicit solvent (48, 49). Zuahar (50) combined the polarization-charge technique with molecular mechanics to minimize effectively a tripeptide in solvent.

One final refinement may be necessary in some situations, the inclusion of electric polarizability, for example, by inclusion of induced dipoles or distributed polarizability (51) in the electrostatic representation of the model. Kuwajima and Warshel (52) examined the effects of this refinement in modeling crystal structures of polymorphs of ice. Models that include polarizability were shown to be useful for predicting the properties of crystalline polymorphs of polymers (53). Caldwell et al. (54) included implicit nonadditive polarization energies in water–ion results, with improved accuracy. At the semiempirical level of quantum theory, Cramer and Truhlar (55–58) added solvation and solvent effects on polarizability to AM1 with impressive agreement between experimental and calculated solvation energies. Rauhut et al. (59) have also introduced an arbitrary shaped cavity model using standard AM1 theory.

2.1.2.2 The Hydrophobic Effect Water has been the nemesis of solvation modeling because of its rather unique thermodynamic properties (60, 61). The biochemical literature discusses at length the "hydrophobic effect" (62). This effect is not "hydrophobic" at all as the enthalpic interaction of nonpolar solutes with water is favorable. This, however, is counterbalanced by an unfavorable entropic interaction that is interpreted as caused by an induced structuring of the water by the nonpolar solute. Water interacts less well with the nonpolar solute than it does with itself due to the lack of hydrogen bonding groups on the solute. This creates an interface similar to the air–water interface, with a resulting surface tension caused by the organization of the hydrogen-bonded patterns available. This is the so-called iceberg formation around nonpolar solutes in water first suggested by Frank and Evans. Studies by both molecular dynamics (63–65) and Monte Carlo simulations (66) support this interpretation (61) although there is still considerable controversy in interpretation of experimental data (67).

2.1.2.3 *Polarizability* The traditional approaches in molecular mechanics have excluded the effects of charge on induced dipoles and multibodied effects. This approximation becomes a serious limitation when dealing with charged systems and molecules like water that are highly polar. A recent paper described nonadditive many-body potential models to calculate ion solvation in polarizable water with good agreement with experimental observation (68). It was necessary to include a three-body potential (ion–water–water) in the molecular dynamics simulation of the ionic solution to obtain quantitative agreement with solvation enthalpies and coordination numbers. Inclusion of a bond dipole model with polarizability in molecular dynamics simulations has given excellent agreement in predicting physical properties of polymers (54).

A novel approach based on the concept of charge equilibration has been suggested

that allows the inclusion of polarizabilities in molecular dynamics calculations (69).

2.1.3 THE POTENTIAL SURFACE. The set of equations that describe the sum of interactions between the ensemble of atoms under consideration is an analytical representation of the Born-Oppenheimer surface, which describes the energy of the molecule as a function of the atomic positions. Many important properties of the molecule can be derived by evaluation of this function and its derivatives. For example, setting the value of the first derivative to zero and solving for the coordinates of the atoms leads one to minima, maxima, and saddle points. Evaluation of the sign of the second derivative can determine which of the above have been found. It is a straightforward procedure to calculate the vibrational frequencies from the force constants by evaluation of the eigenvalues of the secular determinant (the mass-weighted matrix from vibrational spectroscopy). Gradient methods for the location of energy minima and transition states are essential parts of any molecular modeling package. It is important to remember, however, that minimization is an iterative method of geometrical optimization that depends on starting geometry, unless the potential surface contains only one minimum (a condition not found for any system of sufficient complexity to be of real interest).

The ability to locate both minima and transition points enables one to determine the minimum energy reaction path between any two minima. In the case of flexible molecules, these minima could correspond to conformers and the reaction path would correspond to the most likely reaction coordinate. One could estimate the rate of transition by determination of the height of the transition states (the activation energy) between the minima. Elbers (70) developed a new protocol for the location of minima and transition states and applied it to the determination of reaction paths for the conformational transition of a tetra-peptide (71). Huston and Marshall (72) used this approach to map the reaction coordinates of the α- to 3_{10}-helical transition in model peptides.

Despite the limitations that curtail exact quantitative applications, molecular mechanics can provide three-dimensional insight as the geometric relations between molecules are adequately represented. Electrical field potentials can be calculated and compared to give a qualitative basis for rationalizing differences in activity. Molecular modeling and its graphical representation allow the medicinal chemist to explore the three-dimensional aspects of molecular recognition and to generate hypotheses that lead to design and synthesis of new ligands. The more accurate the representation of the potential surface of the molecular system under investigation, the more likely that the modeling studies will provide qualitatively correct solutions.

2.1.4 SYSTEMATIC SEARCH AND CONFORMATIONAL ANALYSIS. Due to the convoluted nature of the potential energy surface of molecules, minimization usually leads to the nearest local minimum (73, 74) and not the global minimum. In addition, many problems in structure–activity studies require geometric solutions that may not be at the global minimum of the isolated molecule. To scan the potential surface with some assurity of completeness, systematic (or grid) search procedures have been developed. To understand the strengths and limitations of this approach, some of the algorithmic details must be considered.

2.1.4.1 *Rigid Geometry Approximation.* A simplifying assumption that is usually invoked to reduce the computational complexity of the problem through elimination of variables is that of rigid geometry. The rationale is based on the high energy cost associated with bond length distortions and the ability to accommodate bond angle

deformations by a reduced set of VDW radii. This approach is compatible with problems for which one is most interested in eliminating conformations that are energetically unlikely, i.e., sterically disallowed, due to VDW interactions that cannot be relieved by bond angle deformation. A successful application requires that one calibrates an appropriate set of VDW radii for the particular application area. Iijima et al. (75) calibrated such a set (Fig. 15.2) for peptide application by comparison with experimental crystallographic data from proteins and peptides.

2.1.4.2 *Combinatorial Nature of the Problem.* Using the rigid geometry assumption, one can analyze the combinatorial complexity of a simplified approach to the problem with some ease. Let us assume a molecule (Fig. 15.3) of N atoms with T torsional degrees of freedom, i.e., rotatable bonds. For each torsional degree of freedom T explored at a given angular increment in degrees A there are $360/A$ values to be examined for each T. This means that $(360/A)^T$ sets of angles, each describing a unique conformation, must be examined for steric conflict. For each conformer, the starting geometry must be modified by applying the appropriate transformation matrices to different subsets of atoms to

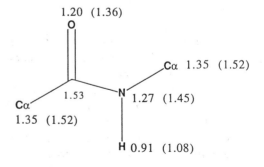

Peptide Bond

Fig. 15.2 Calibrated set of van der Waals radii for peptide backbone for use with rigid geometry approximation (75). Usual radii shown in parentheses. Carbonyl carbon not modified.

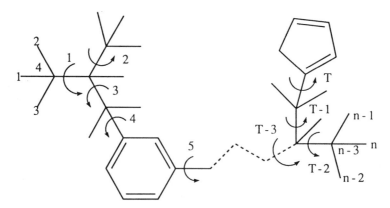

Fig. 15.3   Schematic diagram of molecule with N atoms and T rotatable bonds.

generate the coordinates of the conformation. For each conformation, $N(N-1)/2$ distance determinations to a first approximation (this does not exclude bonded atoms and atoms bonded to the same atom from the check that is necessary) must be calculated and checked against the allowed sum of VDW radii for the two atoms involved. The number of VDW comparisons V is given by:

$$V = (360/A)^T \cdot N(N-1)/2 \quad (15.1)$$

It should be clear that the VDW comparisons are the rate-limiting step by their sheer number, and any algorithmic improvement that reduces the number of such checks or enhances the efficiency of performing such checks is of value.

2.1.4.3 *Pruning the Combinatorial Tree.* From this simplified analysis, systematic search of other than the smallest molecules at a course increment would appear daunting. A hybrid approach with a course grid search followed by minimization has been successfully used to locate minima. There are a number of algorithmic improvements over the "brute force" approach that enhance the applicability of systematic search itself. To understand these improvements, some concepts must be defined. First is the concept of aggregate, which is a set of

atoms whose relative positions are invariant to rotation of the T rotational degrees of freedom (76). *n*-Butane is divided into aggregates (Fig. 15.4). In this simple example, the atoms in an aggregate all are either directly bonded or have a one–three relationship, i.e., are related by a bond angle. Because of the rigid geometry approximation, their relative positions are fixed. Atoms contained within the same aggregate do not, therefore, have to be included in the set of those that undergo VDW checks for each conformation. For linear molecules, there are $n-1$ bonds and the number of one–three interactions depends on the valence of the atom. This simplification leads to a reduction of the number of VDW checks by the factor $N(N-1)/2$, which is multiplied by the number of conformations.

How can one reduce the number of conformations that must be checked? Here the concept of construction becomes useful. One constructs the conformations in a stepwise fashion, starting with an initial aggregate and adding a second aggregate at a given torsional increment for the torsional variable T, which is applied to the rotatable bond connecting the two. If any pair of atoms overlap for that increment, then one can terminate the construction, because no addition operation will relieve that steric overlap. In effect, one has truncated the combinatorial possibilities that

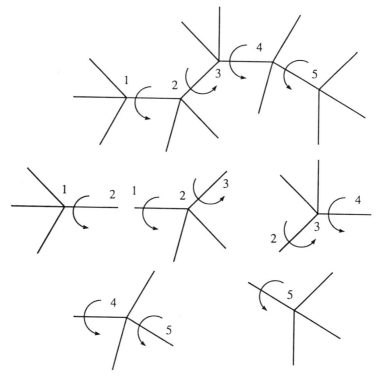

Fig. 15.4 Decomposition of *n*-butane molecule into aggregates.

would have included that subconformation, i.e., one has pruned the combinatorial tree.

2.1.4.4 *Rigid Body Rotations.*

If one constructs the molecule stepwise by the addition of aggregates, then one has two sets of atoms to consider. First are those in the partial molecule (set A) previously constructed, which have been found to be in a sterically allowed partial conformation. For each possible addition of the aggregate, the atoms of the aggregate (set B) must be checked against those in the partial molecule. If one uses the concept of a rigid body rotation, then one can describe the locus of possible positions of any atom in set B as a circle whose center lies on the axis of rotation T_i (the interconnecting bond) at a distance along the axis, which can be calculated. The formula for a circle can be transformed to represent the possible distances between the atom b in set B and any

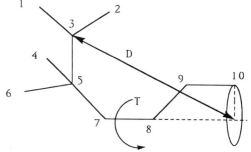

Fig. 15.5 Distance between atoms 1 to 7 and atom 10 separated by a single rotatable bond T can be described with a transformation of the equation of a circle describing the locus of atom 10 as bond T is rotated. Notice that distance D between any atom 1 to 7 and the center of circle of rotation of atom 10, which is on axis of rotation, is fixed regardless of value of T.

atom a in set A as shown in Figure 15.5. An equation with scalar coefficients that describes the variable distance between two atoms as a function of a single torsional variable was derived (77) that has a discriminant whose evaluation can be used to determine if atom *a* and atom *b* will

1. Be in contact despite changes in the value of the torsional rotation of the aggregate, which implies that the current partial conformation must be discarded as there is no possible way to add the aggregate that is sterically allowed.

2. Never come in contact for any value of the torsional rotation so that this pair of atoms can be removed from consideration regarding this aggregate.

3. Come in contact for some values of the torsional rotation that can be calculated for that pair and that removes a segment of the torsional circle from consideration for other atom pairs. If all segments of the torsional circle are disallowed by combinations of the angular requirements of different atom pairs, then the partial conformation of the molecule is disallowed as further construction is not feasible. As a first approximation, this removes a degree of torsional freedom from the problem reducing T to $T-1$ torsional degrees of freedom. At a 10° torsional scan, an approximate reduction in computational complexity of a factor of 36 results.

2.1.4.5 *The Concept and Exploitation of Rings.* Realization that many of the relevant constraints in chemistry can be expressed as interatomic distances, VDW interactions, nuclear Overhauser effect constraints, etc. allows use of the concept of a virtual ring in which the constraint forms the closure bond. Small rings up to six members can be solved analytically (78) so that one can search the torsional degrees of freedom associated with a constraint until only five remain and then solve the problem analytically (Fig. 15.6). The torsional angles for those degrees of freedom are no longer sampled on a grid, thus removing the problem of grid tyranny in

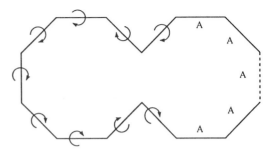

Fig. 15.6 Scheme for combining systematic search with analytical solution for closure. Bonds indicated by arrows are systematically scanned while those indicated by *A* are analytically determined. Dotted bond can represent either chemical bond or experimental distance determination (NOE, etc.).

which valid conformations are missed by the choice of increment and starting conformation. This makes the approach a hybrid, as only part of the conformational space is searched with regular torsional increments. It is, however, much more efficient to solve a set of equations than search five torsional degrees of freedom.

2.1.4.6 *Conformational Clustering and Families.* In a congeneric series, the correspondence between torsional rotation variables is maintained as one compares molecules and a direct comparison of the values allowed for one molecule with those allowed for another is meaningful. Two- or three-dimensional plots (Fig. 15.7) of torsional variables against energy often provide considerable insight into the difference in conformational flexibility between two molecules. Such a plot of the peptide backbone torsional angles (Φ, Ψ) is known as a Ramachandran plot. As more than three torsional variables become necessary to define the conformation of the molecule under consideration, then multiple plots become necessary to represent the variables. Unless special graphical functions are included in the software, then correlations between plots become difficult as each plot is a projection of a multidimensional space. One approach to this problem is to use cluster analysis programs to identify those values of the multidimensional variables that are adjacent in *N*-space. The clusters of conformers that result have been referred to as families. A member of a family is capable of being transformed into another conformer belonging to the same family without having to pass over an energy barrier, i.e., the members of a family exist within the same energy valley.

Because of the combinatorial nature of systematic search, one is often faced with large numbers of conformers that must be analyzed. For some problems, energetic considerations are appropriate, and conformers can be clustered with the closest local minimum, providing to a first approximation an estimate of the entropy associated with each minima, by the number of con-

formers associated, because they can come from a grid search that approximates the volume of the potential well. A single conformer, perhaps the one of lowest energy, can be used with appropriately adjusted error limits in further analyses as representative of the family.

2.1.4.7 Conformational Analysis. While interaction with a receptor will certainly perturb the conformational energy surface of a flexible ligand, high affinity would suggest that the ligand binds in a conformation that is not exceptionally different from one of its low energy minima. Mapping the energy surface of the ligand in isolation to determine the low energy minima will, at the very least, provide a set of candidate conformations for consideration or starting

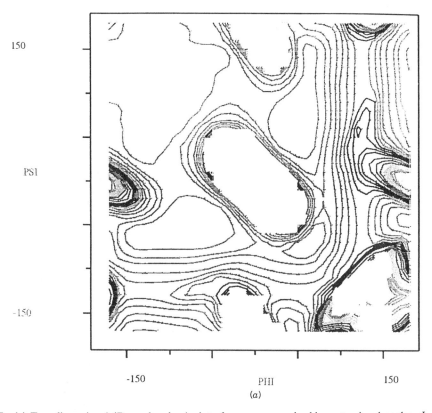

Fig. 15.7 (*a*) Two-dimensional (Ramachandran) plot of energy versus backbone torsional angles, Φ and Ψ, for *N*-acetyl-valine-methylamide. (*b*) Three-dimensional plot of energy versus torsional angles, Φ, Ψ, and $\chi 1$, for *N*-acetyl-valine-methylamide.

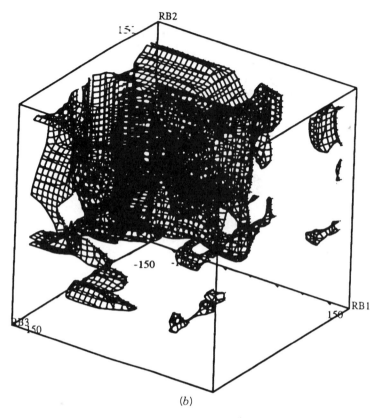

Fig. 15.7 (*Continued*)

points for further analyses. The problem of finding the global minimum on a complicated potential surface is common to many areas and lacks a general solution. Minimization procedures locate the closest local minimum, depending on the starting conformation. Several strategies have developed to map the potential surface and locate minima. Excellent overviews of the different approaches are available (79, 80). Stochastic methods such as Monte Carlo have been advocated for conformational analysis (81, 82), and their usefulness has been demonstrated on carbocyclic ring systems (81, 83–89) (Fig. 15.8). Molecular dynamics can be used to explore the potential energy surface, often with simulated annealing to help overcome activation-energy barriers, but exploration is concen-

trated in local minima and duplication of the surface explored is controlled by Boltzmann's law. Systematic, or grid, search samples conformations in a regular fashion, at least in the parameter space (usually torsional space) that is incremented. Comparisons of a variety of methods were made on cycloheptadecane (84), and it was concluded that the stochastic method was most efficient. In one of the few independent comparisons of the effectiveness of these procedures, Boehm et al. (90) studied the sampling properties on the model system caprylolactam, a nine-membered ring, and concluded that systematic search was both inefficient and ineffective at finding the minima found by the other methods when the number of conformers examined was limited. In an attempt to

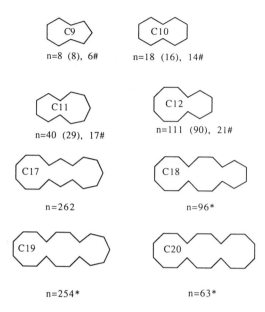

C9   n=8 (8), 6#

C10   n=18 (16), 14#

C11   n=40 (29), 17#

C12   n=111 (90), 21#

C17   n=262

C18   n=96*

C19   n=254*

C20   n=63*

Fig. 15.8 Cycloalkane rings and number of local minima found by various search strategies. n, number of conformers with MM2 (85), parentheses, number of conformers with MM3 (85), #, number of conformers within 25 kJ/mol of global minima (MM2), (82), *, number of minima found within 3 kcal/mol of global minima (81).

repeat these results, Yodo, Kataoka, and Marshall used systematic search on the same problem and found all of the published minima in a single, short run followed by minimization of family representatives.

2.1.4.8 *Other Implementations of Systematic Search.* Numerous other implementations of systematic, or grid, search programs exist in the literature, including those with protein applications (91) and those for small- or medium-size molecules (79, 80). One of the most widely used programs in organic chemistry, MACROMODEL, has a search module coupled to energy minimization for conformational analysis (92). MACROSEARCH was developed as a means of generating the set of conformers consistent with experimental NMR data and has been applied to de-

termine the conformation of a 15-residue peptide antibiotic (93).

2.1.5 STATISTICAL MECHANICS. To understand the relationships between the simulation methods and the desired thermodynamic quantities, a short review of the major concepts of statistical mechanics may be in order (94). This is not meant to be comprehensive, but rather to remind you of the relevant ideas.

The set of configurations produced by the Monte Carlo simulation generates what Gibbs would call an "ensemble," assuming that the number of molecules in the simulation was large and the number of configurations was also large. This ensures that the possible arrangements of molecules that are energetically reasonable have been adequately sampled. One is often interested in the statistical weight W of a particular observable molecule. For example, a particular conformation of a solute molecule (e.g., the staggered rotamer of ethane) could be compared with another conformer (e.g., the eclipsed rotamer) in a simulation with solvent. If more configurations of the surrounding solvent molecules of equivalent energy were available to the staggered than to the eclipsed, then the staggered would have a higher statistical weight. From the inscription on Boltzmann's tomb, we all recall that $S = k \ln W$, where S is entropy and k is Boltzmann's constant. Thus we have a link between statistics and thermodynamics. W in this case would be the number of configurations associated with the particular conformation of ethane under consideration divided by the total number of configurations sampled. The number of configurations would have to be weighted by their energy, of course, unless the distribution was already Boltzmann weighted, as happens when one uses the Metropolis algorithm (95).

Another way of stating this is that the probability P_i of a particular configuration N_i is proportional to its Boltzmann probability divided by the Boltzmann probability of all the other configurations or states:

$$P_i = \exp\left(-E_i/kT\right)\Big/\sum_{i=1}^{N} \exp\left(-E_i/kT\right)$$

The denominator in this equation has been given a special name—partition function—often symbolized by Z, which is derived from the German *Zustandsumme* ("sum over states"). The successive terms in the partition function describe the partition of the configurations among the respective states available. One can express the thermodynamic state functions of an ideal gas in terms of the molecular partition function Z as follows:

$$S = k \ln W = kN \ln Z/N + U/T + kN$$

where N is the number of molecules and U is the internal energy. From this and the assumption of an ideal gas ($pV = NkT$), the Gibbs free energy ($G = U - TS + pV$) leads to:

$$G = -NkT \ln Z/N$$

and similarly, the Helmholtz free energy ($A = U - TS$) leads to the expression

$$A = -kT \ln Z^N/N!$$

all of which may be more familiar if expressed in terms of enthalpy: $H = U + pV$.

In summary, by simulating a relevant statistical sample of the possible arrangements of molecules when they are interacting, one can derive the macroscopic thermodynamic properties by statistical analysis of the results. In this case, one is deriving the partition function not by theoretical analysis of the quantum states available to the molecule but through simulation. In other words, the average properties are valid if the Monte Carlo or molecular dynamics trajectories are ergodic, i.e., constructed such that the Boltzman distribution law is in accord with the relative frequencies with which the different con-

figurations are sampled. (An ergodic system is by definition one in which the time average of the system is the same as the ensemble average.) A basic concept in statistical mechanics is that the system will eventually sample all configurations or microscopic states, consistent with the conditions (temperature, pressure, volume, other constraints) given sufficient time, i.e., a trajectory of sufficient length (in time) would sample configuration space.

2.1.6 MOLECULAR DYNAMICS. Molecular dynamics is a deterministic process based on the simulation of molecular motion by solving Newton's equations of motion for each atom and incrementing the position and velocity of each atom using a small time increment (24, 94, 96). If a molecular mechanics force field of adequate parameterization is available for the molecular system of interest and the phenomena under study occurs within the time scale of simulation, this technique offers an extremely powerful tool for dissecting the molecular nature of the phenomena and the details of the forces contributing to the behavior of the system.

In this paradigm, atoms are essentially a collection of billiard balls, with classical mechanics determining their positions and velocities at any moment in time. As the position of one atom changes with respect to the others, the forces that in experiences also change. The forces on any particular atom can be calculated by evaluation of the energy of the system using the appropriate force field. From physics,

$$F = ma = -\delta V/\delta r = m\delta^2 r/\delta t^2$$

where F is the force on the atom, m is the mass of the atom, a is the acceleration, V is the potential energy function, and r is the Cartesian coordinates of the atom. Using the first derivative of the analytical expression for the force field allows the calculation of the force felt on any atom as a function of the position of the other atoms.

2.1.6.1 Integration.

In this simulation, a numerical integration is chosen, i.e., a time step that is sufficiently small (smaller than the period of fastest local motion in the system) is chosen such that the simulation moves atoms in sufficiently small increments so that the position of the surrounding atoms does not change significantly per incremental move. In general, this means that the time increment is on the order of 10^{-15} s (1 fs). This reflects the need to represent adequately atomic vibrations that have a time scale of 10^{-15} to 10^{-11} s. For each picosecond of simulation, it is necessary to do 1000 iterations of the simulation. For each iteration, the force on each atom must be evaluated and its next position calculated. For simulations involving molecules in solvent, sufficient solvent molecules must be included so that the distance from any atom in the solute to the boundary of the solvent is larger than the decay of the intermolecular interaction between the solute and solvent molecules. This requires several hundred solvent molecules for even small solutes, and the computations to do a single iteration are sufficiently large that simulations of more than several hundred picoseconds for proteins with explicit solvent are still rare. Efforts to increase the time step and thus allow for longer simulations without sacrificing the accuracy of the methodology are under investigation. Combination of normal mode calculations with explicit numerical integration allows time steps up to 50 ps for model systems (97). A similar approach has been shown effective in modeling supercoiling of DNA (98).

Let us attempt a rough trajectory through molecular dynamics. We have a system of N atoms obeying classical Newtonian mechanics. In such a system, we can represent the total energy E_{tot} as the sum of kinetic energy E_{kin} and potential energy V_{pot}:

$$E_{\text{tot}}(t) = E_{\text{kin}}(t) + V_{\text{pot}}(t)$$

where the potential energy is a function of the coordinates $V_i = f(r_i)$ for atoms i to N and r_i is the Cartesian coordinates of atom i. The kinetic energy depends on the motion of the atoms:

$$E_{\text{kin}}(t) = \sum 1/2 M_i V_i^2(t)$$

where M_i is the mass of atom i and V_i is the velocity of atom i.

The energy undergoes constant redistribution because of the movements of the atoms, resulting in changes in their positions on the potential surface and in their velocities. At each iteration $(t \rightarrow t + \Delta t)$, an atom i moves to a new position $(r_i(t) \rightarrow r_i(t + \Delta t))$, and it experiences a new set of forces. The basic assumption is that the time step Δt is sufficiently small that the position of atom i at $t + \Delta t$ can be linearly extrapolated from its velocity at time t and the acceleration resulting from the forces felt by atom i at time t. If Δt is long enough for the atoms surrounding atom i to change their position so that the forces felt by atom i will change during Δt, then the approximation is not valid and the simulation will deviate from that observed with a shorter Δt. After each atom is moved, the forces on the first atom based on the new positions of the other $N - 1$ atoms can be recalculated and a new iteration begun. Several algorithms exist for numerical integration. The ones by Verlet and Gear are in common use, with the one by Verlet being computationally more efficient (94). A variant of the Verlet algorithm in common use is called the leap-frog algorithm. The calculation of the velocity is done at $t - \Delta t/2$ while the calculation of the force occurs at t to derive the new velocity at $t = \Delta t/2$. In other words,

$$V_i(t + \Delta t/2) = V_i(t - \Delta t/2) + F_i(t) \Delta t/M_i$$

The atomic position of atom i is calculated by adding the incremental change in position, $V_i(t + \Delta t/2) \cdot \Delta T$, to the original position $V_i(t)$. By staggering the evaluation of the velocity and force calculations by $\Delta t/2$, an improvement in the simulation performance is obtained.

2.1.6.2 Temperature.

For simulations that can be compared with experimental results, one must be able to control the temperature of the simulation. The temperature of a system is a function of the kinetic energy $E_{kin}(t)$:

$$T(t) = E_{kin}(t)/3/2Nk$$

where k is Boltzmann's constant. One can perform molecular dynamics simulations at a constant temperature T_c by scaling all atomic velocities $V_i(t)$ at each step by a factor t derived from

$$\delta T(t)/\delta t = [T_c - T(t)]/t$$

where T_c is the desired temperature.

2.1.6.3 Pressure and Volume.

Depending on the simulation that one desires to accomplish, either the pressure or volume must be maintained constant. Constant volume is the easiest to perform, as the boundaries of the system are maintained with all molecules confined within those boundaries, and the pressure is allowed to change during the simulation.

2.1.7 MONTE CARLO SIMULATIONS.

The Monte Carlo method is based on statistical mechanics and generates sufficient different configurations of a system by computer simulation to allow the desired structural, statistical, and thermodynamic properties to be calculated as a weighted average of these properties over these configurations (94). The average value $\langle X \rangle$ of the property X can be calculated by the following

formula:

$$\langle X \rangle = \left[\sum_{i=1}^{N} X_i \exp(-E_i/kT) \right] \Big/ \left[\sum_{i=1}^{N} \exp(-E_i/kT) \right]$$

where $N =$ the number of configurations, $E_i =$ the energy of configuration i, $k =$ Boltzmann's constant, and $T =$ temperature. If we have sufficiently sampled the possible arrangements of molecules in the simulation and have an accurate method to calculate their energy E, then the formula above will give a Boltzmann weighted average of the property X.

In practice, one must compromise the number of molecules in the simulation and/or the number of configurations calculated to conserve computer cycles. Two essential techniques that are used are periodic boundary conditions and sampling algorithms, which will be discussed separately.

While it is important to minimize the number of molecules in either Monte Carlo or molecular dynamics simulations for computational convenience, surface effects at the interface between the simulated solvent and the surrounding vacuum could seriously distort the results. To approximate an "infinite" liquid, one can surround the box of molecules by simple translations to generate periodic images. Each atom in the central box has a set of related molecules in the virtual boxes surrounding the central one (Fig. 15.9). The energy calculations for pairwise interactions only consider the interaction of a molecule, or its "ghost," with any other molecule, but not both. In practice, this is accomplished by limiting pairwise interactions to distances less than one half the length of the side of the box. Real concerns often arise regarding convergence of electrostatic terms due to the linear dependence on distance.

For any large nontrivial system, the total number of possible configurations is

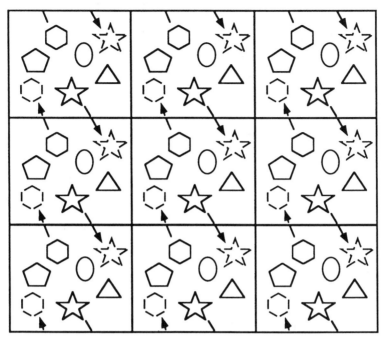

Fig. 15.9 Schematic diagram of simulation with periodic boundary conditions in which adjacent cells are generated by simple translations of coordinates.

beyond comprehension. Consider a set of protons in a magnetic field, the magnetic moments can either be aligned with or opposed to the magnetic field. For only 50 protons, there are 2^{50} combinations, which is a large number. For a small cyclic pentapeptide, there are potentially 36^{10} conformations if one considers a 10° scan of the torsional variables Φ, Ψ. Clearly, some of these are energetically unreasonable because the conformation requires overlap of two or more atoms in the structure. Monte Carlo simulations are successfully performed by sampling only a limited set of the energetically feasible conformations, say 10^6 out of 10^{100} theoretical possibilities. The reason for this success is that the Monte Carlo schemes sample those states that are statistically most important. One could sample all states, calculate the energy of each, and then Boltzmann weight its contribution to the average. Alternatively, one can ignore those states that are energetically high so that they contribute

little, if any, weight to the average and concentrate on those of low energy. In other words, we only look where there are reasonable answers energetically. This is called importance sampling, which is the key to the Monte Carlo procedure.

One aspect shared by Monte Carlo methods and molecular dynamics is the ability to cross barriers. In the case of Monte Carlo, barrier crossing occurs both by random selection of variables as well as acceptance of higher energy states on occasion. Both methods require an equilibration period to eliminate bias associated with the starting configuration. When one considers randomly filling a box with molecules with arbitrary choices for position and orientation, it should be obvious that most examples would result in high energy, especially if the density of such a simulation is made to resemble that of a liquid in which adjacent molecules are often in VDW contact. High energy configurations contribute little to the properties we are trying to evaluate, because they are Boltzmann weighted. It is, therefore, extremely inefficient to calculate configurations randomly. One needs procedures, often referred to as importance sampling, that selectively calculate configurations that will be representative of allowed states. In fact, if one can guarantee that the energy of the configurations actually has a Boltzmann distribution, then one can simply average the properties. In practice, this has been accomplished by an algorithm suggested by Metropolis et al. (95). One essentially uses a Markov process in which the current configuration becomes the basis of generating the next.

1. A molecule in the current configuration is chosen at random, and its degrees of freedom are randomly varied by small increments.

2. The energy of the new configuration is evaluated and compared with that of the starting configuration.

3. If the new energy is lower, the new configuration is accepted and becomes the basis for the next random perturbation.

4. If the energy is higher, $E(\text{new}) > E(\text{old})$, then a random number between 0 and 1 is generated and compared with $\exp(-(E(\text{new}) - E(\text{old}))/kT$. If the number is less, then the configuration is accepted and the process continues by generating a new configuration. If the number is greater, then the configuration is rejected and the process resumes with the old configuration.

In this way, configurations of lower energy are accepted, and the system eventually "minimizes" to sample the higher populated, lower energy configurations; at the same time, higher energy configurations are included but only in proportion to their Boltzmann distribution, which is clearly a function of temperature of the simulation. Because the configurations occur with a probability that depends on their energy

and is proportional to the Boltzmann distribution, one can simply average thermodynamic properties over this distribution of configurations:

$$\langle X \rangle = 1/N \sum_{i=1}^{N} X_i$$

where the sum covers the N configurations generated. As one often does not know an appropriate starting configuration, the initial part of the run may be used to "minimize," or equilibrate, the system, and only the latter part of the simulation is analyzed once the configurational energy has stabilized.

A useful application has combined Monte Carlo sampling with variable temperatures (simulated annealing) to encourage barrier crossing to optimize the docking of ligands into active sites. Random displacements of rigid body translation and rotation and of internal torsional rotations in a substrate within the binding site cavity were performed with Metropolis sampling and a temperature program. This procedure reproduced the crystallographically observed structure of the complex for several test cases (99).

2.1.8 THERMODYNAMIC CYCLE INTEGRATION. Thermodynamic cycle integration is an approach that allows calculation of the free-energy difference between two states (100–102). In this method, one takes advantage of the state-function nature of a thermodynamic cycle and eliminates the paths of the simulation with long time constants, e.g., the formation of a complex that requires diffusion. As an example, the difference in affinity of two ligands (L and M) for the same enzyme or receptor R is described by the following thermodynamic cycle:

$$
\begin{array}{ccc}
R + L & \xrightarrow{\Delta A1} & RL \\
\Delta A3 \downarrow & & \uparrow \Delta A4 \\
R + M & \xrightarrow{\Delta A2} & RM
\end{array}
$$

Because the thermodynamic values of the two states do not depend on the path between the states, one can write the following equation:

$$\Delta\Delta A = \text{the difference in affinity}$$

$$\text{of } L \text{ and } M \text{ for } R$$

$$= \Delta A2 - \Delta A1 = \Delta A4 - \Delta A3$$

By simulating the mutation of L into M, paths $A3$ and $A4$, one can avoid the long simulation required for diffusion of the ligands, paths $A1$ and $A2$, into the receptor. One simply incrementally modifies the potential functions representing ligand L to those representing ligand M during the course of the simulation, making sure that the perturbations are introduced gradually and that the surrounding atoms

have time to relax from the perturbation (Fig. 15.10). Either Monte Carlo or molecular dynamics simulations can use this technique (104). Many interesting applications have appeared in the literature (100, 102, 105, 106). Their success appears directly related to sampling problems and minimal perturbation of the ligand to ensure equilibration.

2.1.9 NON-BOLTZMANN SAMPLING. There are equivalent molecular dynamics and Monte Carlo procedures that allow one to sample regions of configuration space that are not minima (e.g., transition states). One can generate a Monte Carlo trajectory for a system E_v that has energetics similar to that of the Boltzmann system E_0 by sampling in the region associated with a transition barrier and by subtracting a po-

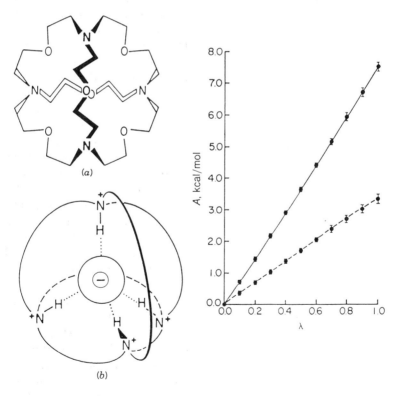

Fig. 15.10 Estimation of difference in affinity ($\Delta\Delta G$) of the two anions Cl$^-$ and Br$^-$ for the cryptand SC24 (*a*, structural formula, *b*, schematic of complex formed with halide ion) as the parameters for Cl$^-$ are slowly mutated into those for Br$^-$ in water (– – – –) as well as in the complex (———). From Ref. 103.

tential V to reduce the barrier

$$E_0 = E_v - V$$

Alternatively, one may want to obtain meaningful statistics for a rare event without oversampling the lower energy states. This can be accomplished by adding a potential W that is zero for the interesting class of configurations and very large for all others (Fig. 15.11)

$$E_0 + E_v + W$$

The details of these sampling procedures that allow one to focus on the aspect of the problem of interest have been reviewed (101). Applications of this approach to determining conformational transitions in model peptides (107–109) are exemplified

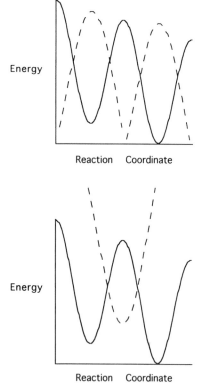

Fig. 15.11 Schematic diagrams of methods for modifying the potential surface to allow adequate sampling during simulations.

in the work of the Elber's group on helix/coil (70, 71, 110), the Brooks group on turn/coil (111–115), and Huston and Marshall (72) and Smythe and co-workers (116) on helical transitions in peptides.

2.2 Quantum Mechanics: Applications in Molecular Mechanics

Detailed discussion of quantum mechanics (117) is clearly beyond the scope of this review; however, its applications to molecular mechanics and modeling will be briefly summarized. Molecular mechanics is based on the laws of classical physics and deals with electronic interactions by highly simplified approximations such as Coulomb's law. All forces operating in intermolecular interactions are essentially electronic in nature. Any effort to quantitate those forces requires detailed information about the nuclear positions and the electron distribution of the molecules involved. At considerable computational cost, quantum mechanics provides information about both nuclear position and electronic distribution. Molecular mechanics is built on the assumption that electronic interactions can be adequately accounted for by parameterization. While most of the systems of interest in biology are too large for the direct application of quantum mechanics, quantum mechanics has at least three essential roles to play in drug design (117): charge approximations, characterization of molecular electrostatic potentials, and parameter development for molecular mechanics.

2.2.1 CHARGE AND ELECTROSTATICS. Estimates of charges in molecular mechanics can be derived, in general, by application of one of the many different quantum chemical approaches, either *ab initio* or semiempirical. Quantum mechanical methods are available for calculating the electron probability distributions for all the electrons in a molecule and then partitioning those distributions to yield representations for the net atomic charges of atoms in the molecule, either as atom-centered charges, or more complex distributed multipole models (26, 28) (Fig. 15.12).

2.2.1.1 *Atom-Centered Point Charges.* In the Mulliken population analysis, all the one-center charge on an atom is assigned to that atom, while the two-center charge is divided equally between the two atoms in the overlap (even if the electronegativities of the two atoms are quite dissimilar). The sum is the gross atomic population, and the net atomic charge is simply this plus the nuclear charge. The result is sensitive to the basis set (the number of atomic orbitals) used. Despite poor fit of the molecular electrostatic potential derived with point charges to the *ab initio* electrostatic po-

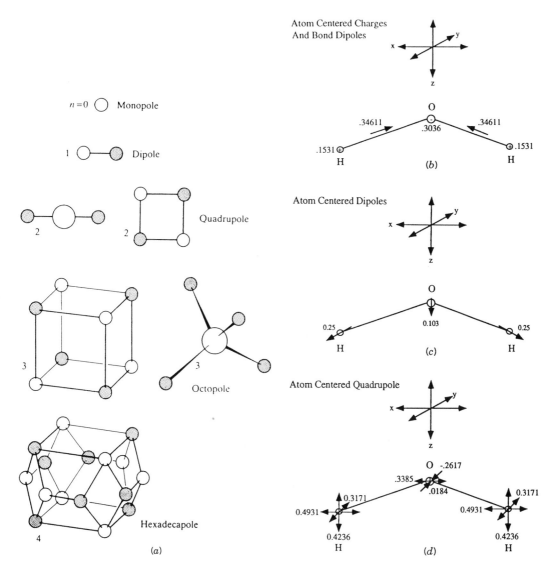

Fig. 15.12 Different approaches to localization of charge used in electrostatic models. (*a*) Atom-centered monopole. (*b*) Atom-centered dipole. (*c*) Atom-centered quadrapole. (*d*) Bond-centered dipole.

tential, or that derived from a distributed multipole analysis (118), widespread use continues because they do reflect chemical trends and are reportedly compatible with known electronegativities. In addition, this option is commonly available in software packages. Unfortunately, poor representation of the electric field surrounding the molecular results from use of atom-centered monopole models (28) even when more careful methods are used to distribute the charge.

2.2.1.2 *Methods to Reproduce the Molecular Electrostatic Potential.*

The molecular electrostatic potential (MEP) surrounding the molecule that is created by the nuclear and electronic charge distribution of the molecule is a dominant feature in molecular recognition. Methods to calculate charge models to represent accurately the MEP as calculated by *ab initio* methods using large basis sets were reviewed (28). The choice between models (Fig. 15.12) depends on the accuracy with which one desires to reproduce the MEP. This desire must be balanced by the increased complexity of the model and its resulting computational costs when implemented in molecular mechanics.

The first problem is to select points where the MEP is to be evaluated and eventually fitted: the position of the shell outside the VDW radii of the atoms in the molecule and the spacing of grid points on that shell. Sampling too close to the nuclei gives rise to anomalies, because the potential around nuclei is always positive. Singh and Kollman (119) reported the use of four surfaces at 1.4, 1.6, 1.8, and 2.0 times the VDW radii with a density of one to five points per Å^2. This paradigm was reported to give an adequate sampling to which the fitted charges were fairly insensitive at least at the higher values. An improved procedure, the restrained electrostatic potential (RESP) fit, was developed by Bayly et al. (27) to enhance trans-

ferability of the resulting point charges. Williams (28) derived a procedure to derive the best fit to a given MEP with a defined set of monopoles, dipoles, etc.

Typically, fragments of molecules of interest are analyzed by *ab initio* techniques to generate their MEPs, which are the reference for parameterization of charge. Recently, Besler et al. (120) have reported fitting atomic charges to the electrostatic potentials calculated by the semiempirical methods AM1 and MNDO. The MNDO charges derived by fitting the MEP can be linearly scaled to agree with results derived from *ab initio* calculations. Among the motivations for semiempirical methods are the facts that semiempirical methods that use high quality basis sets often yield better results than *ab initio* techniques that employ minimal basis sets and that there is a significant reduction in computational time in moving from *ab initio* to semiempirical calculations. Rauhut and Clark (121) used the AM1 wave function to develop a multicenter point-charge model in which each hybrid natural atomic orbital is represented by two charges located at the centroid of each lobe. Thus up to nine charges (four orbitals and one core charge) are used to represent heavy atoms. Results using this approach affirm the observations that distributed charges are more successful in reproducing intermolecular interactions than atom-centered charges (122, 123).

2.2.2 PARAMETER DEVELOPMENT FOR FORCE FIELDS.

Because molecular mechanics is empirical, parameters are derived by iterative evaluation of computational results such as molecular geometry (bond lengths, bond angles, dihedrals), heats of formation, etc. compared with experimental values (10). Lifson coined the expression *consistent* for force fields in which structures, energies of formation, and vibrational spectra have all been used in parameterization by least-squares optimization. In the case of bond lengths, bond angles, and VDW parameters, crystallography have provided most of the essential experimental database. Major efforts to derive general sets of parameters from quantum mechanical calculation have been made, especially for systems for which adequate experimental data are unavailable (124). While quantum mechanics is certainly adequate for initial approximations of parameters and essential for charge approximations, a detailed analysis indicates that *in vacuo* calculations neglect many-body effects and can be misleading. A major effort by Hehre (personal communication) to derive parameters for water from extensive *ab initio* calculations with large basis sets failed even to give a parameter set that reproduced the radial distribution for bulk water. Parameters derived from relevant experimental data in the condensed phase (especially if available in the solvent of theoretical interest) are generally more capable of accurately predicting results, as the many-body effects are implicitly included in the parameterization. The basic assumption is that these "effective" two-body potentials implicitly incorporate many-body interaction energies.

Jorgensen has parameterized by fitting properties of bulk liquids to Monte Carlo simulations to give the AMBER/OPLS force field (125). Conceptually, one is attracted by the use of liquids and their observable properties as constraints during the derivation of a force field that is destined to study the properties of solvated molecules.

2.2.3 MODELING CHEMICAL REACTIONS AND DESIGN OF TRANSITION-STATE INHIBITORS. In cases such as enzyme reactions in which chemical transformations occur, quantum chemical methods must be used to deal with electronic changes in hybridization and bond cleavage (126, 127). Hybrid applications (128–130) for which the reaction core is modeled quantum mechanically and the rest by molecular mechanics would appear a viable option. Alternatively, the geometry of the transition state has been modeled by molecular mechanics with force constants derived from *ab initio* calculations that predict with amazing accuracy the relative selectivity of reactions. Andrews and co-workers (131) pioneered modeling of transition states (132) of enzymatic reactions to design transition-state inhibitors.

3 KNOWN RECEPTORS

A significant challenge is the design of novel ligands for therapeutic targets in which the three-dimensional structure has been determined by either X-ray crystallography, or NMR (5–8). The availability of the coordinates of all the atoms of the target suggests use of modeling of the site and interaction with prospective ligands. Qualitative information can be discerned by simple examination of complexes using molecular graphics, and improvement of known ligands can be made by searching for accessory binding interactions through ligand modification. This approach was pioneered by groups at the Wellcome Research Laboratories (133–135) for designing analogs of 2,3-diphosphoglycerate (Fig. 15.13) to modulate oxygen binding to hemoglobin and at Burroughs-Wellcome (136) for enhancing the affinity of dihydrofolate reductase (DHFR) antagonists. When used in an iterative fashion, novel compounds with improved affinity results (5, 137, 138). Quantification of interactions and design of novel ligands require application of molecular and statistical mechanics to quantify the enthalpy and entropy of binding. In other words, experimental measurements reflect free energies of binding, and both enthalpic and entropic contributions must be estimated for prediction of affinities as part of the design process.

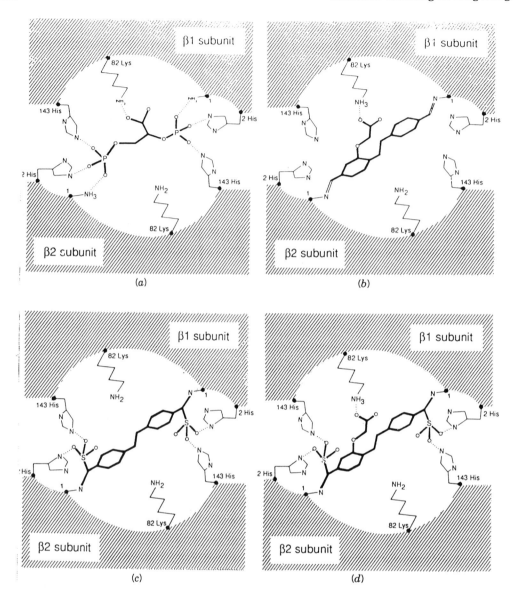

Fig. 15.13 Diphosphoglycerate (*a*) and analogs (*b–d*) designed to optimize interactions bound in schematic model of hemoglobin. From Ref. 135.

3.1 Definition of Site

The availability of three-dimensional structural information on a potential therapeutic target does not guarantee identification of the site of action of the substrate, or inhibitor, unless the structure of a relevant complex has been determined. In fact,

conformational changes often occur during binding of ligands to enzymes that are not reflected in the three-dimensional structure of the enzyme alone. Illustrative examples are the major conformational changes seen in HIV protease on binding the inhibitor MVT-101 (139, 140) (Fig. 15.14) and the changes in domain orientation observed in

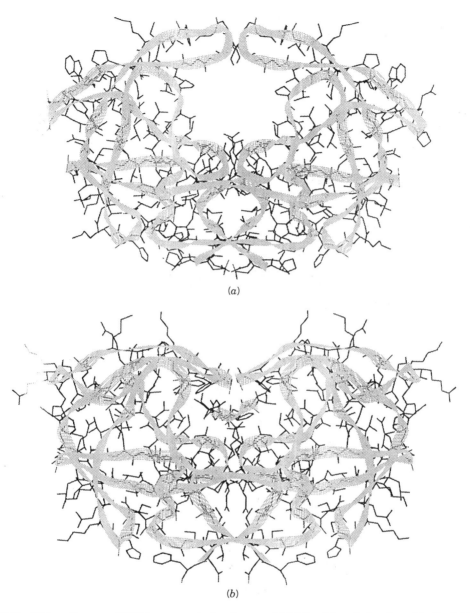

(a)

(b)

Fig. 15.14 Ribbon diagram of HIV-1 protease in the absence of inhibitor (a) and when bound to the inhibitor MVT-101 (b). Diagrams based on crystal structures as reported in Refs. 139 and 140.

the complex of an anti-HIV peptide antibody with the peptide (141). Until the two β-strand flaps have been folded in to complete the active site of HIV protease, many of the important interactions for recognition in this proteolytic system will not have been defined. In other cases of therapeutic targets, allosteric sites are involved in regulation of binding and cannot clearly be discerned from the crystal structure available. Here NMR offers a highly complementary approach, where transfer and isotope-edited NOEs as well as magic-angle spinning NMR on solid samples can help identify those residues of the therapeutic target (Fig.15.15) involved in receptor interaction (1–3).

One significant concern of structure-based design is the dynamics of the target itself. How stable is the active site to modifications in the ligand? Are there alternative potential binding sites that could compete for the ligand? The geometrical identity of serine protease catalytic residues, for example, argues that the specificity essential for biological utility ensures a relatively rigid three-dimensional arrangement of functionality in the active site, which determines molecular recognition and discrimination. The active site has had no evolutionary pressure to optimize binding per se, but rather the rates of interaction and discrimination among the limited chemical repertoire of the biological

milieu. One classic example of the difficulty in interpreting binding as a result of ligand modification occurred when an analog designed to bind to a specific site on hemoglobin actually found a more appropriate site within the packed side chains of the protein molecule (142) (Fig. 15.16). This example emphasizes the importance of protein dynamics. Alternate conformations of the protein that are easily accessible at room temperature may be difficult to characterize experimentally due to relative low abundance and/or lack of resolution of the experimental microenvironment established to favor desolvation and the binding of the ligand despite the entropic cost of fixing the relative geometries of the two molecules. Knowledge of the three-dimensional structure of such cavities can assist the study of binding interactions and the design of novel

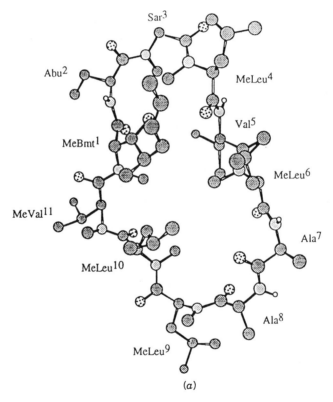

(a)

Fig. 15.15 Bound conformation of cyclosporin (a) as determined by NMR compared with solution conformation (b) (1). Residues involved with interaction with cyclophilin are indicated in bold.

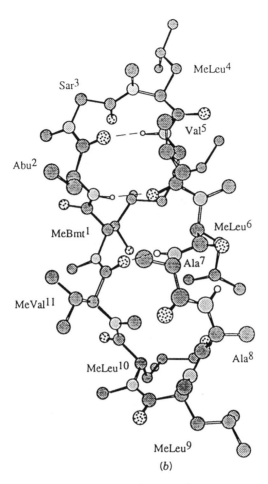

Sar[3]

MeLeu[4]

Val[5]

Abu[2]

MeBmt[1]

MeLeu[6]

Ala[7]

MeVal[11]

Ala[8]

MeLeu[10]

MeLeu[9]

(b)

Fig. 15.15 (*Continued*)

ligands as potential therapeutics. Several algorithms to find, display, and characterize cavity-like regions of proteins as potential binding sites have been developed. Kuntz et al. (7, 144) described the program DOCK, which explores the steric complementarity between ligands and receptors of known three-dimensional structure. Using the molecular surface of a receptor, a volumetric representation of the chosen binding cavity is approximated, using a set of spheres of various sizes that have been mathematically "packed" within it (Fig. 15.17). The set of distances between the centers of the spheres serves as a compact representation of the shape of the cavity. The relative distance paradigm allows com-

parison without the need for orientation of one shape with respect to the other. Potential ligands are characterized in a similar fashion by generating a set of spheres that mimic the shape of the ligand. Matching the distance matrix of the cavity with that of a potential ligand provides an efficient screen for selection of complementary shapes.

Voorinholt et al. (145) used three-dimensional lattices to calculate density maps of proteins. In these maps, lattice points were assigned as a function of the distance to the nearest atom. This technique is effective in delineating regions of low density where channels and cavities exist. Ho and Marshall (146) implemented a search

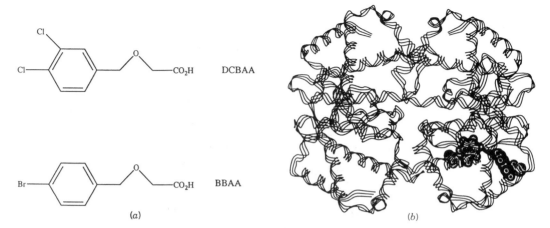

Fig. 15.16 Diagram of crystal structure of hemoglobin in which ((p-bromobenzyl)oxy)acetic acid (BBAA) and ((3,4-dichlorobenzyl)oxy)acetic acid (DCBAA) bind to different sites (142, 143). BBAA shown at lower right with edge-on view of phenyl ring. Coordinates of complexes supplied by Donald J. Abraham, Medical College of Virginia.

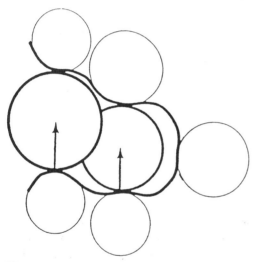

Fig. 15.17 Schematic diagram of small cavity (formed by five atoms with molecular surface indicated by thick line) in which two spheres of different size have been packed according to DOCK program. From Ref. 144.

function in CAVITY to allow the investigator to isolate a single cavity of interest by specifying a seed point. From this seed point, the algorithm systematically explored the entire volume of the cavity, following its borders and effectively filling every crevice within it, i.e., a three-dimen-sional cast of the internal volume was produced using techniques of solid modeling. This cast, or cavity, can be used as a simplified representation of the VDW surface of the receptor for drug design applications (Fig. 15.18). This and many of the techniques discussed below allow a simplified display that focuses of the aspect of the problem under consideration.

3.2 Characterization of Site

3.2.1 HYDROGEN BONDING AND OTHER GROUP BINDING SITES. In evaluating potential ligands, knowledge of the optimal position of particular atoms, or functional groups, within the site can provide valuable insight. The popular program GRID (147) allows a probe atom, or group, to explore the receptor site cavity on a lattice, or grid, while estimating the enthalpy of interaction. A 3-D contour map can be generated from the lattice of interaction energies, which gives a graphical representation of the optimal positions for the atom, or group, in question. Similar ideas are embodied in the field mapping used in the Comparative Molecular Field Analysis (CoMFA)

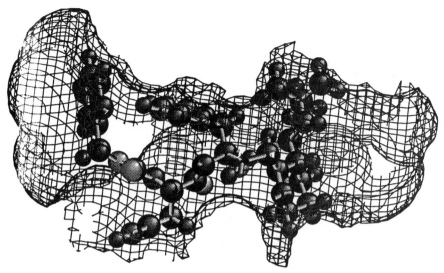

Fig. 15.18 Cast of active site of HIV-1 protease as generated by CAVITY program (146).

paradigm (148) and were first presented in the paradigm's predecessor DYLOMMS (149). Ideal positions for hydrogen-bond donors or acceptors can be mapped in this fashion as a preface to ligand design.

To eliminate the grid that limits the resolution of the local minima found and to orient the functional groups of ligands for optimal connection in generating novel structures, multiple copies of ligands can be distributed in the active site by simulation, and their relative distributions can be examined (150, 151). Miranker and Karplus (150) used molecular dynamics to investigate the interaction of multiple copies of small ligands (such as MeOH, acetonitrile, methylacetamide, etc.) with active-site cavities. After simulated annealing, the quenched populations of ligands concentrated in various orientations at points within the receptor where optimal binding would occur. By connecting the ligands with the most energetically favored binding with fragments from a library of molecular fragments (when the selection is based on overlap with the carbon–carbon bonds of small ligands with fragments), novel compounds could be designed for possible synthesis (Fig. 15.19). This may be an

effective means of designing compounds with high affinity as designs based on natural ligands may be biased towards less optimal interactions.

3.2.2 ELECTROSTATIC AND HYDROPHOBIC FIELDS. As the concept of complementarity underlies much of our design of ligands, surface display of properties such as hydrophobicity and electrostatic potential offer a synopsis of the properties of the active site. Molecular surface displays may be color coded to depict electrostatic potentials (152) and other properties. This can be done with various surface displays (dots, contour, rendered) as well as the cavity display. In the case of CAVITY (146), the loci of filler atoms necessary to pack the cavity is computed, and those present within the outermost layer of the filler solid are identified. These filler atoms essentially form the lining of the cavity. In other words, these points lie along the cavity–pocket interface and are positioned where electrostatic interactions between the pocket and the binding ligand may be represented. At each of these positions, the electrostatic potential of the atoms forming the cavity are calculated using the method

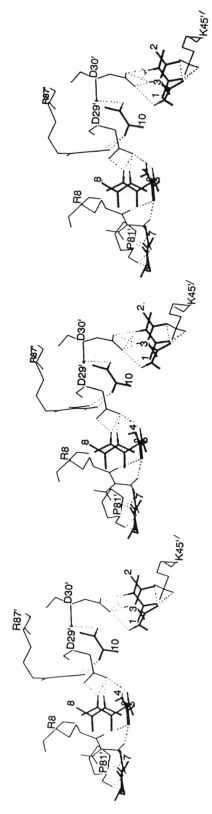

Fig. 15.19 Stereoview of ten minima of *N*-methyl-acetamide bound to open end (S4′) of the active site region of HIV protease by simulation with multiple fragments (150, 151). Left pair for cross-eyed and right pair for wall-eyed viewing.

described by Weiner et al. (153, 154) to compute the electrostatic potential at a specific point in space within a system of charges. These values are then normalized, assigned a color, and displayed.

Researchers interested in studying the electrostatic interactions between binding molecular entities usually do so by color coding the molecular surface of each molecule by electrostatic potential. These surfaces are then docked and visually inspected to note regions of electrostatic complementarity and disparity. Although this method is quite effective, it requires the viewer to scrutinize both electrostatic color surfaces and mentally estimate the degree of electrostatic attraction and repulsion. An effective way to view the electrostatic interaction is to color code the electrostatic complementarity between the ligand and receptor (146). At every cavity–pocket interface point, the electrostatic potential of both the atoms forming the cavity and those of the binding ligand are calculated. A rough approximation of complementarity is computed by multiplying these potentials together. A favorable electrostatic interaction is produced when the electrostatic potentials are opposite in sign. Therefore, favorable interactions are indicated when the product of these values is a negative number. Likewise, unfavorable interactions are indicated when the product of these values is a positive number and the potential of the cavity and that of the binding ligand have the same sign. These products are then normalized, assigned a color, and displayed.

In a similar way, an estimate of the hydrophobic character of a segment of the surface can be quantitated and indicated through color coding. The ability to switch rapidly between these hydrophobic and electrostatic surface representations to integrate visually the optimal complimentarity between site and potential ligand to be designed is helpful.

3.3 Design of Ligands

3.3.1 VISUALLY ASSISTED DESIGN. In the process of optimization of a lead, one needs to ascertain where modification is feasible. Although visualization of the excess space available in the active site cavity by directly examining ligands is useful for locating selected regions where ligand modifications may be made, it is not well suited for fully characterizing the void that exists between the ligand and the receptor (the ligand–receptor gap region); information concerning the relative dimensions of free space is difficult to discern. To facilitate the display of this information, Ho and Marshall (146) developed another algorithm to color code the cavity display by ligand–receptor nearest atom gap distance. The actual VDW surface-to-surface distance (not center to center) between the ligand and enzyme atoms is calculated. When the ligand–receptor distances have been calculated at all cavity–pocket interface lattice points, a user-defined color-coding scale is implemented to generate the displays. This highlights those areas that are less well packed and available for ligand modification.

3.3.2 THREE-DIMENSIONAL DATABASES. Medicinal chemists have recognized the potential of searching three-dimensional chemical databases to aid in the process of designing drugs for known, or hypothetical, receptor sites. Several databases are well known, such as the Cambridge Structural Database (CSD), which contains nearly 90,000 structures of small molecules (155). The crystal coordinates of proteins and other large macromolecules are deposited into the Brookhaven Protein Databank (156). The conformations present in crystallographic databases reflect low energy conformers that should be readily attainable in solution and in the receptor complex. The three-dimensional orientation of the key regions of the drug that are crucial for molecular recognition and binding are termed the pharmacophore. The investigator searches the three-dimensional database using a query for fragments that contain the pharmacophoric functional groups in the proper three-dimensional orientation. Using these fragments as building blocks, completely novel structures may be constructed through assembly and pruning (157). Receptor sites are complex both in geometrical features as well as in their potential energy fields, and many diverse compounds can bind to the same protein by occupying various combinations of subsites. Noncrystallographic databases have also been developed. One example is the three-dimensional database of structures from *Chemical Abstracts* generated using CONCORD (158–161), which contains nearly 700,000 entries. The use of such databases is most applicable when the binding of a particular ligand and its receptor is well understood in terms of functional group recognition and a crystal structure of the complex is known (162). One approach to ligand design is to develop novel chemical architectures (i.e., scaffolds) that position the pharmacophoric groups, or their bioisosteres, in the correct three-dimensional arrangement.

Gund (163, 164) conceived the first prototypic program designed to search for molecules that match three-dimensional pharmacophoric patterns. This program, MOLPAT, performed atom-by-atom searches to verify comparable interatomic distances between pattern and candidate structures. Although rigorous, this approach was tedious and required optimization. Lesk (165) devised a method that used the geometric attributes of the query to screen potential candidates. Similarly, Jakes and Willett (166) proposed that screens based on interatomic distances and atom types could augment search efficiency considerably. Furthermore, Jakes et al.

(167) showed that methods widely used in two-dimensional structure retrieval could be applied to three-dimensional searches to remove the vast majority of compounds before more rigorous comparisons. This was validated in test searches against a subset of the CSD. This concept was furthered by Sheridan et al. (162) who included screens based on aromaticity, hybridization, connectivity, charge, position of lone pairs, and centers of mass of rings. To contain this wealth of information, an inverted bit map (the presence or absence of a feature is encoded as a 1 or zero (bit) at a particular location in a "keyword") was employed for highly efficient screening of hundreds of thousands of compounds in minutes.

Similar database searching methods have been incorporated into a number of current database searching systems. Programs such as CAVEAT (168), ALADDIN (Abbott) (169), 3DSEARCH (Lederle) (170), MACCS-3D (171), CHEM-X (172), UNITY-3DB (173), and others contain considerable functionality useful for such an approach. CAVEAT is designed to assist a chemist in identifying cyclic structures that could serve as the foundation for novel compounds. In particular, it allows an investigator to search rapidly structural databases for compounds containing substituent bonds that satisfy a specific geometric relationship. ALADDIN, 3D-SEARCH, MACCS-3D, and CHEM-X are similar in that geometric relationships between various user-defined atomic components can be used as a query to retrieve matching structures. Features have been included to allow the user to delineate molecular characteristics (atom type, bond angles, torsional constraints, etc.) to ensure the retrieval of relevant compounds. Additional constraints have been incorporated into 3DSEARCH and ALADDIN, including the consideration of retrieved ligand–receptor volume complementarity. Furthermore, CHEM-X performs a rule-based conformational search on each structure in the database to account for conformational flexibility. Comprehensive reviews of three-dimensional chemical database searching are available (174, 175).

Pharmaceutical companies have developed three-dimensional databases for their compound files to help prioritize candidates for screening (172, 176). An essential component in such a system is a method for assessing similarity (174, 177). As most compound databases were entered as two-dimensional structures, this has required conversion to a three-dimensional format. Programs have proven useful in generating plausible three-dimensional structures from the connectivity data (158–161, 178, 179) as reviewed by Sadowski and Gasteiger (180). Because of the inherent flexibility in most compounds, the use of a single conformation to represent the three-dimensional potential for interaction of a molecule is a clear limitation. Development of three-dimensional databases with compact, coded representations of the conformational states available to each compound is a logical next step. Efficient use of such a database requires methods for evaluating three-dimensional similarities. In addition to identification of compounds that can present an appropriate three-dimensional pattern, compounds must also fit within the receptor cavity. Based on a shape-matching algorithm, Sheridan et al. (162) screened candidate compounds to select those whose volumes would fit within the combined volumes of known active compounds. Previously, this group used the same algorithm to help identify potential ligands for papain and carbonic anhydrase by screening compounds from the CSD (181). Screening of the active site of HIV protease identified haloperidol (Fig. 15.20) as an inhibitor of the enzyme and provided a novel chemical lead for further investigation (182). Burt and Richards (184)

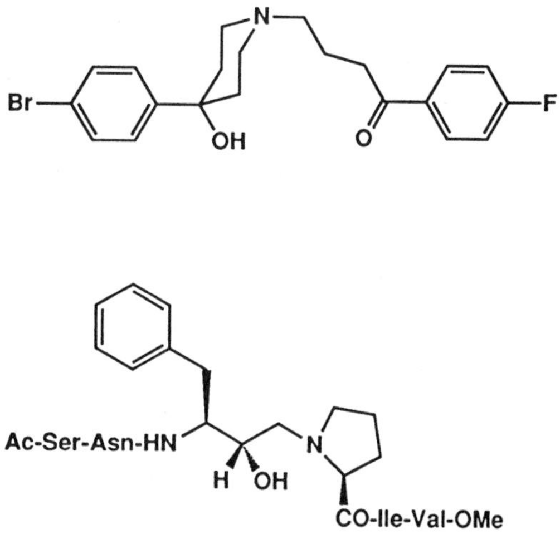

Fig. 15.20 Structure of bromperidol (*top*) found by DOCK program when used on active site of HIV-1 protease compared with structure of JG-365 (*bottom*), a typical substrate-derived inhibitor (182).

introduced flexible fitting of molecules to a target structure with assessment of molecular similarity as a means of dealing with the conformational problem.

The use of preliminary screens can eliminate the vast majority of compounds before more rigorous, and computationally demanding, pattern matching comparisons are made (174, 175). This search strategy is indeed quick and efficient; however, all retrieved compounds must contain every query component as defined in the preliminary screens. As the number and complexity of the query elements increase, one would anticipate fewer true hits but a corresponding rise in the number of near misses. If such near misses could be recovered, effective ligands may simply arise from slight conformational modification to maximize receptor interactions. Furthermore, the retrieval and combinatorial assembly of numerous pharmacophore subcomponents would intuitively produce many more diverse structures than the quest for a single compound in the database incorporating the entire pharmacophore, i.e., all requirements of the query. This suggests an approach that would retrieve compounds containing any combination of a minimum number of matching pharmacophoric elements.

Recently, methods have been developed that employ this divide-and-conquer approach to ligand development. The active site is partitioned into subsites, each containing several pharmacophoric elements. Chemical fragments complementary to each subsite are then designed or retrieved from databases. Finally, fragments are linked to form aggregate ligands. The advantage of this approach is that ligand diversity can be tremendously augmented through the combinatorial assembly of numerous subcomponents. DesJarlais was perhaps the first to employ this philosophy in a novel application (184) of the program DOCK. This well-known program searches three-dimensional databases of ligands and determines potential binding modes of any that will fit within a target receptor (144). However, only a single, static conformation of each database structure is maintained, disregarding ligand flexibility. In DesJarlais's method, conformational flexibility was later introduced by dividing individual ligands into fragments overlapping at rotatable bonds. Each fragment was first docked separately into various receptor regions. Attempts were then made to reassemble the component parts into a legitimate structure. A current example of this approach is the program LUDI (185, 186). In this program, a receptor volume of interest is scanned to determine subsites where hydrogen bonding or hydrophobic contact can occur. Small complementary molecules are then chosen from a database and positioned within these subsites to optimize binding energy. The process concludes with the selection of various bridging fragments to link subsets of small molecules together.

Chau and Dean (187–189) recently published a series of articles addressing whether small molecular fragments with transferable properties could be generated

for further use in automated site-directed drug design. A program was developed to generate combinatorially all three-, four-, and five-atom fragments containing any geometrically allowed combination of hydrogen, carbon, nitrogen, oxygen, fluorine, and chlorine. Aromatic fragments were produced as well. Searches of the Cambridge Structural Database were performed to determine the most frequently occurring fragments (155). To use these fragments as components for ligand assembly, more data were necessary to characterize them better. They were analyzed, therefore, to statistically ascertain bond lengths from the CSD to provide some geometrical constraints for structure assembly. Last, the transferability of atomic residual charges was studied by comparing charges generated for the atoms in each fragment with charges calculated for whole molecules containing the fragment.

Another approach, FOUNDATION searches three-dimensional databases of chemical structures for a user-defined query consisting of the coordinates of atoms and/or bonds (190). All possible structures that contain any combination of a user-specified minimum number of matching atoms and/or bonds are retrieved. Combinations of hits can be generated automatically by a companion program, SPLICE, which trims molecules found from the database to fit within the active site and then logically combines them by overlapping bonds to maximize their interactions with the site (Fig. 15.21) (191). The addition of bridging fragments to those recovered from the database allows generation of many novel ligands for further evaluation.

3.3.3 *DE NOVO* DESIGN. Design of novel chemical structures that are capable of interacting with a receptor of known structure uses methodology that is much more robust as the geometric foundations of molecular sciences are much firmer than the thermodynamic ones. Techniques for

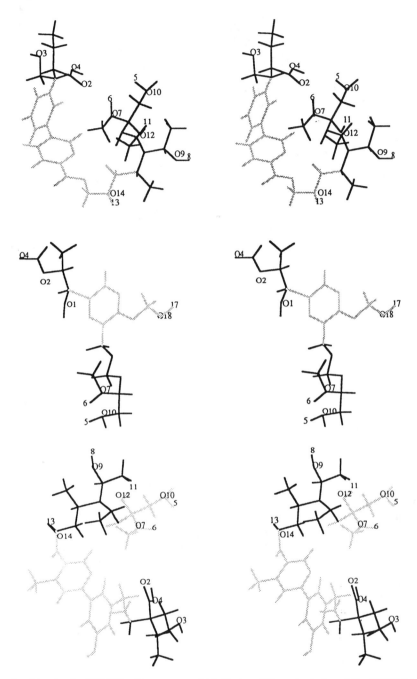

Fig. 15.21 Combination by SPLICE of fragments, which bind to different subsites of the NADP binding site of DHFR to generate a more optimal ligand (191).

the design of novel structures to interact with a known receptor site are becoming more available and show promise. It has become quite evident that much of a molecule acts simply as a scaffold to align the appropriate groups in the three-dimensional arrangement that is crucial for molecular recognition. By understanding the pattern for a particular receptor, one can transcend a given chemical series by replacing one scaffold with another of geometric equivalence. This offers a logical way to change dramatically the side effect profile of the drug as well as its physical and metabolic attributes. Various software tools are already under development to assist the chemist in this design objective.

Lewis and Dean (192, 193) described their approaches to molecular templates. An alternative approach, BRIDGE (Dammkoehler et al., unpublished) is based on the geometric generation of possible cyclic compounds as scaffolds given constraints derived from the types of chemistry the chemist is willing to consider. Nishibata and Itai (194, 195) published a Monte Carlo approach to generating novel structures that fit a receptor cavity. Pearlman and Murko (196) combined a similar approach with molecular dynamics with illustrative applications to HIV protease and FK506 binding protein. CAVEAT is a program developed by Bartlett to find cyclic scaffolds (169) by searching the CSD (156) for the correct vectorial arrangement of appended groups. All of these approaches attempt to help the chemist discover novel compounds which will be recognized at a given receptor. Van Drie (169) have described a program (ALADDIN) for the design or recognition of compounds that meet geometric, steric, or substructural criteria, and Bures et al. (197) have described its successful application to the discovery of novel auxin transport inhibitors. As our knowledge base of receptors grows, such tools will prove increasingly useful. The ability to transcend the

chemical structure of lead compounds while retaining the desired activity should dramatically improve the ability to design away undesirable side effects. The cavity-matching algorithm DOCK (7, 144) has been quite successful in finding noncongeneric molecules of the correct shape to interact with a receptor cavity (198–200).

These approaches implicitly assume that the observed receptor cavity has some physical stability, i.e., a static view, and is not significantly altered by binding of different ligands. While there is no guarantee that this is true for any particular case under study, the specificity seen in biological systems argues that a receptor site has some functional significance in imposing its specific steric and electrostatic characteristics in the molecular recognition and selection process. One must always be prepared, however, for binding to sites other than that targeted and possible exposure of cryptic sites that are not observed in the absence of the ligand (142). The current computational limits in molecular dynamics simulations restrict the chance of uncovering such alternative binding modes in studies. If one can assume the binding mode of the candidate drug is nearly identical to that of a known compound, however, then one has a legitimate basis for thermodynamic perturbation calculations. Multiple or alternate binding modes remain a major fly in the ointment. Naruto et al. (201) have demonstrated a systematic approach to the determination of productive binding modes for mechanism-based inhibitors (Fig. 15.22) that could select starting structures for complexes for molecular dynamics simulations. Combinations of methods, such as Monte Carlo or systematic search, to generate multiple starting configurations for simulations to improve sampling and thermodynamic reliability will increase as adequate computational power to support these hybrid approaches becomes more readily available.

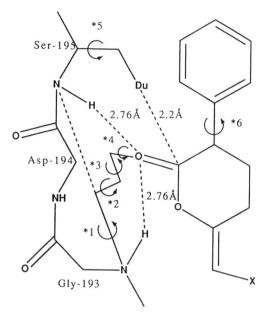

Fig. 15.22 Use of systematic search to explore possible binding modes of mechanism-based inhibitors of chymotrypsin by rotation of six bonds (*) that orient carbonyl of substrate relative to hydroxyl (Du) of Ser-195 (201).

Many technical limitations remain to be overcome before ligand design becomes reliable and routine. Many deficiencies in molecular mechanics previously cited remain that limit reliability. Adequate modeling of electrostatics remains elusive in many experimental systems of interest such as membranes. Newer derivations of force fields, such as MM3 (16, 202), CHARMM (203, 204), AMBER/OPLS (205), ECEPP (206), and others (124, 207) are attempting to represent the experimental data more accurately, while others include a broader spectrum of chemistry such as metals (18–20, 208–212). Combinations of molecular mechanics with quantum chemistry are clearly necessary for problems in which chemical transformations are involved (126, 127, 129, 213). Rather amazing agreement between calculation and experiment have been reported on the relative stabilities of transition-state structures (132, 214), although there is some controversy

regarding this approach (215). In any case, this is another area of rapid growth as adequate computational resources become available.

3.4 Calculation of Affinity

3.4.1 COMPONENTS OF BINDING AFFINITY. The ability to calculate the affinity of prospective ligands based on the known three-dimensional structure of the therapeutic target would allow prioritization of synthetic targets. It would bring quantitation to the qualitative visualization of a potential ligand in the receptor site. While this problem has been solved in principle, in practice, direct application of molecular mechanics has not yet proven to be a reliable indicator. The reasons behind this difficulty become more obvious if one dichotomizes the free energy of binding into a logical set of components.

For example, Williams (216–219) has used a vancomycin-peptide complex (Fig. 15.23) as an experimental system in which to evaluate the various contributions to binding affinity. A similar analysis for antibody mutants was attempted by Novotny (220).

$$\Delta G = \Delta G_{(trans+rot)} + \Delta G_{rotors} + \Delta H_{conform}$$
$$+ \sum \Delta G_i + \Delta G_{vdw} + \Delta G_H$$

where $\Delta G_{(trans+rot)}$ is the free energy associated with translational and rotational freedom of the ligand. This has an adverse effect on binding of 50 to 70 kJ/mol (12 to 16 kcal/mol) at room temperature for ligands of 100 to 300 daltons, assuming complete loss of relative translational and rotational freedom. ΔG_{rotors} is the free energy associated with the number of rotational degrees of freedom frozen. This is 5 to 6 kJ/mol (1.2 to 1.6 kcal/mol) per rotatable bond, assuming complete loss of rotational freedom. $\Delta H_{conform}$ is the strain

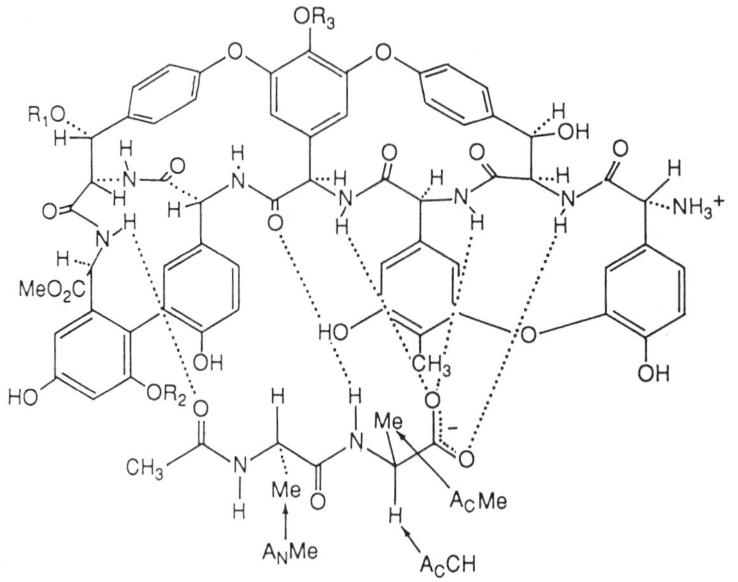

Fig. 15.23 Vancomycin–peptide complex used by Williams et al. (216–219) to investigate components of free energy of binding.

energy introduced by complex formation (deformation in bond lengths, bond angles, torsional angles, etc. from solution states). $\Sigma \Delta G_i$ is the sum of interaction free energies between polar groups. ΔG_{vdw} is the energy derived from enhanced van der Waals interactions in the complex. ΔG_H is the free energy attributed to the hydrophobic effect (0.125 kJ/mol per $\mathring{A}^2$ of hydrocarbon surface removed from solvent by complex formation).

Using this analysis on the vancomycin–dipeptide system, estimates of the contribution of the hydrogen bonds to binding were made that were considerably higher (−24 kJ/mol, −6 kcal/mol) than those derived experimentally (217). The most likely source of error is the assumption of complete loss of relative and internal entropy on binding. In retrospect, Searle and Williams (218) examined the thermodynamics of sublimation of organic compounds without internal rotors, and shown that only 40% to 70% of theoretical entropy loss occurs on crystallization. This provides an estimate of the entropy loss to be expected

on drug-ligand interaction. Applying this correction to the vancomycin–peptide system led to a more conventional view of the hydrogen bond of −2 to −8 kJ/mol (0.5 to −2.0 kcal/mol) (219). As several of the components in the binding energy estimate are directly related to the degree of order of the system (entropy), simulations in solvent may be necessary to quantitate the degree by which the relative motions of the ligand and protein are quenched and the restriction on rotational degrees of freedom on complexation.

3.4.2 BINDING ENERGETICS AND COMPARISONS. Because of the difficulties in calculating binding free energies, attempts to use ΔH as a means of correlation with binding affinities have often appeared in the literature, sometimes meeting with considerable success. These successes are, however, fortuitous and depend on simplifying assumptions as well as the well-known correlation between ΔH and ΔG that has been suggested as an unusual property of the solvent water (221). A similar correlation has been observed in nonaqueous systems and relates to higher entropy loss associated with stronger enthalpic interactions (218). It is a common assumption with congeneric series that the desolvation energies and entropic effects will be approximately the same across members of the series. This, often tacit, assumption may hold for most of the series, but complex formation depends on the total energetics of the complex, and what may appear a relatively innocuous change in a substituent may trigger a different binding mode in which the ligand has reoriented. This will likely impact desolvation as well as entropic effects, as the environments of the majority of interactions of the ligand have changed.

3.4.3 SIMULATIONS AND THE THERMODYNAMIC CYCLE. In a known structure of a drug-receptor complex given a measured affinity of the ligand, the thermodynamic cycle paradigm allows calculation of the difference in affinity ($\Delta\Delta G$) with a novel ligand. Bash et al. (105) successfully calculated the effect of changing a phosphoramidate group (P-NH) to a phosphate ester (P-O) in transition-state analog inhibitors of thermolysin (Fig. 15.24). The difference in free energy between a benzenesulfonamide and its *p*-chloro derivative as an inhibitor of carbonic anhydrase has been calculated (222) as well. This is similar to the original application to enzyme-ligand work on benzamidine inhibitors of trypsin in which the mutation of a proton to a fluorine was calculated (223). Hansen and Kollman (224) calculated differences in the free energy of binding of an inhibitor of adenosine deaminase as one changes a proton to a hydroxyl group using a model of the active site. More recent examples looked at the difference in binding of two stereoisomers of a transition-state inhibitor of HIV protease (225–227) (Fig. 15.25) and

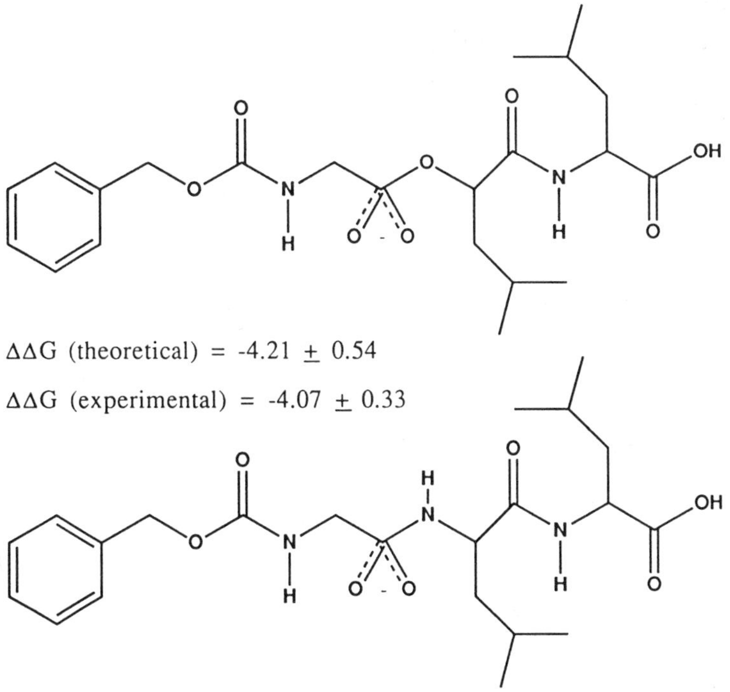

$\Delta\Delta G$ (theoretical) = -4.21 $\pm$ 0.54

$\Delta\Delta G$ (experimental) = -4.07 $\pm$ 0.33

Fig. 15.24 Calculated difference in affinity ($\Delta\Delta G$) compared with experimental value for two inhibitors of thermolysin (105).

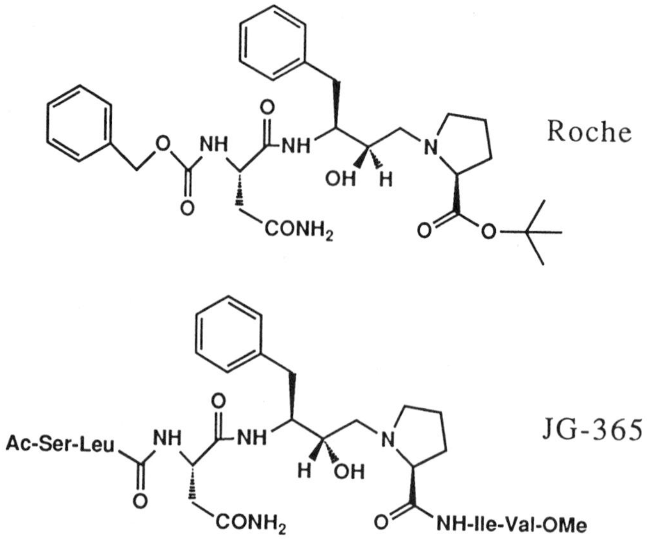

Fig. 15.25 Structures of JG-365 and Ro 31-8959 in which chirality at crucial transition-state hydroxyl is reversed for optimal binding in the two analogues. An alteration in binding mode was predicted to explain this observation, which was subsequently confirmed by crystallography (228).

the affinity of DHFR for methotrexate analogs (229). One obvious conclusion can be drawn: successful applications in the literature deal with relatively minor perturbations to a structure for which there is less chance that the binding mode might be altered. There is at least one example in the literature in which the calculated affini- ty difference did not agree with the experimental date-binding of an antiviral agent to human rhinovirus HRV-14 and to a mutant virus in which a valine was mutated to a leucine (Fig. 15.26) (230). Here a β-branched amino acid (Val) was converted into Leu, which lacks the isopropyl side-chain adjacent to the peptide back-

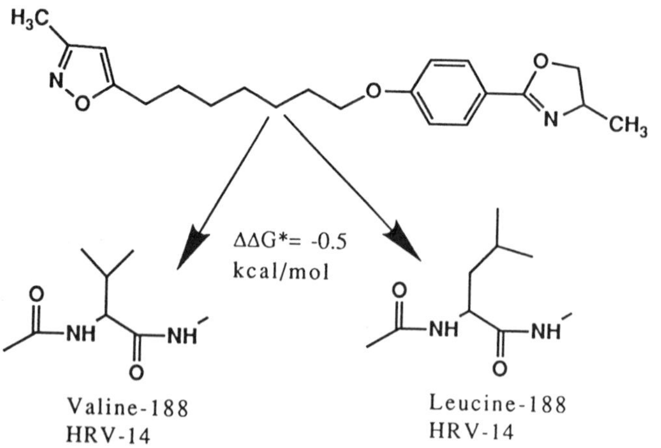

Fig. 15.26 Calculated relative affinity of Sterling-Winthrop antivirals, which bind to a rhinovirus coat protein (HRV-14) and to the V188L mutant. Biological data indicate that the V188L mutant drastically diminishes the activity of the antivirals (230).

bone besides the addition of a methyl group. The differences between calculation and experimental data may be related to rotational isomerism of the side chains, which can be explicitly included (231). Despite the successful examples of this approach that appear in the literature, there exists a growing healthy scepticism regarding its general application. In a discussion of the application of simulations to prediction of the changes in protein stability caused by amino acid mutation, problems in adequate sampling, particularly of the unfolded state, and difficulties with electrostatics were cited (232). A recent review of applications cites numerous other examples (102).

3.4.4 MULTIPLE BINDING MODES.

Realistically, congeneric series, which can be a useful construct, exist only in the mind of the medicinal chemist. The orientation of the drug in the active site depends on a multitude of interactions and a minor perturbation in structure can destabilize the predominant binding mode in favor of another. As examples, detailed analyses of the multiple binding modes shown with thyroxine analogs by transthyretin (a transport protein) (233) and enkephalin analogs by an Fab fragment (234) have been made through crystallography. For this reason, the probability of correct answers with thermodynamic integration studies is directly related to the similarity in structure between the ligand of interest and the reference compound. All three-dimensional methods for predicting affinity require a fundamental assumption about the binding mode (in other words, an orientation rule for aligning compounds in the model). Examination of series of ligands binding to the same site usually includes examples of similar compounds that have different binding modes (for example, the change in orientation (see Fig. 15.25) of the C-terminal portion of the Roche HIV protease inhibitor compared with JG-365) (228).

Molecular modeling is currently capable of distinguishing correctly in many cases between alternate binding modes of the same ligand. Many components (e.g., desolvation and entropy of binding of the ligand) that cloud the issue of direct calculation of affinities are constant when comparing binding modes of the same compound and, therefore, do not have to be evaluated. The computational costs of exploring possible binding modes within the active site are significant, however, expecially when the protein is capable of reorganizing to expose alternative sites, as was the case for a series of ligands for hemoglobin (142).

In a similar fashion, it is generally assumed from the competitive behavior for binding shown by many agonists and antagonists that they bind at the same site on the receptor (certainly, the simplest hypothesis). Recent studies on G-protein coupled receptors indicates that agonists and antagonists often have different binding sites, as mutations in the receptor can affect the binding of one and not the other. An example of such a study on the angiotensin II receptor has been published (235). This story is only beginning to unfold, but appears to be a general phenomenon in G-protein receptors (236, 237). Examples of this phenomenon have been reported with antagonists derived from screening when the structure of antagonist and agonist differ dramatically and also when the antagonists were obtained by minor structural modification of the natural agonist.

3.5 Homology Modeling

Often, the crystal structure of the therapeutic target is not available, but the three-dimensional structure of a homologous protein will have been determined. Depending on the degree of homology between the two proteins, it may be useful to model build the structure of the unknown protein based on the known structure. Many models of the various G-protein coupled receptors have been built based on homology with bacterial rhodopsin (238–240). Models of the three-dimensional structures of human renin (241) and HIV protease (242, 243) were built from crystal structures of homologous aspartyl proteinases as aids to drug design. The known structures of serine proteases have served as templates for models of phospholipase A2 (244) and convertases or subtilases (245). The crystal structure of the MHC class I receptor served to generate a hypothetical model of the foreign antigen binding site of class II histocompatibility molecules (246). Models of human cytochrome P450 have also been built by homology (247).

One of the major difficulties facing construction of such models is the alignment problem, which is compounded by multiple insertions and/or deletions. As the number of known homologous sequences increases, the alignment problem is lessened by consensus criteria. While the interior core of the proteins are often quite similar, significant alterations can occur on surface loops and much effort has been expended to fold these loops (91, 248). In regard to the utility of such models in drug design, one can expect that they will prove useful conceptually but that the molecular details required for optimizing specificity, for example, would be deficient. One is trying to exploit the often subtle differences that arise from sequence changes that are reflected in the three-dimensional structure. Models built by homology would be expected to be weakest in those areas where sequence differences are greatest.

4 UNKNOWN RECEPTORS

Until recently, receptors were hypothetical macromolecules whose existence was postulated on the basis of pharmacological experiments. While recent advances in molecular biology have led to cloning and expression of many of those receptors whose existences were postulated and to a plethora of subtypes, progress in most cases in defining their three-dimensional structure has yet to provide the medicinal chemist with the necessary atomic detail to design novel compounds. Without detailed information about the three-dimensional nature of the receptor, conventional computationally based approaches (i.e., molecular dynamics, Monte Carlo method, etc.) are not possible. One can only attempt to deduce an operational model of the receptor that gives a consistent explanation of the known data and, ideally, provides predictive value when considering new compounds for synthesis and biological testing. The utility of such an approach has been demonstrated by Bures et al. (197) who used the pharmacophoric pattern derived for the plant hormone auxin to find four novel classes of active compounds by searching a corporate three-dimensional database of structures. In many ways, the approach that has evolved is analogous to the American parlor game of twenty questions, in which the medicinal chemist poses the questions in terms of novel three-dimensional chemical structures and attempts to interpret the response of the receptor in a consistent manner. The underlying hypothesis is a structural complementarity between the receptor and compounds that bind. In the same way that the receptor's existence could be deduced based on pharmacological data, some low resolution, three-dimensional schematic of the receptor, at least in regard to the active site or binding pocket, can be deduced by analysis of structure–activity data. It is the purpose of this section to summarize the current approaches in use for receptors of unknown three-dimensional structure and evaluate their utility. For purposes of this section, *receptor* is often used in a completely generic sense (including enzymes, DNA, etc.) as the macromolecular component, i.e., binding site, of recognition of biologically active small molecules.

4.1 Pharmacophore Versus Binding-site Models

4.1.1 PHARMACOPHORE MODELS. It is often useful to assume that the receptor site is rigid and that structurally different drugs bind in conformations that present a similar steric and electronic pattern, the pharmacophore. Most drugs, because of inherent conformational freedom, are capable of presenting a multitude of three-dimensional patterns to a receptor. This pharmacophoric assumption leads to a problem statement that logically is composed of two processes. The first is the determination, by chemical modification and biological testing, of the relative importance of different functional groups in the drug to receptor recognition. This can give some indication of the nature of the functional groups in the receptor that are responsible for binding the set of drugs. Second, a hypothesis is proposed (Fig. 15.27) concerning correspondence, either between functional groups (pharmacophore) in different congeneric series of the drug or between

recognition site points postulated to exist within the receptor (binding-site model).

The intellectual framework for using structure–activity data to extrapolate information regarding the ligand's partner (the receptor) is the concept of the pharmacophore. The pharmacophore, a concept introduced by Ehrlich at the turn of the century, is the critical three-dimensional arrangement of molecular fragments (or the distribution of electron density) that is recognized by the receptor and, in the case of agonists, that causes subsequent activation of the receptor on binding. In other words, some parts of the molecule are essential for interaction, and they must be capable of assuming a particular three-dimensional pattern that is complementary to the receptor to interact favorably. One corollary of the pharmacophoric concept is the ability to replace the chemical scaffold holding the pharmacophoric groups with retention of activity. This is the basis of the current activity in peptidomimetics in which the amide backbone of peptides has been replaced by sugar rings, steroids (249, 250), benzodiazepines (251), or carbocycles (252, 253) (Fig. 15.28). In the pharmacophoric hypothesis, physical overlap of similar functional groups is assumed, i.e., the carboxyl group from compound A physically overlaps with the corresponding

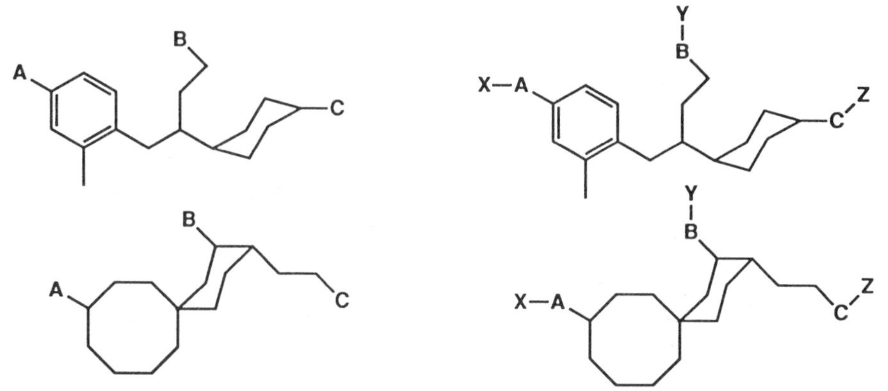

Fig. 15.27 (*a*) Pharmacophore hypothesis with correspondence of functional groups in drugs, A = A′, B = B′, C = C′. (*b*) Binding-site hypothesis using drugs with hypothetical binding sites attached (X, Y, and Z overlap).

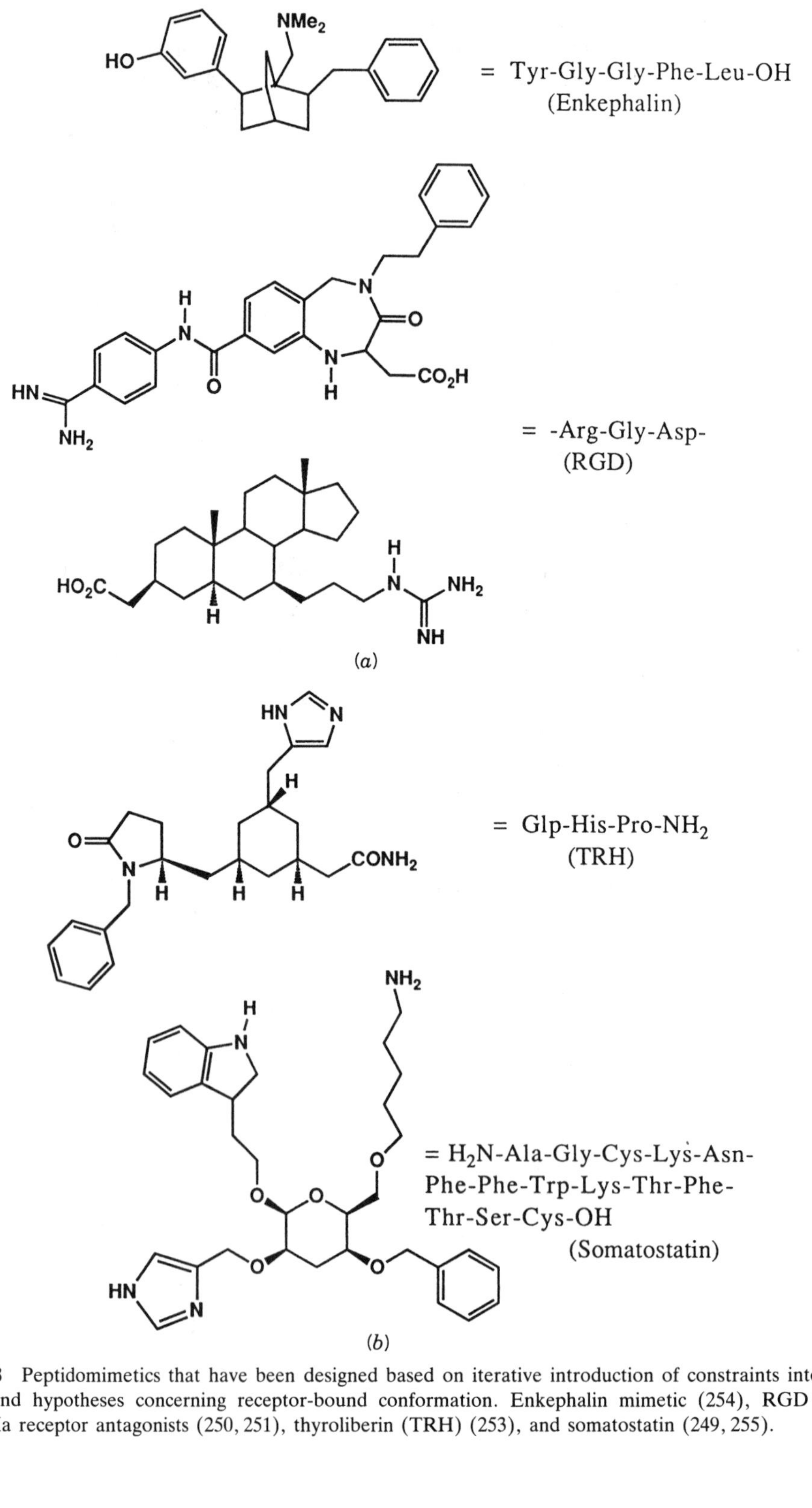

= Tyr-Gly-Gly-Phe-Leu-OH
(Enkephalin)

= -Arg-Gly-Asp-
(RGD)

(a)

= Glp-His-Pro-NH₂
(TRH)

= H₂N-Ala-Gly-Cys-Lys-Asn-
Phe-Phe-Trp-Lys-Thr-Phe-
Thr-Ser-Cys-OH
(Somatostatin)

(b)

Fig. 15.28 Peptidomimetics that have been designed based on iterative introduction of constraints into parent peptide and hypotheses concerning receptor-bound conformation. Enkephalin mimetic (254), RGD platelet GPIIb/IIIa receptor antagonists (250, 251), thyroliberin (TRH) (253), and somatostatin (249, 255).

carboxyl group from compound B and with the bioisosteric tetrazole ring of compound C.

One caveat that must be remembered is the probability of alternate or multiple binding modes. The interaction of a ligand with a binding site depends on the free energy of binding, a complex interaction with both entropic and enthalpic components. Simple modifications in structure may favor one of several nearly energetically equivalent modes of interaction with the receptor and change the correspondence between functional groups that has previously been assumed and supported by experimental data. Changes in the binding mode of an antibody Fab fragment to progesterone and its analogs has been shown by crystallography of the complexes (256, 257). For this reason, analysis of agonists as a class is usually preferred, as the necessity to both bind and trigger a subsequent transduction event is more restrictive than the simple requirement for binding shared by antagonists (235). Compounds that clearly are inconsistent with models derived from large amounts of structure–activity data may be indicative of such changes in binding mode and may require a separate structure–activity study to characterize their interaction.

4.1.2 BINDING-SITE MODELS. One major deficiency in the approach described above is the requirement for overlap of functional groups in accord with the pharmacophoric hypothesis. While it is true that molecules having functional groups that show three-dimensional correspondence can interact with the same site, it is also true that a particular geometry associated with one site is capable of interacting with equal affinity with a variety of orientations of the same functional groups. One has only to consider the cone of nearly equal energetic arrangements of a hydrogen-bond donor and acceptor to realize the problem. Sufficient examples from crystal structures of drug–

enzyme complexes and from theoretical simulation of binding compel the realization that the pharmacophore is a limiting assumption. Clearly, the observed binding mode in a complex represents the optimal position of the ligand in an asymmetric force field created by the receptor that is subject to perturbation from solvation and entropic considerations. Less restrictive is the assumption that the receptor-binding site remains relatively fixed in geometry when binding the series of compounds under study. Experimental support for such a hypothesis can be found in crystal structures of enzyme–inhibitor complexes in which the enzyme presents essentially the same conformation, despite large variations in inhibitor structures; studies of HIV-1 protease complexed with diverse inhibitors support this view (137). In recent years, therefore, there has been an increasing effort to focus on the groups of the receptor that interact with ligands as being the common features for recognition of a set of analogs. When pharmacophore and binding-site hypotheses are compared, the binding-site model is physicochemically more plausible, because overlap of functional groups in binding to a receptor is more restrictive than assuming the site remains relatively fixed when binding different ligands. However, the number of degrees of freedom in binding-site hypotheses (represented by the necessary addition of virtual bonds between groups A and X, B and Y, and C and Z in Figure 15.27) is greater. Additional degrees of freedom complicate subsequent conformational analyses and may preclude any conclusions, unless a sufficiently diverse set of compounds is available.

Other approaches to this problem have emphasized comparison of molecular properties rather than atom correspondences. Kato et al. (258) developed a program that allows construction of a receptor cavity around a molecule, emphasizing the electrostatic and hydrogen-bonding capabilities. Other molecules can then be fit within the cavity to align them. This is similar in concept to the field-fit techniques available in the CoMFA module of SYBYL, in which the molecular field (electrostatic and steric) surrounding a selected molecule becomes the objective criterion for alignment of subsequent molecules for analysis. An example emphasizing molecular properties in pharmacophoric analysis has been given on inhibitors of cAMP phosphodiesterase II (259).

4.1.3 MOLECULAR EXTENSIONS. If one assumes the binding-site points remain fixed and can augment the drug with appropriate molecular extensions that include the binding site (e.g., a hydrogen-bond donor correctly positioned next to an acceptor), one can then examine the set of possible geometric orientations of site points to see if one is capable of binding all the ligands. Here, the basic assumption of rigid site points is more reasonable, at least for enzymes that have evolved to catalyze reactions and must, therefore, position critical groups in a specific three-dimensional arrangement to create the correct electronic environment for catalysis. The program checks this hypothesis by determining if one or more geometrical arrangements of the postulated groups of site points are common to the set of active compounds. Such a geometrical arrangement of receptor groups becomes a candi-

date binding-site model, which can be evaluated for predictive merit.

In a study of the active site of angiotensin-converting enzyme (ACE) (260), this binding site model was used by incorporating the active site components as parts of each compound undergoing analysis. As an example, the sulfhydryl portion of captopril was extended to include a zinc bound at the experimentally optimal bond length and bond angle for zinc–sulfur complexes (Fig. 15.29). The orientation map (OMAP), which is a multidimensional representation of the interatomic distances between pharmacophoric groups (Fig. 15.30), was based on the distances between binding-site points such as the zinc atom with the introduction of more degrees of torsional freedom to accommodate the possible positioning of the zinc relative to ACE inhibitors such as captopril (262). Analyses of nearly 30 different chemical classes (Fig. 15.31) of ACE inhibitors led to a unique arrangement of the components of the active site postulated to be responsible for binding the inhibitors. The displacement of the zinc atom in ACE to a location more distant from the carboxyl-binding Arg seen in carboxypeptidase A is compatible with the fact that ACE cleaves dipeptides from the C-terminus of peptides whereas carboxypeptidase A cleaves single amino acid residues.

Visualization of the OMAP is useful to judge the additional information intro-

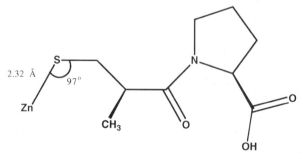

Fig. 15.29 Extension of sulfhydryl group of captopril to include postulated active site zinc, using optimal bond length and angles (260, 261).

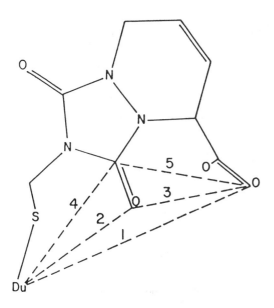

Fig. 15.30 Distances used in five-dimensional OMAP for analysis of ACE inhibitors (260).

duced as each new compound is added (Fig. 15.32). Computationally, it is much more efficient to treat the set of noncongeneric compounds simultaneously (77, 263), but it is reassuring when identical results are obtained if one uses the sequential procedure, introducing each molecule in turn, so that intermediate results may be visually verified. The use of computer graphics to confirm intermediate processing of data in convenient display modes becomes increasingly more important as the individual computations and numbers of molecules under consideration increase.

4.1.4 ACTIVITY VERSUS AFFINITY. Given a consistent model of either type, a limitation is that one can only ask if the compound under consideration can present the three-dimensional electronic pattern (pharmacophore) that is the current candidate. In other words, one is limited to predicting the presence or absence of activity, a binary choice. Even the presence of the appropriate pattern is insufficient to ensure biological activity. For example, competition

with the receptor for occupied space by other parts of the molecule can inhibit binding and preclude activity. One can, therefore, postulate the following conditions for activity:

1. The compound must be metabolically stable and capable of transport to the site for receptor interaction (interpretation of inactive compounds may be flawed by problems with bioavailability).
2. The compound must be capable of assuming a conformation which will present the pharmacophoric or binding-site pattern complementary to that of the receptor.
3. The compound must not compete with the receptor for space while presenting the pharmacophoric or binding-site pattern.

Once these conditions are met, one can attempt to deal with the potency, or binding affinity. This belongs to the domain of three-dimensional quantitative structure–activity relationships (3D-QSAR) (264); the use of the variant CoMFA (148, 265) on ACE inhibitors will be illustrated at the end of this chapter. Condition 3 allows one to use compounds that are capable of presenting the pharmacophoric pattern but incapable of binding to help determine the location of receptor-occupied space in relation to the pharmacophore (receptor mapping) (266). This allows a crude, low resolution map of the position of the receptor relative to the pharmacophoric elements and indicates in which directions chemical modifications may be productive.

The number and diversity of compounds available for analysis determines the methodology to be used. If there is a limited data set, then the pharmacophoric approach should be assessed first, due to its fewer degrees of freedom. If no pharmacophoric patterns are consistent with the

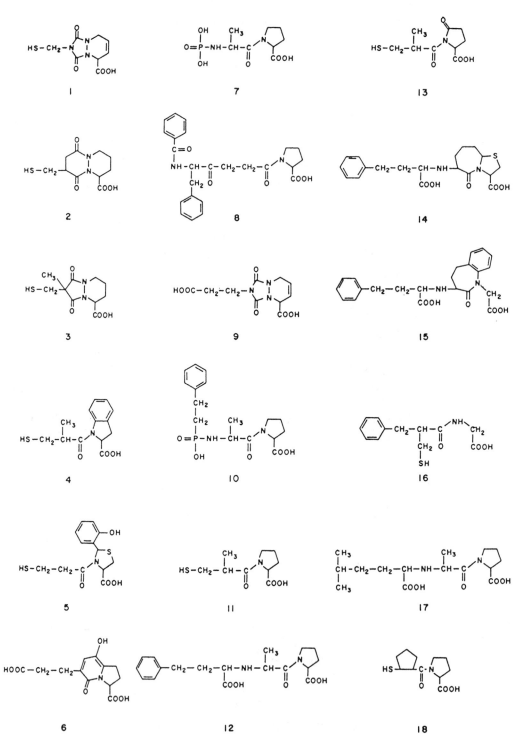

Fig. 15.31 Compounds from different chemical classes of ACE inhibitors used in active site analysis. From Ref. 260.

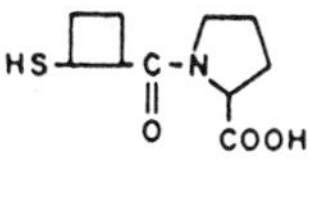

19

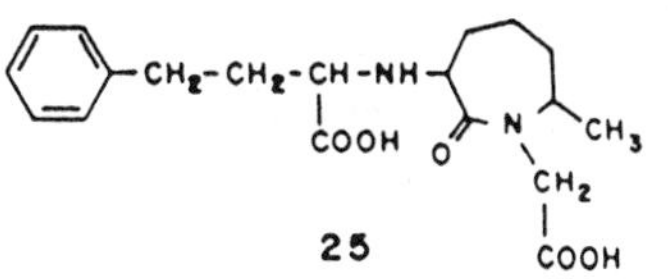

25

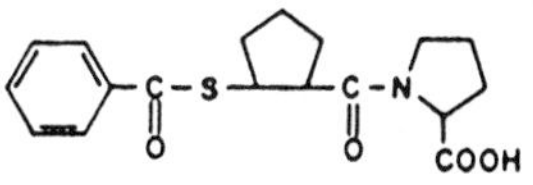

20

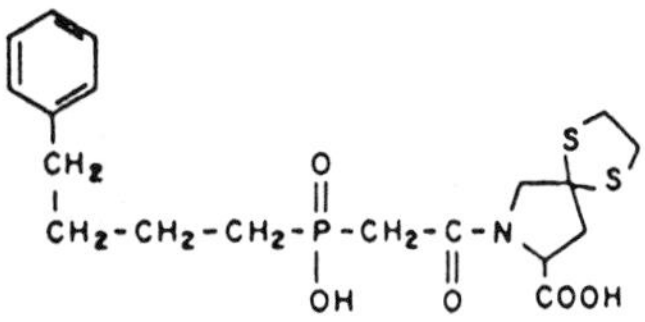

26

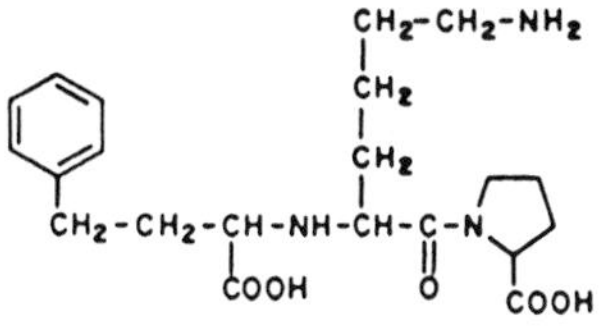

21

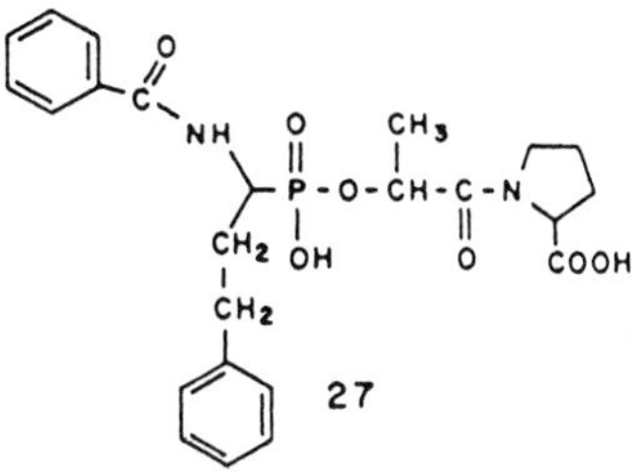

27

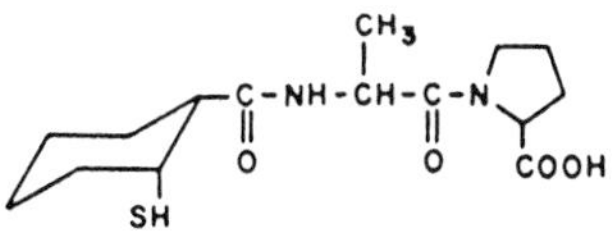

22

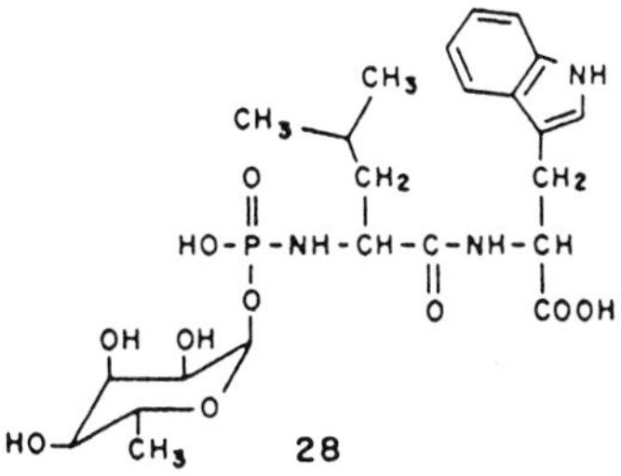

28

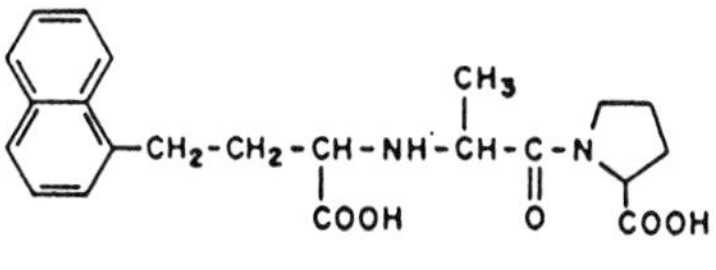

23

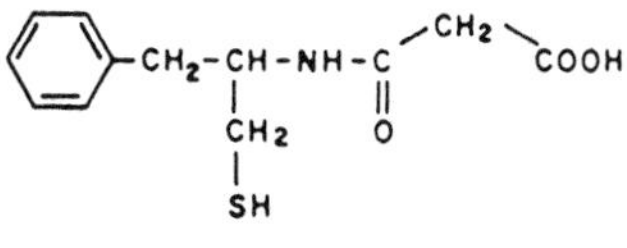

29

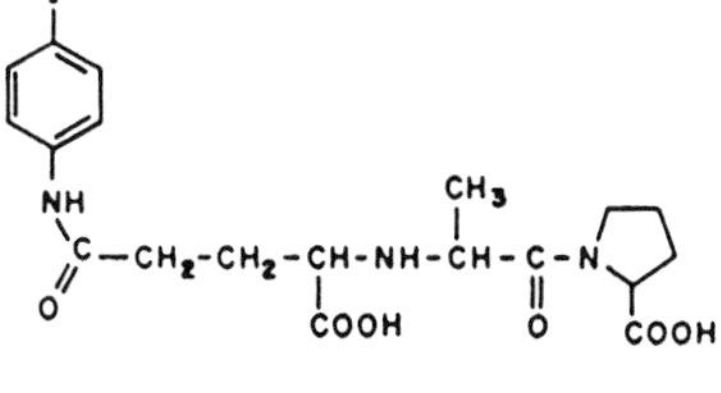

24

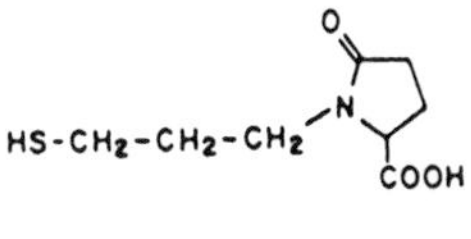

30

Fig. 15.31 (*Continued*)

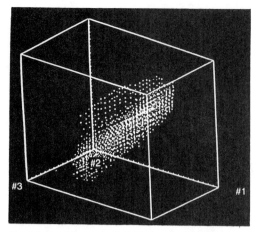

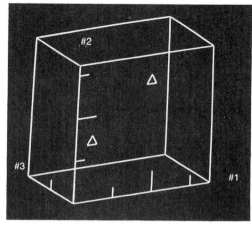

Fig. 15.32 Change in OMAP (projection of three of the five dimensions) as new compounds were introduced to analysis of ACE inhibitors (260). The original OMAP of compound 1 (see Fig. 15.31) is to the left, and the OMAP after completion of analysis is to the right.

set of analogs, then introduction of logical molecular extensions to enable the active site approach is warranted. Operationally, one first determines the set of potential pharmacophoric patterns consistent with the set of active analogs, leading to its name: active analog approach (262). If there are sufficient data, then a unique pharmacophore, or active site model, may be identifiable. The basic assumption behind efforts to infer properties of the receptor from a study of structure–activity relations of drugs that bind is the idea of complementarity. It follows that the stronger the binding affinity, the more likely that the drug fits the receptor cavity and aligns those functional groups that have specific interactions in a way complementary to those of the receptor itself. Certainly, our understanding of intermolecular interactions from studies of known complexes do not dissuade us of this notion but may make us somewhat skeptical of the naive models that often result from such efforts. Andrews et al. (267) have reviewed efforts of this type with regard to CNS drugs.

Clearly, the key to insight relies on chemical modification to determine the relative importance of functional groups for molecular recognition. Often more subtle effects than the simple presence or absence of a group are important, and then comparison of molecular properties becomes of interest. A major impediment to analysis is the definition of a common frame of reference by which to align molecules for comparison. This is equivalent to solving the three-dimensional pharmacophoric pattern and implies that one has distinguished those properties of the molecules under consideration in a manner similar to the receptor. Initial efforts to rationalize structure–activity relationships (SAR) among noncongeneric systems was hampered by an "RMS mentality," i.e., a point of view that required atomic centers to align rather than to overlap with steric and electronically similar groupings. An example would be requiring the six atoms of aromatic benzene rings to overlap at each of the six atoms of the ring vertices rather than the simple requirements for coincidence and coplanarity, which would recognize the torus of electron density that the rings share in common (Fig. 15.33). In congeneric series, the difficulties in assignment of correspondence is less (nonexistent by defini-

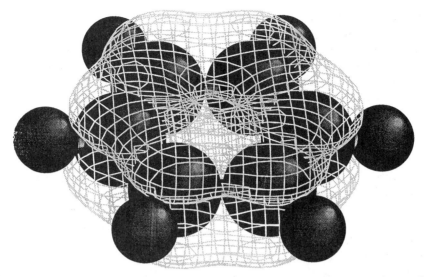

Fig. 15.33 Torus of electron density representing a benzene ring. Atom-to-atom correspondences of ring atoms used in normal fitting routines lead to overconstrained fits.

tion). This allows a variety of approaches, including those based on molecular graph theory (268–271), to detect similarities between molecules, which can form the basis of a correlation analysis. Extrapolation outside of the group of congenerically related compounds on which the analysis was based would appear difficult, if not impossible.

While it is simpler to start an analysis with a congeneric series to identify the recognition elements, diversity in chemical structures implies more information regarding the conformational requirements of the system. A congeneric series requires that the basic chemical framework of the molecule remains constant and that groups on the periphery are either modified (e.g., aromatic substitution) or substituted (e.g., tetrazole for carboxyl functional group). Implicit in this concept is the notion that the compounds bind to the receptor in a similar fashion, and therefore, the changes are localized and comparable for each position of modification. Introduction of degrees of freedom in the substituents and consideration of differences in properties that are conformationally dependent, such

as the electric field, require conformational analysis in an effort to determine the relevant conformation for comparison.

The problem can be divided into two: what are the aspects of the molecules that are in common and that may provide the basis for molecular recognition, and which conformation for each molecule is appropriate to consider? For the first problem, studies on a congeneric series can often yield valuable insight. For determination of the three-dimensional arrangement of the crucial recognition elements, diversity in the chemical scaffolds imposes different constraints on possible three-dimensional patterns and generates an opportunity for determining a unique solution.

4.2 Searching for Similarity

4.2.1 SIMPLE COMPARISONS. To gain insight into molecular recognition, subtle differences in molecules must be perceived. Comparisons can be divided into two categories: those that are independent of the orientation and position of the molecule and those that depend on a known frame of reference. Simple comparisons deal with properties independent of a reference frame. For example, the magnitude of the dipole moment is frame independent, but the dipole itself is a vectorial quantity that depends on the orientation and conformation of the molecule. Similarly, the bond lengths, valence angles, torsion angles, and interatomic distances are independent of orientation. The distance matrix composed of the set of interatomic distances (Fig. 15.34) is a convenient representation of molecular structure that is invariant to rotation and translation of the molecule, but that reflects changes in internal degrees of freedom. The distance range matrix is an extension (see Fig. 15.34) that has two values for each interatomic distance, representing the upper and lower limits or range allowed for a given interatomic distance due to the conformational flexibility of the molecule. Crippen (272) developed a procedure that will generate conformations that conform to the constraints represented by such a distance range matrix. This approach is used to generate structures from experimental mea-

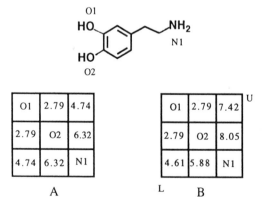

Fig. 15.34 (*a*) Distance matrix in which unique interatomic distances for a particular conformation of a molecule are stored. (*b*) Distance range matrix in which ranges of interatomic distances representing conformational flexibility of molecule are stored. *U*, upper bound; *L*, lower bound.

surements such as nuclear Overhauser effects in NMR experiments. The use of distance range matrices in the identification of pharmacophoric patterns was initially illustrated by Marshall et al. (262) (Fig. 15.35) and has recently been used by Clark (273) in three-dimensional databases for representing the conformational flexibility of molecules. Pepperrell and Willett (274) examined several techniques for comparing molecules, using distance matrices. Other descriptors for comparison of pharmacophoric patterns and retrieval of similar substructures are under active investigation (275).

4.2.2 VISUALIZATION OF MOLECULAR PROPERTIES. Although straightforward displays of molecular structure have proven to be extremely useful tools that enable medicinal chemists to visualize molecules and to compare their structural properties in three dimensions, of even greater potential utility is the display of the various chemical and physical properties of molecules in addition to their structures (276). Such displays allow the comparison not only of molecular shapes and three-dimensional structures but also of molecular properties such as internal energy, electronic charge distribution, and hydrophobic character. A number of different properties have been displayed in this manner in an effort to gain insight into molecular recognition in a series of compounds (276).

Among the more useful properties is the electrostatic potential. Any distribution of electrostatic charge, such as the electrons and nuclei of a molecule, creates an electrostatic potential in the surrounding space that at any given point represents the potential of the molecule for interacting with an electrostatic charge at that point. This potential is a useful property for analyzing and predicting molecular reactive behavior. In particular, it has been shown to be an indicator of the sites or regions of a molecule to which an approaching elec-

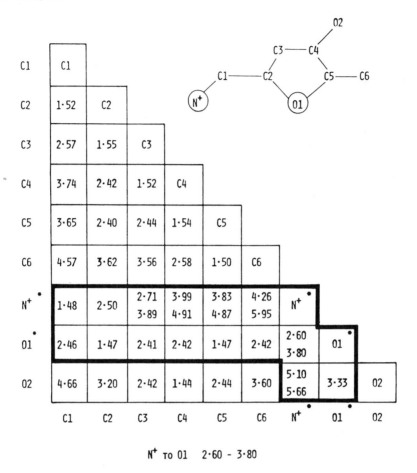

Fig. 15.35 Distance range matrices used for illustration of analysis of muscarinic receptor. From Ref. 262.

trophile or nucleophile is initially attracted or from which it is repelled (Fig. 15.36).

The major obstacle to use of electrostatic potentials in the comparison of different molecules, has been the sheer volume of information produced. The traditional means of displaying such large amounts of data has been to display the electrostatic potential around a molecule as a two-dimensional contour map. The advent of computer graphics techniques have improved the situation by allowing three-dimensional contour maps to be displayed in color on the graphics screen and manipulated in real time along with a display of the molecule itself. An alternative mode

for displaying molecular electrostatic potentials is to employ a dotted surface representation, with the dots taking on an appropriate color according to the electrostatic potential value at the relevant location. Such techniques were initially derived to display empirically determined potentials on the surface of proteins, but have since been used widely to display the electrostatic potentials on sets of small molecules for comparative purposes.

Other graphical uses of the electrostatic potential have been used by Davis et al. (277), who were able graphically to align cAMP and cGMP based on the superimposition of their respective electrostatic

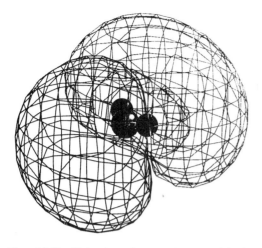

Fig. 15.36 Molecular electrostatic potential for water. Positive potential superimposed on the right surrounds hydrogens, and negative potential on the left surrounds oxygen.

potential minima, and by Weinstein et al. (278) who oriented 5-hydroxytryptamine and 6-hydroxytryptamine based on the alignment of an electrostatically derived orientation vector.

In a similar procedure to that described for the display of electrostatic potential, Cohen and colleagues (279) developed a technique whereby the steric field surrounding a molecule can be displayed on a graphics screen as a three-dimensional isopotential contour map. The map is generated by calculating the VDW interaction energy between the molecule and a probe atom or molecule placed at varying points around the molecule of interest. This interaction energy is then contoured at specific levels to give the most stable VDW contour lines around the molecule, i.e., the contour that represents the most favorable steric position for the probe as it is moved around the target.

A similar three-dimensional contour representation of a molecule can be obtained for both the electronic and steric fields of a molecule within the Comparative Molecular Field Analysis (CoMFA) methodology, which was developed to investigate three-dimensional quantitative structure–activity

relationships (3D-QSARs) (148, 264). In this procedure, the molecule is surrounded by a regular lattice of points, at each point of which a van der Waals and an electrostatic interaction energy between the molecule and a probe atom is computed (Fig. 15.37). Isocontours can then be generated around individual molecules, displayed graphically, and they can be statistically compared throughout a series of molecules in an attempt to generate 3D-QSARs and hence to rationalize activity data. This is similar to the GRID program (147), which uses various probe groups to map potential interactions around a molecule (280).

In situations where, either from previous QSAR work or from experimental evidence, it is known or suspected that differences in the reactivity of a set of molecules are caused primarily by their hydrophobic

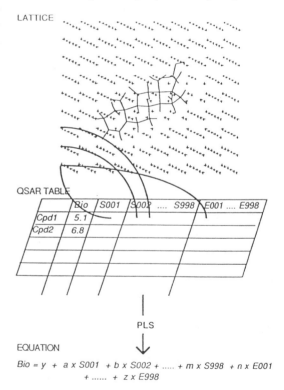

Fig. 15.37 Calculation of electrostatic and VDW fields surrounding a series of molecules in defined orientations are used as a basis for 3D-QSAR correlations in CoMFA. From Ref. 148.

rather than their electrostatic properties, it is probably of more use to compare molecular surfaces that display hydrophobicity or polarity information. Indeed, dotted molecular surfaces color coded by hydrophobic character have been used successfully to rationalize QSARs from several different systems (281, 282). This concept has been extended to calculate the hydrophobic field surrounding a molecule and used in CoMFA studies (283, 284).

4.3 Molecular Comparisons

To compare molecules in a general way, a means of superposition or correctly orienting the molecules in the same reference frame must be available. A procedure for positioning an atom in the molecule at the center of the coordinate frame with other atoms positioned along coordinate axes can be used, or the molecules can be successively fit to one that is used as the standard orientation. An approach that finds geometric similarities in positions of hydrogen-bonded atoms between two molecules has been described (285). Least-squares fitting procedures for designated atoms allows selectivity in orienting the molecules with predetermined conformations in the most appropriate manner. An efficient method for fitting a series of molecules when atom–atom associations have been previously defined between members of the series has also been described (286). In some cases, the use of dummy atoms allows geometric superposition of groups such as aromatic rings without requiring superposition of the atoms composing the ring. By defining the centroid of the ring and erecting a normal to the plane of the ring, the dummy atom at the end of the normal and the centroid dummy atom can be used to superimpose the ring on another ring with similar dummy atoms (Fig. 15.38). This method leads to coincidence and coplanarity of the two ring systems, without requiring the atoms composing the rings to be

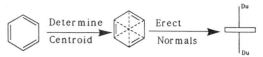

Fig. 15.38 Construction of dummy vector perpendicular to plane of aromatic ring at centroid, which allows superposition and coincidence of aromatic rings by fitting endpoints (Du) of dummy vector without requiring superposition of ring atoms.

coincident. In other words, the rings can be viewed as two tori of electron density without overemphasizing the positions of the atomic nuclei. In numerous studies of biogenic amine ligands, this method of comparison of the aromatic ring components is essential to allow alignment of the nitrogens (267).

4.3.1 VOLUME MAPPING. One method of displaying molecular surfaces that retains the ability to transform the display interactively was developed (287). The procedure involves computing a molecular pseudo-electron density map on a three-dimensional grid that surrounds the molecule, whose atoms are replaced by dummy gaussian atoms. Atom types are characterized by a half-width and an integrated density, chosen so that the Gaussians have a fixed value at a distance equal to the VDW radius (Fig. 15.39). Such density maps may be contoured in three dimensions to provide a chicken-wire envelope around the molecule that corresponds to the van der Waals surface.

A concomitant benefit of this technique is that estimates of the molecular surface area and volume are generated as by-products of the contouring routines, whether the surface is being drawn around one or several molecules. In addition, the generated surfaces and volumes are readily susceptible to logical operations, such as union, intersection, or subtraction, enabling the rapid determination of, e.g.,

Atom	Temperature Factor	Atomic Number
Carbon	60	25
Nitrogen	55	25
Oxygen	50	25
Sulfur	67	35
Phosphorus	70	35
Hydrogen	40	15
Bromine	65	50
Chlorine	60	35
Fluorine	40	40
Iodine	80	53
Sodium	87	85
Potassium	130	85
Calcium	130	85
Lithium	65	50
Aluminum	80	53
Silicon	80	55

Fig. 15.39 Set of parameters to generate pseudoelectron density maps of molecules that can be contoured to represent approximately the VDW surface.

union or difference volumes among a series of molecules.

Once one has fixed the molecules in a common frame of reference, then comparison by a variety of techniques becomes feasible. As an example, difference in volume may be important in understanding the lack of seen activity in compounds that appear to possess all the prerequisites for activity seen in others in the series. In a congeneric series, a significant portion of the molecular structure is common to the molecules under comparison. This common volume, which is shared logically, should not contribute to differences in activity. By subtraction of the volume shared by two molecules, one obtains a difference map in which the volume occupied by one molecule and not the other remains (262). Correlations between the shared volume and the biological activity of a congeneric series of inhibitors of DHFR have been shown by Hopfinger (288). Simon and his colleagues (289) emphasized the use of both overlapping volume and nonoverlapping volume in QSAR studies in the quan-

titative methodology, the minimal steric difference, or the MTD method. This approach has been enhanced to allow comparison of low energy conformers of each molecule and use of those that are sterically most similar. An application to substrates of acetylcholinesterase illustrate this facility (290).

4.3.2 FIELD EFFECTS. Once the frame of reference has been established, other properties of molecules, such as the electrostatic field, can be compared as well. As the electrostatic properties can be sampled on a grid, differences between the values of two molecules can be calculated and a difference map contoured. Such difference maps highlight more clearly the similarities and differences between molecules (291). Hopfinger (292) integrated the difference between potential fields and showed this parameter to be useful in QSAR studies.

An approach to quantifying statistically the similarity between two molecular electrostatic potential surfaces has been developed (177, 293, 294). Here, the previously determined molecular electrostatic potential surfaces are projected outward onto surrounding spheres, which provide a common surface of reference, and then statistical analyses are performed over the points on this common surface in an attempt to quantify the similarities or differences between the two molecules under consideration. Burt and Richards (184) introduced flexibility in the comparison of molecules based on their electrostatic potential fields.

4.3.3 DIRECTIONALITY.
If one is comparing molecules that share interaction at a common site on a biological macromolecule, it is logical to assume that they may do so by interacting with similar sites in the receptor with optimal interaction shown by molecules with correctly oriented functional groups. If one does not have a three-dimensional model of the receptor from which to deduce potential interactive sites, then one can only attempt to deduce the potential interactive receptor-subsites by examination of the molecules that interact with them. Systematically, one can vary the conformation of a molecule and record the relative orientation of groups postulated, or shown experimentally, to play a dominant role in intermolecular interactions. In this way, one can map out the directionality of interactions of each functional group of the ligand in a common frame of reference. Comparison of these maps can often lead to hypotheses regarding pharmacophoric groups and their correspondence between molecules.

4.3.4 LOCUS MAPS.
One can generate a *locus* plot in coordinate space that shows all the potential locations of one group relative to another by fixing one group in a particular orientation as a frame of reference and recording all possible coordinates of the other. An example would be the relative positions of the basic nitrogen to the aromatic ring in compounds such as

dopamine interacting with biogenic amine receptors. One must choose the common fragment (in the example, the aromatic ring) of each molecule and its orientation to generate a similar frame of reference so that the locus of positions of the atom (the basic nitrogen) leads to a meaningful comparison across a series of molecules (Fig. 15.40).

4.3.5 VECTOR MAPS AND CONFORMATIONAL MIMICRY.
Often, one is more interested in accessing the directionality of potential interaction rather than simply looking for overlap of atoms such as the basic nitrogen. In this case, for example, one is interested in determining both the locus of the lone pair of the nitrogen and the nitrogen, as the ordered pair of coordinates determines a vector in the chosen frame of reference. The resulting plot of the locus of all possible vectors of the nitrogen lone pair constitutes a *vector* map. The combination of positional information with relative orientation offers considerable insight into potential interactions with a hypothetical receptor. Lloyd and Andrews's (195) postulation of a common theme in CNS receptors based on an underlying biogenic amine pattern can be rationalized using the vector map approach.

The use of vector maps is essential to the assessment of *conformational mimicry*, in

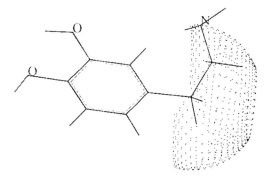

Fig. 15.40 Locus of sterically allowed positions of nitrogen atoms in dopamine relative to the aromatic ring.

which one attempts to determine the statistical probability that the conformation essential for activity will be preserved with a given chemical modification. An example will serve to illustrate this concept and its application. Modification of amide bonds (introduction of amide isosteres) in peptide drugs to increase metabolic stability may alter the potential accessible conformations. This may preclude the compound containing the isostere from adopting the correct orientation for receptor recognition and activation. In the general case, one has no specific information regarding which particular conformation is biologically relevant and can only assess whether the chemical modification mimics the amide bond in its conformational effects. This can be quantitatively assessed by the comparison of the percentage of vectors of the vector map of the parent amide bond, which can be found in a comparable vector map of the analog. Work by Zabrocki et al. (296) on the use of 1,5-disubstituted tetrazole rings as surrogates for the *cis*-amide bond illustrates this application. The linear dipeptide acetyl-Ala-Ala-methylamide (with the amide bond between the two alanine residues in the *cis*-conformation) and the tetrazole analog acetyl-AlaΨ[CN4]Ala-methylamide were modeled using the coordinates derived from diketopiperazines for the *cis*-amide bond or from the crystal structure of the

cyclic tetrazole dipeptide. A systematic, or grid, search that determines the sterically allowed conformations by systematically varying the torsional degrees of freedom was used to generate a Ramachandran plot for each of the pairs of backbone torsional angles (Φ, Ψ) associated with each amino acid residue. The rigid geometry approximation was used with the set of scaled VDW radii shown by Iijima and co-workers (75) to reproduce the experimental crystal data for proteins and peptides. When the *cis*-amide dipeptide model was calculated, the orientations of the $C^\alpha-C^\beta$ bond of Ala-1, with the methylamide fixed as a frame of reference, were recorded for each sterically allowed conformation (Fig. 15.41). Using the same orientation of the methylamide in the tetrazole allowed the program to determine which vectors or orientations of the Ala-1 side chain relative to the methylamide were common to both dipeptides. Alternatively, the acetyl group was used as the fixed frame of reference and the side chain orientation of Ala-2 was used to monitor conformational mimicry. Because the quantitative results were essentially the same, the measurement of mimicry was shown to be independent of the chosen frame of reference. A torsional increment of 10 degrees was used, and a side chain vector was assumed to correspond if both the carbon-α and carbon-β were within 0.2 Å of the coordinates of another vector.

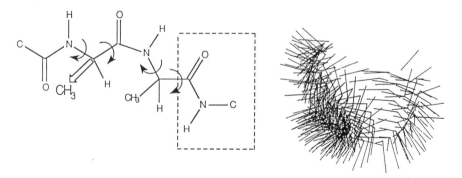

Fig. 15.41 Vector map of the orientations of the C^α-C^β bond of Ala^1; the methylamide is fixed as a frame of reference for the dipeptide Ac-Ala-Ala-NH-CH$_3$, in which the central amide bond was *cis*. From Ref. 296.

The percentage of orientations available to the analog that are also available to the parent is referred to as the conformational mimicry index. For the tetrazole surrogate of the *cis*-amide bond, the conformational mimicry index is 88% (the number of vectors, 747, common to both the tetrazole and *cis*-amide divided by the total number of vectors, 849, allowed for the *cis*-amide). The tetrazole analog has more conformational freedom than the *cis*-amide model with 33,359 conformers allowed compared with 14,912 allowed for the *cis*-amide of the 36^4 (or 1,679,616) possible conformations. This difference was easily visualized in plots of the vector maps for the two dipeptides.

A more recent example of the use of vector maps to evaluate conformational similarity is an application to β-turn mimetics (297, 298). This led to a recognition that many of the various turn types described in peptides based on their backbone dihedral angles lead to quite similar topographical arrangements of the side chains. A new parameter, β (the dihedral angle formed by the backbone atoms $C_{(1)}$-$\alpha C_{(2)}$-$\alpha C_{(3)}$-$N_{(4)}$), was described (Fig. 15.42), which more readily facilitated comparison of the topography of the system.

4.4 Finding the Common Pattern

If one assumes that a common binding mode exists for two or more compounds, then one can use the computer to verify the geometric feasibility of the assumption. One must determine whether it is possible for the two molecules to present a common geometric arrangement of the designated "important" functional groups for recognition. There are two distinct approaches to this problem. The first is associated with minimization methodology and focuses on the existence issue. Is there a conformation that is energetically accessible to each of the molecules under consideration that will place the designated functional groups in a similar orientation? The second approach attempts systematically to enumerate all possible conformations and derive, thereby, all possible orientations or patterns to determine the set of patterns shared by the compounds under study. The latter approach, when it can be applied, addresses the question of uniqueness of the common pattern directly.

The search for the global minimum, or complete set of low energy minima, on a potential surface is a common problem in science and engineering and does not have a general solution. Numerous approaches in chemistry have been used: most commonly, stochastic methods such as distance geometry (272), molecular dynamics, and Monte Carlo sampling. Although distance geometry and molecular dynamics are widely used in the elucidation of solution conformations from NMR data, they have problems in conformational sampling and homogeneous treatment of data from rigid and mobile domains. In general, the difficulties with most methods are similar to

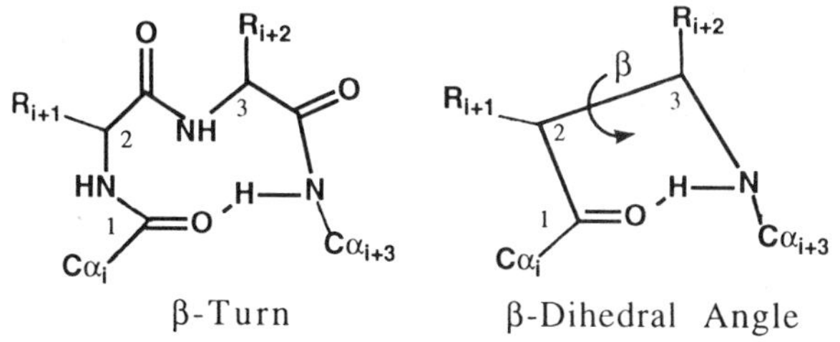

β-Turn β-Dihedral Angle

Fig. 15.42 Definition of new parameter β, the dihedral angle between the backbone atoms $C_{(1)}$-$\alpha C_{(2)}$-$\alpha C_{(3)}$-$N_{(4)}$ of peptides, which is used to describe the topography of reverse turns (297).

those seen with minimization procedures. If one is in the area of the global minimum, then one is likely to converge to that solution. Otherwise, one will be trapped in some local minimum. In contrast, systematic search methods are algorithmic, so that all sterically allowed conformations are generated at the selected torsional grid parameters. Systematic search methods, therefore, do not have problems in sampling and are path independent, but they are combinatorial in complexity, which may limit the fineness of the sample grid and thus compromise the results. Only in small systems such as cycloalkane rings have the potential energy hypersurfaces been mapped (89).

4.4.1 CONSTRAINED MINIMIZATION. In cases where one has internal degrees of freedom, besides the six associated with position and orientation, the use of constrained minimization procedures becomes a useful tech-

nique. Often the standard molecule for comparison has a fixed conformation and the molecule to be fitted has internal degrees of freedom. Several groups have published methods for dealing with this problem. In case one has simultaneous degrees of freedom in both the molecule to be fit and the target, a different approach with simultaneous minimization of all variables is recommended (Fig. 15.43).

The combination of molecular mechanics with flexible minimization routines allows penalty functions to be assigned to force geometrical correspondence of groups, while individual molecules have their internal energy evaluated but are invisible to the other molecules under consideration. A program was described with this capability (299), and its use was illustrated on histamine antagonists (300). Template forcing allows one molecule to be set up as a template and another molecule to be constrained to overlap in a specified

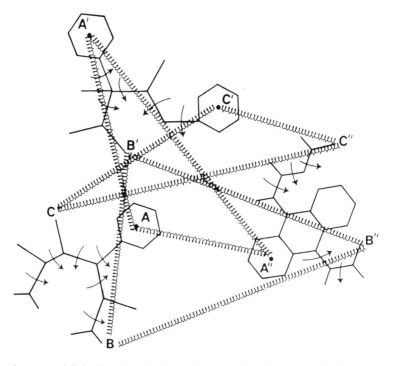

Fig. 15.43 Simultaneous minimization of molecules to force overlap of pharmacophoric groups A, B, and C. Springs represent constraints between groups and only interatomic forces were evaluated.

manner. The strain energy involved in forcing correspondence gives an upper bound estimate of the distortion energy required, as the results depend on the initial problem definition. An alternative approach uses the distance geometry paradigm in which all the constraints are combined to form the distance matrix from which energetically feasible conformations of the set of molecules are sought mathematically. Sheridan and Venkataragharan (301) demonstrated this approach on acetylcholine analogs, which are muscarinic agonists.

Both of these approaches ask the same question and suffer from the same limitations and differ only in computational technique. Each suffers from the local minima problem in that each uses a minimization technique, and the results depend on the starting geometries of the initial set of molecules. Both have the advantage that the unique constraints imposed by particular molecules enter consideration at an early stage and minimize comparison of conformations.

Another variant recently reported uses a Monte Carlo search procedure to generate candidate pharmacophoric patterns (302). A reduced force field parameter set is used initially to lower energy barriers between conformations to ensure greater configurational sampling. Candidate pharmacophores are then refined to produce low energy conformations of molecules overlaid in a common binding mode. Application to antagonists of the human platelet-activating factor led to a consistent binding model for a set of five diverse structures when active site hydrogen-bonding groups were postulated. Barakat and Dean (303, 304) used simulated annealing to optimize structure matching by minimizing the difference matrix between the two molecules. A somewhat similar approach was used by Perkins and Dean (305) who used simulated annealing to search conformational space followed by cluster analysis for each mole-cule with subsequent comparison of a small number of diverse conformers between different molecules.

4.4.2 SYSTEMATIC SEARCH AND THE ACTIVE ANALOG APPROACH. Once the existence of a common pattern has been determined, then the issue of uniqueness must be addressed. The active analog approach uses a systematic search to generate the set of sterically allowed conformations based on a grid search of the torsional variables at a given angular increment (262). For each sterically allowed conformation, a set of distances between the postulated pharmacophoric groups are measured. The set of distances, each of which represents a unique pharmacophoric pattern, constitutes and OMAP. Each point of the OMAP is simply a submatrix of the distance matrix and, as such, is invariant to global translation and rotation of the molecule. If the initial assumption is valid that the same binding mode of interaction, or pharmacophoric pattern, is common to the set of molecules under consideration, then the OMAP for each active molecule must contain the pattern encrypted in the set of distances. By logically intersecting the set of OMAPs, one can determine which patterns are common to all molecules (306). In other words, all potential pharmacophoric patterns consistent with the activity of the set of molecules can be found by this simple manipulation of OMAPs, and the question of uniqueness addressed directly (Fig. 15.44).

A good example is the work of Nelson et al. (307) on the receptor-bound conformation of morphiceptin. Based on structure-activity data, the tyramine portion and phenyl ring of residue three of morphiceptin, Tyr-Pro-Phe-Pro-NH_2, were postulated to be the pharmacophoric groups responsible for recognition and activation of the opioid μ-receptor. It was assumed further that the aromatic rings bound to the receptor in the different analogs were coinci-

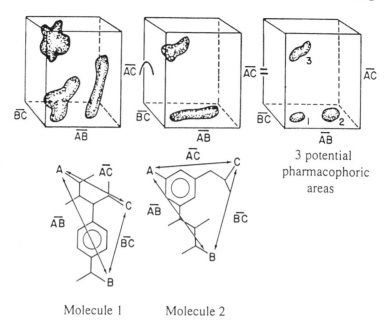

Fig. 15.44 OMAPs generated for two molecules can be logically intersected to determine which three-dimensional patterns are common.

dent and coplanar. A series of active analogs with a variety of conformationally constrained amino acid analogs in positions two and three were analyzed. A unique conformation was found for the two most constrained analogs, which allowed overlap of the Phe and Tyr portions of the molecules (Fig. 15.45). In this case, a five-dimensional orientation map with distances between the nitrogen and normals to the two aromatic rings was used in the analysis.

The active analog approach is appropriate for the unknown receptor problem, as no objective criteria function, such as potential energy, can be used *a priori* in the absence of information regarding the receptor. Adequate sampling of the potential surface to ensure that the complete set of local minima is found is still problematic due to the phenomenon known as "grid tyranny." This relates to the fact that the combinatorial explosion that results by decreasing the increment of the torsion angles scanned limits one to a finite increment for a given problem, let's say 10 degrees for a

seven-rotatable bond problem. Because the energetics of the system is sensitive to interatomic distances, a conformation generated at the 10-degree increment may be sterically disallowed but close to a minimum. Relaxation of the structure might find the relevant conformation, for example, by allowing a torsional angle to vary by 1 degree. Improvements in algorithms described in the following section have helped to overcome this problem.

4.4.3 STRATEGIC REDUCTIONS OF COMPUTATIONAL COMPLEXITY. Logically, the active analog approach can be conceived as sequentially determining all the sterically allowed conformations for each molecule under consideration, generation of an OMAP from those conformations, and logical intersections of the OMAPs to determine the common pharmacophoric patterns. A simple analysis will easily convince one that this is not feasible, due to the computational complexity of the problem. For example, the set of 28 ACE inhibitors

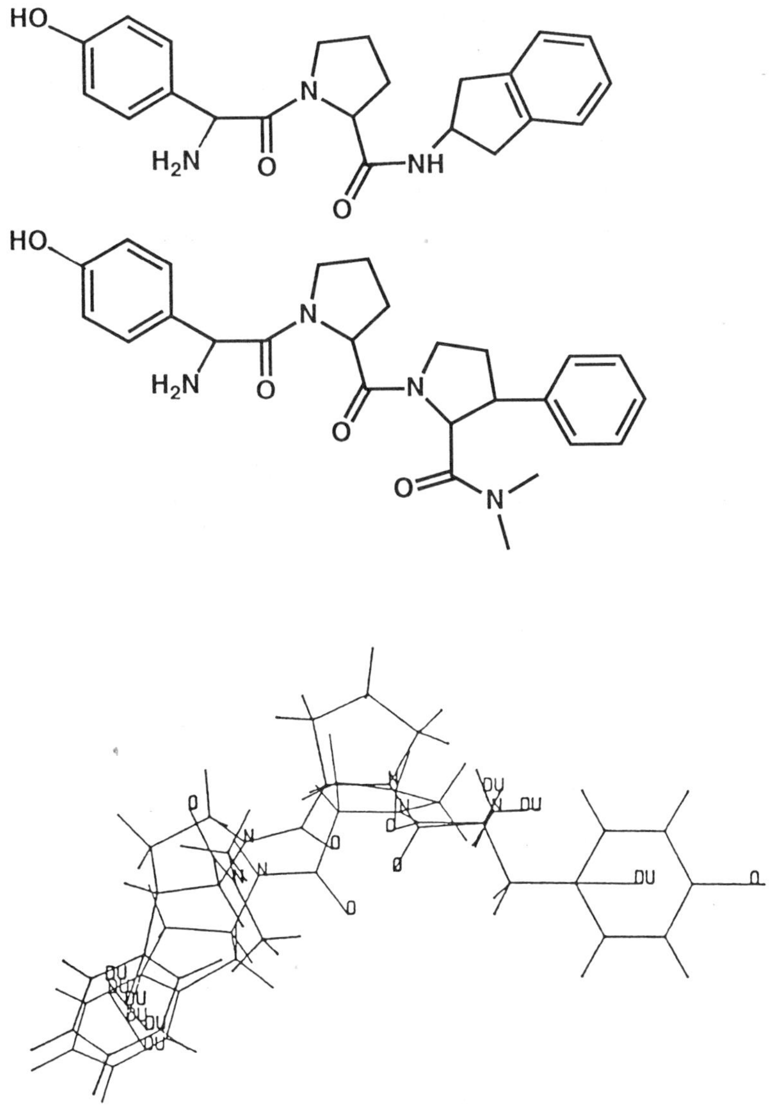

Fig. 15.45 Conformations of two constrained analogs of morphiceptin in which the aromatic rings of Tyr[1] and Phe[3] are overlapped (307).

(see Fig. 15.31) analyzed by Mayer et al. (260) have a total of 163 torsional degrees of freedom, which must be explored to find a common pattern as seen in Table 15.1. If one were to determine all possible conformations for each molecule at 10 degrees of torsional scan, the scan parameter s would be 10 degrees and the number of torsional increments r would be 360 degrees/s, or 36. For each molecule, there are r^n possibilities to be examined. For the set of molecules there are $(6 \times 36^3) + (7 \times 36^5) + (3 \times 36^6) + (5 \times 36^7) + (6 \times 36^8) + (1 \times 36^9)$ possible conformations to be generated and examined. If one compares each conformation of each molecule with all the conformations of the other molecules to find possible correspondences, the combinatorials of the problem explode and one reaches the same level of complexity as a

Table 5.1 Degrees of Torsional Freedom to Specify ACE Active Site Geometry

Degrees of Freedom (n)	Number of Molecules	Total
3	6	18
5	7	35
6	3	18
7	5	35
8	6	48
9	1	9
Totals	28	163

complete conformational search of a peptide of 30 residues at a 10-degree scan (not currently feasible).

One is not interested in the conformational hyperspace of the set of the inhibitors but rather the three-dimensional patterns common to the total set of inhibitors. Many conformations of a molecule often map into one three-dimensional pattern. Transformation of the multidimensional conformational hyperspace in a smaller-dimensioned OMAP space reduces the number of objects for comparison. If one starts with the most constrained inhibitor (fewest torsional degrees of freedom) and determined an OMAP for it, then one can use the upper and lower distance bounds as constraints for searches for the next molecule. In other words, one only looks where there are possible solutions to the problem. A more advanced approach simply examines each candidate solution from the initial OMAP to see if all the other molecules are capable of presenting the same pattern. By changing the focus to the hypothesis of a common three-dimensional pattern, a more efficient approach has been devised (Fig. 15.46). Analysis of this problem at a 10-degree increment takes less than 100 cpu s on a SGI Indigo with the current implementation (263). Clearly, the algorithms that one chooses to do the problem are important.

4.4.4 ALTERNATIVE APPROACHES. A conceptually similar approach to receptor mapping was taken by Ghose and Crippen (308–311) who used the distance geometry method to analyze site points and drug interactions. A site model was postulated with some initial estimates of force constants between the appropriate portion of the ligand and the site point. The binding energy for a particular binding mode can be calculated:

$$E_{\text{calcd}} = cE_c + Sx_{ti,tm}$$

where E_c is the conformational energy, c is a coefficient to be fit, x is the interaction of a site point i with the bound ligand point m, which depends on their types. The novel aspect of this approach was the use of distance geometry to generate a variety of conformers binding within the postulated site and then finding a set of force constants between the postulated site points and ligand points that will predict the affinities of the compounds in the data set when bound in their optimal manner. With a site model of 11 attractive site points and 5 repulsive ones for DHFR, Ghose and Crippen (309) were able to derive force constants that fit 62 molecules with an $R^2 = 0.90$ and predict the activity of 33 molecules with an $R^2 = 0.71$. The compounds, however, are essentially an extended congeneric series, as the core recognition portion of the inhibitor, the pyrimidine ring, is common to all the compounds.

Linschoten et al. (312) extended Crippen's method by using lipophilicity to describe the binding of parts of the ligand to lipophilic areas of the receptor. Using only a nine-point model of the turkey erythrocyte β receptor and six-energy parameters, they successfully modeled 58 compounds. Distance geometry approaches to receptor site modeling have been reviewed (311, 313).

Simon and co-workers (289) developed a quantitative 3-D-QSAR approach: the

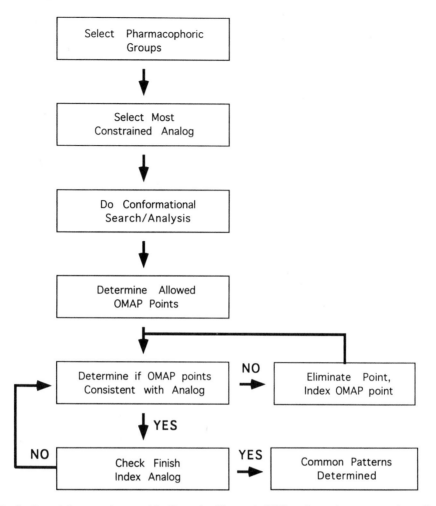

Fig. 15.46 Outline of the procedure used by Dammkoehler et al. (263) to determine common three-dimensional patterns for a set of molecules.

minimal steric (topologic) difference (MTD) approach. Oprea et al. (314) have compared MTD and CoMFA on affinity of steroids for their binding proteins and found similar results. Snyder and Colleagues (315) have developed an automated method for pharmacophore extraction that can provide a clear-cut distinction between agonist and antagonist pharmacophores. Klopman (268, 316) developed a procedure for the automatic detection of common molecular structural features present in a training set of compounds. This was used to produce candidate pharmacophores for a set of antiulcer compounds (268). Extensions of this approach allow differentiation between substructures responsible for activity and those that modulate the activity (316).

Bersuker and Dimoglo (317) described a matrix-based approach that combines geometric and electronic features of a molecule, the electron-topological approach. For each molecule, an electron-topological matrix of congruity (ETMC) is constructed based on a conformer selected by conformational analysis. The ETMC is essentially an interatomic distance matrix

O_1	C_2	C_3	C_4	C_5	C_6	C_7	C_8	C_9	C_{10}	C_{11}	C_{12}	C_{13}	C_{14}	C_{15}	C_{16}	H_{17}
-0.23	5.09	5.22	5.69	6.59	4.22	2.82	2.30	1.75	3.54	4.74	4.96	6.11	6.98	7.09	6.84	1.89
	-0.01	1.00	2.52	2.48	2.54	2.97	4.33	5.14	5.15	4.96	3.79	6.29	6.45	6.79	7.50	6.23
		0.05	0.99	0.99	0.97	2.56	3.86	4.95	4.37	3.89	2.57	5.11	5.38	5.41	6.41	5.95
			-0.01	2.52	2.48	3.24	4.48	5.46	5.04	4.62	3.40	5.79	6.31	5.72	5.09	6.41
				-0.01	2.56	3.85	4.99	6.20	5.17	4.33	2.94	5.21	5.09	5.40	6.68	7.44
					0.05	1.42	2.46	3.69	2.84	2.49	1.42	3.87	4.37	4.38	5.06	4.61
						-0.03	1.40	2.39	2.43	2.83	2.40	4.36	5.07	5.05	5.20	3.40
							0.01	1.09	1.40	2.45	2.78	3.87	4.79	4.75	4.33	2.17
								0.18	2.40	3.69	4.13	4.98	5.94	5.89	5.12	0.93
									-0.03	1.41	2.40	2.58	3.64	3.60	2.92	2.70
										0.05	1.42	0.97	2.51	2.50	2.57	4.10
											-0.04	2.55	3.05	3.07	3.88	4.83
												0.05	0.99	1.00	0.99	5.16
													-0.01	2.53	2.49	6.22
														-0.01	2.49	6.07
															-0.01	4.97
																0.03

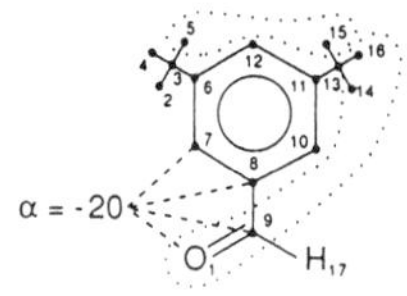

Fig. 15.47 The electron-topological matrix of congruity (ETMC) for a 17-atom fragment proposed by Bersuker and Dimoglo (317) to encode geometrical and electronic features of molecules.

(Fig. 15.47), with the diagonal elements containing an electronic structural parameter (atomic charge, polarizability, HOMO energy etc.). Off-diagonal elements for two atoms that are chemically bonded are used to store information regarding the bond (bond order, polarizability, etc.). Matrices for active compounds in a series are then searched for common features that are not shared by inactive compounds. The successful examples cited are predominately for small, relatively rigid structures where the conformational parameter does not confuse the analysis.

Martin et al. (318) developed a strategy for determining both the bioactive conformation and a superposition rule for each active molecule in a data set. A set of low energy conformers for each molecule is processed by ALADDIN to locate atoms within the molecule and extensions for binding-site points for superposition. A new program, DISCO, that uses a clique-finding algorithm finds superpositions containing at least one conformation of each

molecule and a user-specified minimum number of site points.

4.4.5 RECEPTOR MAPPING. One can attempt to decipher physical properties of the receptor by using data from both active and inactive analogs. Interpretation of results requires some understanding of the interactions between ligand and receptor, which underlie molecular recognition. Oprea and Kurunczi (319) reviewed these interactions in the context of receptor mapping. A basic assumption is that a compound that contains the correct pharmacophoric elements and has the capability of positioning them correctly should be active. Compounds with these attributes that are inactive must be incapable of binding to the receptor in the correct orientation, i.e., steric overlap with the receptor must occur. By calculating the combined volume of the active analogs superimposed in the correct orientation, one has mapped space that cannot be occupied by the receptor and that must be available for binding. Inactive compounds mentioned above should possess novel volume requirements, some portion of which is likely to overlap with that occupied by the receptor. As an example of receptor mapping, Sufrin et al. (266) showed with amino acid analogs of methionine, which inhibited the enzyme methionine : adenosyl transferase, that the data for a set of rigid amino acid inhibitors required the postulation of competition between the inactive analogs and the enzyme for a particular volume of space (Fig. 15.48). Summation of the volume requirements for the set of compounds, when oriented on the amino acid framework, yielded a minimum space from which the

receptor could be excluded. Each amino acid had the necessary binding elements, but several were inactive. Each of the inactive analogs required extra volume not required by the active analogs and shared a small common unique volume whose occupancy by the enzyme would be sufficient to rationalize their inactivity.

Klunk et al. (320) used separate receptor mapping of two different chemical classes of ligands to support the hypothesis that they bound to the same site. Calder et al (321) argued that a successful correlative CoMFA model for 36 compounds of six chemical classes of GABA inhibitors indicated that the alignments used were signifi-

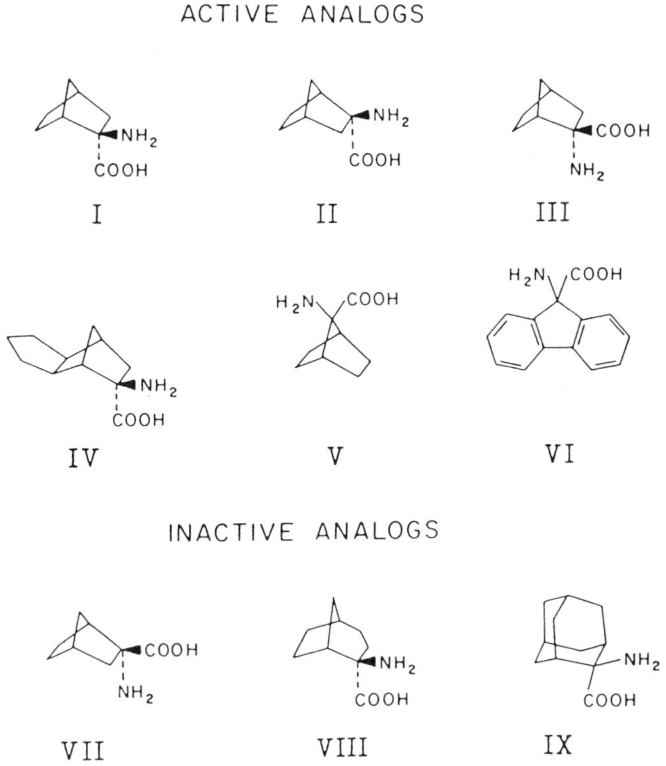

Fig. 15.48 Example of receptor mapping of set of enzyme inhibitors that can be aligned on common amino acid framework. Set of inactive compounds all require common novel volume when compared with active compounds. From Ref. 266 with permission.

cant. In some cases, comparison of volume maps for two receptors have allowed optimization of activity at one receptor with respect to the other. The work of Hibert et al. (322, 323) using receptor mapping to increase the selectivity of a lead compound for the 5-HT$_{1A}$ receptor over the α_1-adrenoreceptor, resulted in clinical trials for a novel chemical class. This steric-mapping approach has become relatively popular and numerous examples appear in current journals on a regular basis (324).

While there are several feasible algorithms to deal with unions of molecular volumes, the use of pseudoelectron density functions calibrated to reproduce VDW radii with three-dimensional contouring to represent the surface has allowed mathematical manipulation of the density associated with each lattice point to allow for union, intersection, and subtraction of volumes (287). Analytical representation of molecular volumes by Connolly (325, 326) and solvent-accessible surfaces by Kundrot et al. (327) may be an alternative that would allow optimization of volume overlap, for example, by minimizing the difference in volume between two structures. The solvent-accessible surface area can be used to approximate the free energy of hydration and a rapid, numerical procedure for its calculation has been reported (328).

4.4.6 MODEL RECEPTOR SITES. One of the first visualizations of a receptor model was that of Beckett and Casey (329) for the opiate receptor published in 1954. Because morphine and many other compounds active at this receptor are essentially rigid, the model did not have to address the interaction of myriad flexible, naturally occurring opioid ligands such as endorphins and enkephalin, which were only subsequently discovered. The model receptor had an anionic site to bind the charged nitrogen, a hydrophobic flat surface with a cleft to bind the phenyl ring, and hydrophobic hydrocarbon bridge seen in mor-

phine. Kier (330) published a number of papers attempting to define the pharmacophore based on semiempirical molecular orbital calculations of *in vacuo* minimum energy conformations. While his basic concepts were valid, his emphasis on the global minima *in vacuo* limited his scope of applicability.

Humber et al. (331) used semi-rigid antipsychotic drugs—the so-called neuroleptics, which antagonize CNS dopamine transmission and displace dopamine from its receptor—to formulate a geometrical arrangement of receptor groups to rationalize their activity. Olson et al. (332) used this model to design a novel stereospecific dopamine antagonist and successfully predicted its stereochemistry.

Because researchers are reasonably convinced the receptor is a protein, construction of hypothetical sites from amino acid fragments and calculation of affinity for these sites should correlate with observed affinity, assuming that the type of interactions and their geometry is represented by the site in some reasonable manner. An individual fragment such as an indole ring from tryptophan does a good job of simulating a flat hydrophobic surface. Holtje and Tintelnot (333) constructed a site for chloramphenecol from arginine and histidine by varying the distances of the amino acid from its postulated binding position and find the optimal distance for correlation with observed affinity for the ribosome. Peptidic pseudoreceptors have been constructed that correctly rank order glutamate NMDA agonists and antagonists (Fig. 15.49) (315).

An intermediate between unknown receptors and ones for which the three-dimensional structure is known are models based on homology. For the medicinal chemist, the G-protein receptors have been of intense interest and numerous models for the various receptor types have been developed based on their presumed three-dimensional homology with bacterior-

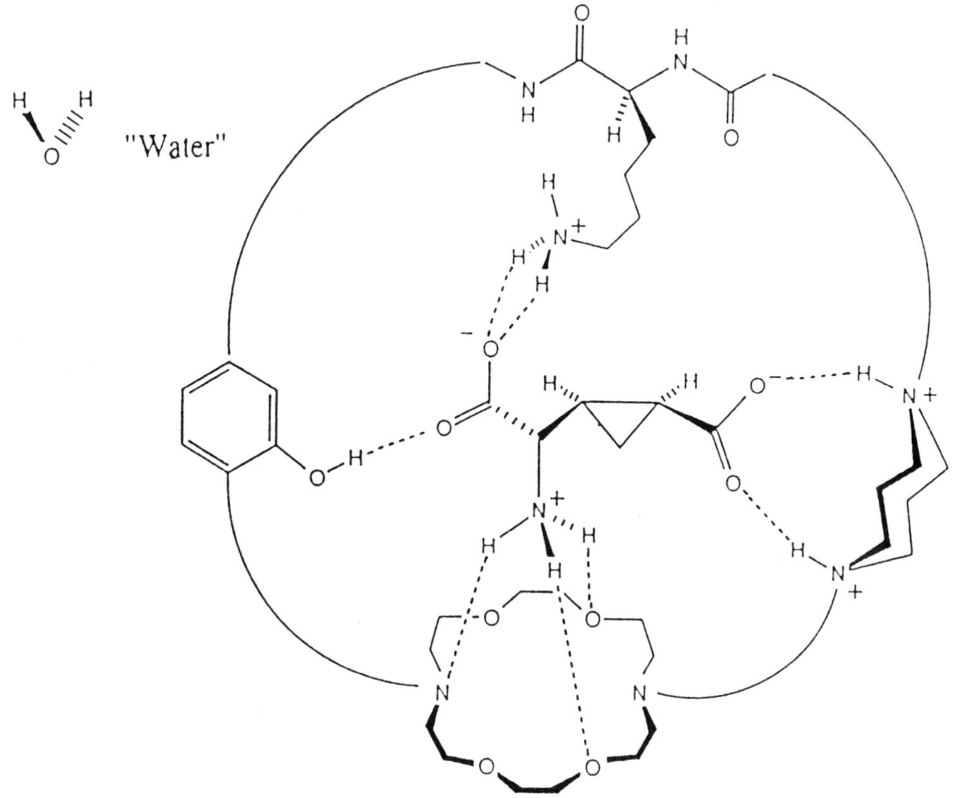

Fig. 15.49 Peptidic pseudoreceptor, which is used to calculate affinity of NMDA agonists and antagonists. From Ref. 315 with permission.

hodopsin (238, 239, 322, 334, 335). Mechanisms of signal transduction (336) and differences between agonists and antagonists (337) have been rationalized based on such models. Nordvall and Hacksell (240) recently combined the construction of such a model for the muscarinic m1 receptor with constraints derived from steric mapping of muscarinic agonists. By adding the experimental constraints from ligand binding, a qualitative model was derived that was able to reproduce experimentally derived stereoselectivities.

4.4.7 ASSESSMENT OF MODEL PREDICTABILITY. As it is unlikely that there will be sufficient structure–activity data to define uniquely a model at atomic resolution in competition with crystallography; justifica-

tion for model building must come from its potential predictive power and possible insight into the receptor–drug interaction before detailed three-dimensional information from either crystal structure or NMR studies. Certainly, the questions regarding the ability of a proposed drug to bind to the active site without steric conflict with the receptor can be addressed by the methods outlined here in a qualitative manner. The resolution of the receptor models is too crude, however, to subject them to molecular mechanics estimates of affinities. There are alternative paradigms based on pattern recognition techniques in which a set of analogs and their activities are used along with their physicochemical parameters to generate a mathematical model that relates the values of the physicochemical parameters for a given analogue with its activity. One such paradigm is Comparative Molecular Field Analysis (CoMFA), which combines the three-dimensional electrostatic and steric fields surrounding the analogs with powerful statistical techniques—e.g., partial least squares (PLS) (338) and cross-validation—to generate predictive models, if a set of orientation rules are available for aligning the molecules for comparison and prediction. Alternative methods for assessing similarity and their use in QSAR schemes have been compared with CoMFA (177). Another approach is the use of neural nets that learn to "see" patterns in much the same way as our own nervous system processes information. Examples of the use of this pattern recognition approach includes classification of the mechanism of action for cancer chemotherapy (339) and QSAR studies of DHFR inhibitors (340, 341) and carboquinones (342). Machine-learning has also been recently applied to the QSAR problem (343). Trimethoprim analogues were successfully analyzed for their inhibition of DHFR, and similar results to the original Hansch results were obtained. It is not clear that this paradigm could be applied to noncongeneric series, at least as outlined.

What appears crucial to such studies is the choice of training set, which encompasses much of parameter space as one is likely to use in the predictive mode as well as tests of the predictive ability of resulting models. Because one is dealing with a situation in which the number of variables is larger (often several times) than the number of observations, linear regression models are not applicable, as chance correlations are highly probable. The use of cross-validation allows selection of correlations that are predictive in a self-consistent manner within the training set. This does not mean to imply that such internally self-consistent models have predictive power outside of the training set of extremely close congeners.

DePriest et al. (344, 345) applied the CoMFA methodology to a series of 68 ACE inhibitors representing 28 different chemical classes. Using the binding-site geometry determined by Mayer et al. (260), a CoMFA model with a statistically significant cross-validated R^2 and considerable predictive ability for inhibitors outside of the training set was derived. Because the geometry of the ACE inhibitors was determined computationally by an active site analysis rather than experimentally, a comparison of the results of the ACE series against thermolysin inhibitors (for which there were crystallographic data to define explicitly the binding-site geometry and the resulting alignment rules) was made, as thermolysin is also a zinc-containing metallopeptidase and shares numerous similarities with ACE. The results give strong support to both the active analog approach (262), used to define the alignment rule for the ACE series, and the CoMFA methodology itself. In the absence of an experimentally known active site geometry, correlations were derived that explain as much as 84% of the variance in activities among a set of 68 diverse ACE inhibitors, using CoMFA steric and electrostatic potentials plus a zinc indicator variable (Fig. 15.50). If the set of 68 ACE inhibitors is divided into 3 classes and correlations are derived for each class, CoMFA parameters alone explain 79% to 99% of the variance in activities. It was notable that statistically significant correlations were found in spite of the fact that CoMFA does not explicitly consider hydrophobicity or solvation. In further support of the active site paradigm, the cross-validated results of the ACE series were equivalent to those of the thermolysin series (cross-validated $R^2 = 0.65$ to 0.70), for which the alignment rule was defined by crystallographic data.

The predictions for molecules outside the training sets are a valid test of the predictive ability of the model, rather than just a confirmation of self-consistency of

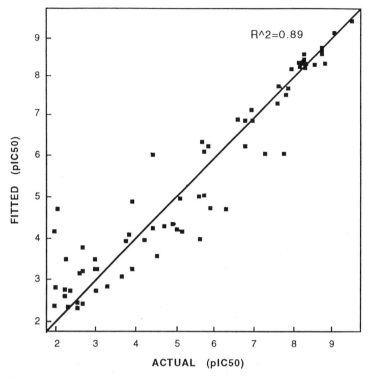

Fig. 15.50 Plot of experimental versus predicted inhibition constants for 68 ACE inhibitors used in derivation of CoMFA model for the ACE active site (345). This plot shows the self-consistency of the model.

the derived model. In other words, statistical analysis alone does not answer the question of a chance correlation for the training set (346). One must investigate lateral correlations such as predictability. The predictive correlations presented by DePriest et al. (344, 345) represent a total of 66 diverse inhibitors that were not chosen as analogs of compounds present in the training set but from published papers on three different chemical classes; they tested all compounds in those papers (predictive $R^2 = 0.46$ for the set of 66 compounds predicted, which had not been included in the training set for the ACE model with a zinc indicator of 10) (Fig. 15.51). The "predictive" R^2 was based only on molecules not included in the training set and was defined as

$$\text{predictive } R^2 = (\text{SD} - \text{"press"})/\text{SD}$$

where SD is the sum of the squared deviations between the affinities of molecules in the test set and the mean affinity of the training set molecules, and "press" is the sum of the squared deviations between predicted and actual affinity values for every molecule in the test set. It should be obvious from the equation that prediction of the mean value of the training set for each member of the test set would yield a predictive R^2 of 0. A total of 35 out of the 66 predicted molecules had residuals less than one log value, with a predictive R^2 for the collective set of these 35 test molecules of 0.90. Of the 31 inhibitors with residuals greater than 1.0, 8 were carboxylates, 12 were phosphates, and 11 were thiols. Clearly, no single class of inhibitors dominated the distribution of residuals. When one considers both the composition and the method of selection of the test data sets

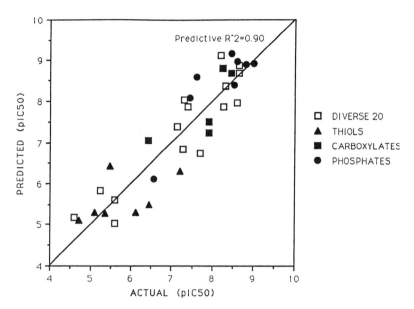

Fig. 15.51 Plot of experimental versus predicted inhibition constants for 35 ACE inhibitors not used in derivation of CoMFA model (345). This plot indicates the predictability of the model. Used with permission.

(range of activities over 7 log units), the fact that more than 50% of the molecules were predicted with correlations greater than $R^2 = 0.90$ lends strong support to the use of CoMFA as a tool for QSAR development.

Use of CoMFA as a predictive tool for receptors of known three-dimensional structure has also been explored. Klebe and Abraham (347) used two enzymes (thermolysin and renin) as well as antiviral activity against human rhinovirus, for which the coat-protein receptor is known, to calibrate CoMFA methodology. They concluded that only enthalpies of binding and not binding affinities could be predicted by CoMFA. Waller et al. (348) have developed a predictive CoMFA model for the binding affinities of HIV-protease inhibitors based on crystal structures of complexes. Initial analysis of the 59 molecules in the training set representing five structurally diverse classes (hydroxyethylamine, statine, norstatine, ketoamide, and dihydroxyethylene) of transition-state protease inhibitors yielded a correlation

with a cross-validated R^2 of 0.786. To evaluate the predictive ability of this model, a test set of 18 additional inhibitors was used, which represented another class of transition-state isostere: hydroxyethylurea (349). The model expressed good predictive ability for the test set of hydroxyethylurea compounds ($R^2_{pred} = 0.624$) with all compounds predicted within 1.096 log unit (1.4 kcal/mol in binding affinity) of their actual activities with an average absolute error of 0.58 log units (0.8 kcal/mol) across a range of 3.03 log units (Fig. 15.52). Predictions from this CoMFA model of HIV protease are being used to prioritize synthesis of *de novo* designed HIV-protease inhibitors not included in development of the model.

Crippen (350) developed a method to model objectively the binding of small ligands to receptors given the experimentally determined affinities of a set of ligands. The procedure Vorom used Voronoi polyhedra to generate the simplest geometrical model of the binding site. In a recent application to DHFR inhibitors, only eight

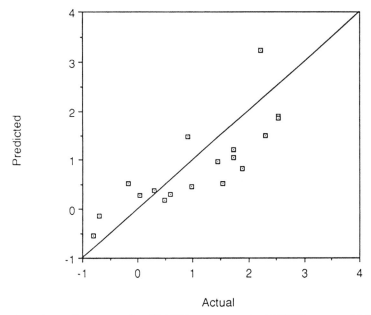

Fig. 15.52 Plot of experimental versus predicted inhibition constants for 18 HIV-1 protease inhibitors not used in derivation of CoMFA model (348). This plot indicates the predictability of the model.

analogues were used in the training set to derive the model, and the affinities of 23/39 of the test set molecules were correctly predicted with an average relative error of 0.83 kcal/mol for the remaining compounds (351).

5 CONCLUSION

Rapid advances in molecular and structural biology have provided ample therapeutic targets characterized in three dimensions. Tools to exploit this information are being rapidly developed and several strategies for *de novo* design of ligands given an active site are under investigation. It is already clear, however, that iterative approaches are necessary due to the lack of precision in predicting affinities for bound ligands. Molecular mechanics and computer graphics are essential components for design of novel ligands, and rapid progress in evolving a useful set of tools is apparent.

The ultimate goal in comparison of molecules with respect to their biological activity is insight into the receptor and its requirements for recognition and activation. Conjecture regarding the receptor is often a necessary part of rationalizing a set of structure–activity data. While the problem of characterizing the active site of an unknown macromolecule indirectly is certainly challenging, the analysis of structure–activity data of a set of ligands, especially if their structural variety is wide, allows useful models of active sites to be developed. There are numerous caveats that must be acknowledged, however, such as flexibility of the receptor, multiple binding modes for ligands, multiple binding modes for ligands, and lack of uniqueness of most models as a result of limited experimental observations. Success in using these methods appears to be increasing. This reflects both technological advances and insight into the problem as well as algorithmic improvements in analytical approaches.

The game of twenty questions with receptors has progressed with experience. Ambiguity in interpretation of results and multiple models clearly reflect the uncertainties inherent in this indirect approach. Nevertheless, the absence of direct experimental data in many biological systems of intense therapeutic interest make this the only game available for many. It is hoped that the next decade will see further progress in the ability to extract three-dimensional information from structure–activity studies on unknown receptors.

This perspective has examined the approaches to molecular modeling and drug design and emphasized their limitations. The reader should be aware, however, that these tools are used daily on many problems of therapeutic interest with increasing success. This is clearly witnessed by publications of such studies in almost every issue of current major journals. For specific application areas, such as RNA (352, 353) DNA (354–358), membrane (359–368), and peptidomimetic modeling (369–374), the reader is referred to the literature.

ACKNOWLEDGMENTS

The work and influence of many talented collaborators as well as the National Institute of Health for grant support (GM 24483) are gratefully acknowledged. While my former colleagues' names are prominent in the references cited, their contributions are numerous and individual citations are avoided due to probable omissions. Current collaborators who have influenced the preparation of this manuscript include Denise Beusen, David Chalmers, Richard Dammkoehler, Chris Ho, Shawn Huston, Gregory Nikiforovich, Mark Smythe, Tudor Oprea, and Chris Waller. A considerable portion of the section on unknown receptors was adapted from a previous review with permission of the publisher (375). The author apologizes to many contributors to the field whose efforts have not been adequately recognized in this review due to a somewhat arbitrary citation of references. Space and time limitations preclude a more thorough discussion of many important aspects.

REFERENCES

1. S. W. Fesik, *J. Med. Chem.*, **34**, 2938–2945 (1991).

2. G. Otting, *Curr. Opin. Struct. Biol.*, **3**, 760–768 (1993).

3. S. O. Smith, *Curr. Opin. Struct. Biol.*, **3**, 755–759 (1993).

4. C. A. Ramsden, Ed., *Quantitative Drug Design Vol. 4 of Comprehensive Medicinal Chemistry*, Pergamon Press, Oxford, UK, 1990, pp. 1–766.

5. K. Appelt, R. J. Bacquet, C. A. Bartlett, C. L. J. Booth, S. T. Freer, M. A. M. Fuhry, M. R. Gehring, S. H. Herrmann, E. F. Howland, C. A. Janson, T. R. Jones, C.-C. Kan, V. Kathardekar, K. K. Lewis, G. P. Marzoni, D. A. Mathews, C. Mohr, E. W. Moomaw, C. A. Morse, S. J. Oatley, R. C. Ogden, M. R. Reddy, S. H. Reich, W. S. Schoettin, W. W. Smith, M. D. Varney, J. E. Villafranca, R. W. Ward, S. Webber, S. E. Webber, K. M. Welsh, and J. White, *J. Med. Chem.*, **34**, 1925–1934 (1991).

6. C. R. Beddell, *The Design of Drugs to Macromolecular Targets*, John Wiley & Sons, Inc., New York, 1992.

7. I. D. Kuntz, *Science*, **257**, 1078–1082 (1992).

8. M. A. Navia and D. A. Peattle, *Trends Pharmacol. Sci.*, **14**, 189–195 (1993).

9. U. Burkert and N. L. Allinger, *Molecular Mechanics*, American Chemical Society, Washington, DC, 1982, pp. 339.

10. J. P. Bowen and N. L. Allinger in K. B. Lipkowitz and D. B. Boyd, Eds., *Review of Computer Chemistry*, VCH Publishers, Inc., New York, 1991, pp. 81–98.

11. M. Clark, I. Cramer, D. Richard, and N. Van Opdenbosch, *J. Comput. Chem.*, **10**, 982–1012 (1989).

12. J. G. Vinter, A. Davis, and M. R. Saunders, *J. Comput. Aided Mol. Des.*, **1**, 31–51 (1987).

13. D. N. J. White and M. J. Bovill, *J. Chem. Soc. Perkin II*, **12**, 1610–1623 (1977).

14. K. Gundertofte, J. Palm, I. Pettersson, and A. Stamvik, *J. Comput. Chem.*, **12**, 200–208 (1991).

15. W. L. Jorgensen and J. Gao, *J. Am. Chem. Soc.*, **110**, 4212–4216 (1988).

16. J.-H. Lii and N. L. Allinger, *J. Comput. Chem.*, **12**, 186–199 (1991).

17. J. Aqvist and A. Warshel, *J. Am. Chem. Soc.*, **112**, 2860 (1990).

18. R. D. Hancock, *Acc. Chem. Res.*, **23**, 253–257 (1990).

19. A. Vedani and D. W. Huhta, *J. Am. Chem. Soc.*, **112**, 4759–4767 (1990).

20. V. S. Allured, C. M. Kelly, and C. R. Landis, *J. Am. Chem. Soc.*, **113**, 1–12 (1991).

21. A. T. Hagler, E. Hugler, and S. Lifson, *J. Am. Chem. Soc.*, **96**, 5319 (1974).

22. S. C. Harvey, *Proteins*, **5**, 78–92 (1989).

23. M. E. Davis and J. A. McCammon, *Chem. Rev.*, **90**, 509–521 (1990).

24. W. F. van Gunsteren and H. J. C. Berendsen, *Angew. Chem. Int. Ed. Engl.*, **29**, 992–1023 (1990).

25. C. E. Dykstra, *Chem. Rev.*, **93**, 2339–2353 (1993).

26. A. J. Stone and M. Alderton, *Mol. Phys.*, **56**, 1047–1064 (1985).

27. C. I. Bayly, P. Cieplak, W. D. Cornell, and P. A. Kollman, *J. Phys. Chem.*, **97**, 10269–10280 (1993).

28. D. E. Williams in Ref. 10, 1991, pp. 219–271.

29. R. J. Loncharich and B. R. Brooks, *Proteins*, **6**, 32–45 (1989).

30. J. Guenot and P. A. Kollman, *J. Comput. Chem.*, **14**, 295–311 (1993).

31. K. Tasaki, S. McDonald, and J. W. Brady, *J. Comput. Chem.*, **14**, 278–284 (1993).

32. J. Shimada, H. Kaneko, and T. Takada, *J. Comput. Chem.*, **14**, 867–878 (1993).

33. H. Schreiber and O. Steinhauser, *Chem. Phys.*, **168**, 75–89 (1992).

34. H. Schreiber and O. Steinhauser, *Biochemistry*, **31**, 5856–5860 (1992).

35. P. E. Smith and B. M. Pettit, *J. Chem. Phys.*, **95**, 8430–8441 (1991).

36. G. E. Marlow, J. S. Perkyns, and B. M. Pettit, *Chem. Rev.*, **93**, 2503–2521 (1993).

37. M. Whitlow and M. M. Teeter, *J. Am. Chem. Soc.*, **108**, 7163–7172 (1986).

38. M. K. Gilson, K. A. Sharp, and B. H. Honig, *J. Comput. Chem.*, **9**, 327–335 (1987).

39. A. Nicholls and B. Honig, *J. Comput. Chem.*, **12**, 435–445 (1991).

40. M. Schaefer and C. Froemmel, *J. Mol. Biol.*, **216**, 1045–1066 (1990).

41. W. G. Richards, P. M. King, and C. A. Reynolds, *Protein Eng.*, **2**, 319–327 (1987).

42. R. A. Pierotti, *Chem. Rev.*, **76**, 717–726 (1976).

43. G. L. Pollack, *Science*, **251**, 1323–1330 (1991).

44. R. J. Zauhar and R. S. Morgan, *J. Comput. Chem.*, **9**, 171–187 (1988).

45. J. Tomasi, R. Bonaccorsi, R. Cammi, and F. J. O. d. Valle, *J. Mol. Struct.*, 24 (1991).

46. K. Sharp, *J. Comput. Chem.*, **12**, 454–468 (1991).

47. W. C. Still, A. Tempczyk, R. C. Hawley, and T. Hendrickson, *J. Am. Chem. Soc.*, **112**, 6127–6129 (1990).

48. C. A. Schiffer, J. W. Caldwell, P. A. Kollman, and R. M. Stroud, *Mol. Simul.*, **10**, 121–149 (1993).

49. P. F. W. Stouten, C. Frommel, H. Nakamura, and C. Sander, *Mol. Simul.*, **10**, 97–120 (1993).

50. R. J. Zauhar, *J. Comput. Chem.*, **12**, 575–583 (1991).

51. A. J. Stone, *Mol. Phys.*, **56**, 1065–1082 (1985).

52. S. Kuwajima and A. Warshel, *J. Phys. Chem.*, **94**, 460–466 (1990).

53. R. A. Sorensen, W. B. Liau, L. Kesner, and R. H. Boyd, *Macromolecules*, **21**, 200–208 (1988).

54. J. Caldwell, L. X. Dang, and P. A. Kollman, *J. Am. Chem. Soc.*, **112**, 9144–9147 (1990).

55. C. J. Cramer and D. G. Truhlar, *J. Am. Chem. Soc.*, **113**, 8305–8311 (1991).

56. C. J. Cramer, *J. Am. Chem. Soc.*, **113**, 8552–8554 (1991).

57. C. J. Cramear and D. G. Truhlar, *J. Comput. Chem.*, **13**, 1089–1097 (1992).

58. C. J. Cramer and D. G. Truhlar, *Science*, **256**, 213–217 (1992).

59. G. Rauhut, T. Clark, and T. Steinke, *J. Am. Chem. Soc.*, **115**, 9174–9181 (1993).

60. F. Franks, *Water, A Comprehensive Treatise*, Plenum Press, New York, 1975.

61. F. H. Stillinger, *Science*, **209**, 451–457 (1980).

62. L. R. Pratt, *Ann. Rev. Phys. Chem.*, **36**, 433–449 (1985).

63. J. P. M. Postma, H. J. C. Berendsen, and J. R. Haak, *Faraday Symp. Chem. Soc.*, **17**, 55–67 (1982).

64. B. G. Rao and U. C. Singh, *J. Am. Chem. Soc.*, **111**, 3125–3133 (1989).

65. I. Ohmine and H. Tanaka, *Chem. Rev.*, **93**, 2545–2566 (1993).

66. W. L. Jorgensen, J. Gao, and C. Ravimohan, *J. Phys. Chem.*, **89**, 3470–3473 (1985).

67. N. Muller, *Trends Biochem. Sci.*, **17**, 459–463 (1992).

68. L. X. Dang, J. E. Rice, J. Caldwell, and P. A. Kollman, *J. Am. Chem. Soc.*, **113**, 2481–2486 (1991).

69. A. K. Rappe and W. A. Goddard III, *J. Phys. Chem.*, **95**, 3358–3363 (1991).

70. R. Czerminski and R. Elber, *Int. J. Quantum Chem. Symp.*, **24**, 167–186 (1990).

71. C. Choi and R. Elber, *J. Chem. Phys.*, **94**, 751–760 (1991).

72. S. E. Huston and G. R. Marshall, *Biopolymers*, **34**, 75–90 (1994).

73. H. A. Scheraga in Ref. 10, 1992, pp. 73–142.

74. T. Schlick in Ref. 10, 1992, pp. 1–71.

75. H. Iijima, J. B. Dunbar Jr., and G. R. Marshall, *Proteins*, **2**, 330–339 (1987).

76. I. Motoc, R. A. Dammkoehler, and G. R. Marshall in N. Trinajstic, Eds., *Mathematic and Computational Concepts in Chemistry*, Ellis Horwood, Chichester, UK, 1986, pp. 222–251.

77. R. A. Dammkoehler, S. F. Karasek, E. F. B. Shands, and G. R. Marshall, *J. Comput. Aided Mol. Des.*, **3**, 3–21 (1989).

78. N. Go and H. A. Scheraga, *Macromolecules*, **3**, 178–187 (1970).

79. A. R. Leach in Ref. 10, 1991, pp. 1–55.

80. S. K. Burt and J. Greer, *Ann. Rep. Med. Chem.*, **23**, 285–294 (1988).

81. D. M. Ferguson and D. J. Raber, *J. Am. Chem. Soc.*, **111**, 4371–4378 (1989).

82. M. Saunders, *J. Am. Chem. Soc.*, **109**, 3150–3152 (1987).

83. M. Saunders, *J. Comput. Chem.*, **10**, 203–208 (1989).

84. M. Saunders, K. N. Houk, Y.-D. Wu, W. C. Still, M. Lipton, G. Chang, and W. C. Guida, *J. Am. Chem. Soc.*, **112**, 1419–1427 (1990).

85. M. Saunders, *J. Comput. Chem.*, **12**, 645–663 (1991).

86. M. Saunders and H. A. Jimenez-Vazquez, *J. Comput. Chem.*, **14**, 330–348 (1993).

87. M. Saunders and N. Krause, *J. Am. Chem. Soc.*, **112**, 1791–1795 (1990).

88. A. V. Shah and D. P. Dolata, *J. Comput. Aided Mol. Des.*, **7**, 103–124 (1993).

89. I. Kolossvary and W. C. Guida, *J. Am. Chem. Soc.*, **115**, 2107–2119 (1993).

90. H.-J. Boehm, G. Klebe, T. Lorenz, T. Mietzner, and L. Siggel, *J. Comput. Chem.*, **11**, 1021–1028 (1990).

91. A. E. Howard and P. A. Kollman, *J. Med. Chem.*, **31**, 1669–1675 (1988).

92. M. Lipton and W. C. Still, *J. Comput. Chem.*, **9**, 343–355 (1988).

93. D. D. Beusen, R. D. Head, J. D. Clark, W. C. Hutton, U. Slomczynska, J. Zabrocki, M. T. Leplawy, and G. R. Marshall, in C. H. Schneider and A. N. Eberle, Eds., *Peptides 1992*, ESCOM Scientific Publishers, Leiden, The Netherlands, 1993, pp. 79–80.

94. M. P. Allen and D. J. Tildesley, *Computer Simulation of Liquids*, Oxford Science Publications, 1989, pp. 385.

95. N. Metropolis, A. W. Rosenbluth, M. N. Rosenbluth, A. H. Teller, and E. Teller, *J. Chem. Phys.*, **21**, 1087 (1953).

96. J. A. McCammon and S. C. Harvey, *Dynamics of Protein and Nucleic Acids*, Cambridge University Press, Cambridge, UK, 1987, pp. 234.

97. G. Zhang and T. Schlick, *J. Comput. Chem.*, **14**, 1212–1233 (1993).

98. T. Schlick and W. K. Olson, *Science*, **257**, 1110–1115 (1992).

99. D. S. Goodsell and A. J. Olson, *Proteins*, **8**, 195–202 (1990).

100. W. L. Jorgensen, *Acc. Chem. Res.*, **22**, 184–189 (1989).

101. D. L. Beveridge and F. M. DiCapua in W. van Gunsteren and P. K. Weiner, Eds., *Computer Simulation of Biomolecular Systems*, ESCOM Science Publishers, Leiden, 1989, pp. 1–26.

102. P. Kollman, *Chem. Rev.*, **93**, 2395–2417 (1993).

103. T. P. Lybrand, J. A. McCammon, and G. Wipff, *Proc. Natl. Acad. Sci. U S A*, **83**, 833–835 (1986).

104. W. L. Jorgensen, *J. Phys. Chem.*, **87**, 5304–5314 (1983).

105. P. A. Bash, U. C. Singh, F. K. Brown, R. Langridge, and P. A. Kollman, *Science*, **235**, 574–576 (1987).

106. P. A. Kollman and K. M. Merz, *Acc. Chem. Res.*, **23**, 246–252 (1990).

107. J. Hermans, R. H. Yun, and A. G. Anderson, *J. Comput. Chem.*, **13**, 429–442 (1992).

108. J. Hermans, *Curr. Opin. Struct. Biol.*, **3**, 270–276 (1993).

109. C. L. Brooks III and D. A. Case, *Chem. Rev.*, **93**, 2487–2502 (1993).

110. R. Elber and M. Karplus, *J. Am. Chem. Soc.*, **112**, 9161–9175 (1990).

111. D. J. Tobias, M. E. Mertz, and C. L. Brooks III, *Biochemistry*, **30**, 6054–6058 (1991).

112. D. J. Tobias and C. L. Brooks III, *Biochemistry*, **30**, 6059–6070 (1991).

113. D. J. Tobias, S. F. Sneddon, and C. L. Brooks III, *J. Mol. Biol.*, **216**, 783–796 (1990).

114. S. F. Sneddon, D. J. Tobias, and C. L. Brooks III, *J. Mol. Biol.*, **209**, 817–820 (1989).

115. D. J. Tobias, S. F. Sneddon, and C. L. Brooks III in R. Lavery, J.-L. Rivail, and J. Smith, eds.,

Advances in Biomolecular Simulations, American Institute of Physics Conference Proceedings No. **239**, Obernai, France, 1991, pp. 174–199.

116. M. L. Smythe, S. E. Huston, and G. R. Marshall, *J. Am. Chem. Soc.*, **115**, 11594–11595 (1993).

117. G. H. Loew and S. K. Burt in Ref. 4, pp. 105–123.

118. S. L. Price and N. G. J. Richards, *J. Comput. Aided Drug Des.*, **5**, 41–54 (1991).

119. U. C. Singh and P. A. Kollman, *J. Comput. Chem.*, **5**, 129 (1984).

120. B. H. Besler, K. M. Merz Jr., and P. A. Kollman, *J. Comput. Chem.*, **11**, 431–439 (1990).

121. G. Rauhut and T. Clark, *J. Comput. Chem.*, **14**, 503–509 (1993).

122. J. G. Vinter and M. R. Saunders in D. J. Chadwick and K. Widdows, Eds., *Host-Guest Molecular Interactions: From Chemistry to Biology*, John Wiley & Sons, Inc., Chichester, UK, 1991, pp. 249–265.

123. C. A. Hunter and J. K. M. Sanders, *J. Am. Chem. Soc.*, **112**, 5525–5534 (1990).

124. U. Dinur and A. T. Hagler in Ref. 10, 1991, pp. 99–164.

125. J. Tirado-Rivese and W. L. Jorgensen, *J. Am. Chem. Soc.*, **112**, 2773–2781 (1990).

126. A. Alex and T. Clark, *J. Comput. Chem.*, **13**, 704–717 (1992).

127. J. Aqvist and A. Warshel, *Chem. Rev.*, **93**, 2523–2544 (1993).

128. M. J. Field, P. A. Bash, and M. Karplus, *J. Comput. Chem.*, **11**, 700–783 (1990).

129. A. Warshel, *Computer Modeling of Chemical Reactions in Enzymes and Solutions*, John Wiley & Sons, Inc., New York, 1991, pp. 236.

130. V. Dagget, S. Schroder, and P. Kollman, *J. Am. Chem. Soc.*, **113**, 8926–8935 (1991).

131. P. R. Andrews and D. A. Winkler in G. Jolles and K. R. H. Wooldridge, Eds., *Drug Design: Fact or Fantasy?* Academic Press, Inc., New York, 1984, pp. 145–174.

132. J. E. Eksterowicz and K. N. Houk, *Chem. Rev.*, **93**, 2439–2461 (1993).

133. P. J. Goodford, *J. Med. Chem.*, **27**, 557–564 (1984).

134. C. R. Beddell, *Chem. Soc. Rev.*, 13, 279–319 (1984).

135. R. Wootton in C. R. Beddell, Ed., *The Design of Drugs to Macromolecular Targets*, John Wiley & Sons, Inc., New York, 1992, pp. 49–83.

136. L. F. Kuyper, B. Roth, D. P. Baccanari, R. Ferone, C. R. Beddell, J. N. Champness, D. K. Stammers, J. G. Dann, F. E. Norrington, D. J. Baker, and P. J. Goodford, *J. Med. Chem.*, **28**, 303–311 (1985).

137. K. Appelt, *J. Comput. Aided Mol. Des.*, **1**, 23–48 (1993).

138. M. von Itzstein, W.-Y. Wu, G. B. Kok, M. S. Pegg, J. C. Dyason, B. Jin, T. V. Phan, M. L. Smythe, H. E. White, S. W. Oliver, P. M. Colman, J. N. Varghese, D. M. Ryan, J. M. Woods, R. C. Bethell, V. J. Hotham, J. M. Cameron, and C. R. Penn, *Nature*, **363**, 418–423 (1993).

139. M. Miller, M. Jaskolski, J. K. M. Rao, J. Leis, and A. Wlodawer, *Nature*, **337**, 576–579 (1989).

140. M. Miller, B. K. Sathyanarayana, A. Wlodawer, M. B. Toth, G. R. Marshall, L. Clawson, L. Selk, J. Schneider, and S. B. H. Kent, *Science*, **246**, 1149–1152 (1989).

141. R. L. Stanfield, M. Takimoto-Kamimura, J. M. Rini, A. T. Profy, and I. A. Wilson, *Structure*, **1**, 83–93 (1993).

142. M. F. Perutz, G. Fermi, D. J. Abraham, C. Poyart, and E. Bursaux, *J. Am. Chem. Soc.*, **108**, 1064–1078 (1986).

143. A. S. Mehana and D. J. Abraham, *Biochemistry*, **29**, 3944–3954 (1990).

144. I. D. Kuntz, J. M. Blaney, S. J. Oatley, R. Langridge, and T. E. Ferrin, *J. Mol. Biol.*, **161**, 269 (1982).

145. R. Voorintholt, M. T. Kosters, G. Vegter, G. Vriend, and W. G. J. Hol, *J. Mol. Graphics*, **7**, 243–245 (1989).

146. C. M. W. Ho and G. R. Marshall, *J. Comput. Aided Mol. Des.*, **4**, 337–354 (1990).

147. P. J. Goodford, *J. Am. Chem. Soc.*, **28**, 849–856 (1985).

148. R. D. Cramer III, D. E. Patterson, and J. D. Bunce, *J. Am. Chem. Soc.*, **110**, 5959–5967 (1988).

149. R. D. Cramer III and M. Milne, In *Abstracts of the 177th National Meeting of the American Chemical Society*, COMP 44, American Chemical Society, 1979.

150. A. Miranker and M. Karplus, *Proteins*, **11**, 29–34 (1991).

151. A. Caflisch, A. Miranker, and M. Karplus, *J. Med. Chem.*, **36**, 2142–2167 (1993).

152. P. K. Weiner, C. Landridge, J. M. Blaney, R. Schaefer, and P. A. Kollman, *Proc. Natl. Acad. Sci. U S A*, **79**, 3754–3758 (1982).

153. S. J. Weiner, P. A. Kollman, D. A. Case, U. C. Singh, C. Ghio, G. Alagona, J. Salvatore Profeta, and P. Weiner, *J. Am. Chem. Soc.*, **106**, 765–784 (1984).

154. S. J. Weiner, P. A. Kollman, D. T. Nguyen, and

D. A. Case, *J. Comput. Chem.*, **7**, 230–252 (1986).

155. D. H. Allen, J. E. Davies, J. J. Galloy, O. Johnson, O. Kennard, C. F. Macrea, E. M. Mitchell, G. F. Mitchell, J. M. Smith, and D. G. Watson, *J. Chem. Inf. Comput. Sci.*, **31**, 187–204 (1991).

156. E. E. Abola, F. C. Bernstein, and T. F. Koetzle in P. S. Glaeser, Ed., *The Role of Data in Scientific Progress*, Elsevier Science Publishing Co., Inc., New York, 1985.

157. P. R. Andrews, E. J. Lloyd, J. L. Martin, and S. L. A. Munro, *J. Mol. Graphics*, **4**, 41–45 (1986).

158. R. S. Pearlman, *Chem. Des. Auto. News*, **2**, 1 (1987).

159. R. S. Pearlman, CONCORD User's Manual, Tripos Associates, Inc., St. Louis, Mo., 1992.

160. R. S. Pearlman, *Chem. Des. Auto. News*, **8**, 3–15 (1993).

161. R. S. Pearlman in H. Kubinyi, Ed., *3D QSAR in Drug Design: Theory, Methods and Applications*, ESCOM Scientific Publishers, Leiden, pp. 41–79 (1993).

162. R. P. Sheridan, A. Rusinko III, R. Nilakantan, and R. Venkataraghavan, *Proc. Natl. Acad. Sci. U S A*, **86**, 8165–8169 (1989).

163. P. Gund, W. T. Wipke, and R. Langridge, *Comput. Chem. Res. Educ. Technol.*, **3**, 5–21 (1974).

164. P. Gund, *Prog. Mol. Subcell. Biol.*, **11**, 117–143 (1977).

165. A. M. Lesk, *Commun. A.C.M.*, **22**, 221–224 (1979).

166. S. E. Jakes and P. Willett, *J. Mol. Graphics*, **4**, 12–20 (1986).

167. S. E. Jakes, N. Watts, P. Willett, D. Bawden, and J. D. Fisher, *J. Mol. Graphics*, **5**, 41–48 (1987).

168. P. A. Bartlett, G. T. Shea, S. J. Telfer, and S. Waterman in S. M. Roberts, Ed., *Molecular Recognition: Chemical and Biological Problems*, Royal Society of Chemistry, London, 1989, pp. 182–196.

169. J. H. Van Drie, D. Weininger, and Y. C. Martin, *J. Comput. Aided Mol. Des.*, **3**, 225–251 (1989).

170. R. P. Sheridan, R. Nilakantan, A. I. Rusinko, N. Bauman, K. S. Haraki, and R. Venkataraghavan, *J. Chem. Inf. Comput. Sci.*, **29**, 255–260 (1989).

171. Molecular Design Ltd., San Leandro, Calif.

172. Chemical Design Ltd., Oxford, UK.

173. Tripos Associates, Inc. *UNITY-3DB User's Manual*, Tripos Associates, Inc., St. Louis, Mo., 1992.

174. Y. C. Martin, M. G. Bures, and P. Willett in Ref. 10, 1990, pp. 213–263.

175. Y. C. Martin, *J. Med. Chem.*, **35**, 2145–2154 (1992).

176. A. I. Rusinko, R. P. Sheridan, R. Nilakantan, K. S. Haraki, N. Bauman, and R. Venkataraghavan, *J. Chem. Inf. Comput. Sci.*, **29**, 251–255 (1989).

177. A. C. Good, S. J. Peterson, and W. G. Richards, *J. Med. Chem.*, **36**, 2929–2937 (1993).

178. D. P. Dolata, A. R. Leach, and K. Prout, *J. Comput. Aided Mol. Des.*, **1**, 73–85 (1987).

179. A. R. Leach, K. Prout, and D. P. Dolata, *J. Comput. Chem.*, **11**, 680–693 (1990).

180. J. Sadowski and J. Gasteiger, *Chem. Rev.*, **93**, 2567–2581 (1993).

181. R. L. DesJarlais, R. P. Sheridan, G. L. Seibel, J. S. Dixon, I. D. Kuntz, and R. Venkataraghavan, *J. Med. Chem.*, **31**, 722–729 (1988).

182. R. L. DesJarlais, G. L. Seibel, I. D. Kuntz, P. S. Furth, J. C. Alvarez, P. R. Ortiz de Montellano, D. L. DeCamp, L. M. Babe, and C. S. Craik, *Proc. Natl. Acad. Sci. U S A*, **87**, 6644–6648 (1990).

183. C. Burt and W. G. Richards, *J. Comput. Aided Mol. Des.*, **4**, 231–238 (1990).

184. R. L. DesJarlais, R. P. Sheridan, J. S. Dixon, I. D. Kuntz, and R. Venkataraghavan, *J. Med. Chem.*, **29**, 2149–2153 (1986).

185. H.-J. Bohm, *J. Comput. Aided Mol. Des.*, **6**, 61–78 (1992).

186. H.-J. Bohm, *J. Comput. Aided Mol. Des.*, **6**, 593–606 (1992).

187. P. L. Chau and P. M. Dean, *J. Comput. Aided. Mol. Des.*, **6**, 385–396 (1992).

188. P. L. Chau and P. M. Dean, *J. Comput. Aided. Mol. Des.*, **6**, 397–406 (1992).

189. P. L. Chau and P. M. Dean, *J. Comput. Aided. Mol. Des.*, **6**, 407–426 (1992).

190. C. M. W. Ho and G. R. Marshall, *J. Comput. Aided Mol. Des.*, **7**, 3–22 (1993).

191. C. M. W. Ho and G. R. Marshall, *J. Comput. Aided Mol. Des.*, **7**, 623–647 (1993).

192. R. A. Lewis and P. M. Dean, *Proc. R. Soc. Lond. [Biol.]*, **236**, 141–162 (1989).

193. R. A. Lewis and P. M. Dean, *Proc. R. Soc. Lond. [Biol.]*, **236**, 125–140 (1989).

194. Y. Nishibata and A. Itai, *Tetrahedron*, **47**, 8985–8990 (1991).

195. Y. Nishibata and A. Itai, *J. Med. Chem.*, **36**, 2921–2928 (1993).

196. D. A. Pearlman and M. A. Murko, *J. Comput. Chem.*, **14**, 1184–1193 (1993).

197. M. G. Bures, C. Black-Schaefer, and G. Gard-

ner, *J. Comput. Aided Mol. Des.*, **5**, 323–334 (1991).

198. D. L. Bodian, R. B. Yamasaki, R. L. Buswell, J. F. Stearns, J. M. White, and I. D. Kuntz, *Biochemistry*, **32**, 2967–2978 (1993).

199. C. S. Ring, E. Sun, J. H. McKerrow, G. K. Lee, P. J. Rosenthal, I. D. Kuntz, and F. E. Cohen, *Proc. Natl. Acad. Sci. U S A*, **90**, 3583–3587 (1993).

200. B. K. Shoichet, R. M. Stroud, D. V. Santi, I. D. Kuntz, and K. M. Perry, *Science*, **259**, 1445–1450 (1993).

201. S. Naruto, I. Motoc, G. R. Marshall, S. B. Daniels, M. J. Sofia, and J. A. Katzenellenbogen, *J. Am. Chem. Soc.*, **107**, 5262–5270 (1985).

202. N. L. Allinger, Z.-Q. S. Zhu and K. Chen, *J. Am. Chem. Soc.*, **114**, 6120–6133 (1992).

203. B. R. Brooks, R. E. Bruccoleri, B. D. Olafson, D. J. States, S. Swaminathan, and M. Karplus, *J. Comput. Chem.*, **4**, 187–217 (1983).

204. F. A. Momany and R. Rone, *J. Comput. Chem.*, **13**, 888–900 (1992).

205. J. Pranata, S. G. Wierschke, and W. I. Jorgensen, *J. Am. Chem. Soc.*, **113**, 2810–2819 (1991).

206. G. Nemethy, M. S. Pottle, and H. A. Scheraga, *J. Phys. Chem.*, **87**, 1883–1887 (1983).

207. T. A. Halgren, *J. Am. Chem. Soc.*, **114**, 7827–7843 (1992).

208. P. S. Charifson, R. G. Hiskey, L. G. Pedersen, and L. F. Kuyper, *J. Comput. Chem.*, **12**, 899–908 (1991).

209. S. C. Hoops, K. W. Anderson, and K. M. Merz Jr., *J. Am. Chem. Soc.*, **113**, 8262–8270 (1991).

210. C. J. Casewit, K. S. Colwell, and A. K. Rappe, *J. Am. Chem. Soc.*, **114**, 10035–10046 (1992).

211. C. J. Casewit, K. S. Colwell, and A. K. Rappe, *J. Am. Chem. Soc.*, **114**, 10046–10053 (1992).

212. A. K. Rappe, C. J. Casewit, K. S. Colwell, W. A. Goddard III, and W. M. Skiff, *J. Am. Chem. Soc.*, **114**, 10024–10035 (1992).

213. Y.-D. Wu and K. N. Houk, *J. Am. Chem. Soc.*, **114**, 1656–1661 (1992).

214. K. Houk, J. A. Tucker, and A. Dorigo, *Acc. Chem. Res.*, **23**, 107–113 (1990).

215. F. M. Menger and M. J. Sherrod, *J. Am. Chem. Soc.*, **112**, 8071–8075 (1990).

216. D. H. Williams, *Aldrichimica Acta*, **24**, 71–80 (1991).

217. A. J. Doig and D. H. Williams, *J. Am. Chem. Soc.*, **114**, 338–343 (1992).

218. M. S. Searle and D. H. Williams, *J. Am. Chem. Soc.*, **114**, 10690–10697 (1992).

219. M. S. Searle, D. H. Williams, and U. Gerhard, *J. Am. Chem. Soc.*, **114**, 10697–10704 (1992).

220. J. Novotny, R. E. Bruccoleri, and F. A. Saul, *Biochemistry*, **28**, 4735–4749 (1989).

221. R. Lumry and S. Rajender, *Biopolymers*, **9**, 1125–1227 (1970).

222. K. M. Merz Jr., M. A. Murcko, and P. A. Kollman, *J. Am. Chem. Soc.*, **113**, 4484–4490 (1991).

223. C. F. Wong and J. A. McCammon, *J. Am. Chem. Soc.*, **108**, 3830–3832 (1986).

224. L. M. Hansen and P. A. Kollman, *J. Comput. Chem.*, **11**, 994–1002 (1990).

225. B. G. Rao, R. F. Tilton, and U. C. Singh, *J. Am. Chem. Soc.*, **114**, 4447–4452 (1992).

226. W. E. Harte Jr. and D. L. Beveridge, *J. Am. Chem. Soc.*, **115**, 3883–3886 (1993).

227. D. M. Ferguson, R. J. Radmer, and P. A. Kollman, *J. Med. Chem.*, **34**, 2654–2659 (1991).

228. D. H. Rich, C.-Q. Sun, J. V. N. Vara Prasad, M. V. Toth, G. R. Marshall, P. Ahammadunny, M. D. Clare, R. D. Mueller, and K. Houseman, *J. Med. Chem.*, **34**, 1222–1225 (1991).

229. J. J. McDonald and C. L. Brooks III, *J. Am. Chem. Soc.*, **114**, 2062–2072 (1992).

230. T. P. Lybrand and J. A. McCammon, *J. Comput. Aided Mol. Des.*, **2**, 259–266 (1988).

231. W. R. Cannon, J. D. Madura, R. P. Thummel, and J. A. McCammon, *J. Am. Chem. Soc.*, **115**, 879–884 (1993).

232. S. Yun-yu, A. E. Mark, W. Cun-Xin, H. Fuhua, J. C. Berendsen, and W. F. van Gunsteren, *Protein Eng.*, **6**, 289–295 (1993).

233. P. De La Paz, J. M. Burridge, S. J. Oatley, and C. C. F. Blake in Ref. 135, pp. 119–172.

234. A. B. Edmundson, J. N. Herron, K. R. Ely, X.-M. He, D. L. Harris, and E. W. Voss Jr., *Philos. Trans. R. Soc. Lond. [Biol.]*, **323**, 495–509 (1989).

235. C. Bihoreau, C. Monnot, E. Davies, B. Teutsch, K. E. Bernstein, P. Corvol, and E. Clauser, *Proc. Natl. Acad. Sci. U S A*, **90**, 5133–5137 (1993).

236. T. M. Fong, R. R. C. Huang, and C. D. Strader, *J. Biol. Chem.*, **267**, 25664–25667 (1992).

237. U. Gether, T. E. Johansen, R. M. Snider, J. A. Lowe, III, S. Nakanishi, and T. W. Schwartz, *Nature*, **362**, 345–348 (1993).

238. M. F. Hibert, S. Trumpp-Kallmeyer, A. Bruinvels, and J. Hoflack, *Mol. Pharmacol.*, **40**, 8–15 (1991).

239. M. F. Hibert, S. Trumpp-Kallmeyer, J. Hoflack, and A. Bruinvels, *Trends Pharmacol. Sci.*, **14**, 7–12 (1993).

240. G. Nordvall and U. Hacksell, *J. Med. Chem.*, **36**, 967–976 (1993).

241. T. L. Blundell, B. L. Sibanda, M. J. E. Stern-

berg, and J. M. Thornton, *Nature*, **326**, 347–352 (1987).

242. L. H. Pearl and W. R. Taylor, *Nature*, **329**, 351–354 (1987).

243. I. T. Weber, *Proteins*, **7**, 172–184 (1990).

244. L. M. Balbes and F. I. Carroll, *Med. Chem. Res.*, **1**, 283–288 (1991).

245. R. J. Siezen, W. M. de Vos, J. A. M. Leunissen, and B. W. Dijkstra, *Protein Eng.*, **4**, 719–737 (1991).

246. J. H. Brown, T. Jardetzky, M. A. Saper, B. Samraoui, P. J. Bjorkman, and D. C. Wiley, *Nature*, **332**, 845–850 (1988).

247. L. M. H. Koymans, N. P. E. Vermeulen, A. Baarslag, and G. M. Donne-op den Kelder, *J. Comput. Aided Mol. Des.*, **7**, 281–289 (1993).

248. R. E. Bruccoleri and M. Karplus, *Biopolymers*, **26**, 137–168 (1987).

249. R. Hirschmann, K. C. Nicolaou, S. Pietranico, J. Salvino, E. M. Leahy, P. A. Sprengeler, G. Furst, and A. B. Smith, III, *J. Am. Chem. Soc.*, **114**, 9217–9218 (1992).

250. R. Hirschmann, P. A. Sprengeler, T. Kawasaki, J. W. Leahy, W. C. Shakespeare, and A. B. Smith III, *J. Am. Chem. Soc.*, **114**, 9699–9701 (1992).

251. T. W. Ku, F. E. Ali, L. S. Barton, J. W. Bean, W. E. Bondinell, J. L. Burgess, J. F. Callahan, R. R. Calvo, L. Chen, D. S. Eggelston, J. S. Gleason, W. F. Huffman, S. M. Hwang, D. R. Jakas, C. B. Karash, R. M. Keenan, K. D. Kopple, W. H. Miller, K. A. Newlander, A. Nichols, M. F. Parker, C. E. Peishoff, J. M. Samanen, I. Uzinskas, and J. W. Venslavsky, *J. Am. Chem. Soc.*, **115**, 8861–8862 (1993).

252. G. L. Olson, H.-C. Cheung, M. E. Voss, D. E. Hill, M. Kahn, V. S. Madison, C. M. Cook, J. Sepinwall, and G. Vincent in *Biotechnology USA 1989*, Conference Management Corp., Norwald, Conn., 1989, pp. 348–360.

253. G. L. Olson, D. R. Bolin, M. P. Bonner, M. Bos, C. M. Cook, D. C. Fry, B. J. Graves, M. Hatada, D. E. Hill, M. Kahn, V. S. Madison, V. K. Rusiecki, R. Sarabu, J. Sepinwall, G. P. Vincent, and M. E. Voss, *J. Med. Chem.*, **36**, 3039–3049 (1993).

254. P. C. Belanger and C. Dufresne, *Can. J. Chem.*, **64**, 1514–1520 (1986).

255. R. Hirschmann, K. C. Nicolaou, S. Pietranico, E. M. Leahy, J. Salvino, B. Arison, M. A. Cichy, P. G. Spoors, W. C. Shakespeare, P. A. Sprengeler, P. Hamley, A. B. Smith III, T. Reisine, K. Raynor, L. Maechler, C. Donaldson, W. Vale, R. M. Friedinger, M. R. Cascieri, and C. D. Strader, *J. Am. Chem. Soc.*, **115**, 12550–12568 (1993).

256. J. H. Arevalo, E. A. Stura, M. J. Taussig, and I. A. Wilson, *J. Mol. Biol.*, **231**, 103–118 (1993).

257. J. H. Arevalo, M. J. Taussig, and I. A. Wilson, *Nature*, **365**, 859–863 (1993).

258. Y. Kato, A. Itai, and Y. Iitaka, *Tetrahedron Lett.*, **43**, 5229–5236 (1987).

259. W. H. Moos, C. C. Humblet, I. Sircar, C. Rithner, R. E. Weishaar, J. A. Bristol, and A. T. McPhail, *J. Med. Chem.*, **30**, 1963–1972 (1987).

260. D. Mayer, C. B. Naylor, I. Motoc, and G. R. Marshall, *J. Comput. Aided Mol. Des.*, **1**, 3–16 (1987).

261. R. J. Hausin and P. W. Codding, *J. Med. Chem.*, **33**, 1940–1947 (1990).

262. G. R. Marshall, C. D. Barry, H. E. Bosshard, R. A. Dammkoehler, and D. A. Dunn in E. C. Olsen and R. E. Christoffersen, Eds., *Computer-Assisted Drug Design*, American Chemical Society, Washington, D.C., 1979, pp. 205–226.

263. R. A. Dammkoehler, S. F. Karasek, E. F. B. Shands, and G. R. Marshall, in *Abstracts of the 204th ACS National Meeting*, American Chemical Society, Washington, D.C., 1992.

264. G. R. Marshall and R. D. Cramer III, *Trends Pharmacol. Sci.*, **9**, 285–289 (1988).

265. U.S. Pat. 5,025,388 (1991), to R. D. Cramer III and S. B. Wold.

266. J. R. Sufrin, D. A. Dunn, and G. R. Marshall, *Mol. Pharmacol.*, **19**, 307–313 (1981).

267. P. R. Andrews, E. J. Lloyd, J. L. Martin, S. L. Munro, M. Sadek, and M. G. Wong in A. S. V. Burgen, G. C. K. Roberts, and M. S. Tute, Eds., *Molecular Graphics and Drug Design*, Elsevier, Amsterdam, The Netherlands, 1986, pp. 216–255.

268. G. Klopman and S. Srivastava, *Mol. Pharmacol.*, **37**, 958–965 (1989).

269. G. Klopman and M. L. Dimayuga, *J. Comput. Aided Mol. Des.*, **4**, 117–130 (1990).

270. G. Rum and W. C. Herndon, *J. Am. Chem. Soc.*, **113**, 9055–9060 (1991).

271. C. Silipo and A. Vittoria in Ref. 4, pp. 153–204.

272. G. M. Crippen, *Distance Geometry and Conformational Calculations*, John Wiley & Sons, Inc., Chichester, UK, 1981.

273. D. E. Clark, P. Willett, and P. W. Kenny, *J. Mol. Graphics*, **10**, 194–204 (1992).

274. C. A. Pepperrell and P. Willett, *J. Comput. Aided Mol. Des.*, **5**, 455–474 (1991).

275. A. R. Poirette, P. Willett, and F. H. Allen, *J. Mol. Graphics*, **11**, 2–14 (1993).

276. G. R. Marshall and C. B. Naylor in Ref. 4, pp. 431–458.

277. A. Davis, B. H. Warrington, and J. G. Vinter, *J. Comput. Aided Mol. Des.*, **1**, 97–120 (1987).

278. H. Weinstein, R. Osman, S. Topiol, and J. P. Green, *Ann. N. Y. Acad. Sci.*, **367**, 434–448 (1981).

279. N. C. Cohen in B. Testa, Ed., *Advances in Drug Research*, Academic Press, Inc., New York, 1985, pp. 40–144.

280. R. C. Wade, K. J. Clark, and P. J. Goodford, *J. Med. Chem.*, **36**, 140–147 (1993).

281. C. Hansch, J. McClarin, T. Klein, and R. Langridge, *Mol. Pharmacol.*, **27**, 493–498 (1985).

282. C. Hansch, T. Klein, J. McClarin, R. Langridge, and N. W. Cornell, *J. Med. Chem.*, **29**, 615–620 (1986).

283. G. E. Kellogg, S. F. Semus, and D. J. Abraham, *J. Comput. Aided Mol. Des.*, **5**, 545–552 (1991).

284. G. E. Kellogg and D. J. Abraham, *J. Mol. Graphics*, **10**, 212–217 (1992).

285. D. J. Danziger and P. M. Dean, *J. Theor. Biol.*, **116**, 215–224 (1985).

286. S. K. Kearsley, *J. Comput. Chem.*, **11**, 1187–1192 (1990).

287. G. R. Marshall and C. D. Barry in *Abstracts of the American Crystal Association, Honolulu, Hawaii*, 1979.

288. A. J. Hopfinger, *J. Med. Chem.*, **2**, 7196–7206 (1980).

289. Z. Simon, A. Chiriac, S. Holban, D. Ciubotariu, and G. I. Mihalas, *Minimum Steric Difference*, Research Studies Press, Letchworth, UK, 1984.

290. D. Ciubotariu, E. Deretey, T. I. Oprea, T. I. Sulea, Z. Simon, L. Kurunczi, and A. Chiriac, *Quant. Struct. Act. Relat.*, **12**, 367–372 (1993).

291. H.-D. Holtje and S. Marrer, *J. Comput. Aided Mol. Des.*, **1**, 23–30 (1987).

292. A. J. Hopfinger, *J. Med. Chem.*, **26**, 990–996 (1983).

293. S. Namasivayam and P. M. Dean, *J. Mol. Graphics*, **4**, 46 (1986).

294. P. L. Chau and P. M. Dean, *J. Mol. Graphics*, **5**, 97 (1987).

295. E. J. Lloyd and P. R. Andrews, *J. Med. Chem.*, **29**, 453–462 (1986).

296. J. Zabrocki, G. D. Smith, J. B. Dunbar Jr., H. Iijima, and G. R. Marshall, *J. Am. Chem. Soc.*, **110**, 5875–5880 (1988).

297. J. B. Ball, R. A. Hughes, P. F. Alewood, and P. R. Andrews, *Tetrahedron*, **49**, 3467–3478 (1993).

298. J. B. Ball and P. F. Alewood, *J. Mol. Recog.*, **3**, 55–64 (1990).

299. J. Labanowski, I. Motoc, C. B. Naylor, D. Mayer, and R. A. Dammkoehler, *Quant. Struc. Act. Relat.*, **5**, 138–152 (1986).

300. S. Naruto, I. Motoc, and G. R. Marshall, *Eur. J. Med. Chem. Chem. Ther.*, **20**, 529–532 (1985).

301. R. P. Sheridan and R. Venkataraghavan, *J. Comput. Aided Mol. Des.*, **1**, 243–256 (1987).

302. E. E. Hodgkin, A. Miller, and M. Whittaker, *J. Comput. Aided Mol. Des.*, **7**, 515–534 (1993).

303. M. T. Barakat and P. M. Dean, *J. Comput. Aided Mol. Des.*, **4**, 295–316 (1990).

304. M. T. Barakat and P. M. Dean, *J. Comput. Aided Mol. Des.*, **4**, 317–330 (1990).

305. T. D. J. Perkins and P. M. Dean, *J. Comput. Aided Mol. Des.*, **7**, 173–182 (1993).

306. I. Motoc, J. Labanowski, C. B. Naylor, D. Mayer, and R. A. Dammkoehler, *Quant. Struc. Act. Relat.*, **5**, 99–105 (1986).

307. R. D. Nelson, D. I. Gottlieb, T. M. Balasubramanian, and G. R. Marshall in R. S. Rapaka, G. Barnett, and R. L. Hawks, Eds., *Opioid Peptides: Medicinal Chemistry*, NIDA Office of Science, Rockville, Md., 1986, pp. 204–230.

308. A. K. Ghose and G. M. Crippen, *J. Med. Chem.*, **27**, 901–914 (1984).

309. A. K. Ghose and G. M. Crippen, *J. Med. Chem.*, **28**, 333–346 (1985).

310. A. K. Ghose and G. M. Crippen in Ref. 4, pp. 716–733.

311. A. K. Ghose and G. M. Chippen, *Mol. Pharmacol.*, **37**, 725–734 (1990).

312. M. R. Linschoten, T. Bultsma, A. P. IJzerman, and H. Timmerman, *J. Med. Chem.*, **29**, 278–286 (1986).

313. G. M. Donne-op den Kelder, *J. Comput. Aided Mol. Des.*, **1**, 257–264 (1987).

314. T. I. Oprea, D. Ciubotariu, T. I. Sulea, and Z. Simon, *Quant. Struct. Act. Relat.*, **12**, 21–26 (1993).

315. J. P. Snyder, S. N. Rao, K. F. Koehler, A. Vedani, and R. Pellicciari in C. G. Wermuth, Ed., *Trends in QSAR and Molecular Modelling 92*, ESCOM Scientific Publishers, Leiden, 1993, pp. 44–51.

316. G. Klopman, *Quant. Struct. Act. Relat.*, **2**, 176–185 (1992).

317. I. B. Bersuker and A. S. Dimogo in Ref. 10, 1991, pp. 423–460.

318. Y. C. Martin, M. G. Bures, E. A. Danaher, J. DeLazzer, I. Lico, and P. Pavlik, *J. Comput. Aided Mol. Des.*, **7**, 83–102 (1993).

319. T. I. Oprea and L. Kurunczi in N. Voiculetz, I. Motoc, and Z. Simon, Eds., *Specific Interactions and Biological Recognition Processes*, CRC Press, Boca Raton, Fla., 1993, pp. 295–326.

320. W. E. Klunk, B. L. Kalman, J. A. Ferrendelli, and D. F. Covey, *Mol. Pharmacol.*, **23**, 511–518 (1982).

321. J. A. Calder, J. A. Wyatt, D. A. Frenkel, and J. E. Casida, *J. Comput. Aided Mol. Des.*, **7**, 45–60 (1993).

322. M. F. Hibert, R. Hoffmann, R. C. Miller, and A. A. Carr, *J. Med. Chem.*, **33**, 1594–1600 (1990).

323. M. F. Hibert, M. W. Gittos, D. N. Middlemiss, A. K. Mir, and J. R. Fozard, *J. Med. Chem.*, **31**, 1087–1093 (1988).

324. A. W. Schmidt and S. J. Peroutka, *Mol. Pharmacol.*, **36**, 505–511 (1989).

325. M. L. Connolly, *Science*, **221**, 709–713 (1983).

326. M. L. Connolly, *J. Appl. Cryst.*, **16**, 548–558 (1983).

327. C. E. Kundrot, J. W. Ponder, and F. M. Richards, *J. Comput. Chem.*, **1991**, 402–409 (1991).

328. S. M. Le Grand and K. M. Merz Jr., *J. Comput. Chem.*, **14**, 349–352 (1993).

329. A. H. Beckett and A. F. Casey, *J. Pharm. Pharmacol.*, **6**, 986–999 (1954).

330. L. B. Kier and H. S. Aldrich, *J. Theor. Biol.*, **46**, 529–541 (1974).

331. L. G. Humber, F. T. Bruderlin, A. H. Philipp, M. Gotz, and K. Voith, *J. Med. Chem.*, **22**, 761–767 (1979).

332. G. L. Olson, H. C. Cheung, K. D. Morgan, J. F. Blount, L. Todaro, L. Berger, A. B. Davidson, and E. Boff, *J. Med. Chem.*, **24**, 1026–1034 (1981).

333. H.-D. Holtje and M. Tintelnot, *Quant. Struct. Act. Relat.*, **3**, 6–9 (1984).

334. W. C. Probst, L. A. Snyder, D. J. Schuster, J. Brosius, and S. C. Sealfon, *DNA Cell Biol.*, **2**, 1–20 (1992).

335. S. Trumpp-Kallmeyer, J. Hoflack, A. Bruinvels, and M. Hibert, *J. Med. Chem.*, **35**, 3448–3462 (1992).

336. D. Timms, A. J. Wilkinson, D. R. Kelly, K. J. Broadley, and R. H. Davies, *Int. J. Quantum Chem. Symp.*, **19**, 197–215 (1992).

337. D. Zhang and H. Weinstein, *J. Med. Chem.*, **36**, 934–938 (1993).

338. B. L. Bush and R. B. Nachbar Jr., *J. Comput. Aided Mol. Des.*, **7**, 587–619 (1993).

339. J. N. Weinstein, K. W. Kohn, M. R. Grever, V. N. Viswanadhan, L. V. Rubinstein, A. P. Monks, D. A. Scudiero, L. Welch, A. D. Koutsoukos, A. J. Chiausa, and K. D. Paull, *Science*, **258**, 447–451 (1992).

340. T. A. Andrea and H. Kalayeh, *J. Med. Chem.*, **34**, 2824–2836 (1991).

341. S.-S. So and W. G. Richards, *J. Med. Chem.*, **35**, 3201–3207 (1992).

342. I. V. Tetko, A. I. Luik, and G. I. Poda, *J. Med. Chem.*, **36**, 811–814 (1993).

343. R. D. King, S. Muggleton, R. A. Lewis, and M. J. E. Sternberg, *Proc. Natl. Acad. Sci. U S A*, **89**, 11322–11326 (1992).

344. S. A. DePriest, E. F. B. Shands, R. A. Dammkoehler, and G. R. Marshall in C. Silipo and A. Vittoria, Eds., *QSAR: Rational Approaches to the Design of Bioactive Compounds*, Elsevier, Amsterdam, The Netherlands, 1991, pp. 405–414.

345. S. A. DePriest, D. Mayer, C. B. Naylor, and G. R. Marshall, *J. Am. Chem. Soc.*, **115**, 5372–5384 (1993).

346. C. Hansch, *Acc. Chem. Res.*, **26**, 147–153 (1993).

347. G. Klebe and U. Abraham, *J. Med. Chem.*, **36**, 70–80 (1993).

348. C. L. Waller, T. I. Oprea, A. Giolitti, and G. R. Marshall, *J. Med. Chem.*, **36**, 4152–4160 (1993).

349. D. P. Getman, G. A. DeCrescenzo, R. M. Heintz, K. L. Reed, J. J. Talley, M. L. Bryant, M. Clare, K. A. Houseman, J. J. Marr, R. A. Mueller, M. L. Vazquez, H.-S. Shieh, W. C. Stallings, and R. A. Stegeman, *J. Med. Chem.*, **36**, 288–291 (1993).

350. G. M. Crippen, *J. Comput. Chem.*, **8**, 943–955 (1987).

351. M. P. Bradley and G. M. Crippen, *J. Med. Chem.*, **36**, 3171–3177 (1993).

352. F. Major, M. Turcotte, D. Gautheret, G. Lapalme, E. Fillion, and R. Cedergren, *Science*, **253**, 1255–1260 (1991).

353. D. Gautheret and R. Cedergren, *FASEB J.*, **7**, 97–105 (1993).

354. P. A. Greenidge, T. C. Jenkins, and S. Neidle, *Mol. Pharmacol.*, **43**, 982–988 (1993).

355. M. G. Cardozo and A. J. Hopfinger, *Mol. Pharmacol.*, **40**, 1023–1028 (1991).

356. M. J. J. Blommers, C. B. Lucasius, G. Kateman, and R. Kaptein, *Biopolymers*, **22**, 45–52 (1992).

357. A. G. Palmer III and D. A. Case, *J. Am. Chem. Soc.*, **114**, 9059–9067 (1992).

358. K. Boehncke, M. Nonella, K. Schulten, and A. H.-J. Wang, *Biochemistry*, **30**, 5465–5475 (1991).

359. J. Xing and H. L. Scott, *Biochem. Biophys. Res. Commun.*, **165**, 1–6 (1989).

360. C. R. Stouch, K. B. Ward, A. Altieri, and A. T. Hagler, *J. Comput. Chem.*, **12**, 1033–1046 (1991).

361. H. L. Scot and S. Kalaskar, *Biochemistry*, **28**, 3687–3691 (1989).

362. P. S. O'Shea and R. Matela, *Biochem. Soc. Trans.*, **14**, 1119–1120 (1986).

363. D. M. Kroll and G. Gompper, *Science*, **255**, 968–971 (1992).

364. L. I. Krishtakik, V. V. Topolev, and Y. I. Kharkats, *Biophysics* **36**, 257–262 (1991).

365. E. Egberts and H. J. C. Berendsen, *J. Chem. Phys.*, **89**, 3718–3732 (1988).

366. R. P. Mason, D. G. Rhodes, and L. G. Herbette, *J. Med. Chem.*, **34**, 869–877 (1991).

367. L. G. Herbette in Ref. 315, pp. 76–85.

368. H. Heller, M. Schaeffer, and K. Schulten, *J. Phys. Chem.*, **97**, 8343–8360 (1993).

369. T. Kataoka, D. D. Beusen, J. D. Clark, M. Yodo, and G. R. Marshall, *Biopolymers*, **32**, 1519–1533 (1992).

370. G. R. Marshall, *Tetrahedron*, **49**, 3547–3558 (1993).

371. G. V. Nikiforovich and G. R. Marshall, *Biochem. Biophys. Res. Commun.*, **195**, 222–228 (1993).

372. G. V. Nikiforovich and V. J. Hruby, *Biochem. Biophys. Res. Commun.*, **194**, 9–16 (1993).

373. G. Nikiforovich and G. R. Marshall, *Int. J. Pept. Protein Res.*, **42**, 171–180 (1993).

374. G. V. Nikiforovich and G. R. Marshall, *Int. J. Pept. Protein Res.*, **42**, 181–193 (1993).

375. G. R. Marshall in Ref. 161.

CHAPTER SIXTEEN

The Role of Recombinant DNA Technology in Medicinal Chemistry and Drug Discovery

MICHAEL C. VENUTI

Parnassus Pharmaceuticals, Inc.
Alameda, California, USA

CONTENTS

1 Perspective, 661
    1.1 Chemistry-driven drug discovery, 662
    1.2 The advent of recombinant DNA
        technology, 664
2 New Therapeutics from Recombinant DNA
   Technology, 664
3 Protein Engineering and Site-directed
   Mutagenesis, 667
    3.1 Second-generation protein therapeutics, 667
    3.2 Epitope mapping, 669
    3.3 Future directions, 672
4 Genetically Engineered Drug Discovery
   Tools, 673
    4.1 Reagents for screening, 673
    4.2 Reagents for structural biology studies, 676
    4.3 Enzymes as drug targets, 676
    4.4 Receptors as drug targets, 681
    4.5 Cellular adhesion proteins, 687
5 Future Prospects, 690

1 PERSPECTIVE

Discovering new drugs has never been a simple matter. From ancient times to virtually the beginning of this century, treatment for illness or disease was based main-

Burger's Medicinal Chemistry and Drug Discovery,
Fifth Edition, Volume 1: Principles and Practice,
Edited by Manfred E. Wolff.
ISBN 0-471-57556-9 © 1995 John Wiley & Sons, Inc.

ly on folklore and traditional curative methods derived from plants and other natural sources. The isolation and chemical characterization of the principal components of some of these traditional medicines, mainly alkaloids and the like, spawned the development of the modern pharmaceutical industry and the production of drugs in mass quantities. Within this century, however, the changes the industry has undergone have been profound. As the companion chapters of this volume describe, the emphasis has changed from isolation of active constituents to creation of new, potent chemical entities. This evolution from folklore to science is responsible for the thousands of pharmaceuticals available worldwide at present (1).

1.1 Chemistry-driven Drug Discovery

The exacting process of discovering new chemical entities that are safe and effective drugs has itself undergone many changes, each of which was prompted by the introduction of some new technology (2, 3). In the 1920s, the first efforts at understanding why and how morphine worked in terms of its chemical structure were initiated. During the 1940s, challenges for mass production of medicinally valuable natural products, like the penicillins, were conquered. By the late 1950s, advances in synthetic organic chemistry enabled the generation of multitudes of novel structures for broad testing into the major focus of the modern pharmaceutical industry. Although serendipitous at best, this approach yielded many valuable compounds, most notably the benzodiazepine tranquilizers chlordiazepoxide (1) and diazepam (2) (4). Even with these successful compounds, however, the process of drug discovery amounted to little more than evaluating available chemical entities in animal models suggestive of human disease.

By the mid-1960s, medicinal chemistry

had clearly become the cornerstone technology of modern drug discovery. Systematic development of structure–activity relationships, even to the point at which predictions about activity might be made, became the hallmark of new drug discovery. Even then, however, an understanding of the actions of drugs at the molecular level was often lacking. Receptors and enzymes were still considered as functional "black boxes" whose structures and functions were poorly understood. The first successful attempts at actually designing a drug to work at a particular molecular target happened nearly simultaneously in the 1970s, with the discovery of cimetidine (3), a selective H_2-antagonist for the treatment of ulcers (5), and captopril (4), an angiotensin-converting enzyme inhibitor for hypertension (6). The success of these two drugs sparked a realignment of chemistry-driven pharmaceutical research. Since then, the art of rational drug design has undergone an explosive evolution, making use of sophisticated computational and structural methodology to help in the effort (7). During the 1980s, mechanism-targeted design and screening combined to produce a number of novel chemical entities. These include the natural product HMG-CoA reductase inhibitor lovastatin (5) for the treatment of hypercholesteremia (8) and the antihypertensive angiotensin II receptor antagonist losartan (6), synthetically optimized from a chemical library screening lead (9).

(1)

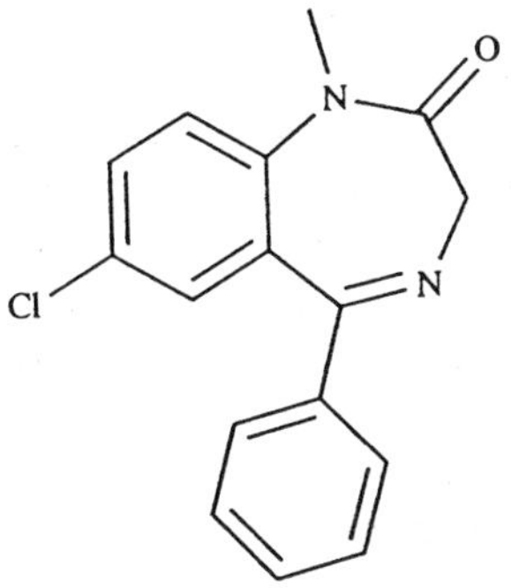

(2)

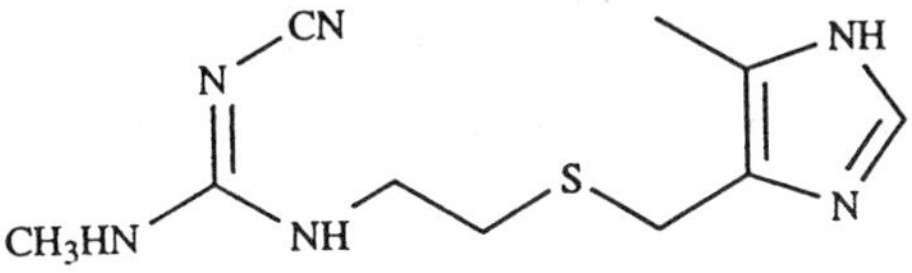

(6)

(3)

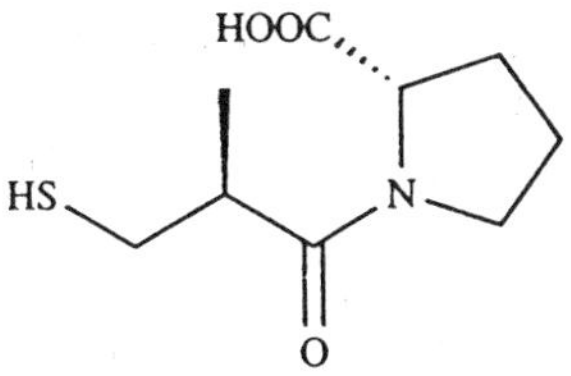

(4)

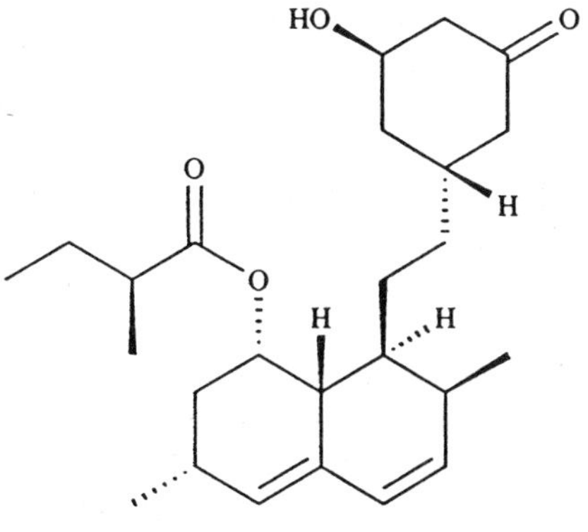

(5)

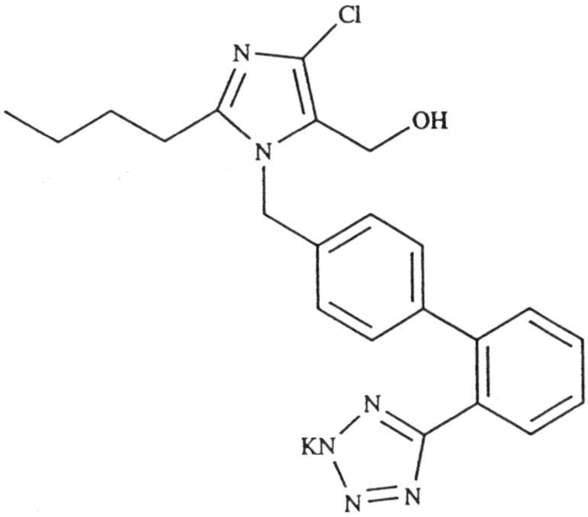

There is little doubt that the task of discovering new therapeutic agents that work potently, specifically, and without side effects has become increasingly important and coincidentally more difficult. Advances in medical research that have provided new clues to the previously obscure etiologies of diseases have revealed new opportunities for therapeutic intervention. This has forced the science of medicinal chemistry, once founded almost solely in near-blind synthesis and screening for *in vivo* effects, to become keenly aware of biochemical mechanisms as an intimate part of the development process. Even with these major advances in the medicinal and pharmaceutical sciences, more fundamental questions remain: What determines a useful biological property? And how is it measured in the discovery process? The answers can determine the discoveries and ultimately the success or failure of any drug discovery program, since both the observation of a useful biological property in a novel molecule and the optimization of structure–activity relationships associated with ultimate clinical candidate selection have rightfully relied heavily on practices, and sometimes prejudices, founded in decades of empirical success (10). Although the task of drug *development* has now been refined into a process without major un-identified obstacles, the challenge to bring the *discovery* of novel compounds to a comparable state of maturity remains. As in the past, another research avenue synergistic with existing discovery technologies is necessary.

1.2 The Advent of Recombinant DNA Technology

The evolution of recombinant DNA technology, from scientific innovation to pharmaceutical discovery process, has occurred in parallel with the development of contemporary medicinal chemistry (11–14). The products of biotechnology research share few of the traits characteristic of traditional pharmaceuticals. These biotechnologically derived therapeutics are large extracellular proteins destined to be, with few exceptions, injectables for use in either chronic replacement therapies or in acute or near-term chronic situations for the treatment of life-threatening indications (15, 16). Many of these products also satisfy urgent and previously unfulfilled therapeutic needs. Their dissimilarity to traditional medicinal agents does not end there, however. Unlike most low molecular weight pharmaceuticals, these proteins were developed not because of their novelty of structure, but because of their novelty of action. Their discovery hinged on recognition of a useful biological activity, its subsequent association with an effector protein, and the genetic identification, expression, and production of the effector by the application of recombinant DNA technology (17, 18).

If modulation of biochemical processes by a low molecular weight compound has been the traditional goal of medicinal chemistry, then association of a biological effect with a distinct protein and its identification and production have been considered the domain of molecular genetics. The application of recombinant DNA technology to the identification of proteins and other macromolecules as drugs or drug targets and their production in meaningful quantity as products or discovery tools, respectively, provide an answer to at least one of the persistent problems of new lead discovery. Because a comprehensive review of the genetic engineering of important proteins is well beyond the scope of this volume, this chapter will instead highlight some novel examples of contemporary advances in recombinant DNA technology, with respect to both exciting new pharmaceuticals and potential applications of recombinantly produced proteins, be they enzymes, receptors or hormones, to the more traditional processes of drug discovery.

2 NEW THERAPEUTICS FROM RECOMBINANT DNA TECHNOLOGY

The traditional role of the pharmaceutical industry, organic synthesis of new chemical entities as therapeutic agents, was suddenly expanded by the introduction of the first biotechnologically derived products in the 1980s. The approval of recombinant human insulin in 1982 broke important ground for products produced by genetic engineering (19). In 1985, another milestone was achieved when Genentech became the first biotechnology company to be granted approval to market a recombinant product, human growth hormone. These events set an entire industry into motion, to produce not only natural proteins for the treatment of deficiency-associated diseases but also true therapeutics for both acute and chronic care.

Industry estimates show the upward trend in biotechnologically derived products continuing into the 1990s. More than 200 products generated by biotechnology are estimated to be somewhere in the development pipeline or approval process. Some important examples of genetically

Table 16.1 Biotechnologically Derived Therapeutics in Clinical Development

Product	Disease Indication	Status
Hormones and Growth Factors		
Human insulin	Diabetes	Approved 1982
Human growth hormone (hGH)	Growth hormone deficiency	Approved 1985
Epidermal growth factor (EGF)	Corneal transplants, cancer, burns, ulcers, wound healing	Phase I/II
Insulin-like growth factor (IGF)	Diabetes, nutritional disorders, wound healing, burns, ulcers	Preclinical/phase II
Platelet-derived growth factor (PDGF)	Postsurgery tissue healing, trauma	Phase I
Transforming growth factor β (TGF-β)	Wound healing, osteoporosis	Preclinical/phase II
TGF-α	Cancer, wound healing	Preclinical
Tissue necrosis factor (TNF)	Cancer, wound healing	Preregistration
Nerve growth factor (NGF)	Neuropathy	Phase I
Brain-derived neurotrophic factor (BDNF)	Alzheimer's disease	Phase I
Erythropoetin (EPO)	Anemia of kidney dialysis	Approved 1989
	AZT-related anemia	Approved 1990
Granulocyte–colony-stimulating factor (G-CSF)	Chemotherapy effects, AIDS, leukemia	Approved 1991
Granulocyte-macrophage–colony-stimulating factor (GM–CSF)	Chemotherapy adjuvant, bone marrow transplant	Approved 1991
Thrombopoeitin (TPO)	Platelet replacement	Preclinical
Relaxin	Cervical ripening in childbirth	Phase II
Enzymes and Inhibitors		
Tissue-type plasminogen activator (t-PA)	Myocardial infarction	Approved 1987
	Pulmonary embolism	Approved 1990
t-PA variants	Myocardial infarction	Phase I/II
Urokinase (recombinant)	Myocardial infarction	Phase II
Factor VII:C	Hemophilia	Phase II
Factor VIII	Hemophilia	Approved 1993
DNase	Cystic fibrosis, bronchitis	Approved 1993
Glucocerebrosidase (GCR)	Gaucher's disease	Approved 1994
Superoxide dismutase (SOD)	Reperfusion injury	Phase II/III
Hirudin	Clot reocclusion	Phase II/III
Cytokines		
Interleukin-1 (IL-1)	Wounds, burns, vaccine adjuvant	Phase I
IL-1β	Bone marrow radio/chemotherapy	Phase II
IL-2	Renal cell carcinoma	Approved 1991
	Malignant melanoma	Phase III
IL-3	Bone marrow failure, platelet deficiencies	Phase I/II
IL-4	Cancer immunomodulator	Phase I/II
Interferon-α (IFN-α)	Hairy-cell leukemia	Approved 1986
	Kaposi's sarcoma	Approved 1988
	Chronic/acute hepatitis	Phase II/III
IFN-α-2b	Genital warts	Approved 1989
	Genital herpes	Application submitted
IFN-β	ARC/AIDS, MS	Approved 1993
	Cancer	Phase I/II

Table 16.1   (*Continued*)

Product	Disease Indication	Status
IFN-γ	Chronic granulomatous disease	Approved 1991
	Leukemias, melanoma	Phase III
	Scleroderma	Phase I
Receptors/Monoclonal Antibodies		
IIbIIa (7E3)	Cardio/thrombolytic	Phase III
TNF	Inflammation/septic shock	Phase II
	Inflammation, RA	Phase II
CD4	AIDS	Suspended
CD4-IgG	AIDS	Phase I/II
MAb-OKT3	Kidney transplant rejection	Approved 1986
	Heart, liver transplants	Application submitted
MAb-anti-CD4	AIDS	Phase I
MAb-ADCC agent	Colorectal cancer	Phase II
MAb-anti-IL-2 receptor	Graft versus host disease	Phase II
MAb-Tc99m	Colorectal cancer	Phase III
MAb-L6	Lung, colon, breast, ovarian cancer	Phase II
MAb-XomaZyme CD5	Graft versus host disease	Application submitted
MAb-anti-CD7	Autoimmune disease	Phase I
MAb-Xomen E5	Gram-negative sepsis	Application submitted
Vaccines		
Hepatitis B	Hepatitis B	Approved 1986
Anti-Leu-3a	HIV infection	Phase II
gp120	HIV infection	Phase I/II
BMY 35047	Melanoma	Phase I
Haemophilus B	Influenza B	Approved 1988

engineered protein therapeutics are summarized in Table 16.1. The variety of products—from hormones and enzymes to receptors, vaccines, and monoclonal antibodies—seeks to treat many diseases thought untreatable just a decade ago. Yet despite this period of phenomenal growth for recombinant DNA–derived therapeutics, the promise of biotechnology, once touted to be limitless, has instead become more realistically defined to include not only the actual recombinant products and the difficulties inherent in their production but also many spinoff technologies, including diagnostics and genetically defined drug discovery tools (20–22).

One particular area of traditional pharmaceutical research in which recombinant DNA technology has made a profound impact has been the engineering of antibiotic-producing organisms (23–25). Always an important source of new bioactive compounds, especially antibiotics (26, 27), fermentation procedures can be directly improved by strain optimization techniques, including genetic recombination and cloning. More exciting is the possibility of producing hybrid antibiotics that combine desirable features of one or more individual compounds for improved potency, bioavailability, or specificity. The art of finding new natural product-based lead compounds by screening fermentation broths, plant sources, and marine organisms by using genetically engineered reagents is becoming of special importance as more of the relevant targets identified by molecular biology operate in obscure or even unknown modes. The structural diversity provided by natural products combined with the ability to test molecular biologically driven biochemical hypotheses has already become an important route for the discovery of new therapeutics (28–30).

3 PROTEIN ENGINEERING AND SITE-DIRECTED MUTAGENESIS

Rapid developments in the technique of site-directed mutagenesis have created the ability to change essentially any amino acid, or even substitute or delete whose domains, in any protein, with the goal of designing and constructing new proteins with novel binding, clearance, or catalytic activities (31, 32). The concomitant changes in protein folding and tertiary structure, protein physiology, binding affinities (for a receptor or hormone), binding specificities (either for substrate or receptor), or catalytic activity (for enzyme active site mutants) are all effects that are measurable against the "wild type" parent, assuming that expression of the gene and subsequent proper folding have successfully occurred. Several surprising observations have been made during the short period that this technology has been available: amino acid substitutions lead, in general, to highly localized changes in protein structure with few global changes in overall folding; substitutions of residues not involved in internal hydrophobic contacts are extremely well accommodated, leading to few unsynthesizable mutants; and proteins seem extremely tolerant of domain substitution, even among unrelated proteins, allowing often even crude first attempts at producing chimeric proteins to be successful. The implications of this technology for the discovery of new pharmaceuticals lie in two areas: second-generation protein therapeutics and site- or domain-specific mutant proteins for structure–function investigations.

Throughout this chapter, amino acids are denoted by their standard one-letter codes; site-specific mutations are represented by the code for the wild type amino acid, the residue number, and the code for the replacement amino acid (31); and the symbol ǂ denotes a proteolytic cleavage site.

3.1 Second-generation Protein Therapeutics

The cloning, expression, and manufacture of proteins as therapeutics involve the same problems encountered in the development and successful clinical approval of any drug. Potency, efficacy, bioavailability, metabolism, and pharmaceutical formulation challenges presented by the natural protein suggest that second-generation products might be engineered to alleviate the particular problem at hand, producing desired therapeutic improvements. The parent proteins to which this technology has been applied extend across the range of recombinant products undergoing clinical evaluation (33).

As an example, for tissue-type plasminogen activator (t-PA), one of the most studied recombinant products (34–36), four properties functioning in concert (i.e., substrate specificity, fibrin affinity, stimulation of t-PA activity by fibrin and fibrinogen, and sensitivity of the enzyme to inhibition by plasminogen activator inhibitors (PAIs)) are responsible for the localization and potentiation of the lytic reaction at a clot surface and are readily analyzed using molecular variants (37). In the absence of crystallographic data, a consensus structure combining the major domains of t-PA has been predicted based on the significant sequence homology with other serum proteins and serine proteases (Fig. 16.1). The complexity of this structure is reflected in

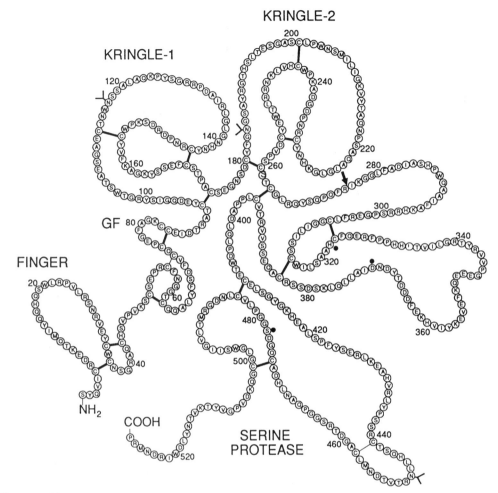

Fig. 16.1 The domain structure of t-PA. Single-letter codes are used to indicate the amino acid residue present in the wild-type protein. ●, active-site residue; Y, glycosylation site; →, "activation" site where hydrolysis causes the one- to two-chain conversion. Reprinted by permission of Annual Reviews, Inc.

its functional multiplicity: efficient production of plasmin by cleavage of the R560–V561 bond of plasminogen, very low binding to plasminogen in the absence of fibrin, moderately high affinity for fibrin, increase in the efficiency of plasminogen activation by 500-fold in the presence of fibrin, rapid inactivation by PAI-1, and rapid hepatic elimination by receptor-mediated endocytosis (38). Point mutations at glycosylation sites (N117Q, N184Q, and N448Q) seemed to confirm the hypothesis that the carbohydrate side chains of t-PA exert

considerable influence on its clearance via the mannose-specific glycoprotein liver receptor. The mutants, which cannot be N-glycosylated, exhibited reduced clearance and prolonged plasma half-life (39). Later studies with multiple mutants have challenged this clearance hypothesis (37–40) and have implicated structural determinants in the EGF-homologous domain instead (41). Prevention of the proteolytic conversion of single- to two-chain t-PA by mutation at the natural cleavage site (R275Q/G-I276) resulted in mutants with significantly increased fibrin binding (42–43) and a dramatic decrease in specific activity (37). The single-chain mutants appear to have the additional advantage of lowered affinity for the PAIs (38). These results are explained by modeling studies that implicate a charge relay system linking the proteolytic cleavage site to the formation of the substrate specificity site. Conservative C- and N-terminal truncations result in little change in specific activity, but the C-terminal truncation yielded a 2-fold increase in stimulation by fibrin. Additional mutagenesis investigations identified a polybasic, charged surface loop consisting of residues 296–302 as the probable site for interaction of t-PA with PAI-1 (44). A number of single-point mutants and one triple-point mutant (K296E/R298E/R299E) within this loop sequence bind ineffectively to PAI-1 (and are thus resistance to its action) (45). BM 06.022, a recombinantly engineered t-PA deletion mutant (t-PA del (V4-E175)), made up of the Kringle 2 and protease domains, has been reported to have the same plaminogenolytic activity but a lower fibrin affinity compared with wild type t-PA (46). Most recently, a new variant of t-PA (T103N, KHRR 296-299 AAAA) was demonstrated to have the combined desirable properties of decreased plasma clearance, increased fibrin specificity, resistance to PAI-1, and in vivo increased potency and decreased systemic activation of plasminogen when administered by bolus dose (47).

Although the systematic changes exemplified by t-PA site-directed mutagenesis studies are the rDNA equivalents of medicinal chemistry (multiple analogue synthesis for structure–activity relationship (SAR) development), more recent applications of this technology bear a less straightforward resemblance to medicinal chemistry–driven drug discovery paradigms. However, these same recombinant techniques can be used to combine artificially domains from different proteins to produce chimeric constructs that incorporate multiple desired properties into a single final product or reagent. For instance, in an effort to overcome the short plasma half-life associated with soluble CD4, the truncated T-cell class II MHC antigen, and HIV-1 gp120 receptor under study as an AIDS therapy, chimeric molecules termed *immunoadhesins* (Fig. 16.2) have been recombinantly constructed from the gp120-specific domains of CD4 and the effector domains of various immunoglobulin classes (48, 49). In addition to dramatically improved pharmacokinetics, these chimeric constructs incorporate functions such as Fc receptor binding, protein A binding, complement fixation, and placental transfer, all of which are imparted by the Fc portion of immunoglobulins. Dimeric constructs from human (CD4-2γ1 and CD4-4γ1) and mouse (CD4-Mγ2a) IgG and a pentameric chimera (CD4-Mμ) from mouse IgM exhibit evidence of retained gp120 binding and anti-HIV infectivity activity. Both CD4-2γ1 and CD4-4γ1 show significantly increased plasma half-lives of 6.7 and 48 h, respectively, compared with 0.25 h for rCD4. Furthermore, the immunoadhesin CD4-2γ1 (CD4-IgG) mediates antibody-dependent–cell-mediated cytotoxicity (ADCC) toward HIV-infected cells and is efficiently transferred across the placenta of primates (50). The practical utility of receptor-IgG chimeric constructs has also been extended to chemical and natural products screening, where they serve as easily detectable biochemical reagents for binding assays.

3.2 Epitope Mapping

Site-directed mutagenesis technology has also been applied to one of the most perplexing problems in structural biochemistry: the nature of the protein–protein interaction. While numerous examples of models of enzyme–ligand complexes have

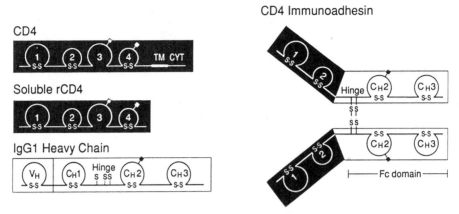

Fig. 16.2 Structure of CD4 immunoadhesin, soluble rCD4, and the parent human CD4 and IgG1 heavy-chain molecules. CD4- and IgG1-derived sequences are indicated by shaded and unshaded regions, respectively. The immunoglobulin-like domains of CD4 are numbered 1 to 4, *TM* is the transmembrane domain, and *CYT* is the cytoplasmic domain. Soluble CD4 is truncated after P368 of the mature CD4 polypeptide. The variable (V_H) and constant (C_H1, Hinge, C_H2, and C_H3) regions of IgG1 heavy chains are shown. Disulfide bonds are indicated by S-S. CD4 immunoadhesin consists of residues 1 to 180 of the mature CD4 protein fused to IgG1 sequences, beginning at D216, which is the first residue in the IgG1 hinge after the cysteine residue involved in heavy–light chain bonding. The CD4 immunoadhesin shown, which lacks a C_H1 domain, was derived from a C_H1-containing CD4 immunoadhesin by oligonucleotide-directed deletional mutagenesis, expressed in Chinese hamster ovary cells cells and purified to >99% purity using protein A-sepharose chromatography (50). Reprinted by permission of Macmillan Magazines Ltd.

been developed based on active-site modifications, this method is only now being extended to the formidable problem of defining the essential elements of a protein–protein (e.g., a protein substrate to a protease or a hormone to its receptor) binding epitope.

An impressive example of a systematic search for a binding epitope is the recent work used to define the human growth hormone–somatogenic receptor interaction (51, 52). First, using a technique termed homologue-scanning mutagenesis, segments of sequences (7 to 30 amino acids in length) from homologous proteins known not to bind to the hGH receptor or to hGH-sensitive monoclonal antibodies (Mab) were systematically substituted throughout the hGH structure, using a working model based on the three-dimensional folding pattern found by crystallographic analysis of the highly homologous porcine growth hormone (53). Using an ELISA-based

binding assay, which measures the affinity of the mutant hGH for its recombinantly derived receptor (54), swap mutations that disrupted binding were found to map within close proximity on the three-dimensional model, even though the residues changed within each subset were usually distant in the primary sequence. By this analysis, three discontinuous polypeptide determinants (the loop between residues 54 and 74, the central portion of helix 4 to the C-terminus, and to a lesser extent, the amino-terminal region of helix 1) were identified as being important for binding to the receptor.

A second technique, termed alanine-scanning mutagenesis, was then applied. Single alanine mutations (62 in total) were introduced at every residue within the regions implicated in receptor recognition. The alanine scan revealed a cluster of a dozen large side chains that, when mutated to alanine, exhibited more than a 4-fold decrease in binding affinity. Many of the residues that constitute the hGH binding epitope for its receptor are altered in close homologues, such as placental lactogen and the prolactins. The overall correct folding of the mutant proteins was determined by cross-reactivity with a single set of conformationally sensitive Mab reagents. Using the receptor-binding determinants identified in these studies, a variant of human prolactin (hPRL) was engineered, containing eight mutations with an association constant for the hGH receptor that was increased by more than 10,000-fold (55).

Finally, biophysical studies, including calorimetry, size-exclusion chromatography, a novel fluorescence quenching binding assay (56), and X-ray crystallography (57), revealed the presence of two overlapping binding epitopes (Fig. 16.3) on growth hormone, by which it actually dimerizes two membrane-bound receptors to induce its effect. The crystal structure confirmed both the 1:2 hormone-to-receptor complex structure and the interface residues identified by the scanning mutagenesis mapping technique. These results indicate that the homologue and alanine-scanning mutagenesis techniques should be generally useful starting points in helping to identify amino acid residues important to any protein–protein interaction (58) and that these techniques have serious potential to provide essential information for rational drug design.

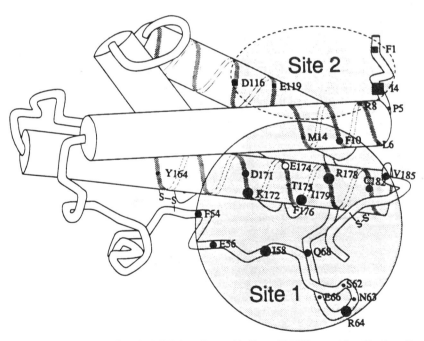

Fig. 16.3 Map of alanine substitutions in hGH that disrupt binding of hGHbp at either Site 1 or Site 2. The two sites are generally delineated by the large shaded circles. Residues for which analine mutations reduce Site 2 binding are shown: ▪, 2- to 4-fold; ▪, 4- to 10-fold; ▪, 10- to 50-fold; and ▪, >50-fold. Sites where analine mutations in Site 1 cause changes in binding affinity for the hGHbp, using an immunoprecipitation assay, are shown: •, 2- to 4-fold reduction; •, 4- to 10-fold reduction; ●, >10-fold reduction; and ●, 4-fold increase. Reprinted from Ref. 56 with permission of The American Association for the Advancement of Science.

3.3 Future Directions

In an intriguing example of what might be termed *reverse* small molecule design, randomized mutagenesis techniques also have been directly applied to the ever-growing problem of antibiotic resistance. Bacterial resistance to increasingly complex antibiotics has become widespread, severely limiting the useful therapeutic lifetime of most marketed antimicrobial agents (59). Using a mutagenesis technique that randomizes the DNA sequence of a short stretch (3 to 6 codons) of a gene, followed by determination of the percentage of functional mutants expressed from the randomized gene, localization of the regions of the protein critical to either structure or function can be accomplished. Application of this technique to TEM-1 β-lactamase (the enzyme responsible for bacterial resistance to β-lactam antibiotics such as penicillins and cephalosporins) over a 66-codon stretch revealed that the enzyme is extremely tolerant of amino acid substitutions: 44% of all mutants function at some level, and

20% function at the level of the wild type enzyme (60). The regions identified as most sensitive to substitution are located either in the active site or in buried positions that likely contribute to the core structure of the protein (Fig. 16.4). Such a library of functional mutant β-lactamases could, in theory, be used to simulate multiple next generations of natural mutations, but at an accelerated pace. Screening of new synthetic β-lactams against such a mutant library might then be used to discover compounds with the potential for increased useful therapeutic lifetimes.

The art of rDNA site-directed mutagenesis, although advancing rapidly, is still limited to the repertoire of the 20 natural amino acids encoded by DNA. To effect more subtle changes in proteins, such as increased or decreased acidity, nucleophilicity, or hydrogen-bonding characteristics, without dramatically altering the size of the residue and without affecting the overall tertiary structure, it has been proposed that site-directed mutagenesis using unnatural amino acids might offer the

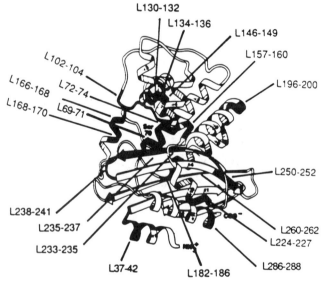

Fig. 16.4 Position of random libraries on a ribbon diagram of the homologous *S. aureus* β-lactamase. Dark regions correspond to the position of random libraries. Lines point to the position of individual libraries. Reprinted by permission from Ref. 60.

needed advantages. In the past, such changes were accomplished semisynthetically on chemically reactive residues such as Cys. However, methodology for carrying out such mutations recombinantly has been successfully used. There are four requirements: (*1*) generation of an amber (TAG) "blank" codon in the gene of interest at the position of the desired mutation, (*2*) identification of a suppressor tRNA that can efficiently translate the amber message but that is not a substrate for any endogenous aminoacyl-tRNA synthetases, (*3*) development of a method for the efficient acylation of the $tRNA_{CUA}$ with novel amino acids, and (*4*) availability of a suitable *in vitro* protein synthesis system to which a plasmid bearing the mutant gene or corresponding mRNA and the acylated $tRNA_{CUA}$ can be added. The first successful demonstration of this methodology involved replacement of F66 with three phenylalanine analogues in RTEM β-lactamase and subsequent determination of the kinetic constants k_{cat} and K_m of the mutants (61). Subsequent applications have centered on the critical issue of the introduction of unnatural amino acid replacements into proteins. The artificial residues can probe effects on stability and folding governed by subtle changes in hydrophobicity and residue side chain packing to a degree not possible using the 20 natural amino acids (62, 63).

4 GENETICALLY ENGINEERED DRUG DISCOVERY TOOLS

4.1 Reagents for Screening

An increasingly important application of recombinant technology lies not in new protein drug product discovery per se but in the ability to provide cloned and expressed proteins as reagents for medicinal chemistry investigations. The common practice of *in vitro* screening for enzyme activity or receptor binding using animal

tissue homogenates (nonhuman, and therefore nontarget) has begun to give way to the use of solid-phase or whole-cell binding assays based on recombinantly produced and isolated or cell-surface expressed reagent quantities of the relevant target protein (64, 65).

The ability to carry out large-scale, high flux screening of chemical, natural products, and recombinantly or synthetically derived diversity libraries (26–29, 66–80) also critically depends on reagent availability and consistency. The inherent differences in these potential sources of drug design information, especially from large combinatorially generated libraries (Table 16.2) requires that assay variations be reduced to the absolute minimum to ensure the ability to analyze data consistently from possibly millions of assay points.

The discovery of the HIV Tat inhibitor Ro 5-3335 (**7**), and its eventual development as the analogue Ro 24-7429 (**8**) are recent successes from screening chemical libraries using recombinant reagents. Tat is a strong positive regulator of HIV expression directed by the HIV-1 long terminal repeat (LTR) and as such constitutes an important and unique target for HIV regulation, because the *tat trans*-activator protein (one of the HIV-1 gene products) has been clearly demonstrated to regulate expression of the complete genome (81). Assays to detect inhibitors of *tat* function by screening (82, 83) presented immediate opportunities to control a key step in the HIV-1 viral replication process. In this instance, to screen for Tat inhibitors, two plasmids were cotransfected into COS cells: a gene for either Tat or the reporter gene for secreted alkaline phosphatase (SeAP) was put under the control of the HIV-1 LTR promoter (84). Because Tat is necessary for HIV expression and SeAP expression is under the control of the HIV LTR, an inhibitor of Tat would necessarily lower the apparent alkaline phosphatase activity. This assay was standardized and used in

Table 16.2   Sources of Chemical and Structural Diversity in Screening

Library	References
Natural products	29
microbial secondary metabolites	26–29
plant extracts	67
marine natural products	68
Chemical and pharmaceutical libraries	
Solid-supported peptides	
on pins	69
on silicon chips	70
on beads	71
on bacteriophage	72
Peptides in solution	73
Peptoid peptidomimetics	74
Antibody diversity	75, 76
PCR-amplified libraries	
DNA	77
RNA	78, 79
Tagged chemical diversity	80

high flux screening to identify structure (**7**), which was then subjected to medicinal chemistry optimization to produce structure (**8**) as the ultimate clinical candidate (85). Such rapid lead discovery highlights the continued importance of highly directed screening to drug discovery, now better enabled by use of recombinant reagents and techniques.

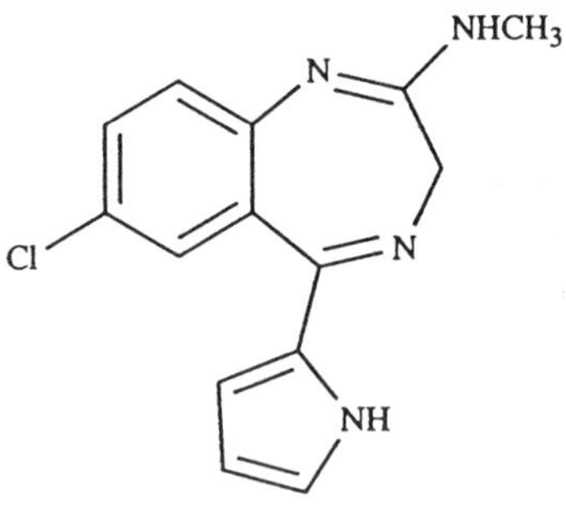

Even more to the point of human pharmaceutical discovery and design, however,

(**8**)

(**7**)

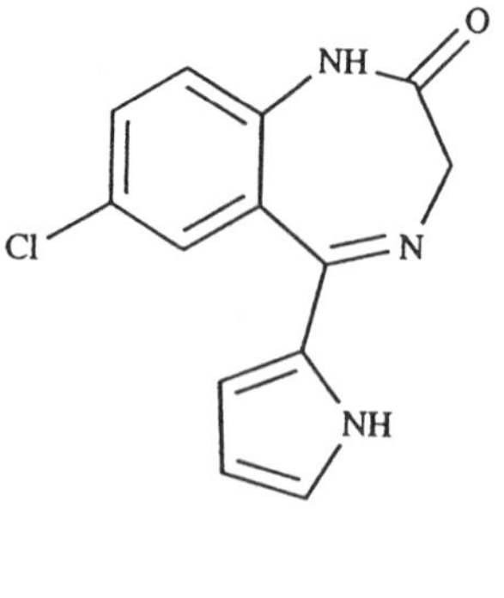

is the issue of species and/or tissue specificities. Sometimes the differences between tissue isolates and recombinant reagent are small; more frequently, however, the sequence homologies and even functional characteristics can vary greatly, providing a distinct advantage in favor of the recombinant protein. When the possibility of achieving subtype specificity, because of either tissue distribution or differential gene expression, pinpoints a particular isoenzyme as a target for selective drug action, it is of obvious importance to be able to test for the desired specificity. The recently developed technique called polymerase chain reaction (PCR), an enzymatic method for the *in vitro* amplification of specific DNA fragments, has revolutionized the search for receptor and enzyme subspecies, making whole families of target proteins available for comparative studies (86). Classic cloning requires knowledge of at least a partial sequence for low stringency screening. This method is unlikely to detect cDNAs corresponding to genes expressed at low levels in the tissue from which the library was constructed. In contrast, the PCR technique can uncover and amplify sequences present in low copy number in the mRNA and offers a greater likelihood of obtaining useful, full-length clones. The selective amplification afforded by PCR can also be used to identify subspecies present

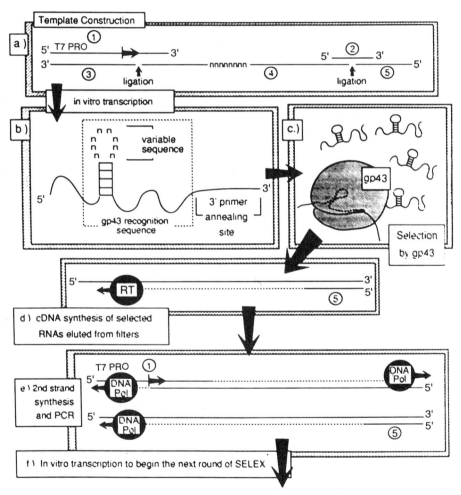

Fig. 16.5 The SELEX experiment. (*a*) Synthetic oligonucleotides ① to ⑤ hybridize as shown and are ligated. (*b*) The 110-base template was purified, annealed, and subjected to *in vitro* transcription. (*c*) The RNA transcripts were gel purified and subjected to selection by gp43 (or the target protein of choice). (*d*) cDNA copies of the RNA were made by RMV reverse transcriptase. (*e*) The cDNAs were amplified using *Taq* DNA polymerase chain extension. (*f*) The resulting double-stranded DNA products of amplification were transcribed *in vitro* and recycled into step c, (79). Reprinted by permission of The American Association for the Advancement of Science.

in tissue in especially short supply, offering yet another advantage over classic methods.

PCR has also been applied to the generation of recombinant diversity libraries of DNA (77), RNA (78, 81), and novel chemical diversity "tagged" for detection and amplification (80). In the systematic evolution of ligands by exponential enrichment (SELEX) procedure (Fig. 16.5), RNA generated by transcription from oligonucleotides with a randomized insert is sorted by binding to the target of choice. The bound RNA is eluted and treated with reverse transcriptase to generate the corresponding cDNA, which is then subjected to PCR using DNA polymerase to produce full-length double-stranded DNA. *In vitro* transcription of this amplified DNA pool yields a new, enriched pool of RNA for the next round of binding selection (78). SELEX and similar PCR-amplified procedures can generate literally millions of potential ligands, structurally diverse yet readily sortable, for receptors or enzymes.

4.2 Reagents for Structural Biology Studies

In combination with molecular genetics, structural biology also has used physical techniques—nuclear magnetic resonance (NMR) spectroscopy and X-ray crystallography—to its advantage in the study of proteins as drug targets, models for new drugs, and discovery tools (87). These two techniques can be used independently, or in concert, to determine the complete three-dimensional structure of proteins. Recent advances in NMR techniques, especially multidimensional heteronuclear studies, offer dramatic improvements in spectral resolution and interpretation (88, 89). Identification of differences in the results from comparative studies on the same protein can reveal important structural or dynamic information (90), possibly rele-

vant to the design of synthetic ligands or inhibitors. Inclusion of such structural biology results into the more traditional synthesis-driven discovery paradigm has become a recognized and important component of drug design in the 1990s (91).

The variety of studies undertaken using these structural biology techniques spans the range of proteins of interest, from enzymes and hormones to receptors and antibodies. Recombinantly produced reagents (accessible as either purified, soluble proteins or cell-surface expressed, functional enzymes and receptors) with potential application to drug discovery fall into a number of general categories: enzymes (with catalytic function), receptors (with signal transduction function), and binding proteins (with cellular adhesion properties). Rather than exhaustively catalog further examples, the next sections will highlight instances in which combinations of directed specific assays and structural biology studies have aided in nonprotein drug discovery.

4.3 Enzymes as Drug Targets

A large number of enzymes have been cloned and expressed in useful quantities for biochemical characterization. The advent of rational drug design paradigms, in particular the methodology surrounding mechanism-based enzyme inhibition (92) and the market success of various enzyme inhibitors such as captopril (**6**) and lovastatin (**8**), have made enzymes of all types more reasonable and accessible targets for medicinal chemistry efforts. Many enzymes either linked to pathologies or known to regulate important biochemical pathways have been extensively cloned for subspecies differentiation and/or access to human isotypes. Pioneering work by Ullrich on protein kinase C (93) set the pace for the continuing investigations into that family, which now includes the protein kinase C subtypes α, β_I, β_{II}, γ, δ, and ε and, more recently, ζ, nPKC-ε, and λ (94). Similar important advances have been made in the molecular biology of other classes of potential medicinal chemistry target enzymes, such as the phosphodiesterase (95) and the phospholipase A_2 (96, 97) families.

The rational basis of enzyme-inhibitor interactions, especially to predict or explain specificity, is among the most intensely active areas of structural biology. One of the most studied therapeutic targets is dihydrofolate reductase (DHFR), an enzyme essential for growth and replication at the cellular level. Inhibitors of DHFR, most notably the antifolates methotrexate (MTX) and trimethoprim (TMP) are used extensively in the treatment of neoplastic and infectious disorders. Some of the observed species selectivities for these inhibitors have been explained in terms of distinctive structural differences at the binding sites of the chicken and *E. coli* enzymes (98, 99), but some of the conclusions made based on the enzyme-inhibitor binding interaction have been challenged by a crystal structure of human recombinant DHFR complexed with folate, the natural substrate (100). Comparisons of the conformations of the conserved human and mouse DHFR side chains revealed differences in packing, most noticeably the orientation of F31. Site-directed mutagenesis studies confirmed the importance of

this observation. The mutant F31L (human F to *E. coli* L mutation) gave equivalent K_i values for inhibition by TMP, but gave a 10-fold increase in K_m for dihydrofolate (101). Similar results were found for the F31S mutant, for which there was also a 10-fold increase in K_m for dihydrofolate and a 100-fold increase in K_d for MTX. The F34S mutant, however, showed greater differences: a 3-fold reduction in K_m for NADPH, a 24-fold increase in K_m for dihydrofolate, a 3-fold reduction in k_{cat}, and an 80,000-fold increase in K_d for MTX, suggesting that phenylalanines 31 and 34 make different contributions to ligand binding and catalysis in human DHFR (102). These results helped to pinpoint major differences among DHFRs of various species and thus suggest ways to design new and more species-specific inhibitors that would preferentially target pathogen versus host DHFR. Such compounds would be expected to be more potent chemotherapeutics, exhibiting less toxicity in humans. The recent design and refinement of inhibitors of *E. coli* thymidilate synthetase such as structure (**9**) attests to the viability and potential cost-effectiveness of this rational design approach (103).

In contrast to the DHFR investigations for which the goal is refinement, problems in *de novo* design of inhibitors require more fundamental help, specifically the availability of the target enzyme in quantity

(9)

(10)

for screening. The ability of rDNA technology to expedite access to quantities of a specific enzyme in a situation in which some indication of specificity would eventually be required of the final inhibitor is no where more evident than in the case of the retroviral aspartic HIV-1 protease (HIV-1 PR) (104). From among the multitude of potential points of intervention into viral replication of the HIV-1 genome, this enzyme was identified as a viable target for anti-AIDS drugs because mutation of the active site aspartic acid (D25) effectively prevents processing of retroviral polyprotein, producing immature, noninfective virions. In addition to the residues DTG at positions 25 to 27, mutations within the sequence GRD/N (positions 86 to 88 in HIV-1 PR)—a highly conserved domain in the retroviral proteases but not present in cellular aspartic proteases—were found to be completely devoid of proteolytic activity, potentially pinpointing a site critical for design of specific inhibitors capable of recognizing the viral, but not the host, proteases.

The search for important tertiary structural differences between HIV-1 PR and known eukaryotic proteases began by determination of the X-ray crystal structure (Fig. 16.6) of recombinantly expressed material at 3 Å resolution (105). Subsequent crystallographic studies on both synthetic (at 2.8 Å) and recombinantly expressed (at 2.7 Å) material helped locate side chains

and resolved some ambiguities in the dimer interface region (106, 107). From this information, a model of the substrate binding site was proposed (108). Far more useful for inhibitor design purposes, complexes of four structurally distinct inhibitors bound to HIV-1 PR were solved (109–112), from which a generalized closest contact map (Fig. 16.7) was developed (104).

With the functional role and tertiary structure of the protease determined, additional studies with both recombinant and synthetic material have yielded automated robotics assays for screening of chemical libraries, fermentation broths, and designed inhibitors using HIV-1 PR cleavage of synthetic pseudosubstrates. Peptide sequences derived from specific retroviral polyprotein substrates and inhibition by pepstatin and other renin inhibitors identified $(S/T)P_3P_2(Y/F)P$ as a consensus cleavage site for HIV-1 PR. One such inhibitor, SGN(FΨ[CH$_2$N]P)IVQ has been used as an affinity reagent for large-scale purification of recombinant HIV-1 PR (113), while Ac-TI(nLΨ[CH$_2$NH]-nL)QR-NH$_2$ was used in the cocrystallization studies mentioned above. From among the large numbers of peptides identified as HIV-1 PR inhibitors, only a limited number have been shown to inhibit effectively viral proteolytic processing and syncytia formation in chronically infected T-cell cultures (114, 115). The most advanced peptidomimetic compound is structure (**10**),

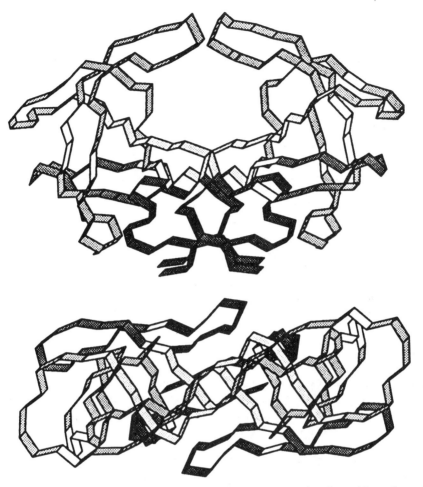

Fig. 16.6 The structure of native HIV-1 protease drawn as a ribbon connecting the positions of α-carbons. The upper structure, in which the pseudo-twofold axis relating one monomer to the other is vertical and in the plane of the page, represents a view along the substrate binding cleft. The lower structure is a top view, with the pseudo-twofold axis perpendicular to the page (104). Reprinted by permission of The American Chemical Society.

which both inhibits HIV-1 PR and exhibits effective and noncytotoxic antiviral activity in chronically infected cells at nanomolar concentrations (116). However, as with other peptidomimetic structures such as inhibitors of another aspartyl protease, renin (117), their transformation into potential drugs will require additional synthetic work. The short interval from identification of the enzyme as a target from among the possibilities presented by the HIV-1 genome to accessing material for

assay and structural purposes has obviously hastened the determination of the viability of HIV-1 PR inhibitors as AIDS therapeutics and also has provided an excellent example of structurally driven rational drug design.

The search for a common mechanism of action of the immunosuppressive drugs cyclosporin (CsA) (**11**) and FK-506 (**12**) highlights another possibility, in which the drug was discovered by screening in cellular or *in vivo* models, but the exact mechanism

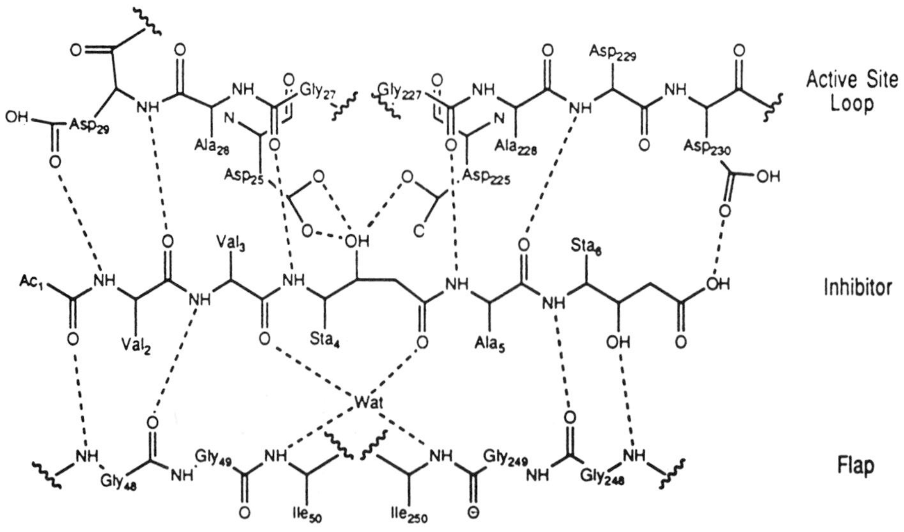

Fig. 16.7 Hydrogen bonds between a prototypical aspartic protease inhibitor (acetyl pepstatin) and HIV-1 protease. The residues are labeled at the C-β position (C-α for glycine). The residues labeled 25 to 50 are from monomer A, those labeled 225 to 250 are from monomer B, and those labeled 1 to 6 are with acetyl pepstatin (104). Reprinted by permission of The American Chemical Society.

or site of action is unknown (118). Using the active molecules, certainly structurally dissimilar but just as certainly related in their effects, two distinct proteins— cyclophilin (CyP) and the FK binding protein (FKBP)—were identified as the specific receptors for cyclosporin and FK-506, respectively. First for CyP (119, 120), then for FKBP (121, 122), these binding proteins were discovered to be distinct and

inhibitor-specific cis-trans peptidyl-prolyl isomerases that, as their name implies, catalyze the slow cis-trans isomerization of proline peptide bonds in oligopeptides and accelerate slow, rate-limiting steps in the folding of some proteins. The biochemical mechanism of inhibition was first proposed to involve a specific covalent adduct between inhibitor and its rotamase (120), but the hypothesis was soon challenged by

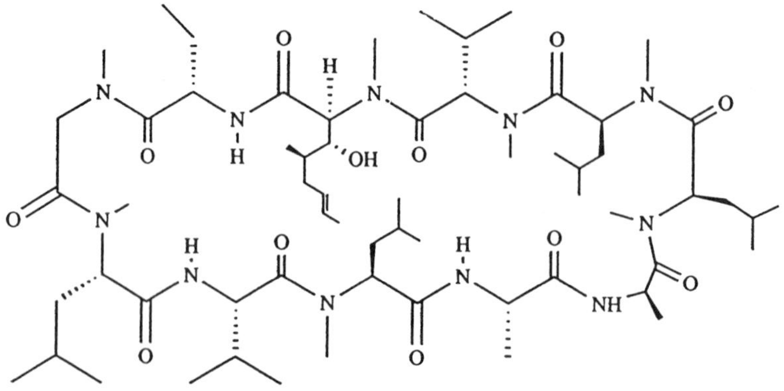

(11)

(12)

evidence that showed that the binding interactions are peptide-sequence specific (123) for both proteins. Using recombinant CyP as standard, four cysteine-to-alanine mutants (C52A, C62A, C115A, and C161A) were shown to retain full affinity for CsA and equivalent rotamase catalytic activity, indicating the cysteines play no essential role in binding or catalysis (124). In the case of FKBP, NMR studies of [8, 9-^{13}C]FK-506 bound to recombinant FKBP, the likely mechanism of inhibition also is noncovalent, suggesting that the α-ketoamide of FK-506 serves as an effective surrogate for the twisted amide of a bound peptide substrate (125). Numerous further NMR, x-ray crystallographic, and computational modeling studies have been carried out on both CsA/CyP and FK-506/FKBP complexes to attempt to discover a structural basis for activity (126, 127).

The exact signal transduction mechanism that triggers the immunosuppressive response in T-cells, however, remained unknown until an elegant set of experiments identified calcineurin, a calcium- and calmodulin-dependent serine/threonine phosphatase, and a complex of calcineurin with calmodulin as the binding targets of the immunophilin-drug complexes (128). The immunosuppressant, displayed by the immunophilin protein, then effectively functions as the critical element that binds the pentapartite complex together, causing inhibition of the phosphatase (Fig. 16.8). The complex seems also to exert two subsequent effects: halting DNA translation in T-lymphocyte nuclei and inhibition of IgE-induced mast cell degranulation. These *in vitro* observations must necessarily be confirmed by further *in vivo* work, but the elucidation of these molecular-level mechanisms will allow the development of more highly tailored and potent immunosuppressive agents (129).

4.4 Receptors as Drug Targets

Even more so than with enzymes, molecular genetics has been primarily responsible for the identification of functional receptor subtypes. Success in the case of cimetidine (**3**), a selective H$_2$-receptor antagonist,

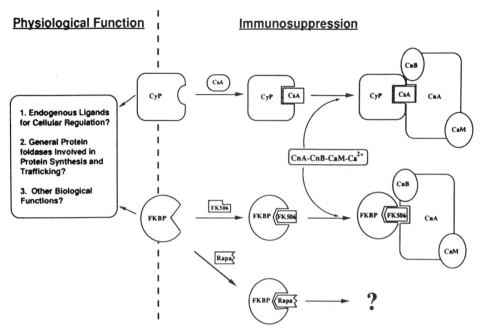

Fig. 16.8 Schematic representation of immunosupressant–immunophilin complex interactions. CyPs bind CsA to form a complex in which both components change in structure. This complex binds to, and inhibits, calcineurin (*CnA*, A subunit; *CnB*, B subunit; *CaM*, Calmodulin) in a calcium-dependent manner. FK506-binding protein complexes with FK506 or rapamycin (*Rapa*). FKBP–FK506 also binds calcineurin. The target of FKBP–rapamycin is unknown but is presumed to be different from calcineurin (129). Reprinted by permission of Cell Press.

made it clear that the design of specific ligands for at least some receptors is a task amenable to medicinal chemistry. The classic tissue-binding pharmacological methods that made distinctions on the basis of ligand selectivity have been supplemented, and in most cases supplanted, by further subtyping made possible by cross-hybridization cloning, using the known receptor genes. Any studies that profile the *in vitro* receptor subtype-specificity of compounds can theoretically help identify potential *in vivo* side effects of the compounds, if the association of subtype to effect is known or suspected. At this point, just the indication of a more specific profile with fewer side effects is enough to help choose one compound over another for preclinical development.

One of the earliest examples of the role of molecular biology in discerning receptor subtype roles was the case of the muscarinic cholinergic receptors (MAChRs).

The two subtypes M_1 and M_2 had been defined pharmacologically by their affinity, or lack thereof, for pirenzepine and were later confirmed by molecular cloning to be distinct gene products *m1* and *m2*, respectively (130–132). Three additional muscarinic receptor genes (*m3* to *m5*) were subsequently isolated (133–135). From this work, a subtype-specific heterologous stable expression system in Chinese hamster ovary (CHO) cells suitable for screening potential subtype-specific ligands was developed. From this assay, pirenzepine, previously thought to bind to *m1* only, was found to have only a 50-fold reduced affinity for *m2*, and an almost equivalent (to *m1*) binding affinity for *m3* and *m4*, suggesting that studies using pirenzepine on tissue homogenate have failed to distinguish adequately among the subtypes (136).

Similar breakthroughs have been realized across the rest of the family of signal transduction G protein–coupled receptors (137, 138), because in addition to the muscarinics, the primary structures of the adrenergic (α_1, α_2, β_1, and β_2), serotonergic, tachykinin, and rhodopsin receptors have been determined (139–141). All of these display the now-familiar homology pattern of seven membrane-spanning domains packed into antiparallel helical bundles (Fig. 16.9). The exceedingly high homology among the large family of G protein–cou-

pled receptors also has allowed the development of three-dimensional models of the proteins to aid in drug refinement (142). For example, mutagenesis studies on the β_2-adrenergic receptor have localized the intracellular domains involved in (*1*) the coupling of the receptor to G proteins (143); (*2*) homologous desensitization by β-adrenergic receptor kinase (β-ARK) (144), itself cloned and a possible target for down-regulation inhibitors (145); (*3*) heterologous desensitization by cAMP-de-

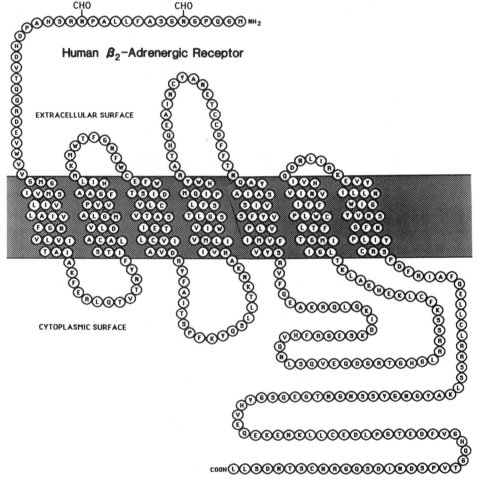

Fig. 16.9 Topographical representation of primary sequence of human β_2-adrenergic receptor, a typical G protein–coupled receptor. The receptor protein is illustrated as possessing seven hydrophobic regions each capable of spanning the plasma membrane, thus creating intracellular and extracellular loops as well as an extracellular amino terminus and a cytoplasmic carboxyl terminal region (141). Reprinted by permission of Pergamon Press plc.

pendent protein kinase (146); and (4) an extracellular domain with conserved cysteine residues implicated in agonist ligand binding (147). A chimeric muscarinic cholinergic: β-adrenergic receptor engineered to activate adenylyl cyclase (a second messenger system not coupled to MAChR agonism) also has helped identify which intracellular loops may be involved in direct G protein interactions (148). The diverse signal transduction functional roles of the many G proteins to which these receptors are coupled (Fig. 16.10) makes them viable drug targets too (149).

The complicated biochemical pharmacology of natriuretic peptides, the regulatory system that acts to balance the renin–angiotensin–aldosterone system (150), has been significantly clarified by the cloning of three receptor subtypes, which revealed the functional characteristics of a new paradigm for second messenger signal transduction via guanylate cyclase (Fig. 16.11). The α-atrial natriuretic peptide (α-ANP) receptor (NPA-R) and the brain natriuretic peptide (BNP) receptor (NPB-R) contain both protein kinase and guanylate cyclase (GC) domains, as determined by both sequence homologies and catalytic activities, while the clearance receptor (ANP-C) completely lacks the necessary intracellular domains for signal

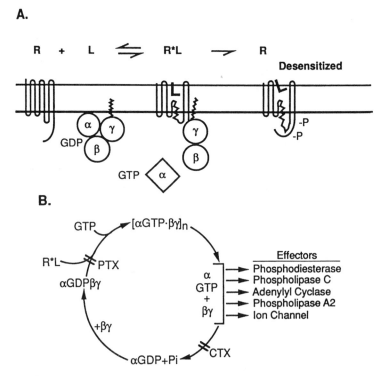

Fig. 16.10 Receptor G protein–mediated signal transduction. A: Receptor (R) associates with a specific ligand (L), stabilizing an activated form of the receptor (R*), which can catalyze the exchange of GTP for GDP bound to the α-subunit of a specific G protein. The βγ-heterodimer may remain associated with the membrane through a 20-carbon isoprenyl modification of the γ-subunit. The receptor is desensitized by specific phosphorylation (−P). B: The G protein cycle. Pertussis toxin (PTX) blocks the catalysis of GTP exchange by the receptor. Activated α-subunits (αGTP) and βγ-heterodimers can interact with different effectors (E). Cholera toxin (CTX) blocks the GTPase activity of some α-subunits, fixing them in an activated form (149). Reprinted by permission of The American Association for the Advancement of Science.

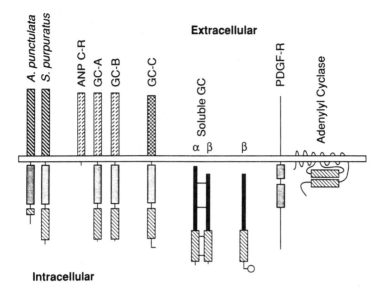

Fig. 16.11 Comparison of various proteins that contain domains homologous to guanylyl cyclase. Homologous domains of two sea urchin guanylyl cyclases (*Arbacia punctulata* and *Strongylocentrotus purpuratus*), the ANPC receptor (ANPC-R), GC-A, GC-B, GC-C, soluble α-subunit, soluble β-subunit, β-like subunit, PDGF receptor, and bovine brain adenylyl cyclase are shaded the same (151). Reprinted by permission of Elsevier Science Publishers, Ltd.

transduction via the guanylate cyclase pathway (151). This system defines the first example of a cell surface receptor that enzymatically synthesizes a diffusible second messenger system in response to hormonal stimulation (152) (Fig. 16.12). Using C-ANP$_{4-23}$, there is now evidence to indicate that the so-called clearance receptor (NPC-R) may be coupled to the adenylate cyclase/cAMP signal transduction system through an inhibitory guanine nucleotide regulatory protein (153). Because the NPs have differential, but not absolute, affinities for their corresponding receptors (154) and because both agonism (155) and antagonism (156) of the GC activity have been demonstrated *in vitro* using ANP analogs, it may be possible to discriminate among the receptor GCs to obtain more subtle structure–activity information for the design of selective NP analogs. Homology between the NP receptors and another guanylate cyclase firmly identified the latter as the elusive heat-stable enterotoxin re-

ceptor St(a)-R (157), which aided in the identification of both the biochemically isolated guanylin (158) and the cloned proguanylin (159) versions of the endogenous natural ligand. This system is presumed to play a role in water retention through cGMP modulation of the CFTR chloride ion channel (160).

The number of receptors of biological significance cloned and expressed for further study continues to grow at an exponential rate (161). These include epidermal growth factor (EGFR); insulin (INSR); insulin-like growth factor-1 (IGF-1R); platelet-derived growth factor (PDGFR) receptors and related tyrosine kinases (162); tumor necrosis factor receptors 1 and 2 (163); subtypes of the GABA$_A$-benzodiazepine receptor complex (164–167); human γ-interferon receptor (168); inositol 1,4,5-triphosphate (IP$_3$)-binding protein P$_{400}$ (169); kainate-subtype glutamate receptor (170); follicle-stimulating hormone receptor (171); multiple mem-

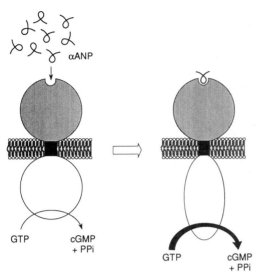

Fig. 16.12 Model for ANP-A and ANP-B receptor function. The unoccupied ANP-A receptor is shown on the left with a basal rate of cGMP synthesis (indicated by a thin arrow). The effect of ligand binding to the amino-terminal extracellular domain is shown on the right. Proposed allosteric modulation of guanylate cyclase by α-ANP is schematically illustrated by a change in shape of the intracellular domain and a thicker arrow to denote an increase in guanylate cyclase–specific activity with greater production of the second messenger cGMP (152). Reprinted permission of Oxford University Press.

bers of the steroid (ER, PR, AR, GR, MR), thyroid hormone (TRα and β), and retinoid (RARα, β and γ, and RXRα) receptor superfamily of nuclear transcriptional factors (172–175); multiple members of the interleukin cytokine receptor family (176); and subtypes of the glutamate (177) and adenosine (178) receptor families. The importance of access to human cloned receptors continues to be underscored, as receptor binding plays an increasingly critical role in modern drug discovery (179).

To make the case for using cloned human receptors for drug discovery even stronger, dramatic evidence that minor amino acid sequence variations inherent in species variability can produce profoundly

different pharmacological effects was recently provided in two instances. In the comparison of rodent versus human analogues of the 5-hydroxytryptamine receptor subtype 5-HT$_{1B}$, the natural receptors were found to bind 5-HT identically, but they differ profoundly in their affinities for many serotonergic drugs (Table 16.3). These striking differences could be reversed by change of a single transmembrane domain residue (T355N), which effectively rendered the two receptors pharmacologically identical (180). A similar study comparing human to chicken and hamster progesterone receptors showed that the steroidal abortifacient RU486 (**13**) shows antagonist activity in humans but not in the two other species, because of the presence of a glycine at position 575. Both the chicken and hamster receptors have a cysteine at this position, and replacement by glycine (C575G) generated a mutant receptor which could bind RU486. Likewise, mutation of the human receptor (G575C) abrogated RU486 binding (181). These and many similar findings emphasize the critical importance of the availability of human clones proteins as potential targets for drug action and as sources of structural information in the discovery of potent and selective therapeutic agents.

(13)

Table 16.3   Comparative Ligand-Binding Properties of Wild-Type and T355N Mutant Human 5-HT$_{1B}$ Receptors Compared with Rodent Receptors

Ligand	K_i(nM)			
	Human (wild type)	Human (T355N)	Rat[14] (5-HT$_{1B}$)	Mouse[15] (5-HT$_{1B}$)
Serotonergic				
5-HT	10 ± 1	8 ± 1	16 ± 1	39
5-CT	4 ± 1	3 ± 1	7 ± 1	10
DHE	6 ± 1	2 ± 1	4 ± 2	NA
RU24969	44 ± 4	2 ± 1	2 ± 1	10
Metergoline	25 ± 3	200 ± 40	129 ± 33	NA
Sumatriptan	38 ± 3	560 ± 100	465 ± 85	NA
Methysergide	130 ± 7	970 ± 130	$1,823 \pm 297$	NA
8-OH-DPAT	$1,600 \pm 100$	$25,000 \pm 1,000$	$>10,000$	30,000
Methiothepin	12 ± 1	38 ± 8	13 ± 4	NA
β-Adrenergic				
(−)Propranolol	$8,100 \pm 400$	17 ± 1	57 ± 4	NA
(−)Pindolol	$11,000 \pm 1,000$	20 ± 3	153 ± 62	69
(−)Alprenolol	$11,000 \pm 800$	13 ± 1	NA	NA

4.5 Cellular Adhesion Proteins

The understanding of the molecular processes that govern cell localization in various pathological conditions has been significantly expanded because of the cloning and expression of some of the major cellular adhesion proteins, especially in the integrin family (Table 16.4), a highly related and widely expressed group of $\alpha\beta$-heterodimeric membrane proteins (182). The interaction in the antigen–receptor cross-linking adhesion of T-cells mediated by the intercellular adhesion molecule (ICAM-1) and the lymphocyte function-associated molecule (LFA-1) was clarified by the cloning and expression of ICAM-1, the major cell surface receptor for rhinovirus (183). A soluble form of human ICAM-1 effectively inhibits rhinovirus infection at nanomolar concentrations (184). As the pivotal interaction in the adhesion of leukocytes to activated endothelium and tissue components exposed during injury (Fig. 16.13), inhibition of ICAM-1/LFA-1 binding represents a potential prime intervention point for new antiinflammatory drugs.

Other members of the integrin family have been also successfully cloned (186). The availability of the individual members of this heterodimer superfamily—characterized by gross similarities in structure (Fig. 16.14), function, and in some cases, avidity for RGD-containing peptides—will allow their individual roles in specific disease pathophysiologies to be ascertained and will provide the means to develop integrin-specific antagonists for a multitude of utilities. Of importance to antithrombotic drug discovery efforts, the integrin $\alpha_{IIb}\beta_3$, also known as GPII$_b$III$_a$ the platelet fibrinogen receptor (187), was successfully expressed as the functional heterodimer, showing that prior association of the endogenous subunits is necessary to produce the

Table 16.4   The Integrin Receptor Family

Subunits		Ligands and Counterreceptors	Recognition Sequence
β_1	a_1	Collagens, laminin	
	α_2	Collagens, laminin	DGEA
	$\alpha_3{}^a$	Fibronectin, laminin, collagens	RGD ± ?'
	α_4	Fibronectin (V25), VCAM-1	EILDV'
	α_5	Fibronectin (RGD)	RGD
	α_6	*Laminin*	
	α_7	Laminin	
	α_8	?	
	α_v	Vitronectin, fibronectin (?)	RGD
β_2	α_1	ICAM-1, ICAM-2	
	α_M	C3b comonent of complement (inactivated), fibrinogen, factor X, ICAM-1	
	α_x	Fibrinogen, C3b component of complement (inactivated)?	GPRP
β_3	α_{IIb}	Fibrinogen, fibronectin, von Willebrand factor, vitronectin, thrombospondin	RGD, KQAGDV'
	α_v	Vitronectin, fibrinogen, von Willebrand factor, thrombospondin, fibronectin, osteopontin, collagen	RGD
β_4	α_6	Laminin ??	
β_5	α_v	Vitronectin	RGD
β_6	α_v	Fibronectin	RGD
$\beta_7(=\beta_P?)$	α_4	Fibronectin (V25), VCAM-1	EILDV
	α_{IEl}	?	
β_8	α_v	?	

cell surface complexes (188). Surface expression of $GPII_bIII_a$ is the common endpoint in platelet activation, initiating the platelet–platelet cross-linking via fibrinogen that is responsible for thrombus formation. A number of compounds, including disintegrin snake venoms, RGD peptides, and organic mimetics, have been shown to inhibit thrombus formation and platelet aggregation in animal and human clinical trials (189, 190).

Lymphocyte and neutrophil trafficking, the first step in the development of an inflammatory response, is known to occur via specific cell surface receptors and ligands, which match the inflammatory cell to the right target. Different receptors and ligands are expressed at different time points during inflammatory processes, from seconds to hours. These protein recognition signals—previously termed homing receptors (HR) and now uniformly called selectins—are membrane-bound proteins, which target circulating lymphocytes to specialized targets, provides one such opportunity for intervention (185, 191). Molecular cloning of the murine HR now called L-selectin revealed that the receptor contains a lectin (carbohydrate binding) domain that is responsible for the binding event (192). The selectin family (Table 16.5) consists of three cell surface receptors that share this affinity for carbohydrate ligands, specifically the tetrasaccharide sialyl Lewis X (**14**). The carbohydrates are likely displayed at multiple O-glycosylation sites on mucin-

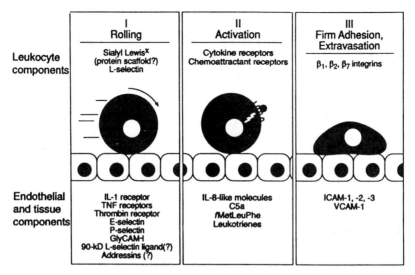

Fig. 16.13 Combinatorial aspects of leukocyte inflammation. Shown are the three major steps that lead to leukocyte inflammation and some of the various adhesion molecules, chemotactic factors, and cell surface receptors that are involved with the process. Step I is the initial low affinity rolling interaction that is mediated by the selectins. Step II is the neutrophil activation event that is mediated by the concentration gradients of various chemotactic factors. C5a is the chemotactic fragment of complement protein C5. Step III is the high affinity adhesion, leukocyte shape change, and extravasation event that is mediated by the binding of various leukocyte integrins to their cognate endothelial ligands (135). Reprinted by permission of The American Association for the Advancement of Science.

like glycoproteins such as Spg50, a novel endothelial ligand for L-selectin discovered by a combination of biochemical isolation, sequencing, and cloning techniques (193). The carbohydrate itself, however, offers a viable starting point for drug design as a structural lead for both carbohydrate analogues and noncarbohydrates (194, 195). Molecular modeling of E-selectin based on antibody mapping and homology to mannose binding protein (196) also suggests drug design possibilities based on proposed analogous structural interactions of the selectin with structure (**14**) (197). Inhibi-

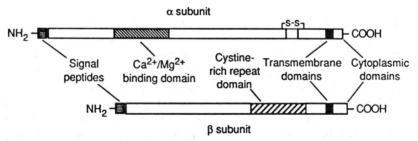

Fig. 16.14 General polypeptide structure of integrins. The α-subunit of the integrins is translated from a single mRNA, and in some cases, it is processed into two polypeptides that remain disulfide bonded to one another. The α-subunit and the β-subunit contain a typical transmembrane domain that is thought to traverse the cell membrane and bring the COOH-termini of the subunits into the cytoplasmic side of the membrane. The α-subunits contain a series of short-sequence elements homologous to known calcium-binding sites in other proteins; the β-subunit is tightly folded by numerous intrachain disulfide bonds (186). Reprinted by permission of The American Association for the Advancement of Science.

(14)

Table 16.5 The Selectin Family

Structure[a]	Name	Location	Expression	Adherent Cell Types	Proposed Function
	L-selectin	Leukocytes (constitutive)	Decreases upon cell activation	PLN endothelium Endothelium adjacent to inflammatory sites (rolling)	Lymphocyte recirculation through PLN Neutrophil (+ other leukocyte?) inflammation
	E-selectin	Endothelium (transcriptionally activated	Increases upon inflammatory activation (IL-1, TNF, LPS) (~hours)	Monocytes Neutrophils (rolling) T-cell subsets (cutaneous?)	Leukocyte inflammation
	P-selectin	Platelets (α-granules) Endothelium (Welbel-Palade bodies)	Increases upon thrombin activation, histamine, substance P, peroxide (~min)	Monocytes Neutrophils (rolling) T-Cell subsets (cutaneous?)	Leukocyte inflammation

[a]L, lectin; E, epidermal growth factor–like; C, complement-binding protein–like; PLN, peripheral lymph node.

tion of selectin-mediated cellular trafficking at specific times might help break a spiraling acute inflammatory cycle, allowing control of acute inflammatory processes, such as shock and adult respiratory distress syndrome (ARDS), and helping in the management of integrin-mediated inflammatory processes that follow (198).

5 FUTURE PROSPECTS

Molecular genetics is only now beginning to identify new targets for drug action. For example, regulation of inducible or tissue-specific gene expression has been an obvious but elusive target for pharmacological intervention (199–201). The tools to monitor such events are now becoming available, as in the case of the low density lipoprotein receptor, for which tissue-specific up-regulation of receptor population may successfully compete with other cholesterol-lowering agents (202, 203). In parallel, another genetic marker for atherosclerotic disease, lipoprotein(a), is a target for selective expression down-regulation (204).

An even more direct method to interfere with gene expression is selectively to bind the gene using sequence-specific recognition elements that prohibit transcription. Antisense oligonucleotides (Chapter 21) are the first sequence-directed molecules designed to inhibit protein expression at the level of translation of mRNA into the undesired protein (205), but this approach has yet to yield viable drugs. The ability to test for inhibition of gene expression or to measure the effects of species-specific agents against relevant pharmacological targets in animal models has also been advanced by the development and use of transgenic (206) or engineered gene knockout animals, such as the CFTR-defective mouse for cystic fibrosis (207), in screening and evaluation procedures.

The power of molecular genetics to provide unique and valuable tools for drug discovery is beginning to be exploited. The prospects for uncovering the molecular etiology of a disease state or for gaining access to a disease-relevant target enzyme or receptor are already being realized. On the horizon are the numerous opportunities that the mapping of the human genome should provide. The acceptance of a "common language" for the actual mapping work (208) has provided new impetus to initiate this decades-long task in earnest (209, 210), making the possibility of rationally intervening in disease states at previously inaccessible or unknown points more of a reality.

The development of recombinant DNA technology into a fully integrated component of the drug discovery process, although only beginning, is inevitable (211, 212). In 1987, Kornberg remarked that "the two cultures, chemistry and biology, [are] growing further apart even as they discover more common ground" (213). However, the broad area of drug development might qualify as one such meeting place for medicinal chemistry and molecular biology where the trend is reversing.

The application of genetic engineering techniques to biochemical and pharmacological problems will facilitate the discovery of novel therapeutics with potent and selective actions. There is little doubt among medicinal chemists that effective collaboration between chemistry and biology is not only needed but is actually growing in importance in drug design (214, 215). The eventual extent of the impact that molecular biology will have on the drug discovery process is, and will be for some time, unknown. However, the reality of recombinant protein therapeutics offers the assurance that this same technology, in conjunction with structural biology, computer-assisted molecular modeling, computational analysis, and medicinal chemistry (216), will help make possible better therapies for those diseases already controllable and new therapies for diseases never before treatable.

REFERENCES

1. J. Liebenau in C. Hansch, P.G. Sammes, and J. B. Taylor, Eds., *Comprehensive Medicinal Chemistry*, Vol. 1, Pergamon Press, Oxford, UK 1990, pp. 81–98.

2. A. Burger in Ref. 1, pp. 1–5.

3. W. Sneader in Ref. 1, pp. 7–80.

4. L. H. Sterbach, *Prog. Drug Res.*, **22**, 229–266 (1978).

5. C. R. Ganellin in J. S. Bindra and D. Lednicer, Eds., *Chronicles of Drug Discovery*, Vol. 1, John Wiley & Sons, Inc., New York, 1982, pp. 1–38.

6. M. A. Ondetti and D. W. Cushman, *J. Med. Chem.*, **24**, 355–361 (1981).

7. J. K. Seydel in E. Mutschler and E. Winterfeldt, Eds., *Trends in Medicinal Chemistry*, VCH Verlagsgesellschaft, New York, 1987, pp. 83–103.

8. J. M. Henwood and R. C. Heel, *Drugs*, **36**, 429–454 (1986).

9. J. V. Duncia, D. J. Carini, A. T. Chiu, A. L. Johnson, W. A. Price, P. C. Wong, R. R. Wexler, and P. B. M. W. M. Timmermans, *Med. Res. Rev.*, **12**, 149–191 (1992).

10. K. R. Freter, *Pharm. Res.*, **5**, 397–400 (1988).

11. J. A. Lowe III and P. M. Hobart, *Annu. Rep. Med. Chem.*, **18**, 307–316 (1983).

12. M. C. Venuti, *Annu. Rep. Med. Chem.*, **25**, 201–211 (1990).

13. A. Harvey, *Trends Pharmacol. Sci.*, **12**, 317–319 (1991).

14. M. C. Venuti in T. Friedmann, Ed., *Molecular Genetic Medicine*, Vol. 1, Academic Press, Inc., New York, 1991, pp. 133–168.

15. W. Szkrybalo, *Pharm. Res.*, **4**, 361–363 (1987).

16. S. Cometta, *Arzneim. Forsch. Drug Res.*, **39**, 929–934 (1989).

17. S. P. Adams in Ref. 1, pp. 409–454.

18. P. Swetly in Y. C. Martin, E. Kutter, and V. Austel, Eds., *Modern Drug Research: Path to Better and Safer Drugs*, Medicinal Research Series, Vol. 12, Marcel Dekker, Inc., New York, 1989, pp. 217–241.

19. I. S. Johnson, *Science*, **219**, 632–637 (1983).

20. C. Hentschel in D. N. Copsey and S. Y. J. Delnatte, Eds., *Genetically Engineered Human Therapeutic Drugs*, Stockton Press, New York, 1988, pp 3–6.

21. S. L. Gordon, in Ref. 20, pp. 137–146.

22. P. Bost, G. Bourat, and A. Jouanneau in Ref. 1, pp. 455–479.

23. C. R. Hutchinson, *Med. Res. Rev.*, **8**, 557–567 (1988).

24. C. R. Hutchinson, C. W. Borell, S. L. Otten, K. J. Stutzmann-Engwall, and Y. Wang, *J. Med. Chem.*, **32**, 929–937 (1989).

25. L. Katz and C. R. Hutchinson, *Annu. Rep. Med. Chem.*, **27**, 129–138 (1992).

26. L. J. Nisbet and J. W. Westley, *Annu. Rep. Med. Chem.*, **21**, 149–157 (1986).

27. P. J. Hylands and L. J. Nisbet, *Annu. Rep. Med. Chem.*, **26**, 259–269 (1991).

28. D. H. Williams, M. J. Stone, P. R. Hauck, and S. K. Rahman, *J. Nat. Prod.*, **52**, 1189–1208 (1989).

29. P. G. Waterman, *J. Nat. Prod.*, **53**, 13–22 (1990).

30. J. D. Coombes, Ed., *New Drugs from Natural Sources*, IBC Technical Services, London, 1992.

31. J. R. Knowles, *Science*, **236**, 1252–1258 (1987).

32. E. T. Kaiser, *Angew. Chem. Int. Ed. Engl.*, **27**, 913–922 (1988).

33. D. J. Livingston, *Annu. Rep. Med. Chem.*, **24**, 213–221 (1989).

34. M. J. Ross, E. B. Grossbard, A. Hotchkiss, D. Higgins, and S. Anderson, *Annu. Rep. Med. Chem.*, **23**, 111–120 (1988).

35. E. Haber, T. Quertermous, G. R. Matsueda, and M. S. Runge, *Science*, **243**, 51–56 (1989).

36. D. L. Higgins and W. F. Bennett, *Annu. Rev. Pharmacol. Toxicol*, **30**, 91–121 (1990).

37. N. L. Haigwood, G. T. Mullenbach, G. K. Moore, L. E. DesJardin, A. Tabrizi, S. L. Brown-Shimer, H. Stauss, H. A. Stöhr, and E.-P. Pâques, *Prot. Eng.*, **2**, 611–620 (1989).

38. J. Krause and P. Tanswell, *Arzneim.-Forsch. Drug Res.*, **39**, 632–637 (1989).

39. A. Hotchkiss, C. J. Refino, C. K. Leonard, J. V. O'Connor, C. Crowley, J. McCabe, K. Tate, G. Nakamura, D. Powers, A. Levinson, M. Mohler, and M. W. Spellman, *Thromb. Haemostas.*, **60**, 255–261 (1988).

40. C. Bakhit, D. Lewis, R. Billings, and B. Malfroy, *J. Biol. Chem.*, **262**, 8716–8720 (1987).

41. G. R. Larson, K. Henson, Y. Blue and P. Horgan, *Fibrinolysis*, **2** (suppl. 1), 29 (1988).

42. K. M. Tate, D. L. Higgins, W. E. Holmes, M. E. Winkler, H. L. Heynecker, and G. A. Vehar, *Biochemistry*, **26**, 338–343 (1987).

43. L. C. Petersen, M. Johannessen, D. Foster, A. Kumar, and E. Mulvihill, *Biochim. Biophys. Acta*, **952**, 245–254 (1988).

44. E. L. Madison, E. J. Goldsmith, R. D. Gerard, M. J. Gething, and J. F. Sambrook, *Nature (London)*, **339**, 721–724 (1989).

45. E. L. Madison, E. J. Goldsmith, R. D. Gerard, M. J. Gething, J. F. Sambrook, and R. S. Bassel-Duby, *Proc. Natl. Acad. Sci. U. S. A.*, **87**, 3530–3533 (1990).

46. U. Kohnert, R. Rudolph, J. H. Verheijen, E. Jacoline, D. Weening-Verhoeff, A. Stern, U. Opitz, U. Martin, H. Lill, H. Prinz, M. Lechner, G.-B. Kreese, P. Buckel, and S. Fischer, *Prot. Eng.*, **5**, 93–100 (1992).

47. C. J. Refino, N. F. Paoni, B. A. Keyt, C. S. Pater, J. M. Badillo, F. M. Wurm, J. Ogez, and W. F. Bennett, *Thromb. Haemostas.*, **70**, 313–319 (1993).

48. D. J. Capon, S. M. Chamow, J. Mordenti, S. A. Marsters, T. Gregory, H. Mitsuya, R. A. Byrn, C. Lucas, F. M. Wurm, J. E. Groopman, S. Broder, and D. H. Smith, *Nature (London)*, **337**, 525–531 (1989).

49. A. Traunecker, J. Schneider, H. Kiefer, and K. Karjalainen, *Nature (London)*, **339**, 68–70 (1989).

50. R. A. Byrn, J. Mordenti, C. Lucas, D. Smith, S. A. Marsters, J. S. Johnson, P. Cossum, S. M. Chamow, F. M. Wurm, T. Gregory, J. E. Groopman, and D. J. Capon, *Nature (London)*, **334**, 667–670 (1990).

51. B. C. Cunningham, P. Jhurani, P. Ng, and J. A. Wells, *Science*, **243**, 1330–1336 (1989).

52. B. C. Cunningham and J. A. Wells, *Science*, **244**, 1081–1085 (1989).

53. S. S. Abdel-Meguid, H. S. Shieh, W. W. Smith, H. E. Dayringer, B. N. Violand, and L. A. Bentle, *Proc. Natl. Acad. Sci. U.S.A.*, **84**, 6434–6437 (1987).

54. G. Fuh, M. G. Mulkerrin, S. Bass, N. McFarland, M. Brochier, J. H. Bourell, D. R. Light, and J. A. Wells, *J. Biol. Chem.*, **265**, 3111–3115 (1990).

55. B. C. Cunningham, D. J. Henner, and J. A. Wells, *Science*, **247**, 1461–1465 (1990).

56. B. C. Cunningham, M. Ultsch, A. M. de Vos, M. G. Mulkerrin, K. R. Klausner, and J. A. Wells, *Science*, **254**, 821–825 (1991).

57. A. M. de Vos, M. Ultsch, and A. A. Kossiakoff, *Science*, **255**, 306–312 (1992).

58. J. A. Wells, B. C. Cunningham, G. Fuh, H. B. Lowman, S. H. Bass, M. G. Mulkerrin, M. Ultsch, and A. M. de Vos, *Recent Prog. Hormone Res.*, **48**, 253–275 (1992).

59. H. C. Nau, *Science*, **257**, 1064–1073 (1992).

60. T. Palzkill and D. Botstein, *Prot. Struct. Function Genet.*, **14**, 29–44 (1992).

61. C. J. Noren, S. J. Anthony-Cahill, M. C. Griffith and P. G. Schultz, *Science*, **244**, 182–188 (1989).

62. J. A. Ellman, D. Mendel, and P. G. Schultz, *Science*, **255**, 197–200 (1992).

63. D. Mendel, J. A. Ellman, Z. Chang, D. L. Veenstra, P. A. Kollman, and P. G. Schultz, *Science*, **256**, 1798–1802 (1992).

64. R. M. Burch and D. J. Kyle, *Pharm. Res.*, **8**, 141–147 (1991).

65. M. D. Walkinshaw, *Med. Res. Rev.*, **12**, 317–372 (1992).

66. W. H. Moos, G. D. Green, and M. R. Pavia, *Annu. Rep. Med. Chem.*, **28**, 315–324 (1993).

67. L. Fellows in J. D. Coombes, Ed., *New Drugs from Natural Sources*, IBC Technical Services Ltd., London, 1992, pp. 93–100.

68. H. C. Krebs, *Prog. Chem. Org. Nat. Prod.*, **49**, 151–363 (1986).

69. H. Geysen, R. Meloen, and S. Barteling, *Proc. Natl. Acad. Sci. U. S. A.*, **81**, 3998–4002 (1984).

70. S. P. Fodor, J. L. Read, M. C. Pirrung, L. Stryer, A. T. Lu, and D. Solas, *Science*, **251**, 767–773 (1991).

71. K. S. Lam, S. E. Salmon, E. M. Hersch, V. J. Hruby, W. M. Kazmierski, and R. J. Knapp, *Nature (London)*, **354**, 82–84 (1991).

72. J. K. Scott, *Trends Biochem. Sci.*, **17**, 241–245 (1992).

73. R. A. Houghten, C. Pinilla, S. E. Blondelle, J R. Appel, C. T. Dooley, and J. H. Cuervo, *Nature (London)*, **354**, 84–88 (1991).

74. R. J. Simon, R. S. Kania, R. N. Zuckermann, V. D. Huebner, D. A. Jewell, S. Banville, S. Ng, L. Wang, S. Rosenberg, C. K. Marlowe, D. C. Spellmeyer, R. Tan., A. D. Frankel, D. V. Santi, F. E. Cohen, and P. A. Bartlett, *Proc. Natl. Acad. Sci. U. S. A.*, **89**, 9367–9371 (1992).

75. M. E. Wolff and A. McPherson, *Nature (London)*, **345**, 365–366 (1990).

76. J D. Marks, H. R. Hoogenboom, A. D. Griffiths, and G. Winter, *J. Biol. Chem.*, **267**, 16007–16010 (1992).

77. L. C. Bock, L. C. Griffin, J. A. Latham, E. H. Vermaas, and J. J. Toole, *Nature (London)*, **355**, 564–566 (1992).

78. C. Tuerk and L. Gold, *Science*, **249**, 505–510 (1990).

79. A. D. Ellington and J. W. Szostak, *Nature (London)*, **346**, 818–822 (1990).

80. S. Brenner and R. A. Lerner, *Proc. Natl. Acad. Sci. U. S. A.*, **89**, 5381–5383 (1992).

81. W. C. Greene, *Annu. Rev. Immunol.*, **8**, 453–475 (1990).

82. L. T. Batcheler, L. L. Strehl, R. H. Neubauer, S. R. Petteway, Jr., and B. Q. Ferguson, *AIDS Res. Hum. Retroviruses*, **5**, 275–278 (1989).

83. J. M. Hasler, T. F. Weighous, T. W. Pitts, D. B. Evans, S. K. Sharma, and W. G. Tarpley, *AIDS Res. Hum. Retroviruses*, **5**, 507–516 (1989).

84. M.-C. Hsu, A. D. Schutt, M. Holly, L. W. Slice, M. I. Sherman, D. D. Richman, M. J. Potash, and D. J. Volsky, *Biochem. Soc. Trans.*, **20**, 525–531 (1992).

85. M. Steinmetz in *Rapid Functional Screening for Drug Development*, IBC USA Conferences, Southborough, Mass., 1992.

86. H. A. Erlich, D. Gelfand and J. J. Sninsky, *Science*, **252**, 1643–1651 (1991).

87. J. W. Erickson and S. W. Fesik, *Annu. Rep. Med. Chem.*, **27**, 271–289 (1992).

88. G. M. Clore and A. M. Gronenborn, *Science*, **252**, 1390–1399 (1991).

89. S. W. Fesik, *J. Med. Chem.*, **34**, 2937–2945 (1991).

90. B. Shaanan, A. M. Gronenborn, G. H. Cohen, G. L. Gilliland, B. Veerapandian, D. R. Davies, and G. M. Clore, *Science*, **257**, 961–964 (1992).

91. I. D. Kuntz, *Science*, **257**, 1078–1082 (1992).

92. R. R. Rando, *Pharmacol. Rev.*, **36**, 111–142, (1984).

93. P. J. Parker, L. Coussens, N. Totty, L. Rhee, S. Young, E. Chen, S. Stabel, M. D. Waterfield, and A. Ullrich, *Science*, **233**, 853–859, (1986).

94. Y. Nishizuka, *Science*, **258**, 607–614 (1992).

95. C. D. Nicholson, R. A. J. Challiss, and M. Shahid, *Trends Pharmacol. Sci.*, **12**, 19–27 (1991).

96. R. M. Kramer, C. Hession, B. Johansen, G. Hayes, P. McGray, E. P. Chow, R. Tizard, and R. B. Pepinsky, *J. Biol. Chem.*, **264**, 5678–5775, (1989).

97. J. L. Seilhamer, W. Pruzanski, P. Vadas, S. Plant, J. A. Miller, J. Kloss, and L. K. Johnson, *J. Biol. Chem.*, **264**, 5335–5338, (1989).

98. D. A. Matthews, J. T. Bolin, J. M. Burridge, D. J. Filman, K. W. Volz, B. T. Kaufman, C. R. Beddell, J. N. Champness, D. K. Stammers, and J. Kraut, *J. Biol. Chem.*, **260**, 381–391, (1985).

99. D. A. Matthews, J. T. Bolin, J. M. Burridge, D. J. Filman, K. W. Volz, and J. Kraut, *J. Biol. Chem.*, **260**, 392–399, (1985).

100. C. Oefner, A. D'Arcy, and F. Winkler, *Eur. J. Biochem.*, **174**, 377–385, (1988).

101. N. J. Prendergast, J. R. Appleman, T. J. Delchamp, R. L. Blakley, and J. H. Freisham, *Biochemistry*, **28**, 4645–4650, (1989).

102. B. I. Schweitzer, S. Srimatkandata, H. Gritsman, R. Sheridan, R. Venkataraghavan, and J. Bertino, *J. Biol. Chem.*, **264**, 20786–20795, (1989).

103. K. Appelt, R. J. Backquet, D. A. Bartlett, C. L. J. Booth, S. T. Freer, M. A. M. Fuhry, J. R. Gehring, S. M. Herrmann, E. F. Howland, C. A. Janson, T. R. Jones, C.-C. Kan, V. Kathardekar, K. K. Lewis, G. P. Marzoni, D. A. Matthews, C. Mohr, E. W. Moomaw, C. A. Morse, S. J. Oatley, R. C. Ogden, M. R. Reddy, S. H. Reich, W. S. Schoettlin, W. W. Smith, M. D. Varney, J. E. Villafranca, R. W. Ward, S. Webber, S. E. Webber, K. M. Welsh, and J. White, *J. Med. Chem.*, **34**, 1925–1934 (1991).

104. J. R. Huff, *J. Med. Chem.*, **34**, 2305–2314 (1991).

105. M. A. Navia, P. M. D. Fitzgerald, B. M. McKeever, C.-T. Leu, J. C. Heimbach, W. K. Herber, I. S. Sigal, P. L. Drake, and J. P. Springer, *Nature (London)*, **337**, 615–620 (1989).

106. A. Wlodawer, M. Miller, M. Jaskólski, B. K. Sathyanarayana, E. Baldwin, I. T. Weber, L. M. Selk, L. Clawson, J. Schneider, and S. B. H. Kent, *Science*, **245**, 616–621 (1989).

107. P. Lapatto, T. Blundell, A. Hemmings, J. Overington, A. Wilderspin, S. Wood, J. R. Merson, P.

J. Whittle, D. E. Danley, K. F. Geoghegan, S. J. Hawrylik, S. E. Lee, K. G. Scheld, and P. M. Hobart, *Nature (London)*, **342**, 299–302 (1989).

108. I. T. Weber, M. Miller, M. Jaskólski, J. Leis, A. M. Skalka, and A. Wlodawer, *Science*, **143**, 928–931 (1989).

109. M. Miller, J. Schneider, B. K. Sathyanarayana, M V. Toth, G. R. Marshall, L. Clawson, L. Selk, S. B. H. Kent, and A. Wlodawer, *Science*, **246**, 1149–1152 (1989).

110. P. M. D. Fitzgerald, B. M. McKeever, J. Van-Middelsworth, J. P. Springer, J. C. Heimbach, C. T. Leu, W. K. Herber, R. A. F. Dixon, and P. L. Darke, *J. Biol. Chem.*, **265**, 14209–14219 (1990).

111. J. Erickson, D. J. Neidhart, J. VanDrie, D. J. Kempf, X. C. Wang, D. W. Norbeck, J. J. Plattner, J. W. Rittenhouse, M. Turon, N. Wideburg, W. E. Kohlbrenner, R. Simmer, R. Helfrich, D. A. Paul, and M. Knigge, *Science*, **249**, 527–533 (1990).

112. A. L. Swain, M. M. Miller, J. Green, D. H. Rich, J. Schneider, S. B. H. Kent, and A. Wlodawer, *Proc. Natl. Acad. Sci. U. S. A.*, **87**, 8805–8809 (1990).

113. J. C. Heimbach, V. M. Garsky, S. R. Michaelson, R. A. F. Dixon, I. S. Sigal, and P. L. Darke, *Biochem. Biophys. Res. Commun.*, **164**, 955–960 (1989).

114. T. D. Meek, D. M. Lambert, G. B. Dreyer, T. J. Carr, T. A. Tomaszek, Jr., M. L. Moore, J. E. Strickler, C. Debouck, L. J. Hyland, T. J. Matthews, B. W. Metcalf, and S. R. Petteway, *Nature (London)*, **343**, 90–92 (1990).

115. T. J. McQuade, A. G. Tomasselli, L. Liu, V. Karacostas, B. Moss, T. K. Sawyer, R. L. Heinrikson, and W. G. Tarpley, *Science*, **247**, 454–456 (1990).

116. N. A. Roberts, J. A. Martin, D. Kinchington, A. V. Broadhurst, J. C. Craig, I. B. Duncan, S. A. Galpin, B. K. Handa, J. Kay, A. Kröhn, R. W. Lambert, J. H. Merrett, J. S. Mills, K. E. B. Parkes, S. Redshaw, A. J. Ritchie, D. L. Taylor, G. J. Thomas, and P. J. Machin, *Science*, **248**, 358–361 (1990).

117. W. Greenlee, *Med. Res. Rev.*, **10**, 173–276 (1990).

118. S. L. Schreiber, *Science*, **251**, 283–287 (1991).

119. N. Takahashi, T. Hayano, and M. Suzuki, *Nature (London)*, **337**, 473–475 (1989).

120. G. Fischer, B. Wittmann-Liebold, K. Lang, T. Kiefhaber, and F. X. Schmid, *Nature (London)*, **337**, 476–478 (1989).

121. J. J. Sieklerka, S. H. Y. Hung, M. Poe, C. S. Lin, and N. H. Sigal, *Nature (London)*, **341**, 755–757 (1989).

122. M. W. Harding, A. Galat, D. E. Uehling, and S. L. Schreiber, *Nature*, (*London*), **341**, 758–760 (1989).

123. R. K. Harrison and R. L. Stein, *Biochemistry*, **29**, 3813–3816 (1990).

124. J. Liu, M. W. Albers, C.-M. Chen, S. L. Schreiber, and C. T. Walsh, *Proc. Natl. Acad. Sci. U. S. A.*, **87**, 2304–2308 (1990).

125. M. K. Rosen, S. Standaert, A. Galat, M. Nakatsuka, and S. L. Schreiber, *Science*, **248**, 863–866 (1990).

126. K. Wüthrich, B. von Freyberg, C. Weber, G. Wider, R. Traber, H. Widmer, and W. Braun, *Science*, **254**, 953–954 (1991).

127. S. Gallion and D. Ringe, *Prot. Eng.*, **5**, 391–397 (1992).

128. J. Liu, J. D. Farmer Jr., W. S. Lane, J. Friedmann, I. Weissman, and S. L. Schreiber, *Cell*, **66**, 807–815 (1991).

129. F. McKeon, *Cell*, **66**, 823–826 (1991).

130. M. Sokolovsky, *Adv. Drug Res.*, **18**, 431–509 (1989).

131. L. Mei, W. R. Roeske, and H. I. Yamamura, *Life Sci.*, **45**, 1831–1851 (1989).

132. E. C. Hulme, N. J. M. Birdsall, and N. J. Buckley, *Annu. Rev. Pharmacol. Toxicol.*, **30**, 633–673 (1990).

133. E. G. Peralta, A. Ashkenazi, J. W. Winslow, D. H. Smith, J. Ramachandran, and D. J. Capon, *EMBO J.*, **6**, 3923–3929 (1987).

134. T. I. Bonner, N. J. Buckley, A. C. Young, and M. R. Brann, *Science*, **237**, 527–532 (1987).

135. T. I. Bonner, A. C. Young, M. R. Brann, and N. J. Buckley, *Neuron*, **1**, 403–410 (1988).

136. E. G. Peralta, J. W. Winslow, A. Ashkenazi, D. H. Smith, J. Ramachandran, and D. J. Capon, *Trends Pharmacol. Sci.*, **9** (suppl.), 6–11 (1988).

139. A. G. Gilman, *Annu. Rev. Biochem.*, **56**, 615–649 (1987).

140. L. Birnbaumer, *Annu. Rev. Pharmacol. Toxicol.*, **30**, 675–705 (1990).

141. H. G. Dohlman, M. G. Caron, and R. J. Lefkowitz, *Biochemistry*, **26**, 2657–2664 (1987).

142. C. Humblet and T. Mirzadegan, *Annu. Rep. Med. Chem.*, **27**, 291–300 (1992).

143. B. F. O'Dowd, M. Hnatowich, J. W. Regan, W. M. Leader, M. G. Caron, and R. J Lefkowitz, *J. Biol. Chem.*, **263**, 15985–15992 (1988).

144. J. L. Benovic, A. DeBlasi, W. C. Stone, M. G. Caron, and R. J. Lefkowitz, *Science*, **246**, 235–240 (1989).

145. M. J. Lohse, R. J. Lefkowitz, M. G. Caron, and J. L. Benovic, *Proc. Natl. Acad. Sci. U. S. A.*, **86**, 3011–3015 (1989).

146. R. B. Clark, J. Friedman, R. A. F. Dixon, and C. D. Strader, *Molec. Pharmacol.*, **36**, 343–348 (1989).

147. C. M. Fraser, *J. Biol. Chem.*, **264**, 9266–9270 (1989).

148. S. K.-F. Wong, E. M. Parker, and E. M. Ross, *J. Biol. Chem.*, **265**, 6219–6224 (1990).

149. M. I. Simon, M. P. Strathmann, and N. Gautam, *Science*, **252**, 802–808 (1991).

150. P. Bovy, *Med. Res. Rev.*, **10**, 115–142 (1990).

151. S. Schultz, P. S. T. Yuen, and D. L. Garbers, *Trends Pharmacol. Sci.*, **12**, 116–120 (1991).

152. D. G. Lowe, M.-S. Chang, R. Hellmiss, E. Chen, S. Singh, D. G. Garbers, and D. V. Goeddel, EMBO J., **8**, 1377–1384 (1989).

153. M. B. Anand-Srivastava, M. R. Sairam, and M. Cantin, *J. Biol. Chem.*, **265**, 8566–8572 (1990).

154. M.-S. Chang, D. G. Lowe, M. Lewis, R. Hellmiss, E. Chen, and D. V. Goeddel, *Nature* (*London*), **341**, 68–72 (1989).

155. P. R. Bovy, J. M. O'Neal, G. M. Ollins, D. R. Patton, P. P. Mehta, E. G. McMahon, M. Palomo, J. Schuh, and D. Blehm, *J. Biol. Chem.*, **264**, 20309–20313 (1989).

156. Y. Kambayashi, S. Nakajima, M. Ueda, and K. Inouye, *FEBS Lett.*, **248**, 28–34. (1989).

157. S. Schultz, C. K. Green, P. S. T. Yuen, and D. L. Garbers, *Cell*, **63**, 941–948 (1990).

158. M. G. Currie, K. F. Fok, J. Kato, R. J. Moore, F. K. Hamra, K. L. Duffin, and C. E. Smith, *Proc. Natl. Acad. Sci., U. S. A.*, **89**, 947–951 (1992).

159. F. J. deSauvage, R. Horuk, G. Bennett, C. Quan, J. P. Burnier, and D. V. Goeddel, *J. Biol. Chem.*, **267**, 6429–6482 (1992).

160. A. C. Chao, F. J. deSauvage, Y. J. Dong, J. A. Wagner, D. V. Goeddel, and P. Gardner, *EMBO J.*, **13**, 1065–1072 (1994).

161. S. Watson and A. Abbott, *Trends Pharmacol. Sci.*, **13** (TiPS Receptor Nomenclature Suppl.) (1992).

162. A. Ullrich and J. Schlessinger, *Cell*, **61**, 203–212 (1990).

163. L. Tartaglia and D. V. Goeddel, *Immunol. Today*, **13**, 151–153 (1992).

164. D. B. Pritchett, H. Lüddens, and P. H. Seeburg, *Science*, **245**, 1389–1392 (1989).

165. R. Sprengel, P. Werner, P. H. Seeburg, A. G. Mukhin, M. R. Santi, D. R. Grayson, A. Guidotti, and K. E. Krueger, *J. Biol. Chem.*, **264**, 20415–20421 (1989).

166. W. Sieghart, *Trends Pharmacol. Sci.*, **10**, 407–411 (1989).

167. R. W. Olsen and A. J. Tobin, *FASEB J.*, **4**, 1469–1480 (1990).

168. V. Jung, C. Jones, C. S. Kumar, S. Stefanos, S. O'Connell, and S. Pestka, *J. Biol. Chem.*, **265**, 1827–1830 (1990).

169. T. Furuichi, S. Yoshikawa, A. Miyawaki, K. Wada, N. Maeda, and K. Mikoshiba, *Nature (London)*, **342**, 32–38 (1989).

170. M. Hollmann, A. O'Shea-Greenfield, S. W. Rogers, and S. Heinemann, *Nature (London)*, **342**, 643–648 (1989).

171. R. Sprengel, T. Braun, K. Nikolics, D. L. Segaloff, and P. Seeberg, *Mol. Endocrinol.*, **4**, 525–530 (1990).

172. R. M. Evans, *Science*, **240**, 889–895 (1988).

173. P. J. Godowski and D. Picard, *Biochem. Pharmacol.*, **38**, 3135–3143 (1989).

174. R. F. Power, O. M. Conneely, and B. W. O'Malley, *Trends Pharmacol. Sci.*, **13**, 318–323 (1992).

175. D. P. McDonnell, B. Clevenger, S. Dana, D. Santiso-Mere, M. T. Tzukerman, and M. A. Gleeson, *J. Clin. Pharmacol.*, **33**, 1165–1172 (1993).

176. T. Kishimoto, S. Akira, and T. Taga, *Science*, **258**, 593–597 (1992).

177. S. Nakanishi, *Science*, **258**, 597–603 (1992).

178. P. J. M. van Galen, G. L. Stiles, G. Michaels, and K. A. Johnson, *Med. Res. Rev.*, **12**, 423–471 (1992).

179. M. Williams, *Med. Res. Rev.*, **11**, 147–184 (1991).

180. D. Oksenberg, S. A. Marsters, B. F. O'Dowd, H. Jin, S. Havlik, S. J. Peroutka and A. Ashkenazi, *Nature (London)*, **360**, 161–163 (1992).

181. B. Benhamou, T. Garcia, T. Lerouge, A. Vergezac, D. Gofflo, C. Bigogne, P. Chambon, and H. Gronemeyer, *Science*, **255**, 206–209 (1992).

182. R. O. Hynes, *Cell*, **69**, 11–25 (1992).

183. T. A. Springer, *Nature (London)*, **346**, 425–434 (1990).

184. S. D. Marlin, D. E. Staunton, T. E. Springer, C. Stratowa, W. Sommergruber and V. J. Merluzzi, *Nature (London)*, **344**, 70–72 (1990).

185. L. Lasky, *Science*, **258**, 964–969 (1992).

186. E. Ruoslahti and M. D. Pierschbacher, *Science*, **238**, 491–497 (1987).

187. D. R. Phillips, I. F. Charo, and R. M. Scarborough, *Cell*, **65**, 359–362 (1991).

188. S. C. Bodary, M. A. Napier, and J. W. McLean, *J. Biol. Chem.*, **264**, 18859–18862 (1989).

189. J. A. Jakubowski, G. F. Smith, and D. J. Sall, *Annu. Rep. Med. Chem.*, **27**, 99–108 (1992).

190. B. K. Blackburn and T. R. Gadek, *Annu. Rep. Med. Chem.*, **28**, 79–88 (1993).

191. T. A. Yednock and S. D. Rosen, *Adv. Immunol.*, **44**, 313–378 (1989).

192. L. A. Lasky, M. S. Singer, T. A. Yednock, D. Dowbenko, C. Fennie, H. Rodriguez, T. Nguyen, S. Stachel, and S. D. Rosen, *Cell*, **56**, 1045–1055 (1989).

193. L. A. Lasky, M. S. Singer, D. Dowbenko, Y. Imai, W. J. Henzel, C. Grimley, C. Fennie, N. Gillett, S. R. Watson, and S. D. Rosen, *Cell*, **69**, 927–938 (1992).

194. K. A. Karlsson, *Trends Pharmacol. Sci.*, **12**, 265–272 (1991).

195. J. H. Musser, *Annu. Rep. Med. Chem.*, **27**, 301–310 (1992).

196. W. I. Weis, K. Drickamer, and W. A. Hendrickson, *Nature (London)*, **360**, 127–134 (1992).

197. D. V. Erbe, B. A. Wolitzky, L. G. Presta, C. R. Norton, R. J. Ramos, D. K. Burns, J. M. Rumberger, B. N. Narasinga Rao, C. Foxall, B. K. Brandley, and L. A. Lasky, *J. Cell Biol.*, **119**, 215–227 (1992).

198. L. Osborn, *Cell*, **62**, 3–6 (1990).

199. T. Maniatis, S. Goodbourn, and J. A. Fischer, *Science*, **236**, 1237–1245 (1987).

200. A. D. Frankel and P. S. Kim, *Cell*, **65**, 717–719 (1991).

201. R. G. Shea and J. F. Milligan, *Annu. Rep. Med. Chem.*, **27**, 311–320 (1992).

202. A. L. Catapano, *Pharmacol. Ther.*, **43**, 187–219 (1989).

203. W. J. Schneider, *Biochim. Biophys. Acta*, **988**, 303–317 (1989).

204. G. Utermann, *Science*, **246**, 904–910 (1989).

205. M. D. Matteucci and N. Bischofberger, *Annu. Rep. Med. Chem.*, **26**, 287–296 (1991).

206. J D. Coombes and M. Evans, *Annu. Rep. Med. Chem.*, **22**, 207–211 (1987).

207. J. N. Snouwaert, K. K. Brigman, A. M. Latour, N. N. Malouf, R. C. Bouchere, O. Smithies, and B. H. Koller, *Science*, **257**, 1083–1088 (1992).

208. M. Olson, L. Hood, C. Cantor, and D. Botstein, *Science*, **245**, 1434–1435 (1989).

209. J. D. Watson, *Science*, **248**, 44–49 (1990).

210. C. R. Cantor, *Science*, **248**, 49–51, (1990).

211. L. H. Hurley, *J. Med. Chem.*, **30**, 7A–8A (1987).

212. F. J. Zeelen, *Trends Pharmacol. Sci.*, **10**, 472 (1989).

213. A. Kornberg, *Biochemistry*, **26**, 6888–6891 (1987).

214. R. H. Hirschmann, *Angew. Chem. Int. Ed. Engl.*, **30**, 1278–1301 (1991).

215. S. L. Schreiber, *Chem. Eng. News*, **70**, 22–32 (1992).

216. P. Knight, *Bio/technology*, **8**, 105–107 (1990).

CHAPTER SEVENTEEN

Mass Ligand Screening as a Tool for Drug Discovery and Development

PAUL M. SWEETNAM

Pfizer Central Research
Groton, Connecticut, USA

CHRISTOPHER H. PRICE

Medical Innovation Partners
Minneapolis, Minnesota, USA

JOHN W. FERKANY

Nova Screen and Oceanix Biosciences Corp.
Baltimore, Maryland, USA

Burger's Medicinal Chemistry and Drug Discovery,
Fifth Edition, Volume 1: Principles and Practice,
Edited by Manfred E. Wolff.
ISBN 0-471-57556-9 © 1995 John Wiley & Sons, Inc.

CONTENTS

1 Drug Discovery and "Systems"
   Pharmacology,   698
   1.1 The black box phenomenon, 698
   1.2 The limited availability of whole animal
       screens, 701
   1.3 Additional problems with "systems"
       screening, 703
   1.4 Future of "systems" screening, 704
2 Drug Discovery and Rational Drug Design
   (RDD)   704
   2.1 Previous RDD successes, 705
   2.2 Future of RDD, 705
3 Drug Discovery Strategies,   706
   3.1 Availability and diversity of radioligand
       binding assays, 707
   3.2 Directed discovery efforts, 707
   3.3 High throughput screening, 709
   3.4 Selectivity screening, 710
   3.5 Future of mass ligand screening, 710

4 The Radioligand Binding Assay,   710
   4.1 Receptor binding theory, 713
   4.2 Practical aspects of high volume receptor
       binding, 714
       4.2.1 Equipment, 715
       4.2.2 Ligand, 716
       4.2.3 Tissue preparation, 716
       4.2.4 Establishing the assay, 717
       4.2.5 Sample preparation, 720
       4.2.6 The assay, 720
       4.2.7 Data analysis, 721
       4.2.8 Role of sample handling, data
             management and automation, 723
5 Chemical Libraries,   724
   5.1 Synthetic libraries, 724
   5.2 Novel libraries (combinatorials), 727
   5.3 Natural product libraries, 728
6 Summary,   730

1 DRUG DISCOVERY AND "SYSTEMS" PHARMACOLOGY

The pharmaceutical industry's role within the health care community is clearly defined: To develop therapeutic agents which prevent, alleviate, or cure human disease states. One of the key elements in this effort is the rapid and reliable discovery of novel compounds that can serve as templates for the development of new agents. Historically, drug discovery has been heavily weighted in the use of "systems" pharmacological (whole animal) screening strategies, astute observations, and serendipity to predict a compound's potential therapeutic utility. In today's pharmaceutical environment (stronger competition, increased research and development costs, and shorter product life cycles) astute observation and serendipidity are still important, but the use of "systems" based high volume screening is lessening. "Systems" screening has been determined to be the rate limiting step in discovery due to the small number of compounds that can be screened and the limited information it can generate on a compound's molecular mechanism of action (MOA). This has produced a shifting of priorities and attitudes from "systems" screening towards mass ligand screening strategies, which offer a rapid, efficient, and reliable means of identifying compounds on the basis of MOA information.

The "systems" approach has been an adequate first line indicator of biological activity in areas such as anti-hypertensive (1,2) and chemotherapeutic research (3), and was responsible for the discovery of a number of important drugs. However, the progress of drug discovery in other therapeutic areas, e.g., central nervous system, has been hindered by a lack of animal models that mimic targeted disease states to serve as first line screens (4). Conversely, there are hundreds of different receptor types, many of which are closely associated with specific disease states, which can be targeted by mass ligand screening (5).

1.1 The Black Box Phenomenon

Conceptually it is not difficult to understand why "systems" screens are difficult to work with. It is the nature of animal models that they are complex and dynamic arrangements of molecular mechanisms which limits their ability to selectively target one MOA (Fig. 17.1). Simply stated, "Whole animal models often identify

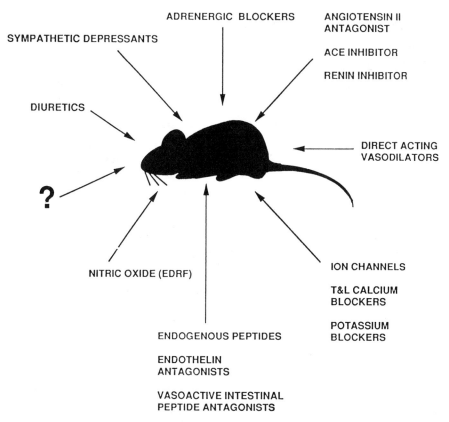

Fig. 17.1 The black box phenomenon. Schematic representation of the standard pharmacological agents used in the treatment of hypertension. Also included are potential areas for the development of new therapeutics. The complex and dynamic processes which regulate blood flow are often interconnected and influenced by a number of indirect mechanisms. This makes the whole animal studies based on "challenge" experiments (artificially induced hypertension followed by drug administration) and simple blood pressure following drug alone administration difficult to interpret.

numerous compounds acting at any number of different sites and can best be described as "Black Box" systems". High throughput assays of limited selectivity tend to be low stringency sieves which maximize the number of compounds that appear to be active. Active compounds are commonly referred to as "hits" or "leads." The criteria defining a "hit" take into account the activity of known reference agents or positive controls in that assay, the concentration of the test compounds to be examined, and the identification of a level of activity which is consistently and significantly above the baseline shift of the assay (Fig. 17.2).

Large numbers of false "hits" complicate subsequent developmental efforts due to the introduction of compounds into the pipeline which do not actually interact with the target of interest. Low stringency can also increase the probability of not detecting actual "hits," termed "false" negatives. Particular care should be taken regarding the area of "false" negatives because there are no strategies available to correct for missed activity, short of a comprehensive rescreening program.

The high degree of selectivity associated with mass ligand screening is a result of the tools used, i.e., the selectivity of the

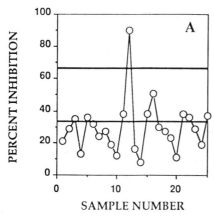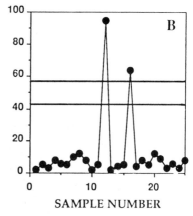

Fig. 17.2 "Hit" criteria. When establishing such criteria it is important to establish the minimal level of activity need to identify a compound as a "hit." This level should be significantly above baseline activity of an assay and at concentration of compound which is great enough to identify weak activity but not great enough to compromise the validity of an assay, e.g., for radioligand binding a "hit" is normally defined as a compound which inhibits activity 50% at a concentration of 10 micromolar. If an assay has a large degree of baseline variability (A) the stringency of the assay is lessened and window defining activity must be broadened accordingly and more compounds are identified as potential "hits." The possibility that activity might be missed resulting from experimental variation can not be ignored. The end result is often a dramatic increase in the percentage of follow up verification work which would be unnecessary if variation of the assay was lessened. A tight baseline (B) affords an assay of greater stringency and reduces the potential to follow up on compounds which are actually inactive.

radioligand for the target receptor, and the position of a receptor in the biological response cascade. Receptors function by transducing a binding phenomenon into the initial response element of a cascade. Monitoring at this position can result in a dramatic increase in the stringency of the screen and a significant decrease in the number of false positives and/or negatives. The small numbers of false positives can be easily eliminated by subsequent verification work. Still, a small number of false positives will consist of compounds that actually inhibit binding through a nonselective MOA, e.g., detergentlike compounds and other membrane perturbating agents. Their elimination can be accomplished by closer examination of their structure, i.e., compounds with long carbon chain moieties (>4 to 5 carbons) following initial screening.

Not all high volume *in vitro* assays selectively target one MOA. Many *in vitro* assays, i.e., cytotoxicity, proliferation, ag-glutination assays, and isolated tissue preparation methodologies, are complicated by multiple mechanistic sites of action like their *in vivo* counterparts (Fig. 17.3). The use of an *in vitro* cell assay to assess anticytotoxic activity, i.e., the search for a tumor necrosis factor alpha (TNFα) antagonist, is complicated by the inability to accurately determine the point in the cytotoxic cascade a "hit" acting to inhibit cytotoxicity. Accurate MOA assessment may be further complicated, as it is with TNF alpha, by lack of information detailing the cytotoxic cascade initiated. The signal transduction mechanism associated with TNFα-induced cytotoxicity is unclear, PLA$_2$ induction and receptor phosphorylation having been suggested as possibilities of transduced activity (6). Conversely, the use of a TNFα radioligand binding will significantly increase the probability of identifying interesting compounds that inhibit TNFα binding to the receptor, i.e., the starting point of the cytotoxic cascade.

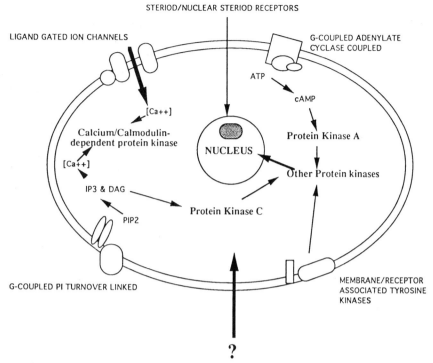

Fig. 17.3 The cellular black box phenomenon. A variety of whole cell assays are best classified as black box. This schematic is a simplified representation of the several very common transduction pathways associated with cellular receptors. In attempting to develop a screen for identifying compounds which inhibit cellular motility as a new generation of chemotherapeutic agents, a selected molecular target, e.g., a specific membrane receptor, would be more appropriate than monitoring actual cellular motility, which could be affected by interaction of a compound with any one of these numerous cellular components.

Certain receptor-based assays are also promiscuous in nature, and care must be taken when adopting them for use in mass ligand screening. The muscarinic receptor subtypes are known to interact with a number of diverse chemical structures at the micromolar concentrations routinely used in mass ligand screening. These weak inhibitory compounds can be eliminated through primary or verification screening at lower concentrations (nanomolar). The recent cloning of these receptor subtypes can increase assay selectivity and possibly lower the number of false positives normally contributed by other contaminating subtypes.

Following the discovery of compounds with "biological/inhibitory" activity from a "systems" screen, another screening effort must be put forth to elucidate the actual MOA for these compounds. This typically employs any number of receptor binding and/or functional assays before an apparent MOA can be proposed. This effort is time consuming, costly, and often unsuccessful. Since the primary goal of drug discovery efforts is rapid addition of significant value to a compound at each level of testing, it is difficult to reconcile the utilization of a "systems" and not a mass ligand approach when possible.

1.2 The Limited Availability of Whole Animal Screens

Knowledge of pharmacology at the molecular level has evolved at a rapid pace, and in certain instances has exceeded knowledge of the "systems" pharmacology. This dichotomy is a direct result of the identification and characterization of numerous receptors and enzymes acting to regulate function at the cellular level. Problems associated with this dichotomy are clearly evident in areas such as psychotropic drug discovery where "systems" approaches have not been developed for areas of CNS research, i.e., depression, Alzheimer's disease, or schizophrenia. In CNS areas where standard "systems" screens are available, they tend to be predisposed towards the identification of compounds similar to existing drugs, i.e., anti-anxiety (sedative) screens/benzodiazepines; antipsychotics (extrapyramidal side effects) screens/dopamine antagonists. They do not offer any advantages over the more selective and expansive menu of receptors offered by mass ligand screening. The lack of "systems" approaches has also hampered the development of leads identified by mass ligand screening and has

ultimately hindered the introduction of new drugs for the treatment of these CNS disorders. This perpetuates the use of therapeutics, many with pronounced side effects, that were introduced clinically over thirty years ago (i.e., tricyclic antidepressants, 1950; monoamine oxidase inhibitors, 1950) (7). Even worse may be the use of drugs, for which the MOAs directly responsible for their therapeutic action are unknown or ambiguous, i.e., the antipsychotics lithium and thorazine (Table 17.1).

The benzodiazepines, widely prescribed anxiolytic drugs, are an example where early stage development was hindered because no known MOA existed to describe to the activities reported in "systems" assays (8). This resulted in the early assessment of the benzodiazepines in animal models originally designed to test drugs for their ability to serve as psychotropic sedatives. Interestingly, this particular action of the benzodiazepines has long been

Table 17.1   Receptor Selectivity Demonstrating Potential Sites Of Action For Thorazine (Chlorpromazine)

Radioligand Binding Assay	Significant Inhibition (nM range)[a]
Adenosine	
Adenosine 1	Yes
Adenosine 2	Yes
Adrenergic	
Alpha 1	Yes
Sigma	Yes
Biogenic amines	
Dopamine 2	Yes
Histamine 1	Yes
Serotonin 2	Yes
Cholinergics	
Muscarinic 1	Yes
Muscarinic 2	Yes
Biogenic amine transporters	
Serotonin	Yes
Dopamine	Yes

[a]Several other activities detected in micromolar range included Phencyclidne, Dopamine 1, Norephinephrine Transporter, Serotonin 1, and Alpha 2.

considered an adverse side effect and many companies now have active chemistry efforts designing "new" benzodiazepinelike drugs which are nonsedating (9). It was not until years following their introduction that the receptor through which the benzodiazepines elicit their effects was identified (10). It could be argued that the introduction of benzodiazepines under the same circumstances, no clearly defined MOA, would be difficult today given the present mind set of the pharmaceutical industry with its emphasis on MOA.

The discovery of a new class of compounds chemically distinct from classical arylacetic acid derivative nonsteroidal antiinflammatories (NSAIDS) was an example of the potential limitations of a systems screening approach (12). These compounds, the leudmedins, were reported to have promise in several animal models of inflammation, but no conclusive studies have been published detailing their actual MOA, and they are now ambiguously classified as inhibitors of leukocyte recruitment (12). Without key information regarding the actual MOA or a dramatic increase in the safety and efficacy of these compounds over existing NSAIDS, "fast track"

Table 17.2 Potential Receptorlike Binding Sites On Endothelial Cells Involved In Leukocyte Adhesion[a]

Selectin molecules
  P-Selectin
  E-Selectin
  GlyCAM-1 (PLN addressins)
Integrin molecules
  ICAM'S
  VCAM-1
  MadCAM-1
  $\alpha 6 \beta 1$
Other molecules
  VAP-1
  CD31

[a]A variety of receptorlike molecules have also been identified on the surface of leucocyte cells.

or standard FDA approval will be difficult. If the leumedins' MOA is related to the inhibition of a cellular adhesion phenomenon, as first proposed, hindsight would suggest that a more selective screening system targeting any one of the numerous adhesion molecules thought to play crucial roles in cellular adhesion, rather than overall event of cellular adhesion and migration, could be more fruitful. (13) (Table 17.2).

1.3 Additional Problems with "Systems" Screening

"Systems" screening's inherent deficiency in detailing MOA is not the only problem. Other problems center around a compound's bioavailability, the rate at which a compound becomes available at the site of drug action (14). Questions such as: what is its solubility and pK_a; does the compound interact with plasma components (silent receptors) in the serum (15); is the compound rapidly metabolized in the liver, and if so are the metabolites active; does the compound cross the blood brain barrier; what dosage regimen is required (acute or chronic administration) to see an effect, need to be answered. These questions are extremely important because certain answers to any one, or combination of the five questions, could result in the masking of a compound's potential activity in a "systems" screen. It is unreasonable to assume that bioavailability data is available for every compound in a given library. Therefore, questions of bioavailability are best addressed once the compound has been determined to be active. At this point studies involving whole animal work and a directed chemistry effort are extremely powerful. Of particular utility is the ability of chemistry support to focus on structural or formulations modifications which increase bioavailability, potency, and, if need be, selectivity. This type of chemistry has long been a strength of the pharmaceutical industry.

Screening strategies that employ radioligand binding or enzyme inhibition assays are run in defined buffering systems and are not constrained by issues of bioavailability. However, they are affected by issues of compound solubility, but these can be corrected for prior to screening by examining the utility of various solubilizing agents or vehicles (see practical aspects of screening). Technically, whole animal studies are costly in both time and materials. To generate one data point for a compound, one or more animals may have to be evaluated over the course of several days. Quantitative interpretation of data generated can be difficult because of animal-to-animal or day-to-day variation. In anti-inflammatory models, e.g., mouse ear or foot edema, which measure tissue swelling, it is not uncommon to report differences in response to reference compounds used to standardize results within individuals of a given test group or between different experimental groups. This is in direct contrast to mass ligand screening approach where intra-experimental variation is limited because thousands of compounds can be tested using a single receptor preparation. Day-to-day variation is significantly reduced because assay components are standardized, i.e., buffer, temperature, proteolytic activity, pH, and incubation times.

In addition to the scientific and technical problems associated with the use of "systems" approaches, scientists must now address ethical questions that have been raised surrounding the use of animals in biomedical research (16). While the evidence supporting the need for such work is overwhelming, scientists should be prepared to accept and comply with stricter governmental regulations restricting the use of animals for certain research purposes. It is the responsibility of the scientific community to design new drug discovery strategies that will not compromise the important contributions made by the pharmaceutical industry in the area of health care. The strategies employed must continue to generate the necessary information to further drug development, while standing up to the sociopolitical scrutiny they are likely to encounter.

1.4 Future of "Systems" Pharmacology

Mention of the limitations associated with utility of "systems" pharmacological strategies for high throughput screening does not suggest that are unimportant in the drug development process. "Systems" approaches need to be positioned in the drug discovery and developmental pipeline where they can have the greatest impact or value addition. For this reason their role in primary screening is lessening. However, there will always be instances where a gap exists between therapeutic need and the availability of a molecular-based screen, and in these instances "systems" approaches may be the only avenue available. Obviously, these approaches will remain valuable tools used to ensure the safety and efficacy of a drug by spanning the gap between activity in a mechanistically driven *in vitro* screen and potential human application. For the foreseeable future, drugs will be tested in animal models before human clinical trials can begin.

2 DRUG DISCOVERY AND RATIONAL DRUG DESIGN

In recent years, a key objective of the drug discovery field has been the development of "Structure-based Rational Drug Design" (RDD), and it would be remiss not to briefly address the practicality of this approach before concentrating on mass ligand screening. In theory, RDD would afford *de novo* drug design using structural information detailing a ligand/receptor or substrate/enzyme interaction at the molecular level. Structural information would be obtained by the integration of numerous technologies, including protein chemistry, molecular biology, x-ray crystallography, high-field NMR spectroscopy, and computational modeling. There are instances where one or more of these pieces have assisted in the development of more selective and potent compounds, e.g., the development of new more potent inhibitors of dihydrofolate reductase (17) and HIV protease (18), but at this point in time completely integrated efforts have not met with the forecasted success. Although the individual components needed for RDD are being developed to a level of sophistication and sensitivity necessary for successful RDD, this approach is still futuristic. The limited information detailing the actual structure conformation of ligand binding domains for the majority of pharmacologically identified receptors is one of the greatest impediments to establishing successful RDD. Molecular techniques, such as site directed mutagenesis, have been touted as one way to assist in the identification of the ligand binding domain of a receptor. However, this technique cannot predict whether an amino acid substitution many Ångstroms from the actual ligand binding domain will significantly alter binding, making pharmacological data generated from these studies difficult to interpret. Recent work has demonstrated that amino acid residues within a transmembrane spanning region can significantly alter a ligand receptor interaction (19). A deletion/substitution of a single proline (rigid) or glycine (flexible) residue can have a profound effect on the three dimensional structure of a receptor and therefore its ability to bind a certain ligand. If a substitution/deletion results in changes of only a few tenths of an Ångstrom it could abort the formation of a hydrogen bond critical to binding (20). Several instances where amino acid substitution/dele-

tion has selectively altered antagonist binding with no apparent alteration of agonist binding have also been reported (21). In addition, it appears that in certain instances the amino acid sequences essential for the binding of synthetic non-peptide ligands are not essential to the binding of natural peptide ligands (20). These findings further complicate the accurate identification of a ligand binding domain utilizing the endogenous peptide, typically an agonist, as the template. It now appears that many of the subtle molecular interactions involved in ligand/receptor interaction must still be detailed in order to afford RRD technologies the opportunity to rapidly and efficiently support the *de novo* design of nonpeptide drugs.

2.1 Previous RDD Successes

The H2 antagonist cimetidine, and the angiotensin converting enzyme (ACE) inhibitors are routinely cited as RDD success stories. In actuality these are not examples of integrated or *de novo* drug design. The actual binding domains of the H2 receptor or ACE have not been accurately modeled, so credit must be given to the strong synthetic chemistry efforts and the existence of excellent starting material or templates, e.g., pit viper toxin in the case of ACE inhibition (22). Even these almost "rational" success stories have not appeared with the frequency to make mass ligand screening obsolete for use in drug discovery.

2.2 Future of RDD

At present many of the technologies which comprise RDD are invaluable tools when used to optimize initial nonpeptide leads identified through mass ligand screening. The identification of a template lessens the necessity of attempting to design synthetic compounds based on the 3-D structure of known peptide or protein ligands which often yield limited 3-D structural information because of their inherent flexibility.

Once a potent peptide or nonpeptide lead has been synthesized it can be used as a starting point for RDD technologies to generate crystallographic analysis of the ligand/receptor complex and computational algorithms that define that interaction. One should not confuse this type of modified RDD drug discovery with the desired goal of *de novo* RDD drug discovery. Unfortunately, original timeline projections for the establishment of integrated RRD in the late 1990s appears to have been overly ambitious, and this approach cannot be counted on to meet the demands of the health care community in the short term. This has resulted in many pharmaceutical companies' "decisions" to re-energize their developmental pipeline by establishing mechanistically driven, high volume screening approaches.

3 DRUG DISCOVERY STRATEGIES

Scientists in the field of drug discovery must constantly recognize the technical and intellectual constraints under which they toil. Therefore they must not only employ proven techniques, but must constantly seek out more innovative approaches. Mass ligand screening is one innovation of biotechnology which when introduced by Nova Pharmaceuticals and others in the early eighties was both praised (23) and panned by various sectors of the scientific community. Detractors argued that rapid advances in biotechnology might bring about the end of the classic pharmaceutical era (24), that proven pharmacological approaches will always be more important than innovative contributions from the biotechnology sector (25), and that mass ligand screening was anti-intellectual when compared to the concept of RDD and

classical "systems." Mass ligand screening was also criticized for its potential to lead researchers down blind alleys. Nova's choice of a nonpeptide bradykinin lead, NPC 12724, has been cited as an example of a trip down a blind alley. In actuality, it was not a failure of mass ligand screening but the improper assumption that a compound with limited ability to inhibited bradykinin binding, 13% at 1 mM, and limited selectivity, e.g., inhibition of 100% of muscarinic binding at the same concentration, was a potential candidate for follow up studies (26).

There are several universally held doctrines in high throughput screening: the first, and most important, is that a compound with less than 50% inhibitory activity at 10 micromolar is not typically a useful candidate. The use of such a high concentration optimizes the chances for the identification of a starting material for chemical modification and development because it will identify both nanomolar and low micromolar activities. However, it should be understood that designing nanomolar inhibitors from these micromolar compounds is a difficult challenge and not always successful (27). The thought that a compound with only mM activity, e.g., NPC 12724, could be chemically modified to break the nanomolar barrier was either very naive or a rather desperate undertaking. Second, not unlike other scientific techniques, it is important to understand the limitations of mass ligand screening in order to correctly interpret the data generated. High throughput screening was not envisioned as a practical method for the identification of compounds with limited inhibitory activity, <20%, at whatever concentration of compound is being tested, whether it be 100 nM or 1 mM. Inhibition of only 10–20% for most assays is within the baseline variation seen in a mass ligand screening assay and will result in generation of false positives. Finally, this strategy was not designed to identify drugs but only the templates from which potential drugs can be developed.

Despite these difficulties the recent successes of mass ligand screening, i.e., Pfizer's substance P antagonist (28), Merck's CCK_B antagonist (29), and Sanofi's neurotensin antagonist (30), suggest that detractors of mass ligand screening were incorrect. It is now clear that the integration of molecular pharmacology and innovative automation and data management strategies are a powerful tool for drug discovery.

3.1 Availability and Diversity of Radioligand Binding Assays

The identification and characterization of numerous receptor and receptor subtypes has resulted in the development of an extensive battery of radioligand binding assays which can be used in mass ligand screening (Table 17.3), positioning this strategy to play an important role in the immediate future of drug discovery. It is not hard to imagine that novel antipsychotic agents will be identified in the short

term by screening against one of the newly cloned dopamine (31) or serotonin (32) receptor subtypes, or other receptors once a link has been established. Not only will the identification of such agents serve as potential therapeutics but also molecular probes necessary for the development of a new generation of "systems" approaches.

3.2 Directed Discovery Efforts

Today, drug discovery efforts reflect the scientific community's emphasis on cellular function at the molecular level. Deciphering a drug's molecular MOA increases the probability of rapid advancement through development and clinical trials. The FDA approval process can also be "fast-tracked" if MOA data for a drug confirms the reduced side effects profiles seen in animal/ human trials. Directed discovery centers around the development of new chemical structures and possibly new drugs by using existing drugs as a templates for aggressive synthetic chemistry effort ("follow the leader" pharmacology). It can be assumed

Table 17.3 Radioligand Binding Assays[a]

Receptor/Selectivity	Reference Radioligand	Compound	K_1 (nM)	Percent Specific Binding
Adenosine				
Adenosine 1	[³H]CPX	2-Chloroadenosine	18.40	90
Adenosine 2	[³H]NECA + CPA[b]	MECA	202.70	85
Adrenergic				
Alpha 1	[³H]Prazosin	Phentolamine	13.00	95
Alpha 2	[³H]RX 781094	Phentolamine	1.70	90
Beta	[¹²⁵]Dihydroalprenolol	Metoprolol	45.00	70
Amino Acids				
Excitatory				
NMDA	[³H]CGS 19755	NMDA	4200.00	70
Quisqualate	[³H]AMPA	AMPA	11.80	90
Kainate	[³H]Kainic Acid	Kainic Acid	35.00	90
Glycine	[³H]Glycine	D-Alanine	895.00	90
PCP	[³H]TCP	PCP	62.30	90
Sigma	[³H]DTG	Haloperidol	11.50	90

Table 17.3 (*Continued*)

Receptor/Selectivity	Reference Radioligand	Compound	K_1 (nM)	Percent Specific Binding
Inhibitory				
Benzodiazepine	[³H]Flunitrazepam	Clonazepam	2.00	90
GABA$_A$	[³H]GABA	Muscimol	2.60	90
GABA$_B$	[³H]GABA + Isoguvacine[b]	GABA	176.00	75
Glycine	[³H]Strychnine	Strychnine Nitrate	52.50	80
Biogenic Amines				
Dopamine 1	[³H]SCH 23390	Butaclamol	37.30	90
Dopamine 2	[³H]Sulpiride	Spiperone	0.10	90
Histamine 1	[³H]Pyrilamine	Triprolidine	1.60	80
Serotonin 1	[³H]5-HT	5-HT	4.60	60
Serotonin 2	[³H]Ketanserin	5-HT	531.00	65
Channel Proteins				
Calcium, T&L	[³H]Nitrendipine	Nifedipine	1.60	90
Calcium, N	[¹²⁵H]Omega-Conotoxin	Omega-Conotoxin	0.10	90
Chloride	[³H]TBOB	TBPS	112.40	70
Potassium, Low Cond.	[¹²⁵H]Apamin	Apamin	0.05	90
Cholinergics				
Muscarinic 1	[³H]Pirenzepine	Atropine	0.30	90
Muscarinic 2	[³H]AF-DX 384	Methoctramine	0.60	98
Nicotinic	[³H]NMCl	Nicotine	0.90	75
Opiate				
Mu	[³H]DAGO	Naloxone	1.60	90
Delta	[³H]DPDPE	Naloxone	42.60	80
Kappa	[³H]U-69593	Cyclazocine	0.20	90
Prostanoids				
Leukotriene B$_4$	[³H]LTB$_4$	LTB$_4$	2.90	70
Leukotriene D$_4$	[³H]LTD$_4$	LTD$_4$	0.60	90
Thromboxane A$_2$	[³H]SQ 29548	U 46619	5.50	75
Reuptake Sites				
Norepinephrine	[³H]DMI	DMI	580.00	87
Serotonin	[³H]Citalopram	Imipramine	20.30	85
Dopamine, Cocaine Site	[³H]WIN	Nomifensine	32.50	75
Second Messenger Systems				
Adenylate Cyclase				
Forskolin	[³H]Forskolin	Forskolin	29.40	85
Protein Kinase C				
Phorbol Ester	[³H]PDBU	PDBU	16.50	90

[a]Abbreviations: 5HT, 5-Hydroxytryptamine; AMPA, Amino-3-hydroxy-5-methylisoxazole-4-propionic acid; CPA, cyclopentyladenosine; CPP, 3,2-carboxypiperazion-4-yl-propyl-phosphonic acid; CPX, Cyclopentyl-1,3-dipropylxanthine; DADLE, 2-D-Alanine-5-D-leucine enkephalin; DAGO, Tyr-D-Ala-Gly-NMe-Phe-Gly-ol; DMI, Desmethylimipramine; GABA, γ aminobutyric acid; LTB$_4$, Leukotriene B$_4$; LTD$_4$, Leukotriene D$_4$; MECA, 5'-N-Methylcarboxamindoadenosine; NECA, 5'-N-Ethylcarboxamidoadenosine; NMCI, N-Methylcarbamyl choline iodide; PCP, Phencyclidine; PDBU, Phorbol-12,13-dibutyrate; QNB, Quinuclidinyl benzilate; TBOB, t-butylbicyclo orthobenzoate; TBPS, t-butylbicyclophosphorothionate; and TCP, N-(1-[2thienyl]cyclohexyl) 3,4-piperidine.

[b]Competing drug added for selectivity.

that since the MOA for the parent drug is well understood, new compound synthesis based on the old drug could identify more efficacious and patentably distinct entities. Dihydropyridines, T + L calcium channel inhibitors used in the treatment of hypertension and angina, are an excellent example of chemistry directed drug development. Nifedipine (Procardia/Pfizer), was introduced in the 1980s (33), and was rapidly followed by the introduction of another patentably distinct group of dihydropyridines (Fig. 17.4) also targeting the identical indication, i.e. nitrendipine/Baypress (Miles) (34). Pharmaceutical involvement in such an endeavor rests on the hope of introducing a more efficacious entity to capture a significant market share from the previously introduced drug or identify a new market, nimodipine for cerebral vasodilation (Nimotop/Miles) (35). FDA approval of "me too" drugs may in part be based on several factors: the new compound (1) has an increase in efficacy, (2) has few side effects, or (3) is equally efficacious but the market for the drug is large and the number of treatment drugs available to the public is limited.

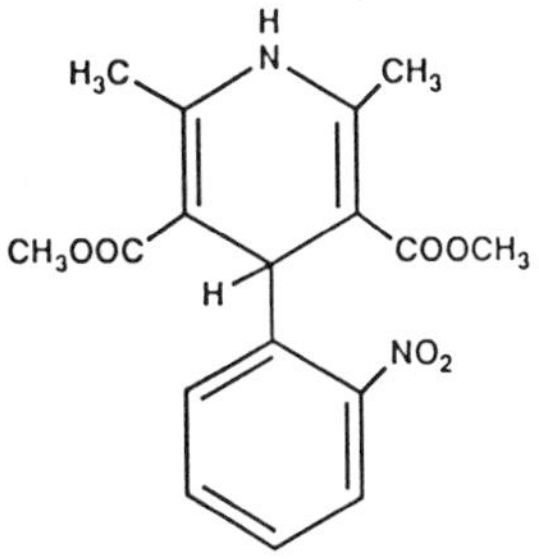

NIFEDIPINE

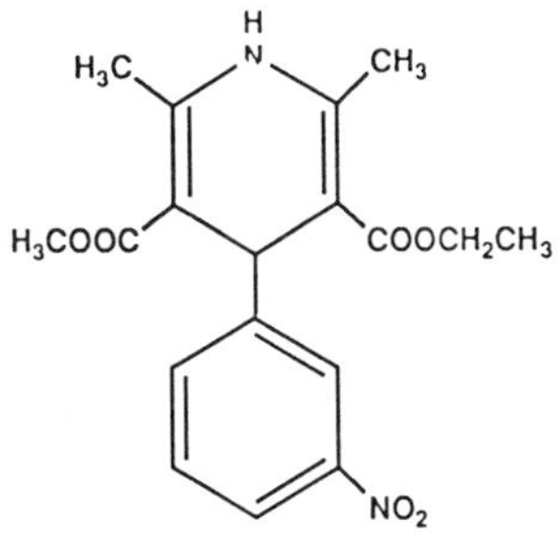

NITRENDIPINE

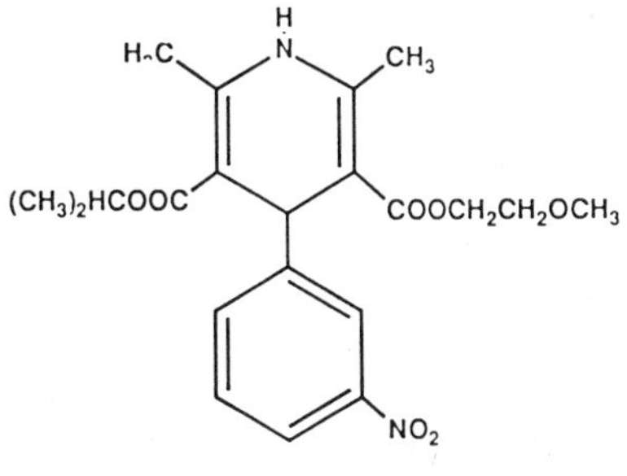

NIMODIPINE

Fig. 17.4 "**Follow the leader pharmaceuticals.**" The modified dihydropyridines first synthesized by Bayer have served as the foundation for the introduction of numerous therapeutic agents that target disease associated with increases in blood pressure through the blockade of T and L calcium channels.

3.3 High Throughput Screening

The second more innovative scheme for drug discovery, which is synergistic with mass ligand screening, requires the identification of a drug which has a MOA unique from those currently used in the treatment of a disease. Recent interest in a novel vasoconstrictive peptide, endothelin, has provided the industry with a potentially new target for antihypertension therapy, the discovery of an endothelin antagonist. The kinetics of endothelin binding show that it is reversible, saturable, and specific and amenable to mass ligand screening approaches (36). The search for an endothelin receptor antagonist (a compound which binds to a receptor but has no intrinsic activity), and not an agonist (a compound which binds to a receptor and activates it), is the most effective utilization of mass ligand screening. The vast majority of "hits" identified in this type of screen will interact with the receptor site but will lack some minor structural detail and therefore the ability to turn that receptor "on." This is analogous to identifying a key that will fit in the lock but not engage the tumblers. A "systems" screen for identification of an endothelin antagonist would not be a logical scientific choice from the multiple mechanisms aspect where the potential for identifying dihydropyridinelike compounds which could attenuate endothelin's hypertensive activity by blocking the recruitment of dihydropyridine sensitive calcium channels is possible (37).

3.4 Selectivity Screening

Selectivity screening is a recent strategy employed by the pharmaceutical industry to deal with the increasing demand for more efficient and cost effective drug development. This type of screening affords the scientist valuable information about potential side effects associated with a compound early in the developmental cycle. This is accomplished by running a lead compound through a large number of different radioligand binding assays, referred to as "profiling." It is often difficult for any one pharmaceutical company to accomplish this task in a meaningful time frame, and to assist them in this effort a number of smaller biotechnology companies have established profiling services. NovaScreen, Baltimore Maryland, offers formats for screening compounds in up to 55 different assays in a rapid (thirty day turnaround) and cost effective manner. Unlike high throughput screening, selectivity screening tests the compounds at pharmacological (nanomolar) as well as nonpharmacological concentration (micromolar) in an attempt to establish the biological significance of any ancillary activity. Such information can guide ongoing synthetic chemistry efforts and allow direct comparison of a potential lead candidate to other products in the development pipeline or on the market, and thus speed the development of drugs and lower the risk of failures.

3.5 Future of Mass Ligand Screening

Over the past decade it has become apparent that mass ligand screening does not appear to be as antediluvian as many scientists had believed. The primary reason for this is the increase in the level of intellectual and technical sophistication required for a high volume screening laboratory to meet the challenge of drug discovery. Scientifically, screening targets are constantly expanding to cover the full range of traditional, e.g., receptor and enzyme assays, and nontraditional, e.g., DNA/ RNA binding proteins, targets. Many of the new biotechnology companies, along with the established companies, view screening technology as an extremely flexible tool capable of taking advantage of new targets and chemical libraries as they become available. This has resulted in a general model of early stage drug discovery that many of the pharmaceutical industries employ (Fig. 17.5).

4 THE RADIOLIGAND BINDING ASSAY

The radioligand binding assay was designed to exploit the fundamental premise that multicellular organisms support life through the regulation and coordination of physiological activities by means of intra- and intercellular chemical communication. Chemical communication at its simplest requires chemical messengers, generically classified as neuronal or hormonal, and "receptive" substances, referred to as receptors (38). Many important aspects of drug/receptor interactions, e.g., the concept of receptor occupancy and efficacy (39) dose–response analysis (40), were elucidated before the direct analysis of ligand/receptor interactions were possible. A major obstacle was the small number of any one receptor type as compared to the total number of different receptors which comprised a target tissue. In the late 1960s

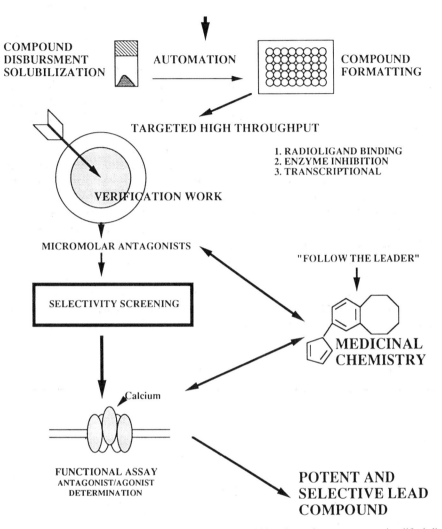

COMPOUND GENERATION/ACQUISITION

COMPOUND
DISBURSMENT   AUTOMATION   COMPOUND
SOLUBILIZATION   FORMATTING

TARGETED HIGH THROUGHPUT

1. RADIOLIGAND BINDING
2. ENZYME INHIBITION
3. TRANSCRIPTIONAL

VERIFICATION WORK

MICROMOLAR ANTAGONISTS

"FOLLOW THE LEADER"

SELECTIVITY SCREENING

MEDICINAL
CHEMISTRY

Calcium

FUNCTIONAL ASSAY
ANTAGONIST/AGONIST
DETERMINATION

POTENT AND
SELECTIVE LEAD
COMPOUND

Fig. 17.5 Pharmaceutical drug discovery development strategy. This schematic represents a simplified discovery/ development strategy where mass ligand screening is used as the primary tool to discover and characterize chemical templates used to develop potential new therapeutic agents.

several laboratories began to investigate the ligand binding interactions using isotopically labeled snake toxins and tissue preparations from electric organs of invertebrate fish rich in acetylcholine receptors (41). The pioneering work performed by Dr. Solomon Synder and his colleagues at Johns Hopkins University, who were able to perfect the competitive radioligand binding assay in their study of receptors in mammalian brain, ushered in a new area of molecular pharmacology. Some estimates suggested that any one receptor type in the central nervous system contributes to as little as one-millionth the total brain weight. A major problem with radioligand binding assays is the use of radioligands that bind nonspecifically to other membrane proteins and lipids which comprise the crude cellular membrane preparations routinely used as the receptor source. This decreases the specific binding signal by increasing the background noise or the nonspecific binding component of an assay. Dr. Snyder's group was able to reduce the nonspecific binding component by terminating the binding reaction using a rapid filtration technique. This technique allows for a simple separation of radioligand from nonspecific sites, while leaving the radioligand bound to the receptor of interest (42,43).

A properly developed radioligand binding assay accurately determines the specific binding of a radioligand to a targeted receptor through the delineation of its total and nonspecific binding components. Total binding is defined as the amount of radioligand that remains following the rapid separation of radioligand bound in a receptor preparation from that which is unbound. The nonspecific binding component is defined as the amount of radioligand that remains following separa-

tion of a reaction mixture consisting of receptor, radioligand, and an excess of unlabeled ligand. Under this condition, the only radioligand that remains represents that which is bound to components other than the receptor. The specific radioligand bound is determined by simply subtracting the nonspecific from total radioactivity bound (Fig. 17.6). The standard means of reporting specific binding is as a percentage of total binding.

The simplicity of this analytical technique and the wide range of physiological systems to which it can be applied, e.g., nervous, cardiovascular, respiratory, gastrointestinal, and immune systems make the radioligand binding assays a powerful tool in any drug discovery effort. Strengthening its utility in drug discovery is the fact that many of the therapeutic agents historically prescribed, e.g., morphine, have been shown to exert their effect by

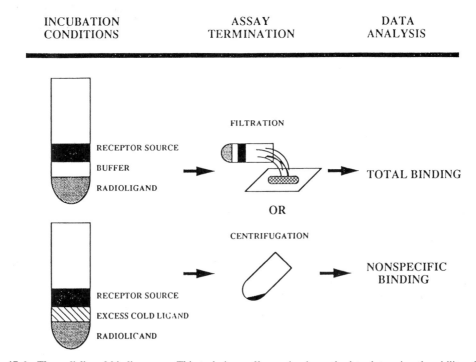

Fig. 17.6 The radioligand binding assay. This technique offers a simple method to determine the ability of a test compound to interact at a targeted receptor. Specific binding in this type of assay is defined as the total radioactivity bound minus the nonspecific binding. Using this technique it is easy to determine if a test compound can inhibit specific binding.

either mimicking or blocking the action of an endogenous chemical messenger/receptor interaction.

4.1 Receptor Binding Theory

The theory of receptor binding is based on the equations that are equivalent to those originally developed to quantify the interactions of enzymes and their substrates (Michaelis-Menton kinetics). There are many excellent reviews which detail the ligand/receptor binding and the reader is referred to them for a more complete discussion of kinetic theories (44,45). Briefly, the binding of a ligand to a receptor must be reversible, saturable, and specific.

Reversibility is defined by the following equation:

$$L + R \underset{K_1}{\overset{K_2}{\rightleftharpoons}} LR \qquad (17.1)$$

L denotes the radioligand, R denotes the receptor, and K_1 and K_2 are rate constants for association (on rate) and dissociation (off rate) for the ligand. In radioligand binding assays, specific binding (i.e., LR concentration) is measured. Assays are run under equilibrium conditions where the "on" and "off" rates are similar. In practical terms equilibrium may be defined as the time it takes specific binding to reach maximal levels. Under equilibrium conditions, the apparent affinity of the receptor for L can be determined by saturation analysis (46) (Fig. 17.7). In these experiments the amount of receptor is held constant and RL is determined as a function of increasing radioligand concentration. Two important pieces of information are derived: K_d, the dissociation constant, and B_{max}, an approximation of receptor density. K_d is simply the concentration of radioligand where 50% of the available receptors are occupied

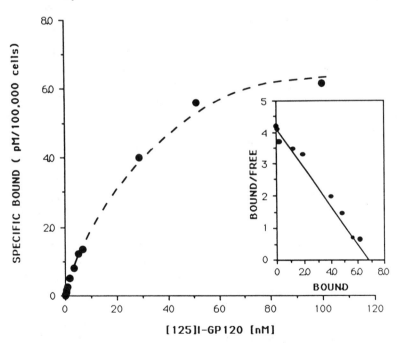

Fig. 17.7 Saturation plot. The envelope glycoproteins of the human immunodeficiency virus (HIV gp120) specifically bound to the CD_4 receptor is plotted as a function of free radioligand concentration. **Scatchard analysis (inset).** Linear analysis of saturation data allows for the easy determination of both apparent K_d ($K_d = -1/$slope) and the apparent B_{max} (intercept of the x-axis).

$$RL = [R + RL][R]/KD + L \quad (17.2)$$

Knowledge of the K_d and the equilibrium conditions for a particular radioligand binding assay will serve as an important internal control to determine the reliability of the assay; i.e., higher affinity drugs should dissociate at a slower rate than those of lower affinity.

Saturability defined by the B_{max} value or receptor density is an important value because it determines the receptor number in the tissue used in the experiment. It will establish that the receptor number is finite and binding should be saturable. In order to obtain an approximate B_{max}, a linear transformation of the equation 17.2 is performed. The transformations most used are the Rosenthal or Scatchard plot (Fig. 17.7 inset), thus:

$$[RL]/[L] = [-1/K_d][RL]$$
$$+ B_{max}/K_d \quad (17.3)$$

Competition/Specificity in a high volume screening assay results in the ability of a test compound to interact with a receptor and will be determined by its ability to compete with the radioligand being used. This competition is the basis for dose-response studies which can be used to determine the potency of a test compound and the specificity of the radioligand binding assay. Dose-response curves are generated by holding the receptor concentration, radioligand concentration (routinely 1/10th the K_d as determined by saturation analysis) and all other experimental conditions constant, while varying the concentration of the test compound (drug). This will result in a decrease of radioligand binding to the receptor as greater concentrations of the test compound (drug) are present. The curves will determine the concentration of the test compound necessary to inhibit 50% (IC_{50}) of the radioligand to the receptor (47) (Fig. 17.8). Using the Cheng-Prusoff equation (48), a K_i can be determined:

$$K_i = IC_{50}/1 + ([L]/K_d) \quad (17.4)$$

Given the $[L] \ll K_d$ the $K_i = IC_{50}$. K_is are similar to a K_ds but are obtained by the dose–response method. Such an equation takes into account variations in the radioligand concentration used in the assay and difference in the apparent K_ds generated between laboratories to standardize results. Using this type of analysis, it is easy to determine the apparent potency of a ligand for a given receptor, and also the selectivity of that assay, by examining other test compounds known to interact with other receptors and other receptor subtypes of the receptor being assayed.

4.2 Practical Aspects of High Volume Receptor Binding

In order to develop a radioligand binding assay as a tool for mass ligand screening, two criteria must be satisfied. The assay must be capable of characterizing the potency and selectivity of the interactions between a radioligand and a targeted receptor, and it must be compatible for a use in a high throughput format. It should be noted that the methodologies for large number of radioligand binding assays reported in the literature must undergo a significant amount of restructuring before they can be used in a high throughput format. In particular, assays being developed for high throughput require careful optimization of aspects not absolutely necessary for low throughput format, i.e., receptor characterization. These include percent specific binding, method of termination of the assay, test compound solubilization effects, and assay volumes.

First, the assay must have a specific binding or signal to noise ratio which is greater than 70%. While numerous radioligand assays have been developed with lower specific binding, e.g., many of the assays targeting the serotonin receptor

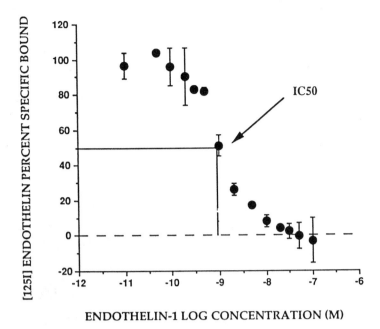

Fig. 17.8 Log-concentration response curve (displacement/inhibition/competition curve). The competition of [125I] endothelin-1 by increasing concentrations of nonradiolabeled endothelin-1. In this experiment the potency of endothelin-1 was determined at the endothelin A receptor expressed in a thoracic smooth muscle cell line (A10). Endothelin is a potent vasoconstricting peptide which regulates smooth muscle contraction. The development of an endothelin antagonist could be useful in the treatment of cardiovascular disorders, including coronary angina, cerebral vasospasm, and hypertension.

subtypes, these are not as amenable to mass ligand screening strategies, due to an increase in experimental variation that is directly proportional to low specific binding. Second, termination of the incubation reaction of binding assays by vacuum filtration over a glass fiber filter allows for rapid and easy handling of a large number of samples. It is not impossible to filter up to 5000 compounds in one hour using a 96 well microtiter plate format by using this method. The termination of 5,000 reactions by centrifugation is far more difficult. Three, the use of microtiter or small assay volumes is amenable to high throughput screening, but not all assays are amenable to volume reduction. Each assay developed for high throughput screening must be developed with these limitations in mind.

4.2.1 EQUIPMENT. The equipment necessary to perform ligand binding assays is

generally available to any laboratory engaged in biomedical research. Although high volume commercial operations may rely heavily on laboratory automation and specialized items (e.g., robotics), the minimal equipment needs make it possible for small laboratories to screen large numbers of compounds successfully in short time frames. Items common to binding assays include the obvious (balances, pH meters, tissue homogenizers, refrigerators/freezers, etc.), as well as high speed centrifuge and a scintillation or beta-plate counter. If iodinated ligands are used, a gamma counter is optimal but not required. Since many binding assays rely on animal tissues as a source of receptors, access to animals and a vivarium is needed. On the other hand, the increasing use of cloned receptors which are transiently or stably expressed frequently necessitates access to a tissue culture facility. Some assays (e.g., TNFα) are performed using plated whole cells. Contingent upon the specific assay, it is sometimes possible to purchase lyophilized receptor preparations or specific tissues from commercial sources.

Although first generation assays were terminated using dialysis or centrifugation, the availability of high affinity ligands makes it possible to stop reactions using vacuum filtration. In this procedure, ligand which is not bound to the receptor is separated from the receptor/ligand complex by trapping the complex on a filter support. Commercial units are available for this purpose, with the most popular models capable of terminating 48–96 individual reactions simultaneously and in a few seconds. Likewise, when whole cells are used, a 96 well microtiter plate prefitted with filter supports is available. Newer models of either device are designed with assay miniaturization in mind, thus allowing reactions to be performed in as little as 250 mL. This lends a considerable reduction in cost since all components of the assay are reduced. Assay miniaturization is also of the utmost importance when the compound of interest is available in limited quantities.

4.2.2   LIGAND.   There are a host of ligands available to label biologically relevant receptors (Table 17.3). Some of these are specific for receptor subtypes, while others

label a heterogeneous family of receptors. Choosing a ligand depends on the purpose of the study; for example, it would be inappropriate to select the generic ligand LSD, which labels all biologically relevant serotonin receptors, if one were interested only in determining if compounds interacted with the $5HT_2$ receptor. In the latter case, selection of [^{3}H]ketanserin would be more appropriate since this compound is selective for the $5HT_2$ receptor subtype (Table 17.4). Conversely, if the object of the study were to identify any compound having serotonergic potential, the use of LSD would be wholly appropriate.

4.2.3   TISSUE PREPARATION.   The preparation of tissue containing the receptor of interest will vary according to the source. Partly because of the range of receptors it contains, the brain/spinal cord axis remains a major source of receptors for binding assays. Assays based on receptors found in tissues, including gut, platelets, lymphocytes, skeletal muscle and endocrine organs, are also well known. The availability of cloned and expressed receptors represents an increasingly important point of departure in developing assays. Likewise, transformed cells remain useful as receptor sources.

The method of receptor preparation depends on the starting material and the

Table 17.4   Radioligand Assay Selectivity in K_i Values for Serotonin Receptor Subtypes[a]

Reference Compound	$5HT_1$	$5HT_2$
Serotonin	4.6	500.0
5-Methoxytrypatamine	45.8	>1,000.0
Methysergide	14.8	6.8
D-LSD	>7,500.0	1.5
Ketanserin	>7,500.0	0.4

[a]The number of serotonin receptor subtypes makes it imperative to demonstrate a particular assay's selectivity. Several major distinctions between $5HT_1$ and $5HT_2$ are the relative potencies of serotoin and ketanserin.

specific assay. Where animal tissues are used, the twin goals of tissue preparation are concentration of receptors and removal of endogenous substances which may interfere with assay sensitivity. Using brain as an example, it is common to homogenize the tissue in a dense liquid (usually $0.32\,M$ sucrose), followed by low speed centrifugation to remove cellular debris. Higher speed centrifugation is performed to concentrate portions of the tissue containing the receptor of interest. Although in most instances only very crude concentration is attempted, in its most extreme form, density gradient centrifugation is employed to isolate relatively pure populations of synaptic membranes containing high densities of receptor protein. In either case, the final material is "washed" several times using sequential resuspension and centrifugation in large amounts of buffer or water in order to remove the bulk of endogenous neurotransmitters which may bind to the receptor population. In some instances, the tissue may be subjected to a series of freeze/thaw cycles to further remove endogenous substances; alternatively, some preparation schemes call for preincubation of the tissue in order to enhance enzymatic or oxidative degradation of endogeneous neurotransmitters.

It is frequently possible to batch prepare tissues and store these frozen for later use. Unfortunately, some assays are best performed using freshly prepared samples, thus necessitating daily preparation. In any event, the use of fresh or frozen tissue will be peculiar to each assay and must be established empirically.

When cultured cells represent the tissue source, preparation is usually simplified and is designed to remove endogenous substances. Typically, cells are nonenzymatically harvested to avoid destroying receptor activity, homogenized to produce a crude membrane preparation, and washed sequentially by centrifugation and resuspension. When whole cells are employed, preparation procedures are generally restricted to replacing culture media with a buffer appropriate to the assay and cell viability.

The availability of cloned and expressed receptors offers advantages over animal tissues of high density, homogeneity and the potential to exclude substances which may interfere with assay sensitivity (Fig. 17.9). Of relevance to drug discovery, clones also offer the opportunity to study compound interactions with human rather than animal proteins, and to enhance the specific binding signal by optimizing the amount of receptor per unit tissue substance through over-expression of the receptor in a host cell. Disadvantages include the possibility that the expressed protein may differ in glycosylation patterns, subunit composition, etc., which may produce a different pharmacological profile, vis-a-vis the native receptor, thus yielding misleading screening results.

4.2.4 ESTABLISHING THE ASSAY. In many instances established assays are employed in random screening programs. More exciting, perhaps, is screening for compounds active at a newly identified receptor or at a receptor for which no appropriate ligand has been previously available. In these cases, it may be necessary to develop a binding assay from scratch.

All useful binding assays have several fundamental characteristics, including linearity, saturability, reversibility, and specificity. When developing an assay each characteristic must be demonstrated prior to using the technique in drug discovery programs.

By linearity, it is implied that the amount of ligand specifically bound to receptors increases in a manner directly proportional to the amount of tissue added to the assay. This makes intuitive sense since increasing the amount of tissue increases the number of receptors present in the incubation. Assays become nonlinear

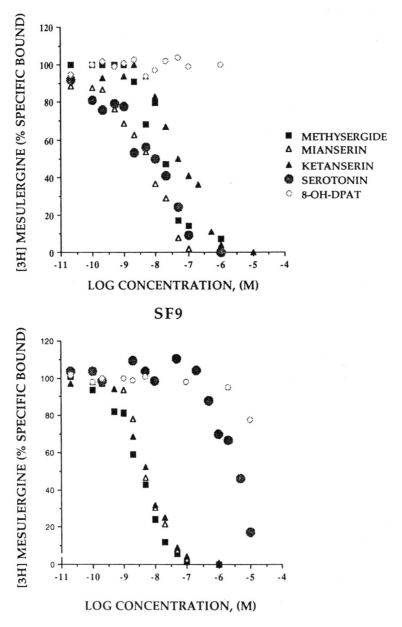

Fig. 17.9   **Characterization of a serotonin receptor subtype (5HT$_{1C}$) cloned from rat.** Log-concentration response curves for 5HT$_{1C}$ receptor using crude membrane preparation, pig choriod plexus, and rat clone expressed in a bacculovirus system (SF9). The characteristic for a number of serotonergic compounds are similar for both types of receptor. However, a major difference between the receptor preparations IC$_{50}$ for the endogenous ligand serotonin. This difference could be the result in actual species differences, alter posttranslational modification patterns, or the contribution of other seretonin subtypes in the crude membrane preparation. It is necessary to rigorously characterize a cloned receptor to establish the pharmacology for that system.

when the number of receptors becomes so great that the concentration of ligand becomes a limiting factor to the reaction. For reasons beyond the scope of this article, it is important that assays are performed in the linear portion of the tissue curve. Likewise, skepticism should prevail if the binding of a ligand is not linear with tissue concentration, as this may indicate non-specific binding of ligand, for example, to filter supports.

Saturability is a corollary of linearity. In the presence of a fixed concentration of receptor, it should be possible to increase the amount of ligand present in the assay so that all receptors are occupied and no further increase in specific binding is observed. When saturation cannot be demonstrated, the assay should probably be discarded because it does not follow the assumption that all tissue contains a finite number of receptors. Memorable to one of us was the "specific" binding of a novel antidepressant to glass fiber filters. While pharmacologically correct, the artifact was recognized when saturation studies were performed.

Most reactions achieve equilibrium, roughly the point where the association and dissociation of the ligand/receptor complex are in balance, in a matter of hours. Determining appropriate equilibrium conditions is done by performing association experiments which measure the amount of ligand specifically bound to the receptor as a function of time. As is the case for saturability, caution should be demonstrated if equilibrium conditions cannot be found, as this may represent sequestration rather than binding of ligand to the receptor.

Equally important to establishing a new binding assay is the demonstration that reactions are reversible. If a ligand irreversibly binds to a receptor (e.g., photoaffinity labeling) (49), the assay would have little value for drug discovery purposes since once bound, no compound could displace the ligand from the receptor. In practice, establishing reversibility is the converse of determining equilibrium conditions. Once a reaction has been brought to equilibrium, a large excess of unlabeled ligand is added to the incubation and the decrease of ligand bound to the receptor is measured as a function of time.

Finally, and of particular importance to random screening programs, a binding assay must be specific. That is, it must only detect compounds which interact with the receptor of interest. In developing a binding assay, the specificity of the system is demonstrated by showing that only reference agents known to interact with the receptor inhibit the binding of ligand. Unfortunately, with the rapid introduction of new ligands, situations may be encountered where the ligand itself is the only agent known to bind to the receptor. In the latter case, it is prudent to be wary of the particular assay since, by default, the specificity of the reaction cannot be demonstrated.

In an ideal world it should be possible to predict assay conditions for binding reactions. Regrettably this is not the case and the characteristics described above must be established on an empirical basis for each system. Likewise, selection of buffers for the reaction must be established on an individual basis; optimal binding may be obtained in a simple Tris buffer, or in a more complex mixture containing multiple salts. Receptor preparations often contain enzymes (proteases, esterases, etc.) which may degrade the ligand or compounds of interest. Assays designed to detect peptides or esters should include appropriate enzyme inhibitors and alternate substrates, e.g., bovine serum albumin, BSA, to minimize enzyme activity. Many peptide ligands are "sticky" and bind in a nonspecific manner to material supports (glass culture tubes, filters, etc.), and these effects must be controlled by pretreating assay supplies with various solvents (e.g., polyethylenemine; PEI).

4.2.5 SAMPLE PREPARATION. Having established the assay, it is necessary to identify a sample preparation scheme compatible with the chemical characteristics of the compounds of interest and the assay itself. A procedure which has proven useful in our own efforts relies upon the initial solubilization of compounds in dimethylsulfoxide (DMSO). DMSO is an effective and routinely used solubilizing agent for mass ligand screening. Typically, more than 75% of synthetic compound libraries are soluble in it (50). In addition, most radioligand binding assays can tolerate relatively high levels of DMSO, up to 10% in the final assay volume, before they are compromised (Fig. 17.10). There are times when more complex or exotic vehicles may be needed and it cannot be assumed that an assay which tolerates DMSO will perform

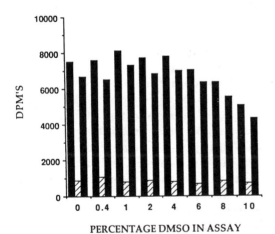

Fig. 17.10 Solubility effects. DMSO, a commonly used solubilizing agent has been shown to alter the characteristics of a radioligand binding assay. The [3H] MK801 binding assay used to study the interaction of compounds with the ion channel associated with an excitatory amino acid receptor subtype (NMDA) is affected minimally by concentrations of DMSO of up to 10% as determined by specific binding. (O) total binding (O) nonspecific binding, and (O) specific binding.

equally well in another solubilizer. If a change of vehicle is needed, the assay may have to be redeveloped to account for minor or major discrepancies, i.e., decreases in the specific binding component, which often result. Only a small percentage of samples should be completely insoluble, and therefore unscreenable, in a compound library if the appropriate vehicle is employed. Partially soluble compounds, if biologically active, should give a "hint" of inhibitory signal in a mass ligand screen. The detectable inhibitory potential, in these instances, could be less than the criteria normally used to define a "hit," e.g., 50% inhibition at 10 uM, but knowing the compound is partially insoluble the "hit" criteria can be adjusted down accordingly.

In the case of mass random screening of libraries including natural products, it is likely that some samples will resist a single standard solubilization routine presenting the option to test partially solubilized compounds or to devote energy to novel solubility schemes. If the library is sufficiently large, the former is generally preferred. While risking false negative results, this decision simplifies testing through the introduction of a common solvent to all assays. In the event that novel schemes are developed, the effects of the required solvents on assay integrity must once again be investigated.

4.2.6 THE ASSAY. The elegance of the binding assay in drug discovery is due to simplicity, sensitivity, precision, high volume and rapid turn-around time. In a typical day it is not unusual for a single individual without automation to process 600–800 individual assay tubes. With automation and miniaturization, 5000 compounds is not unreasonable. The use of high throughput scintillation counters (beta and MicroBeta counters) typically makes data available the following day.

The scheme of a typical binding assay is

straightforward. For assay, tissue preparations containing the receptor of interest are prepared and added to tubes containing the ligand and a small amount of substance being tested. In some tubes, it is useful to include solutions containing various concentrations of a reference agent in order to ensure assay integrity. Likewise, it is useful to generate reference curves on a daily basis using known compounds in order to document the veracity of the test and for comparative reasons.

Final assay volumes are 0.25–1.0 ml, which reduces materials costs and the amount of test compound required. Incubations are routinely performed using duplicate or triplicate tubes, each of which contains identical amounts of ligand, tissue and test agent. Our experience has been that random screening is adequately performed in initial rounds using a single high concentration of test compound. For verification of active compounds, several concentrations are employed, whereas final verification of activity routinely includes a complete (14 point) dose–response evaluation performed on at least two separate occasions. Importantly, verification includes the parallel testing of both the initial solution as well as a new sample prepared on the day of the secondary or tertiary assay.

Following an incubation at the time and temperature appropriate to each assay, reactions are terminated in order to separate bound from free ligand. As mentioned, this is done using one of two methods, centrifugation or filtration. In the former, the incubation mixtures are centrifuged at high speed (e.g., 50,000 g) to pellet the tissue, the incubation solution is decanted, and the pellet is washed rapidly with 5–10 ml of ice-cold assay buffer. The pellet is dissolved in solubilizers, scintillant is added, and the radioactivity contained in the pellet is counted using scintillation spectrophotometry.

In filtration assays, free ligand is separated from the receptor/ligand complex by rapidly filtering the incubation mixtures through an appropriate support, usually a glass fiber filter. The filters are rapidly rinsed with ice cold assay buffer, placed in counting tubes and radioactivity quantified as described above.

From a practical perspective, filtration assays are preferred over centrifugation methods since throughput is increased. Emerging technologies include the development of filter supports which allow direct counting of filters in the absence of scintillation fluor, thus representing a significant cost reduction. When centrifugation assays must be used, commercial equipment and supplies make it possible to perform the entire assay in a centrifugation tube that doubles as a scintillation vial.

4.2.7 DATA ANALYSIS. Output from a typical binding assay is shown in Table 17.5 and is reported as dpm/tube. Tubes 1–3 represent the total amount of ligand bound in the absence of any inhibitory substance. It is assumed to represent the maximum amount of ligand bound under the conditions of the assay. Tubes 4–6 represent the amount of ligand which is nonspecifically bound to components of the assay other than the receptor. This binding may be to filter supports, test tube walls or nonreceptor tissue elements, and is determined by incubating ligand and receptor in the presence of a high concentration of reference agent, typically 1,000-fold the radioligand concentration. Since the concentration of this agent is much greater than the concentration of the ligand, the assumption is made that all receptors are preferentially occupied by the unlabeled material. Tubes 7–33 contain decreasing concentrations of a known reference agent. Note that as the concentration of this agent decreases, the dpm measured correspondingly increases. This results from the mass action principles of equation 17.1, and as the concentration of the reference agent decreases, there is

Table 17.5   Typical Data Report for a High Volume Ligand Binding Assay[a]

Reference Curve

Tube #	[INH]	pico moles IHN/tube	DPM Bound	DPM Specifically Bound	% Inhibition	Log[%INH/(100-%INH)]
1–3	Total		10000			
4–6	Blank (1E-6)	1000	2000	8000	100	
7–9	1E-8	10	2720	720	91	1.005
10–12	7.5E-9	7.5	2720	720	89	0.908
13–15	5E-9	5.0	3320	1320	83.5	0.704
16–18	2.5E-9	2.5	4240	2240	72	0.401
19–21	1E-9	1.0	6000	4000	50	0.0
22–24	7.5E-10	0.75	7760	5760	28	−0.410
24–27	5E-10	0.50	8680	6680	17.5	−0.704
28–30	2.5E-10	0.25	9120	7120	11	−0.908
31–33	1E-10	0.10	9280	7280	9	−1.005

Samples

Tube #	Amount Added	DPM Bound	DPM Specifically Bound	% Inhibition	pmole equivalents sample
34–36	$50\ \mu g$	2160	160	98	
37–39	$5\ \mu g$	7280	6280	66	1.75
40–42	$10^{-5}\,M$	6000	4000	50	
43–45	$10^{-9}\,M$	7760	5760	28	
46–48	$10^{-10}\,M$	8720	6720	16	

[a]The table show an idealized output from a high volume screening assay. Details of data analysis are described in Section 3.

an increasing probability that the radiolabeled ligand will bind to the receptor. The final tubes (34–48) contain the substance/s of interest.

Data analysis begins with the determination of the amount of ligand specifically bund to the receptor. This is the difference in the total and nonspecific (blank) dpm (column 5, row B). Second, nonspecific binding is subtracted from each of the remaining values showed in column 4. Finally, for each concentration of reference agent or sample, the specifically bound dpm are divided by the value for the total specific binding of the ligand (column 5;

row B) and multiplied by 100 to yield the percent inhibition of total binding at each concentration of inhibitor or sample.

As shown in Figure 17.11A, these data are plotted on semi-log paper to yield the sigmoidal curve characteristic of binding reactions. To simplify data analysis, a linear transformation as shown in Figure 17.11B is useful. This is achieved by applying equation 17.2 to the values in column 6 of Table 17.3. Alternatively, the log concentration of the reference agent can be directly plotted against the percent inhibition using log–logit paper (or appropriate software packages are used). As a final

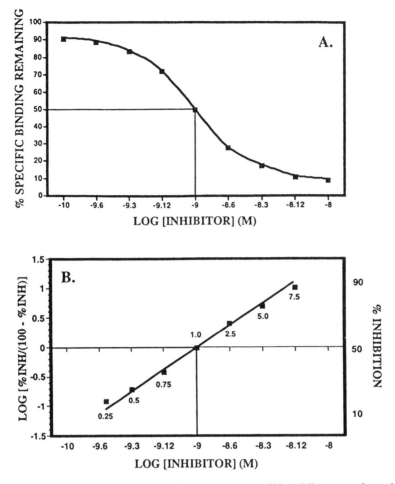

Fig. 17.11 Theoretical log-concentration response curve (A) and linear transformation.

step, it is necessary to determine if test samples inhibited binding. This is done as described above.

As shown in Table 17.5, the amount of reference agent added to each tube of the standard curve can be expressed as either a concentration or absolute amount. If the identity of the substance is unknown, as may be the case when screening natural product extracts, an arbitrary value is assigned to describe compound activity (e.g., mg/mL). If the identity of the tested substance is known, an exact concentration versus inhibition value is determined.

In today's world of high volume screening there are a multitude of software packages available for data reduction purposes. In our own laboratories, information from scintillation counters is fed in real time to a central computing facility. Proprietary software automatically calculates percent inhibition for each compound, reduces and graphs the reference curve, identifies incubation sets with unacceptable variance among triplicate tubes, compares IC_{50}s and ligand concentration to the sum of the historical database, and presents the final results in both tabular and graphical form.

4.2.8   ROLE OF SAMPLE HANDLING, DATA MANAGEMENT AND AUTOMATION.   The mass ligand screening assay is simple and straightforward but not problem free, particularly in the setup stage, posing problems not associated with low volume "systems" approaches. These include the logistics of sample handling and data generation for thousands of compounds screened against a target in rapid succession. To aid in the management of such a task automated or semi-automated work stations have been designed as well as a number of computer support programs. It should be stressed that the types of automation equipment available today have increased productivity by minimizing many of the labor intensive aspects of screening without losing the required accuracy. Much of the automation revolves around methods which can efficiently and accurately weigh compounds, solubilize, and then disburse them in the format required for testing. Such advances can certainly not be characterized as gadget optimization as has been suggested in the past (51).

The actual weighing of 10,000 or more compounds is often the rate limiting step in a mass ligand screening effort. Several short cuts are routinely used to ease the burden on this particular resource. The most obvious is a "scoop" weighing technique in which every compound in a chemical library is assumed to have an identical molecular weight; for a synthetic library the weight choice is usually anywhere between 300 and 1,000. Following disbursement each compound is solubilized using a standardized format. More accurate weighings can be made if any verification work is needed.

There are numerous commercially available software packages which can interpret and collate the large volume of data generated in a mass ligand screen. Most often packages are modified to meet the individual needs of the user. Each data report should detail each compound's solubility, inhibitory activity, and the assays positive control data and specific binding signal. More elaborate and useful information can be obtained by cross referencing to historical parameters of the assay. These measures afford the researcher a means to assess the overall quality of the data being generated. The ability to rapidly determine the activity of a "hit" in other assays it may have been previously run in and the structure of the "hit" are valuable pieces of information when determining potential interest from a pharmacological standpoint. By expanding the structural search to look for similar compounds in the library preliminary structure activity (SAR), studies can be initiated without direct chemistry support.

In the field of drug discovery, mass ligand screening is an approach where pharmacology, technology and serendipity co-exist in a productive manner. This requires that diverse disciplines work together to produce a system which is first and foremost driven by pharmacology. The use of automation must not compromise the scientific validity of the assay solely for the sake of increasing sample throughput. The random nature of high volume screening suggests that the probability of success is directly proportional to the number of compounds screened. However, a successful high volume screening system will be defined by the compounds it places in development not the number of compounds screened. Pharmacology must never be sacrificed solely for the sake of increased throughput.

5 CHEMICAL LIBRARIES

5.1 Synthetic Libraries

Success in drug discovery has often been hindered by limited access to diverse chemical libraries. This limitation was amplified by the advent of mass ligand screening efforts which could examine up to a quarter of a million compounds, entire libraries, in a year. In the early 1900s the need to synthesize and test numerous chemical derivatives of existing drugs as a means to discover new drugs was stressed by pharmacologists. In today's pharmaceutical industry this strategy is often predisposed to the identification of "follows the leader" or "me too" drug discovery, i.e., second generation benzodiazepines and dihydropyridines. These types of success are now often labeled as scientifically undemanding and redundant. More importantly this approach can restrict the number of different structural classes in any one chemical library. Many of these libraries were expanded based on the use of proprietary "biological" heterocycles, i.e., quinazolones, benzodiazepines, and dihydropyridines (Fig. 17.12), and this lack of structural diversity has contributed to the limited number of early successes reported using mass ligand screening at such targets as corticotropin releasing factor, bradykinin, neuropeptide Y antagonist/agonists.

Unfortunately, the problem of increasing the structural diversification of a library cannot be rectified by simply renaming the "me too" chemistry, i.e., "analog research," "directed chemical analysis", "molecular modification," or "secondary structural diversification," and keep pace with the increasing demand for therapeutic

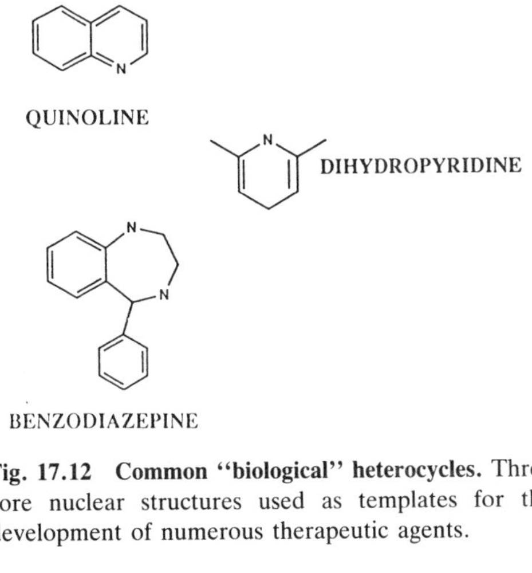

QUINOLINE

DIHYDROPYRIDINE

BENZODIAZEPINE

Fig. 17.12 Common "biological" heterocycles. Three core nuclear structures used as templates for the development of numerous therapeutic agents.

agents targeting novel MOAs. However, this practice will remain a major contributor to library expansion for several very good reasons. Legally, secondary structural diversification is crucial to expanding the breadth of protection provided by a patent before filing. Pharmacologically it aids in the continuing search for chemical backups with enhanced potency, selectivity, and/or bioavailability. Therefore it is easy to understand why many chemical libraries developed solely "in house" will often have a high degree of secondary structural diversity but may lack structural class diversification.

The combination of high throughput screening and the increasing number of novel MOAs being targeted has dramatically increased the demand for new alternatives to increase the number of compounds and the diversity of structural classes within a library. This demand can be met in several ways, including scale up of "in house" synthesis capacities, active chemical acquisition programs, and novel library generation (i.e., peptides and oligonucleotides). Pfizer's substance P (28) and Sanofi's neurotensin (30) antagonists appear to be an example of success through diversification of a library with compounds which are not routinely classified as "biological" heterocycles (Fig. 17.13). "In house" scale up utilizing the traditional pharmaceutical approach may be the least effective option when trying to increase the structural class diversity of a chemical library. The dedication of a chemistry group using traditional methods to generate random structural classes of compounds might seem inappropriate given the limited return that can be expected on the investment. High quality mass ligand screens routinely identify hits in a random screen at a frequency of 1 or 2 per 10,000 compounds screened. A more effective approach envisioned would allow for the rapid generation of hundreds of random structural modifications around a core chemical struc-

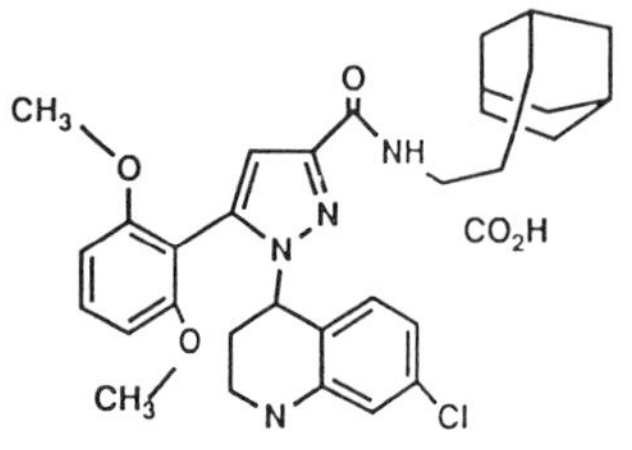

SR 48692

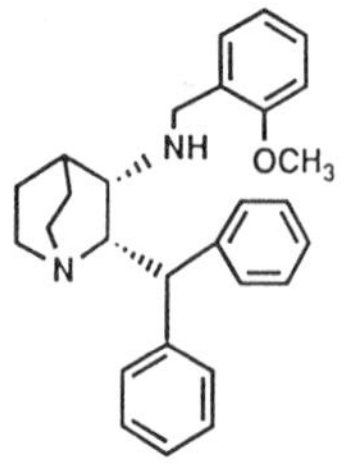

CP 96,345

Fig. 17.13 Unique nonpeptide receptor antagonists. SR 48692, a neurotensin antagonist, and CP 96,345, a substance P antagonist, are nonpeptide structures identified by mass ligand screening of compound libraries consisting of more than "biological" heterocycles.

ture or template. A prototype of this technology has been reported (52) using a benzodiazipine-like core structure and solid state chemistry. Using such a scheme it is possible to envision the rapid expansion, in terms of shear numbers and secondary structural diversity, of a library. Equally important, given the relatively short period of time needed to complete secondary structural diversification, would be the ability to use many different and attractive core structures to increase structural class diversity of a library.

Another approach, a potentially inappropriate one, in dealing with a chemical library of limited structural class diversity is to eliminate redundancy of pre-selection of compounds in an attempt to represent each of the different structural classes or "cores" within a library. Using this approach it is

possible to reduce the number of compounds screened from 100,000 to 10,000. This approach is questionable for several reasons. First, mass ligand screening is a rapid (thousands of compounds can be examined in one week) and cost effective approach (cost per compound screened decreases as sample number increases), eliminating the need for preselection based on logistical/financial concerns. Second, and more importantly, the preselection of compounds may be inappropriate given the limited information compiled on the structural conformation and requirements of the actual ligand binding domains for the vast majority of identified receptors and/or enzymes. The potential for a minor or secondary structural modification having significant impact on pharmacological properties of a core structure should and cannot be ignored. Overall, preselection can be an intellectually naive and time consuming process which will limit the serendipitous nature, and success rate, of a mass ligand screening effort. Serendipity and the law of averages suggests that an increase in the number compounds screened will increase the probability for successfully identifying a biologically active compound, i.e., "hit." Without preselection, compound elimination is more appropriately made only after initial screening data has been reviewed, reducing the chance of intellectual naivete playing a significant and defeating role. This does not mean that certain chemical structures cannot and should not be removed from the screening queue because they have no demonstrated pharmaceutical application, i.e., alkylating agents, but once again, the logistics required to remove them may not be worth the effort from a technical standpoint. In addition, such compounds identified in a screen may serve as first generation molecular tools needed to examine and expand the knowledge about a particular ligand/receptor interaction.

5.2 Novel Libraries (Combinatorials)

Numerous biotechnology companies have been focusing on the generation of combinatorial libraries consisting of small peptides to oligonucleotides as a means of diversifying available libraries to screen. Companies such as AffyMax, Houghton, Gilead, Chiron, and Selectide, are now generating combinatorial libraries using a variety of proprietary technologies. These include supported (53) and nonsupported (54) peptide generation methods and more recently phage expression systems (55). At the present time the feasibility of this approach does not appear to be limited by the generation of the libraries but by the development of mass ligand screens, which are capable of generating useful data. Demonstrated successes of this integration routinely focus on screening based on antibody/antigen interactions, e.g. beta endorphins (53) with only limited success with ligand/receptor interactions (54)

Combinatorial libraries present unique challenges to mass ligand screening approaches because each sample to be tested can be composed of thousands of different entities. Theoretically this format would allow for the examination of tens of millions of peptides without placing undo stress on a screening system with a throughput capacity as low as 1,000 samples per week.

Technically the ability to accurately identify an active compound or hit among thousands of compounds making up any one sample can be a logistic nightmare requiring a comprehensive and time consuming process of iteration, resynthesis, and rescreening. Even if the logistics can be worked out it will remain a difficult process to isolate the actual hit. The actual number of entities generated, as opposed to the theoretical number, in a combinatorial library can be smaller if the foundation, i.e., inorganic bead on which individual peptides or oligonucleotides are synthesized, places conformational restrictions on the synthetic process. In the process of actually screening these combinatorial libraries, nonspecific interactions resulting from possible decreases in solubility and increases in solution viscosity of these primordial soups, could compromise the assay. Most important is the fact that any one peptide or oligonucleotide in these mixtures will have maximal concentration levels below the levels necessary for micromolar detection. Depending on the number of different entities in a single sample it might be impossible to generate concentrations greater then 10–$100 \, nM$ for any one entity in a sample mixture. If 1,000 entities comprise a sample and the absolute concentration of that sample is $100 \, uM$, each individual entity will be present at $100 \, nM$. Taking into account the numerous studies which suggest that IC_{50} values commonly reported for such small linear peptide entities are typically in the uM range, actual hits may go undetected. The antibody/antigen successes and Houghton's potent μ-opioidlike hexapeptide appear to be exceptions to this issue, but may only be the result of screening for particularly favorable examples: the antibody recognition sites for an antigen, and endogenous ligands for the opioid receptors peptide sequences typically consisting of five to ten amino acids. Is a $28 \, nM$ u-opioidlike hexapeptide useful to a drug discovery effort, considering that 1–$5 \, nM$ endogenous pentapeptides were isolated in the late 1970s (56)? More crucial tests of the technology will center around the use of nonpeptide receptors or growth factor receptors for which existing pentamers and hexamers currently do not exist, and the design and implementation of strategies to synthesize peptide analogues, which are structurally more interesting than flexible penta- or hexapeptides. These approaches will more accurately reflect the utility of these libraries for drug discovery efforts supported by mass ligand screening.

It is widely acknowledged that peptides and proteins are not the first choice when designing therapeutic agents for a number of reasons including limitations in oral administration, high doses needed to overcome rapid degradation due to proteolytic activity following administration, and the high cost of production and use. Small peptides often have a high degree of flexibility and proteins are so large it is often difficult to determine the epitope necessary for binding. These factors suggest they can be of limited value in RDD where the stated intent has been to use them as templates for a modeling and computational chemistry effort trying to design nonpeptide drugs. This task is extremely difficult given the limited structural information which can be acquired from these small linear entities. Numerous biotechnology groups have been established on the premise that peptides or their analogs may be good therapeutic agents and possibly templates from which to design more traditional nonpeptide drugs, e.g., Nova, Hoechst, and Cortex Pharmaceutical's bradykinin antagonist programs. However, the majority of reported successes has been in the making of metabolically stable peptidomimetic compounds, and not the discovery of non-peptide leads or drugs. These peptidomimetic successes appear to be the result of traditional peptide chemistry approaches which take into account basic knowledge of protein conformational states and charge interactions before making semirandom amino acid insertions or deletions in a known sequence, and not RRD.

Many pharmaceutical companies are now actively attempting to acquire nonpharmaceutical chemical libraries, e.g., agricultural, photochemical, for the purpose of diversification. However, it is often difficult to gain access to these libraries as their owners become increasingly aware of

what they perceive as their value. It is difficult for nonpharmaceutical companies to establish the true value of their synthetic chemical libraries when their decision process focuses on the reported sales of blockbuster drugs. This often results in the gross overestimation of a library's actual value. The Kodak/Sterling merger is an excellent example of a large and diverse chemical library and a competent pharmaceutical entity, but to date, no blockbuster drug. Therefore, a more sobering and probable scenario which could be used when attempting to determine a synthetic chemical library's value includes in the equation a factor to adjust for the reality that the vast majority of nonpharmaceutical chemical libraries might never yield a blockbuster drug or even a marginally profitable drug.

5.3 Natural Produce Libraries

Natural product libraries can supply high throughput screening efforts with a large number of diverse chemical structures necessary for a successful program. A random, and by no means complete, sampling of drugs which have recently been identified through the screening of natural product libraries illustrates this point quite nicely: Lovastatin (cholesterol lowering), Taxol (certain types of cancer), Cyclosporin A and FK 506 (immunosurpression in transplantation), and the avermectins (anthelmintics). This list, along with the historic examples, such as morphine and aspirin, suggests that natural product libraries are extremely valuable resources which may be underutilized by the pharmaceutical industry. However, there are reasons for this underutilization. Different types of natural product libraries have different levels of value. Such things as the origin of the library are important and medicinal folklore information can add significant value to a library. The logistics of collection must be taken into account, centering on the ability to recollect interesting species for follow up work on compound identification. Compounds of interest may exist as a minute percentage of the biomass of a particular plant and be undetectable, given the sensitivity of the mass ligand screen. This is similar to the problem previously discussed for the synthetic combinatorial libraries with one notable exception: it is not uncommon for natural product entities to have nanomolar IC_{50}s at a receptor site, e.g., morphine.

There are numerous methods for extracting natural products to be screened, and each different procedure often results in a different profile of extracted compounds. The use of the wrong type of extraction could result in eliminating a potentially interesting compound from the screening mixture. Another pitfall of this method is that uncommon chemical structures often found in natural product extracts may limit the ability to synthesize the compounds in the laboratory at the scale necessary for drug development. This problem is compounded when the natural product source is limited. Taxol, a potential anticancer drug, is an excellent example of a limited natural product resource, the Pacific yew tree, taxus brevifola, and a structure which is exceedingly difficult to synthesize in the laboratory (Fig. 17.14)

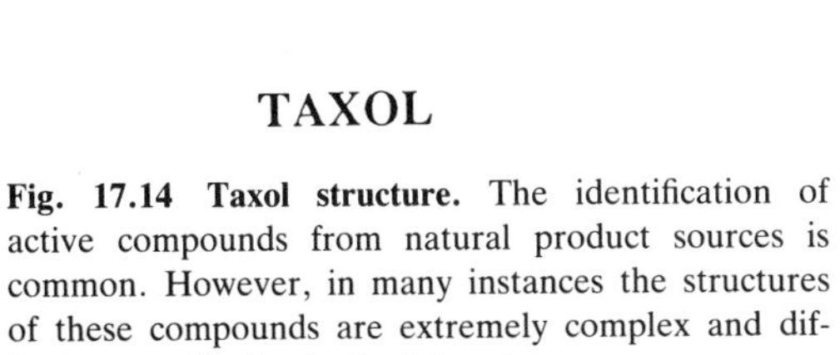

TAXOL

Fig. 17.14 Taxol structure. The identification of active compounds from natural product sources is common. However, in many instances the structures of these compounds are extremely complex and difficult to synthesize in the laboratory.

(57). This has resulted in the search for an alternative source of taxol or a more common compound with a similar enough structure to provide a template from which a simplified synthetic scheme can be designed. Another approach centers around efforts to produce taxol in a plant tissue culture system. A final and crucial problem is the apparent lack of natural product chemists available to meet the growing demands of the pharmaceutical industry.

A number of biotechnology and pharmaceutical companies are focusing on acquiring and screening natural product libraries. Merck has long been considered a leader in natural product drug discovery and has recently solidified their position by entering into agreement with Costa Rica's Institute for Biodiversity. Other industry giants, i.e., Eli Lilly, Smith Kline Beecham, and Glaxo, are attempting to increase the value of their libraries by the addition of unique natural products, i.e., marine microorganisms, amphibian and insect toxins, exotic terrestrial plant extracts, Abbott and Sterling are actively producing microbial fermentation broths or brews, historically excellent sources of antibiotics, on the assumption that these libraries may yield exciting compounds which interact with new and novel target mechanisms now available. A potential problem using microbials centers around the utility of chemical structures classically produced during fermentation, i.e., the macrolides, tetracyclines and beta lactams, to be effective nonantibiotic therapeutics. Once again this type of criticism must be tempered by the level of intellectual naivete concerning the structural requirements of ligand/receptor interactions.

As suggested by the potential therapeutic agents listed above, natural product libraries are indeed an excellent source of potentially novel therapeutics. However, the complexity in dealing with these libraries is a magnitude of order more difficult then dealing with a synthetic library.

This issue should be explained closely before a strong commitment is made to actively screen such libraries.

6 SUMMARY

The sole objective of today's pharmaceutical industry is the identification and introduction of new therapeutics to improve quality of life. The various pressures and constraints being placed on the industry from the various scientific, political and social theaters does not alter the fact that this work must be accomplished in a rapid, reliable, and cost effective manner. To this end, the simplicity of the radioligand binding assay makes it an outstanding and proven resource to aid in the identification of potential lead compounds and assist in monitoring the progress of potential leads through the early stages of drug discovery. Successful mass ligand screening requires the integration of pharmacology, automation, and data management, as well as the efficient management and handling of the chemical library to be screened. The lack of expertise in any of these areas will limit the establishment of a successful program. Equally important is the acceptance and support of mass ligand screening technology by all levels of the organization, i.e., screening, project teams, and management. Certain uses of a mass ligand screening system, e.g., searches for receptor agonists, since they have a greater chance of failure than searches for a receptor antagonists, may be inappropriate uses of this resource. When judging the success of a mass ligand screen one must take into account the objectives being set. The inability of a mass ligand screen to identify a lead following an intensive screening effort should not be judged as a failure, if the assay was pharmacologically valid; in reality a nonsuccessful screen is a direct reflection on the library. Equally dangerous is the thought that mass ligand screening should be judged solely on the rate at which the screening of a library can be completed. It must be emphasized that a successful mass ligand screening program will ultimately be defined by its scientific integrity and the identification of actual lead chemical entities which can be placed in the research and development pipeline, and not theoretical arguments justifying failure or success.

REFERENCES

1. T. F. Blaske and K. L. Melmon in A. G. Gilman, L. S. Goodman, and A. Gilman, Eds., *The Pharmacological Basis of Therapeutics*, Macmillan Publishing Co., Inc., 1980, p. 763.
2. J. A. Oates, L. Gillespie, and S. Undenfriend, *Science* **131**, 1890 (1960).
3. P. Calabresi and R. E. Parks Jr. in Ref. 2, 1980, p. 1256.
4. S. M. Stahl, *Psycho. Pharm. Bull.*, **28**, 3 (1992).
5. J. C. Ventor and L. C. Harrison, Eds., *Molecular and Chemical Characterization of Membrane Receptors*, Alan L. Liss, New York.
6. A. Oliff, *Cell*, **54**, 141 (1988).
7. R. S. Baldessarini, in Ref. 1, 1980, p. 391.
8. W. Haefly in M. J. Parnham and J. Bruinels, Eds., *Discoveries in Pharmacology*, Elsevier, Amsterdam, Vol. 1, 1983, p. 269.
9. E. Usdin in J. B. Malick, S. J. Enna, and H. I. Yamamura, Eds., *Anxiolytics: Neurochemical Behavioral, and Clinical Perspectives*, Raven Press, New York, 1983, p. 1.
10. R. F. Squires and C. Braestrup, *Nature*, **266**, 732 (1977).
11. R. M. Burch, M. Weitzberg, N. Blok, R. Mulhauser, F. Martin, S. G. Farmer, J. M. Bator, J. R. Connor, C. Ko, W. Kuhn, B. A. MacMillan, M. Raynor, B. G. Shearer, C. Tiffany, and D. E. Wilkins, *Proc. Natl. Acad. Sci. USA*, **88**, 355 (1991).
12. R. M. Burch, M. Wietzberg, L. Noronha-Blob, V. C. Lowe, J. M. Bator, J. Perumattam, and J. P. Sullivan, 'Looking ahead,' *Drug News and Perspectives*, 1991.
13. C. R. Mackay and B. A. Imhof, *Immunol. Today*, **14**, 99 (1993).
14. C. T. Easton, F. W. Bonner, and D. V. Parke, *Regulatory Toxicol. and Pharmacol.*, **11**, 288 (1990).
15. E. J. Ariens, *TiPS*, **1**, 11 (1979).

16. P. M. Sweetnam, C. Bauer Jr. and M. Charlton in M. Kapis. Ed. *Non-Animal Techniques in Biomedical and Behavioral Research and Testing*, Lewis Publishers, Boca Raton, Fl., 1993, p. 43.

17. L. F. Kuyper, B. Roth, D. P. Baccanari, R. Ferrone, C. R. Beddell, J. N. Champness. D. K. Stammers, J. G. Dann., F. E. Norrington, D. J. Baker, and P. J. Goodford, *J. Med. Chem.*, **28**, 303 (1985).

18. J. A. Martin, *Antiviral Res.*, **17**, 165 (1992).

19. W. H. J. Ward, D. Timms, and A. R. Fersht, *TiPS*, **11**, 280 (1990).

20. T. M. Fong, M. A. Casieri, H. Yu, A. Bansal, C. Swain, and C. D. Strader, *Nature*, **362**, 350 (1993).

21. A. L. Kopin, Y.-M. Lee, E. W. McBride, L. J. Miller, M. Lu, H. Y. Lin, L. F. Kolakowski, Jr., and M. Beinborn, *Proc. Natl. Acad. Sci. USA*, **89**, 3605 (1992).

22. M. Williams and P. L. Woods C in A. A. Boulton, G. B. Baker, and P. D. Hrdina, Eds., *Neuromethods*, Humana Press, New Jersey, Vol. 4, 1986, p. 543.

23. R. A. Maxwell, *Drug. Develp. Res.*, **4**, 375 (1984).

24. R. N. Re, *The Scientist*, **1**, 19 (Oct. 5, 1987).

25. P. Jannsen, quoted in *Scrip*, **1258**, 9 (1987).

26. R. M. Burch, *J. Receptor Res.*, **11**, 101 (1991).

27. R. M. Snider, D. A. Pereira, K. P. Longo, R. E. Davidson, F. J. Vinick, K. Laitinen, E. Genc-Sehitoglu, and J. N. Crawley, *Bioorg. and Med. Chem. Letts.*, **2**, 1535 (1992).

28. R. M. Snider, J. W. Constantine, J. A. Lowe III, K. P. Longo, W. S. Lebel, H. A. Woody, S. E. Drozda, M. C. Desai, F. J. Vinick, R. W. Spencer, and H.-J. Hess, *Science*, **251**, 435 (1991).

29. R. S. L. Chang, V. J. Lotti, R. L. Monaghan, J. Birnbaum, E. O. Sharply, M. A. Goetz, G. Albers-Schonberg, A. A. Patchett, J. M. Liesch, O. D. Hensens, and J. P. Springer, *Science*, **230**, 177 (1985).

30. D. Gully, M. Canton, R. Boigegrain, F. Jeanjean, J.-C. Molimard, M. Poncelet, C. Guedet, M. Heulme, R. Leyris, A. Brourard, D. Pelaprat, C. Labbe-Jullie, J. Mazella, P. Soubrie, J.-P. Maffrand, W. Rostene, P. Kitabgi, and G. Le Fur, *Proc. Natl. Acad. Sci. U.S.A.*, **90**, 65 (1993).

31. J. R. Buzow, H. H. M. Van Tol, D. R. Grady, P. Albert, J. Salon, M. Christie, C. A. Machida, K. A. Neve, and O. Civelli, *Nature*, **336**, 783 (1988).

32. F. J. Monsma Jr, Y. Shen, R. P. Ward, M. W. Hamblin, and D. R. Sibley, *Mol. Pharm.*, **43**, 320 (1993).

33. T. L. Swanson and C. L. Green, *Gen. Pharmacol.*, **17**, 225 (1986).

34. A. Scriabine, Ed., *New Drugs: Cardiovascular Drugs*, Vol. 2, Raven Press, New York, 1984.

35. B. A. Bunin and G. S. Allen, in R. H. Wilkens, Ed., *Cerebral Atrerial Spasm*, Wilkens and Wilkens, Baltimore, Md, 1980 p. 527.

36. M. J. Cain, R. K. Garlick, and P. M. Sweetnam, *J. Cardiovasc. Pharm.*, **17**, S150 (1991).

37. T. Masaki, *J. Cardiovasc. Pharm.*, **17**, S1 (1991).

38. T. P. Kenakin, *Pharmacologic Analysis of Drug-Receptor Interaction*, Raven Press, New York, 1987.

39. A. J. Clark, *The Mode of Action of Drugs on Cells*, Edward Arnold, London, 1933.

40. E. J. Ariens, *TiPS*, **1**, 11 (1979).

41. J.-P. Changeux, M. Kasai, M. Huchet, and J.-C. Meuneir, *C.R. Acad. Sci. Paris*, **270**, 2864 (1970).

42. S. H. Snyder, *Science*, **224**, 22 (1984).

43. S. H. Snyder, *J. Med. Chem.*, **26**, 1667 (1983).

44. J. P. Bennett Jr. in H. I. Yamamura, S. J. Enna, and M. J. Kuhar, Eds., *Neurotransmitter Receptor Binding*, Raven Press, New York, 1978, p. 57.

45. J. W. Ferkany in A. A. Boulton, G. Baker, and J. Wood, Eds., *Neuromethods*, Humana Press, N.J., 1985, p. 117.

46. L. P. To, V. Balasubramanian, M. E. Charlton, T. A. Franncis, C. Doyle, and P. M. Sweetnam, *J. Immunoassay*, **13**, 61 (1992).

47. L. Weston, M. Connolly, and P. M. Sweetnam, *Soc. Neurosci. Abstr.*, **16**, 286.9 (1990).

48. Y. C. Cheng and W. H. Prusoff, *Biochem. Pharmacol.*, **22**, 3099 (1973).

49. P. M. Sweetnam, E. Nestler, P. A. Gallombardo, S. Brown, H. Bracha, and J. Tallman, *Mol. Brain Res.*, **2**, 223 (1986).

50. P. M. Sweetnam, L. Caldwell, J. Lancaster, C. Bauer Jr., B. McMillam, W. J. Conner, and C. H. Price, *J. Nat. Prod.* **56**, 441 (1993).

51. R. M. Burch and D. J. Kyle, *Pharm. Res.*, **8**, 141 (1991).

52. B. A. Bunin and J. A. Ellman, *J. Amer. Chem. Soc.*, **114**, 10997 (1992).

53. R. W. Barrett, *Rapid Functional Screening for Drug Development*, IC USA Conferences, San Diego, Calif., 1992.

54. R. A. Houghton, J. R. App, S. E. Blondelee, J. H. Cuervo, C. T. Dooley, and C. Pinilla, *Peptide Res.*, **5**, 351 (1992).

55. G. P. Smith, *Science*, **258**, 381 (1992).

56. H. W. Kosterlitz and J. Hughes, *Science*, **17**, 91 (1975).

57. S. Borman, *Chem. and Engineering News*, 30 (Oct. 12, 1992).

CHAPTER EIGHTEEN

Approaches to the Rational Design of Enzyme Inhibitors

ANGELIKA MUSCATE and
GEORGE L. KENYON

Department of Pharmaceutical Chemistry
University of California
San Francisco, California, USA

Burger's Medicinal Chemistry and Drug Discovery,
Fifth Edition, Volume 1: Principles and Practice,
Edited by Manfred E. Wolff.
ISBN 0-471-57556-9 © 1995 John Wiley & Sons, Inc.

CONTENTS

1 Introduction, 734
  1.1 Enzyme inhibitors in medicine, 734
  1.1 Enzyme inhibitors in basic research, 737
2 Rational Design of Noncovalently Binding Enzyme
  Inhibitors, 738
  2.1 Relevant forces for formation of enzyme
    inhibitor complexes, 738
    2.1.1 Electrostatic forces, 739
    2.1.2 Dispersion forces, 739
    2.1.3 Hydrophobic interactions, 739
    2.1.4 Hydrogen bonds, 740
  2.2 Rapid, reversible inhibitors, 740
    2.2.1 Design of rapid, reversible
      inhibitors, 740
    2.2.2 Kinetics, 741
    2.2.3 Types of rapid, reversible inhibitors, 742
    2.2.4 IC_{50} values, 745
    2.2.5 Examples, 746
  2.3 Slow, tight, and slow-tight binding
    inhibitors, 748
    2.3.1 Slow-binding inhibitors, 749
    2.3.2 Examples, 750
  2.4 Transition state analogs, 752
    2.4.1 Examples, 755
  2.5 Multisubstrate inhibitors, 757
    2.5.1 Examples, 759
3 Rational Design of Covalently Binding Enzyme
  Inhibitors, 761
  3.1 Evaluation of the mechanism of inactivation of
    covalently binding enzyme inhibitors, 762

3.2 Mechanism-based inhibitors, 767
   3.2.1 Examples, 767
3.3 Affinity labels, 774
   3.3.1 Examples, 775
3.4 Pseudoirreversible inhibitors, 777
   3.4.1 Examples, 777
4 Conclusions, 779

1 INTRODUCTION

About half of the top 20 drugs sold worldwide are enzyme inhibitors. In recent years, enzyme inhibitors not only have provided an increasing number of potent therapeutic agents for the treatment of diseases, but also have significantly advanced the understanding of enzymatic transformations. The aim of this chapter is to present current approaches to so-called rational inhibitor design, which uses knowledge of enzymic mechanisms and structures in the design process. Rational inhibitor design is intended to complement laborious and resource-consuming screening processes, which consist of testing large numbers of synthetic chemicals or natural products for inhibitory activity against a chosen target enzyme (Chapter 17). Defining criteria for choices of target enzymes for chemotherapy is beyond the scope of this review; many target enzymes are highlighted, however.

1.1 Enzyme Inhibitors in Medicine

Inhibitors of a single enzyme or group of enzymes have great potential as drugs by selectively blocking certain metabolic pathways, decreasing the concentration of enzymatic products, or increasing the concentrations of enzymatic substrates. The effectiveness of an enzyme inhibitor as a drug is dependent upon its potency and specificity towards its target enzyme. High specificity will generally avoid depletion of

the inhibitor concentrations in the host by nonspecific pathways. If the inhibitor reacts only with its target enzyme and not with other sites in the body (and can be given in low doses), toxicity caused by inhibition of other vital enzymes and the formation of toxic decomposition products can often be avoided. Good bioavailability of the drug is also crucial for the drug to reach its site of action in the body in effective therapeutic concentrations. For example, highly polar or charged compounds, such as phosphorylated compounds, frequently cannot readily cross cell membranes and are therefore generally less useful as drugs. Approaches to facilitate the transport of this class of compounds into the cell include the use of liposomes or permeabilizing cell membranes (1–4).

An important area of drug design is the development of agents against microorganisms (bacteria and viruses) and parasites in humans. This can involve the inhibition of an essential enzyme in the pathogen which does not exist in the host, resulting in very little cell toxicity. For example, alanine racemase exists in bacteria but not in humans. Thus, inhibitors of this enzyme serve as good antibacterial agents, such as, for example, L-Ala-P (1) against gram-positive alanine racemases (Fig. 18.1) (5). β-Lactamases, bacterial enzymes also not found in humans, are another important target for drug design. Inhibitors of this enzyme include clavulanic acid (2) (6–10) and sulbactam (penicillanic acid sulfone) (3) (9, 11–14) (Fig. 18.1). These two drugs act by preventing the bacterial degradation of penicillins and cephalosporins by β-lactamases, and have reached the market as synergistic drugs of these commonly prescribed antibacterial agents.

Other target enzymes exist as different isozymes in the pathogen and in the host. A highly specific inhibitor may be able to exploit existing subtle structural differences between these isozymes, yielding an enzyme inhibitor which preferentially binds to the invader's version. Trimethoprim (**4**), for example, an inhibitor of dihydrofolate reductase, is a potent antibacterial agent because of its several thousand-fold stronger binding affinity for the invader's version of the enzyme (Fig. 18.1) (15). Another recent example is acyclovir, (9-(2-hydroxyethyl)-methylguanine, **5a**), an antiviral drug used for the treatment of herpes infections (16) (Fig. 18.1). It binds very tightly to the *Herpes simplex* DNA

polymerase with an estimated half-life of about 40 days. Acyclovir is a prodrug (Chapter 23) because it requires transformation by a viral thymine kinase and cellular phosphotransferases to the corresponding triphosphate (**5b**) in order to serve *in vivo* as an inhibitor of the viral DNA polymerase. Another example is α-difluoromethylornithine (**6**, DMFO), an inhibitor of ornithine decarboxylase, an enzyme found in such organisms as protozoa that cause diseases like the African sleeping sickness. DMFO also inhibits *Pneumocystis carinii*, an infective organism associated with the acquired immune deficiency syndrome (AIDS). DMFO is such a highly specific inhibitor that it can be administered in doses of 30 g per day for several weeks with only minor side affects (17,18).

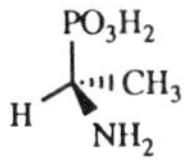

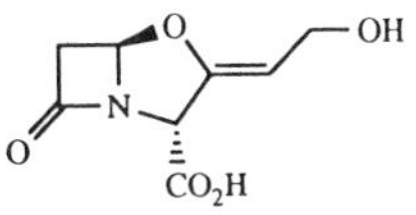

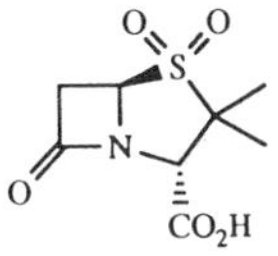

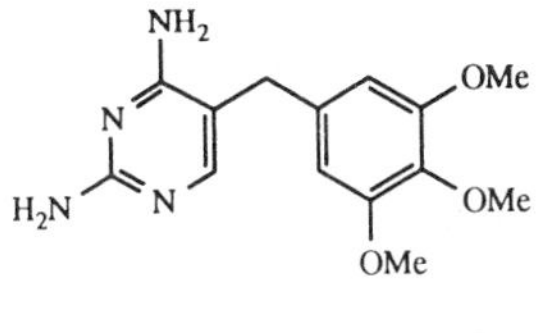

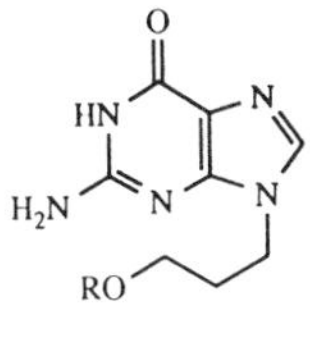

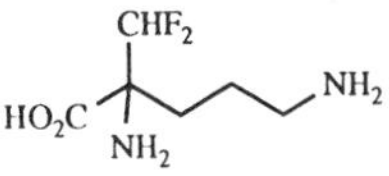

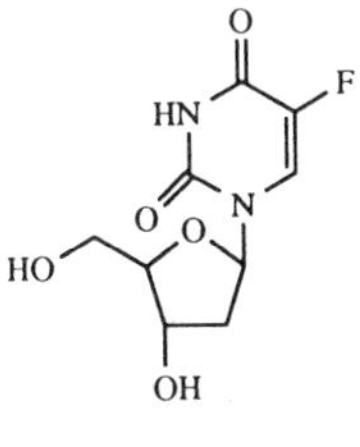

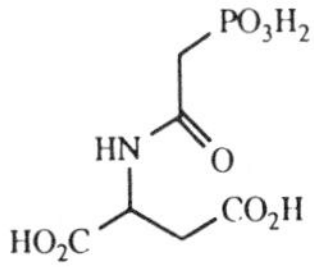

Fig. 18.1 Enzyme inhibitors used as drugs.

Another class of therapeutic agents consists of anticancer agents which are designed to kill tumor cells selectively without harming the normal cells in the organism. Unfortunately, the identification of appropriate target isozymes in tumor cells appears to be quite challenging. Consequently, most of the antitumor agents used today are so-called antiproliferative agents which take advantage of the fact that tumor cells grow and divide much faster than normal cells. Because many normal cells also continue to divide, however, these agents usually show significant cell toxicity. Particularly affected are bone marrow stem and epithelial cells. Antitumor drugs of this class are DMFO (**6**), 5-fluoro-2′-deoxyuridylate (**7**) (19), an inactivator of thymidylate synthase, and phosphonoacetyl-L-aspartate (**8**) (20), an inhibitor of L-aspartate transcarbamoylase (Fig. 18.1).

A number of diseases have been correlated with either the dysfunction of an enzyme or an imbalance of metabolites, and can often be treated by the inhibition of a particular enzyme, either by causing the blockage of a metabolic pathway or by regulating the metabolite concentration in the body. For example, inhibition of angiotension converting enzyme (ACE) has been correlated with the treatment of hypertension and congestive heart failure in humans. Captopril (**9**) (21) and enalapril (**10**) (22) were the first two orally active ACE inhibitors (Fig. 18.2). Inactivators of monoamine oxidase such as tranylcypromine (*trans*-2-phenylcyclopropylamine, **11**) (23, 24) and phenelzine (2-phenylethylhydrazine, **12**) (25,26), are potent antidepressant agents (Fig. 18.2). Compactin (**13a**) and mevinolin (**13b**) are inhibitors of HGM-CoA reductase and act as serum cholesterol lowering agents (27, 28). Catalysis by this enzyme is the rate-determining step in steroid biogenesis. Inhibitors of γ-aminobutyric acid aminotransferase are antiepileptic candidates. An imbalance of the two neurotransmitters, glutamate and γ-aminobutyric acid, is responsible for the epileptic convulsions. Inhibition of γ-aminobutyric acid aminotransferase by vigabatrin (4-amino-4-hexenoic acid, **14**) (29) leads to an increase of the concentration of its substrate, γ-aminobutyric acid, which causes these convulsions to cease (Fig. 18.2).

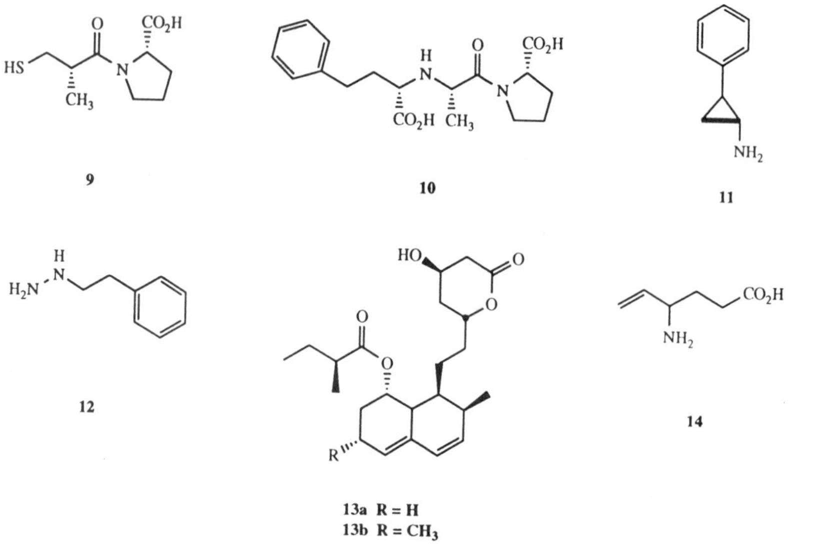

9

10

11

12

13a R = H
13b R = CH₃

14

Fig. 18.2 Enzyme inhibitors used in medicine.

1.2 Enzyme Inhibitors in Basic Research

Enzyme inhibitors have found many exciting applications in basic research. They serve as useful tools for the elucidation of structure and function of enzymes, like probes for chemical and kinetic processes and detection of short-lived reaction intermediates (30). For example, irreversible inhibitors have assisted in the determination of half-site reactivity of enzymes or measurement of enzyme turnover. They have been applied to quantify and localize enzymes in organs *in vivo* (31). Covalently binding enzyme inhibitors have been used to identify active site amino acid residues which could potentially be involved in the catalysis of the enzyme. Reversible enzyme inhibitors have been used to facilitate enzyme purification by using the inhibitor as a ligand for affinity chromatography (32).

Enzyme inhibitors can also be used to mimic genetic disease in animal models. For example, inactivation of γ-cystathionase by propargylglycine mimics a disease state called crystathioninuia. Deficiency of this enzyme leads to the accumulation of cystathionine in the urine and has sometimes been associated with mental retardation. Another application of enzyme inhibitors is the screening of microorganisms for inhibitor-resistant mutants (30). The most common reason for resistance is the increased production of the targeted enzyme which enables these mutant cells to survive. This approach provides mutants, called overproducers, that are capable of generating large amounts of the desired enzyme.

Significant advances have occurred recently in the area of rational enzyme inhibitor design. This chapter will focus on the existing categories of enzyme inhibitors, will discuss approaches to their design as well as their evaluation, and will illustrate some of these principles using recent representative examples from the literature. The reader will be frequently referred to more in-depth descriptions. The enzyme inhibitors discussed in this chapter are classified in Table 18.1. All the enzyme inhibitors described in this chapter are active site-directed. Inhibitors that bind to other than the active site of the enzyme are called allosteric effectors, allosteric inhibitors, or allosteric cofactors and are not included.

Some of the ways that certain enzyme inhibitors have been categorized may appear to be rather arbitrary in that a particular inhibitor may fit into more than one category. This is due to the fact that the different categories commonly used in the field describe nonrelated properties such as kinetic behavior, mechanism of action, or structure. Consequently, we will focus on the design aspect for each category and generally avoid comparisons of the different approaches. Other general reviews of enzyme inhibitors have appeared recently (30, 33–35). In addition, an excellent review by Abeles and Alston (36) on the general use of fluorinated compounds as enzyme inhibitors has appeared recently.

Table 18.1 Classification of Enzyme Inhibitors

Noncovalent Inhibitors	Covalent Inhibitors
Rapid reversible inhibitors	Mechanism-based inhibitors
Tight, slow, slow-tight binding inhibitors	Affinity labels
Transition-state analogs	Pseudoirreversible inhibitors
Multisubstrate analogs	

2 RATIONAL DESIGN OF NONCOVALENTLY BINDING ENZYME INHIBITORS

This class of inhibitors binds to the enzyme's active site in a noncovalent fashion. Based on their kinetics one can distinguish among rapid reversible, tight, slow, slow-tight binding and irreversible inhibitors. Other categories are transition state analogs and multisubstrate inhibitors which mimic the structures of reaction transition states, and intermediates. Traditionally, noncovalently binding enzyme inhibitors were analogs of either substrates, products or reaction intermediates, though numerous examples of nonsubstrate analog inhibitors have been discovered by screening large numbers of natural products or their synthetic analogs for inhibitory activity. Computer-aided inhibitor design is a relatively new and more focused approach to the design and discovery of nonsubstrate analog inhibitors. It is the subject of Chapter 15 in this book. It has also been used to improve the potency of a lead inhibitor, which has been somewhat arbitrarily defined as an inhibitor having a K_i value of less than 10 μM. In order to start a computer-aided drug design project, either the three-dimensional enzyme structure or the pharmacophore structure has to be known. A pharmacophore represents the nature of the chemical groups of a given ligand and their relative orientation important for inhibitor binding. Reviews on the subject are available elsewhere (37–41).

Traditionally, gradual empirical changes in the structure of the analog, such as adding to or exchanging for an existing functional group, lead to an increase of biological activity. Recently, this empirical testing of substrate analogs has become more focused using Quantitative Structure-Activity Relationship (QSAR) methods (Chapter 14). This method uses computer algorithms to correlate the biological activity of a series of inhibitors with their chemical structure, thereby allowing better predictions as to how to change the structure in order to obtain a more potent inhibitor. Reviews on this subject are available (42–44).

2.1 Relevant Forces for Formation of Enzyme Inhibitor Complexes

In order to understand the design concepts of the various types of noncovalently binding enzyme inhibitors, a basic knowledge of the binding forces between an enzyme's active site and its inhibitors is required. A brief overview of the forces involved follows. More comprehensive treatments can be found in Chapter 12 and elsewhere (45–47).

Usually, the binding of an inhibitor is dependent on a variety of interactions, the sum total of which will determine the degree of affinity of an inhibitor for the particular enzyme. The reversible binding process of an inhibitor to an enzyme's active site can be described as shown in equation 18.1:

$$E + I \underset{k_{-1}}{\overset{k_1}{\rightleftharpoons}} E \cdot I \qquad (18.1)$$

The strength of such a noncovalent complex $E \cdot I$ can be quantitatively evaluated by the inhibition constant K_i which describes the state of the equilibrium between the free enzyme (E), inhibitor (I) and the enzyme-inhibitor complex $(E \cdot I)$ (eq. 18.2):

$$K_i = \frac{[E][I]}{[E \cdot I]} \qquad (18.2)$$

The lower the K_i value, the better the inhibitor, since the equilibrium lies more in favor of enzyme-inhibitor complex formation. The Gibbs' free energy (ΔG) is an alternative way of describing the affinity of an inhibitor for the enzyme (eq. 18.3):

$$\Delta G = -RT \ln K_d \qquad (18.3)$$

where K_d is the dissociation constant under consideration, such as the inhibition constant K_i, R is the universal gas constant and T the temperature in degrees Kelvin. The more negative the ΔG values, the smaller the K_i value and therefore, the larger, generally, the attraction forces. The Gibbs' free energy (ΔG) can also be expressed in terms of enthalpy (ΔH) and entropy (ΔS) (eq. 18.4):

$$\Delta G = \Delta H - T\Delta S \qquad (18.4)$$

Therefore, the overall free energy change (ΔG) of a reaction is either lowered by a decrease in the enthalpy or an increase in the entropy.

From a qualitative point of view, the degree of the binding affinity and specificity of a given inhibitor to an enzyme's active site is determined by the sum of all existing (i) electrostatic forces, (ii) dispersion forces, (iii) hydrophobic interactions, and (iv) hydrogen bonds.

2.1.1 ELECTROSTATIC FORCES. These describe interactions between dipolar or charged atoms and molecules, and the magnitude of these forces in turn depends strongly on the dielectric constant of the surrounding medium. Water, for example, has a very large dielectric constant due to its high net permanent dipole moment (dielectric constants: $H_2O = 80$, EtOH = 24, benzene = 2.3). The high polarity of water greatly diminishes the attraction or repulsion forces between any two charged groups owing to the so-called leveling effect of water. Water molecules surrounding any two charged groups become polarized by their charges, resulting in a neutralizing field between the two groups. The formation of buried salt bridges between two charged groups of opposite polarity is an alternative way of looking at ion–ion interactions, as outlined in equation 18.5. It requires desolvation of both ions at the cost of enthalpy, but leads to a significantly

favorable increase of entropy by the freed water molecules. The strength of the ion–ion interaction will depend strongly on the stability of the salt bridge versus the solvated ions in water. In such a complex system, it is very difficult to evaluate the contributions of each of these energies.

$$E - \overset{+}{N}H_3 \cdot (H_2O)_x + I - CO_2^- \cdot (H_2O)_y$$

$$\rightleftharpoons E - \overset{+}{N}H_3{}^- O_2C - I + (H_2O)_{x+y}$$

$$(18.5)$$

2.1.2 DISPERSION FORCES. These attraction forces are also called nonpolar or van der Waals' interactions and are based on induced dipoles between nonpolar molecules. They result from the local fluctuation in the electron density of a given nonpolar compounds, even though these compounds may have no net dipole moment. The magnitude of these forces depends on the polarizability of the particular atoms involved and their distance between each other. The optimal distance between the atoms is the sum of each of their van der Waal's radii. Oxygen has, for example, a much lower polarizability than a methylene group. Therefore, dispersion forces are a lot stronger between nonpolar compounds themselves than between nonpolar compounds and water. These forces are quite weak, but additive. However, dispersion forces usually contribute only a minor part to the attraction forces between hydrophobic regions of the inhibitor and the enzyme's active site, whereas hydrophobic interactions evidently play the major role.

2.1.3 HYDROPHOBIC INTERACTIONS. These describe the partitioning of nonpolar molecules between water and an organic phase as opposed to the interactions of hydrophilic molecules with water. Organic molecules are basically "squeezed out" of the aqueous phase because they lead to interruption of the hydrogen bounding network of water. In order to optimize the number of hydrogen bonds (each of a magnitude of ~25 kJ/mol), water molecules surround the organic molecule with a higher degree of order. Therefore, the hydrophobic effect leads to a decrease in entropy, but no large changes of enthalpy are observed.

2.1.4 HYDROGEN BONDS. This interaction consists of sharing a proton between two electronegative atoms. In general, the distance between the proton and each of the atoms is not equal, with one of the heteroatoms showing a normal covalent bond distance to the proton. The other heteroatom is usually at a distance that is shorter than the van der Waals' contact distance. While these forces can be quite significant in nonpolar solvents, water greatly diminishes their magnitude. In order for a hydrogen bond to form in water between an enzyme and a substrate, the hydrogen bonds between the substrate and water as well as the enzyme and water have to be broken first (eq. 18.6). Overall, this leads to a net retention of the number of hydrogen bonds and, therefore, the net gain in energy is usually either very small or zero. This is based on the assumption that the hydrogen bonds between the inhibitor and enzyme are not significantly more favorable than those between water and the inhibitor or those between water and the enzyme. On the other hand, formation of the enzyme-inhibitor adduct usually leads to an overall increase of entropy. Bound water molecules are released, but only the inhibitor remains fixed in the enzyme's active site.

The contributions of all of these forces to the overall binding affinity of the inhibitor to the enzyme are very difficult to evaluate quantitatively. Hydrophobic interactions, electrostatic forces and hydrogen bonds seem to contribute to a favorable increase in entropy, while an estimation of the enthalpy contributions is considerably more complex. If an inhibitor is "buried,"

i.e., sequestered from water in the active site, all of these forces generally become more potent.

$$
\begin{array}{ccc}
\text{I}\text{-----}\text{H}\text{---}\text{O} & + & \text{E}\text{---}\text{O} \\
\text{I}\text{---}\text{E} & + & \text{O}\text{---}\text{H}\text{-----}\text{O}
\end{array}
$$

(18.6)

2.2 Rapid, Reversible Inhibitors

2.2.1 DESIGN OF RAPID, REVERSIBLE INHIBITORS. These inhibitors act by binding to the target enzyme's active site in a rapid and reversible fashion, thereby blocking the active site and preventing any further substrate binding. The design of potent rapid, reversible inhibitors strives to optimize the noncovalent binding forces, such as electrostatic forces, hydrogen bonds, hydrophobic interactions and dispersion forces, between the inhibitor and the active site of the enzyme. The more information that can be gathered on the shape and chemical nature of the active site and areas in close proximity on the enzyme, the more rational decisions can be made with respect to modifications of a lead inhibitor. The following strategies are commonly used to improve the potency of an inhibitor: (i) Areas of bulk tolerance must be identified to determine the necessary shape complementarity of the inhibitor. In order to optimize the hydrophobic effect, for example, an ideal inhibitor should fit snugly into the active site of the enzyme and maximize contacts between the hydrophobic areas of the enzyme's active site and those of the inhibitor. For example, phenyl groups may increase the hydrophobic effect by slipping into hydrophobic pockets in the active site of the enzyme. (ii) Strategically placed hydrogen bonds and salt-bridges between the active site of the enzyme and the inhibitor may significantly contribute to an increased binding affinity, particularly if they are "buried."

2.2.2 KINETICS. Kinetic evaluation of an inhibitor can provide important information regarding the nature of the enzyme-inhibitor binding, such as the site of binding, the sequence of binding of inhibitor and substrate(s) in multisubstrate-catalyzed reactions and the quantitative effectiveness of binding as expressed in the K_i value. This information can then be used for the rational design of more potent enzyme inhibitors. The reader is referred to other sources for more in-depth reviews of the kinetic equations and mathematical derivations involved (33, 45, 48).

The kinetic evaluation of an inhibitor requires an understanding of the normal catalysis of the enzyme with its substrate(s). In the simplest case, an enzyme-catalyzed reaction involves the conversion of a single substrate to a single product, as shown in equation 18.7:

$$E + S \rightleftharpoons E \cdot S \rightleftharpoons E \cdot P \rightleftharpoons E + P$$

$$(18.7)$$

The enzyme E binds the substrate S in a reversible fashion to form a noncovalent enzyme inhibitor complex E·S, followed by the chemical transformation of substrate S to product P, and subsequent release of the product into the medium. The affinity of the substrate for the enzyme's active site is determined by electrostatic, dispersion and hydrophobic forces and hydrogen bonds as discussed earlier. Enzymatic reactions involving two or more substrates can be simplified, so that the kinetic analysis used for single substrate-catalyzed reactions is justifiable. By keeping all but one of the substrates at fixed, highly saturating con-

centrations, the reaction rate will only be dependent on the concentration of the varied substrate of interest. For the sake of further simplification, the dissociation rate of the E·P complex is considered to be not rate-determining and the re-conversion of product back to substrate is neglected. The latter assumption is valid under so-called initial velocity conditions when less than ~5% of product has formed. Under these conditions, equation 18.7 simplifies to equation 18.8:

$$E + S \underset{k_1}{\overset{k_1}{\rightleftharpoons}} E \cdot S \xrightarrow{k_2} E \cdot P \quad (18.8)$$

The Michaelis-Menten equation (eq. 18.9) is a quantitative description of this process, provided that (i) the concentration of the enzyme involved is negligible compared to the substrate concentration at any time and (ii) steady-state conditions are obeyed. The latter assumption implies equal rates of formation and dissociation of the E·S complex, so that the concentration of E·S can be assumed to be constant under experimental conditions.

$$v = \frac{[S]V_{max}}{K_M + [S]}$$

$$V_{max} = k_2[E] \quad (18.9)$$

The Michaelis-Menten equation states that the initial velocity (v) increases in a linear fashion with low substrate concentrations [S], so that $v = V_{max}[S]/K_M$. At sufficiently high substrate concentrations, the increase in v is less than that of [S]. At high substrate concentrations, v is independent of [S] and directly proportional to the enzyme concentration. The initial velocity is equal to the V_{max} of the enzyme, following $v = V_{max} = k_2[E]$ (Fig. 18.3). The Michaelis-Menten constant K_M is a combination of rate constants and is independent of enzyme concentration under steady-state conditions. It is equivalent to the substrate concentration at which half maximal ve-

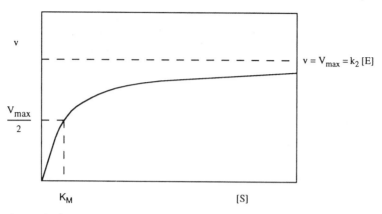

Fig. 18.3 Dependency of substrate concentration on the initial velocity in an enzyme-catalyzed reaction following Michaelis–Menten kinetics.

locity of the enzyme-catalyzed reaction is reached (eq. 18.10).

$$K_M = \frac{k_2 + k_1}{k_1} \quad (18.10)$$

when $[S] = K_M$, then $v = 1/2V_{max}$

It is important to keep in mind, however, that the Michaelis-Menten equation holds true not only for the mechanism as stated above, but for many different mechanisms which are not included in this treatment. Analysis of Michaelis-Menten kinetics is greatly facilitated by a linear representation of the data. Converting the Michaelis-Menten equation into equation 18.11 leads to the popular Lineweaver-Burk plot (Fig. 18.4).

$$\frac{1}{v} = \frac{1}{v_{max}} + \frac{K_M}{V_{max}[S]} \quad (18.11)$$

An alternative method is the commonly preferred Eadie-Hofstee plot (Fig. 18.5) (eq. 18.12)

$$v = V_{max} - \frac{K_M v}{[S]} \quad (18.12)$$

2.2.3 TYPES OF RAPID, REVERSIBLE INHIBITORS. This class of enzyme inhibitors binds to the enzyme in a rapid and reversible fashion, following simple Michaelis-Menten kinetics. Depending on their preference of binding to the free enzyme and/or the enzyme-substrate complex, competitive, uncompetitive and noncompetitive

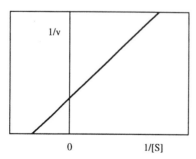

Fig. 18.4 Lineweaver-Burk plot.

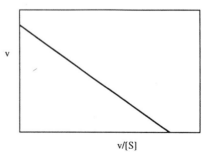

Fig. 18.5 Eadie-Hofstee plot.

inhibition patterns can be distinguished. It will be assumed for further simplicity that the initial equilibrium of free and bound substrate is established significantly faster than the rate of the chemical transformation of substrate to product; therefore, $k_{-1} \gg k_2$, which reduces K_M to the dissociation constant K_S (eq. 18.13):

$$K_S = \frac{k_1}{k_{-1}} \qquad (18.13)$$

Competitive Inhibitors. The binding of a competitive inhibitor and that of the corresponding substrate are mutually exclusive because they compete for the same binding site on the enzyme. A kinetic scheme for competitive inhibition can be outlined as shown in equation 18.14:

$$
\begin{array}{c}
E \overset{S}{\rightleftharpoons} E \cdot S \longrightarrow E + P \\
I \, \big\Updownarrow \\
E \cdot I
\end{array}
\qquad (18.14)
$$

Solving this kinetic scheme for simple Michaelis-Menten kinetics leads to equation 18.15:

$$v = \frac{[S]V_{max}}{[S] + K_M\left(1 + \dfrac{[I]}{K_i}\right)} \qquad (18.15)$$

Competitive inhibitors increase the apparent K_M of the substrate without changing V_{max} by a factor of $(1 + [I]/K_i)$. V_{max} is

reached when sufficiently high concentrations of the substrate can completely displace the inhibitor. However, the affinity of the substrate for the enzyme seems to be decreased in the presence of a competitive inhibitor, because the free enzyme E is not only in equilibrium with the enzyme substrate complex E·S but also with the enzyme inhibitor complex E·I. The evaluation of the kinetics is again greatly facilitated by the conversion of equation 18.15 into a linear form using either Lineweaver-Burk or Eddie-Hofstee plots as presented in Figure 18.6.

Uncompetitive Inhibitors. Uncompetitive inhibitors only have an affinity for the enzyme-substrate complex E·S and do not bind to the free enzyme (eq. 18.16).

$$
\begin{array}{c}
E \overset{S}{\rightleftharpoons} E \cdot S \longrightarrow E + P \\
I \, \big\Updownarrow \\
E \cdot S \cdot I
\end{array}
\qquad (18.16)
$$

Uncompetitive inhibition is frequently observed in multisubstrate-catalyzed reactions and reflects the order of binding of the different substrates. In a bisubstrate-catalyzed reaction, for example, a given inhibitor may be competitive with respect to one of the two substrates and uncompetitive with respect to the other. In a unisubstrate-catalyzed reaction, however, uncompetitive inhibition is rare because all of the sub-

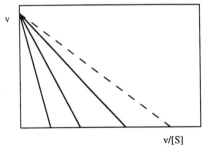
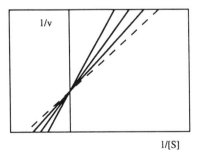

Fig. 18.6 Linear forms of Lineweaver-Burk and Eadie-Hofstee plots exhibiting competitive inhibition pattern. The dotted line indicates a reaction in the absence of inhibitor, while the solid lines represent enzymatic reactions in the presence of an inhibitor.

strate binding sites are already filled. Uncompetitive inhibitors decrease V_{max} by the factor of $(1 + [I]/K_i)$ because some of the enzyme remains in the $E \cdot S \cdot I$ form even at infinite substrate concentration. The apparent K_M for the substrate also decreases by the same factor because the formation of $E \cdot S \cdot I$ will use up some of the $E \cdot S$, thereby shifting the equilibrium further in favor of $E \cdot S$ formation. A plot for a typical uncompetitive inhibition pattern is illustrated in Figure 18.7 and is described by equation 18.17:

$$v = \frac{\dfrac{[S]V_{max}}{1 + [I]/K_i}}{[S] + \dfrac{K_M}{1 + [I]/K_i}} \qquad (18.17)$$

Noncompetitive Inhibitors. Ideal noncompetitive inhibitors bind with the same affinity to the free enzyme and to the enzyme–substrate complex. Both the enzyme–inhibitor complex and the enzyme–inhibitor–substrate complex are rendered catalytically inactive and therefore unable to convert substrate to product. The kinetics are outlined in equation 18.18:

$$\begin{array}{ccc} E & \overset{S}{\rightleftharpoons} E \cdot S & \longrightarrow E + P \\ {\scriptstyle I} \big\Vert & {\scriptstyle I} \big\Vert & \\ E \cdot 5I & \overset{S}{\rightleftharpoons} E \cdot S \cdot I & (18.18) \end{array}$$

Unlike a competitive inhibitor, a noncompetitive inhibitor does not compete for the same substrate binding site on the enzyme. Simple Michaelis-Menten kinetics of noncompetitive inhibitors are described in equation 18.19:

$$v = \frac{\dfrac{[S]V_{max}}{1 + [I]/K_i}}{[S] + K_M} \qquad (18.19)$$

Theoretically, noncompetitive inhibitors do not affect the K_M of the substrate, but decrease V_{max} by a factor of $(1 + [I]/K_i)$ and overall seem to reduce the total amount of enzyme present. A portion of the enzyme will always be bound in the nonproductive enzyme–inhibitor–substrate complex $E \cdot S \cdot I$, causing a decrease of the maximum velocity even at infinite substrate concentrations. However, because noncompetitive inhibitors bind with the same affinity to the free enzyme and the enzyme inhibitor complex, the K_M value of the substrate remains unchanged. Lineweaver-Burk and Eadie-Hofstee plots for noncompetitive behavior are shown in Fig. 18.8. Frequently, the binding constants of the noncompetitive inhibitor for the free enzyme and the enzyme–substrate complex are different. These nonideally behaving noncompetitive inhibitors are called mixed-type inhibitors, and they alter not only V_{max} but also K_M for the substrate.

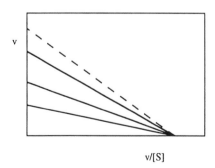

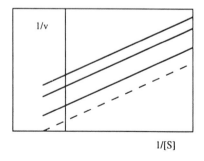

Fig. 18.7 Linear forms of Lineweaver-Burk and Eadie-Hofstee plots exhibiting an uncompetitive inhibition pattern.

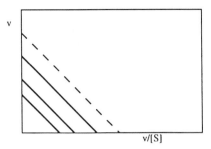 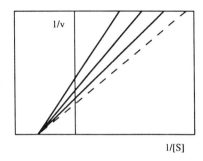

Fig. 18.8 Linear forms of Lineweaver-Burk and Eadie-Hofstee plots exhibiting a noncompetitive inhibition pattern.

In less well-defined situations, steady-state kinetics are insufficient to analyze the mechanism of inactivation for a given inhibitor. For example, irreversible enzyme inhibitors which bind so tightly to the enzyme that the dissociation rate (k_{off}) is equal to zero also exhibit noncompetitive inhibition patters. They act by destroying a portion of the enzyme through irreversible binding, thereby lowering the overall enzyme concentration and decreasing V_{max}. The apparent K_M remains unaffected because irreversible inhibitors do not influence the dissociation constant of the enzyme-substrate complex. A good review describing the kinetic evaluation of irreversibly binding enzyme inhibitors has appeared recently (49). Allosteric effectors may also show noncompetitive kinetic patterns by rendering the enzyme in the $E \cdot S \cdot I$ complex less active than in the $E \cdot S$ complex. Therefore, additional analyses may be necessary in these less well-defined situations, including more in-depth steady-state kinetics, presteady-state kinetics or testing for irreversibly binding enzyme inhibitors. Irreversible covalently binding enzyme inhibitors are discussed extensively later in this chapter.

2.2.4 IC$_{50}$ VALUES. In order to screen a large number of samples quickly, potencies of enzyme inhibitors are frequently compared using IC_{50} values instead of K_i values. IC_{50} values are commonly determined by keeping the concentration of the substrate and the enzyme constant and varying the concentration of the inhibitor in tenfold increments. An IC_{50} value equals the inhibitor concentration that leads to 50% enzyme inactivation. Therefore, an IC_{50} value is not a constant (except in the case of noncompetitive inhibition) and is dependent on the substrate concentration used in the experiment. The dependency of IC_{50} values of competitive inhibitors on the substrate concentration is outlined in equation 18.20:

$$IC_{50} = K_i\left(1 + \frac{[S]}{K_M}\right) \qquad (18.20)$$

It follows from equation 18.20 that substrate concentrations greater than ~0.1 fold of the K_M value lead to an underestimation of the K_i value. This underestimation may become quite significant at high substrate concentrations.

The dependency of the IC_{50} value on the substrate concentration for uncompetitive inhibitors is outlined in equation 18.21:

$$IC_{50} = K_i\left(1 + \frac{K_M}{[S]}\right) \qquad (8.21)$$

At high concentrations of the substrate, the K_i value is comparable to the IC_{50} value, though a significant underestimation may occur at lower substrate concentrations. Therefore, when the type of inhibition is unknown, substrate concentrations close to the K_M value should be used. This minimizes the deviation of the IC_{50} value from the K_i value, in the cases of competitive and uncompetitive inhibitors by a factor of 2. Due to the linear dependency of the initial velocity and the inhibitor concentration for uncompetitive and competitive inhibition, a Dixon plot can provide an estimate of the K_i value and indicate the type of inhibition (48), although more accurate methods such as Lineweaver-Burk

and Eadie-Hofstee plots are preferable. In the case of mixed competitive and irreversible inhibitors, the dependency of the inhibitor concentration and the initial velocity is nonlinear. In those cases, the meaning of the IC_{50} values is limited. IC_{50} values can be quite useful, however, if a large number of samples has to be screened for a preliminary evaluation and if the experimental conditions such as enzyme concentration, inactivation time, and temperature are kept constant.

Representative examples of rapid, reversible inhibitors are given below.

2.2.5   EXAMPLES.

(18.22)

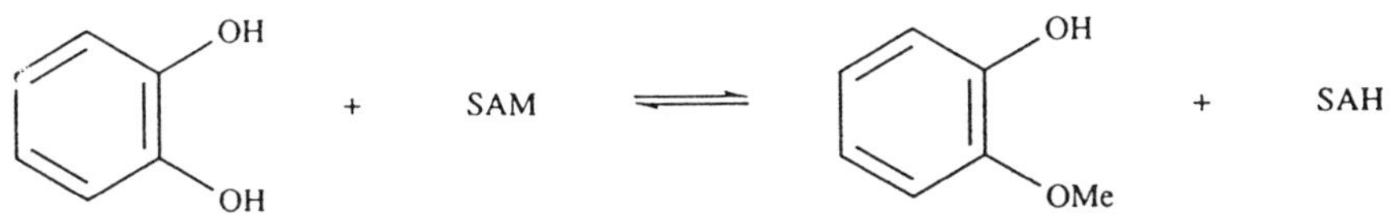

| (23) | (24) | (25) | (26) |

$$(18.23)$$

$$H_2N - Asp - Arg - Val - Tyr - Ile - His - Pro - Phe - His - Leu - CO_2H$$

(27)

$$H_2N - Asp - Arg - Val - Tyr - Ile - His - Pro - Phe - CO_2H \quad + \quad H_2N - His - Leu - CO_2H$$

(28)

$$(18.24)$$

Thymidine $5'$-$[\alpha,\beta$-imido]triphosphate (**15**, TMPNPP) has been reported as a potent, reversible, and competitive inhibitor of human immunodeficiency virus-1 reverse transcriptase (HIV1-RT) with a K_i value of 2.4 μM (Fig. 18.9) (50). Inhibitors of HIV1-RT have potential as drugs for the treatment of AIDS. TMPNPP has been designed as a substrate analog inhibitor of RT by substitution of the α,β-oxygen bridge with an imido functionality. This modification prevents catalytic cleavage at the α,β-P-O-P position, which occurs during normal catalytic cycle using the substrate thymidine triphosphate, for example (**16**, TTP).

13-Desmethyl-13, 14-dihydro-*all-trans*-retinyl trifluoroacetate (**17**, Fig. 18.10) is a substrate analog inhibitor of lecithin retinol acyl transferase (LRAT) which catalyzes the transesterification from dipalmitoyl-phosphatidylcholine (**18**, DPPC) to vitamin A (**19**, eq. 18.22) (51). The enzyme plays an important role in visual pigment regeneration and also the mobilization of vitamin A in the liver and intestine. Shi et al. used (**17**) to further the understanding of the kinetic mechanism of LRAT. The inhibitor was shown to be competitive with respect to DPPC, with a K_i value of 11.4 μM, and uncompetitive with respect to *all-trans*-retinol. This implies that the

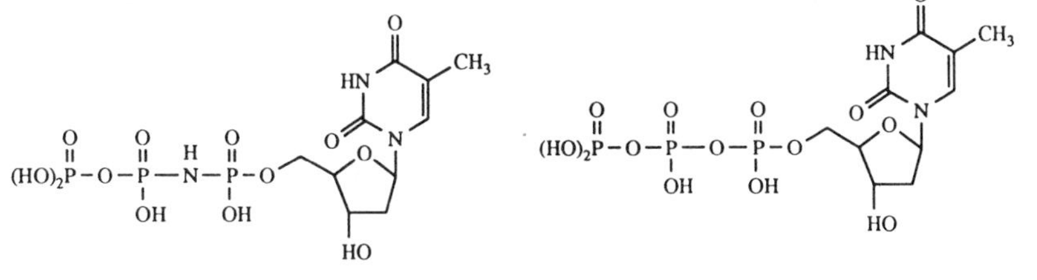

| 15 | 16 |

Fig. 18.9 The substrate TTP and the competitive, substrate analog inhibitor TMPNPP of HIV-RT.

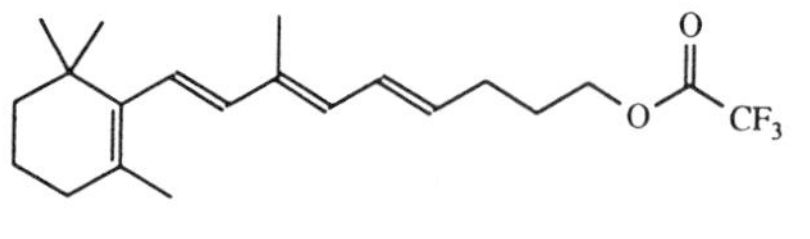

17

Fig. 18.10 Rapid, reversible inhibitor of lecithin retinol acyl transferase.

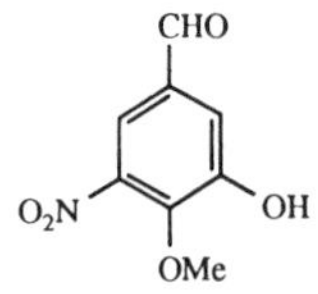

22

Fig. 18.11 Rapid, reversible inhibitor of catechol-*O*-methyltransferase.

inhibitor binds to the same form of the enzyme as DPPC but to a different form than the *all-trans*-retinol.

Perez et al. have developed 3-hydroxy-4-methoxy-5-nitrobenzaldehyde (**22**, Fig. 18.11) as a potent inhibitor of catechol-*O*-methyltransferase (52). This enzyme is involved in the extraneural inactivation of endogenous catecholamines. Disturbances in the normal levels of physiologically active catecholamines are correlated with many diseases, such as Parkinson's disease. The enzyme catalyzes the transfer of a methyl group from *S*-adenosyl-L-methionine (**24**, SAM) to a hydroxy group of a catechol substrate such as (**23**) as outlined in equation 18.23. It was determined that (**22**) was uncompetitive with respect to SAM (**24**) and noncompetitive with respect to (**23**) with K_i values of 13.5 μM and 17.2 μM, respectively.

Angiotensin converting enzyme (ACE) is a carboxydipeptidase which catalyzes the hydrolysis of proangiotensin (**27**) to angiotensin (**28**) as outlined in equation 18.24. (1*S*, 2*R*)-*cis*-2-[[[2-(Hydroxyamino)-2-oxoethyl] methylamino]carbonyl]cyclohexanecarboxylic acid (**29**) has been found to be a potent nonsubstrate analog inhibitor of ACE with a K_i value of 2.7 n*M* (Fig.

18.12) (53). Competitive inhibition was determined with respect to hippurylglycylglycine (**30**).

2.3 Slow, Tight, and Slow-tight Binding Inhibitors

The major assumptions of Michaelis-Menten kinetics do not necessarily hold true for slow, tight and slow-tight binding inhibitors. Unlike rapid reversible inhibitors, the concentration of the inhibitor may not significantly exceed the concentration of the enzyme and the equilibrium may not be established rapidly and reversibly. Slow-binding enzyme inhibitors establish the equilibria among the enzyme, inhibitor, and enzyme-inhibitor complexes slowly, as measured on a steady-state scale of seconds, minutes or longer. The enzyme inhibitor complexes exhibit slow off rates (dissociation rates), while the on rates (association rates) may be either slow or fast. Therefore, slow binding does not reflect on a slow binding process of the inhibitor but rather on a slow equilibrium rate. Simple slow-binding inhibition occurs when a significantly larger concentration of inhibitor

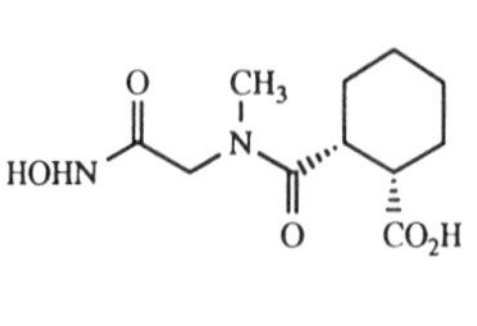

29

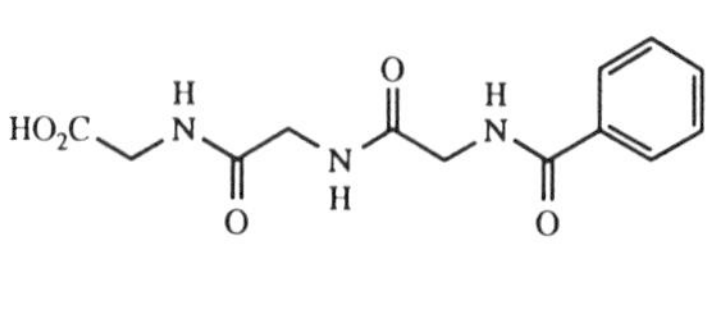

30

Fig. 18.12 Potent nonsubstrate analog inhibitor (**29**) and substrate (**30**) of ACE.

than enzyme is necessary for inhibition. When a slow-binding inhibitor has a very strong affinity for the target enzyme, the inhibitor is characterized as a slow-tight binding inhibitor (Table 18.2). The enzyme is inactivated at inhibitor concentrations comparable to the enzyme concentration. Therefore, the inhibitor concentration is no longer independent of the enzyme concentration as assumed for Michaelis-Menten kinetics, and changes in the inhibitor concentration as a consequence of enzyme-inhibitor complex formation must be considered. Once the off-rate of the inhibitor approaches zero, however, the inhibitor becomes functionally irreversible. The kinetics of covalently binding enzyme inhibitors are covered elsewhere in this chapter. Excellent more in-depth descriptions of slow, tight, and slow-tight binding inhibitors have appeared elsewhere (54, 55) and references therein.

2.3.1 SLOW-BINDING INHIBITORS. For reasons of simplicity, only competitive inhibitors will be discussed in this section. Two different mechanisms have been suggested to rationalize slow-binding behavior. In the one-step Mechanism A, the direct binding process of the inhibitor to the enzyme is slow (equation 18.25). This has been correlated with a barrier to binding at the active site. The inhibitor has to overcome this barrier by correct alignment. Once aligned properly, it binds so tightly that it is released even more slowly from the enzyme. In Mechanism B, the initial

equilibrium between the enzyme E, inhibitor I and the enzyme inhibitor complex $E \cdot I$ is fast, but the subsequent rearrangement to form the final, more stable enzyme-inhibitor complex $E \cdot I^*$ is slow (eq. 18.26). In order to observe the $E \cdot I$ complex, $K_i^* (k_4/k_{-4})$ must be smaller than $K_i(k_3/k_{-3})$ and k_{-4} smaller than k_4. The slow rearrangement step has been correlated with conformational changes of the enzyme upon the initial binding of the inhibitor. The enzyme may be better equipped to accommodate the inhibitor in a transition state than in the ground state. Consequently, slow conformational changes of the enzyme can lead to tight binding of the inhibitor which is then released even more slowly from the enzyme. Alternatively, the slow-binding process has been correlated with the necessary displacement of water molecules at the active site (56). The inhibitor binds loosely to the initial enzyme inhibitor complex. Upon release of water molecules, tighter binding is possible, leading to a more stable $E \cdot I^*$ complex. Overall, Mechanism B appears to be by far the most common mechanism of slow-binding; therefore, the following discussion will be limited to Mechanism B as the potential prototype.

Unfortunately, no general strategies have emerged to allow the design of slow-binding inhibitors. However, slow-binding inhibitors appear to have advantages over rapid, reversible inhibitors for drug development purposes. The rearrangement of $E \cdot I^*$ to $E \cdot I$ is independent of

Table 18.2 Classes of Reversible Inhibitors

Inhibitor Class	I/E Ratio	Attainment of Equilibrium
		$E + I \rightleftharpoons EI$
Rapid reversible	$I \gg E$	Fast
Tight binding	$I \approx E$	Fast
Slow binding	$I \gg E$	Slow
Slow, tight-binding	$I \approx E$	Slow

$$E \underset{k_{-1}}{\overset{S,k_1}{\rightleftharpoons}} E \cdot S \overset{k_2}{\longrightarrow} E + P$$
$$k_{-3} \updownarrow\ I, k_3$$
$$E \cdot I \qquad\qquad (18.25)$$

$$E \underset{k_{-1}}{\overset{S,k_1}{\rightleftharpoons}} E \cdot S \overset{k_2}{\longrightarrow} E + P$$
$$k_{-3} \updownarrow\ I, k_3$$
$$E \cdot I \underset{k_{-4}}{\overset{k_4}{\rightleftharpoons}} E \cdot I^* \qquad (18.26)$$

the substrate concentration, while in the case of rapid, reversible inhibitors, the build-up of substrate upstream of the inhibited enzyme leads to reversal of the inhibition.

A different application of slow-binding enzyme inhibitors is their use as probes for the existence of transition state and reaction intermediates. It is based on the assumption that these intermediates do not bind tightly to the ground state of the enzyme, thereby causing the enzyme to convert to these high affinity complexes slowly. A typical biphasic progress plot for slow-binding inhibitors, obeying Mechanism B, is shown in Fig. 18.13. The initial

burst of the reaction, the linear section of the graph, can be described by competitive Michaelis-Menten kinetics. The higher the concentration of the inhibitor, the shorter the initial linear section of each curve and the slower the subsequent final steady-state-rate, as observed as the asymptotes in Fig. 18.13. If the inhibitor concentration is small, the substrate might be too depleted to permit observation of steady-state rates.

2.3.2 EXAMPLES. Recently, ramiprilat (**31**) has been determined to be a competitive slow-tight binding inhibitor of ACE (Fig. 18.14) (57). The mechanism of ACE is outlined in equation 18.24. K_i and K_i^* values of $10.8\,nM$ and $7\,pM$, a k_4 rate of $2.8 \times 10^{-2}\,s^{-1}$, and a k_{-4} rate of $1.8 \times 10^{-5}\,s^{-1}$ have been determined. The slow-binding process was correlated with Mechanism B.

Compound (**32**) is a slow-binding inhibitor of chymotrypsin with a K_i value of $0.19\,\mu M$ (Fig. 18.15) (58). Chymotrypsin is a serine protease which preferentially catalyzes the hydrolysis of peptide linkages adjacent to the aromatic amino acids phenylalanine, tyrosine, and tryptophan (eq. 18.27).

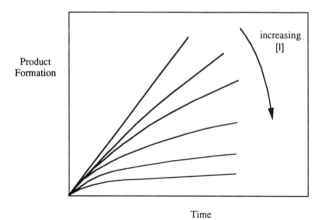

Time

Fig. 18.13 Time dependent enzyme-catalyzed product formation in the presence of a slow-binding inhibitor obeying Mechanism B.

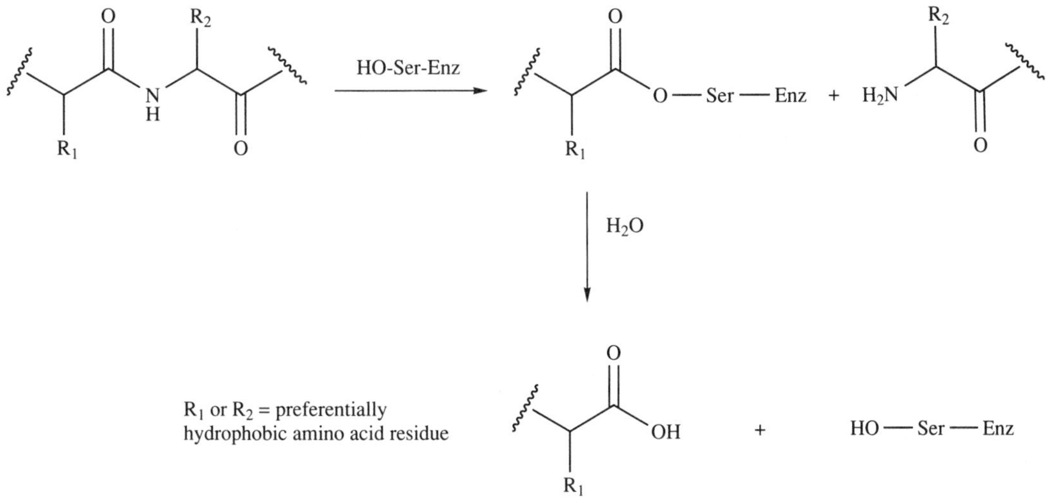

$$(18.27)$$

The authors proposed that the inhibitor (**32**) inhibits the enzyme according to Mechanism A. K_i values of 0.19 and 0.16 μM have been determined by two different methods with k_3 rates of 5509 and 5865 $M^{-1} s^{-1}$, and k_{-3} rates of 1.04×10^{-3} and $9.5 \times 10^{-4} s^{-1}$, respectively. The authors suggested the formation of a covalent tetrahedral intermediate with an active site serine; however, the possibility that fluorinated compound (**32**) was bound as a hydrate could not be excluded.

Bovine lens leucine aminopeptidase was inhibited by the dipeptide bestatin (2S, 3R-3-amino-2-hydroxyphenylbutanyl-L-leucine, **33**) in a slow-binding manner corresponding to Mechanism B (Fig. 18.16) (59). The enzyme catalyzes the hydrolysis of amino-terminal amino acids most effec-

tively if they have a leucine at the N-terminus, although it has a fairly broad specificity. Bestatin is a competitive inhibitor with a K_i value of 0.11 μM and a K_i^* value of 1.3 nM. A k_4 value of $1.5 \times 10^{-2} s^{-1}$ and a k_{-4} value of $2 \times 10^{-4} s^{-1}$ were determined.

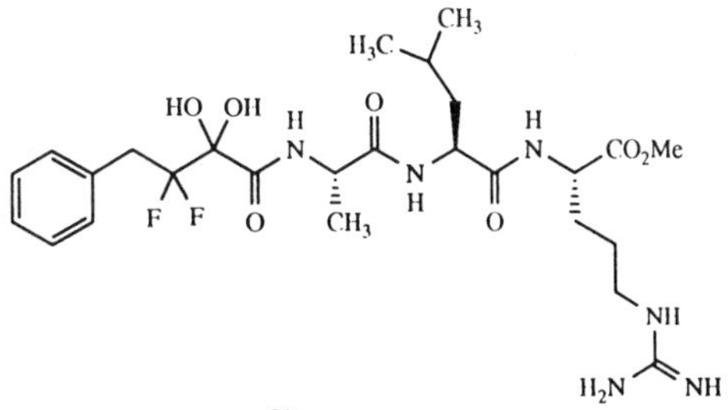

Fig. 18.15 Slow-binding inhibitor of α-chymotrypsin obeying Mechanism A.

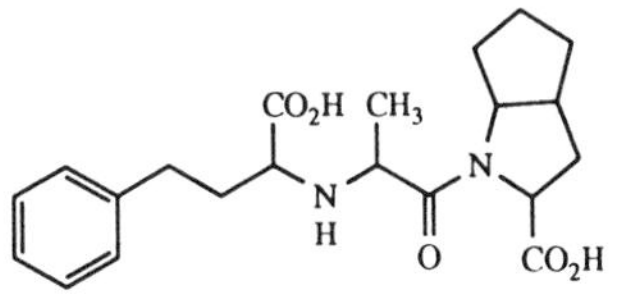

Fig. 18.14 Slow-tight binding inhibitor ramiprilat of ACE following Mechanism B.

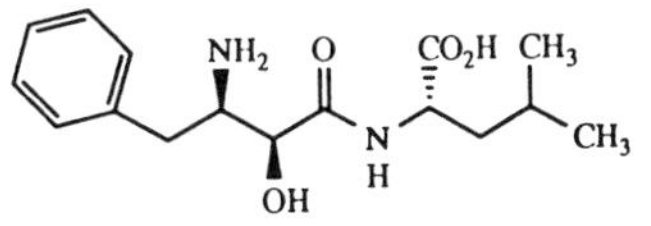

Fig. 18.16 Slow-binding inhibitor bestatin of bovine lens leucine aminopeptidase.

2.4 Transition-State Analogs

Transition-state analogs are stable compounds which mimic the structure of the activated complex during the transition state of an enzymatic reaction. The energy maxima of enzymatic transition states are significantly lower than those of the transition states of the corresponding non-enzyme-catalyzed reactions in solution, in accord with the generally high catalytic rates of enzymatic reactions. Enzymes can stabilize the inherently unstable transition states by reduction of charge separations at relatively nonpolar active sites, extra hydrogen bonds, more effective hydrophobic interactions, and other factors. Therefore, transition state analogs can take advantage of these additional binding energies which are available in the transition state but not in the ground state. In addition, these analogs also have the advantage of reduced molecularity as outlined below for multisubstrate analog inhibitors. General reviews on transition-state analog inhibitors have appeared (30, 60–62).

Simple transition-state theory states that the rate of an enzyme-catalyzed reaction is correlated with the rate of a noncatalyzed reaction by the same factor as the affinity of an enzyme for the transition state to the affinity of an enzyme for a substrate (eq. 18.28) (60).

binding constants of inhibitor to substrate (K_T/K_S) on the order of 10^8 to 10^{14}.

The design of a good transition state mimic is quite challenging. It not only requires a basic knowledge of the mechanism of the target enzyme, but also an understanding of the real energy profile, such as the existence of distinctive chemical steps and transition states (63). In addition, the inherent difficulty in the design of an analog for a metastable structure must be overcome. Activated complexes have partial bonds and are often highly charged, while a transition state analog must be stable and have fully developed bonds. According to the Hammond postulate, high-energy reaction intermediates are much closer in energy to the transition state than to the ground state. Consequently, many so-called transition state analogs are actually analogs of high-energy reaction intermediates. Although a clear distinction exists, the design process is for all practical purposes the same. Both take advantage of binding interactions available in the activated state but not in the ground state of an enzymatic reaction.

Recent insights by Gerlt and Gassman have important implications for the design of transition state analog inhibitors (64). If the reaction mechanism of a target enzyme involves general acid-general base catalysis (eq. 18.29),

$$ E + S \underset{K_N^{\ddagger}}{\rightleftharpoons} E + S^{\ddagger} \xrightarrow{k_N} E + P $$

$$ \frac{K_T}{K_S} = \frac{K_E^{\ddagger}}{K_N^{\ddagger}} = \frac{k_E}{k_N} \qquad (18.28) $$

Therefore, enzymatic catalysis (k_E/k_N) is related to the enhanced binding of the transition state to the enzyme (K_T/K_S). Theoretically, a transition state analog can be very tight binding, with ratios of the

ketone

enol

$$ (18.29) $$

matching the pK_a values of the acidic and basic groups of a transition state analog with those of the general acid and general base catalysts at the active site of the enzyme should lead to very tight binding of the inhibitor. The reaction must also have a late transition state so that the transition state will then look similar to the product. The extra strong binding energies are then rationalized with extra short, strong hydrogen bonds (<2.45 Å), which can be ob-served between two charged heteroatom bases whose conjugate acids have approximately equal pK_a values (65). In addition, solvent effects and changes in bond hybridization may contribute to an enhanced binding affinity for the transition state. This theory was evaluated by Gerlt and Gassman for the reaction catalyzed by mandelate racemase. The mechanism is outlined in equation 18.30.

$$(18.30)$$

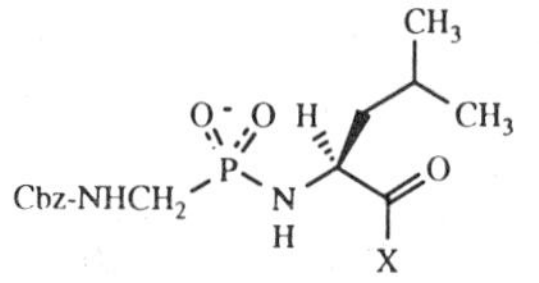

	34 X = D-Ala	
	35 X = NH$_2$	
	36 X = Gly	
	37 X = L-Phe	
	38 X = L-Ala	
	39 X = L-Leu	**40**

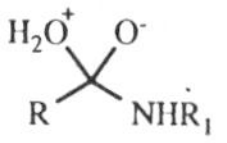

Fig. 18.17 Structures of six proposed transition-state analogs of thermolysin and their corresponding substrates.

They explained the rapid rates of the enzyme-catalyzed proton abstraction alpha to the carboxyl group by the extra tight binding of the enol-like transition state. The pK_a value of the substrate's base (hydroxy group of the enol) matches that of the active site acid catalyst (Glu 317), and the pK_a value of the substrate's acid (α-proton to the carbonyl) matches that of the active site general base catalysts (His 297 and Lys 166).

A careful evaluation is necessary to distinguish between a proposed transition-state analog and a ground state analog. Slow binding, tight binding or structural similarity to the assumed transition state structure alone are not sufficient criteria to establish a transition-state mimic (66). A quantitative evaluation of the earlier correlation between the enhanced rates of enzymatic reactions and the tight binding of transition state analogs as stated in equation 18.28 can be exceedingly difficult because of the fundamental difference in entropy change of a unimolecular enzymatic reaction versus a multimolecular solution reaction (67), and the inaccessibili-

ty of an appropriate rate constant corresponding to the free solution reaction (68, 69).

In an attempt to develop stringent criteria for the distinction between transition and ground state analogs, Bartlett et al. (66) overcame some of these inherent difficulties by comparing the binding affinities of a series of substrate analogs with those of the corresponding transition state analogs. A set of six peptide analog inhibitors was designed as a class of possible transition state inhibitors of thermolysin (Fig. 18.17). The mechanism of catalysis of thermolysin is proposed to proceed via the tetrahedral transition state (**40**), which stimulated the design of these phosphoamidate structural analogs of the transition state. Barlett et al. found that the K_i values for these proposed transition state inhibitors correlated in a linear fashion with the K_M/k_{cat} values of the six corresponding substrates. However, no correlation was found between K_i and K_M (Table 18.3). Therefore, these phosphoamidate analogs must be transition-state analogs and not ground-state analog inhibitors.

Table 18.3　Correlation of the K_i Values of Six Proposed Transition-State Analogs with the K_M/k_{cat} Values of Their Corresponding Substrates

	Inhibitor Data	Corresponding Substrate Data	
Inhibitor	K_i (nM)	K_M (mM)	K_M/k_2 (μM s)
(**34**)	1700	16.6	3200
(**35**)	760	20.6	196
(**36**)	270	10.8	165
(**37**)	78	2.4	20
(**38**)	16.5	10.6	13.6
(**39**)	9.1	2.6	7.0

2.4.1 EXAMPLES. Adenosine deaminase has been a popular target enzyme for the design of transition-state inhibitors, converting adenosine (**41**) into inosine (**43**, eq. 18.31).

(18.31)

The mechanism of catalysis is proposed to proceed via the hydrated, tetrahedral intermediate (**42**). The transition state is in turn proposed to resemble this intermediate. Nebularine (**44**, Fig. 18.18) binds in the form of the nebularine-1,6-hydrate (**45**) to the enzyme's active site with an exceedingly low K_i value of 0.3 pM, approaching the dissociation constant of the transition state of the enzyme-adenosine complex. An additional very potent transition-state analog is the 8R isomer of 2'-deoxycoformycin (**46**) (Fig. 18.18), exhibiting a K_i value of 2.5 pM (70).

Carboxymethyl-CoA (**47**) has been designed and studied as a reaction intermediate inhibitor of citrate synthase (Fig. 18.19) (71). The enzyme catalyzes the Claisen condensation of oxaloacetate and acetyl CoA to give citrate. It exhibited a K_i

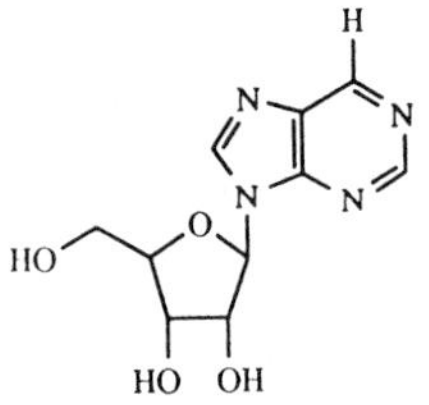

Fig. 18.18 Transition-state inhibitors of adenosine deaminase.

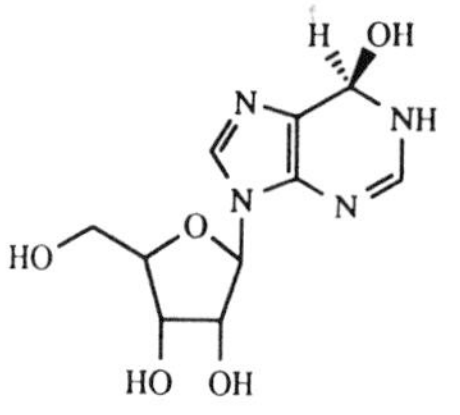

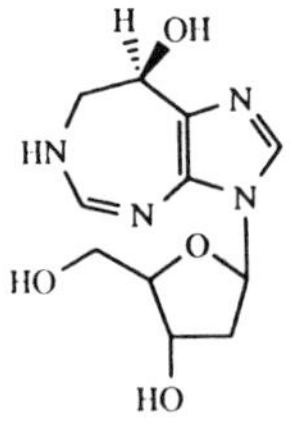

value of ~20 nM in the presence of ox-aloacetate. The reaction is proposed to proceed by concerted acid–base catalysis via the neutral enol-intermediate (**48**) without generating a carbanion bearing a full negative charge. Inhibitor (**47**) is a structural analog of enolic acetyl CoA (**48**), with one of the oxygens mimicking the methylene carbon, and the other being an analog of the hydroxy group of acetyl CoA.

Muehlbacher and Poulter (72) designed 2-(dimethylamino)-1-ethyl diphosphate (**49**) as a reaction intermediate/transition state analog of isopentenyl diphosphate isomerase (Fig. 18.20). The enzyme catalyzes the reversible conversion of isopentenyl diphosphate (**50**) to dimethylallyl diphosphate (**52**, eq. 18.32).

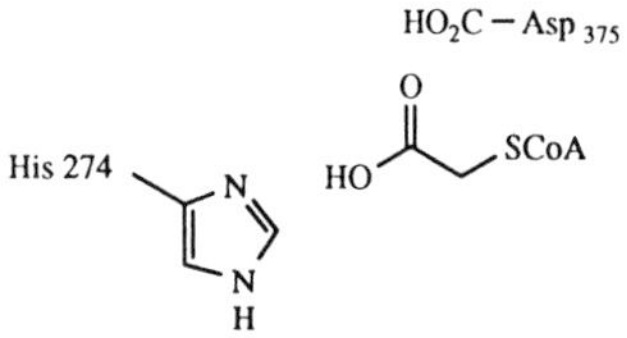

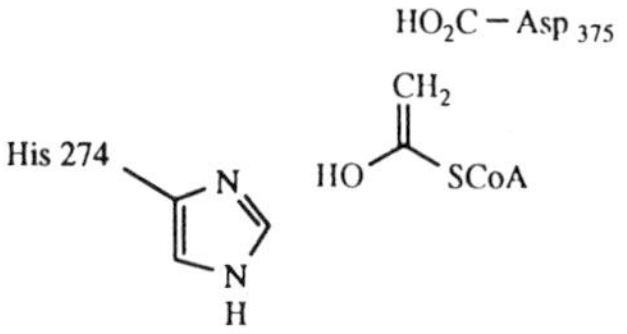

Fig. 18.19 The reaction intermediate inhibitor (**47**) of citrate synthase and the structure of the enolic acetyl CoA (**48**).

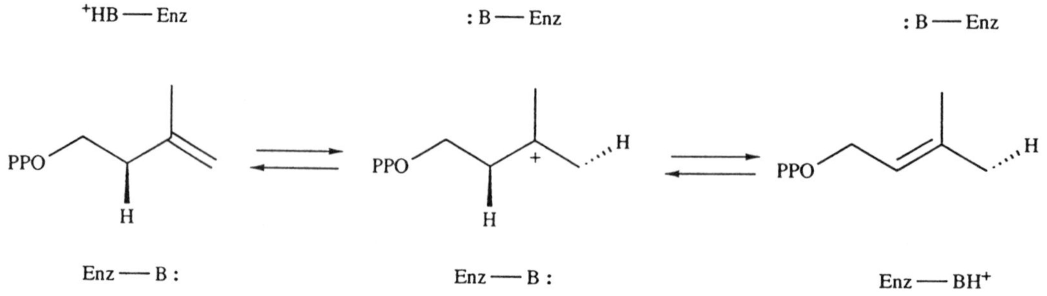

(18.32)

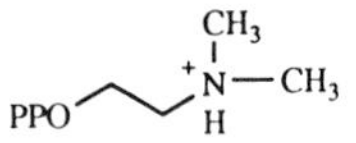

49

Fig. 18.20 A transition-state analog of isopentenyl diphosphate isomerase.

The reaction is proposed to proceed via the carbocationic intermediate (**51**). A K_i value of 15.2 μM was determined for the enzyme from *C. purpurea*.

Boronic acid peptides, such as compound (**53**), have been shown to exhibit good inhibitory activities for serine proteases, such as trypsin. It is proposed that the enzymatic hydrolysis of the peptide proceeds via tetrahedral intermediate (**54**). Tsilikounas and coworkers (73) showed that some boronic peptide derivatives mimic the tetrahedral adduct by forming a complex such as (**55**) with the enzyme as outlined in Fig. 18.21. Inhibitor (**53**) is a slow-binding inhibitor of trypsin with a K_i value of 3.4 nM and a K_i^* value of 0.64 nM.

2.5 Multisubstrate Inhibitors

Many enzymatic reactions require the simultaneous binding of two or more substrates at the active site in order for catalysis to occur. The bound substrates are required to have particular orientations in space and must be in close proximity to each other. The design of multisubstrate analog inhibitors takes advantage of this requirement by mimicking the simultaneous binding of two or more substrates at the active site of the enzyme. Such inhibitors are designed by covalently connecting the corresponding substrates or substrate analogs together, often with a suitable linker group. Inhibitors that combine two substrates are termed bisubstrate analogs, those combining three substrates are termed trisubstrate analogs, etc. In the most common case of a bisubstrate analog inhibitor, two potent single substrate analog inhibitors are first designed as outlined earlier. Potency can be enhanced in a second step, in which the two single substrate inhibitors are connected and the optimal length of the linker is determined. To a first approximation, the K_i value for a bisubstrate analog inhibitor can be ex-

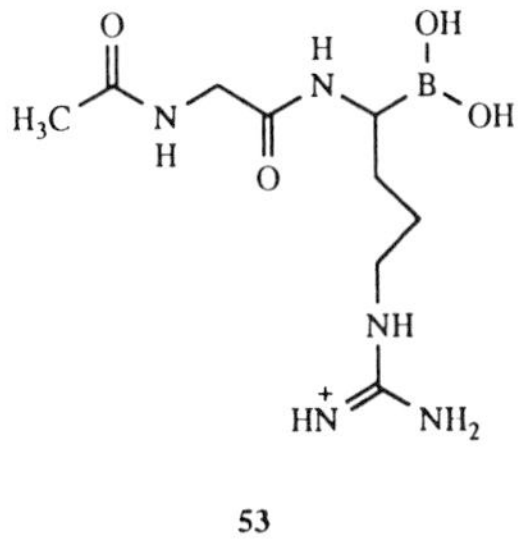

53

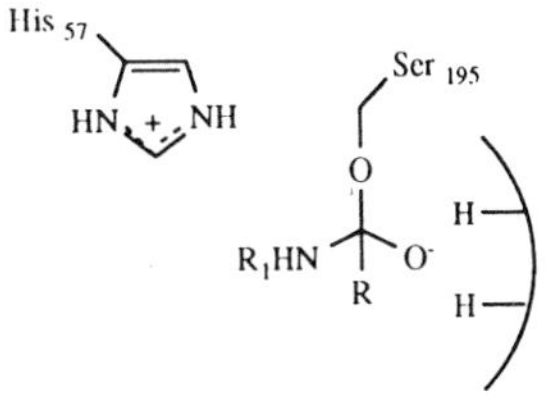

54

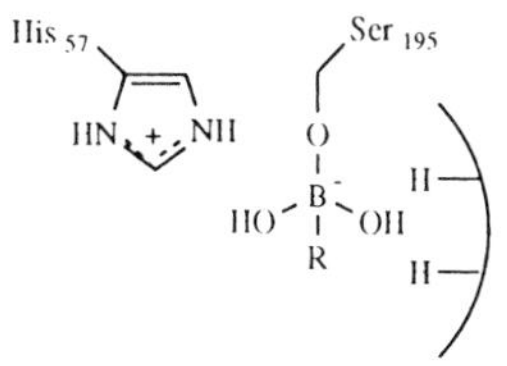

55

Fig. 18.21 Reaction intermediate analog (**55**) of trypsin and the normal tetrahedral reaction intermediate (**54**).

pected to fall in the range of the product of the K_M or K_i values of the two substrates or substrate analogs, respectively. For example, if two substrates of an enzymatic reaction have binding constants in the millimolar range, a bisubstrate analog should have a K_i value in the μM range. Therefore, a multisubstrate analog inhibitor should have much higher binding affinity for the enzyme than a single substrate inhibitor. In fact, an ideal multisubstrate inhibitor can bind up to 10^8 times as tightly as the product of the substrate binding constants, assuming a perfect fit of the bisubstrate analog inhibitor to the two binding sites on the enzyme (46). Such perfection has yet to be observed, however, in practice. An ideal multisubstrate inhibitor is also expected to exhibit competitive inhibition patterns with each of the substrates because the binding of the inhibitor should be mutually exclusive with both substrates. General reviews on multisubstrate inhibitors have appeared (62, 74, 75).

The significantly enhanced binding affinity of a multisubstrate over a single substrate analog inhibitor has been explained by (i) the entropic advantage of reduced molecularity and (ii) the additive binding contributions of each of the substrates. The binding process of two single substrate analog inhibitors is accompanied by the loss of two sets of translational and overall rotational entropies, whereas the corresponding multisubstrate analog inhibitor only suffers the loss of one set of translational and overall rotational entropies (45, 46). However, the gain in entropy in the form of released water molecules from the active site remains unchanged, assuming that the multisubstrate analog binds to the same sites as the two

single substrate analog inhibitors in the ground state of the enzyme. Also, the gain of enthalpy by hydrogen bonds, buried salt bridges, and dispersion forces should remain unchanged. Therefore, a multisubstrate analog inhibitor gains all these extra binding affinities in the form of binding enthalpies (electrostatic, hydrogen bonds, dispersion forces) and entropies (release of water molecules), but does not lose a set of translational and overall rotational entropies. An additional advantage of multisubstrate inhibitors is its expected higher specificity for their target enzyme as compared with a single substrate analog inhibitor because the combination of two substrates makes their structures unique; it is not so likely that they will be recognizable by other enzymes, a frequent drawback in drug design with single substrate inhibitors. Therefore, multisubstrate inhibitors have also been used as an approach to design isozyme-specific inhibitors (76).

It should also be noted that the distinction between a transition state analog and a multisubstrate analog inhibitor is often quite arbitrary. As discussed earlier, so called transition state analogs are often actually more like analogs of reaction intermediates, which may have structures like multisubstrate inhibitors. However, multisubstrate analog inhibitors are not intended to mimic a transition state of the enzymatic reaction.

Another concept related to the class of multisubstrate analog inhibitors is the use of a hydrophobic anchor which takes advantage of the hydrophobic binding interactions near the active site of an enzyme (77). A good example is illustrated with HMG-CoA reductase which catalyzes the reaction shown in equation 18.33.

$$\tag{18.33}$$

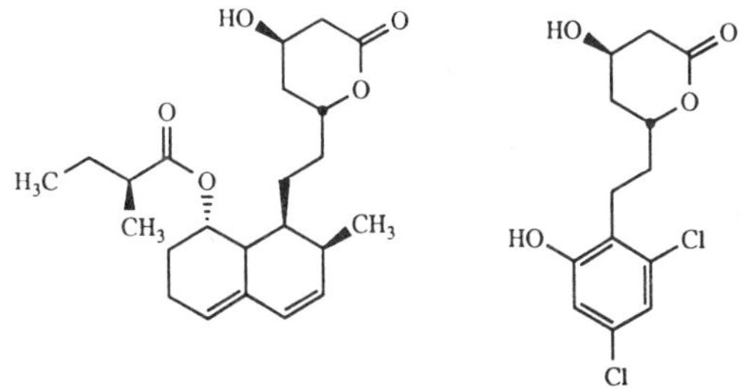

Fig. 18.22 Inhibitors of HMB-CoA reductase, containing a hydrophobic anchor.

Fig. 18.23 The multisubstrate inhibitor β-thioglycinamide ribonucleotide dideazafolate.

Compactin (**13a**) and (**56**) are very potent inhibitors of the enzyme (Fig. 18.22). Based on competition experiments and kinetic inhibition data, the large inhibitory activity was explained by the hydrophobic tails of these inhibitors. Using the upper portions of the inhibitors by themselves in the form of D,L-mevalonate or OH-glutarate resulted in poor inhibitory potency, while using the lower portion of compactin did not lead to any increased inactivation at all. It was determined for (**56**) that the OH-glutarate part of the inhibitor competed with the mevalonate part of the substrate, but did not bind to any other area in the active site. Consequently, it was proposed that the enhanced potency of these two inhibitors was based on the tight binding of the hydrophobic anchor of the lower part of the inhibitors to hydrophobic regions near the active site of the enzyme.

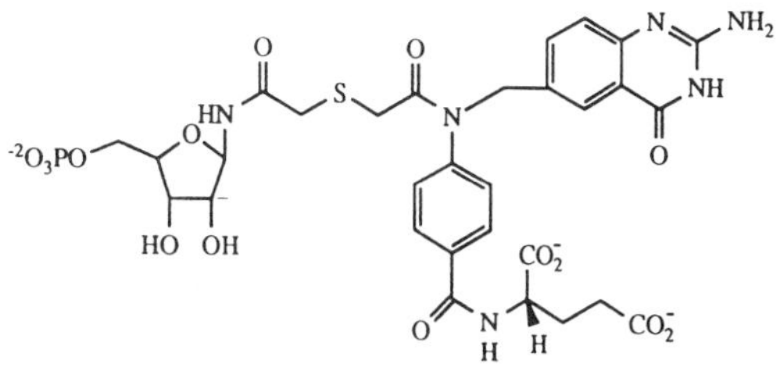

Due to the rather unspecific nature of this interaction, however, the upper portion of the inhibitor was necessary for enzyme specificity. Therefore, this binding behavior is similar to that of a multisubstrate inhibitor by simultaneously binding to two binding sites on the enzyme, leading to greatly enhanced inhibition of the enzyme (47). The anchor in the case of compactin is estimated to provide an entropic advantage by a factor of $\sim 5 \times 10^4$ in binding to the enzyme.

2.5.1 EXAMPLES. Recently, Inglese et al. designed the multisubstrate inhibitor (**57**) for glycinamide ribonucleotide transformylase. It is the most potent known inhibitor of this enzyme, having a K_i value of 250 pM (Fig. 18.23) (78). The enzyme catalyzes the transfer of the formyl group from $(6R, \alpha S)$-10-formyltetrahydrofolate (**59**) to glycinamide ribonucleotide (**58**) (eq. 18.34)

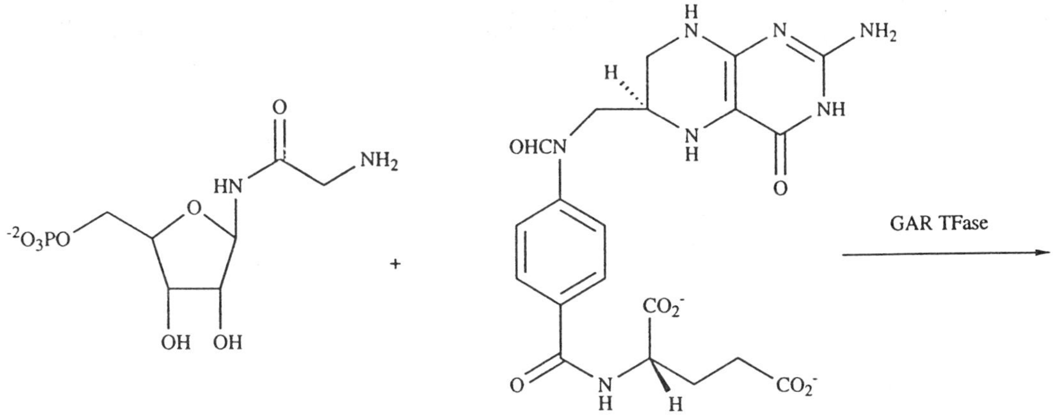

(58)   (59)

(60)   (61)

(18.34)

and has been a target enzyme for the development of antineoplastic agents. The rationale behind the design of multisubstrate inhibitor (**57**) consisted of linking the two substrates of the enzyme via a stable thioether linkage and making a small modification in the folate portion. Inhibitor (**57**) acted as a slow-tight binding inhibitor exhibiting a 1:1 stoichiometry with the enzyme. As expected for a good multisubstrate inhibitor, the product of the K_M values of the two substrates is 3-fold higher than the binding affinity of (**57**).

Kruse et al. (79) have developed multisubstrate inhibitors for dopamine β-hydroxylase. Inhibitors of this enzyme have

been correlated with cardiovascular disorders like hypertension. 1-(4-Hydroxybenzyl)imidazole-2-thione (**62**) and a number of structural analogs were designed to mimic the simultaneous binding of the dopamine moiety (**63**) and oxygen (**64**) at the active site of the enzyme (Fig. 18.24). The sulfur-containing thione is supposed to bind to the soft Cu^{+1} oxidation state of the enzyme like the oxygen molecule during normal catalysis.

Kappler and Hampton (76) have been working on the design of isozyme-specific multisubstrate inhibitors of methionine adenosyltransferase. The reaction catalyzed by the enzyme is shown in equation 18.35.

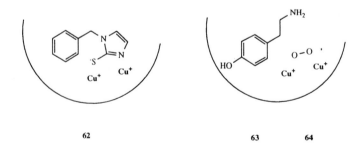

62   63   64

Fig. 18.24 Multisubstrate inhibitor (**62**) of dopamine β-hydroxylase and substrate dopamine (**63**).

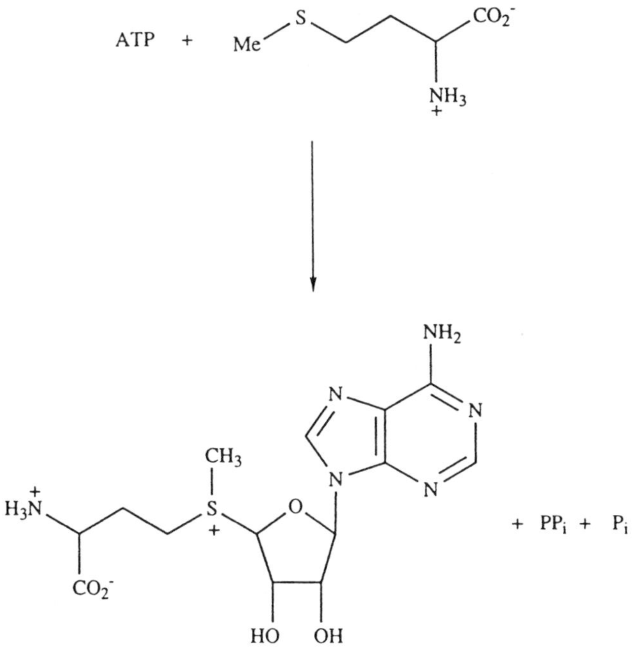

$$(18.35)$$

The structure of the multisubstrate inhibitor (65) is shown in Figure 18.25. The authors tested the inhibitory activity of (65) against two isozymes from kidney (M-2) and Novikoff Ascitic Hepatoma (M-T). Compound (65) exhibited a thirteen-fold higher potency for the M-T isozyme at the methionine binding site, but not at the ATP binding site.

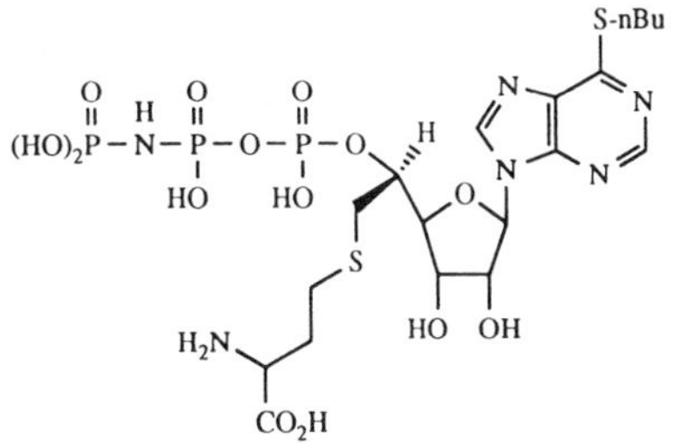

Fig. 18.25 The multisubstrate inhibitor (65) of methionine adenosyltransferase.

3 RATIONAL DESIGN OF COVALENTLY BINDING ENZYME INHIBITORS

Covalently binding enzyme inhibitors can be divided into the categories of mechanism-based inhibitors, affinity labels and pseudoirreversible inhibitors. They are usually substrate or product analogs which first bind to the enzyme's active site in a non-covalent fashion like rapid reversible inhibitors. Upon formation of the enzyme inhibitor complex, however, they react by various mechanisms with one or more amino acid residues resulting in covalent bond formation between the enzyme and the inhibitor. Distinctions among these three categories of enzyme inhibitors are based on this mechanism of covalent bond formation, which generally is the rate-determining step in the enzyme's inactivation. Commonly susceptible amino acid residues are cysteine, histidine, serine, threonine, lysine, aspartic acid, glutamic acid, and tyrosine. In some cases, however, a nucleophilic species is formed which can either react with arginine or any tightly bound organic or inorganic low molecular weight cofactors with electrophilic sites. Arginine is the only common amino acid which has an electrophilic side chain.

Mechanism-based inhibitors (also called suicide substrates, Trojan horse inactivators, enzyme-induced inactivators, k_{cat} inhibitors, and latent inactivators) usually contain a latent functional group which gets activated during the normal catalysis of the enzyme. Upon formation of the initial reversible enzyme inhibitor complex $E \cdot I$, the enzyme starts its normal catalytic cycle leading in a usually rate-determining step to the formation of a highly reactive species $E \cdot I'$ (eq. 18.36a).

$$E + I \underset{k_{-1}}{\overset{k_1}{\rightleftharpoons}} E \cdot I \overset{k_2}{\longrightarrow} E \cdot I' \overset{k_3}{\underset{k_4}{\diagdown}} \begin{array}{c} E - 1'' \\ \\ E + P \end{array}$$

(18.36a)

It can either react with one of the enzyme active-site amino acid residues to form a covalent bond between the enzyme and the inhibitor E-I or be released into the medium to form product P and free active enzyme E.

Affinity labels (or so-called active-site directed, irreversible inhibitors) already contain a reactive, usually electophilic, functional group. Unlike mechanism-based inhibitors, they do not require activation by catalysis at the enzyme's active site. Upon formation of the enzyme inhibitor adduct $E \cdot I$, a nucleophilic amino acid in close proximity in the enzyme's active site reacts with the electrophilic group of the affinity label to form a covalent bond between the enzyme and the inhibitor (E-I) (eq. 18.36b).

$$E + I \underset{k_{-1}}{\overset{k_1}{\rightleftharpoons}} E \cdot I \overset{k_2}{\longrightarrow} E - I' \quad (18.36b)$$

Most often, the covalent bond formation occurs via an S_N2 alkylation-type mechanism, Schiff base formation or acylation.

Pseudoirreversible inhibitors are the least common type of covalently binding enzyme inhibitors. In a first step, they bind to the enzyme's active site in a noncovalent fashion to form an enzyme inhibitor complex $E \cdot I$ (Eq. 18.36c).

$$E + I \underset{k_{-1}}{\overset{k_1}{\rightleftharpoons}} E \cdot I \overset{k_2}{\longrightarrow} E - I' \overset{k_3}{\longrightarrow} E + P$$

(18.36c)

The enzyme starts its catalytic cycle, resulting in a usually rate-determining acylation or alkylation of an active site residue. The covalent reaction intermediate mimics the normal covalent reaction intermediate occurring during catalysis. However, good pseudoirreversible inhibitors form significantly more stable covalent adducts with the enzyme, with half-lives on the order of several hours to days. The inherent lability of the enzyme-inhibitor linkage will eventually lead to hydrolysis or simple reversal of the covalent bond. The half-life of reactivation, as well as the rate of formation of the covalent enzyme inhibitor adduct, will determine its potential as an inhibitor. Pseudoirreversible inactivators are unlike mechanism-based inhibitors in that no highly reactive species is formed during catalysis. They are unlike affinity labels in that they contain no inherently reactive functional groups.

3.1 Evaluation of the Mechanism of Inactivation of Covalently Binding Enzyme Inhibitors

The inherent complexity of the inactivation mechanisms of covalently binding enzyme inhibitors makes it necessary to evaluate their proposed modes of action carefully. An overview of the criteria for the study of mechanism-based inhibitors, affinity labels and pseudoirreversible inhibitors is presented below.

Criteria for the Study of Mechanism-based Inactivators:

1. *Irreversible Inactivation.* Inactivation by mechanism-based inhibitors leads to irreversible covalent bond formation between the enzyme and the inhibitor. In contrast to rapid, reversible inhibitors, the covalent enzyme–inhibitor complex is no longer in equilibrium with free enzyme and inhibitor. Therefore, exhaustive dialysis or gel filtration of the covalent enzyme-inhibitor complex cannot recover free, active enzyme. However, such experiments do not allow distinction between tight-binding, non-covalent inhibitors and mechanism-based inactivators.

2. *Time- and Concentration-dependent Inactivation.* Mechanism-based inhibitors usually exhibit time- and concentration-dependent inactivation, with the rate of inactivation proportional to low inhibitor concentrations. At high inhibitor concentrations, saturation occurs and no further increase in the rate of inactivation is observed. This is based on the assumption that the initial rapid, reversible formation of the enzyme inhibitor adduct E · I is followed by a slower rate-determining catalytic step to form E · I'. Increasing concentrations of the inhibitor should lead to complete enzyme inactivation A typical pseudo first-order plot of log enzyme activity versus time is illustrated in Figure 18.26. Problems, such as nonlinear plots, may become evident while determining the kinetic constants. An in-depth treatment of the potential problems is covered elsewhere (80) and in references cited therein.

3. *Saturation Kinetics and Determination of K_I and k_{inact}.* In order to distinguish the rate and binding constants of rapid reversible inhibitors (K_i and k_{cat}) from the rate and binding constants of mechanism-based inhibitors, the terms of K_I and k_{inact} have been used. Detailed discussions on the kinetics of mechanism-based inhibitors are available elsewhere (80–82) and in references cited therein. In order to determine K_I and k_{inact}, saturation kinetics must be obeyed. Saturation is reached when all of the free enzyme is converted to the reversible enzyme-inhibitor complex E · I. At that point, the rate of inactivation is independent of k_1/k_{-1} (eq. 18.36a), assuming that the rate of formation of the initial reversible enzyme-inhibitor complex is significantly greater than the

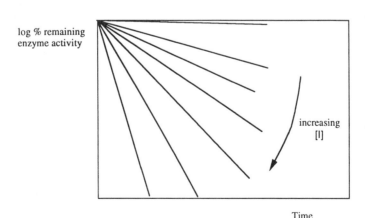

Fig. 18.26 Pseudo first-order inactivation kinetics of a mechanism-based inactivator.

rate of formation of the covalent enzyme-inhibitor complex. Consequently, a higher concentration of inhibitor will not lead to an increased rate of inactivation. The K_I value represents the concentration of inhibitor leading to the half-maximum rate of inactivation, and k_{inact} is the maximum rate of inactivation at the point of saturation. In order to determine the K_I and k_{inact} values, the enzyme is incubated at various subsaturating concentrations of the inhibitor from which the half-life of inactivation at each inhibitor concentration is deduced. Using Kitz and Wilson plots (83), the half-life of inactivation at each inhibitor concentration is plotted against 1/inhibitor concentration. A typical plot is illustrated in Figure 18.27. The intersection of the graph with the y-axis represents the half-life of inhibition at infinite inhibitor concentration, with k_{inact} equal to $0.693/t_{1/2}$. K_I can be determined from the intersection of the graph with the x-axis which is equal to $-1/K_I$. If no saturation occurs with a tested inhibitor, the graph will intercept at the origin of the graph, implying that k_{inact} is much faster than the formation of the initial reversible enzyme-mechanism-based inhibitor complex. If this is observed, one might use a lower temperature or a different pH in order to lower k_{inact}.

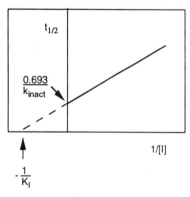

Fig. 18.27 Kitz and Wilson plot.

4. *Substrate Protection.* A mechanism-based inactivator should be active site-directed, thereby competing with the substrate for the same binding site on the enzyme. The enzyme is incubated with increasing amounts of substrate at constant inhibitor concentrations. The higher the substrate concentration, the slower the rate of inactivation because a portion of the enzyme is protected as the $E \cdot S$ complex under initial velocity conditions. A typical plot of log enzyme concentration versus time at different substrate concentrations is shown in Figure 18.28.

5. *Occurrence of a Catalytic Step.* The major difference between the mechanism of inactivation of mechanism-based (and pseudoirreversible) inactivators versus any other type of inhibitor is the necessary involvement of a catalytic step. Upon reversible binding of the mechanism-based inhibitor, the enzyme starts its normal catalytic cycle and converts a latent functional group of the inhibitor into a potent electrophile or nucleophile. The necessary experiments to prove this feature are obviously strongly dependent on the particular catalytic mechanism involved.

6. *No Release of the Activated Species Prior to Enzyme Inactivation.* In order for a mechanism-based inactivator to retain its high specificity during inactivation, a release of the reactive species, followed by rebinding and covalent modification of an active site amino acid residue cannot be part of the normal mechanism of inactivation. Such an inhibitor is termed a metabolically activated affinity label (84) because the nonspecific covalent modification of other than the active site as observed for affinity labels cannot be excluded. The release of an activated species prior to inactivation can be indicated by a time-dependent increase of the inactivation rate, due to the accumulation of free,

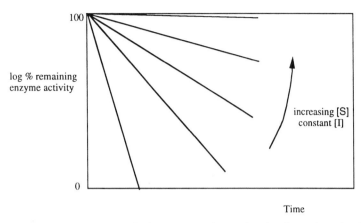

Fig. 18.28 Substrate protection of an enzyme in the presence of an active-site directed covalently binding enzyme inhibitor.

reactive species in solution. Alternatively, a metabolically activated affinity label should inactivate an added second equivalent of fresh enzyme to the incubation buffer at a higher rate than the first equivalent of enzyme. This requires, however, that the reactive species is relatively stable and is not immediately quenched by the incubation buffer. Also, the presence of a free, reactive electrophilic species can be tested by addition of nucleophilic scavengers like thiols (dithiothreitol or β-mercaptoethanol). They should quench all of the free reactive species thereby protecting the enzyme from inhibition. However, this method cannot exclude the possibility that a nucleophilic thiol may even attack the bound reactive species at the active site of the enzyme or that the released reactive species may return and react faster with an active site nucleophile than the added thiol. Due to the obvious complexity of the problem it is advisable to use several different tests in order to avoid misleading conclusions.

7. *Stoichiometry of the Covalent Enzyme-Inhibitor Complex.* In general, complete inactivation of an enzyme requires the binding of one mole of inhibitor per mole of enzyme active site. Exceptions can be certain multimeric enzymes which are inactivated by binding of only one-half mole of inhibitor per mole of enzyme subunit, a phenomenon called half-site reactivity. The stoichiometry of binding is usually determined by incubating an excess of radiolabeled inhibitor with the enzyme to ensure complete irreversible inactivation, followed by exhaustive dialysis or gel filtration. The binding stoichiometry of the obtained enzyme-inhibitor complex in the absence of free inhibitor is then examined for its radiolabel and protein content.

8. *Partition Ratio.* The ratio of the mechanism-based inhibitor molecules converted and released as product relative to each catalytic turnover, leading to enzyme inactivation, has been described by the partition ratio (k_3/k_4, eq. 18.36a). The most efficient inactivators have a partition ratio of zero whereby theoretically every enzymatically processed inhibitor molecule leads to inactivation of a molecule of enzyme. A number of different methods have been used to determine the partition ratio. If the rate of inactivation is relatively fast compared to the chemical stability of the enzyme or the inhibitor under the ex-

perimental conditions, the partition ratio can be determined kinetically by titration of the enzyme activity. Increasing amounts of inhibitor are added to a known amount of enzyme, and the reaction is allowed to go to completion. The excess inhibitor is subsequently removed by gel filtration or dialysis. The amount of inhibitor bound per enzyme active site and the remaining enzyme activity is determined (Fig. 18.29). The intercept with the x-axis represents the minimum number of equivalents of inhibitor necessary to inactivate the enzyme completely. A partition ratio of 5, for example, indicates that on average 5 equivalents of inactivator are converted to product and only every sixth equivalent of inhibitor leads to irreversible covalent bond formation. Alternative methods for determining partition ratios are equilibrium dialysis of the enzyme with radiolabeled inactivator or the determination of k_{cat} and k_{inact}, with k_{cat}/k_{inact} being the partition ratio (80).

9. *Covalent Bond Formation between the Enzyme and the Inhibitor.* In many cases it can be difficult to differentiate between a covalently binding enzyme inhibitor and a very tight but noncovalently binding inhibitor. While even very strong denaturation conditions may not lead to the release of tight, noncovalently bound inhibitors, the covalent linkage

between an enzyme and its inhibitor can sometimes be quite labile to nucleophiles and extremes of pH. A frequently used method to determine the covalently modified amino acid residue of an enzyme's active site is peptide mapping. Enzyme inhibitor complexes, usually prepared from radioactive labeled inhibitor, are treated under denaturating conditions with an appropriate protease. Subsequently, the peptide fragments obtained are usually resolved by high-pressure liquid chromatography and isolated. Analysis of the labeled peptides can be accomplished by Edman degradation. A good description of this method can be found elsewhere (85). Alternatively, electrospray ionization mass spectrometry has been used as a tool to determine the accurate mass of the proteins and enzyme-inhibitor complexes. In a study by Knight and co-workers (86), this method was successfully used to distinguish between covalent and noncovalent complexes, because the latter did not survive the experimental conditions. Excellent more in-depth treatments of the theory and experimental protocols involved have appeared recently for mechanism-based inhibitors (80).

Criteria for the Study of Affinity Labels:
The evaluation of affinity labels is based on the fulfillment of the following criteria: (*1*) irreversible, active site-directed inactivation of the enzyme upon the formation of a stable, covalent linkage with the inhibitor, (*2*) time- and concentration-dependent inactivation showing saturation kinetics, (*3*) a binding stoichiometry of 1:1 of inhibitor to the enzyme's active site, (*4*) determination of the partition ratio, K_I and k_{inact}, and (*5*) verification of covalent bond formation. A more detailed discussion can be found under criteria for mechanism-based inactivators.

Criteria for the Study of Pseudoirreversible Inactivators:

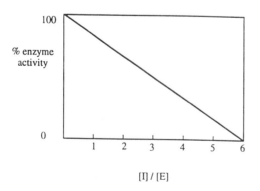

Fig. 18.29 Determination of the partition ratio.

Criteria for the study of pseudoirreversible inhibitors are very similar to those for mechanism-based inhibitors. However, due to the inherent reversibility of pseudoirreversible inhibitors, it may be more difficult to obtain structural evidence for the covalent enzyme inhibitor adduct. In addition, determination of the reactivation rate and characterization of the decomposition products may be of value in understanding mechanisms of the inactivation and recovery processes.

3.2 Mechanism-based Inhibitors

Mechanism-based inactivators have a great potential as drugs because they are commonly quite specific towards their target enzyme. Usually, these fairly unreactive compounds are only converted into highly reactive species upon catalysis by the target enzyme. Consequently, they should show little cell toxicity unless the reactive species fails to bind to the enzyme's active site and is released into solution. This reactive species may then react with other enzymes or turn into a noncovalent inhibitor upon hydrolysis.

The design of mechanism-based inhibitors requires an understanding of the binding specificity requirements for the ligand recognition site of the enzyme in order to promote the formation of the initial noncovalent enzyme inhibitor complex $E \cdot I$. Furthermore, the choice of an appropriate latent functional group requires knowledge of the catalytic mechanism of the target enzyme with its normal substrate. Finally, covalent bond formation of the reactive species E-I' will strongly depend on its inherent chemical reactivity and close proximity to a susceptible amino acid residue or cofactor. The underlying principles in the design of mechanism-based inactivators can be illustrated with the following recent examples. They are also chosen to emphasize the potential of mechanism-based inhibitors as drugs as well as the diversity of their mechanisms of inactivation. All of the following examples have been carefully evaluated on the basis of the above criteria for mechanism-based inhibitors. A number of excellent reviews have appeared lately on the general design of mechanism-based inhibitors (80, 87–95).

3.2.1 EXAMPLES. Pyridoxal phosphate-dependent enzymes have been very successful targets in the design of mechanism-based inhibitors. Good examples are GABA aminotransferase (96), alanine racemase (97) and ornithine aminotransferase (98). Catalysis by these enzymes involves Schiff base-formation of the amino group of the substrate (**66**) with pyridoxal phosphate (**67**) to form complex (**68**). This is followed by abstraction of the alpha proton by an active site base to form a resonance-stabilized carbocation (**69**, eq. 18.37).

(69)   (18.37)

An appropriately positioned latent functional group is subsequently activated and converted into a highly reactive species.

GABA aminotransferase catalyzes the conversion of γ-aminobutyric acid (**70**) to succinic semialdehyde (**73**) and the subsequent transfer of an amino group to pyruvate. The mechanism of the first half of the catalysis is outlined in equation 18.38.

(70)   (71)

(73)   (72)

(18.38)

Z-4-Amino-2-fluorobut-2-enoic acid (**74**) is a mechanism-based inactivator of this en-

zyme (**96**), and the proposed mechanism is shown in equation 18.39.

where Pyr = pyridoxal phosphate ring moiety

$$(18.39)$$

In analogy to the normal catalysis of the enzyme, the inactivation starts with Schiff base-formation of the enzyme-bound pyridoxal phosphate, followed by removal of a γ-proton by an active site base to form the reactive electrophilic intermediate (**76**), which partitions between hydrolysis of the Schiff base linkage and Michael-type addition of an enzyme active site nucleophile, resulting in enzyme reactivation and covalent irreversible inactivation of the enzyme, respectively. The enzyme was inactivated in a time- and concentration-dependent manner, and K_I and k_{inact} values of $0.22\,mM$ and $0.21\,min^{-1}$, respectively, were determined by the method of Kitz and Wilson (83).

S-Adenosylmethionine decarboxylase catalyzes the decarboxylation of *S*-adenosylmethionine and has a covalently

linked pyruvate within the active site which is essential for its catalysis. Pyruvate cofactor (**82**) basically serves the same function as the pyridoxal phosphate during enzyme catalysis by stabilizing the negative charge, formed alpha to the Schiff base. The mechanism of the enzyme is outlined in equation 18.40. *S*-(5'-Deoxy-5'-adenosyl)-1-ammonio-4-(methylsulfonio)-2-cyclopentane (**83**) forms a Schiff base-type complex (**84**) similar to that for the normal substrate equation 18.41 (99). Upon general base catalysis, the highly reactive electrophilic complex (**85**) is formed. Subsequent attack of a nucleophilic active site amino acid residue results in permanent inactivation of the enzyme. Values for K_I and k_{inact} were determined to be $18.3\,\mu M$ and $0.133\,min^{-1}$, respectively.

(18.40)

(18.41)

Alternative approaches for a creation of inhibitors for pyridoxal phosphate-dependent enzymes have involved introduction of an acetylenic group (98) or a halovinyl group (97) alpha to the Schiff base which in both cases lead to the formation of highly electrophilic allenic intermediates and subsequent irreversible, covalent inhibition of each enzyme.

Angiotensin converting enzyme is a zinc protease which catalyzes the hydrolysis of proangiotensin, resulting in the formation of the dipeptide His-Leu and angiotensin (eq. 18.24). However, Spratt and Kaiser determined that ACE also catalyzes the stereospecific enolization of ketonic substrate analogs such as (86) (eq. 18.42), as demonstrated by the α,β elimination of p-nitrothiophenol from this compound (100). Based on this discovery, N-[N-(cyanoacetyl) - L - phenylalanyl] - L - phenyl -

alanine (88) was developed as the first mechanism-based inhibitor of ACE by Ghosh et al. (eq. 18.43). It is proposed that catalytic deprotonation leads to the formation of a highly reactive ketenimine intermediate, which subsequently undergoes covalent bond formation with an active site nucleophile (101).

Uridine diphosphate galactose 4-epimerase contains tightly bound NAD^+ and catalyzes the conversion of UDP-glucose (89) to UDP-galactose (91) via ketonic intermediate 90 (eq. 18.44). First, UDP-glucose is oxidized with concurrent reduction of NAD^+ to NADH. The ketonic intermediate is subsequently non-stereospecifically reduced to either UDP-glucose or UDP-galactose and released from the enzyme. Uridine 5'-diphosphate chloroacetol (UDC, 92) is a substrate analog-inhibitor which is activated by deprotonation by an active site base (eq. 18.45) (102). The highly reactive, nucleophilic enol subsequently attacks the nicotinamide ring of NAD$^+$. The inhibitor–cofactor adduct binds very tightly in a noncovalent fashion to the active site and is not released under nondenaturing conditions. This serves as a good example of the rare case of a mechanism-based inhibitor that inactivates its target enzyme via the formation of a highly reactive nucleophilic species.

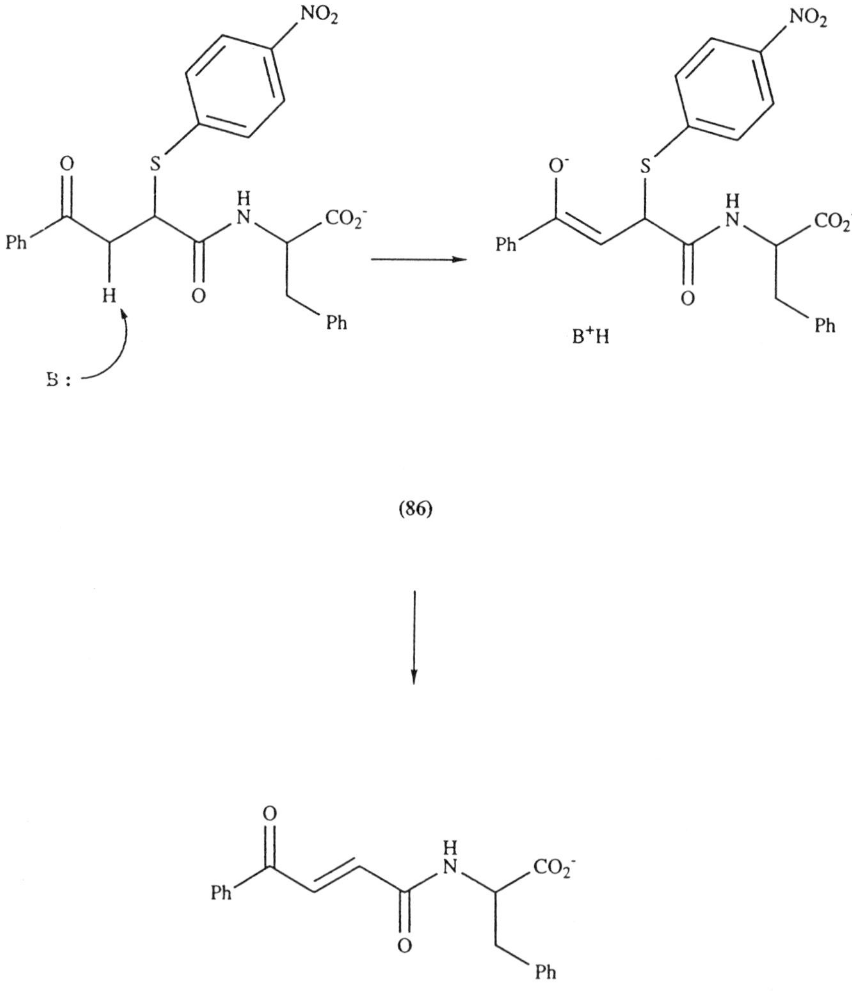

(86)

(87)

$$(18.42)$$

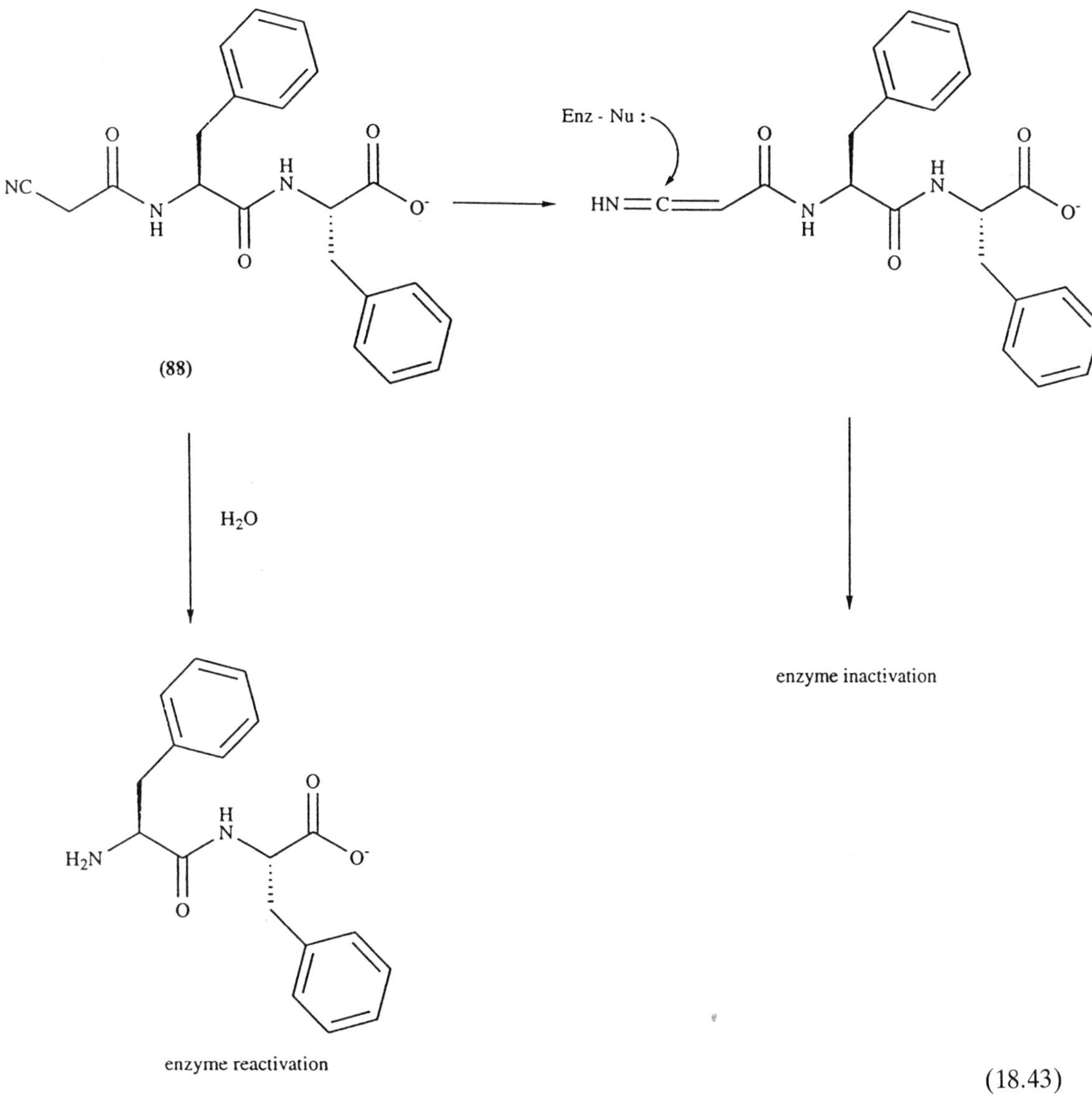

(88)

Enz - Nu :

H₂O

enzyme inactivation

enzyme reactivation

$$(18.43)$$

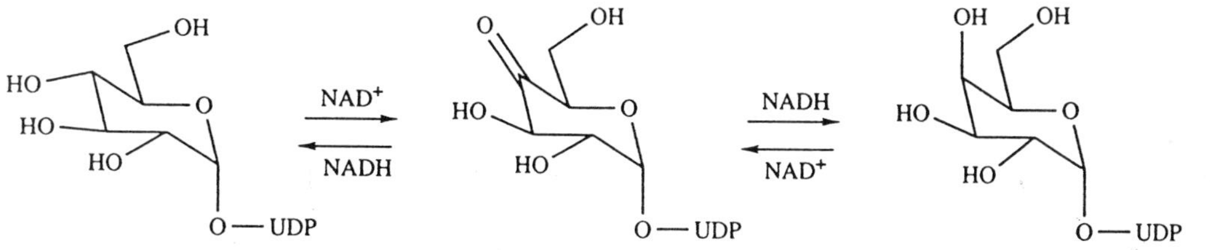

(89)　　　　　　　　(90)　　　　　　　　(91)

$$(18.44)$$

(18.45)

3.3 Affinity Labels

Affinity labels are potentially good drugs, although the presence of a reactive functional group can make then somewhat nonselective and prone towards reaction with other proteins and metabolites. If the affinity label is highly selective towards its target enzyme and has a great affinity for the enzyme's active site, this drawback can be overcome kinetically. Once the inhibitor is bound, the unimolecular reaction between the inhibitor and an amino acid residue in close proximity is entropically quite favorable compared to a bimolecular reaction between two free molecules in solution. More in-depth descriptions have appeared (103–105).

The design of a potent affinity label requires the study of the initial requirements for the inhibitor to bind to the active site. Next, regions of bulk tolerance are determined which are useful for the introduction of a reactive functional group. In some cases, it might be advantageous to place the reactive group at the end of a spacer arm, particularly if no nucleophilic amino acid residue is in close proximity to the reactive group. However, not only are the location and orientation of the reactive functional group critical for its potential as an affinity label, but also the size and inherent reactivity of the functional group. The following recent examples have been

chosen to underscore the principles of the design of affinity labels.

3.3.1 EXAMPLES. Creatine kinase catalyzes the transfer of a phosphoryl group from ATP (**93**) to creatine (**94**), resulting in the formation of phosphocreatine (**96**) and ADP (**95**) (Eq. 18.46). *N*-(2,3-Epoxypropyl)-*N*-amidinoglycine (**97**) was shown to inhibit creatine kinase irreversibly and completely with a 1:1 binding stoichiometry (85). Its mechanism of inactivation is outlined in equation 18.47. It has been postulated that creatine kinase-bound (**97**) is attacked by Cys 282 at the less hindered methylene carbon leading to covalent bond formation. This was supported by model studies. Epoxides have found many applications as reactive groups in affinity label design over the years.

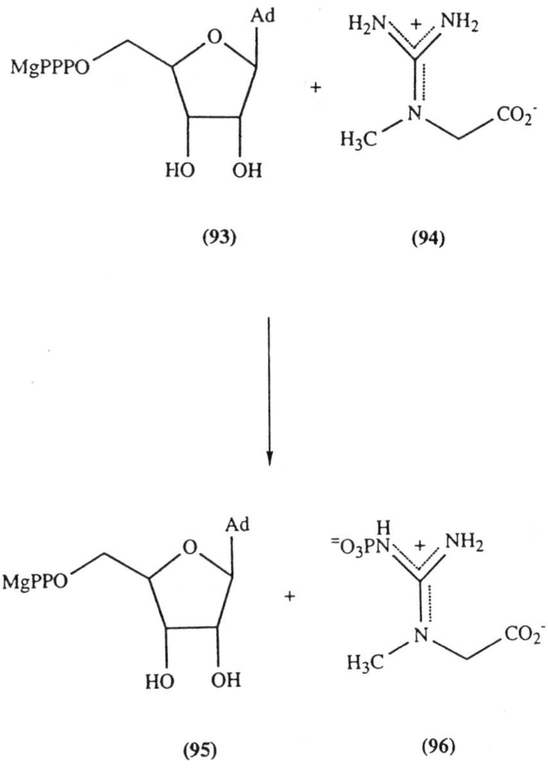

(93)   (94)

(95)   (96)

(18.46)

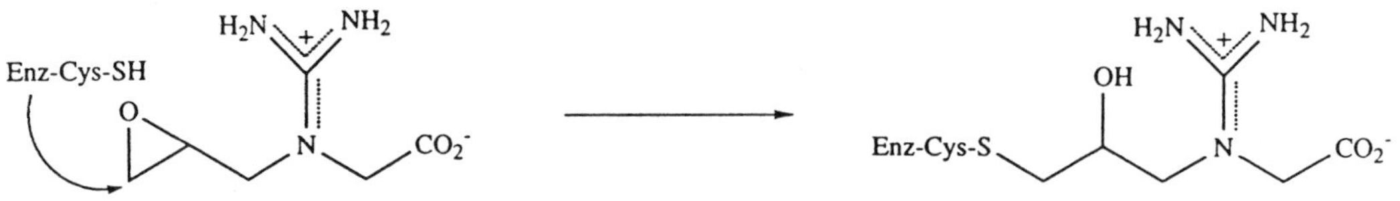

(97)

$$(18.47)$$

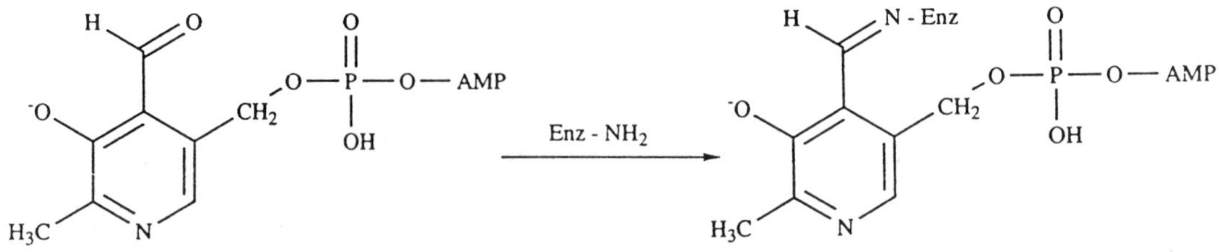

(98)

$$(18.48)$$

3-Phosphoglycerate kinase from yeast was completely and irreversibly inactivated by binding one mole of the substrate analog pyridoxal 5'-diphospho-5'-adenosine (**98**, eq. 18.48) per mole of enzyme subunit.

This enzyme normally catalyzes the conversion of 1,3-diphosphoglycerate (**99**) and ADP (**95**) to 3-phosphoglycerate (**100**) and ATP (**93**) with the equilibrium lying clearly in favor of ATP production (eq. 18.49).

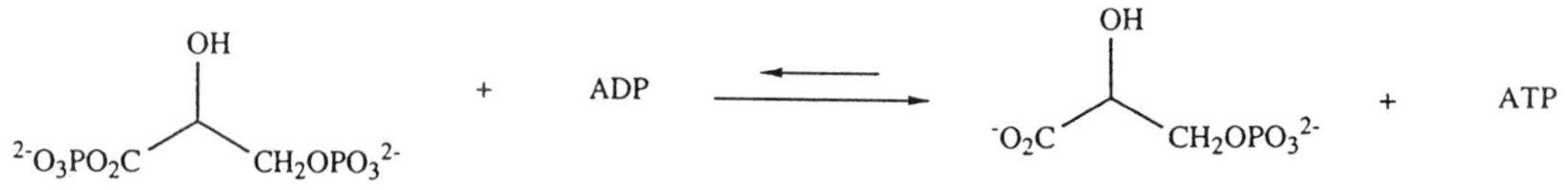

(99)   **(95)**   **(100)**

$$(18.49)$$

The mechanism of inactivation is outlined in equation 18.49. It was shown that Lys 385 underwent Schiff base-formation with the aldehyde of the pyridoxal phosphate analog. The Schiff base-type linkage· was stabilized by borohydride reduction, thereby enabling the analysis of the structure of the complex by peptide mapping (106).

Glycinamide ribonucleotide trans-

formylase catalyzes the transfer of the formyl group from $(6R, \alpha S)$-10-formyltetrahydrofolate (**59**) to glycinamide ribonucleotide **58** (eq. 18.34). N^{10}-Bromoacetyl-5,8-dideazafolate (**101**), a cofactor analog of glycinamide ribonucleotide transformylase, is a potent, active-site directed, irreversible affinity label exhibiting a binding stoichiometry of 1:1 (eq. 18.50).

(101)   (102)

$$(18.50)$$

α-Haloketones have a long tradition as electrophilic reactive groups in the design of affinity labels. It was determined that Asp 144 reacted with the inhibitor, leading to the enzyme-inhibitor adduct (**102**) (107).

3.4 Pseudoirreversible Inhibitors

The potential of pseudoirreversible inhibitors as drugs is strongly dependent on the half-life of the covalent enzyme-inhibitor complex which can be maximized by (i) increasing its rate of formation, and (ii) decreasing its rate of hydrolysis or reversal. In addition, as outlined earlier for mechanism-based inhibitors and affinity labels, a high affinity of the pseudoirreversible inhibitor for the initial reversible enzyme inhibitor adduct E·I will increase its potency. The following approaches to the rational design of this class of inhibitors have been taken.

3.4.1 EXAMPLES. β-Glucosidase catalyzes the hydrolysis of glycosides in a stereospecific, double-displacement mechanism via covalent enzyme-glycosyl intermediate (**104**) (eq. 18.51). Both formation and hydrolysis are proposed to proceed via a transition state with substantial oxocarbocation character (108). In the presence of a given ligand A, transglycosylation may occur as an alternative pathway. Based on this mechanism of catalysis, 2',4'-dinitrophenyl-2-deoxy-2-fluoro-β-D-glucopyranoside (**106**) was developed as a potent inhibitor of the enzyme (eq. 18.52) (109). The authors determined that the covalent 2-deoxy-2-fluoro-α-D-glucopyranosyl enzyme intermediate (**108**) was bound via Glu 358 to the enzyme's active site. The formation of the covalent enzyme intermediate was facilitated by the use of the excellent 2,4-dinitrophenyl leaving group at C-1. Furthermore, the authors were able to correlate the facility of covalent adduct formation with the strength of the leaving group character. The stability of the covalent adduct was increased by replacement of the C-2 hydroxy group with fluorine because it is a more electronegative substituent, smaller than a hydroxy group and also not prone to hydrogen bond formation (36). It is postulated that fluorine sufficiently disrupts the oxocarbocation character of the transition state, leading to increased half-lives of the covalent adduct.

This strategy should be particularly successful for β-glucosidases which appear to exhibit more oxonium ion character in the transition state of the deglycosylation process than that for the glycosylation step.

Chymotrypsin is a serine protease which catalyzes the hydrolysis of a peptidic amide linkage *via* the formation of a covalent enzyme inhibitor adduct with an active site serine (eq. 18.27). 2-Substituted benzoxazinones such as 2-ethoxy-4*H*-3,1-benzoxazin-4-one (**109**) have been shown to inacti-

vate chymotrypsin by the formation of covalent adducts with the active site serine (eq. 18.53) (110). The half-life of inactivation of (**109**) with the enzyme is eleven hours. In the design of these inhibitors, one strives to decrease the rate of deacylation of the covalent enzyme inhibitor adduct without significantly decreasing its rate of formation, thereby leading to an overall increase of the half-life of the covalent adduct. This increase in stability of the enzyme–inhibitor complex is accomplished

$$(18.51)$$

$$(18.52)$$

$$(18.53)$$

by the presence of an electron-donating carbamate ortho to the ester linkage of (111). Unfortunately, an electron-donating group will also decrease the rate of formation of the covalent adduct. This problem was successfully overcome by initial masking of the electron-donating carbamate in the form of (109).

4 CONCLUSIONS

Noncovalently and covalently binding enzyme inhibitors have already found numerous exciting applications in medicine, pharmacology and basic research. Advances in DNA technology have enabled the cloning and overexpression of a significant number of enzymes, thereby providing much larger quantities of the enzymes than were earlier obtainable by traditional methods of enzyme isolation. These advances mean that many new classes of enzymes

will become accessible to the inhibitor design methodologies described in this chapter.

REFERENCES

1. D. K. F. Meijer, R. W. Jansen, and G. Molema, *Antiviral Research* **18**, 215–258 (1992).

2. T. Matsushita, E. K. Ryu, C. I. Hong, and M. MacCoss, *Cancer Research* **41**, 2702–2713 (1981)

3. J. G. Turcotte et al., *Biochim. Biophys. Acta*, **619**, 604–618 (1980).

4. J. G. Turcotte et al., *Biochim. Biophys. Acta*, **619**, 619–631 (1980).

5. F. Artherton et al., *Antimicrob. Ag. Chemother.*, **15**, 696 (1979).

6. S. J. Cartwright and A. F. W. Coulson, *Nature*, **278**, 360 (1979).

7. J. P. Durkin and T. Viswanatha, *J. Antibiot.*, **31**, 1162 (1978).

8. R. L. Charnas and J. R. Knowles, *Biochem.*, **20**, 3214 (1981).

9. R. Labia, V. Lelievre, and J. Peduzzi, *Biochim. Biophys. Acta*, **611**, 351 (1980).

10. C. Reading and T. Farmer, *Biochem. J.*, **199**, 779 (1981).

11. D. G. Brenner and J. R. Knowles, *Biochem.* **23**, 5833 (1984).

12. A. R. English, J. A. Retsema, A. E. Girard, J. E. Lynch, and W. E. Barth, *Antimicrob. Ag. Chemother.*, **14**, 414 (1978).

13. P. S. F. Mezes, A. J. Clarke, G. I. Dmitrienko, and T. Viswanatha, *FEBS Lett.*, **143**, 265 (1982).

14. K. P. Fu and H. C. Neu, *Antimicrob. Ag. Chemother.*, **15**, 171 (1979).

15. L. S. Goodman and A. Gilman, *Pharmacological Basis of Therapeutics*, Macmillan, New York, pp. 1124–1129.

16. P. Furman, M. St. Clair, and T. Spector, *J. Biol. Chem.*, **259**, 9575 (1984).

17. A. Sjoerdsma, J. A. Golden, P. J. Schecter, J. L. R. Barlow, and D. V. Santi, *Trans. Ass. Am. Physns.*, **97**, 70 (1984).

18. E. L. Pritchard, J. E. Seely, H. Poesoe, L. S. Jefferson, and A. E. Pegg, *Biochem. Biophys. Res. Commun.*, **100**, 1597 (1981).

19. W. L. Washtien, *Mol. Pharmacol.*, **25**, 171–177 (1984).

20. H. B. Muss, M. Slavik, B. Bundy, F. B. Stehman, and W. Cressman, *Am. J. Clin. Oncol.*, **7**, 257–260 (1984).

21. D. W. Cushman and M. A. Ondetti, *Prog. Med. Chem.*, **17**, 41 (1980).

22. A. A. Patchett et al., *Nature*, **288**, 280–283 (1980).

23. R. B. Silverman, *J. Biol. Chem.*, **258**, 14766 (1983).

24. E. A. Zeller, S. Sarker, and R. M. Reinen, *J. Biol. Chem.*, **237**, 2333 (1962).

25. D. R. Patek and L. Hellerman, *J. Biol. Chem.*, **249**, 2373 (1974).

26. G. G. S. Collins and M. B. H. Youdim, *Biochem. Pharmacol.*, **24**, 703 (1975).

27. A. Endo, M. Kuroda, and K. Tanzawa, *FEBS Lett.*, **72**, 323–326 (1976).

28. A. Alberts, *Proc. Natl. Acad. Sci.*, **77**, 3957 (1980).

29. B. Lippert, B. W. Metcalf, M. J. Jung, and P. Casara, *Eur. J. Biochem.*, **74**, 441 (1977).

30. G. R. Stark and P. A. Bartlett, *Pharmac. Ther.*, **23**, 45–78 (1983).

31. J. S. Fowler et al., *Science* **235**, 481–485 (1987).

32. H. F. Hixson and A. Nishikawa, *Arch. Biochem. Biophys.*, **154**, 501–509 (1973).

33. D. V. Santi and G. L. Kenyon, in M. E. Wolff, ed., *Burger's Medicinal Chemistry: Approaches to the Rational Design of Enzyme Inhibitors*,

Wiley-Interscience, New York, 1980, pp. 349–391.

34. P. Nuhn and T. Koehler, *Pharmazie*, **46**, 365–382 (1991).

35. A. Muscate, C. L. Levinson, and G. L. Kenyon, *Enzyme Inhibitors*, 4th ed., M. Howe-Grant, Ed., John Wiley & Sons, Inc., New York, in press.

36. R. H. Abeles and T. A. Alston, *J. Biol. Chem.*, **265**, 16705–16708 (1990).

37. K. Appelt et al., *J. Med. Chem.* **34**, 1925–1934 (1991).

38. N. C. Cohen, J. M. Blaney, C. Humblet, P. Gund, and D. C. Barry, *J. Med. Chem.*, **33**, 883–894 (1990).

39. I. D. Kuntz, *Science*, **257**, 1078–1082 (1992).

40. Y. C. Martin, in K. Lipkowitz, D. Boyd, Eds., *Reviews in Computational Chemistry: Searching Databases of Three-Dimensional Structure*, VCH Press, New York, 1990, pp. 213–263.

41. Y. C. Martin, *Methods Enzymol.*, **203**, 587–613 (1991).

42. R. D. Cramer III et al., *J. Med. Chem.*, **22**, 714–725 (1979).

43. J. P. Dirlam et al., *J. Med. Chem.*, **22**, 1118–1121 (1979).

44. Y. C. Martin, *J. Med. Chem.*, **24**, 229–237 (1981).

45. A. Fersht, *Enzyme Structure and Mechanism*, 2nd Ed., W. H. Freeman and Company, New York, 1985.

46. W. P. Jencks, *Adv. Enz. Relat. Areas Mol. Biol.*, **43**, 219–410 (1975).

47. W. P. Jencks, *Proc. Natl. Acad. Sci. U.S.A.*, **78**, 4046–4050 (1981)

48. I. H. Segel, *Enzyme Kinetics: Behavior and Analysis of Rapid Equilibrium and Steady-State Enzyme Systems*, Wiley Interscience, New York, 1975.

49. C. L. Tsou, *Advances in Enzymology and Related Areas of Molecular Biology*, **61**, 381–436 (1988).

50. Q.-F. Ma, I. C. Bathurst, P. J. Barr, and G. L. Kenyon, *J. Med. Chem.*, **35**, 1938–1941 (1992).

51. Y. Q. Shi, I. Hubacek, and R. R. Rando, *Biochem.*, **32**, 1257–1263 (1993).

52. R. A. Perez, E. Fernandez-Alvarez, O. Nieto, and F. J. Piedrafita, *J. Med. Chem.*, **35**, 4584–4588 (1992).

53. L. Turbanti et al., *J. Med. Chem.*, **36**, 699–707 (1993).

54. J. F. Morrison and C. T. Walsh, *Adv. Enzymol. Relat. Areas Mol. Biol.*, **61**, 201–301 (1988).

55. J. F. Morrison, *Trends Biochem. Sci.*, 7, 102–105 (1982).

56. D. H. Rich, *J. Med. Chem.*, 28, 263–273 (1985).

57. P. Buenning, *Journal of Cardiovascular Pharmacology*, 10 (*Suppl. 7*), S31–S35 (1987).

58. M. F. Parisi and R. H. Abeles, *Biochem.*, 31, 9429–9435 (1992).

59. A. Taylor, C. Z. Peltier, F. J. Torre, and N. Hakamian, *Biochem.*, 32, 784–790 (1993).

60. G. E. Lienhard, *Science*, 180, 149–154 (1973).

61. R. Wolfenden, in R. D. Gandour, R. L. Schowen, Eds., *Transition States of Biochemical Processes*, Plenum Press, New York, 1978, pp. 555–578.

62. R. Wolfenden, *Annu. Rev. Biophys. Bioeng.*, 5, 271–306 (1976).

63. P. Bartlett, Y. Nakagawa, C. Johnson, S. Reich, and A. Luis, *J. Org. Chem.*, 53, 3195–3210 (1988).

64. J. A. Gerlt and P. G. Gassmann, *J. Am. Chem. Soc.*, 115, 11552–11568 (1993).

65. W. W. Cleland and M. M. Kreevoy, submitted.

66. P. A. Bartlett and C. K. Marlowe, *Biochemistry*, 22, 4618–4624 (1983).

67. K. Schray and J. P. Klinman, *Biochem. Biophys. Res. Commun.*, 57, 641–648 (1974).

68. L. Frick, R. Wolfenden, E. Smal, and D. C. Baker, *Biochem.*, 25, 1616–1621 (1986).

69. L. Frick, J. P. MacNeela, and R. Wolfenden, *Bioorg. Chem.*, 15, 100–108 (1987).

70. W. M. Kati, S. A. Acheson, and R. Wolfenden, *Biochem.*, 31, 7356–7366 (1992).

71. L. C. Kurz et al., *Biochem.*, 31, 7899–7907 (1992).

72. M Muehlbacher and C. D. Poulter, *Biochem.*, 27, 7315–7328 (1988).

73. E. Tsilikounas, C. A. Kettner, and W. W. Bachovchin, *Biochem.*, 31, 12839–12846 (1992).

74. A. D. Broom, *Fed. Proc.*, 45, 2779–2783 (1986).

75. A. D. Broom, *J. Med. Chem.*, 32, 2–7 (1989).

76. F. Kappler and A. Hampton, *J. Med. Chem.*, 33, 2545–2551 (1990).

77. R. H. Abeles, *Drug Dev. Res.* 10, 221–234 (1987).

78. J. Inglese, R. A. Blatchly, and S. J. Benkovic, *J. Med. Chem.*, 32, 937–940 (1989).

79. L. I. Kruse et al., *J. Med. Chem.*, 33, 781–789 (1990).

80. R. B. Silverman, *Mechanism-Based Enzyme Inactivation: Chemistry and Enzymology*, CRC Press, Boca Raton, 1988.

81. F. Garcia-Canovas, J. Tudela, R. Varon, and A. M. Vazquez, *J. Enzyme Inhibition*, 3, 81–90 (1989).

82. S. G. Waley, *Biochem. J.*, 227, 843–849 (1985).

83. R. Kitz and I. B. Wilson, *J. Biol. Chem.*, 237, 3245–3249 (1962).

84. S. D. Nelson, *J. Med. Chem.*, 25, 753 (1982).

85. D. Buechter, K. Medzihradszky, A. Burlingame, and G. Kenyon, *J. Biol. Chem.*, 267, 2173–2178 (1992).

86. W. B. Knight et al., *Biochem.*, 32, 2031–2035 (1993).

87. R. H. Abeles, *Pure & Applied Chemistry*, 53, 149–160 (1980).

88. R. H. Abeles, *Chem. Eng. News*, 61, 48–56 (1983).

89. T. I. Kalman, *Drug Dev. Res.*, 1, 311–328 (1981).

90. M. G. Palfreyman, P. Bey, and A. Sjoerdsma, *Essays Biochem.*, 23, 28–81 (1987).

91. T. M. Penning, *TIPS*, 212–217 (1983).

92. R. B. Silverman, *J. Enzym. Inhib.*, 2, 73–90 (1988).

93. C. T. Walsh, *Tetrahedron*, 38, 871–909 (1982).

94. C. T. Walsh, *TIBS*, 254–257 (1983).

95. C. T. Walsh, *Ann. Rev. Biochem.*, 53, 493–535 (1984).

96. R. B. Silverman and C. George, *Biochem.*, 27, 3285–3289 (1988).

97. N. A. Thornberry et al., *J. Biol. Chem.*, 266, 21657–21665 (1991).

98. D. De Biase et al., *Biochem.* 30, 2239–2246 (1991).

99. Y. Wu and P. M. Woster, *J. Med. Chem.*, 35, 3196–3201 (1992).

100. T. E. Spratt and E. T. Kaiser, *J. Am. Cheme. Soc.*, 106, 6440–6442 (1984).

101. S. S. Ghosh, O. Nejad-Said, J. Roestamadji, and S. Mobashery, *J. Med. Chem.*, 35, 4175–9 (1992).

102. G. R. Flentke and P. A. Frey, *Biochem.*, 29, 2430–2436 (1990).

103. J. A. Katzenellenbogen, *A. Rep. Med. Chem.*, 222–233 (1974).

104. E. Shaw, *Chemical Modification by Active-site directed Reagents*, 3rd ed., P. D. Boyer, Ed., Academic Press, New York, 1970, pp. 91–147.

105. B. R. Baker, *Design of Active-Site-Directed Irreversible Enzyme Inhibitors*, Wiley Interscience, New York, 1967.

106. T. Pineda, O.-S. Kwon, E. H. Serpersu, and J.

E. Churchich, *Eur. J. Biochem.*, **212**, 719–726 (1993).

107. J. Inglese, J. M. Smith, and S. J. Benkovic, *Biochem.*, **29**, 6678–6687 (1990).

108. S. G. Withers and I. P. Street, *J. Am. Chem. Soc.*, **110**, 8551–8553 (1988).

109. I. P. Street, J. B. Kempton, and S. G. Withers, *Biochem.*, **31**, 9970–9978 (1992).

110. L. Hedstrom, A. Moorman, J. Dobbs, and R. Abeles, *Biochem.*, **23**, 1753–1759 (1984).

CHAPTER NINETEEN

Analog Design

JOSEPH G. CANNON

University of Iowa
Iowa City, Iowa, USA

CONTENTS

1 Introduction, 783

2 Bioisosteric Replacement, 785

3 Rigid Analogs, 788

4 Homologation of Alkyl Chains or Alteration of Chain Branching, Changes in Ring Size, and Ring Position Isomers, 791

5 Alteration of Stereochemistry and Design of Stereosomers and Geometric Isomers, 795

6 Fragments of a Lead Molecule, 797

7 Variations in Interatomic Distance, 799

1 INTRODUCTION

This chapter is limited to nonprotein therapeutic candidates. The rapidly evolving field of peptide analogs and peptidomimetic agents merits and requires separate and extensive consideration. In any strategy aimed at designing new drug molecules or analogs of known biologically active compounds, there are no absolute rules for procedure or guidelines; the knowledge, imagination, and intuition of the medicinal chemist are the most important factors for success. Analog design is as much an art as it is a science. The concept of analog design presupposes that a lead has been obtained, i.e., a chemical compound has been identified that possesses a desirable pharmacological property. The search for and identification of leads is a challenge and is a separate topic. It is sufficient for the present discussion to note that lead compounds are frequently identified as endogenous participants (hormones, neurotransmitters, second messengers, or enzyme cofactors) in the body's biochemistry and physiology, or a lead may result from routine, random biological screening of natural products or of synthetic organic molecules that were

Burger's Medicinal Chemistry and Drug Discovery,
Fifth Edition, Volume 1: Principles and Practice,
Edited by Manfred E. Wolff.
ISBN 0-471-57556-9 © 1995 John Wiley & Sons, Inc.

created for purposes other than for use as drugs.

Analog design is most fruitful in the study of pharmocologically active molecules that are structurally specific: their biological activity depends on the nature and the details of their chemical structure. Hence, seemingly minor modification of the molecule may result in a profound change in pharmacological response (increase, diminish, completely destroy, or alter the nature of the response). In pursuing analog design and synthesis, it must be recognized that the newly created analogs are different chemical entities from the lead compound. It is not possible to retain all and exactly the same solubility and solvent partition characteristics, chemical reactivity and stability, acid or base strength, and/or *in vivo* metabolism properties of the lead compound. Thus, although the new analog may demonstrate pharmacological similarity to the lead compound, it is not likely to be identical to it, nor will its similarities and differences always be predictable.

The goal of analog design is twofold: (*1*) to modify the chemical structure of the lead compound to retain or reinforce the desirable pharmacologic effect while minimizing unwanted pharmacological (e.g., toxicity, side effects, or undesirable metabolism) and physical and chemical properties (e.g., poor solubility and solvent partitioning characteristics or chemical instability), which may result in a superior therapeutic agent; and (*2*) to use target analogs as pharmacological probes (i.e., tools used for the study of fundamental pharmacological and physiological phenomena) to gain greater insight into the pharmacology of the lead molecule and perhaps to reveal new knowledge of basic biology. Studies of analog structure–activity relationships may increase the chemist's ability to predict optimum chemical structural parameters for a given pharmacological effect.

Analog design is greatly facilitated if the chemist can initially define the phar-macophore of the lead compound: that combination of atoms within the molecule that is responsible for eliciting the desired pharmacologic effect. Analog design may be directed toward maintaining this combination of atoms intact in a newly designed molecule or toward a carefully planned, systematic modification of the pharmacophore. If the chemist is uncertain about the composition of the pharmacophoric portion of the molecule, a prime initial goal of analog design should be to define the pharmacophore. The chemist addresses the following questions: What change(s) can be made in the lead molecule that permit(s) retention or reinforcement of the basic pharmacological action? and What change can be made in the molecule that diminishes, destroys, or qualitatively changes the basic pharmacological action? The ideal program of analog design should involve a *single* structural change in the lead molecule with each new compound designed and synthesized. An analog in which multiple changes in the structure of the lead molecule have been made simultaneously may occasionally produce a molecule with highly desirable pharmacologic effects but relatively little useful information will be gained from such a molecule. It cannot be readily determined which change (or which combination of changes) was responsible for the enhancement of the desired pharmacology. On a practical basis, it is frequently chemically impossible to effect only one discrete change in the lead molecule; one simple molecular structural alteration will influence many structural and chemical parameters. Nonetheless, the chemist should be cognizant of the disadvantages inherent in "shotgun" modification of lead molecules.

In analog design, molecular modifications of the lead compound can involve one or more of the following strategies:

1. Bioisosteric replacement.

2. Design of rigid analogs.

3. Homologation of alkyl chain(s) or alteration of chain branching, design of aromatic ring position isomers, and alteration of ring size.

4. Alteration of stereochemistry, or design of geometric isomers or stereoisomers.

5. Design of fragments of the lead molecule that contain the pharmacophoric group (bond disconnection).

6. Alteration of interatomic distances within the pharmacophoric group or in other parts of the molecule.

None of these strategies is inherently preferable to the others; all merit the chemist's attention and consideration. Application of combinations of these strategies to the lead molecule may be highly advantageous. Considering the possible permutations and combinations of these changes that are possible within a single lead molecule, it is obvious that the number of analogs that can be designed from a single lead compound is large. Some structural changes that might be proposed are chemically impossible, e.g., the molecule is incapable of existence, or it represents an overwhelmingly formidable synthetic challenge. These negative factors will diminish the population of possible analogs to be considered for synthesis; nevertheless, the chemist will always be confronted with myriad possible target molecules, resulting from a lead molecule. Rational decisions must be made concerning which compounds should be synthesized, and synthetic priorities must be established for target compounds. It is reasonable that, all other factors being equal, the chemist should synthesize the less challenging targets first. Beyond this truism, the chemist's best resources are his or her intuition and imagination. Selection and application of specific molecular modification strategies depends on the chemical structure of the lead compound and, to a certain extent, on the pharmacologic action to be studied.

All of the strategies of analog design as well as subsequent decisions concerning target compounds to be synthesized can be facilitated by computer-assisted molecular modeling techniques, which may give the chemist further insights into structural, stereochemical, and electronic implications of the proposed molecular modification.

2 BIOISOSTERIC REPLACEMENT

The concept of bioisosterism derives from the observation that certain physical properties of chemically different substances (e.g., carbon monoxide and nitrogen and ketene and diazomethane) are strikingly similar (1). These similarities were rationalized on the basis that carbon monoxide and elemental nitrogen each have 14 orbital electrons, and similarly, diazomethane and ketene each have 22 orbital electrons. Medicinal chemists have expanded and adapted the original concept to the analysis of biological activity. The following definition has been provided: "Bioisosteres are groups or molecules which have chemical and physical properties producing broadly similar biological properties" (2). This definition might be expanded to include the concept that bioisosteres may produce opposite biological effects, and these effects are frequently a reflection of some action on the same physiological process or at the same receptor site. Bioisosteric similarity of molecules is commonly assigned on the basis of the number of valence electrons of an atom or a group of atoms rather than on the number of total orbital electrons, as was originally specified by Langmuir. In a remarkable number of instances, compounds result that have similar (or even diametrically opposite) pharmacologic effects to the parent compound. The significant concept is that the bioisosteres are affecting, in some fashion, the same receptor site or pharmacological mechanism.

Categories of classic isosteres have been illustrated (2) (Table 19.1).

Dihydromuscimol **1** and thiomuscimol **2** are cyclic analogs of γ-aminobutyric acid (GABA) in which the C=N moiety of the heterocyclic ring is bioisosteric with the C=O of GABA. In addition, the -S- moiety of thiomuscimol is bioisosteric with the ring -O- of dihydromuscimol. Both structures (**1**) and (**2**) are highly potent agonists at GABA-A receptors (3). A classic bioiso-

steric replacement study was reported for a methoxytetrahydropyran-derived inhibitor (**4**) of 5-lipoxygenase (4) (Table 19.2). None of the isosteric replacements was as potent as the lead compound (**4**). However, the thio isostere (**5**) approaches the oxygen compound (**4**) in potency, and

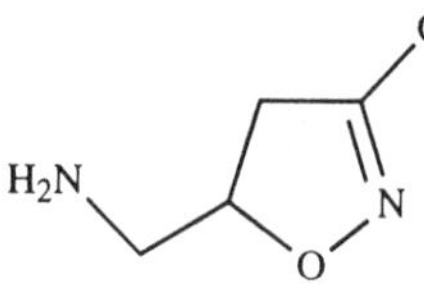

Table 19.2   Inhibition of 5-Lipoxygenase

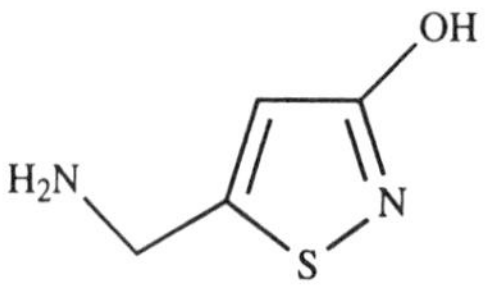

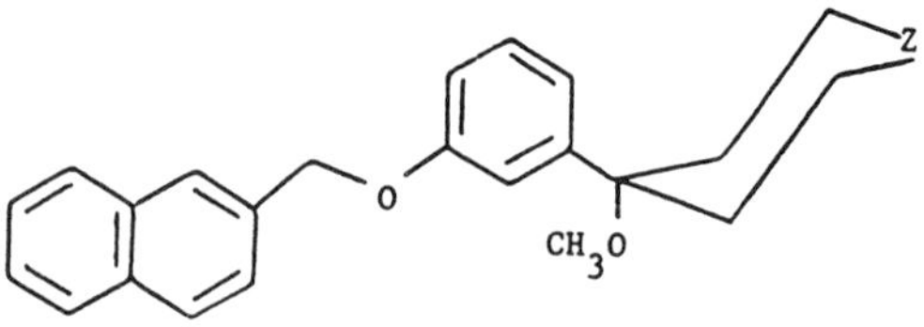

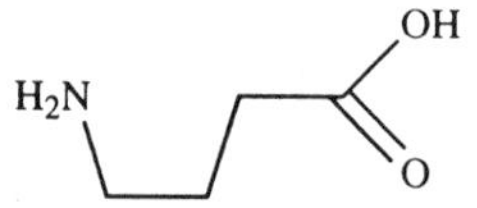

Structure	Z	IC$_{50}$ (μM)
(**4**)	O	0.07
(**5**)	S	0.4
(**6**)	CH$_2$	2.6
(**7**)	C=O	3.4
(**8**)	SO	4.2
(**9**)	SO$_2$	10.6
(**10**)	NCH$_3$	>40

(1)   (2)

(3)

Table 19.1   Bioisosteric Atoms and Groups

1. *Univalent*

–F	—OH	–NH$_2$	–CH$_3$	–Cl
		–SH	PH$_2$	
		–I	t-C$_4$H$_9$	
		–Br	$-i$–C$_3$H$_7$	

2. *Bivalent*

–O–	–S–	–Se–	–CH$_2$–	–NH–
COOR	COSR	COCH$_2$R		CONHR

3. *Tervalent*

–N=	–CH=
–P=	–As=

4. *Quadrivalent*

$$-\overset{|}{\underset{|}{C}}- \qquad -\overset{|}{\underset{|}{Si}}-$$

5. *Ring equivalents*

–CH=CH–	–S– (e.g., benzene-thiophene)
=CH–	=N– (e.g., benzene-pyridine)
–O–	–S– –CH$_2$– –NH–

subsequent studies may reveal other advantages of the sulfur compound as a theraputic agent candidate.

Because of its bioisosteric similarity to the normal substrate L-dopa (**11**), L-mimosine (**12**) inhibits the enzyme tyrosinase (5). These compounds exemplify a situation in which bioisosteres display *opposite* pharmacological effects at the same receptor.

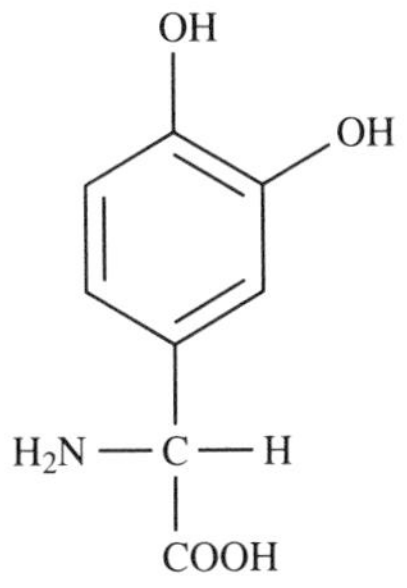

(**14**)

(**11**) 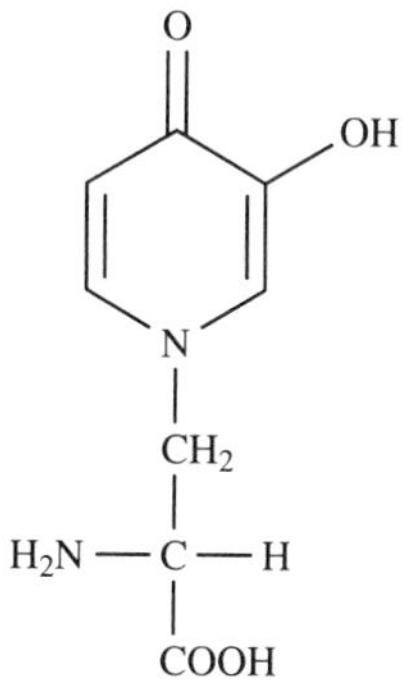   (**12**)

The sulfonium isostere (**13**) of *N,N*-dimethyldopamine (**14**) retains the dopaminergic agonist effect displayed by structure (**14**) (6).

The fact that structure (**13**) bears a permanent unit positive charge was invoked in support of the hypothesis that β-phenethylamines such as structure (**14**) interact with the dopamine receptor(s) in their protonated (cationic) form.

Bioisosteric replacement strategy has

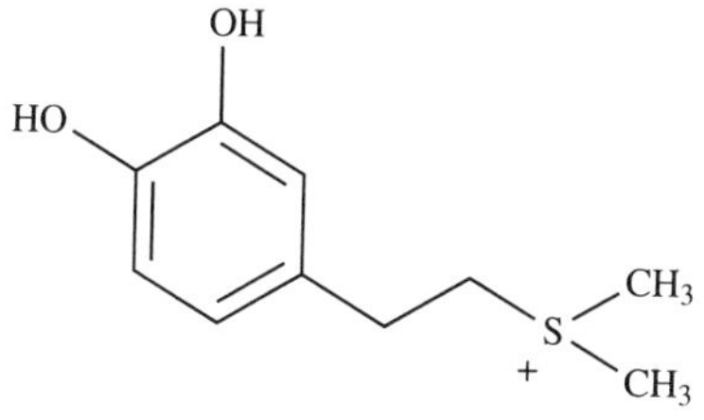

(**13**)

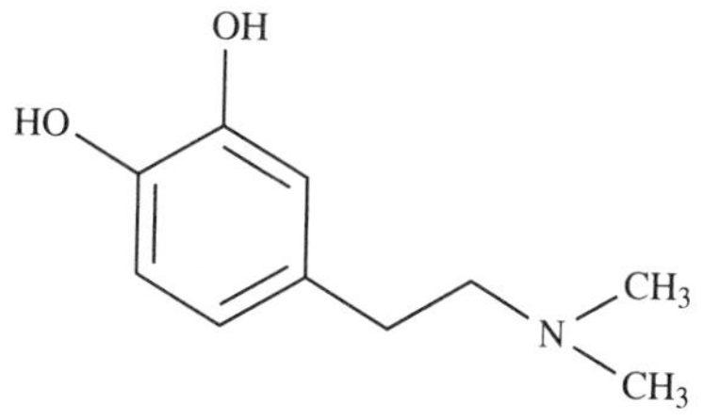

been fruitful in design of tricyclic antidepressants, using the dibenzazepine derivative imipramine (**15**) as the lead.

The structural similarity between imipramine (**15**) and the phenothiazine antipsychotics [typified by chlorpromazine (**16**)] is apparent. Although these two bioisosteric molecules have different pharmacological uses and likely have different mechanism and sites of action in the central nervous system (7), they share the property of being psychotropic agents. In the antidepressant dibenzocycloheptene derivative amitriptyline (**17**), the ring nitrogen of imipramine is replaced by an exocyclic olefinic moiety. Demexiptiline (**18**), doxepin (**19**), and dothiepin (**20**) represent other bioisosteric modifications of imipramine that possess antidepressant activity (8).

While the strategy of bioisosteric replacement may be a powerful and highly productive tool in analog design, Thornber (2) has emphasized that fundamental chemical and physical chemical changes will result from this molecular modification, which may in themselves profoundly affect the pharmacological action of the resulting molecules. Possible modifications include change in size of the atom involved in the bioisosteric replacement, change in the shape of the substituted group and possible resulting change in the shape of the entire molecule, differences in bond angles, change in partition coefficient, change in pK_a of the molecule; alteration of chemical reactivity and chemical stability of the

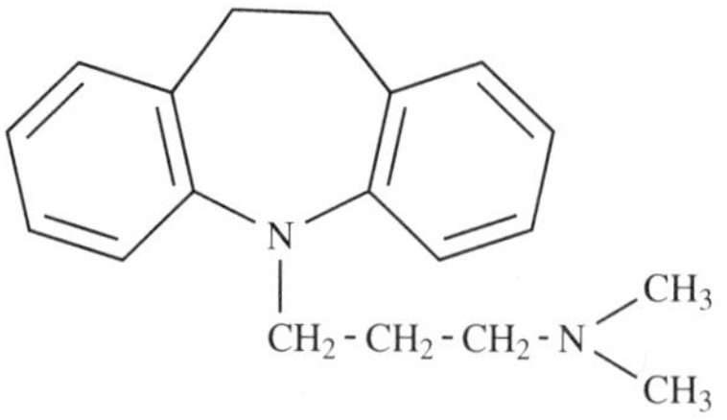

(15)

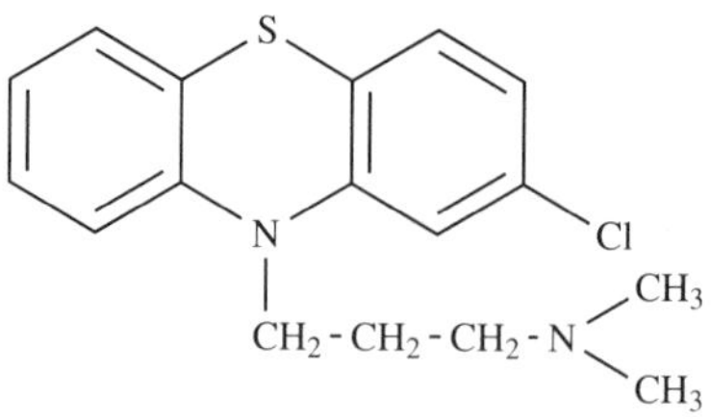

(16)

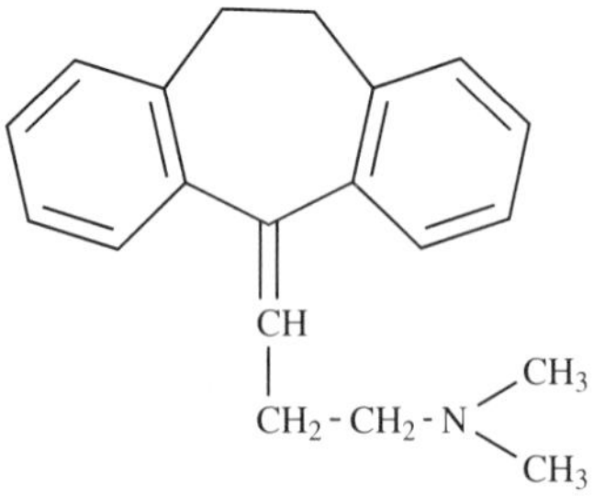

(17)

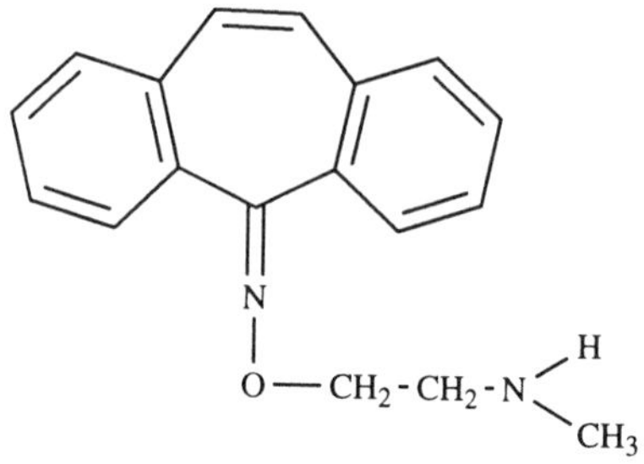

(18)

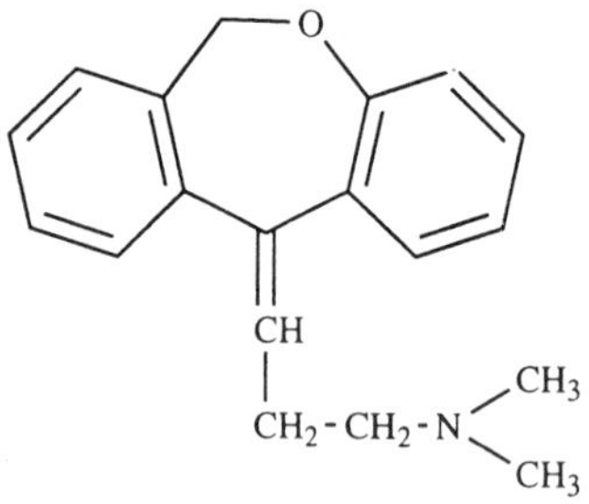

(19)

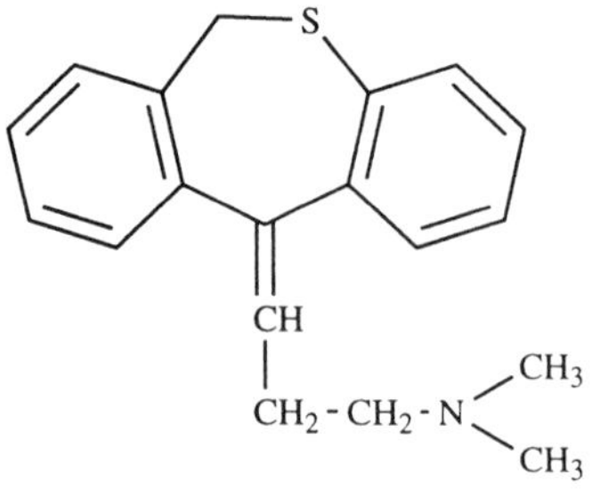

(20)

molecule with accompanying alteration of the nature of *in vivo* metabolism of the molecule, and change in hydrogen bonding capacity. The effect and pharmacological significance of many of these parameters are unpredictable and must be determined experimentally.

3 RIGID ANALOGS

Imposition of some degree of molecular rigidity into a flexible organic molecule (by incorporation of elements of the flexible molecule into a rigid ring system or by introduction of a carbon–carbon double or triple bond) may result in potent, biologically active agents that show a higher degree of specificity of pharmacological effect. There are two possible advantages to this technique (9): the three-dimensional geometry of the pharmacophore can be determined and the key functional groups are held in one position, or in the case of a semirigid structure, these groups are constrained to a limited range of steric dispositions and interatomic distances. By the rigid analog strategy, it is possible to approximate "frozen" specific conformations of a flexible lead molecule, which may provide enhanced pharmacological effect and may assist in defining and understanding structure–activity parameters. Computer-based molecular modeling has been shown to be a useful tool in designing rigid analogs.

The semirigid tetralin congeners (**21**, **22**) of *N,N*-dimethyldopamine (**14**) represent different rotameric conformations of the aromatic ring of dopamine as the aromatic ring relates to the ethylamine side chain when the ring and the side chain are coplanar. Structural constraints of the tetralin ring system impose this restricted geometry on the dopamine moiety. Compounds (**21**) and (**22**) display different spectra of effects at different subpopulations of dopamine receptors (10) which likely reflect different conformations assumed by the flexible dopamine molecule at its various *in vivo* sites of action.

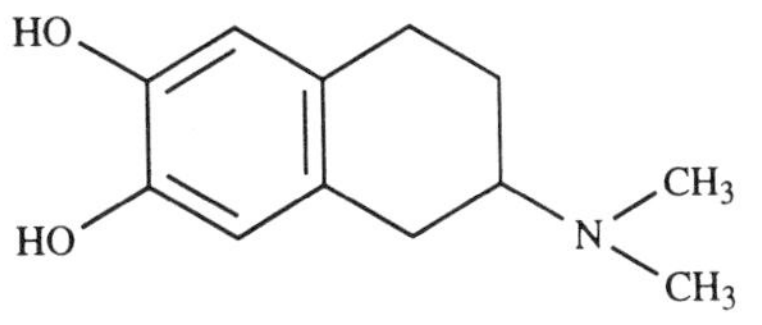

(21)

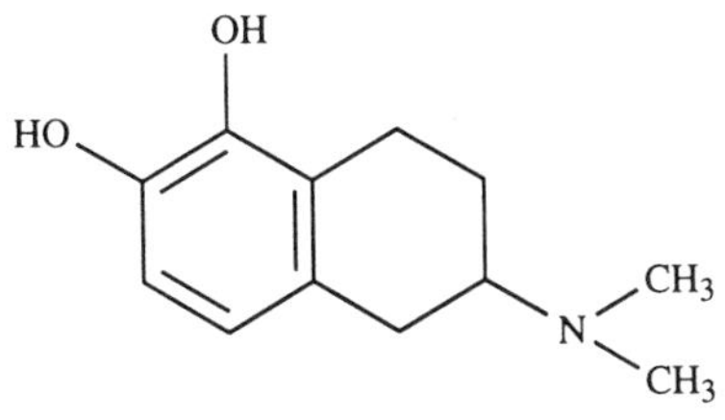

(22)

Restriction of conformational freedom of the acyl moiety in 4-DAMP (**23**) (an antimuscarinic compound displaying higher affinity at ileal M_3 acetylcholine receptors than at atrial M_2-receptors) was imposed by the structure of the spiro-compound (**24**) (11).

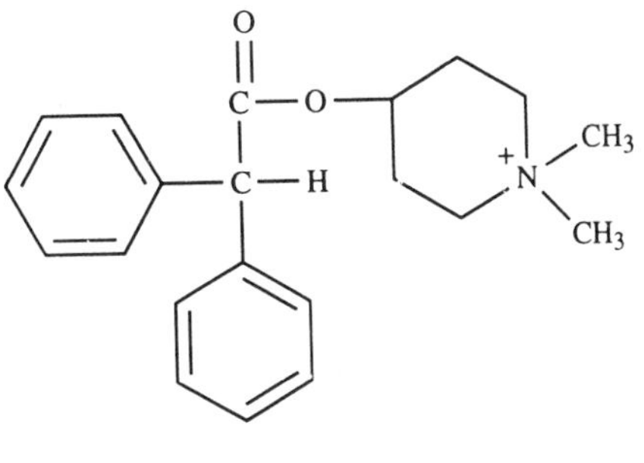

(23)

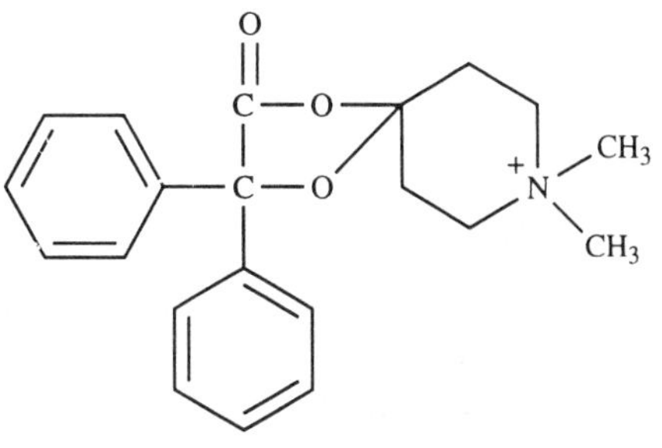

(24)

Spiro-DAMP (**24**) was slightly more potent at M_2 muscarinic receptors than at M_3 receptors. It was proposed that the geometry of the spiro-molecule might reflect the receptor-bound conformation of 4-DAMP (**23**); this conformation differs from that observed in the crystal structure of 4-DAMP.

Imposition of rigidity into the piperidine ring of meperidine (**25**) by introduction of a methylene group between carbons 3 and 6 resulted in the epimers (**26**) and (**27**), frozen conformations of meperidine (12).

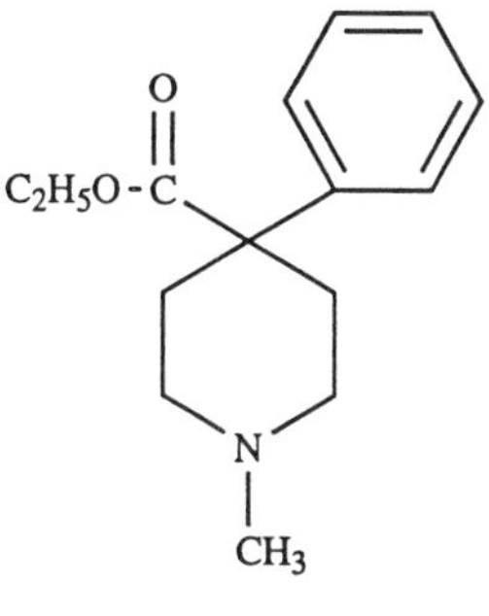

(25)

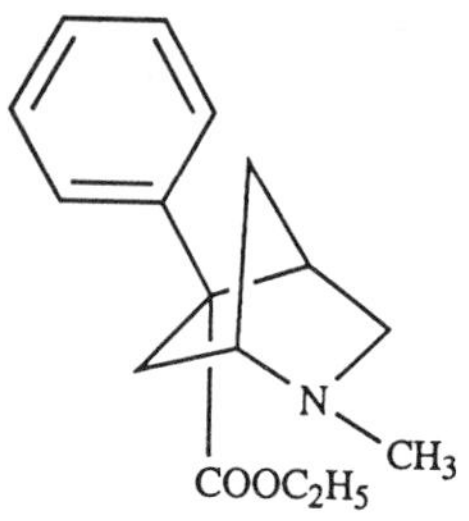

(26) 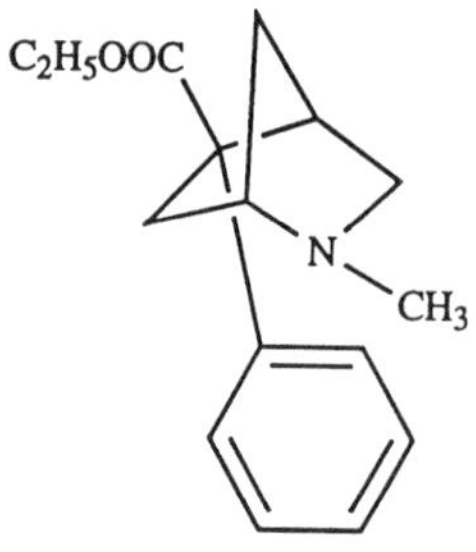   (27)

Isomer (27) was six times as potent as isomer (26), and it was twice as potent as meperidine itself.

Incorporation of the choline portion of the neurotransmitter acetylcholine (28) into a cyclopropane ring system resulted in cis- and trans-1,2-disubstituted molecules (29), (30) in which the acetylcholine molecule is frozen into folded ("cisoid") and extended ("transoid") conformations.

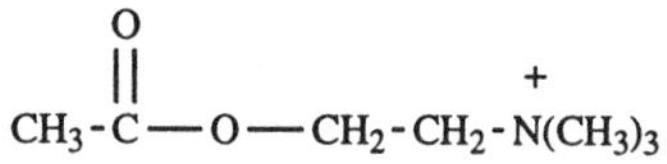

(28)

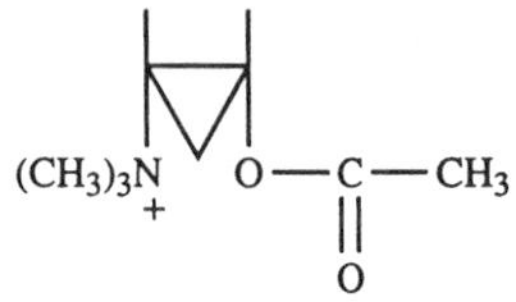

(29) 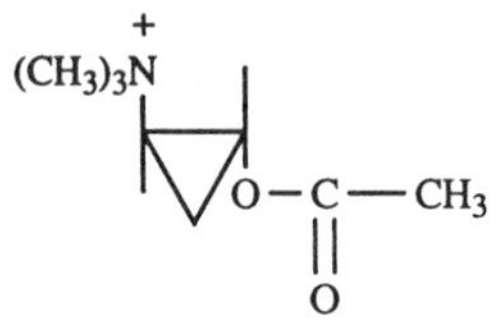   (30)

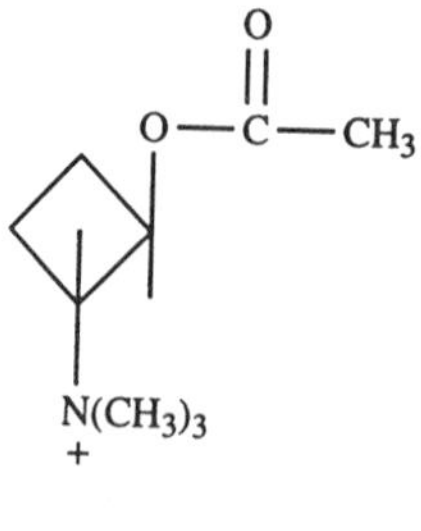

(31)

The (1S), (2S)-(+)-trans-isomer (30) was somewhat more potent than acetylcholine itself in assays for muscarinic agonism (13) and it was an excellent substrate for acetylcholinesterase. The (±)-cis-isomer (29) was almost inert at muscarinic and nicotinic receptors and was a poor substrate for acetylcholinesterase. These data were taken as evidence that the flexible acetylcholine molecule interacts with muscarinic receptors in an extended geometry of the chain of atoms (14). When this semirigid analog strategy for acetylcholine was applied to a cyclobutane ring system [compound (31)], there was a marked loss of pharmacological effect (15). This result is enigmatic; differences in interatomic distances and bond angles in the pharmacophoric moiety as well as differences in the amount of extraneous molecular bulk seem insufficient to account for the dramatic difference in pharmacological potencies between the three- and the four-membered ring systems.

The cyclopropane ring has been employed to impart a degree of rigidity to the side chain of dopamine [structures (32), (33)] (16).

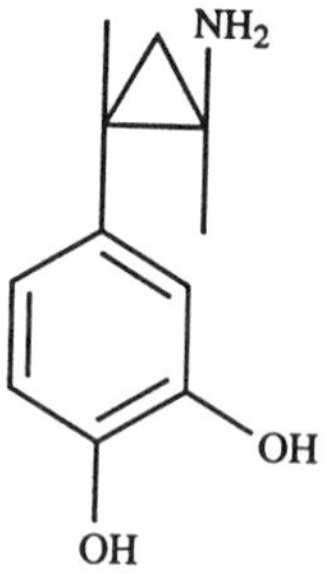

(32) 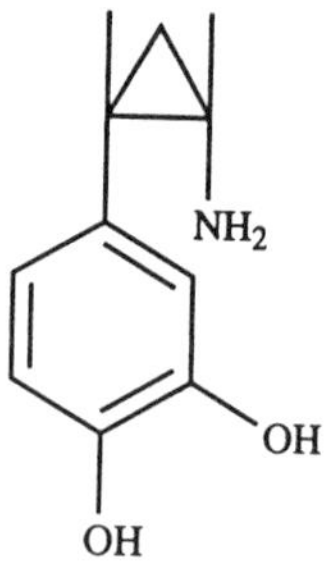   (33)

Neither isomer displayed effects at dopamine receptors, but both were α-adrenoceptor agonists, with the (±)-trans-isomer (32) approximately five times more potent than (±)-cis-isomer (33). It has been suggested (17) that these findings are significant in solving the problem of the preferred conformation of β-phenethyl-amines at the α-adrenoceptor.

The β-phenylethanolamine moiety was incorporated into the *trans*-decalin ring system (**34**) and the racemic modifications of all four possible isomers were prepared as significant frozen conformations of the flexible norepinephrine molecule (18). All four compounds displayed approximately equal (extremely low) potency. The achievement of conformational integrity by incorporation of a flexible pharmacophore into a bulky, complex molecule may be at the expense of biological activity.

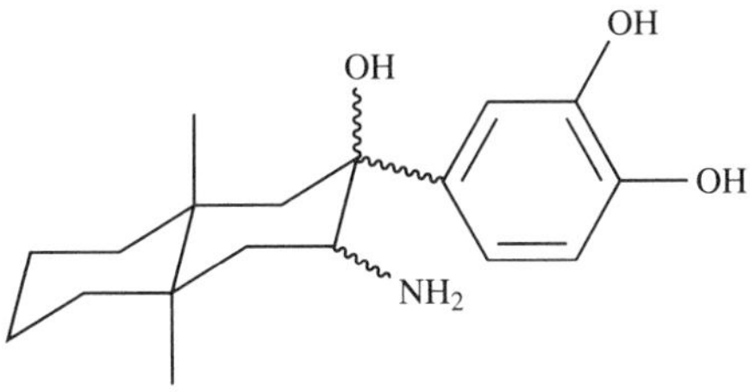

(**34**)

4 HOMOLOGATION OF ALKYL CHAIN OR ALTERATION OF CHAIN BRANCHING, CHANGES IN RING SIZE, AND RING POSITION ISOMERS

Change in the size or branching of an alkyl chain on a bioactive molecule may have a profound (and sometimes unpredictable) effect on physical and pharmacological properties. An increase in the number of carbons in a chain may significantly increase the lipophilic character of the molecule and change the partition coefficient, which may be reflected in the biology of the compound: alteration of absorption, transport, and excretion properties. Alteration of the size and/or shape of an alkyl substituent can affect the conformational preference of a flexible molecule and may alter the spatial relationships of the components

of the pharmacophore, which may be reflected in the ability of the molecule to achieve complimentarity with its receptor or with the catalytic surface of a metabolizing enzyme. The alkyl group itself may represent a binding site with the receptor (via hydrophobic interactions), and alteration of the chain may alter its binding capacity. Conversely, extension of an alkyl chain or branching of it may introduce sufficient extraneous bulk into the molecule to interfere with its optimal interaction with the receptor or with metabolizing enzymes. Position isomers of substituents (even alkyl groups) on aromatic rings may possess different pharmacological properties. In addition to their ability to alter electron distribution in an aromatic ring system, position isomers may differ in their complimentarity to *in vivo* receptors, and a substituent position on a ring may influence the spatial occupancy of the ring system with respect to the remainder of a conformationally variable molecule, What sometimes has been trivialized and denigrated as "methyl group roulette" may indeed be an important parameter in the design of analogs.

Homologation of the *N*-alkyl chain in norapomorphine **35** from methyl (**36**) to ethyl (**37**) to *n*-propyl (**38**) produced increases in emetic action in dogs and in

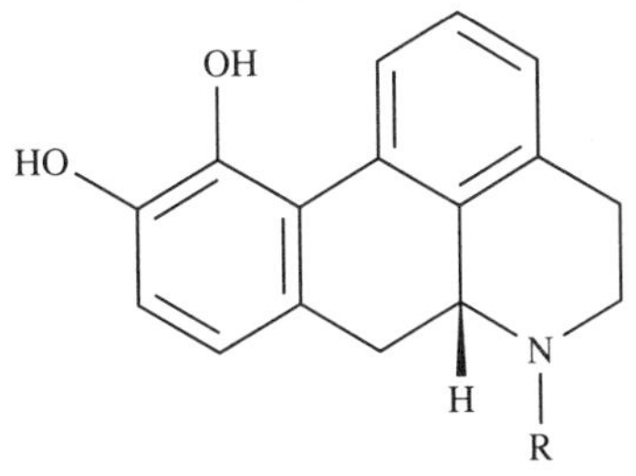

(**35**) R = H   (**38**) R = *n* - C_3H_7

(**36**) R = CH_3 (**39**) R = *n* - C_4H_9

(**37**) R = C_2H_5

stereotypy responses in rodents (19, 20). The homolog, *n*-butyl (**39**) demonstrated a tremendous loss in potency and activity compared with the lower homologs (20). Studies of *N,N*- dialkylated dopamines (**40**)–(**43**) revealed that combinations of alkyl groups may impart a high degree of dopamine agonist effects (21).

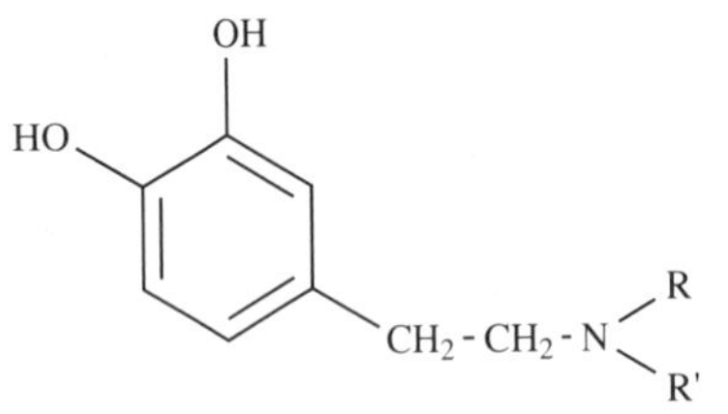

(**40**) R = R′ = CH₃

(**41**) R = R′ = *n*-C₃H₇

(**42**) R = *n*-C₃H₇; R′ = *n*-C₄H₉

(**43**) R = R′ = *n*-C₄H₉

Thus, *N,N*-dimethyldopamine (**40**) is extremely potent in certain assays for dopaminergic agonism, and *N,N*-di-*n*-propyldopamine (**41**) (22) and *N*-*n*-propyl-*N*-*n*-butyldopamine (**42**) (23) are potent dopaminergic agonists, whereas *N,N*-di-*n*-butyldopamine (**43**) is inert (22). It seems likely that the enhanced dopaminergic agonist effects conferred by *N*-ethyl and *n*-propyl groups on aporphine and *β*-phenethylamine-derived molecules are not related merely to enhanced lipophilic character or to partitioning phenomena, but rather to the likelihood that the 2- and 3-carbon chains have a positive affinity for subsites on certain dopamine receptors. These receptor subsites do not accommodate longer chains (e.g., *n*-butyl).

The alkyl linker between the two heterocyclic ring systems in compound (**44**) was modified in studies of the ability of analogs to bind to the cholecystokinin-B receptor (24). When this linking group was ethylene (**45**), extremely potent receptor binding resulted. Introduction of carbon–carbon unsaturation into the linker (**46**) resulted in a 16-fold decrease in binding ability; this suggests a deleterious effect of conformational restriction and limitation of molecular flexibility on biological activity. Branching of the linker chain with a methyl

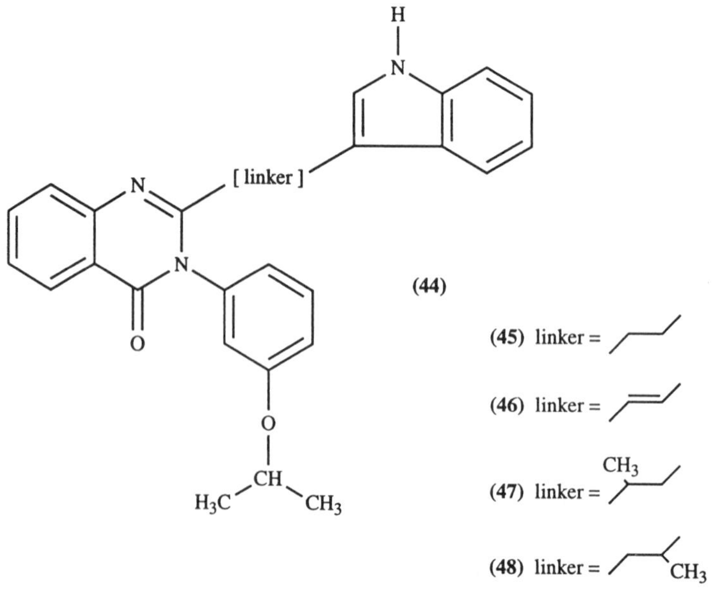

(**44**)

(**45**) linker =

(**46**) linker =

(**47**) linker =

(**48**) linker =

group adjacent to the quinazolinone ring (47) produced a 350-fold decrease in binding potency. However, chain branching with a methyl group in the alternate position on the dimethylene chain produced a compound (48) whose potency was of the same order of magnitude as the extremely potent lead compound (45). The exponential difference in receptor binding ability exhibited by the two isomeric-branched chain-linker compound (47) and (48) was ascribed to unfavorable steric interactions between the receptor and the linker methyl group of structure 47 (24). Isomers such as structures (47) and (48) may generate useful computer-generated molecular modeling data with respect to the preferred conformation of the ligand for optimum receptor interaction and the definition of receptor topography.

A study (25) of (phosphonomethoxy) ethylguanidines (49)–(52) as antiviral agents revealed that branching of the ethylene chain by introduction of a methyl at position 1' (51) diminished antiviral activity 25-fold and diminished toxicity 16-fold compared to the unmethylated system (49).

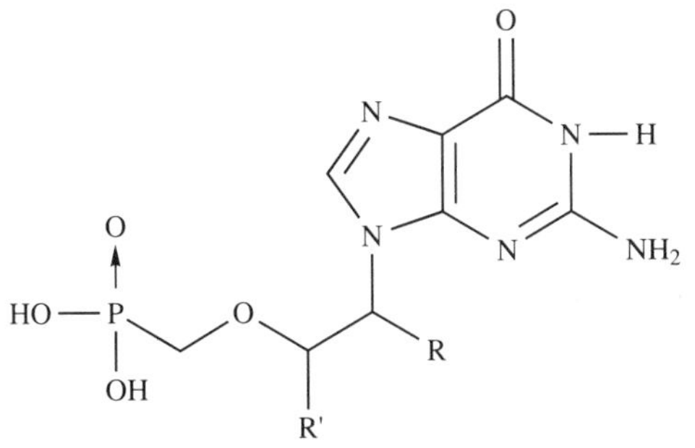

pound (49), but it also exhibited a 30-fold lessening of toxicity to provide a substantial increase in therapeutic index over compound (49). The 2', 2'-gem-dimethyl congener (52) was somewhat less potent than the (R)-2'-monomethyl compound (50) and was markedly more toxic. The (S)-2'-methyl analog (50) exhibited a decidedly lower therapeutic ratio than its (R)-enantiomer, demonstrating pharmacological difference between stereoisomers.

Closely related to the alteration of chain length and/or branching is alteration of ring size. A methoxytetrahydrofuran derivative (53) (Table 19.3) showed activity as an inhibitor of 5-lipoxygenase (4). The size of the oxygen-containing ring as well as the position of the oxygen member with respect to the methoxy and aryl substituents was varied, as shown in Table 19.3. The (seven-membered) oxepane ring derivative (58) and the (six-membered) tetrahydropyran ring derivative (57) showed enhanced potency over the tetrahydrofuran lead compound (53).

In a series of arylsulfonamidophenethanolamines (59) (26), derivatives bearing the sulfonamido group meta to the ethanolamine side chain displayed properties of a β-adrenoceptor partial agonist, whereas those bearing the sulfonamido group in the para position were β-antagonists (26).

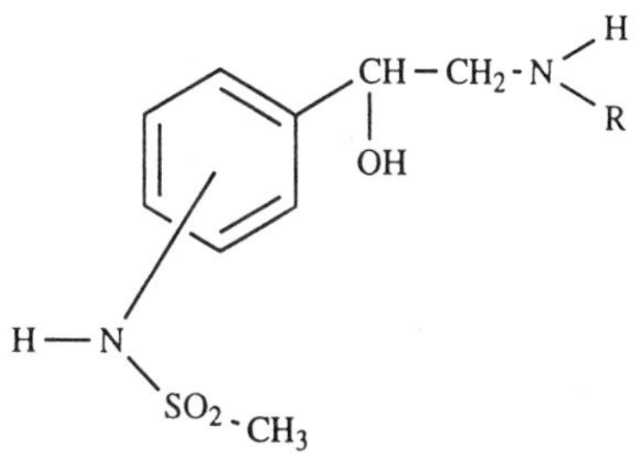

(49) R = R' = H

(50) R = H ; R' = CH$_3$

(51) R=CH$_3$; R' = H

(52) R = H ; R' = gem - di - CH3

(59)

In contrast, (R)-(50), the 2'-methyl congener, exhibited only a 5-fold decrease in antiviral potency as compared to com-

The phenolic group of serotonin (60) was incorporated into a pyran ring (61) (27), which represents an alkyl substituent at position 4 of the indole ring system.

Table 19.3   Inhibition of Lipoxygenase

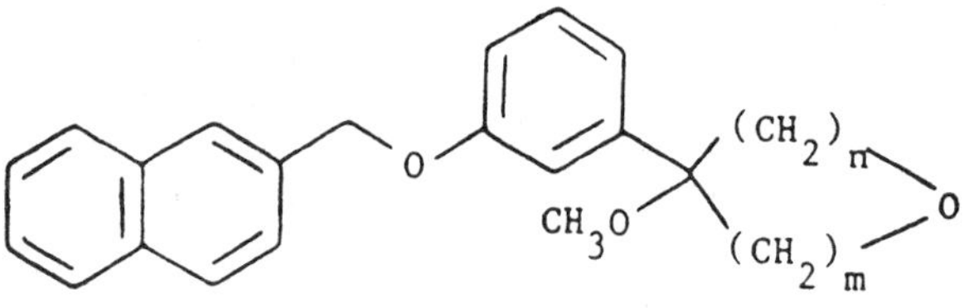

Structure	n	m	IC$_{50}$ (μM)
(53)	1	2	0.7
(54)	1	1	2.5
(55)	1	3	1.7
(56)	1	4	2.5
(57)	2	2	0.07
(58)	2	3	0.2

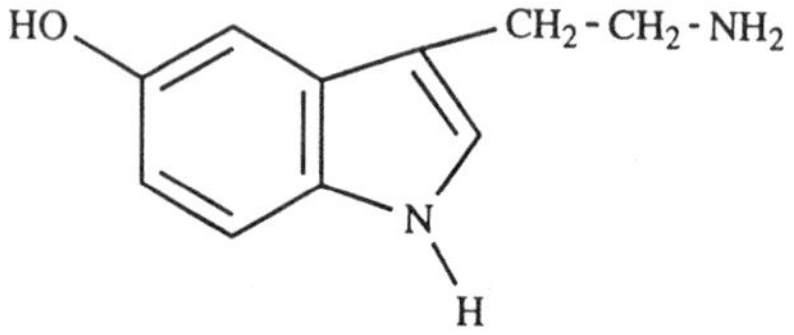

(60)

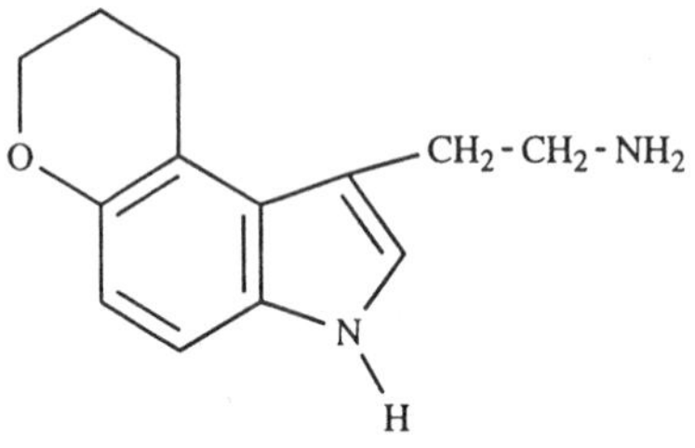

(61)

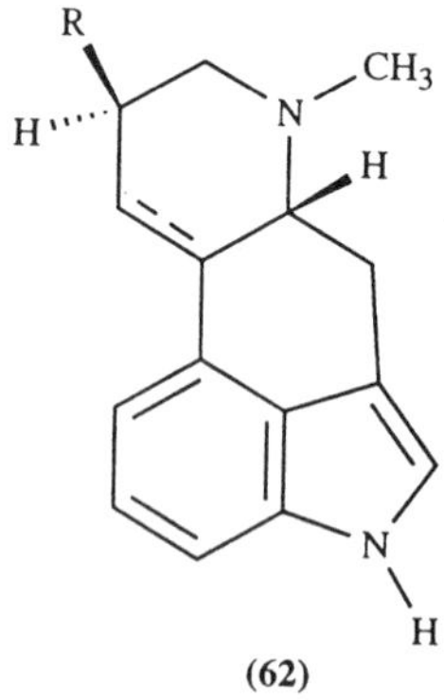

(62)

This analog lost serotonin-like affinity for 5-HT$_1$ receptors, but it is potent and selective for 5-HT$_2$ receptors. The low affinity for 5-HT$_1$ receptors was rationalized, in part, on the basis of steric interference between the dihydropyran ring and the aminoethyl side chain which inhibits the tryptamine system from assuming the folded "ergot alkaloid-like" conformation, as illustrated in structure (62), which probably approximates the conformation of serotonin at 5-HT$_1$ receptors.

5 ALTERATION OF STEREOCHEMISTRY AND DESIGN OF STEREOISOMERS AND GEOMETRIC ISOMERS

The earlier, almost universally accepted, opinion that, in the case of chiral molecules one enantiomer would be expected to demonstrate pharmacological activity and the other enantiomer should be expected to be pharmacologically inert is not valid. It must be anticipated that all stereoisomers of an organic molecule will exhibit frequently widely different and unpredictable pharmacological effects.

$(\pm)$ - 3 - (3 - Hydroxyphenyl) - N - n - propylpiperidine ("3-PPP") (**63**) was described (28) as having highly selective action at dopaminergic autoreceptors.

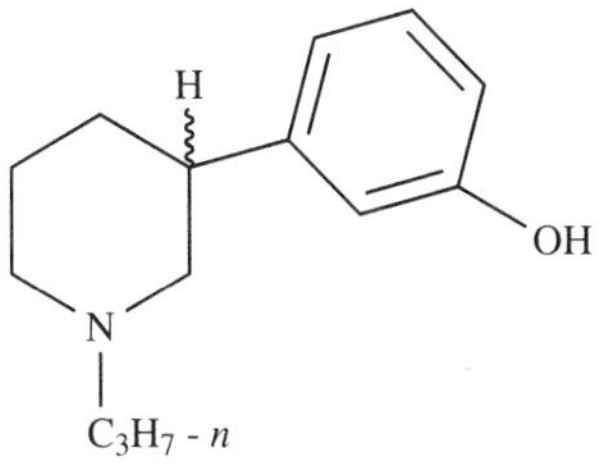

(63)

This racemate was resolved (29). At high doses the (R)-enantiomer selectively stimulated presynaptic dopaminergic receptor sites, while at lower doses, it selectively stimulated postsynaptic receptor sites. In contrast, the (S)-enantiomer stimulated presynaptic dopamine receptors and at the same dose level, it blocked postsynaptic dopamine receptors. Thus this enantiomer exhibits a bifunctional mode of dopaminergic attenuation, that of presynaptic agonism and postsynaptic antagonism. The pharmacological effects of the racemic modification are the sum total of the complex activities of the two enantiomers, and the observed pharmacology of racemic 3-PPP is not an accurate reflection of the pharmacological potential of the individual enantiomers. Pharmacological testing of only a racemic modification is inadequate and may be misleading.

(R) - $(-)$ - 11 - Hydroxy - 10 - methylaporphine (**64**) is a highly selective serotonergic 5-HT$_{1A}$ agonist (30).

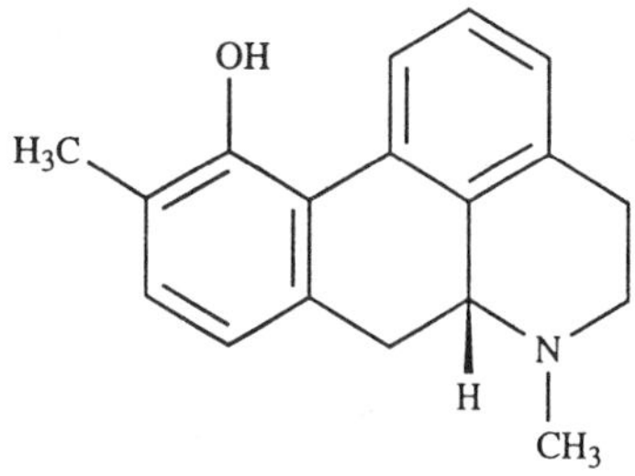

(64)

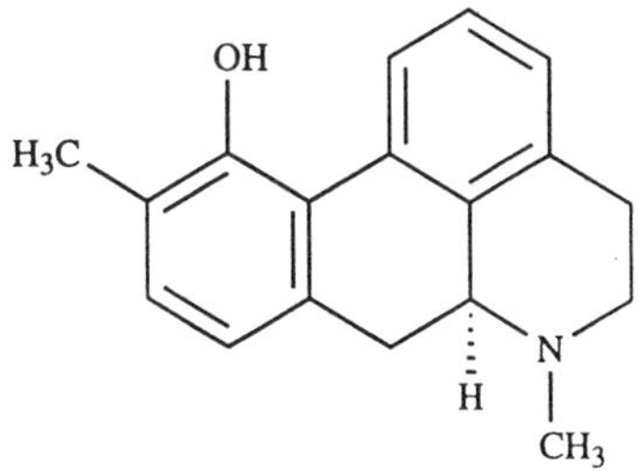

(65)

Remarkably, the (S)-enantiomer (**65**) is a potent antagonist at this same subpopulation of serotonin receptors (31). The phenomenon of enantiomers which possess opposite effects (agonist–antagonist) at the same receptor, once considered to be extremely rare, has recently been noted more often, probably due to the increasing recognition by chemists and pharmacologists that each member of an enantiomeric pair may possess its own unique and unpredictable pharmacology.

In addition to stereochemistry about a carbon center, other potentially chiral atoms offer possibilities for pharmacological significance. A gastroprokinetic compound (**66**) with serotonergic activity bears a chiral sulfoxide moiety (32). The enantiomers are equipotent, but the (*S*)-isomer demonstrates a greater intrinsic activity than the (*R*).

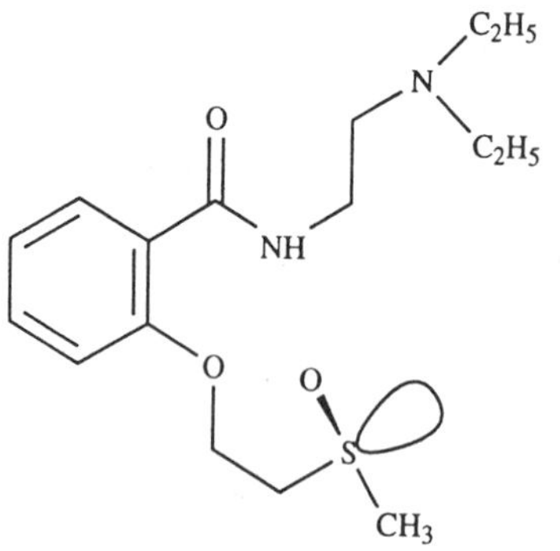

(**66**)

cis- and *trans*-4-Aminocrotonic acids (**67**), (**68**) were prepared (33) as congeners of γ-Aminobutyric acid (GABA) (**3**).

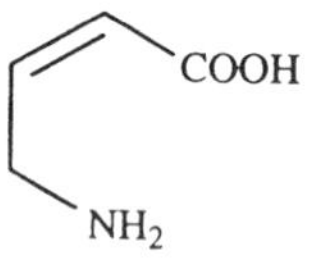

(**67**)

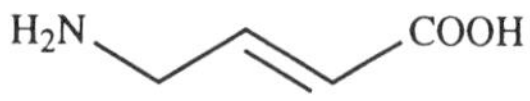

(**68**)

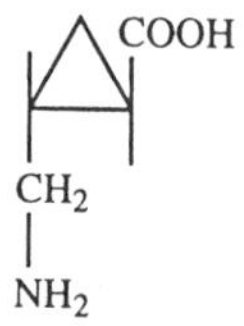

(**69**)

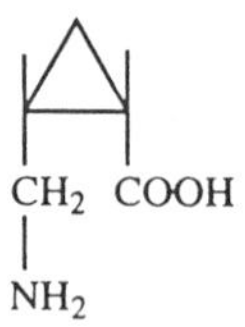

(**70**)

The folded *cis*-isomer (**67**) was inert in assays for GABA agonism, whereas the extended *trans*-isomer (**68**) was active. These data demonstrate biological differences of geometric isomers, which in turn involve yet another structural parameter: imposition of a degree of structural rigidity upon the molecule. A parallel strategy to

the *cis/trans* GABA congeners (**67**) and (**68**) addressed *cis*- and *trans*-1,2-disubstituted cyclopropane derivatives (**69**) and (**70**) whose relative effects at GABA receptors paralleled those of the olefinic derivatives (34).

Hexestrol (**71**), the saturated congener of diethylstilbestrol (**72**), is the *meso*-form of the molecule. It has the greatest estrogenic potency of the three possible stereoisomers (35). In diethylstilbestrol (**72**), the E-isomer (trans), has 10 times the estrogenic potency of the Z-isomer (cis); this effect has been rationalized because the E-geometric isomer is an open chain analog of the natural estrogen estradiol (**73**) (36). In dienestrol (**74**), the geometric isomerism possible with olefinic moieties has been invoked to achieve a similar kind of open chain analogy to the steroid ring system as in diethylstilbestrol, and a high level of estrogenic activity results.

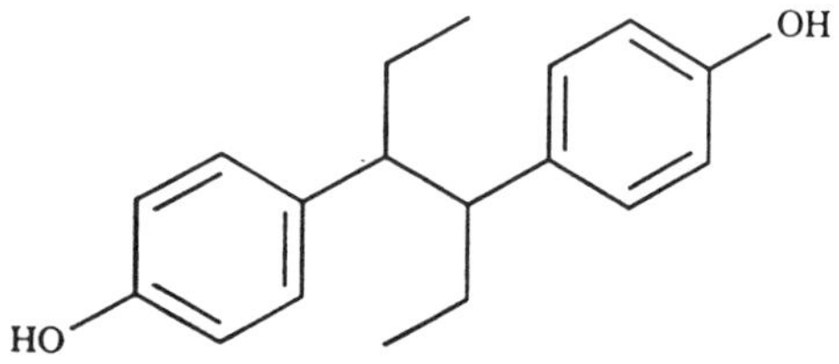

(**71**)

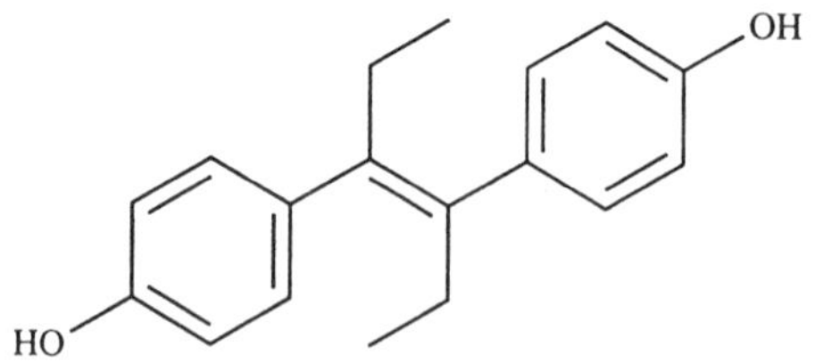

(**72**)

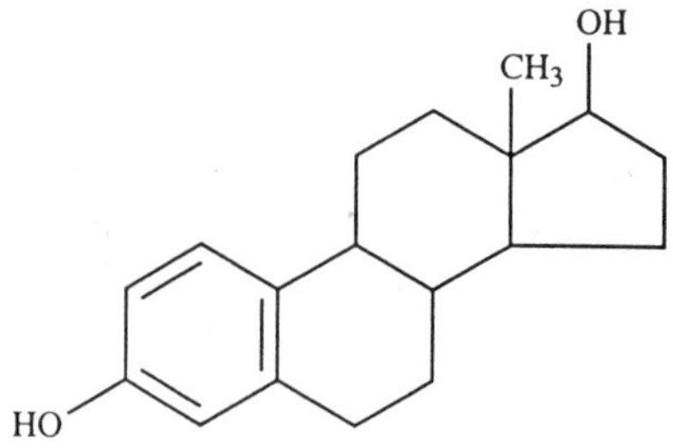

(**73**)

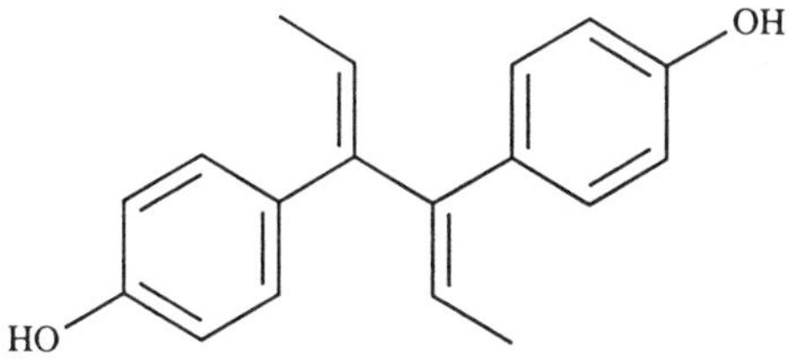

(74)

6 FRAGMENTS OF THE LEAD MOLECULE

Design of fragments of a lead molecule is based on the premise that lead molecules, especially polycyclic natural products, may be more structurally complex than is necessary for optimal pharmacologic effect. Buried within the structure of such a lead compound is a pharmacophoric moiety that, if it can be clearly defined, may be "dissected out" to result in a biologically active, simpler molecule that may itself be used as a lead in further analog design. A bond disconnection strategy may be employed, in which bonds in the chemical structure are broken or removed to destroy one or more of the rings. The result may be a valuable drug that is more accessible (through chemical synthesis) than the original lead molecule. A disadvantage to this strategy of drug design is that greater flexibility may be introduced into a rigid molecule, and the conformational integrity of the pharmacophore that may have existed in the original lead molecule is compromised or lost, sometimes at the expense of activity/potency. There may be a similar destruction of chiral centers, which may be undesirable.

Morphine (75) can be cited as a lead molecule to illustrate fragment analog design.

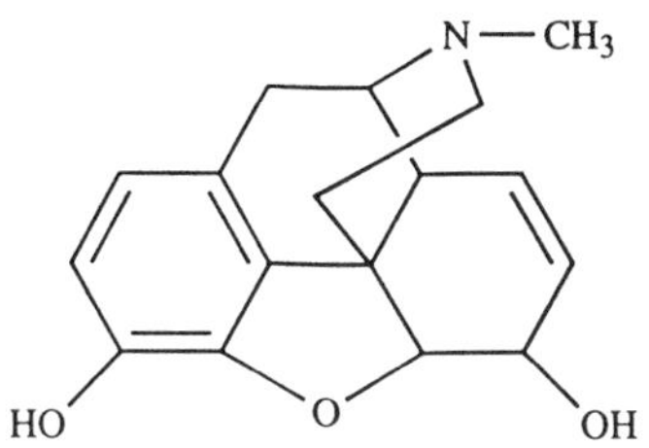

(75)

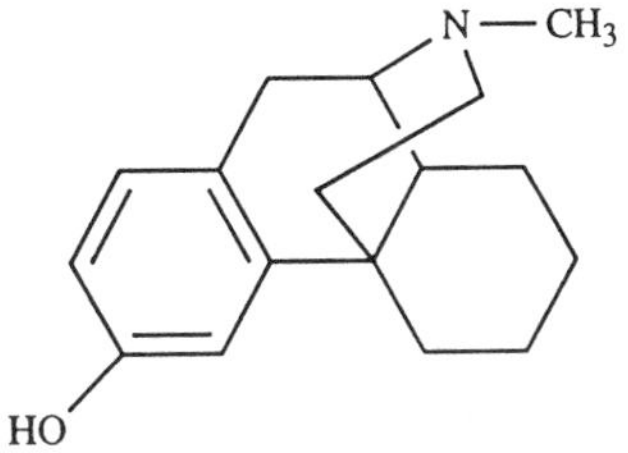

(76)

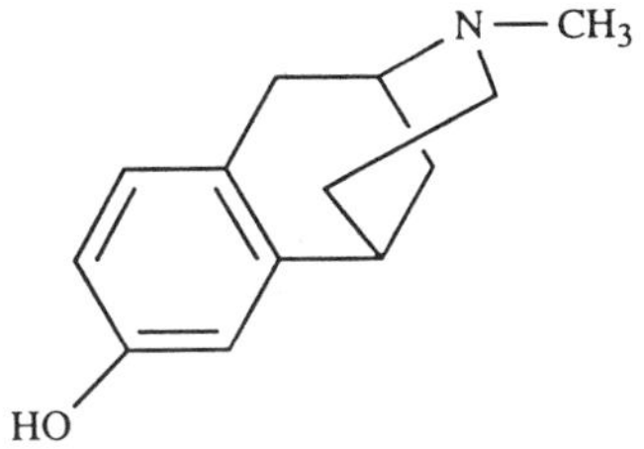

(77)

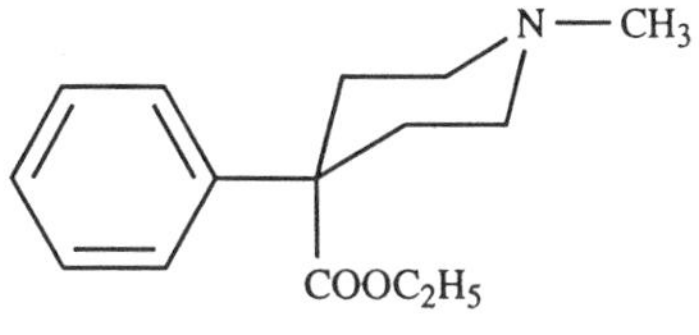

(78)

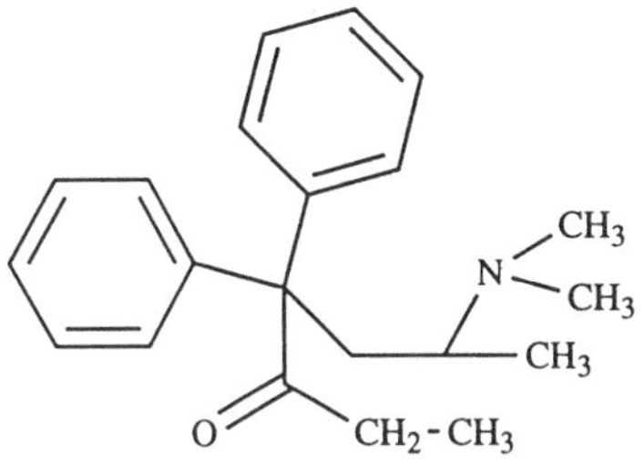

(79)

The analgestic pharmacophore of morphine has been defined (37) as the basic nitrogen, an aromatic ring (the "A" ring) three carbon atoms removed from the nitrogen, and a quaternary carbon adjacent to the aromatic ring, which provides a region of molecular bulk (37). A bond disconnection strategy involved disruption of the hydrofuran ring to give rise to morphinan ring derivatives, e.g., levorphanol (**76**), whose pharmacological effects closely parallel those of morphine (38). Further simplification of the morphine ring system led to benzomorphan derivatives, typified by metazocine (**77**) in which morphine like narcotic analgesic activity is retained. Final-

ly, 4-phenylpiperidine derivatives typified by meperidine (**78**) and the noncyclic system methadone (**79**) present the putative analgesic pharmacophore with a seemingly minimal number of extraneous atoms. These simple compounds retain narcotic analgesic activity. It must be noted, however, that the discovery of analgesic activity in 4-phenylpiperidine derivatives was not a result of a systematic structure-activity study of the morphine molecule, but was serendipitous (39).

Asperlicin (**80**), a potent cholecystokinin-A antagonist, was subjected to two different bond disconnection strategies, as indicated (40).

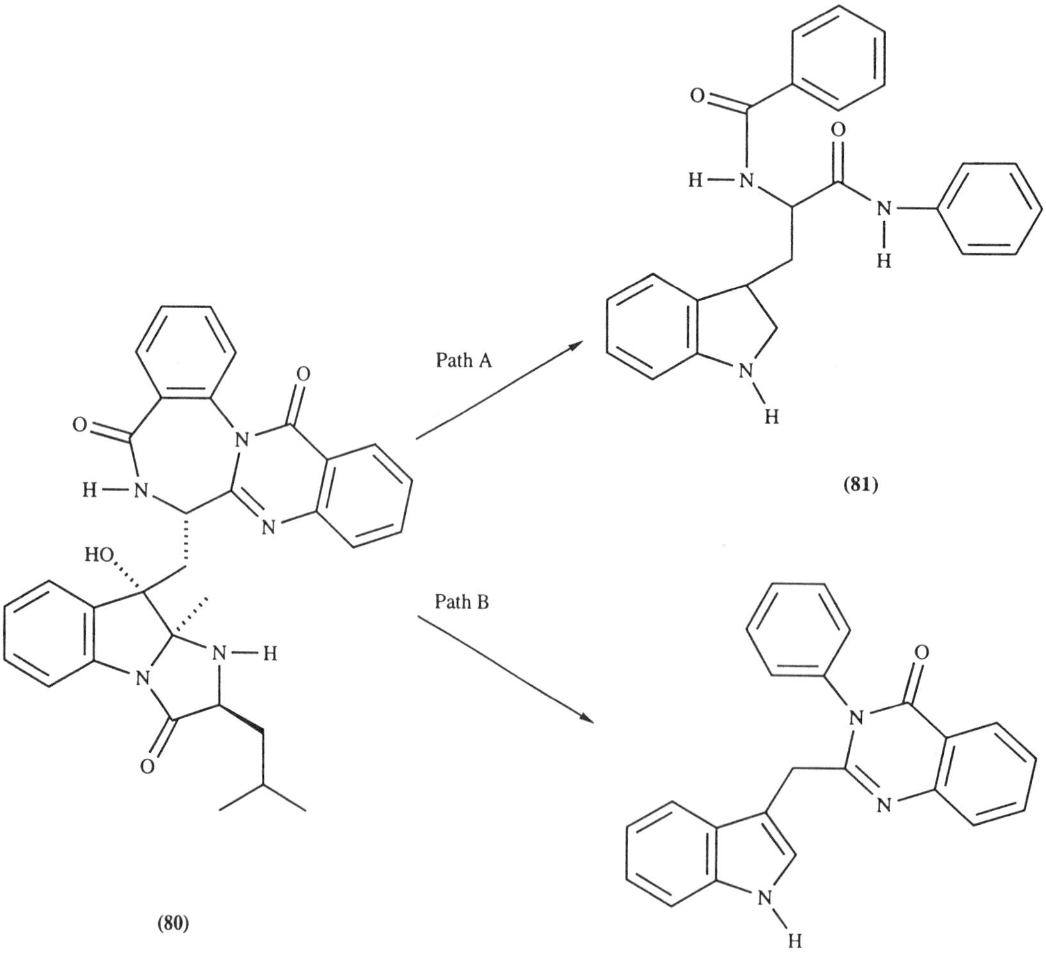

Path A

(81)

Path B

(80)

(82)

Path A leads to tryptophan derivatives (**81**), some of which are potent cholecysto-kinin antagonists (41). Some quinazolinone derivatives (**82**) of disconnection pathway B showed extremely high potency and excellent selectivity as cholecystokinin-B receptor subtype ligands (24). A combination of X-ray crystallography and computer-based molecular modeling was utilized in the decision making process in the bond disconnection (24) and in the design of specific target molecules.

The myoneural blocking pharmacophore in *d*-tubocurarine (**83**) includes the two cationic heads (a quaternary ammonium group and a protonated tertiary amine); the cationic heads are separated by ten atoms (nine carbons and one oxygen).

(**83**)

$$(CH_3)_3\overset{+}{N} - (CH_2)_{10} - \overset{+}{N}(CH_3)_3$$

(**84**)

Based on these parameters, a simple molecule, (decamethonium) (**84**), in which two trimethylammonium heads are separated by 10 methylene groups to approximate the internitrogen distance in *d*-tubocurarine, was designed independently by two groups of investigators (42, 43). This synthetic fragment/analog of *d*-tubocurarine exhibits a high degree of potency and activity in production of flaccid paralysis of skeletal

muscles, superficially like that of the lead compound. However, *d*-tubocurarine's myoneural blockade is of the nondepolarizing type whereas decamethonium produces a depolarizing type of skeletal muscle blockade. This fundamental difference in mechanism of action is due in part to the flexibility of the decamethonium molecule compared with *d*-tubocurarine. The difference in mechanism of action of the two myoneural blocking agents results in a considerable difference in the spectrum and severity of side effects and in the technique of employment in clinical practice. In all types of analog design, changes in chemical structure may result in changes in mechanism of action, even though the chemical nature of the pharmacophoric group may not be altered.

7 VARIATION IN INTERATOMIC DISTANCES

Alteration of distances between portions of the pharmacophore of a molecule (or even between other portions) may produce profound qualitative and/or quantitative changes in pharmacological actions. In a series of congeners of hemicholinium (**85**), the central biphenyl portion of the molecule was changed to terphenyl (**86**) and to *p*-phenylene (**87**). Both changes resulted in profound loss of myoneural blocking activity (44). This result was ascribed to alteration of the interquaternary nitrogen distance of 14.4 Å in hemicholinium (**85**) (which was assumed to be the optimum for myoneural blockade) to 18.4 Å in the terphenyl analog and to 10.2 Å in the *p*-phenylene analog. The central biphenyl "spacer" in hemicholinium (**85**) was changed to a 2,7-disubstituted phenanthrene (**88**), *trans,trans*-4,4-bicyclohexyl (**89**), and 2,2'-dimethylbiphenyl (**90**). In all three of these systems the 14.4-Å interquaternary distance in hemicholinium (**85**) was maintained; all of these congeners were quali-

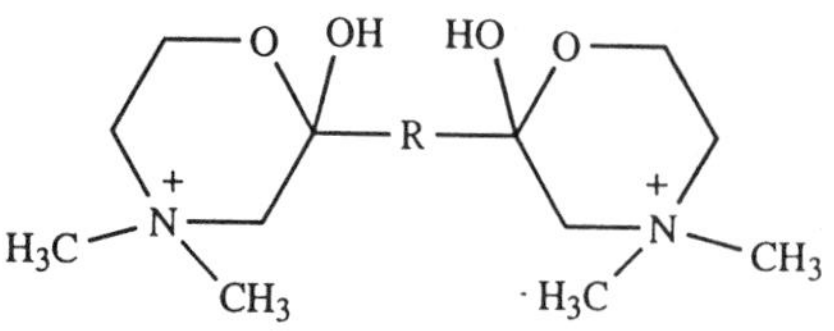

(85) R =

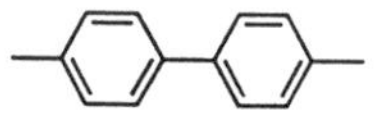

(86) R =

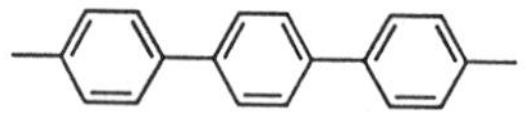

(87) R =

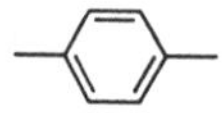

(88) R =

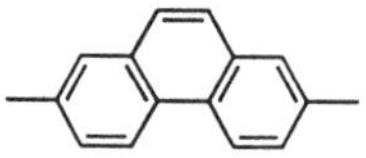

(89) R =

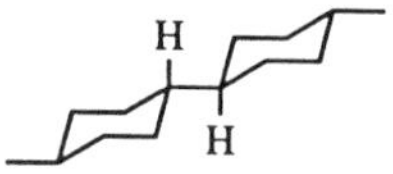

(90) R =

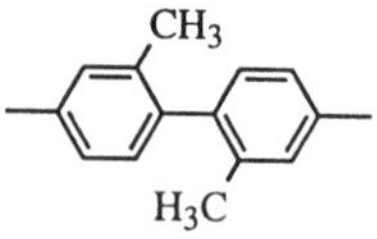

(91) R =   —(CH$_2$)$_6$—

(92) R =   —(CH$_2$)$_7$—

(93) $n = 1$

(94) $n = 2$

(95) $n = 3$

tatively and quantitatively similar to hemicholinium in inhibition of neuromuscular transmission. Conformational analysis of the polyalkylene congeners (91 and 92) demonstrated that when the flexible polyalkylene chain is maximally extended and in a staggered conformation, the interquaternary distance in the hexamethylene congener (91) is approximately 14 Å, and in the heptamethylene congener (92) it is approximately 15 Å. Both compounds exhibited hemicholinium-like inhibition of neuromuscular transmission, although they were less potent than hemicholinium (45). This diminution of potency might be ascribed to the compromising of another structural parameter in the hemicholinium molecule: the rigidity of the central biphenyl spacer unit that maintains the internitrogen distance.

In a series of phenylalkylenetrimethylammonium derivatives (93)–(95), nicotinic agonism is maximal when $n = 3$ [compound (95)].

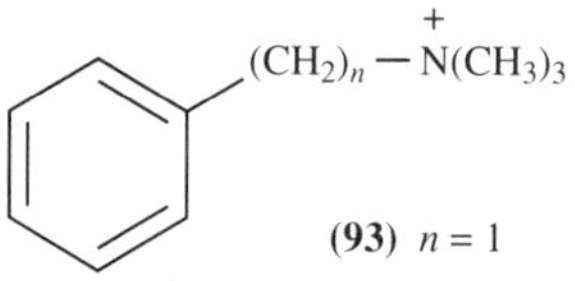

It was concluded (46) that a moiety (benzene ring) with high electron density three or four single bond lengths (approx. 6 Å) from the cationic center is a requirement for nicotinic agonism in the series (46).

In α,ω-bis-trimethylammonium polymethylene compounds (96–99), maximal activity for blockade of autonomic ganglia resides in those derivatives where $n = 5$ or 6 (96 and 97) (47, 48)

$$(CH_3)_3\overset{+}{N} - (CH_2)_n - \overset{+}{N}(CH_3)_3$$

(96) $n = 5$ (98) $n = 16$

(97) $n = 6$ (99) $n = 18$

Ganglionic effects drop drastically when $n = 4$ or 7. These observations have been rationalized on the basis of attainment of optimal interquaternary distance in the penta- and hexamethylene congeners for optimal interaction with ganglionic receptor subsites. Remarkably, as the number of methylene groups in compound (96) is further greatly expanded, a high level of ganglionic blocking potency returns. The hexadecyl and octadecyl congeners (98) and (99) are approximately four times as potent at autonomic ganglia as the penta- and hexamethylene compounds. As was mentioned previously, polymethylene bis-quaternary systems, in which the cationic heads are separated by 10 methylene groups, have potent effects at myoneural junctions and little action at autonomic ganglia. Thus extension of a *bis*-quaternary polyalkylene molecule from 5 or 6 methylenes to 10 produces a pharmacological change from ganglionic blockade to myoneural blockade, and further extension to 16 or 18 methylenes results in loss of myoneural effects and a return of ganglionic blocking action.

REFERENCES

1. I. Langumuir, *J. Am. Chem. Soc.*, **41**, 868, 1543 (1919).

2. C. W. Thornber, *Chem. Soc. Rev.*, **8**, 563 (1979).

3. P. Krogsgaard-Larsen, H. Hjeds, D. R. Curtis, D. Lodge, and G. A. R. Johnston, *J. Neurochem.*, **32**, 1717 (1979).

4. C. G. Crawley, R. I. Dowell, P. N. Edwards, S. J. Foster, R. M. McMillan, E. R. H. Walker, D. Waterson, T. G. C. Bird, P. Bruneau and J. -M. Girodeau, *J. Med. Chem.*, **35**, 2600 (1992).

5. H. Hashiguchi and H. Takahashi, *Mol. Pharmacol.*, **13**, 362 (1977).

6. K. Anderson, A. Kuruvilla, N. Uretsky, and D. D. Miller, *J. Med. Chem.*, **24**, 683 (1981).

7. R. J. Baldessarini in A. G. Gilman, L. S. Goodman, T. W. Rall and F. Murad, Eds., *Goodman and Gilman's the Pharmacological Basis of Therapeutics*, 7th ed., Macmillan, New York, 1985, pp. 393–397, 414–418.

8. S. I. Ankier in G. P. Ellis, and G. B. West, Eds., *Progress in Medicinal Chemistry*, Vol. 23, Elsevier, Amsterdam, The Netherlands, 1986, pp. 121–185.

9. E. Mutschler and G. Lambrecht, in E. J. Ariëns, W. Soudijn, and P. B. M. W. M. Timmermans, Eds., *Stereochemistry and Biological Activity of Drugs*, Blackwell, Oxford, UK, 1983, p. 65.

10. J. G. Cannon in E. Jucker, Ed., *Progress in Drug Research*, Vol. 29, Birkhäuser Verlag, Basel, 1985, pp. 324–334.

11. C. Melchiorre, A. Chiarini, M. Gianella, D. Giardina, W. Quaglia and V. Tumiatti, in V. Claassen, Ed., *Trends in Drug Research*, Vol. 13, Elsevier, Amsterdam, The Netherlands, 1990, pp. 37–48.

12. P. S. Portoghese, A. A. Mikhail, and H. J. Kupferberg, *J. Med. Chem.*, **11**, 219 (1968).

13. C. Y. Chiou, J. P. Long, J. G. Cannon, and P. D. Armstrong, *J. Pharmacol. Exp. Ther.*, **166**, 243 (1969).

14. J. G. Cannon, and P. D. Armstrong, *J. Med. Chem.*, **13**, 1037 (1970).

15. J. G. Cannon, T. Lee, V. Sankaran, J. P. Long, *J. Med. Chem.*, **18**, 1027 (1975).

16. P. W. Ehrhardt, R. J. Gorczynski and W. G. Anderson, *J. Med. chem.* **22**, 907 (1975).

17. R. R. Ruffolo Jr. in G. Kunos, Ed., *Adrenoceptors and Catecholamine Action, Part B*, Wiley-Interscience, New York, 1983, pp. 10–11.

18. E. E. Smissman, and W. H. Gastrock, *J. Med. Chem.*, **11**, 860 (1968).

19. M. V. Koch, J. G. Cannon, and A. M. Burkman, *J. Med. Chem.*, **11**, 977 (1968).

20. E. R. Atkinson, F. J. Bullock, F. E. Granchelli, S. Archer, F. J. Rosenberg, D. G. Teiger, and F. C. Nachod, *J. Med. Chem.*, **18**, 1000 (1975).

21. J. G. Cannon in Ref. 10, pp. 309–310.

22. J. G. Cannon, F.-L. Hsu, J. P. Long, J. R. Flynn, B. Costall, and R. J. Naylor, *J. Med. Chem.*, **21**, 248 (1978).

23. J. Z. Ginos, and F. C. Brown, *J. Med. Chem.*, **21**, 155 (1978).

24. M. J. Yu, J. R. McCowan, N. R. Mason, J. B. Deeter and L. G. Mendelsohn, *J. Med. Chem.*, **35**, 2534 (1992).

25. K.-L. Yu, J. J. Bronson, H. Yang, A. Patick, M. Alam, V. Brankovan, R. Datema, M. J. M. Hitchcock, and J. C. Martin, *J. Med. Chem.*, **35**, 2958 (1992).

26. R. H. Uloth, J. R. Kirk, W. A. Gould, and A. A. Larsen, *J. Med. Chem.*, **9**, 88 (1966).

27. J. E. Macor, C. B. Fox, C. Johnson, B. K. Koe, L. A. Label, and S. H. Zorn, *J. Med. Chem.*, **35**, 3625 (1992).

28. S. Hjorth, A. Carlsson, H. Wikström, P. Lindberg, D. Sanchez, U. Hacksell, L.-E. Arvidsson, U. Svensson, and J. L. G. Nilsson, *Life Sci.*, **28**, 1225 (1981).

29. H. Wikström, D. Sanchez, P. Lindberg, U. Hacksell, L.-E. Arvidsson, A.M. Johansson, S.-O. Thorberg, J. L. G. Nilsson, K. Svensson, S. Hjorth, D. Clark, and A. Carlsson, *J. Med. Chem.*, **27**, 1030 (1984).

30. J. G. Cannon, P. Mohan, J. Bojarski, J. P. Long, R. K. Bhatnagar, P. A. Leonard, J. R. Flynn, and T. K. Chatterjee, *J. Med. Chem.*, **31**, 313 (1988).

31. J. G. Cannon, S. T. Moe, and J. P. Long, *Chirality*, **3**, 19 (1991).

32. B. T. Butler, G. Silvey, D. M. Houston, D. R. Borcherding, V. L. Vaughn, A. T. McPhail, D. M. Radzik, H. Wynberg, W. Ten Hoeve, E. Van Echten, N. K. Ahmed, and M. D. Linnik, *Chirality*, **4**, 155 (1992).

33. G. A. Johnston, D. R. Curtis, P. M. Beart, C. J. A. Game, R. M. McColloch, and B. Twitchin, *J. Neurochem.*, **24**, 157 (1975).

34. R. D. Allan, D. R. Curtis, P. M. Headley, G. A. Johnson, D. Lodge, and B. Twitchen, *J. Neurochem.* **34**, 652 (1980).

35. D. T. Witiak, D. D. Miller, and R. W. Brueggemeier, in W. O. Foye, Ed., *Principles of Medicinal Chemistry*, 3rd Ed., Philadelphia, Lea & Febiger, 1989, p. 461.

36. D. S. Fullerton, in R. F. Doerge, Ed., *Wilson and Gisvold's Textbook of Organic Medicinal and Pharmaceutical Chemistry*, 8th ed., Philadelphia, J. B. Lippincott, 1982, p. 670.

37. T. Nogrady, *Medicinal Chemistry*, 2nd ed., New York, Oxford University Press, 1988, p. 457.

38. J. H. Jaffe, and W. R. Martin, in Ref. 7, p. 513.

39. A. Korolkovas, *Essentials of Medicinal Chemistry*, 2nd ed., Wiley-Interscience, New York, 1988, p. 238.

40. M. J. Yu, K. J. Thrasher, J. R. McCowan, N. R. Mason and L. G. Mendelsohn, *J. Med. Chem.*, **34**, 1505 (1991).

41. F. W. Hahne, R. T. Jensen, G. F. Lemp, and J. D. Gardner, *Proc. Natl. Acad. Sci. U. S. A.*, **78**, 6304 (1981).

42. R. B. Barlow, and H. R. Ing, *Nature*, **161**, 718 (1948).

43. W. D. M. Paton, E. J. Zaimis, *Nature*, **161**, 718 (1948).

44. J. G. Cannon, T.-L. Lee, A. M. Nyanda, B. Bhattacharyya, and J. P. Long, *Drug Des. Deliv.* **1**, 209 (1987).

45. J. G. Cannon, T. M.-L. Lee, Y.-A. Chang, A. M. Nyanda, B. Bhattacharyya, J. R. Flynn, T. Chatterjee, R. K. Bhatnagar, and J. P. Long, *Phar. Res.*, **4**, 359 (1989).

46. W. C. Holland in E. J. Ariëns, Ed., *Proceedings of the International Pharmacology Meeting*, Vol. 7, Pergamon Press, Oxford, UK, 1966, p. 295.

47. D. J. Triggle, *Neurotransmitter-Receptor Interactions*, Academic Press, New York, 1971, p. 360.

48. V. Trcka in D. A. Kharkevich, Ed., in *Handbook of Experimental Pharmacology*, *Vol. 53: Pharmacology of Ganglionic Transmission*, Springer-Verlag, New York, 1980, p. 138.

CHAPTER TWENTY

Peptidomimetics for Drug Design

MURRAY GOODMAN

Department of Chemistry, University of California
   at San Diego
San Diego, California

SEONGGU RO

Research and Development Park of LUCKY Ltd.
Biotechnology Science Town
Daejon, Korea

CONTENTS

1 Introduction, 804

2. Cyclization of Peptides, 805
   2.1 General features, 805
   2.2 Constrained units for cyclization of peptides, 809
   2.3 Various cyclic linkages, 811·
   2.4 Backbone cyclization and bicyclic structures, 813

3 Constrained Amino Acids, 814
   3.1 α-Methylated amino acids, 814
   3.2 α,α-Dialkylglycine and α-aminocycloalkane carboxylic acids, 817
   3.3 N^{α}–C^{α} Cyclized amino acids, 818
      3.3.1 Proline mimetics with different ring sizes, 819
      3.3.2 Highly constrained proline mimetics, 820
      3.3.3 Pyroglutamic acids and hydroxy proline analogs, 823
   3.4 N^{α}-Methylated amino acids, 823
   3.5 β- and γ-Amino cycloalkane carboxylic acids, 825
   3.6 α,β-Unsaturated amino acids, 826
   3.7 β,β-Dimethyl and β-methyl amino acids, 828
   3.8 β-Substituted-2,3-methano amino acids, 829

Burger's Medicinal Chemistry and Drug Discovery,
Fifth Edition, Volume 1: Principles and Practice,
Edited by Manfred E. Wolff.
ISBN 0-471-57556-9 © 1995 John Wiley & Sons, Inc.

3.9   N–C$^\delta$ and C$^\alpha$–C$^\delta$ cyclized amino acids, 831

3.10 Substituted proline, 832

3.11 Miscellaneous mimetics for amino acids, 832

4 Molecular Mimics for Secondary Structures, 833

5 Amide Bond Isosteres, 838

5.1   The retro-inverso modifications [NH–C(O)], 838

5.2   The reduced amide bonds (methyleneamine: CH$_2$–NH), 838

5.3   Methylenethioether (CH$_2$–S) and methylenesulfoxide [CH$_2$–S(O)], 840

5.4   Methylene ether (CH$_2$–O), 841

5.5   Ethylene ("Carba": CH$_2$–CH$_2$), 842

5.6   Thioamide [C(S)–NH], 842

5.7   *trans*-Olefin (CH=CH, *trans*) and *trans*-fluoroolefin (CH=CF, *trans*), 843

5.8   1,5-Disubstituted tetrazole ring [CN$_4$], 844

5.9   Ketomethylene [C(O)–CH$_2$] and fluoroketomethylene [C(O)–CFR, R=H or F], 845

5.10 Miscellaneous amide isosteres, 846

6 Nonpeptide Ligands for Peptinergic Receptors, 847

7 Conclusions, 848

1 INTRODUCTION

In the past two decades, a wide variety of naturally occurring bioactive peptides have been discovered. These peptides function as hormones, enzyme inhibitors or substrates, growth promoters or inhibitors, neurotransmitters, and immunomodulators. Most of these peptides exhibit their biological activities through binding to corresponding acceptor molecules (receptors or enzymes). Each acceptor molecule plays a unique biological role, allowing the interaction of bioactive peptides with acceptor molecules to control specific physiological events. This characteristic can allow bioactive peptides to act as therapeutic agents. Extensive studies have been undertaken in an effort to understand the physiological effects of these bioactive peptides. Unfortunately, the use of native peptides for clinical applications has been limited by intrinsic properties of peptides.

One of the most important considerations which limits the clinical application of native peptides is rapid degradation of peptides by peptidase enzymes. There are many specific and nonspecific peptidases in biological systems which rapidly metabolize peptides. Such metabolic instability complicates oral delivery of peptides. Passage through the blood–brain-barrier is an additional problem for peptides which act in the central nervous system (CNS).

Bioactive peptides act on specific acceptor molecules. However, because of the inherent flexibility of peptides, they may adopt different conformations required for recognition by multiple acceptor molecules. For example, receptors often have subtypes related to different physiological phenomena. Each subtype may require different conformations of peptides for binding. In many cases, native peptides can bind to more than one receptor subtype and this property may lead to undesirable side effects.

In an effort to counteract these detrimental properties, numerous modifications of peptide structure have been considered. These modified structures are referred to as peptidomimetics; chemical structures derived from bioactive peptides which imitate natural molecules. It is widely believed that such modifications will enhance the desirable properties and avoid undesirable properties of native peptides. Many analogs incorporating peptidomimetic components have exhibited improved pharmacological and pharmacokinetic properties, including increased bioactivity, selectivity, metabolic stability, absorption, and lower toxicity. Some of these peptidomimetic analogs are currently used as therapeutic agents.

Since bioactive peptides must adopt a specific conformation to bind to an acceptor molecule, the exploration of a binding conformation is one of the most important processes involved in the effort to obtain potent and selective therapeutic agents. For this purpose, constrained peptidomimetics based on cyclic structures, constrained amino acids or amide isosteres, and mimics of peptide secondary structures have been employed. These peptidomimetics cause the resulting peptides to adopt distinct preferred conformations by removing the flexibility of the parent linear peptides. In many cases, such conformational changes are accompanied by alterations in the bioactivity profiles of the resulting analogs. Thus, the comparison of bioactivities and the effects of peptidomimetics on the overall conformations of peptides (obtained from conformational studies using modern techniques of spectroscopy and molecular modeling) can provide insight into the structures required for bioactivity. The resulting structural information can be used for the design of more effective peptidomimetics in an effort to generate the required conformations for high selectivity and potency.

To improve the metabolic stability of native peptides, amide isosteres have been incorporated into peptide bonds which are particularly susceptible to enzymatic degradation. In many cases, these modifications, as well as the incorporation of constrained peptidomimetics can enhance metabolic stability. The transformation of a peptide structure to a completely nonpeptidic molecule (retaining pharmacophores and the required three-dimensional array) is an attractive approach to the development of therapeutic agents from native peptides. These types of drug candidates can incorporate metabolic stability and oral bioavailability. In addition, these molecules, which are relatively rigid compared with peptides, can provide desirable selectivities. Other pharmacokinetic properties (solubility, hydrophobicity, transport characteristics, etc.) can also be enhanced from small changes in peptidomimetic structures.

This chapter will focus on the general features of representative peptidomimetic strategies including: cyclization of peptides, incorporations of unnatural amino acids, linkages between consecutive residues, replacements of peptide bond with amide isosteres and transformations of the secondary structure of peptides to nonpeptidic molecules. Conformational preferences, physical properties, and applications to drug design of the above peptidomimetics will be described.

2 CYCLIZATION OF PEPTIDES

2.1 General Features

Cyclization of peptides reduces the degrees of freedom for each constituent within the ring. This modification can substantially reduce the flexibility of parent linear molecules and stabilize specific secondary structures of peptides. Furthermore, if the conformation stabilized by the cyclization closely resembles the structure responsible for the bioactivity, this modification can increase potency and selectivity of the resulting peptides. Cyclic structures have been observed in many native peptides such as somatostatin, oxytocin, cyclosporin A, atrial natiuretic peptides, calcitonin and peptide antibiotics. However, the size of the cyclic rings of these peptides are too large to generate conformationally constrained structures. Thus, smaller cyclic structures (11 to 18 membered rings) have been considered in peptidomimetic design. Cyclic structures have been incorporated into numerous bioactive peptides leading to highly potent and selective analogs.

One of the most important applications of this modification is in the studies of opioid peptides. From X-ray crystallographic studies of enkephalins (Tyr-Gly-Gly-Phe-Leu/Met-OH), two different types of structures were reported (1, 2). One of these structures adopts a β-turn stabilized by two antiparallel hydrogen bonds between Tyr[1] and Phe[4] (1). The other structure contains the fully extended conformation (2). The spectroscopic and computational studies of enkephalins support these results by showing the existence of several different conformations in equilibrium (3–5). To avoid the fully extended structure in the conformational equilibrium of enkephalins, Schiller et al. have cyclized an enkephalin analog (6).

There are four different ways to cyclize linear peptides: connection of the amino terminus to the carboxyl terminus; the amino terminus to a side chain; a side chain to the carboxyl terminus; and one side chain to another side chain. However, since the free amine of Tyr[1] is required for opioid activity, only the side chain to carboxyl terminus and the side chain to side-chain cyclizations can be used, leading to three series of analogs: Tyr-c[D-X-Gly-Phe-Leu] [X = Lys, Orn, A_2bu (diaminobutyric acid) and A_2pr (diaminopropionic acid)] (6–9), Tyr-c[D-Cys/Pen-Gly-Phe-(D/L)-Cys/Pen]-OH/NH$_2$ (10–12) (Pen stands for penicillamine which is β,β-dimethyl cystein) and Tyr-c(D-Lys-Gly-Phe-Glu)-OH (Fig. 20.1) (13).

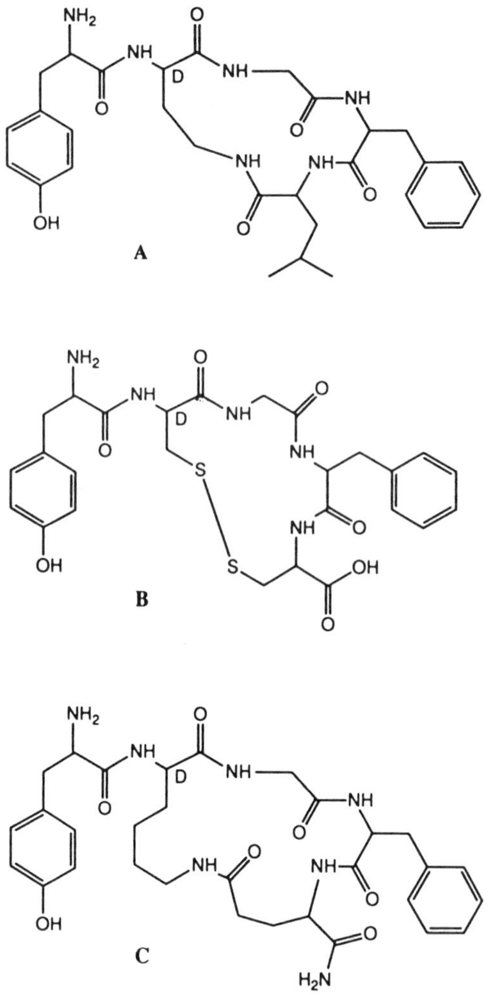

The cyclic structures of the Tyr-c(D-X-Gly-Phe-Leu) series are formed through the lactam bridge between the side chain of the second residue and the carboxyl terminus of Leu (5). The resulting analogs

Fig. 20.1 The typical cyclic enkephalin analogs, A, Tyr-c[D-A$_2$bu-Gly-Phe-Leu]; B, Tyr-c[D-Cys-Gly-Phe-Cys]-OH; and C, Tyr-c[D-Lys-Gly-Phe-Glu]-NH$_2$.

show higher activities than enkephalins in the GPI (guinea pig ileum) assays which represent bioactivities of opioids at the μ or morphine-binding opioid receptor. On the contrary, lower activities are observed in the MVD (mouse vas deferens) tests which represent bioactivities at the δ or enkephalin-binding opioid receptor (Table 20.1) (6–9). Namely, the resulting cyclic analogs are highly μ-receptor selective. These bioactivity profiles are different from parent enkephalins which show δ-receptor selective activities (Table 20.1). These profiles are also different from those of Tyr-Xaa-Gly-Phe-NH$_2$ [Xaa = D-Ala, D-Nva (norvaline) and Nle (norleucine)] which are the real parent analogs of this cyclic peptide series (9). All of these linear parent analogs are nonselective. The results indicate that the cyclization of δ-selective or nonselective enkephalins leads to μ-selective analogs. The cyclization reduces the possibility that linear enkephalins will adopt the conformations which can be recognized by the δ opioid receptor.

Another cyclic enkephalin series, Tyr-c[D-Cys/Pen-Gly-Phe-(D,L)-Cys/Pen]-OH/NH$_2$, has been synthesized through the disulfide bridge formation between Cys/Pen residues in positions 2 and 5 (10–12). The Cys containing analogs are superactive at both the μ- and δ-receptors and the Pen containing analogs are highly δ-receptor selective (Table 20.1) (10). These results demonstrate that β,β-dimethylation of Cys residues excludes the

conformation for μ opioid receptor recognition in this cyclic peptide system. The Pen containing analogs will be discussed again later. The Tyr-c(D-Lys-Gly-Phe-Glu)-NH$_2$ analog was also prepared by lactam formation between the free amine of the Lys sidechain and the carboxylic acid of the Glu side chain. This analog is active at both μ- and δ-receptors (Table 20.1) (13). These results indicate that the bioactivities of analogs can be varied by means of cyclization, changes in ring sizes, and conformational constraints.

Another peptide opioid dermorphin (Tyr-D-Ala-Phe-Gly-Tyr-Pro-Ser-NH$_2$) (14), was also cyclized in the laboratories of Goodman (15–19), Schiller (20–22) and Spatola (23). The linear N-terminal tetrapeptide and pentapeptide of dermorphin retain the bioactivity of dermorphin (24). Since the size of the cyclic structure must be small in order to obtain highly constrained structures, these sequences have been employed for the cyclization of dermorphin. Among the resulting analogs,

Table 20.1 Various Cyclic Enkephalins and their Bioactivities

Analog	Cyclization and Ring Size	GPI[a] IC$_{50}$/nM	MVD[b] IC$_{50}$/nM	MVD/GPI IC$_{50}$-Ratio	Reference
Tyr-c(D-A$_2$pr-Gly-Phe-Leu)	(sm[c], 13)	23.4 ± 4.2	73.1 ± 14.5	3.12	9
Tyr-c(D-A$_2$bu-Gly-Phe-Leu)	(sm, 14)	14.1 ± 2.9	81.4 ± 5.8	5.77	9
Tyr-c(D-Orn-Gly-Phe-Leu)	(sm, 15)	48 ± 4.3	475 ± 99	9.90	9
Tyr-c(D-Lys-Gly-Phe-Leu)	(sm, 16)	4.80 ± 1.79	141 ± 28	29.4	9
Tyr-c(D-Cys-Gly-Phe-Cys)-OH	(ss[d], 14)	3.06	0.19	0.062	11
Tyr-c(D-Cys-Gly-Phe-D-Cys)-OH	(ss, 14)	1.48	0.12	0.081	11
Tyr-c(D-Cys-Gly-Phe-Cys)-NH$_2$	(ss, 14)	1.51 ± 0.03	0.760 ± 0.086	0.503	11
Tyr-c(D-Cys-Gly-Phe-D-Cys)-NH$_2$	(ss, 14)	0.780 ± 0.010	0.298 ± 0.037	0.382	11
Tyr-c(D-Pen-Gly-Phe-Pen)-OH	(ss, 14)	10000	2.5	0.00025	12
Tyr-c(D-Pen-Gly-Phe-D-Pen)-OH	(ss, 14)	25250	3.40	0.00014	12
Tyr-c(D-Lys-Gly-Phe-Glu)-NH$_2$	(ss, 18)	1.13 ± 0.14	0.648 ± 0.132	0.573	13
Tyr-Gly-Gly-Phe-Leu-OH		246 ± 39	11.4 ± 1.1	0.0463	

[a]The GPI stands for guinea pig ileum which is a muscle preparation for the *in vitro* assay to measure bioactivities at the μ opioid receptor.

[b]The MVD stands for mouse vas deferens which is a muscle preparation for the *in vitro* assay to measure bioactivities at the δ opioid receptor.

[c]The sm denotes the side chain to main chain cyclization.

[d]The ss denotes the side chain to side chain cyclization.

Table 20.2   Various Cyclic Dermorphin Analogs and their Biological Activities

Analog	Cyclization and Ring Size	GPI[a] IC$_{50}$/nM	MVD[b] IC$_{50}$/nM	MVD/GPI IC$_{50}$-Ratio	Reference
Tyr-c(D-Orn-Phe-Asp)-NH$_2$	(ss[c], 13)	36.2 ± 3.7	3880 ± 840	107	22
Tyr-c(D-Cys-Phe-Cys)-NH$_2$	(ss, 11)	64.7 ± 11.9	740 ± 187	11.4	22
Tyr-c(D-Orn-Phe-Gly)	(sm[d], 12)	8.60 ± 0.78	145 ± 15	16.9	15
Tyr-c(D-Lys-Phe-Ala)	(sm, 13)	0.19	0.51	2.7	23
Tyr-c(D-A$_2$bu-Phe-Ala-Leu)	(sm, 14)	0.63 ± 0.049	1.72 ± 0.27	2.71	15
Tyr-D-Ala-Phe-Gly-NH$_2$		45.2 ± 3.19	510 ± 31.82	11.3	24

[a]The GPI stands for guinea pig ileum which is a muscle preparation for the *in vitro* assay to measure bioactivities at the μ opioid receptor.

[b]The MVD stands for mouse vas deferens which is a muscle preparation for the *in vitro* assay to measure bioactivities at the δ opioid receptor.

[c]The ss denotes the side chain to main chain cyclization.

[d]The sm denotes the side chain to main chain cyclization.

Tyr-c(D-Orn-Phe-Asp)-NH$_2$ (20–22), Tyr-c(D-Cys-Phe-Cys)-NH$_2$ (22) and Tyr-c(D-Orn-Phe-Gly) (15, 17, 18) are μ-receptor selective. The analog Tyr-c[D-Orn-Phe-Asp)-NH$_2$ is active only at the μ-receptor. On the other hand, Tyr-c(D-Lys-Phe-Ala) and Tyr-c(D-A$_2$bu-Phe-Ala-Leu) show superactivity at both the μ- and δ-receptors (Table 20.2) (16). The cyclic dermorphin analogs with the tetrapeptide sequence are highly constrained because of the small size of the ring.

Cyclic somatostatins are another representative example of cyclic peptides. The native somatostatin contains a large cyclic structure formed by a disulfide bridge (Fig. 20.2) (25). The structure–activity relationship studies of this molecule indicate that the Phe-Trp-Lys-Thr (26–30) sequence is important for the bioactivity of somatostatin. Replacement of Trp with D-Trp increases activity (31). Furthermore, conformational analysis of somatostatin and its analogs proposed that a β-turn within the

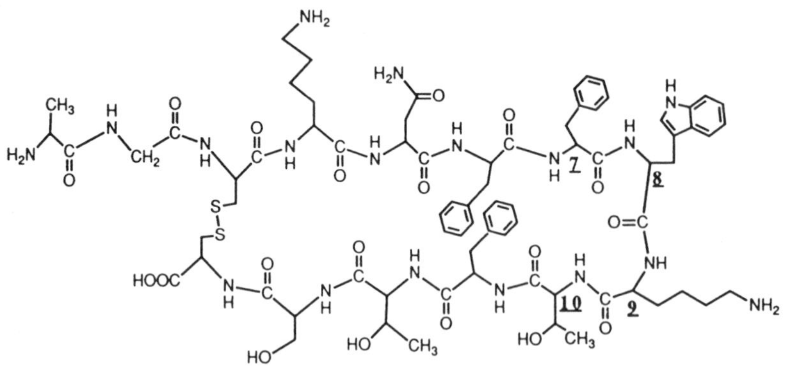

H$_2$N-Ala-Gly-Cys-Lys-Asn-Phe-Phe^7-Trp^8-Lys^9-Thr^{10}-Phe-Thr-Ser-Cys-H

Fig. 20.2   Structure and sequence of native somatostatin.

Table 20.3   Growth Hormone Release Inhibition by Cyclic Somatostatin Analogs

Analog	Relative Potency[a]	Reference
D-Phe-c(Cys-Phe-D-Trp-Lys-Thr-Cys)-Thr-ol	5	34
c(Pro-Phe-D-Trp-Lys-Thr-Phe)	1.7	27, 28
c[(NMe)-α-benzyl-O-AMPA-Phe-D-Trp-Lys-Thr](I)	<0.0001	37
c[(NMe)-α-benzyl-O-AMPA-Phe-D-Trp-Lys-Thr](II)	0.013	37

[a]A ratio between the IC_{50} value for the inhibition of growth hormone release by cyclic somatostatin analog and the IC_{50} value for the inhibitin of growth hormone release by native somatostatin.

above sequence is required for receptor recognition (31, 32). To stabilize such a secondary structure around the pharmacophoric sequence of somatostatin, analogs with smaller ring size were synthesized. Such efforts resulted in the highly active lead analogs D-Phe-c(Cys-Phe-D-Trp-Lys-Thr-Cys)–Thr-ol (33, 34) and c(Pro-Phe-D-Trp-Lys-Thr-Phe) (26) (Table 20.3). The former analog is synthesized by a side chain to side chain cyclization while the cyclic structure of the latter analog is formed by an amino terminus to carboxyl terminus cyclization of a hexapeptide derivative.

2.2 Constrained Units for Cyclization of Peptides

Specific functional units have been utilized to enhance the stability of specific molecular conformations. The conformational analyses of the somatostatin analogs based on the structure c(Pro[6]-Phe[7]-D-Trp[8]-Lys[9]-The[10]-Phe[11]) (the superscript numbers show the relative positions of amino acids with respect to native somatostatin) indicate that a cis peptide bond between Phe[11]–Pro[6] is important for high bioactivity (26). To mimic such a cis amide bond, Van Binst et al. (35, 36) have incorporated the o, m, or p-aminomethylphenylacetic acids (o, m, or p-AMPA) into the bridging region to replace the Phe[11]-Pro[6] dipeptide se-

quence. However, all of these analogs are inactive. The conformational studies of these analogs indicated that the inactivity arose from the absence of the aromatic ring corresponding to the side chain of Phe[11] and distortions on the conformation of the pharmacophoric sequence as well as the bridging region. These conformational studies also showed that hydrogen-bonding between the NH and C(O) groups of o-AMPA may explain the inactivity of these analogs. To avoid this hydrogen-bonding, N-methylation on the amine of o-AMPA has been considered. Since the side chain aromatic ring of Phe[11] was important for bioactivity, the introduction of benzyl group was also considered. Thus, N-methyl-α-($R\&S$)-benzyl-o-AMPA (37) (Fig. 20.3A) has been incorporated into the bridging region. One of the two isomers has shown substantial bioactivity (Table 20.3). A similar constrained unit, p-aminomethylbenzoic acid (p-AMBA) was incorporated into a arginyl-glycinyl-aspatyl sequence containing peptide (RGD peptide) leading to an active inhibitor of cell adhesion (Fig. 20.3B) (38). Recently, the incorporation of o- and m-aminobenzoic acid into inactivators of trypsinlike proteinases was also reported (39).

Sulfhydryl containing constrained units are useful to provide constraints and increase hydrophobicities. Derivatives of desaminocystein (Fig. 20.4) such as β,β-pentamethylene-β-mercaptopropionic acid (Ppa), 2-mercaptobenzoic acid (Mba),

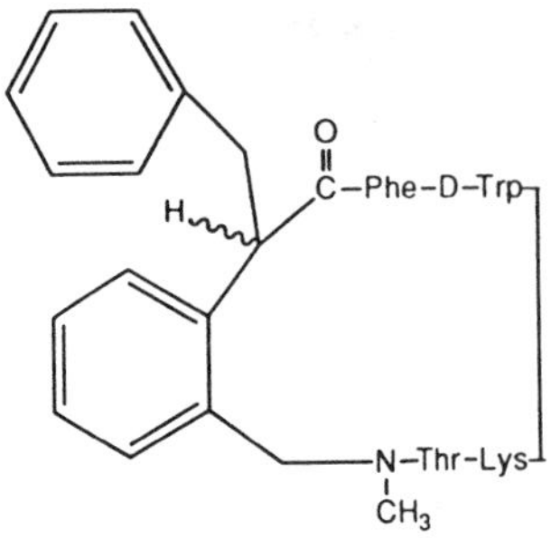

Fig. 20.3 Structures of A, a somatostatin analog c[(N-Methyl)-α-benzyl-o-AMPA-Phe-D-Trp-Lys-Thr]; and B, a modified RGD peptide c[Arg-Gly-Asp-pAMBA].

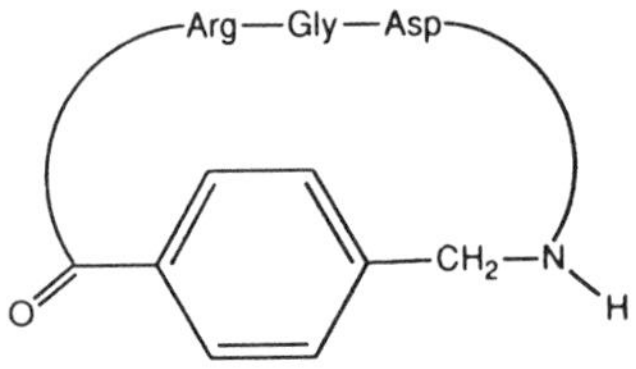

β,β-dimethyl-β-mercaptopropionic acid (Dmpa), and β,β-diethyl-β-mercaptopropionic acid (Depa) have also been incorporated into bioactive peptides including antagonists of vasopressin, oxytocin, RGD peptides, and others (40–44). When the Ppa, Mba, Dmpa, and Depa were incorporated into position X of a vasopressin analog [X-Phe(NO$_2$)-Phe-Val-Asn-Cys]-Pro-Lys-D-Tyr-NH$_2$, the resulting analogs were active (Table 20.4) (40). The Dmpa containing analog shows higher activity than any other analogs which contain Ppa, Mba, and Depa (Table 20.4). Since these four units have functional groups with different sizes and hydrophobicities, the bioactivity results can be used to understand optimal redundant properties for binding.

A methylated derivative of Ppa, β,β-(4-methylpentamethylene)-β-mercaptopropionic acid (4-MePpa) was also synthesized (Fig. 20.5). The two isomers (cis and trans) of this unit were incorporated into the place of Ppa in c[Ppa-D-Tyr(Et)-Phe-Val-Asn-Cys]-Pro-Arg-NH$_2$ (SK&F 101926). The resulting analogs are potent vasopressin V$_2$ receptor antagonists which also show some agonist activity (45). The resulting trans-isomer analog exhibited more agonist activities than the cis-isomer. However, the agonist activities of cis-isomer containing analogs were considerably less than the corresponding unsubstituted analogs. These results indicated that small changes in the structure of constrained units could provide desirable pharmacological properties.

Table 20.4   Binding Assays of Vasopressin Analogs

Analog	K_d (nM)^a
c[Ppa-Phe(NO$_2$)-Phe-Val-Asn-Cys]-Pro-Lys-D-Tyr-NH$_2$	3.2 ± 0.7
c[Mab-Phe(NO$_2$)-Phe-Val-Asn-Cys]-Pro-Lys-D-Tyr-NH$_2$	27 ± 4.6
c[Dmpa-Phe(NO$_2$)-Phe-Val-Asn-Cys]-Pro-Lys-D-Tyr-NH$_2$	1.8 ± 0.6
c[Depa-Phe(NO$_2$)-Phe-Val-Asn-Cys]-Pro-Lys-D-Tyr-NH$_2$	2.55 ± 0.12

^{a}The K_d denotes the dissociation constant calculated from the binding assays of vasopressin analogs to the V_1 receptor.

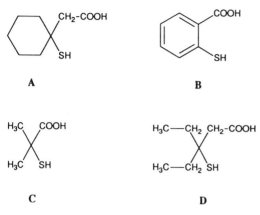

Fig. 20.4 Desaminocysteine derivatives, A, β,β-pentamethylene-β-mercaptopropionic acid (Ppa); B, 2-mercaptobenzoic acid; C, β,β-dimethyl-β-mercaptopropionic acid (Dmpa) and β,β-diethyl-β-mercaptopropionic acid (Depa).

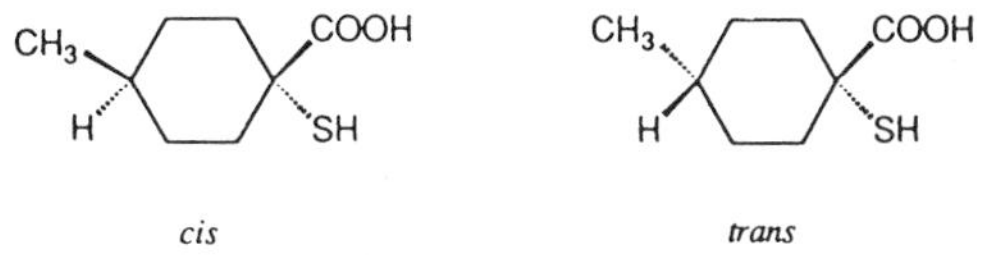

CH₃ ... H / SH ... COOH (cis)   CH₃ ... H / SH ... COOH (trans)

cis   *trans*

Fig. 20.5 Structures of *cis*- and *trans*-β,β-(4-methylpentamethylene)-β-mercaptopropionic acid (*cis*- and *trans*-4-MePpa).

2.3 Various Cyclic Linkages

The lactam and disulfide bridge formations have been the most popular linkages for cyclic structures. Several linkages have also been devised to connect various types of sidechain functional groups to peptide termini or other side chains. For example, to form a cyclic structure using two side-chain hydroxyl groups, a phosphodiester linkage (Fig. 20.6A) was proposed (46). In fact, this linkage occurs naturally in a protein, flavodoxin, isolated from *azotobacter*. Since the P(O) moieties can act as hydrogen-bonding or metal-binding acceptors, this linkage affects the conformational features of the resulting analogs. A disiloxane bridge has also been employed for linking two hydroxyl groups (47) and has been

introduced into an enkephalin analog. The resulting cyclic enkephalin (Fig. 20.6B) has shown opioid activity.

A urethane linkage can be useful for connecting an amine to a side-chain hydroxyl group. Furthermore, the C(O)–NH bond of urethane has a high tendency to assume a cis configuration which can facilitate the formation of cyclic peptides. Wu and Kohn have synthesized Tyr-urethane containing pseudopeptides (Fig. 20.7) (48). An ester linkage connecting a carboxyl group and a hydroxyl group has been observed in many naturally occurring antibiotics. This linkage was used for the synthesis of a series of human renin inhibitors (49).

Cyclic linkages with aromatic rings also occur in nature. For example, an aryl ether linkage has been found in glycopeptide antibiotics (vancomycin) (50) and in the

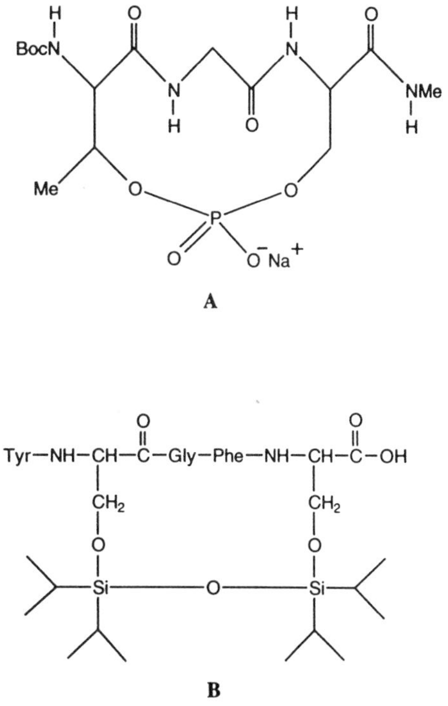

A

Tyr—NH—CH—C(=O)—Gly—Phe—NH—CH—C(=O)—OH with CH₂—O—Si and CH₂—O—Si linked by Si—O—Si

B

Fig. 20.6 Structures of A, a model peptide containing phosphodiester linkage; and B, disiloxane containing cyclic enkephalin.

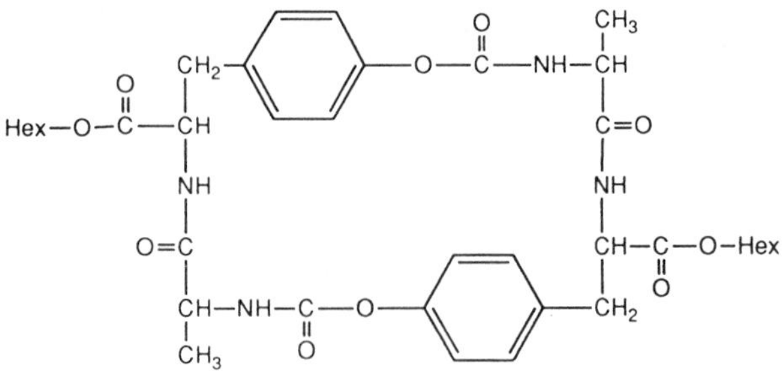

Fig. 20.7 Structure of urethane linkage-containing peptide.

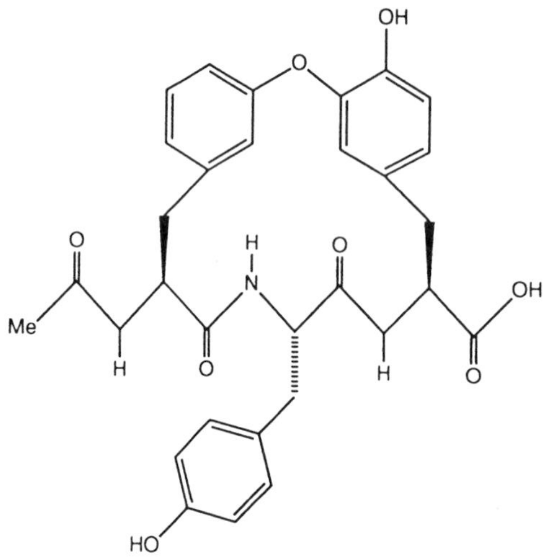

Fig. 20.8 Naturally occurring angiotensin converting enzyme inhibitor K-13.

naturally occurring angiotensin-converting enzyme inhibitor K-13 (Fig. 20.8) (51). Recently, Thaisrivongs et al. reported the connection of a histidine side chain to the

N-terminus of a renin inhibitor by using the $-CH_2-C(O)-$ unit (Fig. 20.9) (52). The resulting analogs exhibited high binding affinity.

Recently, the lanthionine (monosulfide) bridge (53) which is observed in nisin and other peptide antibiotics, has been incorporated in the place of disulfide bridges in several bioactive peptides (54). The resulting analogs are more constrained than their disulfide-bridged counterparts because of their decreased ring size. Additionally, this modification increases the metabolic stability of the resulting analogs. When this modification was incorporated into cyclic enkephalins [i.e., Tyr-c(D-Ala$_L$-Gly-Phe-Ala$_L$)-NH$_2$ (55): Fig. 20.10], the resulting analogs showed bioactivities similar to those of their disulfide bridged counterparts [i.e., Tyr-c(D-Cys-Gly-Phe-Cys)-NH$_2$]. However, the half-life of the lanthionine enkephalin in the rat brain homogenates is much longer than that of the parent disul-

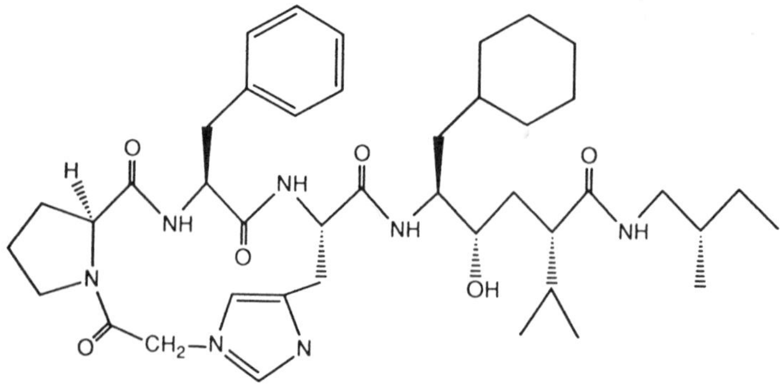

Fig. 20.9 A renin inhibitor in which the side chain of His is linked to N-terminus by $-CH_2-C(O)-$ unit.

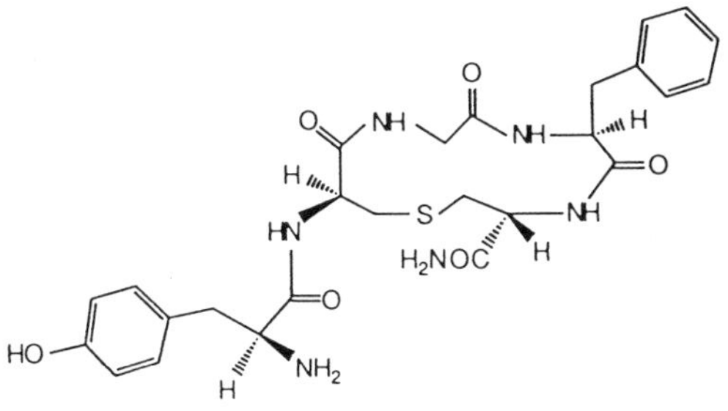

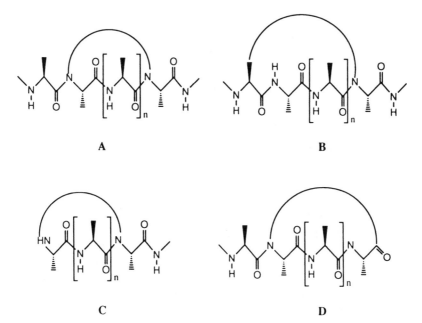

Fig. 20.10 Chemical structure of Tyr-c(D-Ala$_L$-Gly-Phe-Ala$_L$)-NH$_2$. This analog contains a lanthionine (monosulfide) bridge.

fide compounds. This structure is presently being incorporated into disulfide bridge containing peptides that include oxytocin and calcitonin as well as opioids.

2.4 Backbone Cyclizations and Bicyclic Structures

Gilon et al. have achieved the cyclization of peptides by linking an N$^\alpha$ atom to either another N$^\alpha$ atom, other side chains, the amino terminus or the carboxyl terminus using an appropriate linker (56). The possible cyclic structures are depicted in Figure 20.11. They also introduced this structure into a Substance P analog, Ac-Arg-Phe-Phe-Phe-Pro-Leu-Met-NH$_2$, leading to the structures shown in Figure 20.12. The analogs have similar biological profiles and show protracted activity in various tissues when compared to the parent analog (56). In the NMR studies of these two analogs, isomers containing a cis structure about the substituted amide bond were observed (57).

Bicyclic structures have been studied to avoid the flexibility of large cyclic peptides (58). When a bicyclic structure was formed in the oxytocin sequence, the resulting peptides showed high antagonist activity (59, 60). Also the parent monocyclic precursor possessed very little agonist activity. Multicyclic structures have also been considered as a method to stabilize an amphiphilic α-helical structure (61).

Fig. 20.11 Four possible backbone cyclizations, A, an N$^\alpha$ atom to another N$^\alpha$ atom; B, an N$^\alpha$ atom to a side chain; C, an N$^\alpha$ atom to amino terminus; or D, an N$^\alpha$ atom to carboxylic terminus.

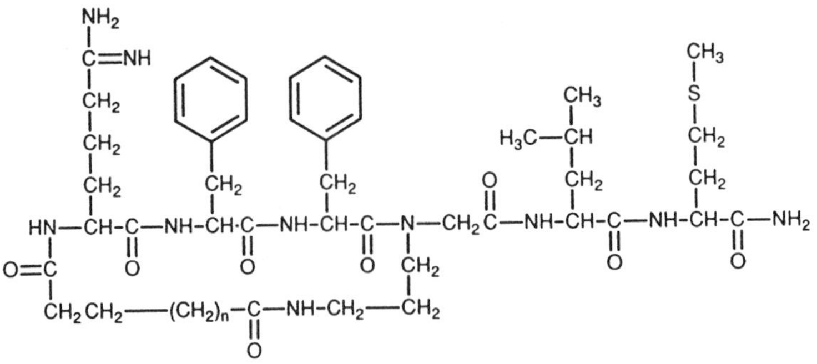

Fig. 20.12   Backbone cyclized substance P analogs. One analog has $C^\gamma H_2$ ($n = 1$) and another analog does not have this methylene ($n = 0$).

3 CONSTRAINED AMINO ACIDS

Constrained amino acids have been introduced into the sequences of bioactive peptides in order to obtain local constraints. Incorporation of these amino acids specifically restricts the rotation of N^α–C^α, C^α–C(O), C(O)–NH bonds, and side-chain conformations by covalent or noncovalent steric interactions. Thus, these amino acids can be used as conformational probes in an effort to understand local conformations responsible for the bioactivity of a particular peptide.

3.1 α-Methylated Amino Acids

Amino acids which are α-methylated have a structure in which the α-hydrogen atom is replaced by a methyl group. Methylation severely restricts rotation around the N–C^α (ϕ) and C^α–C(O) (ψ) bonds of amino acids. Figure 20.13 displays the changes in the allowed (ϕ) and (ψ) regions upon the α-methylation of glycine (Ala) (62). About 70% of the conformational space available to Gly cannot be adopted by Ala. Furthermore, about 90% of this conformational space is not available to α-aminoisobutyric acid [Aib or α-methylalanine (MeA); Fig. 20.14 (A) (63–64).]

Among the α-methylated amino acids, Aib (observed in native channel peptides) is the most extensively studied. The conformational behaviors of Aib containing peptides were summarized in reviews by Venkataram Prasad, Balaram, and Karle (65, 66). Further studies have also been published (67–85). The conformational space preferentially adopted by Aib residues includes both the regions of left- and right-handed α and 3_{10} helices (86). This amino acid rarely exhibits extended structures (87). The Aib residue has been incorporated into numerous bioactive peptides including enkephalin (15, 88–91), angiotensin (92), bradykinin (93), chemoattractants (94), and substance P (95) in order to obtain highly active and selective analogs and to understand the conformations responsible for the recognition of their receptors.

Unlike Aib, all other α-methylated amino acids are chiral. Toniolo et al. reviewed the conformational preferences of isolvaline [Iva or L-α-ethyl-alanine (EtA); Fig. 20.14B], α-methylvaline [(αMe)Val], α-methylleucine [(αMe)Leu], and α-methylphenylalanine [(αMe)Phe; Fig 20.14C)] in peptides (96). The conformational preferences were determined by X-ray crystallographic analyses, ^{1}H-NMR spectroscopic studies, and conformational

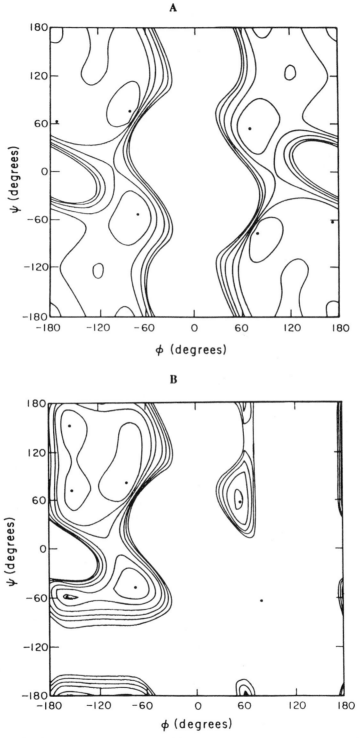

Fig. 20.13 Conformational energy contour map of (A), *N*-acetyl-*N'*-methyl-glycineamide; (B) *N*-acetyl-*N'*-methyl-alanineamide; and (C) *N*-acetyl-*N'*-methyl-*α*-amino-isobutyric acid amide.

C

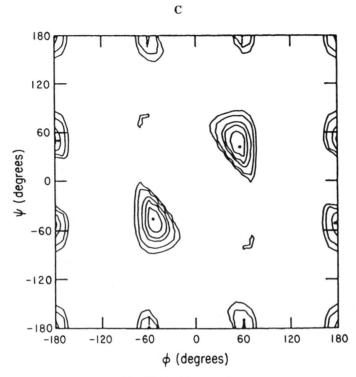

Fig. 20.13 (*Continued*)

energy calculations. In general, tripeptides and longer peptides containing these amino acids are folded in β-turns or in a 3_{10}-helical array. Furthermore, these amino acids rarely adopt the fully extended structure ($\phi = 180°$, $\psi = 180°$). Recently, the crystal state conformational analysis of homopeptides from [D-(αMe)Phe]$_n$ ($n = 1$, 2, 3, and 4) was reported (97). All of the

(αMe)Phe residues were found to prefer torsion angles in the helical region of ϕ, ψ conformational map.

These amino acids have also been incorporated into bioactive peptides. For example, the (αMe)Phe containing cyclic dermorphin analog, Tyr-c[D-Orn-(αMe)-Phe-Glu]-NH$_2$, shows activities similar to the Phe containing parent analog (98). On

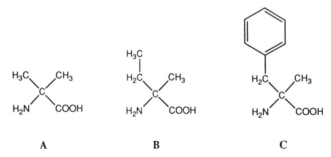

Fig. 20.14 Structures of α-methylated amino acids, A, α-aminoisobutyric acid (Aib); B, isovaline (Iva) (α-ethylalanine); and C, α-methylphenylalanine (αMePhe).

the contrary, the incorporation of (αMe)Tyr into enkephalin leads to an inactive analog (99). When (αMe)Phe is incorporated into a chemoattractant, the resulting compound shows reduced activity (100).

In addition, other α-methylated amino acids were studied resulting in the syntheses of (αMe)Arg (101), (αMe)Pro (102), (αMe)Orn (102), and (αMe)Ser (103). The X-ray studies of a (αMe)Ser-containing peptide indicated that this residue favorably adopts a conformation in which $\phi = -55°$ and $\psi = -32°$ (104).

3.2 α,α'-Dialkylglycines and α-Aminocycloalkane Carboxylic Acids

The replacement of the two hydrogens on the C^α atom of a glycine residue with two identical alkyl or aryl groups results in α,α-disubstituted glycines (Fig. 20.15) (105, 106) with the Aib residue having the simplest structure among this type of amino acids. As mentioned in the previous section, allowable ϕ and ψ angles for this residue are restricted to the α- or 3_{10}-helix regions. However, diethylglycine (Deg) and dipropylglycine (Dpg) residues exhibit different conformational preferences (Fig. 20.15A). These residues preferentially adopt fully extended structures where ϕ and ψ angles are both 180° (107, 108). A similar extended structure was also ob-

served as a minimum energy conformation from the conformational studies of diphenylglycine (Dφg; Fig. 20.15B (109). The dibenzylglycine (Dbg; Fig. 20.15C) residue of the tripeptide Gly-Dbg-Gly readily adopts conformations where the ϕ and ψ angles are (180°, 90°) and (180°, 270°) (110).

The α-aminocyclcloalkanecarboxylic acids (Ac^{n}c, $n = 3$–7) are also α,α-dialkylglycines with cyclized side chains incorporated into a cyclic structure (Fig. 20.16A). For example, α-aminocyclopropane carboxylic acid (Ac^{3}c) (111) contains a three-membered ring including the α-carbon. Several peptides containing Ac^{3}c were examined by X-ray crystallography. In the solid state, this residue assumes a β-turn conformation or a distorted 3_{10} helix (112, 113). The conformational preference of other aminocycloalkane carboxylic acids such as α-aminocyclopentane carboxylic acid (Ac^{5}c) (114, 115), α-aminocyclohexane carboxylic acid (Ac^{6}c) (116), and α-aminocycloheptane carboxylic acid (Ac^{7}c) (117) are also similar.

It is interesting that although dialkylglycines and aminocycloalkane carboxylic acids have the same number of side-chain carbons, they show different conformational preferences. For example, Ac^{5}c and Ac^{7}c prefer a folded conformation, whereas Deg and Dpg favor a fully extended structure. This comparison demonstrates the substantial effects of cyclic side chains

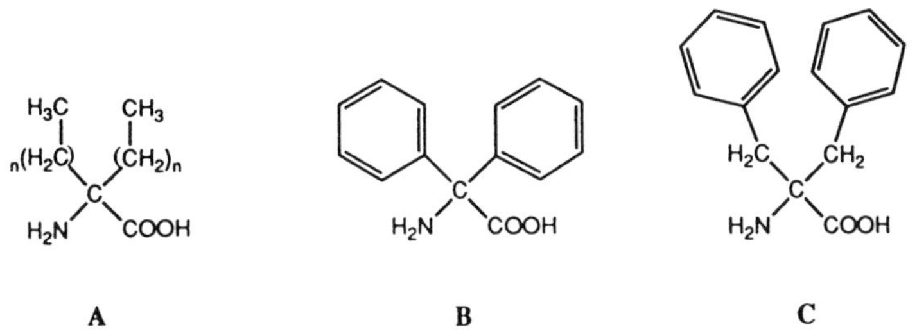

A   **B**   **C**

Fig. 20.15 Structures of α,α-dialkylated glycines, A, α-aminoisobutyric acid ($n = 0$, Aib); α,α-diethylglycine ($n = 1$, Deg) and α,α-dipropylglycine ($n = 2$, Dpg); B, α,α-diphenylglycine (Dφg); and C, α,α-dibenzylglycine (Dbg).

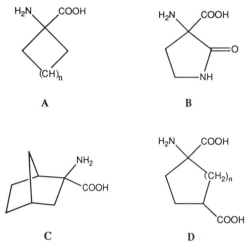

Fig. 20.16 Structures of A, aminocycloalkane carboxylic acids; α-aminocyclopropane carboxylic acid (Ac^3c, $n = 0$), α-aminocyclobutane carboxylic acid (Ac^4c, $n = 1$), α-aminocyclopentane carboxylic acid (Ac^5c, $n = 2$), α-aminocyclohexane carboxylic acid (Ac^6c, $n = 3$) and α-aminocycloheptane carboxylic acid (Ac^7c, $n = 4$); and their modifications B, α-aminopyrrolidone carboxylic acid (Apc); C, α-amino-norborane carboxylic acid; and D, 1-aminocyclopentane-1,3-dioic acid ($n = 1$) and 1-aminocyclohexane-1,4-dioic acid ($n = 2$).

on the conformation of the amino acid in peptides.

The α-aminocycloalkanecarboxylic acids were incorporated into bioactive peptides including opioid peptides, chemotactic peptides, and sweeteners. When Ac^5c was incorporated into various positions of enkephalins, the resulting peptides showed higher *in vivo* activity than the parent enkephalin amide (15). The chemotactic analogs (HCO-Met-X-Phe-OMe) containing Ac^5c, Ac^6c, and Ac^7c showed higher activity than their parent peptides (94). The Aib containing analog is slightly less active and the Ac^3c containing analog is inactive. Aspartame analogs in which Ac^nc ($n = 3$–8) residues are incorporated (Asp-Ac^n-OMe) have been synthesized. The analogs with Ac^nc ($n = 3$–5) retained a sweet taste (118). On the contrary, Ac^6c and Ac^7c containing analogs are bitter and the Ac^8c containing analog is tasteless.

Recently, aminopyrrolidone carboxylic acid has been synthesized (Apc: Fig. 20.16B) (119). The structure of Apc is similar to Ac^5c except that one ethylene ($C^\beta H_2$-$C^\alpha H_2$) of the five-membered ring is replaced with an amide bond. Thus, the Apc residue contains a stereogenic center and the side-chain can be involved in hydrogen-bonding. When Apc was incorporated into valmuceptin, one of the resulting analogs, Tyr-(D,L)-Apc-Phe-Val-NH$_2$, showed opioid activity. On the other hand, the Ac^5c containing analog was inactive (120).

The α-aminonorborane carboxylic acids (Fig. 20.16C) can be classified as aminocycloalkane carboxylic acids (121, 122). Since these residues are bulky and highly constrained, they may be expected to show highly preferred conformations. In addition, analogs of glutamic acid were synthesized by placing the carboxyl group at the γ-position of Ac^5c and Ac^6c (Fig. 20.16D) (123).

3.3 N^α-C^α Cyclized Amino Acids

The N^α–C^α cyclized amino acids have been devised as modifications of proline. One of the most important characteristics of these amino acids is the occurrence of cis/trans isomerism (Fig. 20.17) (124). The tertiary amide bond of N^α–C^α cyclized amino acids leads to the cis and trans amide bonds with approximately 2 kcal/mole energy difference (125). This value is much lower than that of a normal peptide bond (approx. 10 kcal/mol). This type of cis/trans isomerization can be detected by NMR. The NMR studies of morphiceptin (Tyr-Pro-Phe-Pro-NH$_2$) have shown four different isomers generated from cis/trans isomerization of the Tyr-Pro and Phe-Pro amide bonds (126).

Since the N^α–C^α bond of prolinelike amino acids is included in the pyrrolidine ring, the ϕ angle of these amino acids is

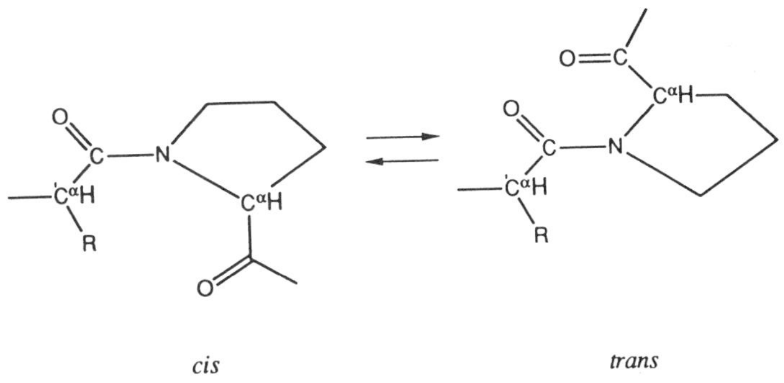

Fig. 20.17 A cis/trans isomerization of proline.

highly restricted. The rotation of the $C^\alpha-$C(O) bond is also constrained by the steric interaction between the pyrrolidine ring and C(O). These amino acids can affect the conformation of the preceding residue. The ψ angle rotation for the preceding L-residue is restricted to between 60 and 180°. When the Pro residue assumes a trans configuration, the steric interaction occurs between the side chain of the preceding L-residue and the $C^\delta H_2$ attached to the nitrogen of the Pro residue. In a cis isomer of proline, a steric overlap occurs between the side chain of the preceding L-residue and the C^α group of the Pro residue (127).

3.3.1 PROLINE MIMETICS WITH DIFFERENT RING SIZES. Structures such as Azy (azyline or aziridine-2-carboxylic acid), Aze (azetidine-2-carboxylic acid), and Pip

(pipecolic acid) are proline analogs or mimetics with different ring sizes (Fig. 20.18A). The Azy and Aze have 3- and 4-membered rings, respectively, whereas the Pip contains a 6-membered ring. When one of the methylene groups in the cyclic structure is replaced by an oxygen or a sulfur, (O)Pro (oxazolidine-4-carboxylic acid), (O)Pip (perhydro-1,4-oxazine-3-carboxylic acid or 3-morpholinecarboxylic acid), (S)Pro (or Thz; thiozolidine-4-carboxylic acid), and (S)Pip (perhydro-1,4-thioxazine-3-carboxylic acid) are obtained (Fig. 20.18B). The conformational behavior of these amino acids is well-summarized in a review written by Toniolo (128). Recently, piperazic acid (Piz; Fig. 20.18C) was found as a component of the naturally occurring oxytocin antagonist c[Pro-D-Phe-(NOH)Ile-D-Piz-Piz-D-(NMe)Phe] (129).

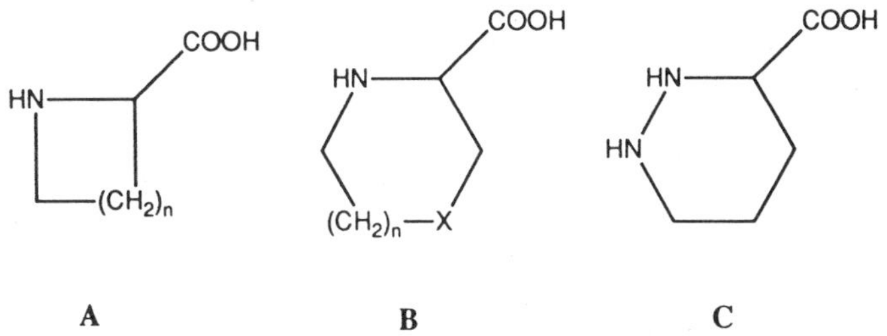

Fig. 20.18 Proline mimetics with different ring size. A, aziridine-2-carboxylic acid (Azy, $n = 0$), azetidine-2-carboxylic acid (Aze, $n = 1$), proline (Pro, $n = 2$) and pipecolic acid (Pip, $n = 3$) and their modified forms; B, oxazolidine-4-carboxylic acid [$n = 0$, $X = O$; (O)Pro or Oxz], thiozolidine-4-carboxylic acid [$n = 0$, $X = S$; (S)Pro or Thz], perhydro-1,4-oxazine-3-carboxylic acid or 3-morpholine carboxylic acid [$n = 1$, $X = O$; (O)Pip and perhydro-1,4-thioxazine-3-carboxylic acid [$n = 1$, $X = S$; (S)Pip]; and C, piperazic acid (Piz).

The Aze residue was incorporated into collagen, the fibrous protein whose structure is characterized by a large population of proline and hydroxyproline. From theoretical calculations peptides containing Aze are somewhat more flexible than the corresponding peptides containing Pro (130–132). This occurrence can be explained by a decrease in repulsive noncovalent interactions between the rings of neighboring residues. Since the Aze residue is smaller than the Pro residue, the steric interaction between Aze residues is weaker than those between Pro residues. Thus, the replacement of Pro with Aze destabilizes the collagenlike triple helix (130–132).

Veber et al. incorporated Aze, Thz, and Pip in place of Pro in a somatostatin analog c(Pro-Phe-D-Trp-Lys-Thr-Phe) (133). The resulting analogs exhibited higher activity than the parent analog. The incorporation of (O)Pro, (S)Pro, and Pip in place of Pro in morphiceptin provided analogs with reduced activities (134). When D-Pip was incorporated at the same position, the resulting Tyr-D-Pip-Phe-Pro-NH$_2$ showed opioid activity (135), unlike Tyr-D-Pro-Phe-Pro-NH$_2$ (136). This result suggests that the Pip residue can adopt conformations not allowed for the Pro residue.

3.3.2 HIGHLY CONSTRAINED PROLINE MIMETICS.

Highly constrained Pro analogs have been devised incorporating additional functional groups (Fig. 20.19). Methanoprolines, containing [5,3,0] and [5,4,1] bicyclic systems, have been prepared, including 2,4-methanoproline (2,4-MePro; Fig. 20.19A (137–139) 2,3-methanoproline (2,3-MePro; Fig. 20.19B (140) and 3,4-methanoproline (3,4-MePro; Fig. 20.19C (141). Methylation on a carbon of the proline ring produced 2-methylproline [(αMe)Pro; Fig. 20.19D] (142) and 3-methylproline [(βMe)Pro; Fig. 20.19E] (142). The ethylene group was incorporated in the structures of 4-aza-

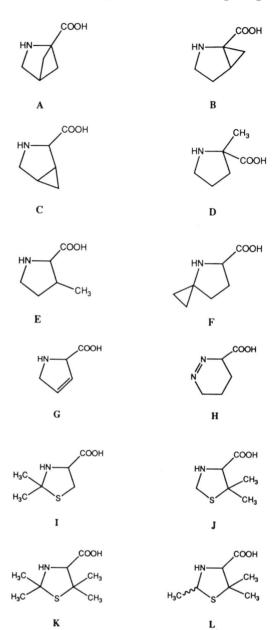

Fig. 20.19 Constrained proline mimetics. A, 2,4-methanoproline (2,4-MePro); B, 2,3-methanoproline (2,3-MePro); C, 3,4-methanoproline (3,4-MePro); D, 2-methylproline [(αMe)Pro]; E, 3-methylproline [(βMe)Pro]; F, 4-azaspiro[2.4]heptane carboxylic acid; G, 3,4-dehydroproline (3,4-ΔPro); H, dehydropiperazic acid (ΔPiz); I, 2,2-dimethylthiazolidine-4-carboxylic acid (2,2-Dtc); J, 5,5-dimethylthiazolidine-4-carboxylic acid (5,5-Dtc); K, 2,2,5,5-tetramethylthiazolidine-4-carboxylic acid; and L, 2,5,5-trimethylthiazolidine-4-carboxylic acid.

spiro[2,4]heptane carboxylic acid (Fig. 20.19F) (141). In 3,4-dehydroproline (3,4-ΔPro; Fig. 20.19b (134) and dehydropiperazic acid (ΔPiz; Fig. 20.19H) (129, 143–145), one of the bonds in the ring was replaced with a double bond. In addition, methyl groups were introduced into the thiazolidine structure and the resulting 2,2- or 5,5 -dimethylthiazolidine -4- carboxylic acid (Dtc; Fig. 20.19I, J) have been extensively studied (146). Recently, 2,2,5,5 - tetramethylthiazolidine - 4 - carboxylic acid was synthesized (Fig. 20.19K) and two isomers of 2,5,5-trimethylthiazolidine-4-carboxylic acid (Fig. 20.19L) (120) were synthesized.

Scheraga et al. carried out conformational studies of 2,4-MePro containing peptides using NMR, X-ray crystallographic, and computational techniques (138, 139). The NMR studies of Ac-2,4-MePro-NHMe and Ac-Tyr-2,4-MePro-NHMe in aqueous solution indicate that the Ac-2,4-MePro and Tyr-2,4-MePro amide bonds adopt a trans structure to an overwhelming extent. This result suggests that the bicyclic structure generated by the incorporation of a methylene group into a Pro residue stabilizes the trans amide bond. The energy difference between cis- and trans-forms was calculated to be 5.9–8.8 kcal/mol. The additional methylene group also perturbs backbone conformational angles. The calculation of the interior torsion angle ϕ of this amino acid showed two minima at $\pm 29°$, rather than one at $-70°$, as seen with the Pro residue. Similarly, optimal values for the ψ torsional angle are also perturbed. The average ψ values of this amino acid are $-50°$ and $90°$, whereas those of the Pro residue are $-19°$, $75°$, and $160°$. In the crystalline state, the observed (ϕ, ψ) angles for Ac-2,4-MePro-NHMe and its enantiomer are $(-29°, 114°)$ and $(29°, -114°)$, respectively.

Marshall and his associates incorporated this amino acid in place of each of three Pro residues in bradykinin (Arg-Pro-Pro-Gly-Phe-Ser-Pro-Phe-Arg), one at a time. In spite of the desirable effects of 2,4-MePro which stabilize the trans configuration of the Pro-Pro and Ser-Pro amide bonds, the resulting analogs showed significantly reduced activities (137). An explanation for the reduced activities can be suggested by postulating that the additional methylene of the 2,4-MePro is involved in conformational changes of the residue and the steric interactions with the receptor. Marshall's group also incorporated this amino acid into angiotensin II (Asp-Val-Try -Val-His-Pro-Phe) providing an analog with 26% of potency of the parent molecule.

Stammer et al. synthesized 2,3-MePro and carried out conformational studies (140). In the X-ray structure of Ac-(2R,3S)-MePro-NHMe, the ϕ and ψ torsion angles are $76°$ and $7°$, respectively, and the Ac-(2R,3S)-MePro bond is in a cis conformation. The ϕ and ψ angles were found to be essentially the same as those of Ac-D-Pro-NHMe. The NMR studies of this model compound indicate the existence of the two stereoisomers. A somewhat greater preference for the cis form of the Ac-2,3-MePro amide bond was observed. This result was supported by the above X-ray structure and the relative energies of two isomers. The cis isomer of Ac-2,3-MePro-NHMe was favored over the trans isomer by 1.4 kcal/mol from the calculations. When a taste ligand was synthesized using this amino acid, the resulting compound [Asp-(2S,3R) -2,3-MePro-OPr] was bitter (147). The NMR studies of this compound suggest that the Asp-(2S,3R)-MePro amide bond adopts only a cis configuration. The comparison of the relative energies of the fully minimized cis and trans isomers of Asp-(2S,3R)-MePro-OPr demonstrate a 2.1 kcal/mol energy difference favoring the cis conformation.

Delaney and Madison carried out conformational studies of Ac-(αMe)Pro-NHMe and Ac-(βMe)Pro-NHMe (142). In the NMR studies, the Ac-(αMe)Pro-NHMe did not exhibit a cis isomer in any solvent, while both *anti*- and *syn*-(βMe)Pro-NHMe (*anti*; the methyl group is on the opposite side of the proline ring from the carboxamide, *syn*; on the same side) exhibited 15% to 25% of the cis isomer in different solvents. The absence of a cis isomer of Ac-(αMe)Pro-NHMe may be caused by the steric interactions between the α-methyl and acetyl–methyl groups.

The conformational behaviors of Ac-*anti*-(βMe)Pro-NHMe are nearly identical with those of Ac-Pro-NHMe in the same solvents (142). Specifically, the C_7 conformer (γ-turn; $\phi = -80°$, $\psi = 80°$) dominates the conformational populations in nonpolar solvents. A mixture of C_7, right-handed α helix, and polyproline II ($\phi = -80°$, $\psi = 150°$) conformers was observed in acetonitrile. On the other hand, in water, the polyproline II conformation predominated. For Ac-*syn*-(βMe)Pro-NHMe, the γ-turn can be destabilized by steric interactions between the methyl group and the carbonyl oxygen of the Pro residue.

In addition, the hydrogen-bonding in the C_7 conformer of Ac-(αMe)Pro-NHMe (between C(O) of the acetyl group and NH of the terminal methylamide) is unusually strong as shown by IR spectroscopy (142). A significant amount of this intramolecular hydrogen-bonding is retained in aqueous solution. These results indicate that the α-methyl group stabilizes the γ-turn of this model peptide by inducing a fold of the mainchain to avoid methyl eclipsing interactions. The α-methylated structure also shields the peptide hydrogen bond from solvent. The stabilization of the γ-turn by the α-methylation of Pro was also observed in the conformational studies of (αMe)Pro containing bradykinin (148) and other bioactive peptides (149). The (αMe)Pro was incorporated into a renin inhibitor producing a highly active analog, Boc-(αMe)Pro-Phe-His-Leuψ[CHOHCH$_2$]Val-Ile-Amp (150).

Samanen et al. examined the conformational preferences of 5,5-dimethylthia-

zoline-4-carboxylic acid (Dtc) (146). The ^{1}H-NMR spectrum of Boc-Dtc-Ile-OMe displayed two stereoisomers resulting from the cis/trans isomerization of the Boc-Dtc bond. On the other hand, the X-ray crystal structure of Boc-Dtc-OH showed only a cis configuration of the urethane amide bond. Conformational studies using Ac-Dtc-NHMe suggest that the steric interaction between the *syn*-β-methyl group and the carbonyl group of Dtc destabilized hydrogen-bonding between the Boc C(O) and the NH of the terminal amide of the C_7 conformation. This γ-turn conformation is the predominant conformation for Ac-Pro-NHMe. Instead, the Dtc residue adopts conformations in which ψ is 110–150° or 320–360°. These results suggest that the substitution of Dtc for Pro may test the functional importance of the C_7 conformation in a position of a bioactive peptide. When this amino acid was incorporated into position 5 of an angiotensin II (Sar-Arg-Val-Tyr-X-His-Pro-Ile-OH) analog (92, 151) the resulting analog showed higher activity than the Pro containing analog. This residue was also introduced into cholecystokinin. An R-Dtc containing analog showed high bioactivity (152).

Other constrained Pro analogs have been incorporated into bioactive peptides. For example, 3,4-dehydroproline (ΔPro) was introduced into somatostatin (133), morphiceptin (134), and oxytocin (153) in place of Pro. The resulting analogs displayed higher activity than the parent compounds. When ΔPiz was incorporated in place of Piz of the naturally occurring oxytocin antagonist, the resulting analog was highly active (115–117, 121).

The introduction of additional groups into the proline structure also provides substantial preferences for their conformations and cis/trans structures at the preceding amide bond. Thus, these proline mimetics can be useful in the design of biologically active peptide analogs since they affect local conformations and cis/trans preferences of the amide bonds.

3.3.3 PYROGLUTAMIC ACIDS AND HYDROXY PROLINE ANALOGS. Pyroglutamic acid (pGlu) also contains a N^α–C^α cyclized structure, but it is formed by *N*-acylation (Fig. 20.20A). This novel amino acid derivative is present in many naturally occurring peptides and has been incorporated into bioactive peptide analogs (154–158). Molecular mechanical calculations for L-pGlu-NHMe indicate that this residue adopts a folded conformation (159). However, the X-ray structure of L-pGlu-NHMe has displayed an extended conformation. A highly constrained derivative of this residue, 2,3-MepGlu: Fig. 20.20B) was also prepared to increase the metabolic stability of thyrotrophin releasing hormone (TRH). The resulting 2,3-MepGlu containing TRH analog is significantly more stable to enzymatic degradation than TRH. The X-ray crystal structure of 2,3-MepGlu-NHMe displayed that the (ϕ, ψ) angles of this residue are ($-143°$, $-16°$) (159).

Naturally occurring hydroxyproline has also been modified. These synthetic studies include the introduction of an additional hydroxyl group (i.e., 3,4-dihydroxy proline; Fig. 20.20C), changes in ring size (i.e., 3,4-dihydroxy pipercolic acid: Fig. 20.20D) (160) and alkylation of a hydroxy group (alkoxy proline: Fig. 20.20E) (161).

These analogs represent interesting mimetics which can be incorporated into bioactive peptides.

3.4 N^α-Methylated Amino Acids

The N^α-methylated amino acids are commonly found in naturally occurring peptide antibiotics. Since the methylation of N^α eliminates the hydrogen on the N^α atom, the hydrogen-bonding pattern of peptides containing these amino acids are different from that of the unmethylated peptides. The *N*-methylated amide bond often adopts a cis as well as a trans geometry as with the N^α–C^α cyclized amino acid derivatives above. Conformational calculations and NMR studies on Sar-Sar (Sar: sarcocine or N-methylglycine) dipeptide showed that the two forms are nearly isoenthalpic; the cis isomer is higher in energy only by 0.6 kcal/mol (162). Amino acid *N*-methylation also affects the rotation of ϕ and ψ angles. The allowed conformational space of Ac-Ala-NHMe in a trans configuration is reduced when a methyl group is incorporated (Fig. 20.21A). The allowed conformational space for the cis isomer of Ac-(NMe)Ala-NMe is also depicted (Fig. 20.21B). The ϕ and ψ angles of the two

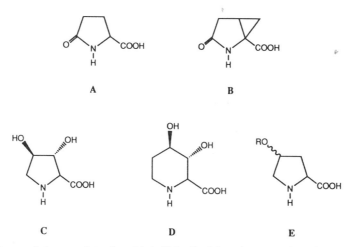

Fig. 20.20 Structures of A, pyroglutamic acid (pGlu); B, 2,3-methanopyroglutamic acid (2,3-MepGlu); C, 3,4-dihydroxyproline; D, 3,4-dihydroxypipercolic acid; and E, 4-alkoxyproline.

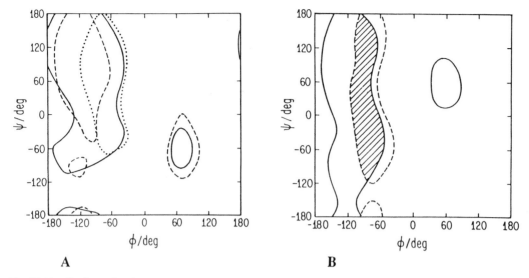

Fig. 20.21 Conformational energy contour map of **A** Ac-Ala-NHMe (solid), Ac-(NMe)Ala-NHMe (dashed) and Ac-Pro-NHMe (dotted) in a trans configuration of the amide bond; and **B**, Ac-(NMe)Ala-NHMe (solid) and Ac-Pro-NHMe (dashed) in a cis configuration of the amide bond.

lowest energy conformations for this isomer are approximately ($-70°$, $140°$) and ($-70°$, $-40°$), respectively. These are similar to those for the Pro residue (163, 164).

The N-methylated amino acid can affect the rotation of the C^α–C(O) bond of the preceding residue. The ψ angle of any L-amino acid residue which immediately precedes a N^α-methylamino acid is restricted to a range from $60°$ to $180°$. When the N-methylated amino acid assumes a trans configuration, a range of $-180° < \psi < 0°$ is precluded by steric overlap involving the side chain of the preceding L-residue with the methyl group attached to the nitrogen. The same ψ angle range is also precluded for the L-residue followed by a cis conformer of the N-methylated amino acid because of steric overlaps between the side chain of the L-residue and the C^αH group of the N-methyl amino acid. In addition, when the residue preceding the N-methyl amino acid is a β-substituted or branched amino acid, the torsion angle for the side chain conformation (χ) is also severely restricted by the N^α-methylated residues (163, 164).

The above conformational restrictions of N-methylated amino acids has been used to help understand the molecular basis of the bioactivities of morphiceptin and dermorphin (163, 165). The biologically important functional groups of these two peptide opioids involve the amino and phenolic groups of the Tyr[1] residue and the aromatic group of the Phe[3] residue. The relative spatial arrangements of these functional groups can be defined by a set of eight torsion angles: ψ^1, χ_1^1 and ω^1 of Tyr[1], ϕ^2, ψ^2, and ω^2 of Pro[2] or D-Ala[2], ϕ^3 and χ_1^3 of Phe[3]. To estimate each of these angles for morphiceptin bioactivity, a series of analogs were designed in which N-methyl amino acids were systematically incorporated into morphiceptin and dermorphin tetrapeptides. The resulting analogs have showed a correlation between bioactivity and distinct conformational preferences. The biologically meaningful value of each torsion angle was specifically identified by comparing its accessible space and bioactivities of the corresponding analog. Similar methods were applied for dermorphin. From these studies, conformations that are responsible for the bioactivities of morphiceptin and dermorphin have been postulated (163, 165).

Aubry and Marraud studied the effects of N-methylation on the β-turn structure by examining crystal structures of ten N-methylated R-C(O)-X-(NMe)Y-NHR dipeptides (Table 20.5) (166). Five of these analogs contained homochiral X and Y residues, two contained a heterochiral sequence and three contained one or two Gly residues. The distances between the α-carbons of the X and Y residues of methylated peptides in the trans configuration were found to be similar to those of the non-N-methylated peptides. However, the distances of the cis isomer are about 1 Å shorter. Aubry and Marraud also found that the β-turn of heterochiral dipeptide sequences are not perturbed by N-methylation and retain the same extent of β-folding. On the other hand, homochiral sequences preferentially have adopted a different β-turn conformation upon N-methylation.

In addition to peptide opioids (163, 165, 167, 168), these amino acids were incorporated into other bioactive peptides such as bradykinin (169), an opioid antagonist (CTOP) (170), TRH (164), angiotensin II (92), luteinizing hormone-releasing hormone (LHRH) (171), and CCK$_5$ (172).

3.5 β- and γ-Amino Cycloalkane Carboxylic Acids

The Pro residue allows a cis/trans isomerization at the preceding amide bond. There is difficulty in analyzing conformations where two or more distinct but interchanging structures are made up of all-trans isomer and isomers with at least one cis amide bond coexist. To avoid the possibility of such cis/trans isomerization, β-aminocyclopentane carboxylic acid (β-Ac^{5}c: Fig. 20.22A) was incorporated into peptides (173–175). This amino acid is similar to Pro but the preceding amide bond can adopt only a trans configuration since it contains an exocyclic amine. The residue contains an extra stereogenic center. Thus, four different isomers (1S,2R, 1S,2S, 1R,2R, and 1R,2S) are available. When these isomers are incorporated, each isomer imparts conformational effects on the peptide structure. Thus, the comparisons between the results of conformational analyses and bioassays of the four analogs containing these isomers can provide useful

Table 20.5 Conformations of N-Methylated Amino Acid-Containing Dipeptides

Compound	$\phi_1{}^a$	$\psi_1{}^a$	$\omega_1{}^a$	$\phi_2{}^a$	$\psi_2{}^a$	Conformation
tBu-C(O)-Pro-(NMe)Ala-OMe	−70	153	176	−92	157	
tBu-C(O)-Pro-(NMe)Ala-NHiPr	−62	135	−13	119	60	βVI-turn
tBu-C(O)-Pro-(NMe)Leu-NHMe	−66	146	−4	−108	55	βVI-turn
tBu-C(O)-Pro-(NMe)Phe-NHMe	−63	146	4	−113	52	βVI-turn
tBu-C(O)-Ala-(NMe)Ala-NHiPr	−66	137	−1	−113	48	βVI-turn
tBu-C(O)-Pro-D-(NMe)Ala-NHMe	−58	136	−178	97	−19	βII-turn
tBu-C(O)-Ala-D-(NMe)Ala-NHMe	−61	129	179	99	−23	βII-turn
tBu-C(O)-Pro-(NMe)Gly-NHiPr	−56	135	−178	96	−17	βII-turn
tBu-C(O)-Ala-(NMe)Gly-NHiPr	−71	153	171	103	−148	
iPr-C(O)-Gly-(NMe)Gly-NHiPr	−73	163	174	−90	−176	

^{a}The unit for all the torsion angles is degrees.

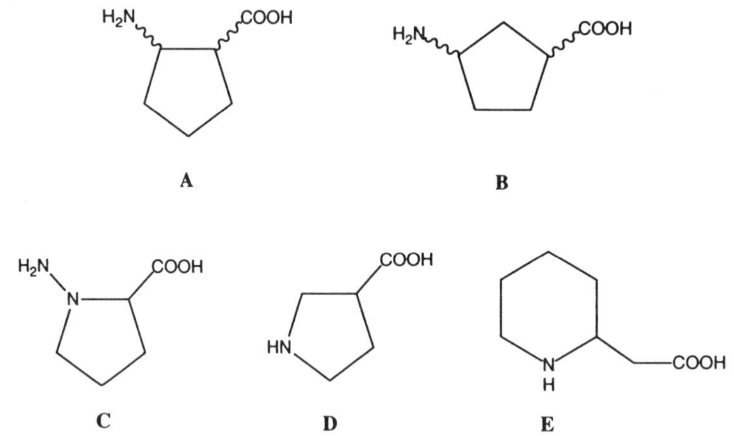

Fig. 20.22 Structures of A, β-aminocyclopentane carboxylic acid (β-Ac^{5}c); B, γ-aminocyclopentane carboxylic acid (γ-Ac^{5}c); C, aminoproline (aminoPro; D, β-proline (βPro); and E, piperidineacetic acid.

information about the conformations responsible for bioactivity.

When β-Ac^{5}c was incorporated into the second position of morphiceptin, only the (1S,2R) isomer containing analogs were active (173, 175). The conformational analysis of these analogs provided a preferred conformation which is similar to the structure suggested from the studies of other morphiceptin analogs (163, 165). Also these amino acids have been incorporated into somatostatin and taste ligands (174). Although the resulting somatostatin analogs were inactive, their conformational analyses provided useful information about the molecular basis for somatostatin bioactivity. The taste of Asp-β-Ac^{5}c-OMe is dependent on the configurations of the β-Ac^{5}c. For the trans-β-Ac^{5}c containing molecules, the 1R,2R-analog is sweet, where the 1S,2S-analog is bitter. For the analogs with cis-β-Ac^{5}c, the 1S,2R-analog is sweet, whereas the 1R,2S-analog is tasteless. The results of the conformational studies for these taste ligands were consistent with our model for the molecular basis of taste (174).

Also synthesized was γ-aminocyclopentane carboxylic acid (γ-Ac^{5}c; Fig. 20.22B) (173), 1-aminoproline (aminoPro; Fig.

20.22C), and β-proline (β-Pro; Fig. 20.22D) (120, 176). These proline analogs have been incorporated into morphiceptin. The γ-Ac^{5}c and aminoPro containing analogs are inactive., but the bioactivity of β-Pro-containing analogs are dependent on the configuration of that residue (120). Piperidineacetic acid (Fig. 20.22E) has also been synthesized and is also useful as a peptidomimetic residue in constrained peptides (177).

3.6 α,β-Unsaturated Amino Acids

In α,β-unsaturated amino acids (dehydro amino acids) (178), a double bond exists between C$^\alpha$ and C$^\beta$ (Fig. 20.23). These residues have been found naturally in antibiotics of microbial origin and in some proteins. Singh et al. extensively studied a number of small peptides containing dehydrophenylalanine(s) (ΔPhe) and dehydroleucine (ΔLeu) using X-ray crystallography (179–184). In most cases, these dehydro residues induce β-turn structures in the peptide backbone by promoting hydrogen-bonding between C(O) of the residue i and NH of the residue $i + 3$ (Fig. 20.24) (185). The values of ϕ and ψ are close to 80 and

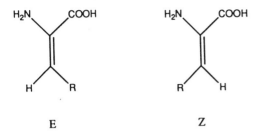

Fig. 20.23 Structures of dehydroamino acid in E and Z forms.

0°, respectively, when the ΔPhe residue is placed in the $(i + 2)$ position of the β-turn. If these residues occur at the $(i + 1)$ position, the ϕ and ψ are centered around −60 and 120°, respectively.

In the cases of Ac-ΔPhe-OH or Ac-ΔPhe-OEt, the ϕ values are close to either −60 or 80°. These values suggest a marked preference of ΔPhe for the two conformations in which ϕ and ψ are −60 and 120° or 80 and 0° (180). Similar results were obtained from the NMR and IR spectroscopic studies of Boc-X-ΔPhe-NHMe (X = Ala, Gly, Pro, Val) (186). From the X-ray-crystallographic studies of Ac-Pro-ΔVal-NHMe, a slightly different β-turn was observed. This peptide adopts the torsion angles, $\phi_1 = -68.3°$, $\psi_1 = -20.1°$, $\phi_2 = -73.5°$ and $\psi_2 = -14.1°$ (187). This conformation is characterized as a β-turn structure between the type I and the type III conformations. The NMR and IR studies of model peptides, homochiral Ac-Pro-Y-NHMe (Y = Val, Phe, Leu, Abu), and heterochiral Ac-Pro-D-Y-NHMe, as well as α,β-unsaturated Ac-Pro-ΔY-NHMe [ΔY = ΔVal, (Z)-ΔPhe, (Z)-ΔLeu, (Z)-ΔAbu] were carried out (188). The homochiral compounds are conformationally flexible and display an inverse γ-turn, a β-turn and open forms in an equilibrium depending on the nature of the Y residue side chain. However, the heterochiral and α,β-dehydropeptides display type II β-turns as the dominating secondary structures (188).

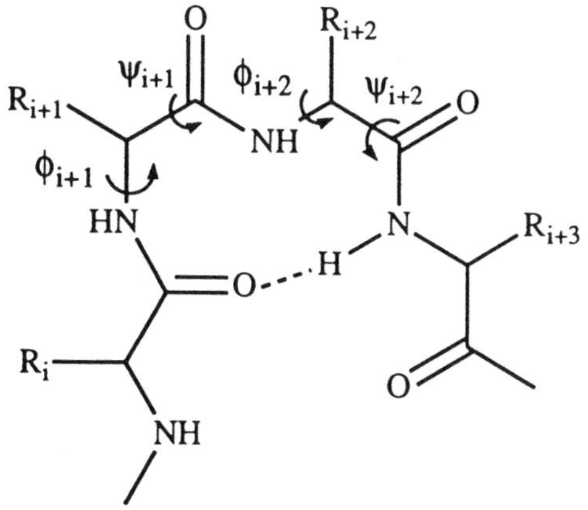

The crystal structure of the linear tetrapeptide, Boc-Leu-ΔPhe-Ala-Leu-OCH₃, exhibits a double turn in which the type III and type I β-turns occur consecutively using ΔPhe as a common corner residue (189). This structure contains Leu ($\phi = -54.1°$, $\psi = -34.5°$) and ΔPhe ($\phi = -59.9$, $\psi = -17.1°$) as the corner residues of the type III β-turn, and ΔPhe ($\phi = -59.9°$, $\psi = -17.1°$) and Ala ($\phi = -80.4°$, $\psi = 0.5°$) as the corner residues for the type I β-turn. Furthermore, two intramolecular 4-1 type hydrogen bonds were observed to stabilize this turn structure. The above torsion angles indicate that the overall structure of this peptide is helical. Similar 3_{10} helical structures induced by consecutive β-turns are observed in other peptides containing ΔPhe, including Z-D-Ala-ΔPhe-Gly-NH₂ (190) and Ac-ΔPhe-Val-OH (191).

When peptides contained two ΔPhe residues, such helical structures were more clearly observed. For example, the peptide Ac-ΔPhe-Ala-ΔPhe-NHMe adopts a right-handed 3_{10}-helical conformation (192). The two consecutive 10-membered rings are formed by two hydrogen bonds between acetyl C(O) and NH of ΔPhe[3] and between C(O) of ΔPhe[1] and NH of the N-methyl amide. In the solid state, the conformation of Boc-D-Ala-ΔPhe-Gly-ΔPhe-D-Ala-OMe is characterized by the presence of two type III β-turns. Thus, this peptide assumes a

Fig. 20.24 Typical β-turn structure.

left-handed 3_{10}-helical conformation. The left-handed sense is due to the D-Ala residues (193). In the crystal structures of Boc-Gly-ΔPhe-Leu-ΔPhe-Ala-NHMe (194) and Boc-Ala-ΔPhe-ΔPhe-NHMe (195), 3_{10}-helical structures were observed. Recently, Chauhan et al. reported a crystal structure of Boc-Val-ΔPhe-Ala-Phe-Ala-Phe-ΔPhe-Val-ΔPhe-Gly-OMe (196) which showed seven consecutive type III β-turns formed by seven 4-1 intramolecular hydrogen bonds. Thus, the overall conformation is a right-handed 3_{10} helix with three complete helical turns.

The ΔAla residue has different conformational preferences from those observed in ΔPhe and ΔLeu. In the crystal structure of Boc-Phe-ΔAla-OMe, the ϕ and ψ angles of the ΔAla residue are -170 and 178° (197). The NMR studies of the other ΔAla containing peptide, Boc-X-ΔAla-NHMe (X = Ala, Val and Phe), indicate that the ΔAla induces an inverse γ-turn around the preceding residue of the ΔAla (X residue) (198). The ϕ and ψ angles of the preceding residue of ΔAla are -70 and 70°, respectively. The interproton distance between $C^\alpha H$ of the $i + 1$ residue and N$\overline{H}$ of the $i + 2$ residue is 2.5 Å. Unlike the structure of Boc-Val-ΔAla-NHMe in solution, the corresponding saturated analog, Boc-Val-Ala-NHMe, does not show any intramolecular hydrogen-bonding. A similar inverse turn structure of ΔAla was observed in the conformational studies of nisin (199).

In addition to restricting the peptide backbone, the dehydrostructure fixes the side chain conformation. The side chain conformation is one of the most important factors in generating a favorable interaction between peptides and acceptor molecules (receptors or enzymes). The Newman projections about the C^α–C^β bond in three classical low energy conformations of β-substituted amino acids in a peptide are depicted in Fig. 20.25. When these conformers of an L-amino acid are examined by standard steric factors, the gauche$^-$ (g^-; $\chi_1 = -60°$) and trans (t; $\chi_1 = 180°$) conformers show similar stability; the gauche$^+$ (g^+; $\chi_1 = 60°$) is the least stable. In the C^α–C^β dehydro structure, only two forms (Z and E: Fig. 20.23) are possible. The χ_1 of the Z-isomer is 0°, whereas that of E-isomer is fixed at 180°.

Because of the difficulty involved in the syntheses of (E)-dehydroamino acids (200, 201), the (Z) isomers have been studied more extensively. The dehydroamino acids have been incorporated into various bioactive peptides including peptide opioids (202–207), thyroliberin (208), TRH (209), bradykinin (210) and inhibitors of the N-acetylated α-linked acidic dipeptidase (211).

3.7 β,β-Dimethyl and β-Methyl Amino Acids

Side-chain dimethyl substitution strongly affects the conformation of a given residue. The global topology and dynamic prop-

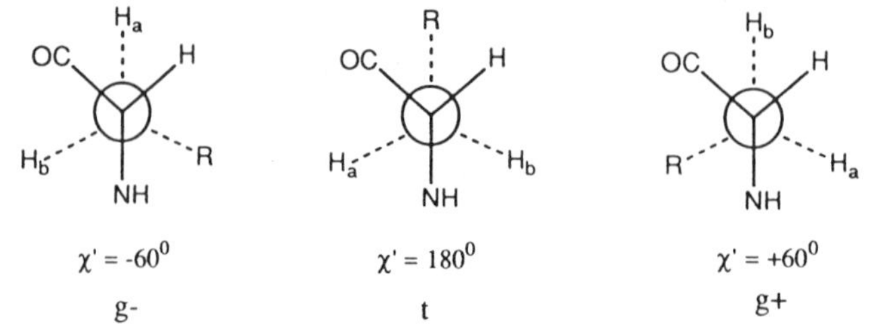

Fig. 20.25 Newman projections about C^α–C^β bond of β-substituted amino acids.

erties of cyclic peptides are influenced by the bulkiness of geminal methyl groups. A β,β-dimethyl amino acid, penicillamine (Pen, β,β-dimethylcysteine) has been used for many disulfide bridged cyclic peptides including angiotensin II (212), oxytocin antagonists (213), peptide opioids (214, 215), RGD peptides (44), and others (216, 217). The incorporation of Pen affects the disulfide bond angles through steric constraints. When this amino acid was incorporated into cyclic enkephalins [i.e., Tyr-c(D-Pen-Gly-Phe-D-Pen)-OH: DPDPE], the resulting peptides were highly δ opioid receptor selective (Table 20.1) (218). These results indicate that the Pen can stabilize the conformation responsible for recognition at the δ-receptor. However, these peptides were less active than Tyr-c(D-Cys-Gly-Phe-D-Cys)-OH (218). It is possible that the extra methyl groups sterically hinder the interaction of the peptide with its receptor.

Monomethylation on the β-carbon (219) of amino acids can bias sidechain conformations by virtue of steric interactions. A β-methylated-β-substituted amino acid can have four different stereochemical structures because it contains two chiral carbons ($2S,3R$, $2S,3S$, $2R,3S$ and $2R,3R$). Each isomer favorably adopts one of the three different side-chain conformations (g^-, t and g^+) as mentioned in the previous section (Fig. 20.25). The $2S,3R$ isomer favors the g^- conformation and the $2S,3S$ isomer favors the *trans* conformation (Fig. 20.26). In addition, the $2R,3S$ isomer stabilizes the g^+ conformation while the $2R,3R$ isomer prefers the *trans* conformation.

This modification has been applied to the aromatic residues of a somatostatin analog, [c(Pro-Phe-D-Trp-Lys-Thr-Phe)] (220). The population of three side-chain conformations (g^-, t and g^+) was calculated from NMR studies (221). As speculated in Figure 20.26, the $2S,3R$- and $2R,3S$-aromatic residues contain a higher

population of g^- and g^+, respectively. The $2S,3S$- and $2R,3R$-residues adopt a t conformation with increased populations compared to those of the parent analogs. The resulting analogs have shown different bioactivities, which were clearly dependent on the configuration at the α- and β-carbons. From the conformational analyses of these analogs, a model responsible for the bioactivity of somatostatin can be suggested. In addition, molecular dynamics calculations of these analogs permit the proposal of a pharmacophoric array which is dependent on the configuration of β-methyl groups.

Hruby et al. incorporated (βMe)Tyr and (βMe)Phe into positions 1 and 4 of DPDPE, respectively (222, 223). The resulting (βMe)Tyr-containing analogs were completely inactive at the opioid receptors. Among the analogs containing four isomers of (βMe)Phe, only the L-(βMe)Phe containing analogs were active but their activities were lower than those of DPDPE. The preference of L-amino acid at position 4 was also observed in the structure-bioactivity relationship study on their parent analogs. A possible explanation for the lower activities is the unfavorable interaction between these analogs and opioid receptors caused by steric hinderance due to the methyl group. Recently, 3,2'-dimethylphenylalanine was synthesized. This residue contains an additional methyl group on the 2 position of phenyl ring. When the stereo isomers of this residue were incorporated into oxytocin, all of the resulting analogs were active (224).

3.8 β-Substituted-2,3-Methano Amino Acids

These amino acids contain the structure of β-substituted $\mathrm{Ac^3c}$ (Fig. 20.27). They restrict the rotation of the N^α–C^α and C^α–$C(O)$ bonds in a manner similar to $\mathrm{Ac^3c}$. The calculated global energy minimum of

2S,3S Isomer

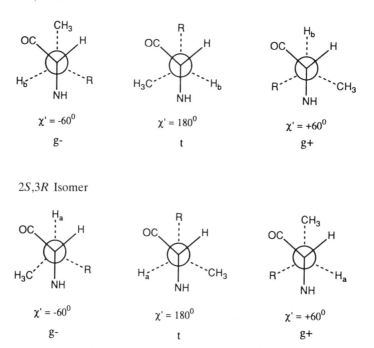

Fig. 20.26 Newman projections of the side chain conformations of (2S,3S)- and (2S,3R)-β-methylated-β-substituted amino acids.

the (1S,2S)-(E)-β-methyl-α,β-methanoalanine [or (1S,2S)-(E)-1-amino-2-methylcyclopropane carboxylic acid; (βMe)Ac³c] was found to occur at $\phi = -90°$ and $\psi = 90°$ (225). Another minimum energy well was found to occur at $\phi = 90°$, $\psi = -60°$. The allowed ϕ, ψ conformational map of (1S,2R)-(Z)-(βMe)Ac³c was also calculated. The results indicated that the minimum energy occurs at $\phi = -90°$ and $\psi = 90°$ (225).

Since (βMe)Ac³c has two chiral carbons, four stereo isomers of this amino acid are available. All of these stereo isomers have been incorporated into taste ligands leading to Asp-(βMe)Ac³c-OMe (226). The 1R,2R isomer containing compound is sweet, whereas the other analogs containing the other stereo isomers are tasteless. In addition, dimethyl and trimethyl Ac³c were also synthesized and incorporated into taste ligands (226). Conformational analyses were carried out for all of the above taste ligands using ¹H-NMR and molecular modeling techniques (226). Their taste properties were explained on the basis of a previously reported topochemical model for taste response (227–231).

These 2,3-methanoamino acids severely restrict the rotation of C^α–C^β (χ_1) and C^β–C^γ (χ_2). The χ_1 of the (Z)-isomers are fixed at $+120°$ or $-120°$ while those of the (E)-isomers are restricted to $0°$ (Fig. 20.27). The X-ray crystallographic study of the dipeptide, (Z)-(+)-(βPh)Ac³c-Leu-OH [(βPh)Ac³c denotes 1-amino-2-phenylcyclopropane carboxylic acid (or 2,3-methanophenylalanine)], indicates that the (βPh)Ac³c residue adopts the conformation where $\phi = 88.4°$, $\psi = 21.5°$, $\chi_1 = -132°$ and $\chi_2 = 99°$ (232). The χ_2 angle of this structure can be explained by the ability of cyclopropane to restrict side-chain rotation.

These 2,3-methano amino acids have

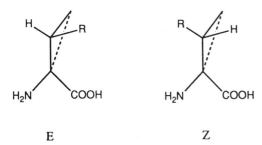

E   **Z**

Fig. 20.27 Structures of *E*- and *Z*-isomers of β-substituted-2,3-methano amino acids.

also been incorporated into bioactive peptides. For example, four possible stereoisomers of (βPh)Ac^{3}c and (βHO-Ph)Ac^{3}c [1-amino-2-(4-hydroxy) phenylcyclopropane carboxylic acid or 2,3-methanotyrosine] were incorporated into the (D-Ala^2, Leu^5)-enkephalin sequence. Only one of the (*Z*)-(βPh)Ac^{3}c containing analogs showed bioactivity at the μ and δ opioid receptors while the others were inactive. Interestingly, among the inactive analogs, one of the (*E*)-(βPh)Ac^{3}c containing analogs exhibited antagonistic activity at the δ-receptor (233, 234). Most of the (βHO-Ph)Ac^{3}c (235) containing analogs were active only at the δ-receptor without any antagonistic activity (236).

Other 2,3-methano amino acids have been synthesized. These amino acids include 2,3-methanomethionine (237), 2,3-methanohomoserine (238) and others (239, 240). In addition, 3,4-methano amino acids such as 3,4-methanoglutamic acid (241, 242) and 3,4-methanohomophenylalanine (243) have been reported.

3.9 N–C^δ and C^α–C^δ Cyclized Aromatic Amino Acids

The cyclization between N and C^δ or between C^α and C^δ of Phe and Tyr has led to highly constrained amino acids such as 1,2,3,4 -tetrahydroisoquinoline -3-carboxylic acid (Tic) (98, 244, 245) 2-aminoindane -2-carboxylic acid (Aic) (98) 1-aminotetralin-2-carboxylic acid (Atc) (98), 7-hydroxy-1,2,3,4-tetrahydroisoquinoline carboxylic acid (HO-Tic) (246, 247), 2-amino-5-hydroxyindane carboxylic acid (Hai) (248), and 2-amino-6-hydroxytetralin-2-carboxylic acid (Hat) (Fig. 20.28) (248, 249). These amino acids are particularly effective for fixing the rotation around C^α–C^β (χ$_1$) and C^β–C^γ (χ$_2$) bonds. The Tic residue restricts χ$_1$ to either −60° (g$^-$) or 60° (g$^+$). The χ$_1$ = 180° (*t*) side-chain rotamer is excluded. The χ$_2$ for this residue is about 160° (98, 244, 235). In the Aic or Hai residues (Fig. 20.28B), χ$_1$ and χ$_2$ are restricted to −80 and −20° or −160 and 20°

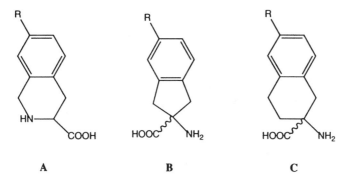

A   **B**   **C**

Fig. 20.28 Structures of C^δ–N^α and C^δ–C^α cyclized amino acids. A, 1,2,3,4-tetrahydroisoquinoline-3-carboxylic acid (Tic, R = H) and 7-hydroxy-1,2,3,4-tetrahydroisoquinoline-3-carboxylic acid (HO-Tic, R = OH); B, 2-aminoindane-2-carboxylic acid (Aic, R = H) and 2-amino-5-hydroxyindane-2-carboxylic acid (Hai, R = OH); and C, 2-aminotetralin-2-carboxylic acid (Atc, R = H) and 2-amino-6-hydroxytetralin-2-carboxylic acid (R = OH).

(98). The Atc and Hat residues (Fig. 20.28C) can adopt only two side-chain conformations. These conformations are characterized by torsion angles [$\chi_1 = 180°$ (t), $\chi_2 = 25°$] or [$\chi_1 = -60°$ (g^+), $\chi_2 = -25°$] for the L-residue and [$\chi_1 = 180°$ (t), $\chi_2 = -25°$] or [$\chi_1 = 60°$ (g^+), $\chi_2 = 25°$] for the D-residue (98).

The Tic, Aic, and Atc compounds were incorporated into a dermorphin analog Tyr-c(D-Orn-Phe-Glu)-NH$_2$ as modifications of Phe by Schiller et al. (98). The resulting analogs, which contained Aic, D-Atc and L-Atc showed bioactivities at the receptor binding assays, whereas the Tic containing analog was totally inactive. Hruby et al. incorporated the Tic residue into μ opioid receptor selective antagonists to examine the side-chain conformations for bioactivity (250). A new series of δ opioid receptor selective antagonists have been obtained using the Tic residue by Schiller et al. (251). The Tic residue has also been incorporated into bradykinin (161). When the Hai and Hat were incorporated into positions 1 and 4 of the enkephalin sequence, respectively, the resulting analog with Hat showed μ-receptor selective activity, whereas the analog with Hai was inactive (248). In addition, the Aic^3-containing chemotactic peptide analog, HCO-Met-Leu-Aic-OMe, was highly active (252).

3.10 Substituted Proline

All three types of amino acids described in Section 3.9 are effective in the restriction of the conformations around the $C^\alpha - C^\beta$ bond because of the inclusion of this bond in a 5- or 6-membered ring. However, because of their bicyclic structures, these modifications also limit the allowed values of χ_2. Thus, β substituted prolines are attractive as mimetics since they allow for conformational freedom in the χ_2 rotation of the side chain. In this structure, the χ_1 rotation is limited in range from -85 to $-150°$.

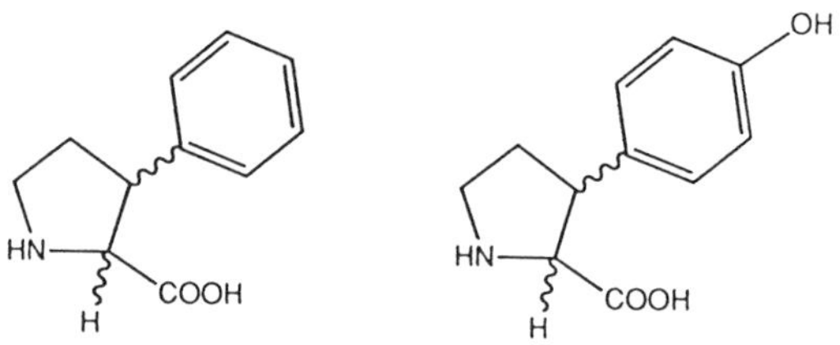

Fig. 20.29 Structures of A, β-phenylproline [(βPh)Pro] and B, β-(4-hydroxyphenyl)proline (Hpp).

The β-phenylproline [(βph)Pro: Fig. 20.29A (253)] and β-(4'-hydroxyphenyl)-proline (Hpp: Fig. 20.29B (254) residues were synthesized and incorporated into opioid peptides. These proline analogs can be considered as $N^\alpha - C^\beta$ cyclized phenylalanine or tyrosine. When the enantiomeric mixture of *trans*-β-phenylproline was incorporated into Tyr-Pro-X-N(CH$_3$)$_2$, only one of the resulting analogs was active (253). The *trans*-Hpp containing cyclic dermorphin analog *t*-Hpp-c(D-Cys-Phe-D-Pen)-OH showed activity similar to that of the parent analog, whereas the D-*t*-Hpp containing analog was completely inactive (254).

Other functional groups, for example, the propyl and carboxyl groups, have been incorporated into the β position of Pro (255). Various α and γ-substituted prolines were also synthesized and are likely candidates to be incorporated into bioactive peptides (256–258).

3.11 Miscellaneous Mimetics for Amino Acids

The incorporation of a bulky side chain can provide conformational constraints for a peptide. The bulky groups can restrict the movements of the other side chains of the peptide. This steric interaction may lead to changes in the conformation of peptide backbones. Naphthylalanine [βNal(1) or βNal(2)] (259, 260) and O-t-butylserine or O-t-butylthreonine (261, 262) were incorporated into cyclic and linear enkephalins. The resulting analogs were more constrained and showed higher bioactivities than the parent analogs (260, 263).

The incorporation of a D-amino acid is one of the most popular modifications. In naturally occurring peptides, D-amino acids are often observed as a critical residue for bioactivity. For example, the D-amino acids at position 2 of dermorphin and deltorphins are required for opioid activities (218). In many cases, the incorporation of a D-amino acid increases bioactivities of peptides including enkephalins (218), somatostatin (31), and oxytocin (264). When the second residue of enkephalin (Gly) was replaced with D-Ala, the resulting analog showed a higher bioactivity and metabolic stability than the parent. The replacement with L-Ala generated an inactive analog. In addition, incorporation of the D-residue can affect the secondary structure of peptides. If the central residues of a β-turn ($i + 1$ and $i + 2$ residues) have the L-configuration, a type I turn is often formed. If the residue at the $i + 1$ position is L and the residue at position $i + 2$ is D (an L,D-pair), then a type II form is stabilized. A D,L-pair at the central position will stabilize a type II$'$ turn. These results are well summarized in a review by Rose et al. (185).

Combinations of amino acid modifications have also been considered. The (NMe)Aib and (NMe)Ac^{5}c have been synthesized in which N-methylation and α-alkylation are combined. An attempt was made to incorporate these residues in place of Pro^6 of the cyclic somatostatin analog [c(Pro^6-Phe^7-D-Trp^8-Lys^9-Thr^{10}-Phe^{11})] (265, 266). After the partially protected linear hexapeptides H-D-Trp-Lys(Boc)-Thr(tBu)-Phe-(NMe)Aib / (NMe)Ac^{5}c-Phe-OH were assembled, they were cyclized. During the removal of the Boc and tBu protecting groups in the presence

of trifluoroacetic acid, half of the (NMe)Aib containing cyclic molecule was ring-opened. In case of the (NMe)Ac^{5}c structure, all of the protected cyclic peptide was ring-opened. The cleavage sites are identified as the amide bond of (NMe)Aib and (NMe)Ac^{5}c to the succeeding phenylalanyl residue by NMR spectroscopy. Preliminary results of conformational studies for the protected (NMe)Aib and (NMe)Ac^{5}c containing cyclic peptides indicated that the amide bond between (NMe)Aib/(NMe)Ac^{5}c and the succeeding residue Phe is highly constrained.

The β-amino-tetrahydronaphthyl carboxylic acid (βAtnc) has also been synthesized as a constrained Phe analog on the basis of the β-amino acid structure (120). The α-benzylproline is a new type of constrained amino acid which incorporates the N–C$^\alpha$ cyclization on the Phe structure (256).

4 MOLECULAR MIMICS OF PEPTIDE SECONDARY STRUCTURES

The secondary structures of most peptides and proteins show well-defined conformational features. It is well known that these structures are critical for the bioactivities of peptides. The secondary structures of peptides can be interchanged because of inherent flexibility. Thus, efforts have been made to fix specific secondary structures in peptides by use of peptidomimetic structures. A recent issue of *Tetrahedron* was devoted to the studies of peptidomimetics for peptide secondary structures (267).

One of the most important structural features of peptides and proteins is the β-turn. In many proteins, β-turn structures are exposed and may be part of ligand recognition sites (185, 268). Furthermore, β-turns are common conformations for many bioactive peptides. In Figure 20.30, representative nonpeptidic β-turn mimics are depicted. When these structures were

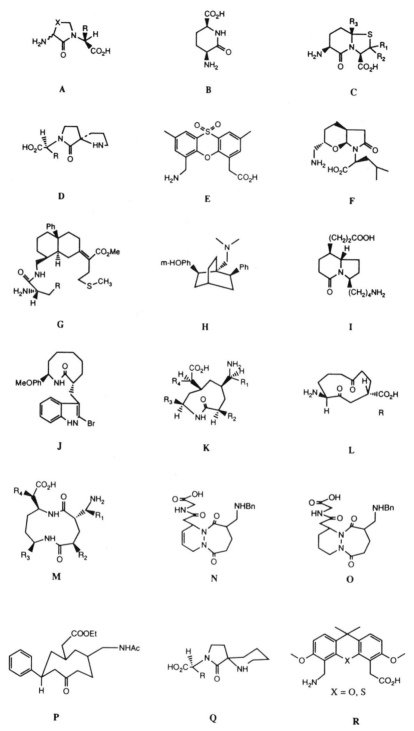

Fig. 20.30 Structures of β-turn mimics. The structure C was originally proposed but the modeling studies indicated that the structure with reversed configuration of the carbon substituted by R_3 is closer to the β-turn. Personal communication with Dr. Klaus Muller.

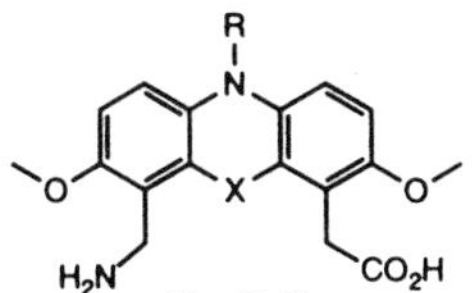

S 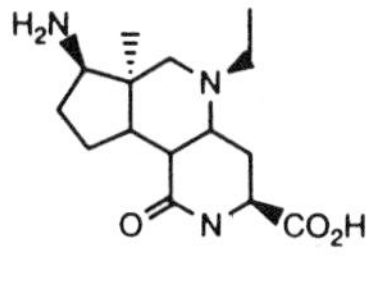   T 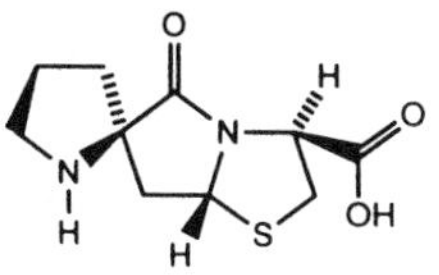   U

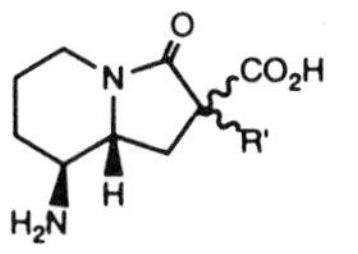

V 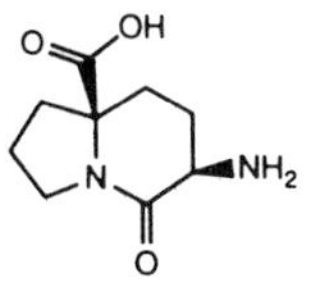   W

Fig. 20.30 *(Continued)*

incorporated into bioactive peptides, some of the resulting analogs showed high activity. The studies on the nonpeptidic β-turn mimics were reviewed by Ball and Alewood (Fig. 20.31A–M) (269), and their modified forms or new β-turn mimics were reported (Fig. 20.31N–W) (270–279).

A γ-turn mimic has been synthesized by Huffman et al. (280). In the Figure 20.31, the generalized γ-turn (A) and Huffman's mimic (B) are depicted. Compared to an idealized γ-turn, where torsional angles are $\psi_i = 120°$, $\phi_{i+1} = 80°$, $\psi_{i+1} = -65°$, and $\phi_{i+2} = -120$, the corresponding angles determined by X-ray crystallography of the mimic are $\psi_i = 128°$, $\phi_{i+1} = 56°$, $\psi_{i+1} = -67°$ and $\phi_{i+2} = -123°$ (280). When this mimic

was incorporated into RGD antagonists, the resulting analogs were highly active but, interestingly, enkephalin analogs were inactive (281). It may be that γ-turn destroys the enkephalin recognition at the receptor. Kahn et al. synthesized another γ-turn mimic (Fig. 20.31C). When this structure was incorporated into bradykinin, the resulting analog exhibited bioactivity (282). Kemp and Carter also suggested two structures as γ-turn templates (Fig. 20.32) (283).

In addition, mimics or templates of β-sheet structure have been studied. In the conformational studies of a naturally occurring antitumor agent bouvardin, it is indicated that the β-sheet structure of this

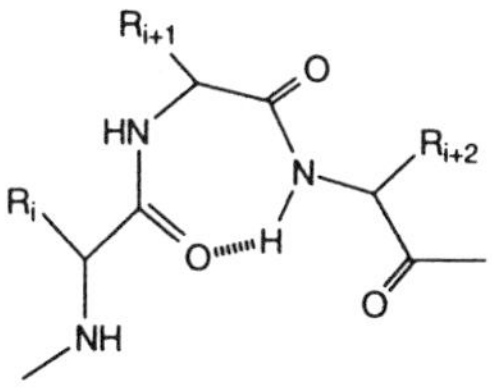

A 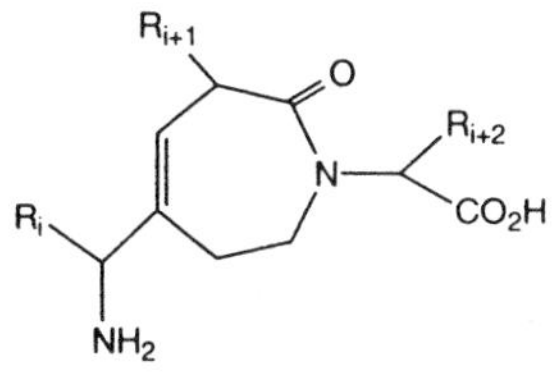   B 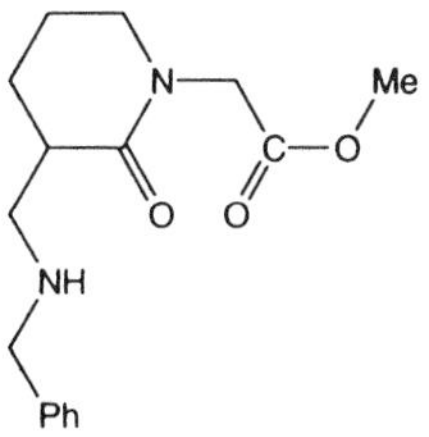   C

Fig. 20.31 Typical γ-turn structure; and B, C, its mimetic structures.

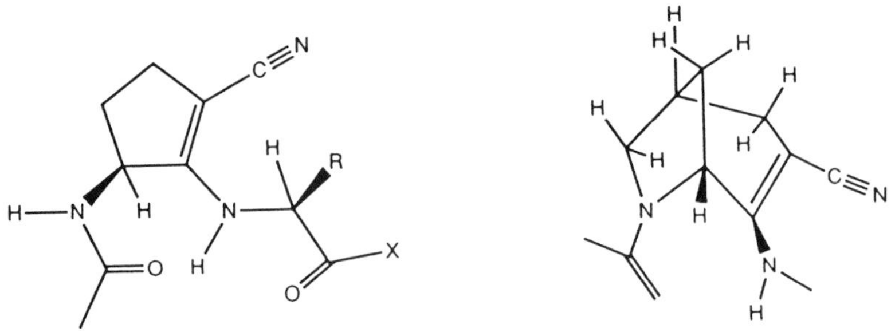

Fig. 20.32 Structures of γ-turn templates.

compound can be stabilized by the structure depicted in Figure 20.33A (284). Kemp et al. mimicked and induced β-sheet structure by using epindolidione derivatives (Fig. 20.33B) (285, 286). When this structure was incorporated into a peptide, the NMR parameters (temperature coefficients for amide proton, coupling constant for α- and amide proton and NOEs measured in DMSO) of the peptide indicated that the resulting peptide adopted β-sheet structure. The compound 2'-aminomethylbiphenyl-2-carboxylic acid (Fig. 20.33C) was devised for the same purpose (287). However, it was found to generate a conformation between the geometries of an idealized β-sheet and γ-loop (287). Recently, two new structures which can stabilize a β-strand were reported by Diaz et al. (Fig. 20.34D) (288) and by Smith et al. (Fig. 20.34E) (289). In the study by Diaz et al. (288) 4-(2-aminoethyl)-6-dibenzofuranpropionic acid (Fig. 20.34D) was incorporated in place of D-Phe-Pro in the linear gramicidin S octapeptide analog Val-Lys-Leu-D-Phe-Pro-Val-Lys-Leu-NH$_2$. It was also incorporated into a larger related peptide, Lys-Val-Lys-Val-Lys-Val-[4-(2-aminoethyl)-6-dibenzofuranpropionic acid]-Val-Lys-Val-Lys-Val-Lys-NH$_2$. The NMR and CD studies of these peptides in aqueous solution indicated that the mimetic (Fig. 20.33D) can stabilize the antiparallel β-sheet structure. The mimic reported by Smith et al. (Fig. 20.33E) is characterized

by the pyrrolin-4-ones (289). The X-ray analysis of a model compound including this structure (Fig. 20.33E) indicated the presence of an antiparallel β-pleated-sheet structure (289).

Helical structure can also be stabilized by peptidomimetic structures. Kemp et al. synthesized mimetic structures in which the pyrrolidine rings of two consecutive Pro residues were connected by a thiomethylene. The resulting units could act as templates nucleating helical conformations (290, 291). Muller et al. incorporated derivatives of diacyl-azabicyclo[2,2,2]octane (Fig. 20.34A) and Kemp's triacid (Fig. 20.34B) into the N-terminus of peptides as templates for α-helical structure. The resulting peptides exhibited substantially increased helicity compared to the peptides without such templates (275).

In addition, dipeptide structures can be designed as constraints to restrict the conformational flexibilities of the backbone and side chains. The resulting units display unique conformational preference and can thus stabilize the secondary structures of peptides. Toniolo has reviewed these types of constrained units extensively (128). Also, several subsequent reports on the same structures described in the review article (128) have been published (292–297). Recently, new types of constrained dipeptide units have also been reported (298, 299).

R = H, OH

A

B

C

D

E

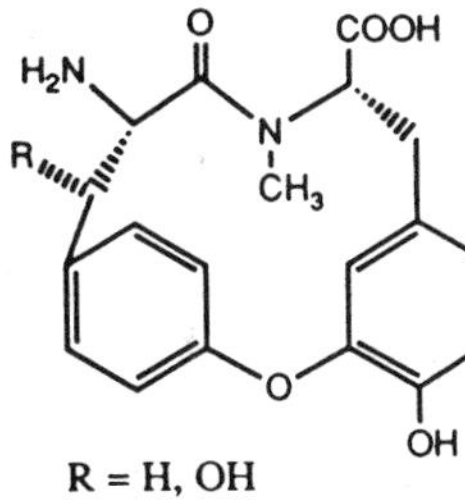

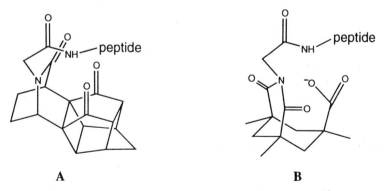

Fig. 20.33 Mimics of secondary structures.

A

B

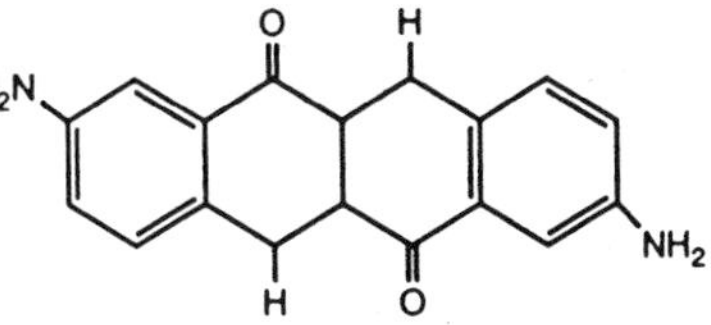

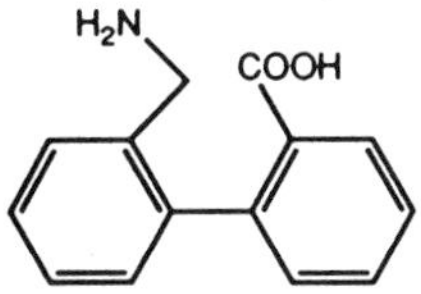

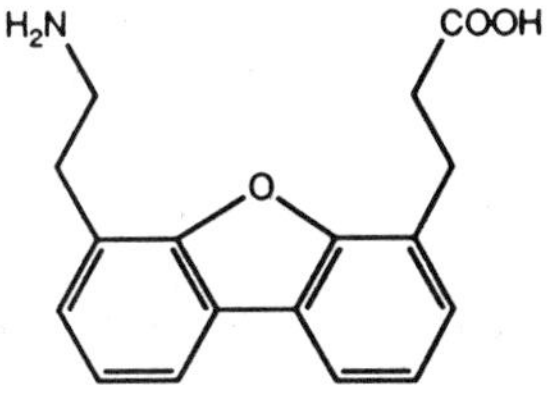

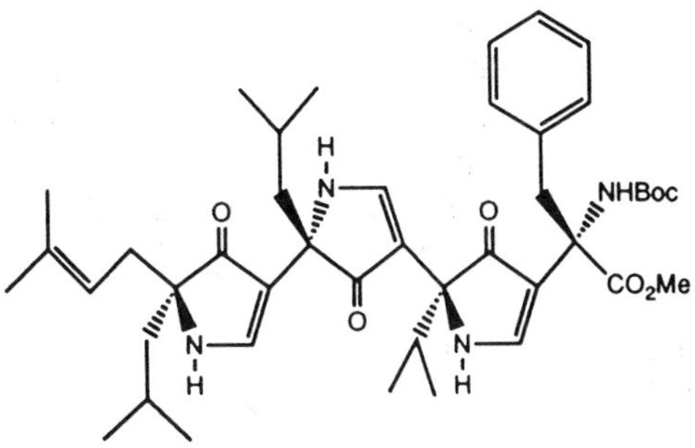

Fig. 20.34 Derivatives of A, diacyl-azabicyclo[2,2,2]octane; and B, Kemp's triacid as templates for α-helical structure.

5 AMIDE BOND ISOSTERES

Peptides are rapidly and specifically degraded by enzymes in biological systems. For example, the (Leu^5)-enkephalin in a rat-brain homogenate degraded in a matter of minutes. To increase metabolic stability of biologically active peptides, many amide bond isosteres have been devised. These peptide bond surrogates resemble the amide bond but are more resistant to enzymatic cleavage. Most of these modifications are accompanied by changes in geometric or topochemical structure, electronic distributions, and hydrophilic or lipophilic properties. The introduction of amide isosteres results in local and global changes in dipole moments and in the pattern of intramolecular as well as peptide-receptor hydrogen-bond formation. Thus, peptide bond modifications not only increase metabolic stability but can improve selectivity towards the receptor subtypes, change pharmacological functions and enhance pharmacokinetic properties such as oral bioavailability, transportability across the blood–brain barrier and duration of action at the target tissues.

As in the case of constrained amino acids, isosteric modifications at selected sites of a peptide sequence can act as conformational probes by allowing different degrees of rotational freedom in the backbone. Selected properties of the amide bond can be removed through the peptide backbone modifications, which may allow the examination of the specific requirements for bioactivity. These characteristics make the amide bond isosteres attractive tools for studying bioactive peptides and designing new drug molecules.

5.1 The Retro-Inverso Modifications [NH–C(O)]

As a means of protection against enzymatic cleavage as well as preservation of amide geometry, the retro–inverso modification has been one of the most widely used amide isosteres (300, 301). In this modification, specific peptide bonds are reversed in direction resulting in a *gem*-diaminoalkyl residue (gAA) on the amino-terminal end and a 2-alkylmalonyl residue (mAA) on the carboxyl-terminal end of each reversal (Fig. 20.35). This one-bond reversal is referred to as the "pairwise" retro–inverso modification because it affects pairs of adjacent residues. If the reversal operation is repeated for two or more successive amide bonds in a peptide, the modification is referred to as an "extended" retro–inverso modification. The sequence-direction of central residue(s) in the altered segment should be reversed to give retro-amino acids (rAA: Fig. 20.35). These modifications have been incorporated into numerous bioactive peptides. Many of the resulting analogs are highly active, selective, and metabolically stable. Recently these results have been reviewed by Chorev and Goodman (302) and the review also includes the development of synthetic methods and numerous conformational studies of these modifications.

In addition, the retro–inverso modification is useful for designing new cyclic structures. For example, cyclization by connecting two carboxylic groups is facilitated by using the *gem*-diaminoalkyl residue. To connect two amine groups, dicarboxylic acids are the most appropriate. These concepts were applied for cyclizing bioactive peptides including opioid peptides (303) and others (304).

5.2 The Reduced Amide Bond (Methyleneamine: CH_2–NH)

Methyleneamine is a reduced form of amide bond. This amide isostere ($-CH_2-NH-$) does not have the double bond character. Thus, the reduced peptide bond offers free rotation around the C–N bond

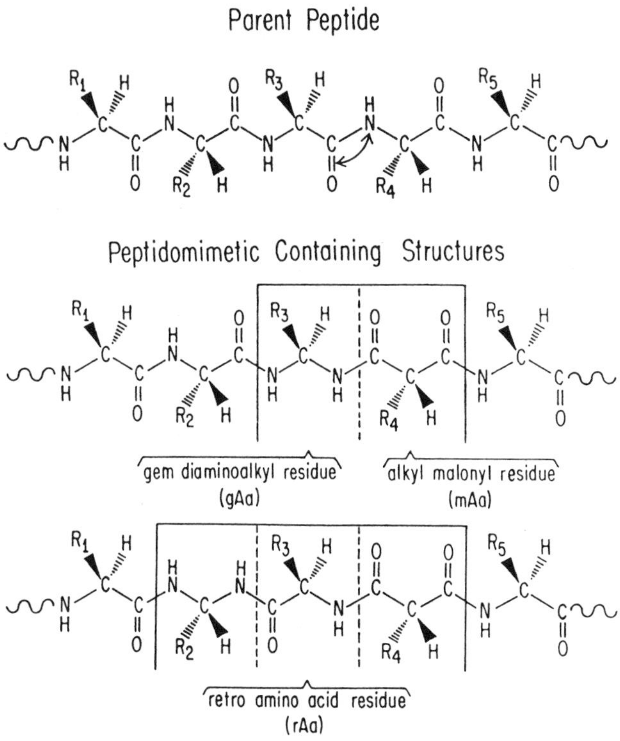

Parent Peptide

Peptidomimetic Containing Structures

gem diaminoalkyl residue
(gAa)

alkyl malonyl residue
(mAa)

retro amino acid residue
(rAa)

Fig. 20.35 Structures of retro-inverso modifications.

(ω angle). In addition, since the amino group of methyleneamine is protonated at physiological pH, the methylene cannot act as a H-bonding acceptor.

The influence of a protonated methyleneamine bond on the secondary structure of peptides was studied by Marraud et al. (166, 305, 306) using the reduced bond modified dipeptides, tBuC(O)-Pro-Glyψ-[CH$_2$-N$^+$H$_2$Et]*B$^-$Ph$_4$ and tBuC(O)-Pro-Glyψ[CH$_2$-N$^+$H$_2$Me]*B$^-$Ph$_4$ (where ψ denotes a pseudopeptide or surrogate bond), the effects of this modification on the ability to form a β-turn were studied. In solution, IR and ^{1}H-NMR experiments showed evidence of strong hydrogen-bonding between N$^+$–H and C(O) of the t-butylcarbonyl groups. The protonation of an amine in the reduced bond facilitated the formation of a 10-membered ring, similar in structure to β-turns. This result indicated that a reduced amide bond in

pseudopeptide analogs can retain β-folding tendencies at physiological pH.

When the amine of the reduced amide bond is not protonated, the overall conformation of the pseudopeptide unit can be very different. Van Binst et al. studied Pro-Leu-Gly-NH$_2$, which is potentially useful in the treatment of mental depression and Parkinsonism (307). This peptide adopts a preferred C$_{10}$ β-turn conformation in DMSO or acetonitrile and in the crystalline state. When an amide bond is replaced by a methyleneamine, the conformation of the resulting peptides shows a dependence on protonation status. The HCl*Pro-Leuψ[CH$_2$-NH]Gly-NH$_2$ adopts a similar conformation to the parent whereas the HCl* Pro-Leuψ[CH$_2$-NH*HCl]Gly-NH$_2$ does not display a β-turn structure.

When one of the amide bonds in bombesin (308–310), secretin (311), peptide opioids (312–316), substance P (317, 318), gastrin (319), and growth-hormone releasing factor (320) is replaced by this modification, the resulting peptides show either agonistic or antagonistic activities. The reduction of an amide bond in a peptide altered the pharmacological role from agonist to antagonist as well as changed agonistic potencies. Bioactivities (either agonistic or antagonistic) were found to be dependent on the position of the modification. This modification has also been incorporated into other bioactive peptides including cholecystokinin (321, 322), oxytocin (323), somatostatin (324), human renin inhibitors (325, 326) and HIV protease inhibitors (327) leading to active analogs. Spectroscopic studies of several peptides with this modification (morphiceptin (313), gastrin (328) and bombesin (329) have also been reported.

Since the reduced amide bond is relatively flexible compared to the amide, the introduction of constraints has been investigated. Examples include alkylmethyleneamine [CH(R)–NH; Fig. 20.36A] (330), amidomethyleneamine (CH[C(O)–NH$_2$]–NH; Fig. 20.36B (331), methylene-N-acetylamine [CH$_2$–N(Ac); Fig. 20.36C]

(332, 333), methylene-N- formylamine [CH$_2$–N(For); Fig. 20.37] (332) and methylenealkylamine [CH$_2$–N(R); Fig. 20.36D (334). The methylenealkylamine modified neurokinin analogs show bioactivities similar to or higher than those of amide- or methyleneamine-containing analogs (334). When amidomethyleneamine is incorporated into the angiotensin II analog, the resulting peptide is inactive (331).

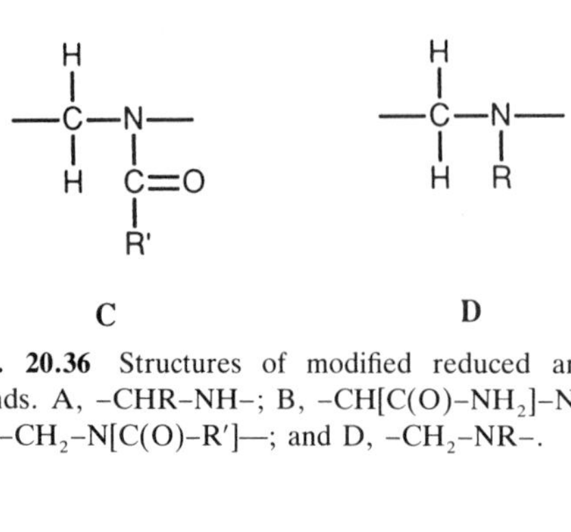

5.3 Methylenethioether [CH$_2$–S] and Methylenesulfoxide [CH$_2$–S(O)]

The methylenethioether modification was considered as an amide isostere which could offer polarity, flexibility, and metabolic stability. Spatola et al, incorporated this modification into LH–RH (335) and peptide opioids (315, 336–339). The stability of the methylenethioether modified analog in biological systems was examined using a linear enkephalin analog, Tyr-Gly-Gly-Pheψ[CH$_2$–S]Leu-OH (340). This analog showed a 21-fold longer half-life than leucine enkephalin when it was subjected to blood serum. Incorporation of this modification has generated highly active analogs. For example analogs with this modification, Tyr-D-Ala-Gly-Pheψ[CH$_2$–S]Leu - NH$_2$ and Tyr - c[D - Lys - Gly - Pheψ [CH$_2$–S]Leu], show higher activity at both μ and δ opioid receptors than their corresponding all-amide parent peptides (315, 337). When this modification was introduced into a somatostatin analog, the activity of the resulting c[Proψ[CH$_2$–S]Phe-D-Trp-Lys-Thr-Phe] exceeded somatostatin tetradecapeptide (341). However, it is only six percent of the activity of their parent analog c(Pro-Phe-D-Trp-Lys-Thr-Phe). An LH-RH analog, [Gly$^6\psi$[CH$_2$S]-Leu^7]LH-RH, displayed low potency when compared to its all amide bond counterpart, possibly because the CH$_2$S moiety imparted increased flexibility at the β-turn centered at 6–7 position (335). In addition,

Fig. 20.36 Structures of modified reduced amide bonds. A, –CHR–NH–; B, –CH[C(O)–NH$_2$]–NH–; C, –CH$_2$–N[C(O)–R']—; and D, –CH$_2$–NR–.

these modifications have been incorporated into oxytocin (323), CCK-B dipeptide antagonists (333), and a renin inhibitor (326).

Molecular modeling studies suggest that the methylenethioether modification is compatible with secondary structures of peptides and proteins. To investigate this point, Spatola et al. studied c(Gly^1-Pro^2-Gly^3-D-Phe^4-Pro^5) and its methylenethioether modified analogs using NMR spectroscopy (342, 343). The parent peptide contains a β-turn and a γ-turn through a hydrogen bond between Gly^{1}C(O) and D-Phe^{4}NH and another hydrogen bond between D-Phe^{4}C(O) and Gly^{1}NH (344–347). A single conformer whose amide bonds are all in a trans configuration is observed in CDCl$_3$. However in DMSO, this peptide displays 10% of a second conformer in which a cis amide bond is included. A methylenethioether modified model compound, c(Gly-Proψ[CH$_2$–S]Gly-D-Phe-Pro), can adopt both β- and γ-turns in CDCl$_3$, as assessed by chemical shift data temperature coefficients and solvent dependence data. In DMSO, the ratio of the two isomers is 3:2. The major conformer contains a cis amide bond at the Gly-Pro bond, but retains the intramolecular γ-turn hydrogen bond (343). Another pseudopeptide, c(Proψ[CH$_2$-S]-Gly-Pro-Gly-D-Phe), shows similar phenomena in both solvents. The population of the all trans conformer in DMSO is 55%. This result is interesting because the pseudopeptide retains the same overall conformation as its parents though the C(O) for the γ-turn hydrogen bond was replaced with methylene (342). In summary, the model peptide and its analogs modified with methylenethioether can adopt the same conformation as the parent peptide. In the above case, steric restrictions on the backbone are retained upon replacement of an amide bond by a methylenethioether surrogate group.

The thioether is easily oxidized to generate R- and S-sulfoxide. The resulting methylenesulfoxide is also a useful amide bond isostere because of the fact that it contains an additional stereogenic center, a highly constrained structure and relatively strong hydrogen bond-accepting capacity (as compared with the methylenethioether). Thus, Spatola et al. studied c(Gly-Pro-ψ[CH$_2$-(R/S)-S(O)]-Gly-D-Phe-Pro) and compared the results with the studies of its all-amide parent and methylenethioether-modified precursor (348). The NMR studies indicate that the methylene sulfoxide-modified pseudopeptide induces conformational changes that are distinctly different from its parent and precursor molecules. When this modification was incorporated into cyclic enkephalin, both isomers of the resulting analog, Tyr-c(D-Lys-Gly-Pheψ[CH$_2$-(R/S)-S(O)]Leu), have shown similar bioactivities to the all-amide parent analog and methylenethioether-modified precursors (337).

5.4 Methylene Ether (CH$_2$–O)

The methylene ether bond (–CH$_2$–O–) (349, 350) has some advantages over the methylenethioether. The nucleophilicity and oxidation possibility of oxygen are negligible compared with sulfur. The ether has higher polarity and can form stronger hydrogen bonds. Furthermore, the CH$_2$–O- group possesses closer geometric resemblance to an amide than the methylenethioether linkage (351). Chorev et al. introduced this modification into substance P and Leu-enkephalinamide (352). The resulting pGlu-Phe-Pheψ[CH$_2$–O] Gly-Leu-Met-NH$_2$ retains the activity of the parent analog. The Tyrψ[CH$_2$–O]Gly -Gly-Phe-Leu-NH$_2$ is twice as active as its all-amide parent analog at the μ opioid receptor and shows reduced activity in the δ opioid receptor. This modification has also been incorporated into a renin inhibitor (326, 353), and the CCK-B dipeptide antagonist (333) to produce active analogs.

5.5 Ethylene ("Carba": CH₂–CH₂)

Although the carba replacement (354–356) is a modification of the reduced amide bond (similar to methylene thioether or methylene ether), it possesses different characteristics because the whole "carba" surrogate is nonpolar. This modification does not allow for the possibility of intramolecular hydrogen-bonding. This characteristic leads to more flexible backbone conformations. When this modification is incorporated into Tyr-Gly of Met-enkephalinamide, it displays an order of magnitude decrease in activity (312). However, Tyr-Glyψ[CH₂–CH₂]Gly-Phe-Met-OH shows higher activity than Met-enkephalin in *in vivo* tests (357). A "carba" modified cholecystokinin shows activity similar to its all-amide parent molecule (321), while a renin inhibitor with this modification shows only minimum activity (326).

5.6 Thioamide [C(S)–NH]

With the introduction of facile thionating reagents such as Lawesson's reagent (358, 359), thioamides have been easily incorporated into peptides as amide isosteres. Spectroscopic and X-ray studies of di- and trithiopeptides, using various spectroscopic techniques, revealed that a thioamide adopts a Z planar configuration similar to that of an amide (360–365). The bond length of the thiocarbonyl (1.64 Å) and the covalent radius of sulfur (1.04 Å) are much longer than those of carbonyl and oxygen (1.24 Å and 0.74 Å, respectively) (366). Thus, the larger volume of the thioamide can restrict the allowed torsional angles in the vicinity of the thioamide more than in that of the amide. The computational studies of the thioamide bond containing small peptides have indicated that the allowed ϕ, ψ conformational space for thioamide containing residue is reduced

(367, 368). However, the regions where experimentally most protein conformational angles are observed are not drastically affected except in the area with high ψ values. Studies of the hydrogen-bonding properties of thioamides have shown that the NH of a thioamide is a stronger H-bond donor (higher acidity) and the thiocarbonyl is a weaker H-bond acceptor than the corresponding amide (369). Thus, hydrogen-bonding between C(O) and HN–C(S) is stronger while the H-bonding between C(S) and HN–C(O) is weaker as compared to the hydrogen-bond between C(O) and HN–C(O) (360–363, 370). The incorporation of the thioamide isostere in key positions of peptide analogs can lead to compounds with either enhanced or reduced conformational flexibility depending on whether steric or hydrogen bonding forces prevail.

Spatola and coworkers carried out studies to examine the compatibility of a thioamide with reverse turn features using the specific sequences of model peptides (371) as they did in the studies of methylenethioether (342, 343) and methylenesulfoxide (348). The NMR studies of the model compound, c(Proψ[C(S)-NH] Gly-Pro-Gly-D-Phe), have shown that this molecule can adopt the same general conformation (in CDCl₃ and DMSO) as its all-amide parent (344–347). The model compound c(Gly-Proψ[C(S)-NH]-Gly-D-Phe-Pro) retained the same conformations as the parent in CDCl₃ but exhibited two conformers in DMSO with a ratio 2:1. The minor conformation contains a cis amide bond at the Gly–Pro bond. The strength of the intramolecular hydrogen-bonding for β- and γ-turns, estimated from the temperature coefficients of an amide proton, are equal to and a little weaker than those of the parent molecule, respectively. Thus, the overall conformational effects of the thioamide modification may not be dramatic.

Many bioactive peptide analogs incorporating this modification have been synthesized. When thioamides were incorporated into oxytocin (372), the activity of the resulting analogs was not high. Thioamide analogs of the thyrotropin-releasing hormone (i.e., *p*Glu-His-Proψ[C(S)-NH]H) were synthesized and showed a similar potency to the parent analog (373–375). A C-terminal growth hormone releasing hexapeptide analog with this modification (His-D-Trp-Ala-D-Phe-Lysψ[C(S)-NH]H) was completely inactive (376). In analogs of Leu-enkephalin, modification of the amide bond between residue 1 and 2 produced an inactive compound, whereas modification of the amide bond between residue 2 and 3 led to an analog that was more potent and selective for the δ-receptor than Leu-enkephalin (377, 378). This modification was also incorporated into cyclic enkephalins (379), CCK-B dipeptide antagonists (333), peptide-substrates of carboxypeptidase A (380), substance P (381), gastrin (382), chemotactic peptide (383), bombesin (384) and leucine aminopeptidase (385). The resulting analogs were found to be more stable against enzymatic degradation than their amide counterparts. In addition, to examine the conformation responsible for the bioactivities, the X-ray studies of thioamide containing chemotactic peptides (286) and protected Leu-enkephalin were carried out (387).

5.7 *trans*-Olefin (CH=CH, *trans*) and *trans*-Fluoroolefin (CF=CH, *trans*)

The peptide bond in polypeptides and proteins generally assumes a trans configuration since its cis counterpart induces unfavorable steric interactions. Among the mimics of amide bonds which have been reported, the *trans* carbon–carbon double bond (olefin: Fig. 20.37A) is most suitable to mimic the linkage in terms of geometry, bond angle and bond length. Whereas the amide bond has some degree of flexibility

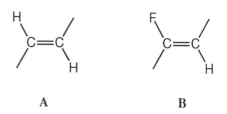

Fig. 20.37 Structures of A, *trans*-olefin; and B, *trans*-fluoroolefin.

and possesses hydrogen-bonding capability, the trans olefin fixes the replaced peptide linkage in a trans configuration and eliminates all possibility of hydrogen-bonding. This modification can provide valuable information concerning the role of an amide bond at a specific site in a peptide, in its bioactivity profiles and conformational behavior. Furthermore, the substitutions of an amide bond with a trans olefin increases the hydrophobicity of the resulting peptides and thus potentially facilitates biotransportability through cell membranes, including passage through the blood brain barrier. Improved metabolic stability is also observed. A number of synthetic methods for this modification have been developed and applied towards the synthesis of bioactive peptide analogs (388–392).

Dermorphin and its tetrapeptide analogs which incorporated this modification between Phe and Gly, showed activity comparable to the parent molecules (393). The conformational behavior of the trans olefin bond was examined using these analogs. All of the olefin modified analogs exhibited essentially the same ^{1}H-NMR parameters: chemical shifts, temperature coefficients for amide protons, and coupling constants between NH and C^αH and between C^αH and C^βH. The sets of NOE observed from dermorphin and Tyr-D-Ala-Pheψ (CH=CH, *trans*) Gly-Tyr-Pro-Ser-NH$_2$ are also the same in terms of their pattern and intensity. The incorporation of a trans olefin bond in place of the amide bond between residue 3 and 4 did not alter the conformational characteristics of the peptides, in DMSO solution. These results are in agreement with those of the theoretical studies of Ac-Ala-NHMe, Ac-ψ[CH=CH, *trans*] Ala-NHMe, Ac-Alaψ[CH=CH, *trans*]-CH$_3$ and Ac-ψ[CH=CH, *trans*] Alaψ[CH=CH, *trans*]-CH$_3$ (394, 395). In these studies, a single substitution of the peptide bond with trans-olefin bond does not introduce dramatic changes in conformational preferences. This modification was incorporated into other bioactive peptides including linear and cyclic enkephalin analogs (396–398), substance P (397), angiotensin-converting enzyme inhibitors (399), renin inhibitors (326), inhibitors of protein kinase (389, 391, 400) and others (323, 333).

Recently, a fluoroolefinic isostere [ψ(CF=CH, *trans*): Fig. 20.37B] was designed and utilized (401). Because the electronic properties of fluorine are similar to those of oxygen, this modification seems to resemble amide more than the simple olefin. This modification has already been incorporated into the amide bond between Phe and Gly of the full length of substance P (Arg-Pro-Lys-Pro-Gln-Gln-Phe-Phe-Phe-Gly-Leu-Met-NH$_2$) and *p*Glu-Phe-Phe-Gly-Leu-Met-NH$_2$. The bioactivity of the fluoroolefin modified substance P analog with this modification is similar to that of the natural peptide. The *p*Glu-Phe-Pheψ[CF=CH, *trans*]-Leu-Met-NH$_2$ is ten times more active than the analog with a *trans* ethylene group. The ^{1}H, ^{13}C and ^{15}N chemical shifts, temperature coefficients, and coupling constants of substance P and its fluoroolefin modified analog are very similar. These results suggest an overall similarity between amide and fluoro olefin bonds. This amide isostere has also been incorporated into opioids leading to an active analog (402).

5.8 1,5-Disubstituted Tetrazole Ring (CN$_4$)

To mimic a cis amide bond, Hann et al. attempted to synthesize a cis-olefin. How-

ever, the resulting olefin quickly isomerized to a more stable trans-olefin (403). Thus, Marshall et al. proposed a tetrazole (404) ring as an amide isotere in order to lock an amide bond into a cis configuration (Fig. 20.38) (405). The possible conformations available to the linear dipeptide, Ac-Ala-Ala-NHMe, in which the central amide bond was fixed in the cis configuration was compared with Ac-Alaψ[CN$_4$]Ala-NHMe, in which the central amide bond was replaced with the 1,5-disubstituted tetrazole ring (406). A novel procedure for assaying conformational mimicry showed that approximately 88% of the conformations accessible to the cis isomer of the parent dipeptide were also available to the tetrazole analog (406). This index of conformational mimicry represents the percentage of conformations available to the parent peptide which the analog is capable of adopting as measured by the ability to orient the peptide chain and side chains, on either side of the modification in a similar manner to that of the parent peptide (406, 407).

During these studies, the tetrazole analog was found to have more conformational freedom than the cis amide model. This result is explained by the increased valence angle between the C$^\alpha$–C=N of tetrazole analog corresponding to the C$^\alpha$–C=O angle of the cis amide. However, the increase in steric bulk in the tetrazole analog where the amide hydrogen is replaced by nitrogen can cause some constraints. Thus, the conformational flexibility is dependent on the relative importance of these two opposing effects (406). Since another conformational study using Cbz-Proψ[CN$_4$]Ala-OBzl has

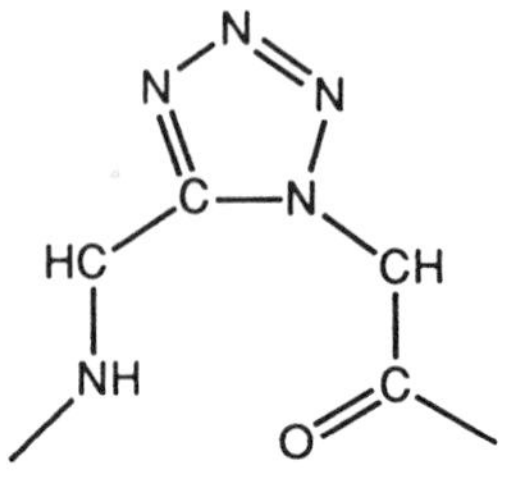

Fig. 20.38 Structure of cyclotetrazole.

also provided similar results (407), the tetrazole ring can be a conformational mimic for the cis amide bond.

Since proline and N-alkylated amino acids can adopt a cis configuration at their preceding amide bonds in bioactive peptides to bind and recognize their receptors, the tetrazole modified analog can be a useful probe to understand the receptor bound conformation of these peptides. This modification does not contain an adjacent hydrogen-bond donor and acceptor of the cis amide and steric bulk could prevent binding to the receptor. Consequently, activities of tetrazole containing analogs can be strong evidence of the role of a cis amide in receptor recognition while lack of activity will not exclude the cis amide from this consideration.

This modification has been incorporated as a replacement of the Phe-(NMe)Ala bond of a cyclic somatostatin hexapeptide analog to produce c[D-Trp-Lys-Val-Pheψ (CN$_4$)Ala-Thr] (408). From the conformational studies of this type of somatostatin analogs, it has been suggested that a cis configuration of this bond is required for recognition at the receptors. Since the resulting analog has shown nearly equivalent activity compared to the parent analog, the tetrazole modification functions as a conformational mimic of the cis amide bond in this system. This modification has also been incorporated into the Leu^8-Gly^9 amide bond of deaminooxtocin (409), the Pro^2-Pro^3 and Ser^6-Pro^7 amide bonds of bradykinin (410, 411) and the scissile Phe-Pro bond of HIV protease substrate (412). The bioactivities of these analogs were greatly diminished. If the tetrazole does not grossly distort the topology of the peptide, these results indicate that the cis conformer of the amide bond may not be biologically relevant; or the increased steric hindrance generated from the tetrazole ring and the lack of a hydrogen bond donor, as compared with the cis amide bond, precluded binding of these analogs to the receptors and enzymes.

5.9 Ketomethylene [C(O)–CH$_2$] and Fluoroketomethylene [C(O)-CFR, R=H or F]

The ketomethylene (Fig. 20.39) unit is observed in the structure of the naturally occurring aminopeptidase inhibitor called arphamenines [Argψ(C(O)–CH$_2$)Phe-OH] and Argψ[C(O)-CH$_2$] Tyr-OH (413–415). This modification is conformationally different from the amide bond because the bond between the carbonyl carbon and methylene carbon does not possess any double-bond character. Furthermore, the hydrogens of the methylene cannot be donated to form a hydrogen bond. When ketomethylene replaced the amide bond (416, 417) between Phe and Gly of the angiotensin converting enzyme inhibitor, Bz-Phe-Gly-Pro-OH, the resulting analog is a hundred times more active than the parent peptide (418). This modification has also been incorporated into inhibitors of pepsin (419), aminopeptidase (420), renin (326), and porcine pancreatic elastase (PPE) (421). The mechanism of inhibition for serine protease (i.e., PPE) most likely involves interaction between a serine residue of the enzyme and the ketone carbonyl group of the inhibitor to form a hemiketal structure which resembles the tetrahedral intermediate involved in peptide bond hydrolysis. The replacement of the Met^{28}-Gly^{29} bond of C-terminal octapeptide of cholecystokinin (321) and the Phe^8–Gly^9 bond of the C-terminal hexapeptide of substance P (422, 423) with ketomethylene produced analogs which retained the activity of their respective parent analogs.

The increased potency of fluorinated

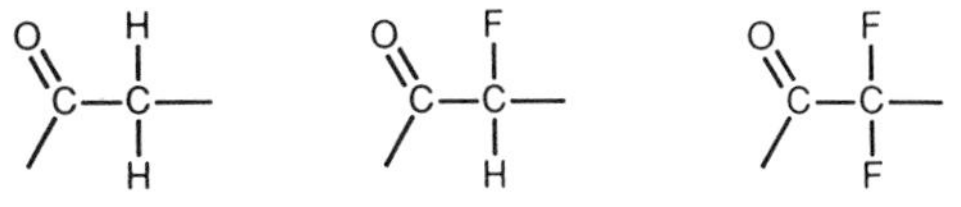

Fig. 20.39 Structures of A, ketomethylene; B, ketofluoromethylene; and C, ketodifluoromethylene.

enzyme inhibitors led to the replacement of the hydrogen(s) of ketomethylene with fluorine (424, 425). The readily hydrated fluoroketone is proposed to mimic the tetrahedral intermediate that forms during the enzyme-catalyzed hydrolysis of a peptide bond. Thus, the ketofluoromethylenes (Fig. 20.39) were considered as a steric replacement of the amide bond. Since the atomic radius of fluorine is similar to that of hydrogen, the steric hindrance of this modification can be minimized. In addition, fluorination can increase the aqueous solubility of the resulting analogs, and with this result that incorporation of these modifications into enzyme inhibitors is now in progress.

5.10 Miscellaneous Amide Isosteres

In addition to the representative amide isosteres described above, many others have been incorporated into bioactive peptides and studied by spectroscopic and computational techniques. Since the planar amide bond in the enzyme substrates must be transformed to a tetrahedral species in the transition state of peptide bond cleavage, various mimics of such intermediates have generated highly active enzyme inhibitors (426). These studies have been extensively reviewed by Rich (427) and Greenlee (428) among others (429, 430). These mimics include methyleneamine, ketomethylene (431) (described in the previous section), phosphonate, phosphonaminate (426, 432), hydroxyethylene (433–435), and dihydroxyethylene (326, 436, 437). Currently, these modifications are widely used for the inhibitors of renin (326, 438, 439), HIV-protease (436, 440–444) and other enzymes (420, 431). Other structures such as epoxides (426), cis-olefins (333), methylene sulfones (323, 326), methylene hydroxyamines (326) and

Table 20.6 Physicochemical Properties of Amide Isosteres[a]

Compound	d $(\text{Å})^b$	α $(\text{degree})^c$	β $(\text{degree})^d$	v $(\text{Å}^3)^e$
$CH_3-C(O)-NH-CH_3$	3.8	119	120	69.3
$CH_3-NH-C(O)-CH_3$	3.8	119	120	69.3
$CH_3-CH_2-O-CH_3$	3.7	107	113	67.0
$CH_3-C(O)-O-CH_3$	3.7	116	113	65.8
$CH_3-CH_2-NH-CH_3$	3.8	111	115	71.6
$CH_3-C(O)-CH_2-CH_3$	3.9	118	110	75.6
trans-$CH_3-CH=CH-CH_3$	3.9	122	122	68.2
cis-$CH_3-CH=CH-CH_3$	3.0	125	236	68.5
$CH_3-CH_2-CH_2-CH_3$	3.9	111	112	76.0
$CH_3-CH(OH)-CH_2-CH_3$	4.0	111	113	83.3
$CH_3-CH_2-S-CH_3$	4.2	110	98	76.2
$CH_3-C(S)-NH-CH_3$	3.8	115	116	82.0
$CH_3-C(O)-N(CH_3)-CH_3$	3.9	119	119	85.5

    [a]The estimation was carried out using the N-methylacetamide $[CH_3-C(O)-N(CH_3)-CH_3]$ and its analogs in which the amide $[-C(O)-NH-]$ of N-methylacetamide was replaced with amide isosteres as model compounds. Each model was built to mimic the *trans* form of the amide.

    [b]The d denotes the distance between the two methyl groups.

    [c]The α denotes the angles for $CH_3-C(O)-NH$ of N-methylacetamide and counterparts of the other model compounds.

    [d]The β denotes the angles for $C(O)-NH-CH_3$ of N-methylacetamide and counterparts of the other model compounds.

    [e]The v denotes the volume of the space occupied by the entire model molecules.

sulfone amides (445, 446) have also been reported as amide isosteres.

Rees et al. systematically quantified some of the amide isosteres using N-methylaceamide and its derivatives (Table 20.6) (333). These steric factors were calculated with the molecular modeling package SYBYL in terms of distance (d) between the two methyl groups, angles for $CH_2{}^C$–NH (α) and C–NH–CH$_3$ (β) and the volume of the space occupied by the entire molecule (v).

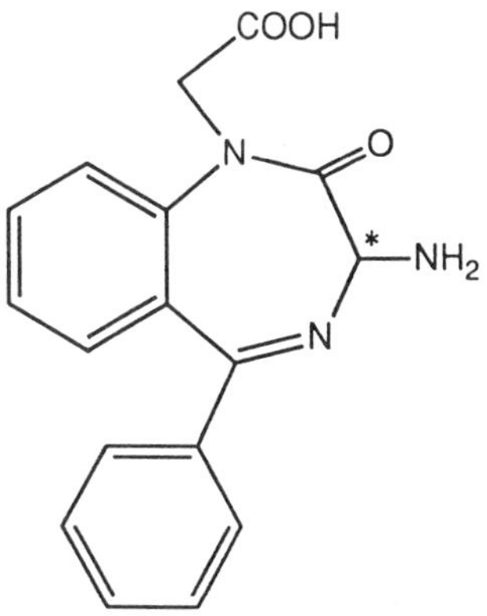

6 NONPEPTIDE LIGANDS FOR PEPTINERGIC RECEPTORS

In the previous sections, the considerable progress in obtaining peptide analogs with improved pharmacological properties using peptidomimetics have been described. These peptidomimetic modifications of native peptides have generated many important therapeutic agents. Another approach to peptidomimetics, which could be one of the most important, involves the transformation of peptide structures into nonpeptide structures while retaining the bioactivities at the peptinergic receptors (447). In the opioid area, numerous nonpeptide structures have been devised on the basis of morphine which binds to the same receptors of peptide opioids (448). These efforts have led to many useful analgesics. Portoghese et al. used the message-address concept (449, 450) developed in the peptide area to modify morphine structures (451, 452). The resulting analogs have shown antagonistic activities with high selectivities and potencies.

There has been rational design of nonpeptide analogs based on the structure of native peptides. One of the earliest studies was carried out on the angiotensin converting enzyme inhibitors. Wyvratt and Patchett have reviewed this process (429). Other peptides (CCK, LH-RH, etc.) have also been transformed to nonpeptidic structures. The results are well-described in

Fig. 20.40 A derivative of bezodiazepine.

Freidinger's review (453) and other reports (454, 455). Interestingly, 1,4-benzodiazepine and its derivatives (Fig. 20.40) (456) were often used to generate useful therapeutic agents or promising candidates in various categories of peptides showing agonistic and antagonistic activities (453).

Recently, Hirschmann et al. used β-D-glucose as a spacer to arrange the pharmacophoric groups of somatostatin (Fig. 20.41) (457). These nonpeptide analogs are characterized by the rearrangement of the pharmacophores of the corresponding peptides on a glucose scaffold. The resulting analogs show somatostatin activities.

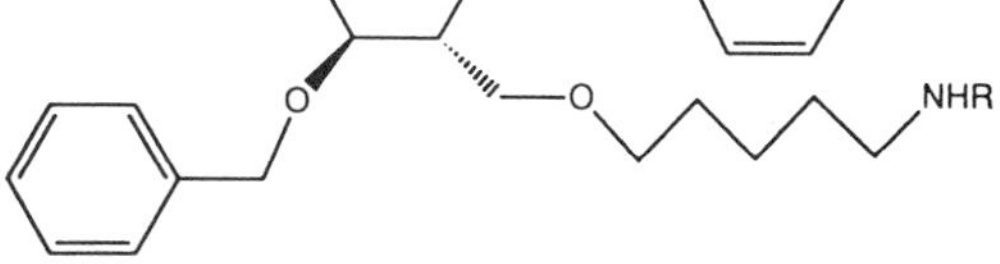

II R = H, R' = OBn
III R = R' = H
IV R = Ac, R' = OBn

Fig. 20.41 A somatostatin analog in which a β-D-glucose is used as a scaffold for the array of pharmacophoric groups.

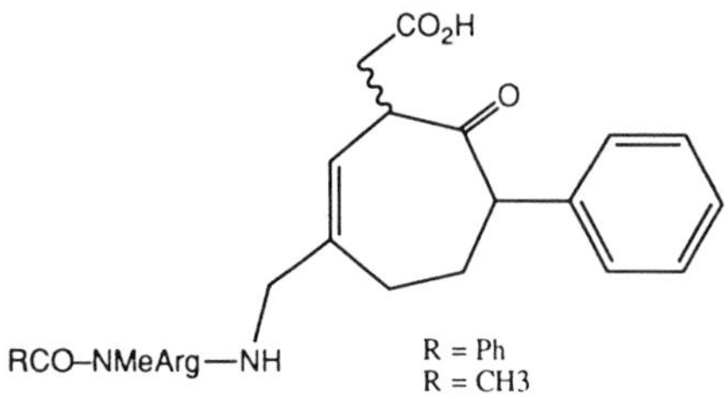

Fig. 20.42 RGD peptide analogs in which A, a γ-turn mimic is incorporated; and B, a steroid structure is used as a scaffold to arrange side chains of Arg and Asp.

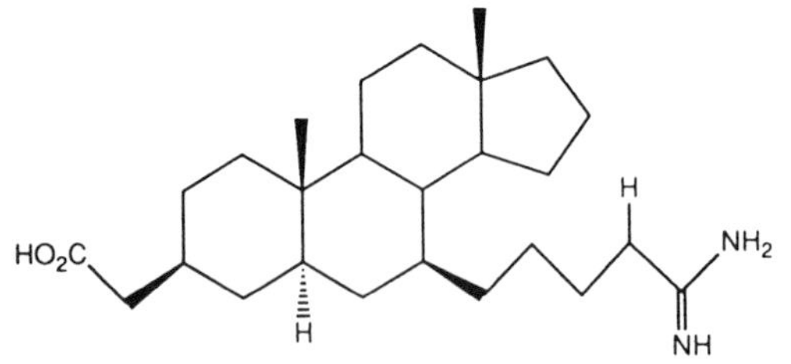

Because of the development of molecular modeling techniques, the importance of conformational features for such designs have been emphasized. As mentioned, a nonpeptide mimic of turn structure (Fig. 20.32B) was used by Callahan et al. as a spacer for the pharmacophores of RGD peptides providing highly active analogs (Fig. 20.42) (281). Recently, Hirschmann et al, used a steroid as a conformationally restricted spacer leading to an analog with substantial activity (Fig. 20.42B) (458).

7 CONCLUSIONS

In this chapter, various modifications of general peptide structures have been described. The intention has not been to cover chemical methods for each modification and bioactivity profiles completely. However, the general features, conformational preferences and representative appli-

cations for many peptidomimetics have been discussed.

Some peptidomimetics are designed as place holders whereas others are isosteric replacements. The effects of these mimetic structures on bioactivity are not generalized for all bioactive peptides. There are cases where a modification in one system leads to bioactive analogs while the same peptidomimetic structure in another peptide family results in inactive analogs. The bioactivities of the resulting analogs vary according to the position of modification. In addition, since each peptidomimetic has unique conformational effects and physicochemical properties, the bioactivities of modified analogs depend on modifications which are incorporated.

The varied bioactivity profiles caused by incorporation of constrained peptidomimetics have been useful in the establishment of conformation-bioactivity relationships of various peptide families. Using such approaches, some laboratories have proposed conformations responsible for the bioactivities and selectivities of many bioactive peptides such as opioids, somatostatins and taste ligands, among others. In addition, these constrained peptidomimetics can be used for the design of peptinergic receptor ligands with higher affinity and structural resemblance.

Other pharmacological properties including metabolic and chemical stability, oral bioavailability and solubility have also been obtained as a result of the introduction of peptidomimetics. For example, incorporation of amide isosteres and other modifications have led to analogs with longer half-lives in biological systems.

It is clear that modified peptides and nonpeptidic analogs represent the present and future in drug design. Hopefully, this chapter has provided insight into the chemistry currently used to explore and design novel drug structures. From such chemistry, new and useful therapeutic agents will emerge.

ACKNOWLEDGMENTS

The authors wish to thank Noriyuki Kawahata for his help and discussions and to acknowledge Todd Romoff and Dr. Anna Toy-Palmer for their helpful comments. This work has been accomplished with support from the National Institute of Health (DA 05539, DA 06254, GM 18694, DE 05476 and DK 15410).

REFERENCES

1. G. D. Smith and J. F. Griffin, *Science*, **199**, 1214–1216 (1978).
2. I. L. Karle, J. Karle, D. Mastropaolo, A. Camerman and N. Camerman, *Acta Crystallogr. Sect. B*, **39**, 625–637 (1983).
3. J. L. DeCoen, C. Humblet, and M. H. J. Koch, *FEBS Lett.*, **73**, 38–42 (1977).
4. S. Premilat and B. Maigret, *Biochem. Biophys. Res. Commun.*, **91**, 534–539 (1979).
5. P. Manavalan and F. A. Momany, *Int. J. Peptide Protein Res.*, **18**, 256–275 (1981).
6. J. DiMaio and P. W. Schiller, *Proc. Natl. Acad. Sci. U.S.A.*, **77**, 7162–7166 (1980).
7. P. W. Schiller and J. DiMaio, *Nature*, **297**, 74–76 (1982).
8. J. Dimaio, C. Lemieux, and P. W. Schiller, *Life Sci.*, **31**, 2253–2256 (1982).
9. J. Dimaio, T. M-D. Nguyen, C. Lemieux, and P. W. Schiller, *J. Med. Chem.*, **25**, 1432–1438 (1982).
10. P. W. Schiller, B. Eggimann, J. Dimaio, C. Lemieux, and T. M-D. Nguyen, *Biochem. Biophys. Res. Commun.*, **101**, 337–343 (1981).
11. P. W. Schiller, J. DiMaio, and T. M.-D. Nguyen, in *Proceedings of 16th FEBS Congress* (Part B), Y. A. Ovchinnikov, Ed., UNU Science Press, Utrecht, 1985, pp. 457–462.
12. H. I. Mosberg, R. Hurst, V. J. Hruby, J. J. Galligan, T. F. Burks, K. Gee, and H. I. Yamamura, *Life Sci.*, **32**, 2565–2569 (1983).
13. P. W. Schiller, in *The Peptides*, Vol. 6, S. Udenfriend and J. Meienhofer, Eds., Academic Press, Orlando, 1984, pp. 219–268.
14. P. C. Montecucchi, R. De Castiglione, S. Piani, L. Gozzini and V. Erspamer, *Int. J. Peptide Protein Res.*, **17**, 275–283 (1981).
15. S. Ro, *Thesis Dissertation*, University of California, San Diego, 1991.
16. S. Ro, Q. Zhu, C-. W. Lee, M. Goodman, K. Darlak, A. F. Spatola, N. N. Chung, P. W. Schiller, A. B. Malmerg, T. L. Yaksh, T. F. Burks, *J. Peptide Science*, in press.
17. M. Goodman, S. Ro, G. Ösapay, T. Yamazaki and A. Polinsky, in *Medications Development: Drug Discovery, Databases and Computer-Aided Drug Design*, R. S. Rapak and R. L. Hawkes, Eds, U.S. Dept. of Health and Human Services, Rockville, Maryland, pp. 195–209, 1993.
18. M. Goodman, S. Ro, T. Yamazaki, J. R. Spencer, A. Toy, Z. Huang, Y.-B. He, and T. Reisine, *Bioorg. Chem.*, **18**, 1375–1393 (1992).
19. M. Goodman, S. Ro, T. Yamazaki, G. Ösapay, and A. Polinsky, in N. Yanaihara, Ed., *Proceedings of 2nd Japanese Peptide Symposium*, ESCOM, Leiden, 1993, pp. 239–242.
20. P. W. Schiller, T. M-D. Nguyen, L. Maziak, and C. Lemieux. *Biochem. Biophys. Res. Commun.*, **127**, 558–564 (1985).
21. P. W. Schiller, T. M-D. Nguyen, C. Lemieux, and A. Maziak, *J. Chem.*, **28**, 1766–1771 (1985).
22. P. W. Schiller, T. M-D. Nguyen, L. A. Maziak, B. C. Wilkes, and C. Lemieux, *J. Med. Chem.*, **30**, 2094–2099 (1987).
23. K. Darlak, T. F. Burks, W. S. Wire, and A. F. Spatola, in *Peptides 1990, Proceedings of the 21st European Peptide Symposium*, E. Giralt and D. Andreu, Eds., ESCOM, Leiden, 1991, p. 401.
24. S. Salvadori, G. Sarto, and R. Tomatis, *Int. J. Peptide Protein Res.*, **19**, 536–542 (1982).
25. P. Brazeau, W. Vale, R. Burgus, N. Ling, M. Bucher, J. Rivier, and R. Guillemin, *Science*, **179**, 77–79 (1973).
26. D. F. Veber, R. M. Freidinger, D. S. Perlow, W. J. Paleveda, Jr., F. W. Holly, R. G. Strachan, R. F. Nutt, B. J. Arison, C. Homnick, W. C. Randall, M. S. Glitzer, R. Saperstein and R. Hirschmann, *Nature*, **292**, 55–58 (1981).
27. D. F. Veber, in *Peptides: Chemistry and Biology, Proceedings of the 12th American Peptide Symposium*, J. A. Smith and J. E. Rivier, Eds., ESCOM, Leiden, 1992, pp. 1–14.
28. D. F. Veber, R. Saperstein, R. F. Nutt, R. M. Freidinger, S. F. Brady, P. Curley, D. S. Perlow, W. J. Paleveda, C. D. Colton, A. G. Zacchei, D. J. Tocco, D. R. Hoff, R. K. Vandlen, J. E. Gerich, L. Hall, L. Mandarino, E. H. Cordes, P. S. Anderson, and R. Hirschmann, *Life Sci.*, **34**, 1371–1378 (1984).
29. J. Rivier, M. Brown, and W. Vale, *Biochem. Biophys. Res. Commun.*, **65**, 746–751 (1975).
30. W. Vale, J. Rivier, N. Ling, and M. Brown, *Metabolism*, **27**, 1391–1401 (1978).

31. D. F. Veber, F. W. Holly, W. J. Palaveda, R. F. Nutt, S. J. Bergstrand, M. Torchia, M. W. Glitzer, R. Saperstein, and R. Hirschmann, *Proc. Natl. Acad. Sci. U.S.A.*, **75**, 2636–2640 (1978).

32. H. Kessler, M. Bernd, H. Kogler, J. Zarbock, O. W. Sorensen, G. Bodenhausen, and R. R. Ernst, *J. Am. Chem. Soc.*, **105**, 6944–6952 (1983).

33. W. Bauer, U. Briner, W. Doepfner, R. Haller, R. Huguenin, P. Marbach, T. J. Petcher, and J. Pless, *Life Sci.*, **31**, 1133–1140 (1982).

34. C. Wynants, D. H. Coy, and G. Van Binst, *Tetrahedron*, **44**, 941–973 (1988).

35. P. Vander Elst, E. Van Den Berg, H. Pepermans, L. V. Auwera, R. Zeeuws, D. Tourwe, and G. Van Binst, *Int. J. Pepide Protein Res.*, **29**, 318–330 (1987).

36. P. Vander Elst, D. Gondol, C. Wynants, D. Tourwe, and G. Van Binst, *Int. J. Peptide Protein Res.*, **29**, 331–346 (1987).

37. M. Elseviers, L. Van Der Auwera, H. Pepermans, D. Tourwe, and G. Van Binst, *Biochem. Biophys. Res. Commun.*, **154**, 515–521 (1988).

38. T. J. Lobl, S-L. Chiang, C. Mikos, F. Gorcsan, and P. M. Cardarelli, presented as a poster of the Protein Society Meeting, 1992.

39. M. Wakselman, J. Xie, J.-P. Mazaleyrat, N. Boggetto, A.-C. Vilain, J.-J. Montagne, and M. Reboud-Ravaux, *J. Med. Chem.*, **36**, 1539–1547 (1993).

40. D. Barbeau, S. Guay, W. Neugebauer, and E. Escher, *J. Med. Chem.*, **35**, 151–157 (1992).

41. M. Manning, S. Stoev, K. Bankowski, A. Misicka, and B. Lammek, *J. Med. Chem.*, **35**, 382–388 (1992).

42. M. Manning, J. Przyblski, Z. Grzonka, E. Nawrocka, B. Lammek, A. Misicka, and L. L. Cheng, *J. Med. Chem.*, **35**, 3895–3904 (1992).

43. Manning, M. Kruszynski, K. Bankowski, A. Olma, B. Lammekl, L. L. Chen, W. A. Klis, J. Seto, J. Haldar, and W. H. Sawyer, *J. Med. Chem.*, **32**, 382–391 (1989).

44. C. E. Peishoff, F. E. Alo, J. W. Bean, R. Calvo, C. A. D'Ambrosio, D. S. Eggleston, S. M. Hwang, T. Kline, P. F. Koster, A. Nichols, D. Powers, T. Romoff, J. M. Samanen, J. Stadel, J. A. Vasko, and K. D. Kopple, *J. Med. Chem.*, **35**, 3962–3969 (1992).

45. W. F. Huffman, C. Albrightson-Winslow, B. Brickson, H. G. Bryan, N. Caldwell, G. Dytko, D. S. Eggleston, L. B. Kinter, M. L. Moore, K. A. Newlander, D. B. Schmidt, J. S. Silverstri, F.

46. L. Stassen, N. C. F. Yim, *J. Med. Chem.*, **32**, 880–884 (1989).

46. A. H. van Oijen, C. Erkelens, J. H. Van Boom, and R. M. J. Liskamp, *J. Am. Chem. Soc.*, **111**, 9103–9105 (1989).

47. J. S. Davies, E. J. Tremeer, and R. C. Treadgold, in *Peptides 1986, Proceedings from the 19th European Peptide Symposium*, D. Theodoropoulos, Ed., Walter de Gruyter, Berlin, 1987, pp. 401–405.

48. Y. Wu and J. Kohn, *J. Am. Chem. Soc.*, **113**, 687–688 (1991).

49. A. E. Weber, T. A. Halgren, J. J. Doyle, R. J. Lynch, P. K. S. Siegl, W. H. Parsons, W. J. Greenlee, and A. A. Patchett, *J. Med. Chem.*, **34**, 2692–2701 (1991).

50. D. A. Evans, J. A. Ellman, and K. M. DeVries, *J. Am. Chem. Soc.*, **111**, 8912–8914 (1989).

51. H. Kase, M. Kaneko, and K. Yamada, *J. Antiobiot.*, **40**, 450–454 (1987).

52. S. Thaisrivongs, J. R. Blinn, D. T. Pals, and S. R. Turner, *J. Med. Chem.*, **34**, 1276–1282 (1991).

53. G. Ösapay, S. Wang, H. Shao, and M. Goodman, in *Proceedings of 2nd Japanese Peptide Symposium*, N. Yanaihara, Ed., ESCOM, Leiden, 1993, pp. 152–154.

54. G. Jung, in *Nisin and Novel Lantibiotics*, G. Jung and H.-G. Sahl, Eds., ESCOM, Leiden, 1990, pp. 1–34.

55. A. Polinsky, M. G. Cooney, A. Toy-Palmer, G. Ösapay, and M. Goodman, *J. Med. Chem.*, **35**, 4185–4194 (1992).

56. C. Gilon, D. Halle, M. Chorev, Z. Selinger, and G. Byk, *Biopolymers*, **31**, 745–750 (1991).

57. J. Saulitis, D. F. Mierke, G. Byk, C. Gilon, and H. Kessler, *J. Am. Chem. Soc.*, **114**, 4818–4827 (1992).

58. G. C. Zanotti, B. E. Campbell, K. R. K. Easwaran, and E. R. Blout, *Int. J. Peptide Protein Res.*, **32**, 527–535 (1988).

59. P. S. Hill, D. D. Smith, J. Slaninova, and V. J. Hruby, *J. Am. Chem. Soc.*, **112**, 3110–3113 (1990).

60. D. D. Smith, J. Slaninova, and V. J. Hruby, *J. Med. Chem.*, **35**, 1558–1563 (1992).

61. G. Ösapay, J. W. Taylor, *J. Am. Chem. Soc.*, **112**, 6046–6051 (1990).

62. S. S. Zimmerman, M. S. Pottle, G. Nemethy, and H. A. Scheraga, *Macromolecules*, **10**, 1–9 (1977).

63. W. F. Degrado, *Adv. Protein. Chem.*, **39**, 51–124 (1988).

64. Y. Paterson, S. M. Rumsey, E. Benedetti, G. Nemethy, and H. A. Scheraga, *J. Am. Chem. Soc.*, **103**, 2947–2955 (1981).

65. B. V. Venkataram Prasad and P. Balaram, *CRC Critical Rev.*, **16**, 307–348 (1984).

66. I. L. Karle and P. Balaram, *Biochemistry*, **29**, 6747–6756 (1990).

67. S. Gupta, S. B. Krasnoff, D. W. Roberts, J. A. A. Renwick, L. S. Brinen, and J. Clardy, *J. Org. Chem.*, **57**, 2306–2313 (1992).

68. U. Slomczynska, D. D. Beusen, J. Zabrocki, K. Kociolek, A. Redlinski, F. Reusser, W. C. Hutton, M. T. Leplawy, G. R. Marshall, *J. Am. Chem. Soc.*, **114**, 4095–4106 (1992).

69. G. Valle, M. Crisma, C. Toniolo, R. Beisswenger, A. Rieker, and G. Jung, *J. Am. Chem. Soc.*, **111**, 6828–6833 (1989).

70. E. E. Hodgkin, J. D. Clark, K. R. Miller, and G. R. Marshall, *Biopolymers*, **30**, 533–546 (1990).

71. G. Basu and A. Kuki, *Biopolymers*, **32**, 61–71 (1992).

72. G. Basu, K. Bagghi, and A. Kuki, *Biopolymers*, **31**, 1763–1774 (1991).

73. I. L. Karle, J. L. Flippen-Anderson, M. Sukumar, and P. Balaram, *Proteins: Struct. Func. Gent.*, **12**, 324–330 (1992).

74. C. Toniolo, M. Crisma, G. M. Bonora, E. Benedetti, B. Di Blasio, V. Pavone, C. Pedone, and A. Santini, *Biopolymers*, **31**, 129–138 (1991).

75. I. L. Karle, J. L. Flippen-Anderson, K. Uma, M. Sukumar, and P. Balaram, *J. Am. Chem. Soc.*, **112**, 9350–9356 (1990).

76. C. Aleman, J. A. Subirana, and J. J. Perez, *Biopolymers*, **32**, 621–631 (1992).

77. I. L. Karle, J. L. Flippen-Anderson, K. Uma, H. Balaram, and P. Balaram, *Biopolymers*, **29**, 1433–1442 (1990).

78. T. Taga, M. Itoh, K. Machida, T. Fujita, and T. Ichihara, *Biopolymers*, **29**, 1057–1064 (1990).

79. G. Basu, M. Kubasik, D. Anglos, B. Secor, and A. Kuki, *J. Am. Chem. Soc.*, **112**, 9410–9411 (1990).

80. M. Grimaldi, F. Rossi, M. Saviano, E. Benedetti, V. Pavone, and C. Pedone, *Biopolymers*, **30**, 197–204 (1990).

81. G. R. Marshall, E. E. Hodgkin, D. A. Langs, G. D. Smith, J. Zabrocki, and M. T. Leplawy, *Proc. Natl. Acad. Sci. USA*, **87**, 487–491 (1990).

82. B. Di Blasio, F. Rossi, E. Benedetti, V. Pavone, M. Saviano, C. Pedone, G. Zanotti, and T. Tancredi, *J. Am. Chem. Soc.*, **114**, 8277–8283 (1993).

83. R. Gessmann, H. Brueckner, and M. Kokkinidis, *Pep. Res.*, **4**, 239–244 (1991).

84. K. Otoda, Y. Kitagawa, S. Kimura, and Y. Imanishi, *Biopolymers*, **33**, 1337–1345 (1993).

85. I. L. Karle, J. L. Flippen-Anderson, K. Uma, and P. Balaram, *Biopolymers*, **33**, 401–407 (1993).

86. C. Toniolo and E. Benedetti, *TIBS*, **16**, 350–353 (1991).

87. C. Toniolo, *Biopolymers*, **28**, 247–257 (1987).

88. R. Nagaraj and P. Balaram, *FEBS Lett.*, **96**, 273–276 (1978).

89. R. Nagaraj, T. S. Sudha, and P. Balaram, *FEBS Lett.*, **106**, 271–274 (1979).

90. P. Balaram and T. S. Sudha, *Int. J. Peptide Protein Res.*, **21**, 381–388 (1983).

91. R. Cotton, M. G. Giles, L. Miller, J. S. Shaw, and D. Timms, *Eur. J. Pharmacol.*, **97**, 331–332 (1984).

92. J. Samanen, T. Cash, D. Narindray, E. Brandeis, W. Adams, Jr., H. Weideman, and T. Yellin, *J. Med. Chem.*, **34**, 3036–3043 (1991).

93. R. E. London, J. M. Stewart, and J. R. Cann, *Biochem. Pharmacol.*, **40**, 41–48 (1990).

94. C. Toniolo, M. Crisma, G. Valle, G. M. Bonora, S. Polinelli, E. L. Becker, R. J. Freer, Sudhanand, R. B. Rao, P. Baiaram, and M. Sukumar, *Pep. Res.*, **2**, 275–281 (1989).

95. M. Tallon, D. Ron, D. Halle, P. Amodeo, G. Salviano, P. A. Temussi, Z. Selinger, F. Naider, M. Chorev, *Biopolymers*, **33**, 915–926 (1993).

96. C. Toniolo, M. Crisma, F. Formaggio, G. Valle, G. Cavicchioni, G. Precigoux, A. Aubry, J. Kamphuis, *Biopolymers*, **33**, 1061–1072 (1993).

97. G. Valle, M. Pantano, F. Formaggio, M. Crisma, C. Toniolo, and G. Precigoux, G. Sulzenbacher, W. H. J. Boesten, Q. B. Broxterman, H. E. Schoemaker, and J. Kamphuis, *Biopolymers*, **33**, 1617–1625 (1993).

98. P. W. Schiller, G. Weltrowska, T. M.-D. Nguyen, C. Lemieux, N. N. Chung, B. J. Marsden, and B. C. Wilkes, *J. Med. Chem.*, **34**, 3125–3132 (1991).

99. D. H. Coy and A. J. Kastin, *Peptides*, **1**, 175–177 (1980).

100. C. Toniolo, M. Crisma, S. Pegoraro, G. Valle, G. M. Bonora, E. L. Becker, S. Polinelli, W. H. J. Boesten, H. E. Schoemaker, E. M. Meijer, J. Kamphuis, and R. Freer, *Pep. Res.*, **4**, 66–71 (1991).

101. Z. Tian, P. Edwards, and R. W. Roeske, *Int. J. Peptide Protein Res.*, **40**, 119–126 (1992).

102. J. J. Ellington and I. L. Honigberg, *J. Org. Chem.*, **39**, 104–106 (1974).

103. J. D. Aebi and D. Seebach, *Tetrahedron Lett.*, **25**, 2545–2548 (1984).

104. V. Pavone, B. Di Blasio, A. Lombardi, O. Maglio, C. Isernia, C. Pedone, E. Benedetti, E. Altmann, and M. Mutter, *Int. J. Peptide Protein Res.*, **41**, 15–20 (1993).

105. R. M. Williams and M.-N. Im, *J. Am. Chem. Soc.*, **113**, 9276–9286 (1991).

106. M. Sahebi, P. Wipf, and H. Heimgartner, *Tetrahedron*, **45**, 2999–3010 (1989).

107. G. R. Marshall, J. D. Clark, J. B. Dunbar, G. D. Smith, J. Zabrocki, A. S. Redlinski, and M. R. Leplawy, *Int. J. Peptide Protein Res.*, **32**, 544–555 (1988).

108. E. Benedetti, C. Toniolo, P. Hardy, V. Barone, A. Bavoso, B. Di Blasio, P. Grimaldi, F. Lelj, V. ,Pavone, C. Pedone, G. M. Nonora, I. Lingham, *J. Am. Chem. Soc.*, **106**, 8146–8152 (1984).

109. M. Crisma, G. Valle, G. M. Bonora, E. De Menego, C. Toniolo, F. Lelj,, V. Barone, and F. Fraternali, *Biopolymers*, **30**, 1–11 (1990).

110. A. M. Freitas and H. L. S. Maia, in *Peptides 1988, Proceedings fromn the 20th European Peptide Symposium*, G. Jung and E. Bayer, Eds., Walter de Gruyter, Berlin, 1989, pp. 13–15.

111. A. M. P. Koskinen and L. Munoz, *J. Org. Chem.*, **58**, 879–886 (1993).

112. E. Benedetti, B. Di Blasio, V. Pavone, C. Pedone, and A. Santini, *Biopolymers*, **28**, 175–184 (1989).

113. G. Valle, M. Crisma, C. Toniolo, E. M. Holt, M. Tamura, J. Bland, and C. H. Stammer, *Int. J. Peptide Protein Res.*, **34**, 56–65 (1989).

114. A. Santini, V. Barone, A. Bavoso, E. Benedetti, B. Di Blasio, F. Fraternali, F. Lelj, V. Pavone, C. Pendone, M. Crisma, G. M. Bonora, and C. Toniolo, *Int. J. Biol. Macromol.*, **10**, 292–299 (1988).

115. R. Bardi, A. M. Piazzesi, C. Toniolo, M. Sukumar, and P. Balaram, *Biopolymers*, **25**, 1635–1644 (1986).

116. G. Di Blasio, A. Lombardi, F. Nastri, M. Saviano, C. Pedone, T. Yamada, M. Nakao, S. Kuwata, and V. Pavone, *Biopolymers*, **32**, 1155–1161 (1992).

117. G. Valle, M. Crisma, C. Toniolo, Sudhanand, R. B. Rao, M. Sukumar, and P. Balaram, *Int. J. Peptide Protein Res.*, **38**, 511–518 (1991).

118. J. W. Tsang, B. Schmied, R. Nyfeler, and M. Goodman, *J. Med. Chem.*, **27**, 1663–1668 (1984).

119. V. V. Antonenko, T. Yamazaki, and M. Goodman, presented in 13th American Peptide Symposium as a poster (P-202), 1993.

120. M. Goodman and S. Ro, unpublished results of our laboratories.

121. C. Cativiela, P. Lopez, and J. A. Mayoral, *Tetrahedron: Asymmetry*, **1**, 379–388 (1990).

122. *Ibid.*, 61–64 (1990).

123. F. Trigalo, D. Buisson, F. Acher, and R. Azerad, in *Second Forum on Peptides: Proceedings of the Second Forum on Peptides*, A. Aubry, M. Marraud, B. Vitous, Eds., Colloque INSERM/John Libbey Eurotext, 1989, Vol. 174, pp. 297–300.

124. T. E. Creighton, in *Proteins*, W. H. Freeman and Co., New York, 1984, p. 163.

125. M. Vasquez, G. Memethy, and H. A. Sheraga, *Macromolecules*, **16**, 1043–1049 (1983).

126. M. Goodman and D. F. Mierke, *J. Am. Chem. Soc.* **111**, 3486–3489 (1989).

127. C. R. Cantor and P. R. Schimmel, in *Biophysical Chemistry* Part I, W. H. Freeman and Co., San Francisco, Calif., 1980, p. 270.

128. C. Toniolo, *Int. J. Peptide Protein Res.*, **35**, 287–300 (1990).

129. D. J. Pettibone, B. V. Clineschmidt, P. S. Anderson, R. M. Freidinger, G. F. Lundell, L. R. Koupal, C. D. Schwartz, J. M. Williamson, M. A. Goetz, O. D. Hensens, J. M. Liesch, and J. P. Springer, *Endocrinology*, **125**, 217–222 (1989).

130. A. Zagari, G. Nemethy, and H. A. Scheraga, *Biopolymers*, **30**, 951–959 (1990).

131. *Ibid.*, 961–966 (1990).

132. *Ibid*, 967–974 (1990).

133. M. Goodman and D. F. Veber, unpublished results.

134. K.-J. Chang, in R. S. Rapaka, G. Barnett, and R. L. Hawks, Eds., *NIDA Research Monographs*, Vol. 69, U.S. Government Printing Office, Washington, 1986, pp. 101–111.

135. C. Liebmann, M. Szucs, K. Neubert, B. Hartrodt, H. Arold, and A. Barth, *Peptides* **7**, 195–199 (1986).

136. K.-J. Chang, A. Killian, E. Hazum, P. Cuatrecasas, and J.-K. Chang, *Science*, **212**, 75–77 (1981).

137. P. Juvvadi, D. J. Dooley, C. C. Humblet, G. H. Lu, E. A. Lunney, R. L. Panek, R. Skeean, G. R. Marshall, *Int. J. Peptide Protein Res.*, **40**, 163–170 (1992).

138. S. Talluri, G. T. Montelione, G. van Duyne, L. Piela, J. Clardy, and H. A. Scheraga, *J. Am. Chem. Soc.*, **109**, 4473–4477 (1987).

139. G. T. Montelione, P. Hughes, J. Clardy, H. A. Scheraga, *J. Am. Chem. Soc.*, **108**, 6765–6773 (1986).

140. F. L. Switzer, H. Van Halbeek, E. M. Holt, and C. H. Stammer, *Tetrahedron*, **45**, 6091–6100 (1989).

141. R. C. Petter, *Tetrahedron Lett.*, **30**, 399–402 (1989).

142. N. G. Delaney and V. Madison, *J. Am. Chem. Soc.*, **104**, 6635–6641 (1982).

143. M. G. Bock, R. M. DiPardo, P. D. Williams, D. J. Pettibone, B. V. Clineschmidt, R. G. Ball, D. F. Veber, R. M. Freidinger, *J. Med. Chem.*, **33**, 2321–2323 (1990).

144. D. S. Perlow, J. M. Erb, N. P. Gould, R. D. Tung, R. M. Freidinger, P. D. Williams, and D. F. Veber, *J. Org. Chem.*, **57**, 4394–4400 (1992).

145. R. M. Freidinger, P. D. Williams, R. D. Tung, M. G. Bock, D. J. Pettibone, B. V. Clineschmidt, R. M. DiPardo, J. M. Erb, V. M. Garsky, N. P. Gould, M. J. Kaufman, G. F. Lundell, D. S. Perlow, W. L. Whitter, D. F. Veber, *J. Med. Chem.*, **33**, 1845–1848 (1990).

146. J. Samanen, G. Zuber, J. Bean, D. Eggleston, T. Romoff, K. Kopple, M. Sounders, and D. Regoli, *Int. J. Peptide Protein Res.*, **35**, 501–509 (1990).

147. S. Matsui, V. P. Srivastava, E. M. Holt, E. W. Taylor, and C. H. Stammer, *Int. J. Peptide Protein Res.*, **37**, 306–314 (1991).

148. J. H. Welsh, O. Zerbe, W. von Philipsborn, and J. A. Robinson, *FEBS Lett.*, **297**, 216–220 (1992).

149. M. G. Hinds, J. H. Welsh, D. M. Brennand, J. Fisher, M. J. Glennie, N. G. Richards, D. L. Turner, and J. A. Robinson, *J. Med. Chem.*, **24**, 1777–1789 (1991).

150. S. Thaisrivongs, D. T. Pals, J. A. Lawson, and S. R. Turner, *J. Med. Chem.*, **30**, 536–541 (1987).

151. J. Samanen, D. Narindray, T. Cash, E. Brandeis, W. Adams, Jr., T. Yellin, D. Eggleston, C. DeBrosse, D. Regoli, *J. Med. Chem.*, **32**, 466–472 (1989).

152. J. W. Tiley, W. Danho, V. Madison, D. Fry, J. Swistok, R. Makofske, J. Michalewsky, A. Schwartz, S. Weatherford, J. Triscari, and D. nelson, *J. Med. Chem.*, **35**, 4229–4252 (1992).

153. A. Buku, N. Yamin, and D. Gazis, *Peptides*, **9**, 783–786 (1988).

154. C. Prasad, in *Handbook of Neurochemistry*, Vol. 8, A. Lathja, Ed., Plenum, New York, 1984, pp. 175–200.

155. D. B. Lacky, *J. Biol. Chem.*, **267**, 17508–17511 (1992).

156. R. J. Ashworth, F. M. Morrell, A. Aitken, Y. Patel, S. M. Cockle, *J. Endocrinol.*, **129**, 1–4 (1991).

157. U. Wormser, R. Laufer, M. Chorev, C. Gilon, and Z. Selinger, *Neuropeptides*, **16**, 41–49 (1990).

158. M. Suzuki, H. Sugano, K. Matsumoto, M. Yamamura, and R. Ishida, *J. Med. Chem.*, **33**, 2130–2137 (1990).

159. C. Mapelli, L. F. Elrod, F. L. Switzer, C. H. Stammer, and E. M. Holt, *Biopolymers*, **28**, 123–128 (1989).

160. G. W. J. Fleet and D. R. Witty, *Tetrahedron: Asymmetry*, **1**, 119–136 (1990).

161. D. J. Kyle, J. A. Martin, R. M. Burch, J. P. Carter, S. Lu, S. Meeker, J. C. Prosser, J. P. Sullivan, J. Togo, L. Noronha-Blob, J. A. Sinsko, R. F. Walters, L. W. Whaley, R. N. Hiner, *J. Med. Chem.*, **34**, 2649–2653 (1991).

162. J. C. Howard, F. A. Momany, R. H. Andreatta, H. A. Scheraga, *Macromolecules*, **6**, 535–541 (1973).

163. T. Yamazaki, S. Ro, M. Goodman, N. N. Chung, P. W. Schiller, *J. Med. Chem.*, **36**, 708–719 (1993).

164. P. Manavalan and F. A. Momany, *Biopolymers*, **19**, 1943–1973 (1980).

165. T. Yamazaki, S. Ro, and M. Goodman, *Biochem. Biophys. Res. Commun.*, **181**, 664–670 (1991).

166. A. Aubry and M. Marraud, *Biopolymers*, **28**, 109–122 (1989).

167. J. Morley, *Annu. Rev. Pharmacol. Toxicol.*, **20**, 81–110 (1980).

168. M. Kawai, N. Fukuta, N. Ito, T. Kagami, Y. Butsugan, M. Maruyama, and Y. Kudo, *Int. J. Peptide Protein Res.*, **35**, 452 (1990) (and references therein).

169. M. P. Filatova, N. A. Dri, N. A. Komarova, O. M. Orfkkchovich, V. M. Reiss, I. T. Liepinya, G. V. Nikiforovich, *Bioorg. Khim.* **12**, 59–70 (1986).

170. W. Kaznierski, W. S. Wire, G. K. Lui, R. J. Knapp, J. E. Shook, T. F. Burks, H. I. Yamamura, V. J. Hruby, *J. Med. Chem.*, **31**, 2170–2177 (1988).

171. F. Haviv, T. D. Fitzpatrick, R. E. Swenson, C. J. Nichols, N. A. Mort, E. N. Bush, G. Diaz, G. Bammert, A. Nguyen, N. S. Rhutasel, H. N. Nellans, D. J. Hoffman, E. S. Johnson, and J. Greer, *J. Med. Chem.*, **36**, 363–369 (1993).

172. V. J. Hruby, F. S. Knapp, W. Kazmierski, G. K. Lui, and H. I. Yamamura, in *Peptides: Chemistry, Structure and Biology, Proceedings of 11th American Peptide Symposium*, J. E. Rivier and G. R. Marshall, Eds., ESCOM, Liedin, 1990, pp. 53–55.

173. D. F. Mierke, G. Nößner, P. W. Schiller, and M.

Goodman, *Int. J. Peptide Protein Res.*, **35**, 35 (1990).

174. T. Yamazaki, Z. Huang, A. Pröbstl, M. Goodman, in *Peptides 1990, Proceedings from the 21st European Peptide Symposium*, E. Giralt and D. Andreu, Eds., ESCOM, LEIDEN, 1991, pp. 389–392.

175. T. Yamazaki, A. Pröbstl, P. W. Schiller, and M. Goodman, *Int. J. Peptide Protein Res.*, **37**, 364–381 (1991).

176. G. Johnson, J. R. Drummond, P. A. Boxer, and R. F. Bruns, *J. Med. Chem.*, **35**, 233–241 (1992).

177. C. Morley, D. W. Knight, A. C. Share, *Tetrahedron: Asymmetry*, **1**, 147–150 (1990).

178. U. Schmidt, A. Lieberknecht, and J. Wild, *Synthesis*, 159–172 (1988).

179. T. P. Singh, P. Narula, V. S. Chauhan, A. K. Sharma, and W. Hinrichs, *Int. J. Peptide Protein Res.*, **33**, 167–172 (1989).

180. T. P. Singh, P. Narula, and H. C. Patel, *Acta Cryst.*, **B46**, 539–545 (1990).

181. P. Narula, H. C. Patel, T. P. Singh, V. S. Chauhan, and A. K. Sharma, *Biopolymers*, **27**, 1595–1606 (1988).

182. P. Narula, H. C. Patel, T. P. Singh, and V. S. Chauhan, *Biopolymers*, **29**, 935–941 (1990).

183. T. P. Singh, P. Narula, V. S. Chauhan, and P. Kaur, *Biopolymers*, **28**, 1287–1294 (1989).

184. H. C. Patel, T. P. Singh, V. S. Chauhan, and P. Kaur, *Biopolymers*, **29**, 509–515 (1990).

185. G. D. Rose, L. G. Gierasch, and J. A. Smith, *Adv. Pro. Chem.*, **37**, 1–109 (1985).

186. P. Kaur, K. Uma, P. Balaram, and V. S. Chauhan, *Int. J. Peptide Protein Res.*, **33**, 103–109 (1989).

187. E. Ciszak, G. Pietrzynski, B. Rzeszotarska, *Int. J. Peptide, Protein*, **39**, 218–222 (1992).

188. G. Pietrazinski, B. Rzeszotarska, and Z. Kubica, *Int. J. Peptide Protein Res.*, **40**, 524–531.

189. V. S. Chauhan and K. K. Bhandry, *Int. J. Peptide Protein Res.*, **39**, 223–228 (1992).

190. V. Busetti, M. Crisma, C. Toniolo, S. Salvadori, and G. Balboni, *Int. J. Biol. Macromol.*, **14**, 23–28 (1992).

191. S. Dey, P. Sharma, B. Khandelwal, and T. P. Singh, *Int. J. Peptide Protein Res.*, **38**, 440–444 (1991).

192. M. R. Ciajolo, A. Tuzi, C. R. Pratesi, A. Fissi, and O. Pieroni, *Biopolymers*, **32**, 717–724 (1992).

193. M. R. Ciajolo, A. Tuzi, C. R. Pratesi, A. Fissi, and O. Pieroni, *Biopolymers*, **30**, 911–920 (1990).

194. K. K. Bhandry, and V. S. Chauhan, *Biopolymers*, **33**, 209–217 (1993).

195. A. Tuzi, M. R. Ciajolo, G. Guarino, P. A. Temussi, A. Fissi, and O. Pieroni, *Biopolymers*, **33**, 1111–1121 (1993).

196. K. R. Rajashankar, S. Ramakumar, and V. S. Chauhan, *J. Am. Chem. Soc.*, **114**, 9225–9226 (1992).

197. B. Padmanabhan, S. Dey, B. Khandelwal, G. Subba Rao, and T. P. Singh, *Biopolymers*, **32**, 1271–1276 (1992).

198. A. Gupta and V. S. Chauhan, *Biopolymers*, **30**, 395–403 (1990).

199. D. E. Palmer, C. Pattaroni, K. Nunami, R. K. Chadha, M. Goodman, T. Wakamiya, K. Fukase, S. Horimoto, M. Kitazawa, H. Fujita, A. Kubo, and T. Shiba, *J. Am. Chem. Soc.*, **114**, 5634–5642 (1992).

200. M. Makowski, B. Tzeszotarska, Z. Kubica, G. Peitrzynski, and J. Hetper, *Liebigs Ann. Chem.*, 980–991 (1986).

201. C. Shin, Y. Yonezawa, and M. Ikeda, *Bull. Chem. Soc. Jpn.*, **59**, 3573–3579 (1986).

202. Y. Shimohigashi, J. W. Dunning, A. J. Kolar, and C. H. Stammer, *Int. J. Peptide Protein Res.* **21**, 202–208 (1983).

203. Y. Shimohigashi, C. H. Stammer, T. Costa, and P. F. Von Voightlander, *Int. J. Peptide Protein Res.*, **22**, 489–494 (1983).

204. T. J. Nitz, Y. Shimohigashi, T. Costa, H. C. Chen, and C. H. Stammer, *Int. J. Peptide, Protein Res.*, **27**, 522–529 (1986).

205. S. Salvadori, M. Marastoni, G. Balboni, G. Marzola, and R. Tomatis, *Int. J. Peptide Protein Res.*, **28**, 254–261 (1986).

206. *Ibid.*, 262–273 (1986).

207. M. A. Castiglione-Morelli, G. Saviano, P. A. Temussi, G. Balboni, S. Salvadori, and R. Tomatis, *Biopolymers*, **28**, 129–138 (1989).

208. M. D. Grim, V. Chauhan, Y. Shimohigashi, A. J. Kolar, C. H. Stammer, *J. Org. Chem.*, **46**, 2671–2673 (1981).

209. A. M. Felix, C. T. Wan, C. T. Liebman, C. M. Delaney, T. Mowles, B. A. Berrghardt, A. M. Charnecki, and J. Meienhofer, *Int. J. Peptide Protein Res.*, **10**, 299–310 (1977).

210. G. H. Fisher, P. Berryer, J. W. Ryan, V. Chauc, and C. V. Stammer, *Arch. Biochem. Biophys.*, **211**, 269–274 (1981).

211. N. Subasinghe, M. Schulte, M. Y.-M. Chan, R. J. Roon, J. F. Koerner, and P. L. Johnson, *J. Med. Chem.*, **33**, 2734–2744 (1990).

212. K. L. Spear, M. S. Brown, E. J. Reinhard, E. G. McMahon, G. M. Olins, M. A. Palomo, D. R. Patton, *J. Med. Chem.*, **33**, 1935–1940 (1990).

213. M. Kruszynski, B. Lammek, M. Manning, J. Seto, J. Haldar, and W. H. Sawyer, *J. Med. Chem.*, **23**, 364–368 (1980).

214. H. I. Mosberg, R. Hurst, V. Hruby, K. Gee, H. I. Yamamura, J. J. Galligan, and T. F. Burks, *Proc. Natl. Acad. Sci. USA*, **80**, 5871–5878 (1983).

215. H. I. Mosberg, D. L. Heyl, R. C. Haaseth, J. R. Omnaas, F. Medzihrasky, and C. B. Smith, *Mol. Pharmacol.*, **38**, 924 (1990).

216. D. F. Dyckes, J. J. Nestor, Jr., M. F. Ferger, and V. du Vigneaud, *J. Med. Chem.*, **17**, 250–252 (1974).

217. H. I. Mosberg, R. Hurst, V. J. Hruby, J. J. Galligan, T. F. Burks, K. Gee, H. I. Yamamura, *Biochem. Biophys. Res. Commun.*, **106**, 506–512 (1983).

218. V. J. Hruby and A. Gehrig, *Med. Res. Rev.* **9**, 343–401 (1989) and references therein.

219. Y. Kataoka, Y. Seto, M. Yamamoto, T. Yamada, S. Kuwata, and H. Watanabe, *Bull. Chem. Soc. Jpn.*, **49**, 1081–1084 (1976).

220. Z. Huang, Y.-B. He, K. Raynor, M. Tallent, T. Reisine, M. Goodman, *J. Am. Chem. Soc.*, **114**, 9390–9401 (1992).

221. M. T. Cung and M. Marraud, *Biopolymers*, **21**, 953–967 (1982).

222. G. Toth, K. C. Russell, G. Landis, T. H. Kramer, L. Fang, R. Knapp, P. Davis, T. F. Burks, H. I. Yamamura, and V. J. Hruby, *J. Med. Chem.*, **35**, 2384–2391 (1992).

223. V. J. Hruby, G. Toth, C. A. Gehrig, L-F. Kao, R. Knapp, G. K. Lui, H. I. Yamamura, T. H. Kramer, P. Davis, T. F. Burks, *J. Med. Chem.*, **34**, 1823–1830 (1991).

224. M. Lebl, G. Toth, J. Slaninova, and V. J. Hruby, *Int. J. Peptide Protein Res.*, **40**, 148–151 (1992).

225. K. I. Varughese, A. R. Srinivasan, and C. H. Stammer, *Int. J. Peptide Protein Res.*, **26**, 242–251 (1985).

226. Y.-F. Zhu, T. Yamazaki, J. W. Tsang, S. Lok, and M. Goodman, *J. Org. Chem.*, **57**, 1074–1081 (1992).

227. M. Goodman, J. Coddington, D. F. Mierke, and W. D. Fuller, *J. Am. Chem. Soc.*, **109**, 4712–4714 (1987).

228. E. Benedetti, B. Di Bassio, V. Pavone, C. Pedone, W. D. Fuller, D. F. Mierke, and M. Goodman, *J. Am. Chem. Soc.*, **112**, 8909–8912 (1990).

229. M. Goodman, D. F. Mierke, and W. D. Fuller, in *Peptide Chemistry: Proceedings of the Japan Symposium on Peptide Chemistry*, T. Shiba and S. Sakakibara, Eds., Protein Research Foundation, Japan, 1988, pp. 699–704.

230. R. D. Feinstein, A. Polinsky, A. J. Douglas, C. M. G. F. Beijer, R. K. Chadha, E. Benedetti, M. Goodman, *J. Am. Chem. Soc.*, **113**, 3467–3473 (1991).

231. T. Yamazaki, Y.-F. Zhu, A. Pröbstl, R. Chadha, and M. Goodman, *J. Org. Chem.*, **56**, 6644–6656 (1991).

232. K. I. Varughese, C. H. Wang, H. Kimura, and C. H. Stammer, *Int. J. Peptide Protein Res.*, **31**, 299–300 (1988).

233. Y. Shimohigashi, T. Costa, A. Pfeiffer, A. Herz, H. Kimura, C. H. Stammer, *FEBS Lett.*, **222**, 71–74 (1987).

234. C. Mapelli, H. Kimura, and C. H. Stammer, *Int. J. Peptide Protein Res.*, **28**, 347–359 (1986).

235. C. Mapelli, G. Turocy, F. L. Switzer, and C. H. Stammer, *J. Org. Chem.*, **54**, 145–149 (1989).

236. C. H. Stammer, C. Mapelli, and V. P. Srivastava, in *Peptides: Chemistry, Structure and Biology, Proceedings of 11th American Peptide Symposium*, J. E. Rivier and G. R. Marshall, Eds., ESCOM, Leiden, 1990, 344–345.

237. K. Burgess and K.-K. Ho, *J. Org. Chem.*, **57**, 5931–5936 (1992).

238. D. J. Aitken, J. Royer, and H.-P. Husson, *J. Org. Chem.*, **55**, 2814–2820 (1990).

239. P. K. Subramanian, D. M. Kalvin, K. Ramalingam, and R. W. Woodard, *J. Org. Chem.*, **54**, 270–276 (1989).

240. N. De Kimpe, P. Sulmon, and P. Brunet, *J. Org. Chem.*, **55**, 5777–5784 (1990).

241. K. Shimamoto, M. Ishida, H. Shinozaki, and Y. Ohfune, *J. Org. Chem.*, **56**, 4167–4176 (1991).

242. R. Pellicciari, B. Natalini, M. Marinozzi, J. B. Monahan, and J. P. Snyder, *Tetrahedron Lett.*, **31**, 139–141 (1990).

243. Y. Zelechonok and R. B. Silverman, *J. Org. Chem.*, **57**, 5787–5790 (1992).

244. G. Valle, W. M. Kazmierski, M. Crisma, G. M. Bonora, C. Toniolo, and V. J. Hruby, *Int. J. Peptide Protein Res.*, **40**, 222–232 (1992).

245. V. J. Hruby, *Biopolymers*, **33**, 1073–1082 (1993).

246. P. Sipos, G. Peintler, and G. Toth, *Int. J. Peptide Protein Res.*, **39**, 207–210 (1992).

247. D. Tourwe, G. Toth, M. Lebl, K. Verschueren, R. J. Knapp, P. Davis, G. Van Binst, H. I. Yamamura, T. F. Burks, T. Kramer, V. J. Hruby, in *Peptides: Chemistry and Biology, Proceedings of the Twelfth American Peptide Symposium*, J. A. Smith and J. E. Rivier, Eds., ESCOM, Leiden, 1992, pp. 307–308.

248. T. Deeks, P. A. Crooks, and R. D. Waigh, *J. Med. Chem.*, **26**, 762–765 (1983).

249. J. S. Shaw and M. J. Turnbull, *Eur. J. Pharmacol.*, **49**, 313–317 (1978).

250. W. M. Kazmierski, H. I. Yamamura, and V. J. Hruby, *J. Am. Chem. Soc.*, **113**, 2275–2283 (1991).

251. P. W. Schiller, T. M.-D. Nguyen, G. Weltrowska, B. C. Wilkes, B. J. Marsden, C. Lemieux, and N. N. Chung, *Proc. Natl. Acad. Sci. USA*, **89**, 11871–11875 (1992).

252. E. Gavuzzo, G. Lucente, F. Mazza, G. P. Zecchini, M. P. Paradisi, G. Pochetti, and I. Torrini, *Int. J. Peptide Protein Res.*, **37**, 268–276 (1991).

253. R. D. Nelson, D. I. Gottlieb, T. M. Balasubramanian, and G. R. Marshall, in *NIDA Research Monographs*, Vol. 69, R. S. Rapaka, G. Barnett, and R. L. Hawks, Eds., U.S. Government Printing Office, Washington, D.C., 1986, pp. 204–230.

254. H. I. Mosberg and H. B. Kroona, *J. Med. Chem.*, **35**, 4498–4500 (1992).

255. J. Y. L. Chung, J. T. Wasicak, W. A. Arnold, C. S. May, A. M. Nadzan, and M. W. Holladay, *J. Org. Chem.*, **55**, 270–275 (1990).

256. M. W. Holladay and A. M. Nadzan, *J. Org. Chem.*, **56**, 3900–3905 (1991).

257. A. M. Koskinen and H. Rapoport, *J. Org. Chem.*, **54**, 1859–1866 (1989).

258. T. R. Webb and C. Eigenbrot, *J. Org. Chem.*, **56**, 3009–3016 (1991).

259. D. F. Mierke, O. E. Said-Nejad, P. W. Schiller, and M. Goodman, *Biopolymers*, **29**, 179–196 (1990).

260. T. Yamazaki, O. E. Said-Nejad, P. W. Schiller, and M. Goodman, *Biopolymers*, **31**, 877–898 (1991).

261. G. Gacel, V. Dauge, P. Breuze, P. Delay-Goyet, and B. P. Roques, *J. Med. Chem.*, **31**, 1891–1897 (1988).

262. P. Delay-Goyet, C. Seguin, G. Gacel, and B. P. Roques, *J. Biol. Chem.*, **263**, 4124–4130 (1988).

263. J. Belleney, G. Gacel, M. C. Fournie-Zaluski, B. Maigret, and B. P. Roques, *Biochemistry*, **28**, 7392–7400 (1989).

264. G. Flouret, T. Majewski, and W. Brieher, *J. Med. Chem.*, **36**, 747–749 (1993).

265. J. R. Spencer, N. G. J. Delaet, A. Toy-Parmer, V. V. Antonenko, and M. Goodman, *J. Org. Chem.*, **58**, 1635–1638 (1993).

266. J. R. Spencer, *Thesis Dissertation*, University of California, San Diego, 1993.

267. *Tetrahedron*, **49** (17), (1993).

268. J. B. Ball, P. R. Andrews, and P. J. Alewood, *FEBS Lett.*, **273**, 15–18 (1990).

269. J. B. Ball and P. F. Alewood, *J. Mol. Recogn.*, **3**, 55–64 (1990).

270. M. G. Hinds, J. H. Welsh, D. M. Brennand, J. Fisher, M. J. Glennie, N. G. J. Richards, D. L. Turner, J. A. Robinson, *J. Med. Chem.*, **34**, 1777–1789 (1991).

271. G. L. Olson, M. E. Voss, D. E. Hill, M. Kahn, V. S. Madison, and C. M. Cook, *J. Am. Chem. Soc.*, **112**, 323–333 (1990).

272. M. Kahn and S. Bertenshaw, *Tetrahedron Lett.*, **30**, 2317–2320 (1989).

273. M. J. Genin, W. B. Gleason, and R. L. Johnson, *J. Org. Chem.*, **58**, 860–866 (1993).

274. M. J. Genin, W. H. Ojala, W. B. Gleason, R. L. Johnson, *J. Org. Chem.*, **58**, 2334–2337 (1993).

275. K. Muller, D. Obrecht, A. Knierzinger, C. Stankovic, C. Spiegler, W. Bannwarth, A. Trzeciak, G. Englert, A. M. Labhardt, and P. Schonholzer, in *Perspectives in Medicinal Chemistry*, B. Testa, E. Kybuiz, W. Fuhrer, and R. Giger, Eds., Verlag Helvetic Chimica Acta, Basel, Switzerland, 1993, pp. 513–531.

276. M. J. Genin and R. L. Johnson, *J. Am. Chem. Soc.*, **114**, 8778–8783 (1992).

277. D. G. Mullen and P. A. Bartlett, in *Peptides 1990, Proceedings from the 21st European Peptide Symposium*, E. Giralt and D. Andreau, Eds., ESCOM, Lieden, 1991, pp. 364–365.

278. R. Gonzalez-Muniz, M. J. Domingues, M. T. Garcia-Lopez, I. Gomez-Monterrey, and J. R. Harto, in *Peptides 1990, Proceedings from the 21st European Peptide Symposium*, E. Giralt and D. Andreau, Eds., ESCOM, Lieden, 1991, pp. 366–367.

279. J.-P. Dumas and J. P. Germanas, *Tetrahedron Lett.*, **35**, 1493–1496 (1994).

280. W. F. Huffman, J. F. Callahan, D. S. Eggleston, K. A. Newlander, D. T. Takata, E. E. Codd, R. F. Walker, P. W. Schiller, C. Lemieux, W. S. Wire, T. F. Burks, in *Peptides: Chemistry and Biology, Proceedings of 10th American Peptide Symposium*, G. R. Marshall, Ed., ESCOM, Leiden, 1988, pp. 105–108.

281. J. F. Callahan, J. W. Bean, J. L. Burgess, D. S. Eggleston, S. M. Hwang, K. D. Kopple, P. F. Koster, A. Nichols, C. E. Peishoff, J. M. Samanen, J. A. Vasko, A. Wong, and W. F. Huffman, *J. Med. Chem.*, **35**, 3970–3972 (1992).

282. M. Sato, J. Y. H. Lee, H. Nakanish, M. E. Jojnson, R. A. Chrusciel, and M. Kahn, *Biochem. Biophys. Res. Commun.*, **187**, 999–1006 (1992).

283. D. S. Kemp and J. S. Carter, *J. Org. Chem.*, **54**, 109–115 (1989).

284. S. D. Jolad, J. J. Hoffmann, S. J. Torrance, R. M. Wiedhopf, J. R. Cole, S. K. Arora, R. B.

Bates, R. L. Gargiulo, G. R. Kriek, *J. Am. Chem. Soc.*, **99**, 8040–8044 (1977).

285. D. S. Kemp and B. R. Bowen, *Tetrahedron Lett.*, **40**, 5081–5082 (1988).

286. D. S. Kemp and B. R. Bowen, *Tetrahedron Lett.*, **40**, 5077–5080 (1988).

287. V. Brandmeier, M. Feigel, and M. Bremer, *Angew. Chem. Int. Ed. Engl.*, **28**, 486–488 (1989).

288. H. Diaz, K. Y. Tsang, D. Choo, J. R. Espina, and J. W. Kelly, *J. Am. Chem. Soc.*, **115**, 3790–3791 (1993).

289. A. B. Smith, III, T. P. Keenan, R. C. Holcomb, P. A. Sprengeler, M. C. Guzman, J. L. Wook, P. J. Carroll, R. Hirschmann, *J. Am. Chem. Soc.*, **114**, 10672–10674 (1992).

290. D. S. Kemp, T. P. Curran, W. M. Davis, J. G. Boyd, and C. Muendel, *J. Org. Chem.*, **56**, 6672–6682 (1991).

291. D. S. Kemp, T. P. Curran, J. G. Boyd, and T. J. Allen, *J. Org. Chem.*, **56**, 6683–6697 (1991).

292. Y. Kojima, Y. Ikeda, E. Kumata, J. Maruo, A. Okamoto, K. Hirotsu, K. Shibata, and A. Ohsuka, *Int. J. Peptide Protein Res.*, **37**, 468–475 (1991).

293. R. L. Baxter, S. S. B. Glover, E. M. Bordon, R. O. Gould, M. C. McKie, A. I. Scott, and M. D. Walkinshaw, *J. Chem. Soc. Perkin Trans. 1*, 365–371 (1988).

294. D. K. Sukumaran, M. Prorok, and D. S. Lawrence, *J. Am. Chem. Soc.*, **113**, 706–707 (1991).

295. M. J. Deal, R. M. Hagan, S. J. Ireland, C. C. Jordan, A. B. McElroy, B. Porter, B. C. Ross, M. Stephens-Smith, and P. Ward, *J. Med. Chem.*, **35**, 4195–4204 (1992).

296. P. Ward, G. B. Ewan, C. C. Jordan, S. J. Ireland, R. M. Hagan, and J. R. Brown, *J. Med. Chem.*, **33**, 1848–1851 (1990).

297. S. Capasso and C. A. Mattia, L. Mazzarella, F. Sica, and A. Zagari, *Pep. Res.*, **3**, 262–270 (1990).

298. D. J. Kempf and S. L. Condon, *J. Org. Chem.*, **55**, 1390–1394 (1990).

299. J. P. Wolf and H. Rapoport, *J. Org. Chem.*, **54**, 3164–3173 (1989).

300. M. Chorev, R. Shavitz, M. Goodman, S. Minick, and R. Guillemin, *Science*, **204**, 1210–1214 (1974).

301. M. Goodman and M. Chorev, *Acct. Chem. Res.* **12**, 1–7 (1979).

302. M. Chorev and M. Goodman, *Acc. Chem. Res.*, **26**, 266–273 (1993).

303. J. Berman, M. Goodman, T. Nguyen and P. W. Schiller, *Biochem. Biophys. Res. Commun.*, **115**, 864–870 (1983).

304. A. S. Dutta, J. J. Gormley, P. F. McLachlan, and J. S. Major, *J. Med. Chem.*, **33**, 2560–2568 (1989).

305. L. El Masdouri, A. Aubry, C. Sakarellos, E. J. Gomez, M. T. Cung, and M. Marraud, *Int. J. Peptide Protein Res.*, **31**, 420–428 (1988).

306. M. Marraud, V. Dupont, V. Grand, Zerkout, A. Lecoq, G. Boussard, J. Vidal, A. Collet, and A. Aubry, *Biopolymers*, **33**, 1135–1148 (1993).

307. P. Vander Elst, M. Elsevier, E. De Cock, M. Van Marsenille, D. Tourwe, and G. Van Binst, *Int. J. Peptide Protein Res.*, **27**, 633–642 (1986).

308. R. T. Jensen and D. H. Coy, *Trends Pharm. Sci.*, **12**, 13–19 (1991).

309. D. H. Coy, P. Heinz-Erian, N.-Y. Jiang, Y. Sasaki, J. Taylor, J.-P. Moreau, W. T. Wolfrey, J. D. Gardner, and R. T. Jensen, *J. Biol. Chem.*, **263**, 5056–5060 (1988).

310. D. H. Coy, J. E. Taylor, N.-Y. Jiang, S. H. Kim, L. Wang, S. Huang, J.-P. Moreau, J. D. Gardner, and R. T. Jensen, *J. Biol. Chem.*, **264**, 14691–14697 (1989).

311. B. M. Haffar, S. J. Hocart, D. H. Coy, S. Mantey, H.-C. V. Chiang, and R. T. Jensen, *J. Biol. Chem.*, **266**, 316–322 (1991).

312. D. Hudson, R. Sharpe, and M. Szelke, *Int. J. Peptide Protein Res.*, **15**, 122–129 (1980).

313. N. G. J. Delaet, P. M. F. Verheyden, D. Tourwe, G. Van Binst, P. Davis, and T. F. Burks, *Biopolymers*, **32**, 957–969 (1992).

314. S. Salvadori, R. Guerrini, P. A. Borea, and R. Tomatis, *Int. J. Peptide Protein Res.*, **40**, 437–444 (1992).

315. A. F. Spatola, F. Formaggio, P. W. Schiller, W. S. Wire, and T. F. Burks, in *Second Forum on Peptides*, A. Aubry, M. Marraud, and B. Vitoux, Eds., Colloque INSERM/John Libbey Eurotext, 1989, Vol. 174, pp. 45–54.

316. P. W. Schiller, G. Weltrowska, T. M.-D. Nguyen, B. C. Wilkes, N. N. Chung, and C. Lemieux, *Med. Chem.*, **36**, 3182–3187 (1993).

317. J.-M. Qian, D. H. Coy, N.-Y. Jiang, J. D. Gardner, and R. T. Jensen, *J. Biol. Chem.*, **264**, 16667–16671 (1989).

318. S. Zacharia, W. J. Rossowski, N.-H. Jiang, P. Hrbas, A. Ertan, and D. H. Coy, *Eur. J. Pharmacol.*, **203**, 353–357 (1991).

319. J. Martinez, J.-P. Bali, M. Rodriguez, B. Castro, R. Magous, J. Laur, and M. F. Lignon, *J. Med. Chem.*, **28**, 1874–1879 (1985).

320. S. J. Hocart, W. A. Murphy, and D. H. Coy, *J. Med. Chem.*, **33**, 1954–1958 (1990).

321. C. Mendre, M. Rodriguez, M. F. Lignon, M. C. Galas, C. Gueudet, P. Worms, and J. Martinez, *Eur. J. Pharmacol.*, **186**, 213–222 (1990).

322. C. Mendre, M. Rodriquez, J. Laur, A. Aumelas, and J. Martinez, *Tetrahedron*, **44**, 4415–4430 (1988).

323. E. D. Nicolaides, F. J. Tinney, J. S. Kaltenbronn, J. T. Repine, D. A. DeJohn, E. A. Lunney, W. H. Roark, J. G. Marriott, R. E. Davis, and R. E. Voigtman, *J. Med. Chem.*, **29**, 959–971 (1986).

324. Y. Sasaki, W. A. Murphy, M. L. Heiman, V. A. Lance, and D. H. Coy, *J. Med. Chem.*, **30**, 1162–1166 (1987).

325. M. Szelke, B. Leckie, A. Hallett, D. M. Jones, J. Sueiras, B. Atrash, and A. F. Lever, *Nature*, **299**, 555–557 (1982).

326. J. S. Kaltenbronn, J. P. Hudspeth, E. A. Lunney, B. M. Michnikewicz, E. D. Nicolaides, J. T. Repine, W. H. Roark, M. A. Stier, F. J. Tinney, P. D. W. Woo, and A. D. Essenburg, *J. Med. Chem.*, **33**, 838–845 (1990).

327. M. Cushman, Y. Oh, T. D. Copeland, S. Oroszlan, and S. W. Snyder, *J. Org. Chem.*, **56**, 4161–4167 (1991).

328. A. Aumelas, M. Rodriguez, A. Heitz, B. Castro, and J. Martinez, *Int. J. Peptide Protein Res.*, **30**, 596–604 (1987).

329. C. Di Bello, A. Scatturin, G. Vertuani, G. D'Auria, M. Gargiulo, L. Paolillo, E. Trivellone, L. Gozzini, R. De Castiglione, *Biopolymers*, 1397–1408 (1991).

330. S. K. Davidsen and M. Y. Chu-Moyer, *J. Org. Chem.*, **54**, 5558–5567 (1989).

331. R. Mohan, Y. Chou, R. Bihovsky, W. C. Lumma, Jr., P. W. Erhardt, and K. J. Shaw, *J. Med. Chem.*, **34**, 2402–2410 (1991).

332. Y. S. Oh, T. Yamazaki, M. Goodman, *Macromolecules.*, **25**, 6322–6331 (1992).

333. C. I. Fincham, M. Higginbottom, D. R. Hill, D. C. Horwell, J. C. O'Toole, G. S. Ratcliffe, D. C. Rees, E. Roberts, *J. Med. Chem.*, **35**, 1472–1484 (1992).

334. S. L. Harbeson, S. A. Shatzer, T. B. Le, and S. H. Buck, *J. Med. Chem.*, **35**, 3949–3955 (1992).

335. A. F. Spatola, N. S. Agarwal, A. L. Bettag, J. A. Yankeelov, C. Y. Bowers, and W. W. Vale, *Biochem. Biophys. Res. Commun.*, **97**, 1014–1023 (1980).

336. A. F. Spatola and J. V. Edwards, *Biopolymers*, **25**, S229–244 (1986).

337. A. F. Spatola, K. Darlak, W. S. Wire, and T. F. Burks, in *Peptides: Chemistry, Structure and Biology, Proceedings of 11th American Peptide Symposium*, J. E. Rivier and G. R. Marshall, Eds., ESCOM, Leiden, 1990, p. 334.

338. K. Darlak, Z. Grzonka, A. F. Spatola, D. E. Benovitz, T. F. Burks, and W. S. Wire, in G. Jung and E. Bayer, Eds., "Peptides 1988," *Proceedings from the 20th European Peptide Symposium*, Walter de Gruyter: Berlin, 1989, pp. 634–636.

339. A. F. Spatola, H. Saneii, J. V. Edwards, A. L. Bettag, M. K. Anwer, P. Rowell, B. Browne, R. Lahti, and P. Von Voigtlander, *Life Sci.*, **38**, 1243–1249 (1986).

340. D. E. Benovitz and A. F. Spatola, *Peptides*, **6**, 257–261 (1985).

341. T. W. Gero, A. F. Spatola, I. Torres-Aleman, and A. V. Schally, *Biochem. Biophys. Res. Commun.*, **120**, 840–845 (1984).

342. M. K. Anwer, D. B. Sherman, and A. F. Spatola, *Int. J. Peptide Protein Res.*, **36**, 392–399 (1990).

343. A. F. Spatola, M. K. Anwer, A. L. Rockwell, and L. M. Gierasch, *J. Am. Chem. Soc.*, **108**, 825–831 (1986).

344. L. G. Pease and C. Watson, *J. Am. Chem. Soc.*, **100**, 1279–1286 (1978).

345. A. C. Bach, II, A. A. Bothner-By, and L. M. Gierash, *J. Am. Chem. Soc.*, **104**, 572–576 (1982).

346. M. D. Bruch, J. H. Noggle, and L. M. Gierash, *J. Am. Chem. Soc.*, **107**, 1400–1407 (1985).

347. I. L. Karle, *J. Am. Chem. Soc.*, **100**, 1286–1289 (1978).

348. S. Ma, J. F. Richardson, and A. F. Spatola, *J. Am. Chem. Soc.*, **113**, 8529–8530 (1991).

349. R. E. TenBrink, *J. Org. Chem.*, **52**, 418–422 (1987).

350. P. Breton, M. Monsigny, and R. Mayer, *Int. J. Peptide Protein Res.*, **35**, 346–351 (1990).

351. E. Rubini, C. Gilon, D. Levian-Teitelbaum, Z. Selinger, M. Weinstock-Rosin, and M. Chorev, in *Peptides 1984, Proceedings of the 18th European Peptide Symposium*, U. Ragnarson, Ed., Almqvist & Wiksell International, Stockholm, Sweden, p. 337.

352. E. Roubini, R. Laufer, C. Gilon, Z. Selinger, B. P. Roques, and M. Chorev, *J. Med. Chem.*, **34**, 2430–2438 (1991).

353. R. E. TenBrink, D. T. Pals, D. W. Harris, and G. A. Johnson, *J. Med. Chem.*, **31**, 671–677 (1988).

354. M. Rodriguez, A. Heitz, and J. Martinez, *Int. J. Peptide Protein Res.*, **39**, 273–277 (1992).

355. M. Rodriguez, A. Heitz, and J. Martinez, *Tetrahedron Lett.*, **31**, 5153–5156 (1990).

356. M. Rodriguez, A. Heitz, and J. Martinez, *Tetrahedron Lett.*, **31**, 7319–7322 (1990).

357. K. Kawasaki and M. Maeda, *Biochem. Biophys. Res. Commun.*, **106**, 113–116 (1982).

358. S. Shceibye, B. S. Pedersen, and S. O. Lawesson, *Bull. Soc. Chim. Belg.*, **87**, 229 (1978).

359. K. Clausen, M. Thorsen, and S. O. Lawesson, *Tetrahedron*, **37**, 3635–3639 (1981).

360. M. Kajtar, M. Hollosi, T. Kajtar, Zs. Majer, and K. E. Kover, *Tetrahedron*, **42**, 3931–3942 (1986).

361. M. Hollosi, Z. Majer, M. Zewdu, F. Ruff, M. Kajtar, and K. E. Kover, *Tetrahedron*, **44**, 195–202 (1988).

362. D. J. S. Guthrie, C. H. Williams, and D. T. Elmore, *Int. J. Peptide Protein Res.*, **28**, 208–211 (1986).

363. L. Maziak, G. Lajoie, and B. Belleau, *J. Am. Chem. Soc.*, **108**, 182–183 (1986).

364. R. Bardi, A. M. Piazzesi, C. Toniolo, O. E. Jensen, R. S. Omar, and A. Senning, *Biopolymers*, **27**, 747–761 (1988).

365. M. Hollosi, E. Kollat, J. Kajtar, M. Kajtar, and G. D. Fasman, *Biopolymers*, **30**, 1061–1072 (1990).

366. W. Walter and J. Voss, in *The Chemistry of Amides*, J. Zabicky, Ed., Interscience, New York, 1970, p. 383.

367. T. F. M. la Cour, *Int. J. Peptide Protein Res.*, **30**, 564–571 (1987).

368. O. E. Jensen, S. O. Lawensson, R. Bardi, A. M. Piazzesi, and C. Toniolo, *Tetrahedron*, **41**, 5595–5606 (1985).

369. E. P. Dudek and G. Dudek, *J. Org. Chem.*, **32**, 823–826 (1967).

370. M. Hollosi, M. Zewdu, E. Kollat, Z. Majer, M. Kajtar, G. Batta, K. Kover, and P. Sandor, *Int. J. Peptide Protein Res.*, **36**, 173–181 (1990).

371. D. B. Sherman and A. F. Spatola, *J. Am. Chem. Soc.*, **112**, 433–441 (1990).

372. W. C. Jones, Jr., J. J. Nestor, Jr., and V. du Vigneaud, *J. Am. Chem. Soc.*, **95**, 5677–5679 (1973).

373. M. Kruszynski, G. Kupryszewski, U. Ragnarsson, M. Alexandrova, V. Strbak, M. C. Tonon and J. Vaudry, *Experientia*, **41**, 1576–1577 (1988).

374. L. Lankiewicz, C. Y. Bowers, G. A. Reynolds, V. Labroo, L. A. Cohen, S. Vonhof, A. L. Siren, and A. F. Spatola, *Biochem. Biophys. Res. Commun.*, **184**, 359–366 (1992).

375. M. Alexandrova, V. Strbak, M. Kruszynski, J. Zboinska, and G. Kupryszewski, *General Physiology and Biophysics*, **10**, 287–297 (1991).

376. Z. Majer, M. Zewdu, M. Hollosi, J. Seprodi, Z. Vadasz, and I. Teplan, *Biochem. Biophys. Res. Commun.*, **150**, 1017–1020 (1988).

377. G. LaJoie, F. Lepine, S. LeMarie, F. Jolicoeur, C. Aube, A. Turcotte, and B. Belleau, *Int. J. Peptide Protein Res.*, **24**, 316–327 (1984).

378. K. Clausen, A. F. Spatola, C. Lemieux, P. Schiller, and S. O. Lawesson, *Biochem. Biophys. Res. Commun.*, **120**, 305–310 (1984).

379. D. B. Sherman, A. F. Spatola, W. S. Wire, T. F. Burks, T. M. D., and P. W. Schiller, *Biochem. Biophys. Res. Commun.*, **162**, 1126–1132 (1989).

380. P. Campbell and N. T. Nashed, *J. Am. Chem. Soc.*, **104**, 5521–5226 (1982).

381. M. Kruszynski, G. Kupryszewski, K. Misterek, and S. Gumulka, *Pol. J. Pharmacol. Pharmacy*, **42**, 483–490 (1990).

382. S. E. Haugen, A. J. Douglas, B. Ronning, B. Walker, A. K. Sandvik, R. F. Murphy, D. T. Elmore, and H. L. Waldum, *Scand. J. Gastroenterol.*, **24**, 577–580 (1989).

383. B. Belleau, G. Lajoie, G. Sauve, V. S. Rao, and A. di Paola, *Int. J. Immunopharmacol.*, **11**, 467–471 (1987).

384. M. Cushman and J. Jurayj, *Tetrahedron*, **48**, 8601–8614 (1992).

385. R. E. Beattie, D. T. Elmore, C. H. Williams, and D. J. S. Guthrie, *Biochem. J.*, **245**, 285–288 (1987).

386. A. G. Michel, G. Lajoie, C. A. Hassani, *Int. J. Peptide Protein Res.*, **36**, 489–498 (1990).

387. M. Doi, S. Takehara, T. Ishida, M. Inoue, *Int. J. Peptide Protein Res.*, **34**, 369–373 (1989).

388. Y. K. Shue, G. M. Carrera, M. D. Tufano, A. M. Nadzan, *J. Org. Chem.*, **56**, 2107–2111 (1991).

389. L. S. Lehman de Gaeta, M. Czarniecki, *J. Org. Chem.*, **54**, 4004–4005 (1989).

390. T. Ibuka, H. Habashita, A. Otaka, N. Fujii, Y. Oguchi, T. Uyehara, and Y. Yamamoto, *J. Org. Chem.*, **56**, 4370–4382 (1991).

391. A. Spaltenstein, P. A. Carpino, F. Miyake, and P. B. Hopkins, *J. Org. Chem.*, **52**, 3759–3766 (1987).

392. M. T. Cox, D. W. Heaton, and J. Horbury, *J. Chem. Soc. Chem. Comm.*, 799–802 (1980).

393. H. Jaspers, D. Tourwe, G. Van Binst, H. Pepermans, P. Borea, L. Ucelli, and S. Salvadori, *Int. J. Peptide Protein Res.*, **39**, 315–321 (1992).

394. P. Deschrijver and D. Tourwe, *FEBS Lett.*, **146**, 353–356 (1982).

395. M. Baginsky, L. Piela, J. Skolnick, *J. Comp. Chem.*, **14**, 471–477 (1993).

396. M. M. Hann, P. G. Sammes, P. D. Kennewell and J. B. Taylor, *J. Chem. Soc. Chem. Commun.*, 234–235 (1980).

397. M. T. Cox, J. J. Gormley, C. F. Hayward, N. N.

Petter, *J. Chem. Soc. Chem. Commun.*, 800–802 (1980).

398. D. Tourwe, J. Couder, M. Ceusters, D. Meert, T. F. Burds, T. H. Kramer, P. Davis, R. Knapp, H. I. Leysen, and G. Van Binst, *Int. J. Peptide Protein Res.*, **39**, 131–136 (1992).

399. R. L. Johnson, *J. Med. Chem.*, **27**, 1351 (1984).

400. A. Spaltenstein, P. A. Carpino, F. M. Miyake, and P. B. Hopkins, *Tetrahedron Lett.*, **27**, 2095–2098 (1986).

401. E. Felder, T. Allmendinger, H. Fritz, E. Hugerbuler, and M. Keller, in *Peptides: Chemistry and Biology, Proceedings of the Twelfth American Peptide Symposium*, J. A. Smith and J. E. Rivier, Eds., ESCOM, Leiden, 1992, pp. 161–162.

402. N. S. Chandrakumar, P. K. Yonan, A. Stapelfeld, M. Savage, E. Rorbacher, P. C. Contreras, and D. Hammond, *J. Med. Chem.*, **35**, 223–233 (1992).

403. M. M. Hann, P. G. Sammes, P. D. Kennewell, and J. B. Taylor, *J. Chem. Soc., Perkin Trans. 1*, 307–314 (1982).

404. K. L. Yu and R. L. Johnson, *J. Org. Chem.*, **52**, 2051–2059 (1987).

405. G. R. Marshall, C. Humblet, N. Van Opdenbosch, and J. Zabrocki, in *Peptides: Synthesis-Structure-Function, Proceedings of the Seventh American Peptide Symposium*, D. H. Rich and E. Gross, Eds., Pierce, Rockford, 1981, pp. 669–672.

406. J. Zabrocki, G. D. Smith, J. B. Dunbar, H. Iijima, and G. R. Marshall, *J. Am. Chem. Soc.*, **110**, 5875–5880 (1988).

407. G. D. Smith, J. Zabrocki, T. A. Flak, and G. R. Marshall, *Int. J. Peptide Protein Res.*, **37**, 191–197 (1991).

408. J. Zabrocki, U. Slomczynska, and G. R. Marshall, in *Peptides: Chemistry and Biology, Proceedings of 11th American Peptide Symposium*, J. E. Rivier and G. R. Marshall, Eds., ESCOM, Leiden, 1990, p. 195.

409. M. Lebl, J. Slaninova, and R. L. Johnson, *Int. J. Peptide Protein Res.*, **33**, 16–21 (1989).

410. J. Zabrocki, J. B. Dunbar, Jr., K. W. Marshall, M. V. Toth, and G. R. Marshall, *J. Org. Chem.*, **57**, 202–209 (1992).

411. J. Zabrocki, G. D. Smith, J. B. Dunbar, Jr., K. W. Marshall, M. Toth, and G. R. Marshall, in *Peptides 1988, Proceedings from the 20th European Peptide Symposium*, G. Jung and E. Bayer, Eds., Walter de Gruyter, Berlin, 1989, pp. 295–297.

412. A. Garopalo, C. Tarnus, J. M. Remy, R. Leppik, F. Piriou, B. Harris, and J. T. Pelton, in *Peptides: Chemistry, Structure and Biology, Proceedings of 11th American Peptide Symposium*, J. E. Rivier and G. R. Marshall, Eds., ESCOM, Leiden, 1990, p. 833.

413. H. Umezawa, T. Nakamura, S. Fukatsu, T. Aoyagi, and K. Tatsuta, *J. Antibiot.*, **36**, 1787–1788 (1983).

414. S. Ohuchi, H. Suda, H. Naganawa, T. Takita, T. Aoyagi, H. Umezawa, H. Nakamura, and Y. Iitaka, *J. Antibiot.*, **36**, 1576–1580 (1983).

415. H. Umezawa, T. Aoyagi, S. Ohuchi, A. Okuyama, H. Suda, T. Takita, M. Hamada, and T. Takeuchi, *J. Antibiot.*, **36**, 1572–1575 (1983).

416. C. Jennings-White and R. G. Almquist, *Tetrahedron Lett.*, **23**, 2533–2534 (1982).

417. J. V. N. Vara Prasad and D. H. Rich, *Tetrahedron Lett.*, **31**, 1803–1806 (1990).

418. R. G. Almquist, W-R. Chao, M. E. Ellis, and H. L. Johnson, *J. Med. Chem.*, **23**, 1392–1398 (1980).

419. D. H. Rich, F. G. Salituro, M. W. Holladay, and P. G. Schmidt, in J. A. Vuda and M. Gordon, Eds., *Conformationally Directed Drug Design, ACS Symposium Series 251*; American Chemical Society, Washington, D.C., 1984, pp. 211–237.

420. S. L. Harbeson and D. H. Rich, *J. Med. Chem.*, **32**, 1378–1392 (1989).

421. H. Hori, A. Yasutake, Y. Minematsu, and J. C. Powers, in *Peptides: Structure and Function," Proceedings of the Ninth American Peptide Symposium*, D. M. Deber, V. J. Hruby, and K. D. Kopple, Eds., Pierce, Rockford, Il., 1985, pp. 812–822.

422. A. Ewenson, R. Laufer, M. Chorev, Z. Selinger, and C. Gilon, *J. Med. Chem.*, **29**, 295–299 (1986).

423. A. Ewenson, R. Laufer, M. Chorev, Z. Selinger, and C. Gilon, *J. Med. Chem.*, **31**, 416–421 (1988).

424. G. S. Garrett, T. J. Emge, S. C. Lee, E. M. Fischer, K. Dyehouse, and J. M. McIver, *J. Org. Chem.*, **56**, 4823–4826 (1991).

425. D. B. Damon and D. J. Hoover, *J. Am. Chem. Soc.*, **112**, 6439–6442 (1990).

426. P. A. Bartlett and C. K. Marlowe, *Science*, **235**, 569–571 (1987).

427. D. H. Rich, in C. Hansch, P. G. Sammes, and J. B. Taylor, Eds., *Comprehensive Medicinal Chemistry*, Pergamon, Oxford, UK, pp. 391–441.

428. W. J. Greenlee, *Med. Res. Rev.*, **10**, 173–236 (1990).

429. M. J. Wyvratt and A. A. Patchett, *Med. Res. Rev.*, **5**, 483–531 (1985).

430. T. K. Sawyer, in *Peptide-Based Drug Design: Controlling Transport and Metabolism*, in press.

431. M. W. Holladay, F. G. Salituro, and D. H. Rich, *J. Med. Chem.*, **30**, 374–383 (1987).

432. S. R. Bertenshaw, R. S. Rogers, M. K. Stern, and B. H. Norman, *J. Med. Chem.*, **36**, 173–176 (1993).

433. A. K. Ghosh, S. P. McKee, and W. J. Thompson, *J. Org. Chem.*, **56**, 6500–6503 (1991).

434. B. E. Evans, K. E. Rittle, C. F. Homnick, J. P. Springer, J. Hirshfield, and D. F. Veber, *J. Org. Chem.*, **50**, 4615–4625 (1985).

435. D. M. Jones, B. Nilsson, and M. Szelke, *J. Org. Chem.*, **58**, 2286–2290 (1993).

436. S. Thaisrivongs, A. G. Tomasselli, J. B. Moon, J. Hui, T. J. McQuade, S. R. Turner, J. W. Strohbach, W. J. Howe, W. G. Tarpley, and R. L. Heinrikson, *J. Med. Chem.*, **34**, 2344–2356 (1991).

437. W. R. Baker and S. L. Condon, *J. Org. Chem.*, **58**, 3277–3284 (1993).

438. P. Raddatz, A. Jonczyk, J. O. Minck, C. J. Schmitges, and J. Sombroek, *J. Med. Chem.*, **34**, 3267–3280 (1991).

439. D. E. Epps, J. Cheney, H. Schostarez, T. K. Sawyer, M. Prairie, W. C. Krueger, and F. Mandel, *J. Med. Chem.*, **33**, 2080–2086 (1990).

440. W. J. Thompson, P. M. D. Fitzgerald, M. K. Holloway, E. A. Emini, P. L. Darke, B. M. McKeever, W. A. Schleif, J. C. Quintero, J. A. Zugay, T. J. Tucker, J. E. Schwering, C. F. Homnick, J. Nunberg, J. P. Springer, and J. R. Huff, *J. Med. Chem.*, **35**, 1685–1701 (1992).

441. S. D. Young, L. S. Payne, W. J. Thompson, N. Gaffin, T. A. Lyle, S. F. Britcher, S. L. Graham, T. H. Schultz, A. A. Deana, P. L. Darke, J. Zugay, W. A. Schleif, J. C. Quintero, E. A. Emini, P. S. Anderson, and J. R. Huff, *J. Med. Chem.*, **35**, 1702–1709 (1992).

442. T. K. Sawyer, D. J. Staples, L. Liu, A. G. Tomasselli, J. O. Hui, K. O'Connell, H. Schostarez, J. B. Hester, J. Moon, J. W. Howe, C. W. Smith, D. L. Decamp, C. S. Craik, B. M. Dunn, W. T. Lowther, J. Harris, R. A. Poorman, A. Wlodawer, M. Jaskolski, and R. L. Heinrikson, *Int. J. Peptide Protein Res.*, **40**, 274–281 (1992).

443. T. J. Tucker, W. C. Lumma, Jr., L. S. Payne, J. M. Wai, S. J. de Solms, E. A. Giuliani, P. L. Darke, J. C. Heimbach, J. A. Zugay, W. A. Schleif, J. C. Quintero, E. A. Imini, J. R. Huff, and P. S. Anderson, *J. Med. Chem.*, **35**, 2525–2533 (1992).

444. P. Ashorn, T. J. McQuade, S. Thaisrivongs, A. G. Tomasselli, W. G. Tarpley, and B. Moss, *Proc. Natl. Acad. Sci. USA*, **87**, 7472–7476 (1990).

445. A. Calcagni, E. Gavuzzo, G. Lucente, F. Mazza, F. Pinnen, G. Pochetti, and D. Rossi, *Int. J. Peptide Protein Res.*, **34**, 471–479 (1989).

446. A. Calcagni, E. Gavuzzo, G. Lucente, F. Mazza, G. Pochetti, and D. Rossi, *Int. J. Peptide Protein Res.*, **34**, 319–324 (1989).

447. G. L. Olson, D. R. Bolin, M. P. Bonner, M. Bos, C. M. Cook, D. C. Fry, B. J. Graves, M. Hatada, D. E. Hill, M. Kahn, V. S. Madison, V. K. Rusiecki, R. Sarabu, J. Sepinwall, G. P. Vincent, and M. E. Voss, *J. Med. Chem.*, **36**, 3039–3049 (1993).

448. G. R. Lenz, S. M. Evans, D. E. Walters, and A. J. Hopfinger, Eds., *Opiates*, Academic Press, Inc., Orlando, Fla., 1986.

449. R. Schwyzer, *Ann. N.Y. Acad. Sci.*, **297**, 3–27 (1977).

450. R. Schwyzer, *Biopolymers*, **31**, 785–792 (1991).

451. P. S. Portoghese, *J. Med. Chem.*, **34**, 1757–1762 (1991).

452. S. L. Olmsted, A. E. Takemori, and P. S. Portoghese, *J. Med. Chem.*, **36**, 179–180 (1993).

453. R. M. Freidinger, *Trends Pharm. Sci.*, **10**, 270–274 (1989).

454. B. E. Evans, J. L. Leighton, K. E. Rittle, K. F. Gilbert, G. F. Lundell, N. P. Gould, D. W. Hobbs, R. M. DiPardo, D. F. Veber, D. J. Pettibone, B. V. Clineschmidt, P. S. Anderson, and R. M. Freidinger, *J. Med. Chem.*, **35**, 3919–3927 (1992).

455. R. M. Keenan, J. Weinstock, J. A. Finkelstein, R. G. Franz, D. E. Gaitanopoulos, G. R. Girard, D. T. Hill, T. M. Morgan, J. M. Samanen, and J. Hempel, *J. Med. Chem.*, **35**, 3858–3872 (1992).

456. B. A. Bunin and J. A. Ellman, *J. Am. Chem. Soc.*, **114**, 10997–10998 (1991).

457. R. Hirschmann, K. C. Nicolaou, S. Pietranico, J. Salvino, E. M. Leahy, P. A. Sprengeler, G. Furst, A. B. Smith, III, C. D. Strader, M. A. Cascieri, M. R. Candelor, C. Donaldson, W. Vale, and L. Maechler, *J. Am. Chem. Soc.*, **114**, 9217–9218 (1992).

458. R. Hirschmann, P. A. Sprengeler, T. Kawasaki, L. W. Leahy, W. C. Shakespeare, and A. B. Smith, III, *J. Am. Chem. Soc.*, **114**, 9699–9701 (1992).

CHAPTER TWENTY-ONE

Oligonucleotide Therapeutics

STANLEY T. CROOKE

Isis Pharmaceuticals
Carlsbad, California, USA

CONTENTS

1 Introduction, 864
2 Pharmacodynamics, 864
  2.1 Interactions with nucleic acids, 865
    2.1.1 RNA intermediary metabolism, 865
    2.1.2 Affinity, 865
    2.1.3 Specificity, 866
    2.1.4 Nucleic acid selectivity, 867
    2.1.5 RNA structure, 867
  2.2 Mechanisms of action of oligonucleotides interacting with nucleic acid targets, 869
    2.2.1 Occupancy-only mediated mechanisms, 869
      2.2.1.1 Transcriptional arrest, 869
      2.2.1.2 Inhibition of splicing, 871
      2.2.1.3 Translational arrest, 871
      2.2.1.4 Disruption of necessary RNA structure, 872
    2.2.2 Occupancy activated destabilization, 872
      2.2.2.1 5' Capping, 872
      2.2.2.2 Inhibition of 3' polyadenylation, 873
      2.2.2.3 Other mechanisms, 873
      2.2.2.4 Activation of RNase H, 873
    2.2.3 Covalent modification of the target nucleic acid by the oligonucleotide, 874
    2.2.4 Oligonucleotide induced cleavage of nucleic acid targets, 875
  2.3 Influence of receptor sequences in RNA on activity, 876
  2.4 Interactions with Nonnucleic Acid Targets, 877
3 Pharmacokinetics, 877
  3.1 Nuclease stability, 877
  3.2 Intracellular stability, 878
  3.3 Cellular uptake and distribution, 879

Burger's Medicinal Chemistry and Drug Discovery,
Fifth Edition, Volume 1: Principles and Practice,
Edited by Manfred E. Wolff.
ISBN 0-471-57556-9 © 1995 John Wiley & Sons, Inc.

3.4 *In vivo* pharmacokinetics, 881
3.5 Toxicology, 882
4 Medicinal Chemistry, 883
    4.1 Heterocycle modifications, 884
        4.1.1 Pyrimidine modifications, 884
        4.1.2 Purine modifications, 885
        4.1.3 Oligonucleotide conjugates, 885
        4.1.4 Nuclease stability, 886
    4.2 Enhanced cellular uptake, 887
    4.3 Cleavage reagents, 888
    4.4 Sugar modifications, 888
    4.5 Backbone modifications, 888
    4.6 Activities of oligonucleotides, 890
        4.6.1 Activities in cells in tissue culture, 891
        4.6.2 *In vivo*, 893
5 Conclusions, 894

1 INTRODUCTION

Recently, considerable interest in the therapeutic application of oligonucleotides has developed. Although the initial interest in oligonucleotides focused on their interactions with nucleic acid receptors, as the chemical and biological properties of the array of novel oligonucleotides have been better appreciated, interest has broadened to include the use of oligonucleotides as ligands to interact with non-nucleic acid receptors as well.

Conceptually, oligonucleotides can be designed to hybridize with single or double-stranded nucleic acids. Hybridization with single-stranded nucleic acids occurs via Watson-Crick patterns of hydrogen bonding. These interactions are well understood and provide a framework for the facile design of highly specific oligonucleotides. Interactions with double-stranded nucleic acids and oligonucleotides comprised of natural bases occur via non-Watson-Crick hydrogen bonding motifs and require regions in which the targeted double-stranded nucleic acid has stretches of purine bases on one strand complemented to pyrimidine bases on the opposite strand. This obviously poses significant limitations on the therapeutic utility of such approaches as design

of oligonucleotides is limited to stretches of polypurines and polypyrimidines. However, recent progress suggests that even this limitation is yielding to medicinal chemistry approaches (see medicinal chemistry section).

The demonstration that oligonucleotides may interact with non-nucleic acid targets, e.g., proteins, with sequence, nucleic acid type and secondary structure specificity was, of course, predicted by the behavior of natural nucleic acids. However, the creation of libraries of oligonucleotide analogs greatly facilitates the exploration of these potential interactions for therapeutic purposes.

The chapter attempts to summarize the recent progress on oligonucleotides that may have therapeutic activity by interacting with any of the potential targets yet considered. The objective is to place oligonucleotide therapeutics in the context of modern drug discovery and development.

2 PHARMACODYNAMICS

Conceptually, oligonucleotide drug effects can be rationalized by traditional receptor theory and basic concepts concerning drug action.

2.1 Interactions with Nucleic Acids

2.1.1 RNA INTERMEDIARY METABOLISM. Oligonucleotides are designed to modulate the information transfer from gene to protein—in essence, to alter the intermediary metabolism of RNA. Figure 21.1 summarizes the processes.

RNA intermediary metabolism is initiated with transcription. The transcription initiation complex contains proteins that recognize specific DNA sequences and locally denature double-stranded DNA, thus allowing a member of the RNA polymerase family to transcribe one strand of the DNA (the antisense strand) into a sense pre-mRNA molecule. Usually during transcription, the 5′ end of the pre-mRNA is capped by adding a methyl-guanosine and most often by methylation of one or two adjacent sugar residues. This enhances the stability of the pre-mRNA and may play a role in a number of key RNA processing events (1). Between the 5′ cap and the site at which translation is initiated is usually a stretch of nucleotides; this area

may play a key role in regulating mRNA half-life (2).

2.1.2 AFFINITY. The affinity of oligonucleotides for their receptor sequences results from hybridization interactions. The two major contributors to the free energy of binding are hydrogen bonding (usually Watson-Crick base pairing) and base stacking in the double helix that is formed. Affinity is affected by ionic strength. Affinity results from hydrogen bonding between complementary base pairs and the reduction in entropy resulting from the stacking of the coplanar bases. Consequently, affinity increases as the length of the oligonucleotide receptor complex increases. Affinity also varies as a function of the sequence in the duplex. Nearest neighbor rules allow the prediction of the free energy of binding for DNA–DNA and RNA–RNA hybrids with relatively high precision (3, 4).

Recent progress has resulted in more precise characterization of the affinities of DNA–RNA duplexes. As a general rule,

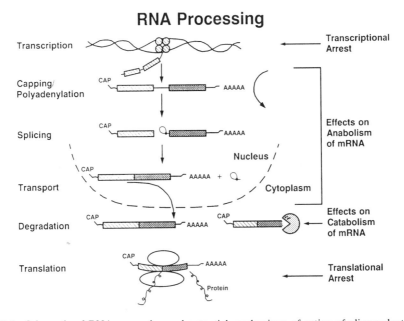

Fig. 21.1 Schematic of RNA processing and potential mechanisms of action of oligonucleotides.

RNA–RNA duplexes are more stable than DNA–RNA duplexes, but the stabilities of duplexes are affected by the sequences (5).

As will be discussed in considerable detail later in this review, numerous modifications have been introduced into oligonucleotides. Based on the substantial amount of medicinal chemistry performed in the recent past, it is clear that modifications can be introduced into bases, sugars and/or the backbone that have no effect on or enhance affinity for single-stranded DNA or for RNA. Of course, there are modifications that are not tolerated and result in significant losses of affinity. As an example, Figure 21.2 provides a summary of a few modifications in the 2′ position and their effects on the affinity of oligonucleotides for DNA or RNA.

2.1.3 SPECIFICITY. Specificity derives from the selectivity of Watson–Crick or other types of base pairing. The decrease in affinity associated with a mismatched base pair varies as a function of the specific mismatch, the position of the mismatch in a region of complementarity, and the sequence surrounding the mismatch. The $\Delta\Delta G^0 37$, or change in Gibbs free energy of binding induced by a single mismatch, varies from $+0.2$ to $+4.9\,kcal/mol$ per modification at $100\,mM$ NaCl. Thus, on average, a single base mismatch results in a change in affinity of approximately 500 fold (6). Modifications of oligonucleotides can alter specificity.

Based on the differences in affinity of oligonucleotides for their complementary target sequence, calculations suggest that unmodified oligodeoxynucleotides between 11–15 in length should be able to selectively bind to a single RNA species in the cell (7). Studies in our laboratories have demonstrated that affinities predicted by nearest neighbor analyses are useful in rational drug design (6). For example, using strategies based on nearest neighbor predictions, it is possible to selectively inhibit the production of mutant RAS containing a single base change in the mRNA vs. normal RAS in cells in tissue culture (8).

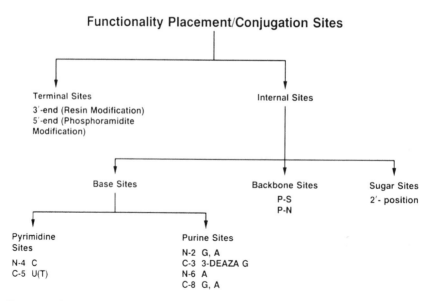

Fig. 21.2 Summary of a few modifications in the 2′ position and then effects on the affinity of oligonucleotides for DNA or RNA.

2.1.4 NUCLEIC ACID SELECTIVITY. The 2'-hydroxyl in RNA results in the sugar assuming a different conformation from that in DNA. RNA–RNA duplexes assume an A-form double helix, whereas DNA–DNA duplexes assume an A-form double helix, whereas DNA–DNA duplexes assume a B-form double helix. Consequently, it is possible to modify oligonucleotides so that they bind more tightly to RNA or DNA sequences (9). For example, in Table 21.1, 2'-F, 2'-methoxy and 2'-propoxy all increase the affinity of oligonucleotides for RNA while having minimal effects on binding to DNA.

2.1.5 RNA STRUCTURE. RNA can assume a variety of secondary structures deriving from intramolecular base pairing. The simplest structures are stemloops in which double-stranded regions are interspersed with loops and random coils. More complex structures, described as pseudoknots, also form (10). These structures are

Table 21.1 Qualitative Comparison of Backbone Modifications

Natural phosphodiester linkage   Synthetic backbone modifications

		$3' \rightarrow 5'$ Linker Atoms			
	L_1	L_2	L_3	$T_M{}^b$	Nuclease Resistance[b]
Phosphate	O	PO_2	P	+ +	−
Carbonate	O	C = O	O		+
Carbamate	O	C = O	NH	− / +	+ +
Silyl	O	SiR	O	?	+ +
Sulfur	CH_2	S(O)N	CH_2	+ + + ?	X
Sulfonate	O	SO_2	CH_2	X	X
Sulfonamide	O	SO_2	NH	+ +	+ +
Formacetal	O	CH_2	O	X	+ +
Thioformacetal	O	CH_2	S	−	+ +
Oxime	CH_2	=N	O	− / +	+ +
Methyleneimino	CH_2	NH	O	+ +	+ +
Methylene (methylimino) MMI	CH_2	NCH_3	O	+ +	+ +
Methylene (dimethylhydrazo) MDH	CH_2	NCH_3	CH_3	+ +	+ +
Methyleneoxy (methylimino) MOMI	CH_2	O	NCH_3	+	+ +

[a](Modified from ref. 196).
[b]X indicates data not available.

profoundly important in determining RNA function and influencing the ability of oligonucleotides to bind to their RNA targets. The types of effects of bound oligonucleotides on RNA function are affected by RNA structure as well.

Some of the types of structures that RNA can assume are shown in Figure 21.3. The stability of such structures varies as a function of the length of double-stranded stem, the sequence and other factors, and it is likely that in the cell, RNA molecules assume structures that represent equilibria between various potential, relatively stable structures. It is also likely that the secondary structures of RNA are very dynamic and, of course, RNA is often complexed with proteins.

Recent laboratory studies provide insights that support that promulgation of rules that facilitate the design of oligonucleotides that can interact with structures RNA (11, 12), and these are shown below.

1. Optimization begins with analysis of the structured target. Binding strategies should minimize the energy required to break structure in the target RNA by exploiting its weakest elements, such as loop regions, short stems and bulged bases, and by avoiding long continuous stems.

2. Affinity is increased by maximizing the *total* number of binding interactions in the hybrid complex, including base pairs between the oligonucleotide and target, and new base pairs in the rearranged target.

3. Topological considerations are essential to maximize stem lengths in the complex and minimize loop lengths.

4. The most stable heteroduplexes are formed by targeting sequences that maximize base stacking.

5. In contrast to "linear" RNA targets, the number of base pairs that can be complemented in structured RNA is often limited. Therefore, an oligonucleotide with the highest affinity per base pair should be used. 2'-*O*-methyl oligonucleotides are currently one of the highest affinity analogs available. In addition, they are resistant to nucleolytic degradation and can be used in cell culture experiments (13).

6. The oligonucleotide should not have strong internal structure or form stable dimers.

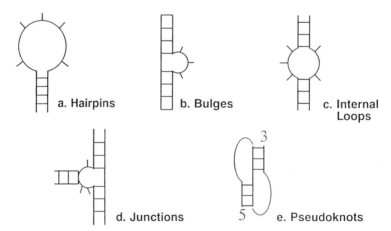

Fig. 21.3 Examples of structured RNAs. In each example, there are both single-stranded regions that are constrained by being contained within a more complex structure. Experimental evidence has shown that in some cases these regions can be used to initiate hybridization with an oligonucleotide which then propagate heteroduplex formation into the double-stranded regions, resulting in disruption of existing base pairing. This figure was redrawn from Puglisi et al. (10).

7. All bases in the oligomer should be involved in binding. Unpaired bases (as in the ATWA-17-mer) cause loss of specificity by increasing the likelihood of hybridization at non-target sites while not contributing to affinity at the target site. Moreover, longer oligonucleotides have greater potential for internal structure.

8. Biological utility of the structured RNA must be compromised by oligonucleotide binding.

More complicated structures can also be formed with DNA-like oligonucleotides and RNA. NMR studies suggest that, in DNA–RNA duplexes, the RNA assumes an A-like quality, and the DNA strand assumes a non-A-like conformation. Triple stranded structures can also be formed. Triple helical structures can be formed between DNA and RNA strands. When formed, the strands adopt a conformation intermediate between A-form and B-form. Moreover, significant variations in stability of the triplex have been noted such that a triplex comprised of a single-stranded RNA and a double-stranded DNA or double-stranded DNA–RNA hairpin loop is much more stable than triplexes formed from other components (14).

2.2 Mechanisms of Action of Oligonucleotides Interacting with Nucleic Acid Targets

The mechanisms by which interactions of oligonucleotides with nucleic acids may induce biological effects are complex and potentially numerous. Furthermore, very little is currently understood about the roles of various mechanisms or the factors that may determine which mechanisms are involved after oligonucleotides bind to their receptor sequences. Consequently, a discussion of mechanisms remains largely theoretical.

2.2.1 OCCUPANCY-ONLY MEDIATED MECHANISMS. Classic competitive antagonists are thought to alter biological activities because they bind to receptors preventing natural agonists from binding and inducing normal biological processes. Binding of oligonucleotides to specific sequences may inhibit the interaction of the RNA or DNA with proteins, other nucleic acids or other factors required for essential steps in the intermediary metabolism of the RNA or its utilization by the cell.

2.2.1.1 *Transcriptional Arrest.* Oligonucleotides may bind to DNA and prevent either initiation or elongation of transcription by preventing effective binding of factors required for transcription, thus producing transcriptional arrest. Although it is possible that oligonucleotides could bind to segments of DNA that are partially denatured by the transcription complex, this is highly unlikely. The initiation and elongation of transcription require a complex set of proteins and other factors, and it is difficult to conceive of a mechanism by which oligonucleotides might compete effectively against the transcriptional machinery for these single-stranded regions. Nevertheless, there are reports of activities that can be explained most simply by this mechanism (15, 16). Additionally, Helene and colleagues (17) reported that hexanucleotides to nonanucleotides with acridine derivatives at the 3′-terminus inhibited transcription of the β-lactamase gene. However, they also reported that when the RNA polymerase was preincubated with the oligonucleotide-acridine adducts, nonspecific inhibition was observed (18).

More recently, Neilson et al. (19) have reported on a highly modified oligonucleotide structure that appears to bind to DNA with very high affinity, via a mechanism whereby one of the DNA duplex strands is displaced by the incoming ligand. This ligand consists of an achiral polyamide backbone of aminoethylglycyl units linked to thymine. This class of structures, known as peptidelike nucleic acids (PNA), may provide extremely useful pharmacophores for designing molecules to bind specifically and tightly to DNA and other natural nucleic acid structures.

The alternative to seeking a transient single-stranded region, or to attempting to denature a double-stranded region of DNA is to inhibit transcription by interacting with double-stranded DNA, i.e., forming triple-stranded structures. To form triple-stranded structures, hydrogen bonds, other than Watson-Crick, must be formed. In most current triple-strand motifs, the oligonucleotide becomes the third strand by recognizing hydrogen bonding donor/acceptor sites on a purine reference strand and lying in the major groove, i.e., Hoogstein binding motif (20–28). Alternative motifs have also been proposed. For example, Hogan and colleagues (29) proposed that a purine rich oligonucleotide can form a triplex structure based upon the purines in the oligonucleotide base pairing in parallel fashion with the purines in the duplex DNA. However, other studies by Dervan's group (30) suggested that the purine rich oligonucleotide bound to the duplex DNA with an antiparallel orientation.

The formation of triple-stranded structures using natural nucleosides requires runs of purines Watson-Crick hydrogen bonded to their complementary pyrimidines. When cystidine is used to form a triple strand with a G-C base pair, it must be protonated, and this occurs at nonphysiological acid conditions (25). Furthermore, all motifs employ one or more "weak" hydrogen bonds, and thus to achieve sufficient stability, relatively long triple-strand structures are required.

The principal theoretical advantage of triple helical inhibition schemes is that transcription represents the first step in the intermediary metabolism of RNA and may, therefore, provide substantial leverage for drug therapy. The other advantages that have been suggested are much more speculative. For example, it has been sug-

gested that the smaller number of genes (one or two) compared to the number of mRNA molecules (usually less than 1000) per cell is an advantage for approaches that inhibit transcription. However, this ignores the kinetics of the targets. Genes have an infinite half-life relative to cell life. RNA molecules are synthesized and degraded with varying kinetics. Furthermore, a variety of mechanisms exist to assure that even covalent modifications of DNA are repaired. Another concept has been that triple helixes in DNA might produce permanent biological effects. That this is entirely specious is shown by the fact that even alkylating and DNA cleaving anticancer drugs do not produce permanent effects.

A number of theoretical disadvantages of triple helical inhibition of transcription have also been enumerated. It is thought that homopurine–homopyrimidine sequences may play important regulatory roles in DNA as they are much more abundant than statistically predicted (31). Longer term, a more substantial problem may simply be gaining sequence-specific access to DNA in chromatin. Additionally, deliberate interactions with the genome raise concerns about mutagenicity, carcinogenicity and teratogenicity which, in most therapeutic settings, are of considerable importance.

Several strategies have been developed to circumvent the requirement for purine–pyrimidine runs and other limitations. For example, purine oligonucleotides form triplex structures at higher pH values than pyrimidine rich oligonucleotides (29, 30). Similarly, pyrimidine rich oligonucleotides in which 2'-O-methyl pseudoisocytidine was substituted for 2'-deoxycytidine formed triplex structures at neutral pH (32). Oligonucleotides with linkers that allow crossover of the oligopyrimidine from one strand of the duplex to the other have been reported, and this motif suggested to be a solution to the creation of a broader sequence repertoire (33). To enhance the stability of triple helices, intercalators and photoactivable crosslinkers and alkylators have been conjugated to oligo pyrimidines (34–36). To increase potency and enable identification of sites of binding, a number of cleavage moieties have been conjugated to oligopyrimidines (37–42). Finally, to enhance nuclease stability, methylphosphonates (43) and α-oligonucleotides (41) have been shown or suggested to form triple helices.

In addition to cleavage of DNA *in vitro* by triplex-forming oligonucleotides coupled to cleavage reagents and alkylation induced by oligonucleotide-coupled alkylators, several other methods have been used to show triplex formation. These include agarose affinity column purification (44), NMR (45), protection from UV dimerization (46), solution hybridization (47), inhibition of binding of DNA binding proteins (48), inhibition of restriction endonucleases (49), and repression of c-myc transcription *in vitro* (29). Recently, a 28-mer phosphodiester stabilized at the 3' end by propylamine directed to enhancer elements for the IL-2 receptor gene was shown to inhibit the transcription of the gene when incubated with human lymphocytes. The authors reported evidence for selectivity as well (50).

Obviously, triple helix-based inhibition of transcription is of potential therapeutic importance, particularly for targets, that for a variety of reasons may be difficult to inhibit at the post-transcriptional level. However, substantial medicinal chemistry must be completed to create oligonucleotides that can interact with duplex structures in a sequence-specific fashion without requiring special motifs. Once this is accomplished, of course, additional studies must show that the other theoretical limitations previously discussed can be overcome.

2.2.1.2 *Inhibition of Splicing.*

A key step in the intermediary metabolism of most mRNA molecules is the excision of introns.

These "splicing" reactions are sequence specific and require the concerted action of splicesomes. Consequently, oligonucleotides that bind to sequences required for splicing may prevent binding of necessary factors or physically prevent the required cleavage reactions. This then would result in interactions of the production of the mature mRNA. Although there are several examples of oligonucleotides directed to splice junctions, none of the studies presented data showing inhibition of RNA processing, accumulation of splicing intermediates or a reduction in mature mRNA. Nor are there published data in which the structure of the RNA at the splice junction was probed and the oligonucleotides demonstrated to hybridize to the sequences for which they were designed (51–54). Activities have been reported for anti-c-myc and antiviral oligonucleotides with phosphodiester, methylphosphonate and phosphorothioate backbones.

2.2.1.3 *Translational Arrest.*

The mechanism for which the majority of oligonucleotides have been designed is translational arrest by binding to the translation initiation codon. The positioning of the initiation codon within the area of complementarity of the oligonucleotide and the length of oligonucleotide used have varied considerably. Again, unfortunately, only in relatively few studies have the oligonucleotides, in fact, been shown to bind to the sites for which they were designed and other data that support translation arrest as the mechanism been reported.

Target RNA species that have been reported to be inhibited include HIV (55), vesicular stomatitis virus (VSV) (56), n-myc (57) and a number of normal cellular genes (58–61).

A significant number of targets may be inhibited by binding to translation initiation codons. For example, ISIS 1082 hybridizes to the AUG codon for the UL13 gene of herpes virus types 1 and 2. RNase H studies confirmed that it binds selectively in this area. In vitro protein synthesis studies confirmed that it inhibited the synthesis of the UL13 protein, and studies in HeLa cells showed that in inhibited the growth of herpes type 1 and type 2 with IC_{50} of 200–400 nM by translation arrest (62). Similarly, ISIS 1753, a 30-mer phosphorathioate complementary to the translation initiation codon and surrounding sequences of the E2 gene of bovine papilloma virus, was highly effective, and its activity was shown to be due to translation arrest. ISIS 2105, a 20 mer phosphorothioate complementary to the same region in human papilloma virus, was shown to be a very potent inhibitor. Compounds complementary to the translation initiation codon of the E2 gene were the most potent of the more than 50 compounds studied complementary to various other regions in the RNA (63).

In conclusion, translation arrest represents an important mechanism of action for antisense drugs. A number of examples purporting to employ this mechanism have been reported and recent studies on several compounds have provided data that unambiguously demonstrate that this mechanism can result in potent antisense drugs.

2.2.1.4 Disruption of Necessary RNA Structure.

RNA adopts a variety of three-dimensional structures induced by intramolecular hybridization, the most common of which is the stem loop. These structures play crucial roles in a variety of functions. They are used to provide additional stability for RNA and as recognition motifs for a number of proteins, nucleic acids and ribonucleoproteins that participate in the intermediary metabolism and activities of RNA species. Thus, given the potential general activity of the mechanism, it is surprising that occupancy-based disruption RNA has not been more extensively exploited.

As an example we designed a series of oligonucleotides that bind to the important step-loop present in all RNA species in HIV, the TAR element. We synthesized a number of oligonucleotides designed to disrupt TAR, showed that several indeed did bind to TAR, disrupt the structure, and inhibit TAR- mediated production of a reporter gene (64). Furthermore, general rules useful in disrupting stem-loop structures were developed as well (11).

Although designed to induce relatively non-specific cytotoxic effects, two other examples are noteworthy. Oligonucleotides designed to bind to a 17 nucleotide loop in Xenopus 28 S RNA required for ribosome stability and protein synthesis inhibited protein synthesis when injected into Xenopus oocytes (65). Similarly, oligonucleotides designed to bind to highly conserved sequences in 5.8 S RNA inhibited protein synthesis in rabbit reticulocyte and wheat germ systems (66).

2.2.2 OCCUPANCY ACTIVATED DESTABILIZATION.

RNA molecules regulate their own metabolism. A number of structural features of RNA are known to influence stability, various processing events, subcellular distribution and transport. It is likely that, as RNA intermediary metabolism is better understood, many other regulatory features and mechanisms will be identified.

2.2.2.1 5′ Capping.

A key early step in RNA processing is 5′ capping (Fig. 21.1). This stabilizes pre-mRNA and is important for the stability of mature mRNA. It also is important in binding to the nuclear matrix and transport of mRNA out of the nucleus. As the structure of the cap is unique and understood, it presents an interesting target.

Several oligonucleotides that bind near the cap site have been shown to be active, presumably by inhibiting the binding of proteins required to cap the RNA. However, again, in no published study has this putative mechanism been rigorously demonstrated. In fact, in no published study have the oligonucleotides been shown to bind to the sequences for which they were designed. For example, the synthesis of SV40 T-antigen was reported to be most sensitive to an oligonucleotide linked to polylysine and targeted to the 5′ cap site of RNA (67).

In studies in our laboratory, we have designed oligonucleotides to bind to 5′ cap structures and reagents to specifically cleave the unique 5′ cap structure (68).

2.2.2.2 Inhibition of 3′ Polyadenylation.
In the 3′ untranslated region of pre-mRNA molecules are sequences that result in the post-transcriptional addition of long (hundreds of nucleotides) tracts of polyadenylate. Polyadenylation stabilizes mRNA and may play other roles in the intermediary metabolism of RNA species. Theoretically, interactions in the 3′ terminal region of pre-mRNA could inhibit polyadenylation and destabilize the RNA species. Although there are a number of oligonucleotides that interact in the 3′ untranslated region and display antisense activities (69), to date, no study has reported evidence for alterations in polyadenylation.

2.2.2.3 Other Mechanisms.
In addition to 5′ capping and 3′ adenylation, there are clearly other sequences in the 5′ and 3′ untranslated regions of mRNA that affect the stability of the molecules. Again, there are a number of antisense drugs that may work by these mechanisms.

Zamecnik and Stephenson (70) reported that 13 mer targeted to untranslated 3′ and 5′ terminal sequences in Rous sarcoma viruses was active. Oligonucleotides conjugated to an acridine derivative and targeted to a 3′-terminal sequence in type A influences viruses were reported to be active (71–73). Against several RNA targets, studies in our laboratories have shown that

sequences in the 3′ untranslated region of RNA molecules are often the most sensitive. For example, ISIS 1939 is a 20 mer phosphorothioate that binds to and appears to disrupt a predicted stem-loop structure in the 3′ untranslated region of the mRNA for ICAM is a potent antisense inhibitor. However, inasmuch a 2′-O-methyl analog of ISIS 1939 was much less active, it is likely that, in addition to destabilization to cellular nucleolytic activity, activation of RNase H (see below) is also involved in the activity of ISIS 1939 (69).

2.2.2.4 Activation of RNASE H.
RNase H is an ubiquitous enzyme that degrades the RNA strand of an RNA–DNA duplex. It has been identified in organisms as diverse as viruses to human cells (for review see ref. 74). At least two classes of RNase H have been identified in eukaryotic cells. Multiple enzymes with RNase H activity have been observed in prokaryotics (74). Furthermore, there are data that suggest that in eukaryotic cells there are multiple isozymes.

Although RNase H is involved in DNA replication, it may play other roles in the cell and is found in the cytoplasm as well as the nucleus (75). However, the concentration of the enzyme in the nucleus is thought to be greater and some of the enzyme found in cytoplasmic preparations may be due to nuclear leakage.

RNase H activity is quite variable. It is absent or minimal in rabbit reticulocytes (76), but present in wheat germ extracts (74). In HL60 cells, for example, the level of activity in undifferentiated cells is greatest, relatively high in DMSO and Vitamin D differentiated cells, and much lower in PMA-differentiated cells (77).

The precise recognition elements for RNase H are not known. However, it has been shown that oligonucleotides with DNA-like properties as shown as tetramers can activate RNase H (78). Changes in the sugar influence RNase H activation as sugar modifications that result in RNA-like oligonucleotide, e.g., 2'-fluoro or 2'-O-methyl, do not appear to serve as substrates for RNase H (79–80). Alterations in the orientation of the sugar to the base can also affect RNase H activation as α-oligonucleotides are unable to induce RNase H or may require parallel annealing (81–82). Additionally, backbone modifications influence the ability of oligonucleotides to active RNase H. Methylphosphonates do not activate RNase H (48, 83). In contrast, phosphorothioates are excellent substrates (62, 77, 84, 85). More recently, chimeric molecules have been studied as oligonucleotides to bind to RNA and activate RNase H (86, 87). For example, oligonucleotides comprised of wings of 2'-O-methyl phosphonates and a five-base gap of deoxyoligonucleotides bind to their target RNA and activate RNase H (86, 87). Furthermore, a single ribonucleotide in a sequence of deoxyribonucleotides was shown to be sufficient to serve as a substrate for RNase H when bound to its complementary deoxyoligonucleotide (88).

That it is possible to take advantage of chimeric oligonucleotides designed to activate RNase H only at relatively limited lengths of RNA receptors to enhance specificity has also been demonstrated (89–90). In a recent study, RNase H mediated cleavage of target transcript was much more selective when deoxyoligonucleotides comprised of methylphosphonate deoxyoligonucleotide wings and phosphodiester gaps were compared to full phosphodiester oligonucleotides.

Despite the information about RNase H and the demonstrations that many oligonucleotides may activate RNase H in lysate and purified enzyme assays (91–93), relatively little is yet known about the role of structural features in RNA targets in activating RNase H and direct proof that RNase H activation is, in fact, the mechanism of action of oligonucleotides in cells.

Recent studies in our laboratories pro-

vide additional, albeit indirect, insights into these questions. ISIS 1939 is a 20 mer phosphorothioate complementary to a sequence in the 3' untranslated region of ICAM-1 RNA (69). It inhibits ICAM production in human umbilical vein endothelial cells, and northern blots demonstrate that ICAM-1 mRNA is rapidly degraded. A 2'-O-methyl analog of ISIS 1939 displays higher affinity for the RNA than the phosphorothioate, is stable in cells, but inhibits ICAM-1 protein production much less potently than ISIS 1939. It is likely that ISIS 1939 destabilizes the RNA and activates RNase H. In contrast, ISIS 1570 and 18 mer phosphorothioate that is complementary to the translation initiation codon of the ICAM-1 message inhibited production of the protein, but caused no degradation of the RNA. Thus, two oligonucleotides that are capable of activating RNase H had different effects, depending on the site in the mRNA at which they bound (69).

2.2.3 COVALENT MODIFICATION OF THE TARGET NUCLEIC ACID BY THE OLIGONUCLEOTIDE. A large number of oligonucleotides conjugated to alkylating and photoactivable alkylating species have been synthesized and tested for effects on purified nucleic acids and intracellular nucleic acid targets (93–98). The potential disadvantages are equally obvious: nonspecific alkylation may occur *in vivo* and result in toxicities.

A variety of alkylating agents have been used to covalently modify single stranded DNA and shown to induce alkylation at sequences predicted by the complementary oligonucleotide to which they were attached (94–98). Similar alkylators have been employed to covalently modify double-stranded DNA after triplex formation (29, 42, 99, 100).

Photoactivable cross-linkers and platinates have been coupled to oligonucleotides and shown to crosslink sequence specifically as well. Photoactivable cross-linkers coupled to phosphodiesters, methylphosphonates and phosphorothio-ates have been shown to produce sequence-specific cross-linking (35, 101–107). Photo reactive cross-linking has also been demonstrated for double stranded DNA after triplex formation (41, 106).

Preliminary data suggesting that covalent modifications of nucleic acids in cells is feasible and may enhance the potency of oligonucleotides have also been reported. Psoralen-linked methylphosphonate oligonucleotides were reported to be significantly more potent than methylphosphonate oligonucleotides in inhibiting rabbit globin mRNA in rabbit reticulocyte lysate assay (109). Psoralen-linked methylphosphonates were also reported to be more potent in inhibiting herpes simplex virus infection in HeLa cells in tissue culture (52). Additionally, although not producing covalent modification, a 9 mer phosphodiester conjugated with an intercalator inhibited mutant Ha-ras synthesis in T-24 bladder carcinoma cells (110).

2.2.4 OLIGONUCLEOTIDE INDUCED CLEAVAGE OF NUCLEIC ACID TARGETS. Another attractive mechanism by which the potency of oligonucleotides might be increased is to synthesize derivatives that cleave their nucleic acid targets directly. Several potential chemical mechanisms are being studied and positive results have been reported.

The mechanism that has been most broadly studied is to conjugate oligonucleotides to chelators of redox-active metals and generate free radicals that can cleave nucleic acids. Dervan and colleagues have developed EDTA-conjugated oligonucleotides that cleave double-stranded DNA sequence specifically after triplex formation (28, 42). Dervan and others have also employed EDTA-oligonucleotide conjugates to cleave single-stranded DNA (111,112). It is thought that EDTA-chelated iron generates hydroxyl radicals via a fentonlike

reaction that cleave the DNA. However, the cleavage occurs at several several oligonucleotides near the nucleotide at which EDTA is attached rather than with absolute specificity.

In the presence of copper, oligonucleotides conjugated to 2,10-phenanthroline also cleave DNA via a free radical mechanism with some sequence specificity (38–40, 113–114), as do porphyrin-linked oligonucleotides oligonucleotides when exposed to light (115–117). Porphyrin-linked oligonucleotides, however, oxidize bases and induce crosslinks as well as cleave the phosphodiester backbone.

To date, no reports have demonstrated selective cleavage of an RNA or enhanced potency of oligonucleotides in cells using oligonucleotides and cleaving moieties that employ these mechanisms. However, it seems likely that studies in progress in a number of laboratories will explore this question shortly.

Another mechanism that may be intrinsically more attractive for therapeutic applications, particularly for cleavage of RNA targets, is a mechanism analogous to that used by many ribonucleases, nucleotodiyltransferases, phosphotransferases and ribozymes.

Ribozymes are oligoribonucleotides or RNA species capable of cleaving themselves or other RNA molecules (118). Furthermore, the Tetrahymena ribozyme has been shown to cleave DNA, but at a slower range than RNA (113). Although several classes of ribozymes have been identified and differ with regard to substrate specificity, the use of internal or external guanosine and other characteristics, they all employ similar enzymatic mechanisms. Cleavage and ligation involve a Mg^{2+}-dependent transesterification with nucleophilic attack by the 3′-hydroxyl of guanosine (119).

The notion that a relatively small oligonucleotide could be designed that could interact with desired sequences as ribozyme therapeutics was given impetus by studies that showed activity for ribozymes as short as a 19 mer (120), and the demonstration that ribozyme activity can be retained after substitutions, such as phosphorothioates, are introduced (119).

Consequently, creating oligonucleotides that cleave RNA targets by synthesizing oligonucleotides with appropriate tethers and functionalities positioned to catalyze degradation via acid-base mechanisms (121) is an attractive possibility.

In conclusion, an array of potential post-binding mechanisms has already been identified for oligonucleotides. However, for specific oligonucleotides, insufficient data are available to draw firm conclusions about mechanism, and it is likely that more than one mechanism may play a role in the activity of a given oligonucleotide.

Perhaps more importantly, it is clear that many additional mechanisms are likely

to be identified as progress continues. It is important to consider the structure and function of receptor sequences in designing oligonucleotides, and to continue to study potential mechanisms in detail. Clearly, RNase H may play a role in the mechanisms of many oligonucleotides, but equally clearly, it is not critical for the activity of others. In the future, the mechanisms (and resulting efficacy) for which oligonucleotides are designed will probably be optimized for each drug target and chemical class of oligonucleotide.

2.3 Influence of Receptor Sequences in RNA on Activity

The selection of the optimal site for binding of an oligonucleotide in a specific pre-mRNA or mRNA molecule is complex and still largely empirical. A number of factors,

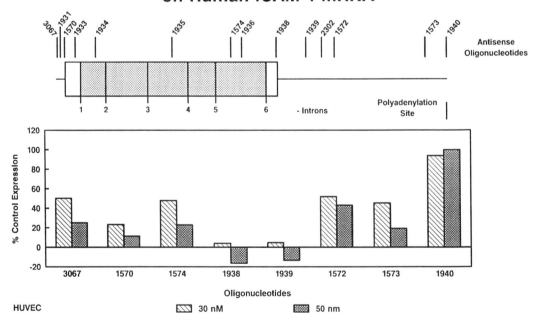

Fig. 21.4 cDNA map of human intercellular adhesion molecule 1 (ICAM-1) and the activities of several oligonucleotides. Each oligonucleotide was a 20 mer phosphorothioate deoxyoligonucleotide. For detailed methods, see reference 69.

including the chemistry of the oligonucleotide, the local structure of the RNA target, the functions of the site to which the oligonucleotide binds, the terminating mechanism, and cell type influence the relative potency derived from interactions at different sites in an RNA molecule.

Figure 21.4 shows a map of the cDNA for human ICAM and the activities of a few exemplary oligonucleotides. All of the oligonucleotides shown are deoxyoligonucleotides with phosphorothioate backbones and of equal length. All should activate RNase H. Clearly, however, there are wide variations in potency that cannot be explained simply by differences in affinity or other relatively simple notions.

In our laboratory, we have made qualitative comparisons of the sites in various RNA targets that display greatest sensitivity to phosphorothioate deoxyoligonucleotides and whether reduction in the mature mRNA content is noted in cells treated with the most active oligonucleotides. At present, no generic patterns have emerged, although more detailed analyses on target sequences within specific mRNA species suggest that oligonucleotides that bind to sites that induce greater loss of mRNA are more potent. For example, the most potent inhibitor of ICAM production is ISIS 1939, a compound that binds to a site in the 3' untranslated region and results in an extensive degradation of ICAM mRNA that is due to RNase H activation and other mechanisms (69).

2.4 Interactions with Non-Nucleic Acid Targets

Conceptually, oligonucleotides can be used to bind to non-nucleic acid targets and most attention has been focused on interactions with proteins. Although considerable information concerning protein–nucleic acid interactions deriving from studies on nucleic acid binding proteins is available,

compared to the understanding of the factors contributing to nucleic acid–nucleic acid interactions, much less is still understood. Consequently, several combinatorial methods that support directed screening of oligonucleotides have been developed and promising results have been reported.

Two papers describing very similar methods that employ the polymerase chain reaction to generate and screen RNA or DNA libraries have been published (122–125). Furthermore, potential therapeutic utility has been suggested by identifying a phosphodiester oligonucleotide that binds to thrombin.

Several combinatorial methodologies have also been developed. Because other strategies use the polymerase chain reaction to generate and screen oligonucleotides, the techniques are not satisfactory for screening modified oligonucleotides and, therefore, their use in cellular-based assays in which nuclease digestion of oligonucleotides is a problem is limited. In the methods developed in our laboratory, as no enzymes are used, it is possible to screen diverse chemical libraries and to use cell-based, or even *in vivo* assays (126).

3 PHARMACOKINETICS

As with any other class of drugs, oligonucleotide drugs must attain a sufficient concentration at their receptor for a sufficient period of time to display activity. Inasmuch as most of the targets for oligonucleotides are intracellular, oligonucleotides must be relatively stable in and outside the cell and must be able to traverse the cellular membrane.

3.1 Nuclease Stability

Oligonucleotides may be degraded by nucleases. Nucleases that degrade DNA or RNA from either the 5' or 3' terminus are known as exonucleases; those that cleave internally, endonucleases. Numerous nucleases exist and have been shown to degrade oligonucleotides. Although in serum, the dominant nuclease activity is 3′ exonuclease, in cells and other bodily fluids, 3′ and 5′ exonucleases and endonucleases are present.

3.2 Intracellular Stability

The nuclease activity of sera derived from different species varies. Fetal calf serum is more active than mouse serum, and human serum appears to have the least nuclease activity (77). However, all sera display substantial nuclease activity and there are significant lot-to-lot variations. In all sera tested, 3′ exonucleases constitute the primary nuclease activity (9, 31, 127). In a number of publications, fetal calf serum used in tissue culture experiments has been heated to inactivate nucleases. Again, however, conditions were not standardized and in some lots of sera, heating to 65°C for 30 minutes does not inactivate all nucleases (31).

Another factor that has contributed to confusion is that a variety of labeling methods and analytical techniques have been employed. Studies have employed $3'^{32}P$- and $5'^{32}P$-labeled oligonucleotides, $5'^{32}P$-labeled oligonucleotides and oligonucleotides labeled with fluorescent pendant groups at the 5′ terminus (128–130). Relatively few studies have used uniformly labeled oligonucleotides. Furthermore, relatively few studies have rigorously separated intact oligonucleotides from degradation products and even fewer have performed careful kinetic studies.

Phosphodiester oligodeoxynucleotides are rapidly degraded in biological systems such as serum. Work from many laboratories has demonstrated that a wide range of modifications may be used to enhance the stability of oligonucleotides. Phosphate

modifications have been shown to result in marked increases in stability. Phosphorothioate oligonucleotides have been shown t be extremely stable in media, cells and cell extracts, serum, various tissues, urine and stable to most nucleases (131–133). The non-ionic methylphosphonate analogs have also been shown to be extremely stable to nucleases (134–140). As with phosphorothioates, these oligonucleotides are diastercomeric at each modified phosphate and the R isomer is slightly more sensitive than the S isomer to degradation by nucleases (31, 141). Other classes of modifications that have been reported to result in substantial nuclease stability include the phosphoramidates (55, 109) and isoropyl phosphate triesters (142–143). Interestingly, ethylphosphate triesters were shown to be cleaved after being deethylated in cells (136, 144). Oligonucleotides containing α-anomers in the sugar moiety are substantially more stable in serum and cells than natural phosphodiesters (129, 145–148). Modifications at the 2′-position of the sugar and various positions of the bases have also been shown to enhance nuclease stability (9, 79, 149–150).

In addition to uniform modifications, a number of pendant groups at the 5′ and/or 3′ termini and more recently in internal positions of oligonucleotides, have been reported to enhance nuclease stability. Modifications include intercalating agents (101, 151–153) and poly-L-lysine (154–155) at the 5′ or 3′ terminus and a number of modifications such as amino–alkoxy (156), anthraquinone (157) and alkyl groups (150). Moreover, heterocycle modifications, including pendant groups from the N_2 site of guanine (158–159), pendant groups from 3-deazaguinine (1600, and 5 and 6 position modifications of deoxycytidine and thymidine (161), have shown increased stability to nucleases of varying levels.

In conclusion, numerous medicinal chemistry strategies can be employed to create oligonuncleotides with varying degrees of nuclease stability. The choice of the modification(s) employed is dictated by the level of stability desired and other desired properties of the oligonucleotides. It is now possible to design oligonucleotides that display excellent hybridization characteristics and half lives when incubated with nucleases, serum, cells or cell extracts that range from minutes to several days.

Studies in our laboratory have employed either phosphodiester oligonucleotides uniformly labelled with ^{32}P, or phosphorothioate oligonucleotides uniformly labeled with ^{5}S. The kinetics of degradation have been studied using several cell lines *in vitro* and cytoplasmic and nuclear extracts derived from HeLa cells. In contrast to a number of studies, in all cells studied to date, phosphodiester oligonucleotides were degraded within 15–30 minutes of incubation (127, 162). In contrast, phosphorathioate oligonucleotides of 15, 21 and 30 nucleotides in length and various sequences were stable for at least 24 hours when incubated with various cells. In fact, in studies in HeLa cells in which ISIS 1082, a 21 mer phosphorothioate, was incubated with the cells, then extracted from cells at various time points and analyzed on polyacrylamide gels, the compounds was stable for more than four days.

3.3 Cellular Uptake and Distribution

Antisense oligonucleotides typically are 15–30 nucleotides long and, thus, have molecular weights that range from 4500–9000 daltons. The charge carried by phosphodiesters is negative and they are highly water soluble. The charge and hydrophilicity of modified oligonucleotides vary depending on the modifications. Consequently, it is likely that membrane transport and cellular distribution will vary widely as a function of the modifications introduced into oligonucleotides. For the two classes of

modified oligonucleotides for which significant data have been reported, methylphosphonates and phosphorothioates, this is clearly the cases, and for both classes of oligonucleotides, the evidence is compelling that they do enter many cells at pharmacologically relevant concentrations.

Methylphosphonates are unchanged and lipophilic. Although thought to be taken up by most cells in tissue culture via passive diffusion, detailed studies of the kinetics of cellular uptake, distribution and metabolism of uniformly labeled methylphosphonates have not been reported. Studies in Syrian hamster fibroblasts on oligonucleotides 3–9 nucleotides in length showed linear cell association for 1 hour, then reduced uptake. At equilibrium, the intracellular concentration of oligonucleotide was reported to be equivalent to the extracellular concentration of oligonucleotide was reported to be equivalent to the extracellular concentration (83, 136). In another study, a 21 mer methylphosphonate labeled with ^{32}P at the 5′ terminus was reported to be taken up by CV-1 cells. Cell association was linear for two hours. In contrast, one study suggested that methylphosphonates may be taken up by fluid phase endocytosis (163).

Unfortunately, however, studies proving that the cell-associated radioactivity represented intact oligonucleotide have not been reported. Nor were detailed studies on characteristics of uptake or intracellular distribution presented (164).

Phosphorothioates are negatively charged but because of the sulfur, atoms may be slightly more lipophilic than phosphodiesters and tend to bind non-specifically to serum proteins. Studies in our laboratories have shown that phosphorothioate oligonucleotides bind to serum albumin and, in the presence of serum albumin, cell-associated is reduced (77, 162).

Studies employing a 28 mer phosphorothioate deoxycytidine that was uniformly labeled with ^{32}P demonstrated that when

HeLa cells were incubated with $1 \mu M$ of the drug, significant intracellular concentrations were achieved. Cellular uptake was linear, reaching a plateau of $60 \, \text{p-mole}/10^6$ cells in six hours. Adsorption t the cell membrane was minimal. Uptake was also concentration-dependent, reaching a plateau at approximately $1 \mu M$. The drug associated with HeLa cells was intact for 24 hours and was located in both nuclei and cytoplasm. Infection with herpes virus type 2, but nt type 1, increased cellular uptake (165).

Laboratory studies have confirmed and extended the observations on phosphorothioate oligonucleotides. The cellular uptake, distribution and metabolism of ISIS 1082, a uniformly ^{35}S-labeled 21 mer phosphorothioate with a mixed antisense sequence, have been characterized in HeLa cells and a variant line conditioned to growth in suspension, HeLa S_3 cells. Incubation of HeLa cells with $5 \mu M$ of the drug resulted in approximately 8% of input radioactivity being associated with the cells. Cell association was linear for approximately eight hours, and approximately 20% of the cell-associated radioactivity appeared to be adsorbed to the membrane. Uptake was temperature dependent, required viable cells and was inhibited by metabolic poisons. Uptake was concentration dependent, being linear to $10 \mu M$. Uptake was influenced slightly by calcium and magnesium and was saturable. Natural oligonucleotides and methylphosphonates did not compete for uptake while other phosphorothioates were competed. However, different length and sequence phosphorothioates competed differentially (162, 166).

Other phosphorothioates of various lengths and other cell lines have also been studied. HL 60 cells appear to take up less phosphorothioate oligonucleotides of varying size and sequences, these drugs have been shown to be stable in cells and cytoplasmic and nuclear extracts. In HeLa cells, no degradation of intracellular ISIS 1082

was observed for four days (162). Preliminary studies confirmed that these oligonucleotides distributed to both cytoplasma and nuclei and showed that there is an active temperature-dependent efflux process as well (167–168).

Pendant modifications of phosphodiester oligonucleotides have also been studied. A 9 mer labeled with acridine at the 3′ terminus was reported to be taken up by Trypanosome brucei (152). More recently, the same group has reported that a 9 mer coupled at the 3′ terminus to acridine via a dodecanal linker was more active in cells expressing mutated RAS than 1 9 mer with a 3′ acridine only (110) 3′-Poly-L-lysine oligonucleotides have been reported to be stable to serum nucleases and to have enhanced activity as compared to phosphodiesters. However, uptake was not studied (56, 154, 168). In a later publication, the uptake of a poly-L-lysine oligonucleotide conjugate was enhanced compared to the unmodified oligonucleotide (169). However, it should be noted that when used to treat cells other than L929 cells, poly-L-lysine conjugates were inactive (154).

A number of lipid conjugates have also been studied. 5′ linked thriethylammonium 1, 2-di-O-hexadecyl-rac-glycerol-3-H-phosphonate oligonucleotides ere taken up 8–10 fold more than unmodified oligonucleotides by L929 cells and were more active against varicella zoster viral infections, albeit at high concentrations (170). An oligonucleotide linked at the 5′ terminus to an undecyl residue was reported to be active, but no uptake or stability studies were reported (171).

Liposomes and related formulations have been shown to enhance cellular uptake of oligonucleotides $in \, vitro$. Like et al. (172) compared the uptake of phosphodiester and phosphorothioate deoxythymydine heptamers into HL-60 cells using oligonucleotides coupled to 2-methoxy-6-chloro 9-(5-hydroxypentyl) amino acridine and monitoring with flow cytometry. They did not determine the integrity of the oligonucleotides, but reached the conclusion that phosphodiester dT_7 was taken by HL-60 cells much more effectively than phosphorothiate $d-T_7$ was, and that uptake plateaued at 50 hours. They reported increased anti-c-myc activity of phosphorothioate oligonucleotides after loading them in phosphatidyl serine liposomes. The uptake of a tetramer 2',5' deoxyadenylate into L1210 cells was reported to 2,5 deoxyadenylate into L1210 cells was reported to be increased by loading the oligo-adenylate into Staphyloccus aureus protein crosslinked phospholipid vesicles (173). In our laboratories, we have shown that a cationic lipid mixture of DOTMA and DOPE can significantly increase the uptake and activity of phosphorothioate oligonucleotides in several cell lines. It also alters the intracellular distribution of these oligonucleotides (167).

With the exception of methylphosphonates, the conclusion from studies that have addressed the mechanisms of uptake of oligonucleotides is that the most likely mechanism is receptor mediated endocytosis. In fact, in one study, an 80 kilodalton protein that appeared to bind oligonucleotides was partially purified and postulated to be a "receptor" (174). However, the evidence supporting this mechanism is limited and there are insufficient data to conclude that receptor mediated endocytosis is the most common mechanism of uptake of charged oligonucletodies in most cells.

In conclusion, although many questions remain to be answered, it appears that many cells in tissue culture may take oligonucleotides up at pharmacologically relevant concentrations. Clearly, oligonucleotides of different types behave differently, and there are substantial variations as a function of cell type. Moreover, length and specific sequences may alter uptake and pendant modifications may profoundly influence cellular uptake.

Once in the cell, it would seem that oligonucleotides distribute to the cytoplasma and the nuclei. In most, if not all cells, phosphodiester oligonucleotides are rapidly degraded while methylphosphonates and phosphorothioates are much more stable. Again, pendant modifications may alter the rate of intracellular degradation and distribution.

Mechanisms of uptake and distribution are poorly understood. However, it is clear that multiple mechanisms may play a role, and that different types of oligonucleotides may behave very differently.

Novel formulations may enhanced cellular uptake. Liposomes and cationic lipids significantly enhance uptake and may alter the mechanisms of uptake and intracellular fate of oligonucleotides.

3.4 In Vivo Pharmacokinetics

Preliminary *in vivo* pharmacokinetic data are available on methylphosphonate and phosphorothioate oligonucleotides. A 12 mer ^{3}H-labeled methylphosphonate injected in the tail vein of mice demonstrated a pharmacokinetic pattern of rapid distribution and elimination (175). The plasma elimination half-life was less than two hours. While the kinetics of distribution and elimination were rapid, a pattern of broad tissue distribution was observed. No radiolabel was recovered in the brains of treated animals. Analysis of certain tissues containing radiolabeled material suggested that a significant extent of metabolism of the oligonucleotide occurred within hours of administration.

Studies have been performed on ^{35}S-labeled phosphorothioates in rats. A true distribution phase of 15–25 minutes was observed after a single intravenous dose of a 27 mer followed by prolonged elimination phase of 20–40 hours (176). The prolonged elimination phase may result from the binding of phosphorothioates to serum proteins. Phosphorothioates distributed broadly to all tissues except the brain and were eliminated in the urine intact. Phosphorothiates were rapidly and extensively absorbed after IM and IP administration (176).

Repeated daily doses of 50 mg/kg of a 27 mer phosphorothioate to mice resulted in similar distribution and elimination kinetics, but slight differences in tissue concentrations from single-dose studies. Liver, kidney, spleen and lung were the organs with highest concentrations. Again, the drug was excreted intact in the urine (176).

Continuous osmotic pump administration of the same compound subcutaneously for four weeks at doses of 50–150 mg resulted in similar pharmacokinetics (176).

Recently, a series of pharmacokinetic studies was performed on a 20-mer phosphorothioate oligonucleotide, ISIS 2105 (177). This compound is targeted to bind to a site within the E2 gene product of human papillomavirus. Following intravenous administration in rabbits, the pharmacokinetic behavior of the compound fit a 2-compartment model with an elimination half-life of approximately 100 hours and a majority of radiolabel recovered in the urine. Studies of the intradermal pharmacokinetics of this compound demonstrated 70–80% bioavailability relative to intravenous administration.

Additional studies in the rabbit and mouse with ISIS 2105 following intradermal administration demonstrate that the phosphorothioate has prolonged residence time in the skin (measured in days).

Studies with ISIS 1082, a 21 mer phosphorothioate, in mice showed that when applied to the cornea in a sodium acetate buffer, a significant adsorption t the cornea and absorption into the aqueous and vitreous humors occurred (177). Moreover, significant systemic bioavailability was observed. In rabbit, as much as 25% of an applied ocular dose was systemically bio-

available. Post-absorption pharmacokinetics were equivalent to I.V. pharmacokinetics.

Taken together, these studies (i.e., those regarding phosphorothioates) demonstrate an absorption distribution and elimination profile that is consistent with effective systemic drug therapy. The value of other approaches to chemical modifications or formulation of oligonucleotides in order to enhance theory pharmacokinetics and bioavailability remain to be determined.

3.5 Toxicology

Very little information has been published on the toxicology of oligonucleotides. As with any other group of pharmacologic ligands, toxicity of oligonucleotides will be defined by both interactions with "intended" and "unintended" receptors. For example, a particular phosphorothioate oligonucleotide might produce toxicities as a result of interactions with its intended RNA sequence target and sites on other RNAs with similar sequences or other macromolecules. These can be defined as pharmacologic and chemical toxicities respectively.

The *in vitro* toxicological effects of a significant number of oligonucleotides have recently been described (162). Although considerable variability has been reported, in general, it appears that neither phosphodiesters, phosphorothioates or methylphosphonate oligonucleotides are significantly toxic to most cells *in vitro* at concentrations less than 100 μM.

The nature and extent of the toxicological effects as well as mechanism vary as a function of the chemical class. Phosphodiester oligonucleotides have been reported to result in cytotoxicity in some cells, and it is thought that this may be due to degradation to nucleosides followed by uptake and alteration of nucleotide pools. Methylphosphonates have been reported to be minimally toxic at concentrations below 150 μM against most cell lines (179).

A large number of phosphorothioates using several cell lines and various measures of toxicity have been evaluated. Again, minimal toxicological effects were observed at concentrations less than 200 μM. Toxicity increased as the duration of exposure increased, but even after 96 hours, minimal toxicity was observed. Toxicity was slightly greater for longer oligonucleotides (30 mers), and was greater in experiments in which no fetal calf serum was added. This is possibly due to the fact that phosphorothioates bind to albumin. Toxicity also varied as a function of the cell line studies, but no cell line was sensitive to concentrations below 10 μM (162). There was also a suggestion of sequence dependency but not clear pattern emerged. Minimal effects on macromolecular synthesis were observed, with DNA synthesis being the most sensitive (162).

Although there are very limited published data on the *in vivo* toxicology of oligonucleotides, given the number of compounds in preclinical and clinical development, it is likely that a number of publications will issue in the near future.

4 MEDICINAL CHEMISTRY

The core of any rational drug discovery program is medicinal chemistry. Although the synthesis of modified nucleic acids has been a subject of interest for some time, the intense focus on the medicinal chemistry of oligonucleotides dates perhaps to no more than four years prior to this chapter. Consequently, the scope of medicinal chemistry has recently expanded enormously, but the biological data to support conclusions about synthetic strategies are only beginning to emerge.

Modifications in the base, sugar and phosphate moeties of oligonucleotides have been reported. The subjects of medicinal chemical programs include approaches to create enhanced affinity and more selective affinity for RNA or duplex structures, the ability to cleave nucleic acid targets, enhanced nuclease stability, cellular uptake and distribution, and *in vivo* tissue distribution, metabolism and clearance.

Figure 21.5 shows the structure of an oligonucleotide, a number of design features and various design strategies that have been implemented at Isis and in other

Oligonucleotide Medicinal Chemistry Program

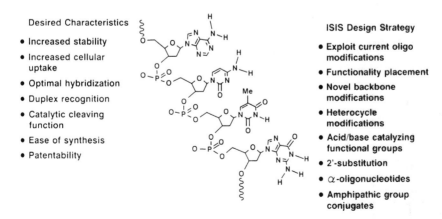

Fig. 21.5 Structure of an oligonucleotide showing a number of design features and strategies implemented at Isis and other laboratories.

laboratories. (With regard to this class of molecules, as with all others. Increase potency and selectivity by improving pharmacokinetic and pharmacodynamic properties.

Although substantial progress in the medicinal chemistry oligonucleotides has been made in the past three years, it is not yet possible to reach conclusions about the therapeutic ability of the novel modifications. Preliminary data on effects on nuclease stability and hybridization properties and, for a few modifications, activity *in vitro* suggest that the next generation of oligonucleotides may display substantially improved potencies and selectivity.

4.1 Heterocycle Modifications

4.1.1 PYRIMIDINE MODIFICATIONS. A selectively large number of modified pyrimidines have been synthesized and now evaluated in oligonucleotides. The principle sites of modification are C-2, C-4, C-5 and C-6 (Fig. 21.6). These and other nucleoside analogs have recently been thoroughly reviewed (177). Consequently, a very brief summary of the analogs that displayed interesting properties is incorporated here.

Inasmuch as the C-5 position is involved in Watson-Crick hybridization, C-2 modified pyrimidine containing oligonucleotides

have shown unattractive hybridization properties. An oligonucleotide containing 2-thiothymidine was found to hybridize well to DNA and, in fact, the T_m increased by approximately 0–5°C per modification (180).

In contrast, several modifications in the 4 position that have interesting properties have been reported. 4-thiopyrimidines have been incorporated into oligonucleotides with no significant negative effect on hybridization (181). A bicyclic and a *N*4-methoxy analog of cytosine was shown to hybridize with both purine bases in DNA with T_m is approximately equal t natural base pairs (182). Finally, a fluorescent base (Fig. 21.7a) has been incorporated into oligonucleotides and shown to enhance duplex stability (183).

A large number of modifications at the C-5 position have also been reported, including halogenated nucleosides. (Although the stability of duplexes may be enhanced by incorporating 5-halogenated nucleosides, the occasional mispairing with G and the potential that the oligonucleotide might degrade may cause the release of toxic nucleosides analogs (see ref. 177 for review).)

In general, as expected, modifications in the C-6 position of pyrimidines are highly duplex destabilizing (184). Oligonucleotides containing 6-aza pyrimidines (Fig.

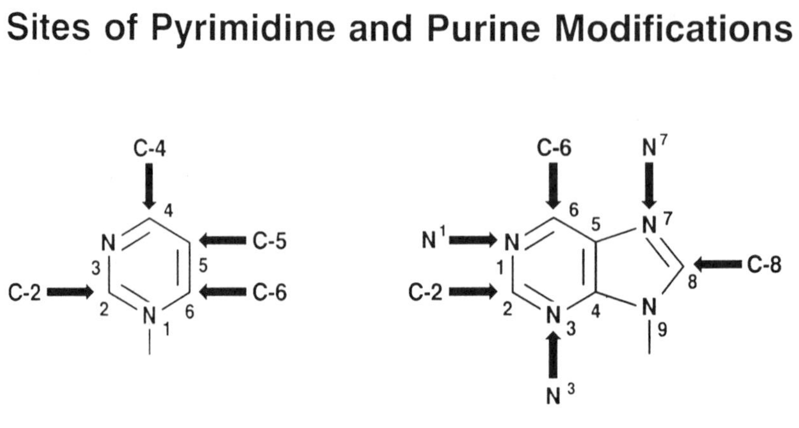

Sites of Pyrimidine and Purine Modifications

Fig. 21.6 Sites of pyrimidine and purine modifications. Arrows indicate the site(s) of modification.

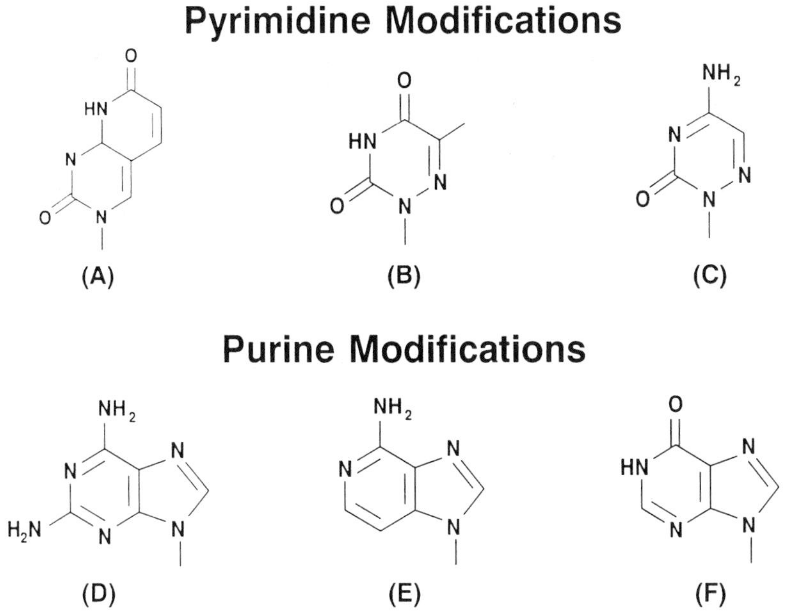

Pyrimidine Modifications

(A)   (B)   (C)

Purine Modifications

(D)   (E)   (F)

Fig. 21.7 Pyrimidine and purine modifications.

21.7b–c) have been shown to reduce T_m by 1–2 ≠ C per modification, but to enhance the nuclease stability of oligonucleotides and to support RNase H induced degradation of RNA targets (177).

4.1.2 PURINE MODIFICATIONS. Although numerous purine analogs have been synthesized, when incorporated into oligonucleotides, they normally have resulted in destabilization of duplexes, so they have been of little interest. For example, modifications at the N1 site of urines destabilize duplexes as would be expected (185). Similarly, C2 modifications have usually resulted in destabilization. However, 2-6-diaminopurine (Fig. 21.7d) has been reported to enhance hybridization by approximately 1°C per modification when paired with T (1986). Of the 3-position substituted bases reported to date, only 3-deaza, an adenosine analog (Fig. 21.7c) has been shown to have no negative effective on hybridization.

Modifications at the C-6 and C-7 positions have likewise resulted in only a few interesting bases from the point of view of

hybridization. Inosine (Fig. 21.6f) has been shown to have little effect on duplex stability, but because it can pair and stack with all four normal DNA bases, it behaves as a universal base and creates an ambiguous position in an oligonucleotide (187). Similarly, modifications at N^7 have resulted in destabilization of duplexes (177).

In contrast, some C8 substituted bases have yielded improved hybridization properties when incorporated in oligonucleotides (177).

Finally, very recently, Dervan and colleagues (188, 189) have reported the synthesis of novel nucleosides that recognize G–C base pairs. These modifications may be quite important as they provide the means to create triplex forming oligonucleotides that can be targeted to mixed sequences.

4.1.3 OLIGONUCLEOTIDE CONJUGATES. The introduction of functionality at specific sites in an oligonucleotide has been the subject of substantial investigation. Conceptually, introduction of various functionalities at one or more sites in an oligonucleotide could result in enhancement of pharmacodynamic or pharmacokinetic properties or both. As the extensive literature on oligonucleotide conjugates has recently been reviewed in detail this chapter presents only an overview (190).

Figure 21.8 adapted from reference 190, shows a general scheme describing the sites that have been modified. In addition to modifications at the 3′ and 5′ termini, it is now possible to introduce modifications internally at a number of positions without

adversely affecting the stability of duplexes formed with DNA or RNA targets.

Although conjugation of various functionalities to oligonucleotides has been reported to achieve a number of important objectives, the data supporting some of the claims are limited and generalizations are not possible based on the data presently available.

4.1.4 NUCLEASE STABILITY. As discussed earlier, numerous 3′ modifications have

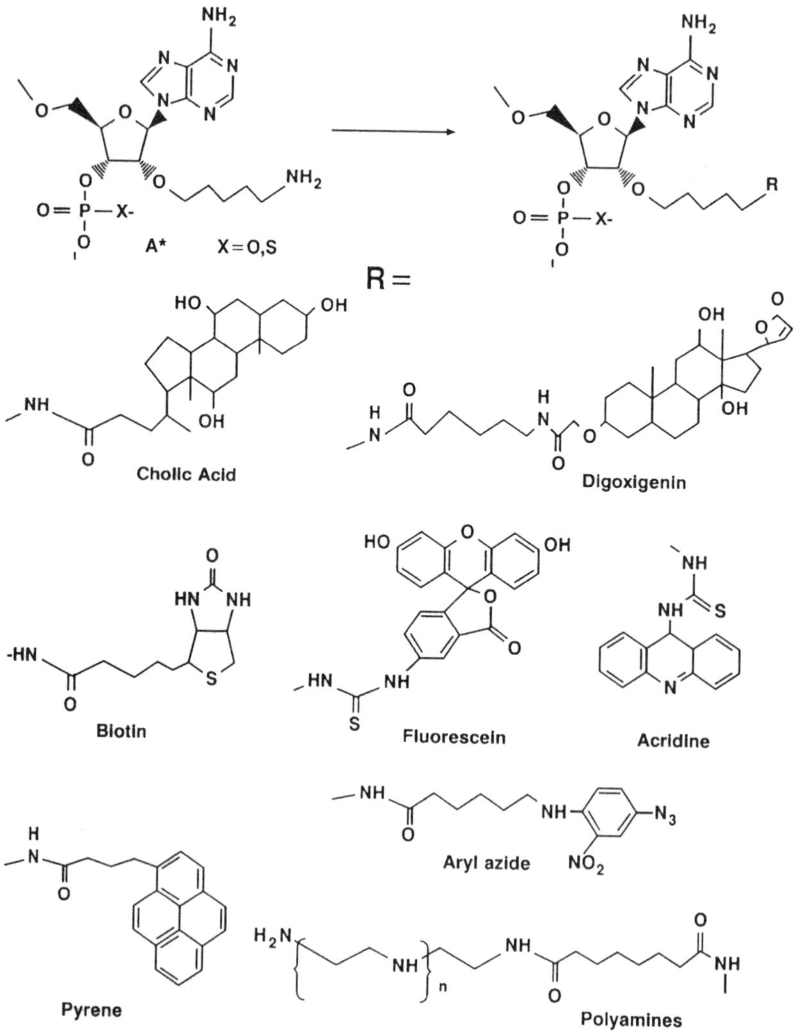

Fig. 21.8 General scheme describing sites of oligonucleotide modification.

been reported to enhance the stability of oligonucleotides in serum (190). Both neutral and charged substituents have been reported to stabilize oligonucleotides in serum and, as a general rule, the stability of a conjugated oligonucleotide tends to be greater as bulkier substituents are added. Inasmuch as the principle nuclease in serum is a 3′ exonuclease, it is not surprising that 5′ modifications have resulted in significantly less stabilization. Internal modifications of base, sugar and backbone have also been reported to enhance nuclease stability at or near the modified nucleoside (190).

The demonstration that modifications may induce nuclease stability sufficient to enhance activity in cells, in tissue culture, and in animals has proven to be much more complicated because of the presence of 5′ exonucleases and endonucleases. 3′ modification and internal point modifications have not provided sufficient nuclease stability to demonstrate pharmacological activity in cells (191). In fact, even a 5′ nucleotide long phosphodiester gap in the middle of a phosphorothioate oligonucleotide resulted in the sufficient loss of nuclease resistance to cause complete loss of pharmacological activity (192).

4.2 Enhanced Cellular Uptake

Although oligonucleotides have been shown to be taken up by a number of cell lines in tissue culture, with perhaps the most compelling data relating to phosphorothioate oligonucleotides, a clear objective has been to improve cellular uptake of oligonucleotides. Inasmuch as the mechanisms of cellular uptake of oligonucleotides are still very poorly understood, the medicinal chemistry approaches have been largely empirical and based on many unproven assumptions.

Because phosphodiester and phosphorothioate oligonucleotides are water soluble, the conjugation of lipophilic substituents to enhance membrane permeability has been a subject of considerable interest. Uniformly, studies in this area have not been systematic and, at present, there is precious little information about the changes in physicochemical properties of oligonucleotides actually effected by specific lipid conjugates.

As previously discussed, phospholipids, cholesterol and cholesterol derivatives, cholic acid and simply alkyl chains have been conjugated to oligonucleotides at various sites in the oligonucleotide. The effects of these modifications on cellular uptake have been assessed using fluorescent, or radiolabeled, oligonucleotides, or by measuring pharmacological activities.

From the perspective of medicinal chemistry, very few systematic studies have been performed. The activities of short alkyl chains, adamantine, daunomycin, fluorescein, cholesterol and porphyrin conjugated oligonucleotides were compared in ne study (193). The cholesterol modification was reported to be more effective at enhancing uptake than the other substituents.

It also seems likely that the effects of various conjugates on cellular uptake may be affected by the cell type and target studied. For example, we have studied cholic acid conjugates of phosphorothioates, deoxyoligonucleotides or phosphorothioate 2′-O methyl oligonucleotides, and observed enhanced activity against HIV and no effect on the activity of ICAM directed oligonucleotides.

Additionally, polycationic substitutions and various groups designed to bind to carrier systems have been synthesized. Although many compounds have been synthesized (see ref. 190 for review), the data reported to date are insufficient to draw firm conclusions about the value of such approaches or structure activity relationships.

4.3 Cleavage Reagents

As previously discussed, a large number of potential DNA or RNA cleavage reagents have been conjugated to oligonucleotides. In addition to the substituents previously mentioned, bleomycin (194) phenazone-5,10,di-N-oxide (195), and a wide range of redox active substituents (190) have been conjugated and shown to cleave DNA or RNA with ·some evidence of specificity. However, again the value of such agents as therapeutics remains to be defined.

4.4 Sugar Modifications

A growing number of oligonucleotides in which the pertofuranase ring is modified or replaced have been reported (4). Uniform modifications at the 2′ position have been shown to enhance hybridization to RNA (Fig. 21.2), and in some cases, to enhance nuclease resistance (4). Chimeric oligonucleotides containing 2′ deoxyoligonucleotide wings have been shown to be more potent than parent molecules (191).

Other sugar modifications include α oligonucleotides, carbocyclic oligonucleotides and hexapyranosyl oligonucleotides (4). Of these, α-oligonucleotides have been most extensively studied. They hybridize in parallel fashion to single stranded DNA and RNA and are nuclease resistant. However, they have been reported to be incapable of activating RNase H.

4.5 Backbone Modifications

Substantial progress in creating new backbones for oligonucleotides that replace the phosphate or the sugar–phosphate unit has been made. The objectives of these programs are to improve hybridization by removing the negative charge, enhance stability and potentially improve pharmacokinetics.

Table 21.1 presents a number of backbone modifications that have been reported in which the phosphate has been modified or replaced (196). The table presents qualitative comparisons with regard to nuclease stability and affinity. However, only limited data have been reported for any of these backbones and most of the data are derived from homopolymers with mixed backbones. Studies in our laboratories have shown that the hybridization of mixed sequences differ substantially from results obtained with homopolymers and that fully modified oligomers behave quite differently from oligomers in which more than one backbone is incorporated into an oligonucleotide. Consequently, even preliminary conclusions about the relative merits of particular backbones with regard to hybridization are not possible.

Despite the caveats, the range of backbone replacements and the preliminary data are causes of considerable optimism that oligonucleotides in which all phosphates are replaced and in which the charge can be optimized are feasible. In our laboratories, we have been particularly interested in a series of backbone modifications in which the phosphate is replaced by a nitrogen–oxygen bridge (Fig. 21.9). Figure 21.10 shows the hybridization of an oligonucleotide in which increasing numbers of the phosphates are replaced with one of the several modified backbones units shown in Figure 21.8. The N-methyl aminohydroxy and the N,N-dimethyl hydrazino backbones appear to provide excellent affinity, specificity and nuclease resistance (196).

Replacement of the entire sugar-phosphate unit has also been accomplished and the oligonucleotides produced have displayed very interesting characteristics. Figure 21.11 compares the structures of the peptide nucleic acid (PNA) backbone and DNA (19,197–198). PNA oligonucleotides have been shown to bind to single-stranded DNA and RNA with extraordinary affinity and high sequence specificity. They have

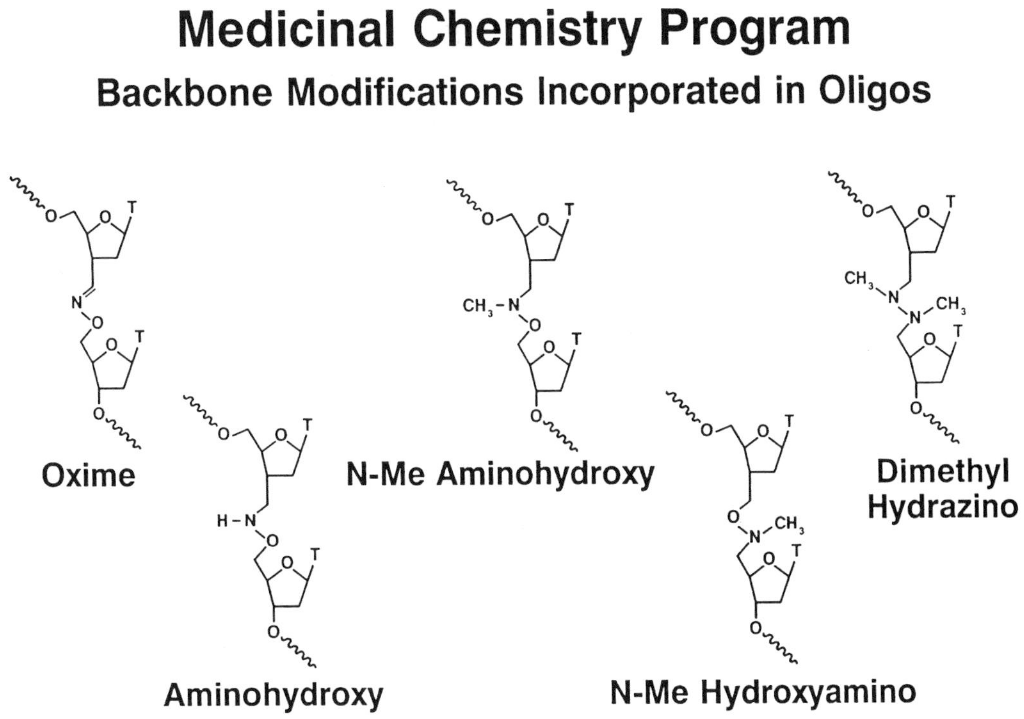

Medicinal Chemistry Program
Backbone Modifications Incorporated in Oligos

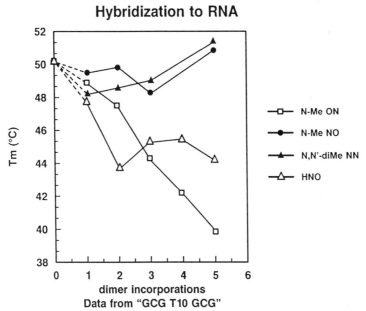

Fig. 21.9 Backbone modifications in which the phosphate is replaced by non-ionic and achiral linkages.

Backbone Modification Chemistry
Hybridization to RNA

Data from "GCG T10 GCG"

Fig. 21.10 Hybridization of oligonucleotide in which increasing numbers of phosphate linkages are replaced with backbone linkages in Figure 21.8.

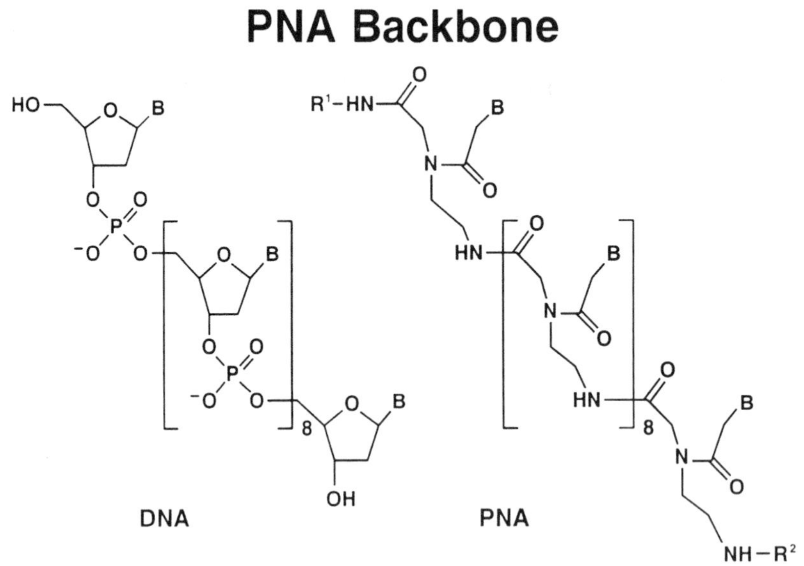

PNA Backbone

Fig. 21.11 Comparison of the structures of PNA backbone and DNA.

been shown to be able to invade double-stranded nucleic acid structures. PNA oligonucleotides can form triple-stranded structures with DNA or RNA.

Very recently, PNA oligonucleotides were shown to be able to act as antisense and transcriptional inhibitors when microinjected in cells (199). PNA oligonucleotides appear to be quite stable to nucleases and peptidases as well.

In summary, then, in the past five years, enormous advances in the medicinal chemistry of oligonucleotides have been reported. Modifications at nearly every position in oligonucleotides have been attempted and numerous potentially interesting analogs have been identified. Although it is far too early to determine which of the modifications may be most useful for particular purposes, it is clear that a wealth of new chemicals are available for systematic evaluation, and the these studies should provide important insights into the SAR of oligonucleotide analogs.

4.6 Activities of Oligonucleotides

In the past several years, scores of articles have been published demonstrating the activity of a large number of oligonucleotides in a variety of systems. A number of excellent reviews have summarized the activities of these compounds (31,62,200–201).

4.6.1 ACTIVITIES IN CELLS IN TISSUE CULTURE. To date, oligonucleotides have been reported to inhibit the growth of a large number of viruses in tissue culture, the expression of numerous oncogenes, a variety of normal cellular genes, and a number of transfected reporter genes controlled by several regulatory elements. The oligonucleotides used, the cells employed, the receptor sequences, concentrations and conditions have differed widely. Only a few of the studies have reported detailed dose response curves and conditions. Studies for which sufficient information was presented are summarized in Table 21.2.

Table 21.2 Summary of Antisense Oligonucleotides[a]

Target	Cell Type	Serum	Oligo Types	Length	Concentration	Reference
Viruses						
HTLV-III	H9 cells	−	P	12–26	5–50 mg/mL	53
HIV	H–T cells	+	PS	14–28	0.51 μM	129
HIV (gag/pol)	H–T cells	+	PS	18–24	1–10 μM	207
HIV	H9 cells	+	PS, others	20	4–20 μg/mL	55
HIV	CZM cells	+	PS	18–28	10 μM	64
Herpes simplex	Vero cells	+	CH_3P	7	50–100 μM	54
Herpes simplex	HeLa Cells	+	PS	28	1–10 μM (nonantisense)	165
Herpes simplex	Vero cells	+	CH_3P	12	20–50 μM	142
Herpes simplex	Vero cells	+	CH_3P psoralen	12	5 μM	142
Herpes simplex	HeLa cells	+	PS	21	0.2–4 μM	208
Vesicular stomatitis	L929 cells	+	CH_3P	9	25–50 μM	179
Vesicular stomatitis	L929 cells	+	P-lipid	11	50–150 μM	170
Vesicular	L929 cells	+	*p*-poly L-lysine	10–15	0.1 μM	56
Influenza	MDCK cells	+	P-acridine	11	50 μM	71
Tick-born encephalitis		+	Various	Various	0.1–1 μM	209
SV40	MDCK cells	+	CH_3P	6–9	25 μM	210
Rous	Chicken fibreblasts	+	Various	Various	10 μM	70
Hepatitis B	Alexander	+	P	15	8.5 μM	211
Bovine papalloma virus	C-127 cells	+	PS	4–30	0.01–1 μM	63
Oncogenes						
c-myc	T-lymphocytes	+	P	15	30 μM	178
c-myc	HL-60 cells	+	P, PS	15	10 μM	212
c-myc	Burkitt cells	−	P	21	100 μM	51
c-myb	PMBC	+	P	18	40 mg/mL	213
BCL-2	L697 cells	−	P, PS	20	25–150 μM	214
N-myc	Neuroblastoma cells	+	P	15	1–5 μM	208
N-ras	T15 cells	+	CH_3P	9	Inactive	215
Host Genes						
Multiple drug resistance	MCF-1 cells	+	PS	15		216
PCNA (cyclin)	3T3	+	P	18	30 μM	217
Prothymosin	Human myeloma cells	−	P	16–21	40 μM	59
T cell receptor	T cell	+	P	22		60
Gm CSF	Endothelial cells	−	P	15, 18	$10^{-5} M$	60
CSF-1	FL-ras/myc cells	+	P	?	?	218

Table 21.2   (*Continued*)

Target	Cell Type	Serum	Oligo Types	Length	Concentration	Reference
Host Genes						
EGF receptor		+	P	13	30 μM	219
BFGH	Human astrocytes	−	P	15	10–75 μM	220
β Globin	Rabbit reticulocytes	+	CH_3P	9	100 μM	221
TAU	Neurons	−	P	20–25	3–50 μM	222
cAMP-Protein Kinase II β	HL-60 cells	+	P	21	15 μM	223
Myeloblastin	HL-60 cells	+	P	18	?	224
Phospholipase A$_2$ activating protein	BC3H$_1$	+	P	25	25 μM	225
ICAM-1	A549 HVEC tymphocytes	−	PS	18–20	0.01–1 μM	226
IL-2	T-lymphocytes	−	P	15	5 μM	161
IL-1α	HUVEC	+	P	18	10 μM	226
IL-1β	Monocytes	+	PS	15	0.1–2.5 μM	227
IFG-1	Myoblasts	−	P	15	10 μM	228
Perforin	T-lymphocytes	−	P	18	5–35 μM	229
Other						
Chloramphenicol acetyl transferase	CV-1 cells	+	P, PS, CH_3P	21	5–30 μM	164
Placental alkaline Phosphatase Driven by HIV TAR	SK-mel-2 cells	+	PS	18–28	0.25–5 μM	64
Chloramphenicol Acetyl transferase Driven by human Papilloma virus E2 responsive Element	C-127 and CV-1 cells	+	PS	14–20	1–10 μM	63

[1]cAMP, cyclic AMP; CH_3P, methylphosphonate oligonucleotides; EGF, epidermal growth factor; G-CSF, granulocyte colony-stimulating factor; GM-CSF, granulocyte macrophage colony-stimulating factor; HB, hepatitis B; HIV, human immunodeficiency virus; HSV, herpes simplex virus; HTLV, human T-cell lymphotrophic virus; IV, influenza virus; P, phosphodiester oligonucleotides; P-acridine, phosphodiester oligonucleotide conjugated with acridine moiety; P-lipid, phosphodiester oligonucleotide conjugated with lipid moiety; P–S phosphorothioate oligonucleotides; PCNA, proliferating cell nuclear antigen; PMA, phorbol mysteric acid; RSV, Rous sarcoma virus; TAR, Tat response element; TBE, tick-borne encephalitis; VSV, vesicular stomatitis.

The data presented in Table 21.2 support only a few generalizations as follows:

1. Even though phosphodiesters are relatively rapidly degraded, a number of laboratories have reported activities for unmodified phosphodiester oligonucleotides in cells incubated in the absence of serum. The concentrations required to display activity were typically greater than 10 μM.

2. A variety of modified oligonucleotides have been reported to be active. Methylphosphonates appear to be less potent than phosphorothioates, but considerable variation has been reported depending on the system. Conjugation of alkylators and intercalators to phosphodiesters and methylphosphates has been reported to increase potency. Lipophilic and poly-lysine conjugates have also displayed enhanced activities.

3. Oligonucleotides have demonstrated a broad array of activities against viral targets, oncogenes, normal host gene products and various transfected genes. Thus, there is clear evidence of the broad potential applicability of these drugs.

4. Although the data from studies incorporated in Table 21.2 are limited, when combined with the *in vitro* toxicologic data, the therapeutic indexes of phosphorothioates appear to be quite high *in vitro*. methylphosphonates appear to have lower therapeutic indexes, and too little data are available to draw conclusions about other classes of oligonucleotides.

5. Very little data that support putative mechanisms of action have been reported, and generalizations concerning desired mechanisms of action are not possible. Nevertheless, it would see that a variety of mechanisms of action may be employed by oligonucleotides to result in significant biological activities.

4.6.2 IN VIVO. There are now emerging data supporting the notion that oligonucleotides may be administered to animals and demonstrate pharmacological activity. Although many controls need to be added and much remains to be learned, In aggregate the data suggesting in vivo activity are progressively more compelling.

Table 21.3 summarizes the published reports (abstracts and full publications) demonstrating *in vivo* activity of oligonucleotides. Local antiviral effects have been reported for phosphorothioate oligonucleotides and methylphosphonate oligonucleotides. Intraperitoneal administration of a phosphorothioate oligonucleotide design to inhibit expression of the p120 protein inhibited growth of an intraperitoneal tumor (202). Additionally, a phosphorothioate oligonucleotide designed to inhibit c-myb

Table 21.3 Reported Activities Of Antisense Drugs In Animals

Target	Animal	Reference
HSV-1	Mouse	52
HSV-1	Mouse	230
Tick-Borne Encephalitis Virus	Mouse	209
p120 Oncogene	Mouse	202
c-myb	Rats	203
Interleukin 1	Mouse	204
NF-^{K}B	Mouse	205

production and injected locally was shown in inhibit internal accumulation in the rat carotid artery (203).

Systemic activity of oligonucleotides has also been reported. A phosphorothioate oligonucleotide designed to inhibit interleukin 1 production was shown to be effective after systemic administration in mice (204). Very recently, a phosphodiester oligonucleotide with a 3′ terminal phosphorothioate designed to inhibit NF-KB production was shown to inhibit growth of tumors dependent on this factor when administered systemically to mice (205).

5 CONCLUSIONS

Oligonucleotides designed to interact with nucleic acid receptors represent a potentially revolutionary advance in pharmacotherapy. Advances in the recent past and the intense focus directed to the area at present assure that the paradigm will be fully explored.

Key to continued progress in the field of antisense therapeutics is the realization that oligonucleotides and their RNA targets via the same principals of pharmacology that govern the actions of all other classes of drugs. Considering the properties of drugs that define their pharmacologic value, such as ligand–receptor binding affinity and fidelity, and realizing the intrinsic properties of oligonucleotides, it is very clear that these compounds have enormous potential value in treating human diseases.

During the next few years, a number of oligonucleotide compounds will enter into clinical trials. These first generation antisense drugs (e.g., phosphorothioates) will encounter many of the same issues and hurdles that confront all novel pharmaceutical agents; large-scale process development of adequate methods and tools to define clinical pharmacokinetics and metabolism, etc. Another important component of this process is the continued examination and definition of the molecular pharmacodynamics and pharmacokinetics of these drugs. We need to better understand how the structure and function of RNA defines the sensitivity of specific target sites to antisense oligonucleotides, the precise role of RNase H and other intracellular enzymes and proteins in the mechanism of action in oligonucleotides, the processes by which oligonucleotides penetrate the cellular membranes and distribute within cells, the non-sequence specific interactions that oligonucleotides can engage in both in and out of cells, and the metabolic pathways (both nuclease and non-nuclease) and metabolites that are likely to play a role in the metabolism of antisense drugs. The combination of this molecular, cellular and clinical information will allow us to better determine the specific molecular targets and diseases that can be successfully treated with the first generation of antisense drugs. As importantly, additional studies will define the biology, chemistry and pharmacology of second and third generation antisense drugs. Oligonucleotides that work by interacting with nonnucleic acid targets may also be of considerable interest. The development of combinatorial screening methodologies facilitates the identification of novel oligonucleotide pharmacophores.

ACKNOWLEDGEMENTS

The author appreciates the contributions by Drs. Chris Mirabelli, Dan Cook, Muthiah Manoharan, Yogesh Sanghvi and Frank Bennett and appreciates the use of their unpublished data. The author thanks Drs. Muthiah Manoharan, Yogesh Sanghvi and Frank Bennett for their helpful review of the manuscript and Mrs Colleen Matzinger for her excellent administrative and typographical support.

REFERENCES

1. K. Mizumoto and Y. Kaziro, In *Progress in Nucleic Acid Res. and Mol. Biol.*, Vol. 34, Academic Press, 1987, p. 1.

2. J. Ross, *Mol. Biol. Med.*, **5**, 1 (1988).

3. S. M. Freier, R. Kierzek, J. A. Jaeger, N. Sugimoto, M. H. Caruthers, and T. Neilson, *Proc. Natl. Acad. Sci. USA* **83**, 9373 (1986).

4. K. J. Breslauer, R. Frank, H. Blocker, and L. A. Marky, *Proc. Natl. Acad. Sci. USA* **83**, 8746, (1986).

5. S. M. Freier, in *Antisense Research and Applications*, S. T. Crooke and B. Lebleu, Eds., CRC Press, Boca Raton, Fla, 1993, p. 67.

6. S. M. Freier, W. F. Lima, Y. S. Sanghvi, T. Vickers, M. Zounes, P. D. Cook, and D. J. Ecker, in *Gene Regulation by Antisense Nucleic Acids*, J. Ivant and R. Erickson, Eds., Raven Press, Ltd., New York, 1992, p. 95.

7. C. Cazenave and C. Helene, in *Antisense Nucleic Acids and Proteins Fundamentals and Applications*, J. N. M. Mol and A. R. van der Krol, Eds.), Marcel Dekker, Inc., 1991, p. 47.

8. B. P. Monia, J. F. Johnston, D. J. Ecker, M. Zounes, W. Lima, and S. M. Freier, *J. Biol. Chem.*, **267**, 19954 (1992).

9. P. D. Cook, *Anti-Cancer Drug Design*, **6**, 585 (1991).

10. J. D. Puglisi, J. R. Wyatt, and I. Tinoco, Jr., *J. Mol. Biol.*, **214**, 437 (1990).

11. D. J. Ecker, T. A. Vickers, T. W. Bruice, S. M. Freier, R. D. Jenison, M. Manoharan, and M. Zounes, *Science*, **257**, 958 (1992).

12. W. F. Lima, B. P. Monia, D. J. Ecker, and S. Freier, *Biochem.*, **31**, 12055 (1992).

13. D. J. Ecker, in *Antisense Research and Applications* S. T. Crooke and B. Lebleu, Eds.), CRC Press, Inc., Boca Raton, Fla, 1993, p. 387.

14. R. W. Roberts and D. M. Crothers, *Science*, **258**, 1463 (1992).

15. F. Gasparro, M. O'Malley, L. Amici, and R. Edelson, *J. Invest. Derm.*, **95**, 527 (1990) (abstract).

16. F. P. Gasparro, H. H. Wong, S. J. Ugent, M. E. O'Malley and R. L. Edelson, *Clin. Res*, **37**, 30A (1989) (abstract).

17. C. Helene, T. Montenay-Garestier, T. Saison, M. Takasugi, J. J. Toulme, U. Asseline, G. Lancelot, J. C. Maurizot, F. Toulme and N. T. Thoung *Biocheimie*, **67**, 777 (1985).

18. C. Helene, in DNA-Ligand Interactions, W. Buschlbauer and W. Saenger, Eds., Plenum Press, 1987, p. 127.

19. P. E. Nielson, M. Egholm, R. H. Berg, O. Buchardt, *Science*, **254**, 14971 (1991).

20. G. Felsenfeld, D. R. Davies, and A. Rich, *J. Am. Chem. Soc.*, **79**, 2023 (1957).

21. M. N. Lipsett, *Biochem. Biophys. Res. Commun.*, **11**, 224 (1963).

22. F. B. Howard, J. Frazier, M. N. Lipsett, and H. T. Miles *Biochem. Biophys. Res. Commun.*, **17**, 93 (1964).

23. J. H. Miller and H. M. Sobell *Proc. Natl. Acad. Sci. USA*, **55**, 1201 (1966).

24. J. S. Lee, D. A. Johnson, and A. R. Morgan, *Nucl. Acids. Res.*, **6**, 3073 (1979).

25. A. R. Morgan and R. D. Wells, *J. Molec. Biol.*, **37**, 63 (1968).

26. S. Arnott, P. J. Bond, E. Selsin, and P. J. C. Smith, *Nucleic Acids Res.*, **3**, 2459 (1976).

27. K. Hoogsteen, *Acta Cryst.*, **12**, 822 (1959).

28. P. B. Dervan, In *Oligodeoxynucleotide: Antisense Inhibitors of Gene Expression*, J. S. Cohen, Ed., CRC Press, Inc., 1989, p. 197.

29. M. Cooney, G. Czernuszewicz, E. H. Postel, S. J. Flint, and M. E. Hogan, *Science*, **241**, 456 (1988).

30. P. A. Beal and P. B. Dervan, *Science*, **251**, 1360 (1991).

31. E. Uhlmann and A. Peyman *Chemical Reviews*, **90**, 543 (1990).

32. A. Ono, P. O. P. Ts'o, and L. Kan, *J. Am. Chem. Soc.*, **113**, 4032 (1991).

33. D. A. Horne, and P. G. Dervan, *J. Amer. Chem. Soc.*, **112**, 2435 (1990).

34. J. S. Sun, J. C. Francois, T. Montenay-Garestier, T. Saison-Behmoaras, V. Roig, N. T. Thuong, and C. Helene, *Proc. Natl. Acad. Sci. USA.*, **86**, 9198 (1989).

35. D. Praseuth, L. Perrouault, T. LeDoan, M. Chassignol, N. Thuong and C. Helene, *Proc. Natl. Acad. Sci. USA*, **85**, 1349 (1988).

36. V. V. Vlassov, S. A. Gaidamakov, V. F. Zarytova, D. G. Knorre, A. S. Levina, A. A. Nikonova, L. M. Podust, and O. S. Fedorova. *Geme*. **72**, 313 (1988).

37. J. C. Francois, T. Saison-Behmoaras, M. Chassignol, N. T. Thuong, and C. Helene *C.R. Acad. Sci. Paris*, **307(III)**, 849 (1988).

38. J. C. Francois, T. Saison-Behmoaras, C. Barbier, M. Chassignol, N. T. Thuong, and C. Helene, *Proc. Natl. Acad. Sci. USA*, **86**, 9702 (1989).

39. J. C. Francois, T. Saison-Behmoaras, M. Chassignol, N. T. Thuong, and C. Helene, *J. Biol. Chem.*, **264**, 5891 (1989).

40. J. C. Francois, T. Saison-Behmoaras, M. Chassignol, N. T. Thuong, J S. Sun, and C. Helene, *Biochemistry*, **27**, 2272 (1988).

41. L. Perrouault, U. Asseline, C. Rivalle, N. T. Thuong, E. Bisagni, C. Giovannangeli, T. Le Doan, and C. Helene, *Nature*, **344**, 358 (1990).

42. H. E. Moser and P. B. Dervan, *Science*, **238**, 650 (1987).

43. F. H. Hausheer, U. C. Singh, J D. Saxe, O. M. Colvin, and P. O. P. T'so, *Anti-Cancer Drug Design*, **5**, 159 (1990).

44. A. G. Letai, M. A. Palladine, E. Fromm, V. Rizzo and J. R. Fresco, *Biochemistry*, **27**, 9108 (1988).

45. V. Sklenar and J. Feigon, *Nature*, **345**, 836 (1990).

46. V. I. Lyamichev, M. D. Frank-Kamenetskii, and V. N. Soyfer, *Nature*, **344**, 568 (1990).

47. S. L. Broitman, D. D. Im, and J. R. Fresco, *Proc. Natl. Acad. Sci. USA*, **84**, 5120 (1987).

48. J. L. Maher, III, B. Wold, and P. G. Dervan, *Science*, **245**, 725 (1989).

49. J. C. Hanvey, M. Shimizu, and R. D. Wells, *Nucleic Acids Res.*, **18**, 157 (1989).

50. F. M. Orson, D. W. Thomas, W. M. McShan, D. J. Kessler, and M. E. Hogan *Nucleic Acids Res.*, **19**, 3435 (1991).

51. M. E. McManaway, L. M. Neckers, S. L. Loke, A. A. Al-Nasser, R. L. Redner, B. T. Shiramizu, W. L. Goldschmidts, B. E. Huber, K. Bhatia, and I. T. Magrath, *Lancet*, **335**, 808 (1990).

52. M. Kulka, C. Smith, L. Aurelian, R. Fishelevich, K. Meade, P. Miller, and P. Ts'o, *Proc. Natl. Acad. Sci. USA*, **86**, 6868 (1989).

53. P. C. Zamecnik, J. Goodchild, Y. Taguchi and P. S. Sarin, *Proc. Natl. Acad. Sci. USA*, **83**, 4143 (1986).

54. C. C. Smith, L. Aurelian, M. P. Reddy, P. A. Miller and P. O. P. Ts'o, *Proc. Natl. Acad. Sci. USA*, **83**, 2785 (1985).

55. S. Agrawal, J. Goodchile, M. P. Civeira, A. T. Thornton, P. M. Sarin and P. C. Zaecnik, *Proc. Natl. Acad. Sci. USA*, **85**, 7079 (1988).

56. M. Lemaitre, B. Bayard, and B. Lebleu, *Biochem*, **84**, 648 (1987).

57. A. Rosolen, L. Whitesell, M. Olegalo, R. H. Lennett, and L. M. Neckers, *Cancer Res.*, **50**, 6316 (1990).

58. G. Vasanthakumar and N. K. Ahmed, *Cancer Commun.*, **1**, 225 (1989).

59. A. R. Sburlati, R. E. Manrow and S. L. Berger, *Proc. Natl. Acad. Sci. USA*, **88**, 253 (1991).

60. H. Zheng, B. M. Sahai, P. Kilgannon, A. Fotedar, and D. R. Green, *Proc. Natl. Acad. Sci. USA*, **86**, 3758 (1989).

61. J. A. M. Maier, P. Voulalas, D. Roeder, and T. Maciag, *Science*, **249**, 1570 (1990).

62. C. K. Mirabelli, C. F. Bennett, K. Anderson, and S. T. Crooke, *Anti-Cancer Drug Design*, **6**, 649 (1991).

63. L. M. Cowsert, M C. Fox, G. Zon, and C. K. Mirabelli, *Antimicrobial Agents and Chemotherapy*, **37**, 171 (1993).

64. T. Vickers, B. F. Baker, P. D. Cook, M. Zounes, R. W. Buckheit, Jr., J. Germany, and D. J. Ecker, *Nucleic Acids Res.*, **19**, 3359 (1991).

65. S. K. Saxena and E. J. Ackerman, *J. Biol. Chem.*, **265**, 3263 (1990).

66. K. Walker, S. A. Elela, and R. N. Nazar, *J. Biol. Chem.*, **265**, 2428 (1990).

67. P. Westerman, B. Gross, and G. Honkis, *Biomed. Biochim. Acta*, **48**, 85 (1989).

68. B. Baker, *J. Am. Chem. Soc.*, **115**, 3378 (1993).

69. M. Y. Chiang, H. Chan, M A. Zounes, S. M. Freier, W. F. Lima, and C. F. Bennett, *J. Biol. Chem.*, **266**, 18162 (1991).

70. P. C. Zamecnik and M. L. Stephenson, *Proc. Natl. Acad. Sci. USA*, **75**, 280 (1978).

71. A. Zerial, N. T. Thuong, and C. Helene, *Nucleic Acids Res.*, **15**, 9909 (1987).

72. N. T. Thuong, U. Assenine, and T. Monteney-Garestier, in *Oligodeoxynucleotides: Antisense Inhibitors of Gene Expression*, CRC Press, Inc., Boca Raton, Fla, 1989, p. 25.

73. C. Helene and J.-J. Toulme, in *Oligodeoxynucleotides: Antisense Inhibitors of Gene Expression*, J. S. Cohen, Ed., CRC Press, Inc., Boca Raton, Fla, 1989, p. 137.

74. R. J. Crouch and M-L. Dirksen, in *Nucleases*, S. M. Linn and R. J. Roberts, Eds., Cold Spring Harbor Laboratory, Cold Spring Harbor, N.Y. 1985, p. 211.

75. C. Crum, J D. Johnson, A. Nelson, D. Roth, *Nucleic Acids. Res.*, **16**, 4569 (1988).

76. M. T. Haeuptle, R. Frank and B. Dobberstein, *Nucleic Acids Res.*, **14**, 1427 (1986).

77. G. Hoke, Unpublished data, 1991.

78. H. Doris-Keller, *Nucleic Acid Res.*, **7**, 179 (1979).

79. A. M. Kawasaki, M. D. Casper, S. M. Freier, E. A. Lesnik, M. C. Zounes, L. L. Cummins, C. Gonzalez, and P. D. Cook, *J. Med. Chem.*, **36**, 831 (1993).

80. B. S. Sproat, A. L. Lamond, B. Beijer, P. Neuner, and U. Ryder, *Nucleic Acids Res.*, **17**, 3373 (1989).

81. F. Morvan, B. Rayner, and J-L. Imbach, *Anti-Cancer Drug Design*, **6** 521 (1991).

82. C. Gagnor, B. Rayner, J.-P. Leonetti, J.-L. Imbach, and B. Leubleu *Nucleic Acids Res.*, **17**, 5107 (1989).

83. P. S. MIller, in *Oligodeoxynucleotides: Antisense Inhibitors of Gene Expression*, J. S. Cohen, Ed., CRC Press, Inc. Boca Raton, Fla, 1989, p. 79.

84. C. A. Stein and J. S. Cohen, in *Oligodeoxynucleotides: Antisense Inhibitors of Gene Expression*, J. S. Cohen, Ed., CRC Press, Inc., Boca Raton, Fla., p. 97.

85. C. Cazenave, C. A. Stein, N. Loreau, N. T. Thuong, L. M. Neckers, C. Subasinghe, C. Helene, J. S. Cohen, and J.-J. Toulme, *Nucleic Acids Res.*, **17**, 4255 (1989).

86. R. Quartin, C. Brakel, and J. Wetmur, *Nucleic Acids Res.*, **17**, 7253 (1989).

87. P. Furdon, Z. Dominski, and R. Kole, *Nucleic Acids Res.*, **17**, 9193 (1989).

88. P. S. Eder and J. A. Walder, *J. Biol. Chem.*, **206**, 6472 (1991).

89. B. P. Monia, E. A. Lesnik, C. Gonzalez, W. F. Lima, D. McGee, C. J. Guinosso, A. M. Kawasaki, P. D. Cook, and S. M. Freier, *J. Biol. Chem.*, **268**, 4514 (1993).

90. R. V. GIles and D. M. Tidd, *Nucleic Acids Res.*, **20**, 763 (1992).

91. R. Y. Walder and J. A. Walder, *Proc. Natl. Acad. Sci. USA*, **85**, 5011 (1988).

92. J. Minshull and T. Hunt, *Nucleic Acids Res.*, **14**, 6433 (1986).

93. C. Gagnor, J. Bertrand, S. Thenet, M. Lemaitre, F. Morvan, B. Rayner, C. Malvy, B. Lebleu, J. Imbach and C. Paoletti, *Nucleic Acids Res.*, **15**, 10419 (1987).

94. D. G. Knorre, V. V. Vlassov, and V. F. Zarytova, in *Oligodeoxynucleotides: Antisense Inhibitors of Gene Expression*, J. S. Cohen, Ed., CRC Press, Inc., Boca Raton, Fla., 1989, p. 173.

95. D. G. Knorre, V. V. Vlassov, and V. F. Zarytova, *Biochimie*, **67**, 785 (1985).

96. V. V. Vlassov, V. F. Zarytova, I. V. Kutyavin, and S. V. Mamave, *FEBS Lett.*, **231**, 352 (1988).

97. J. Summerton and P. A. Bartlett, *J. Molec. Biol.*, **122**, 145 (1978).

98. T. R. Webb and M. D. Matteucci, *Nucleic Acids, Res.*, **14**, 7661 (1986).

99. T. Le Doan, L. Perrouault, D. Praseuth, N. Habhoub, J. Decout, N. T. Thuong, J. Lhomme, and C. Helene, *Nucleic Acids Res.*, **15**, 7749 (1987).

100. O. S. Federova, D. G. Knorre, L. M. Podust, and F. V. Zarytova, *FEBS Lett.*, **228**, 273 (1988).

101. D. Praseuth, T. L. Doan, M. Chassignol, J. L. Decrout, N. Habhoub, J. Lhomme, N T. Thuong, and C. Helene, *Biochemistry*, **27**, 3031 (1988).

102. T. Le Doan, L. Perrouault, M. Chassignol, N. T. Thuong, and C. Helene, *Nucleic Acids Res.*, **15**, 8643 (1987).

103. T. Le Doan, L. Perrouault, N. T. Thuong, C. Helene, *J. Inorg. Biochem.*, **36**, 274 (abstract) (1989).

104. T. Le Doan, D. Praseuth, L. Perrouault, M. Chassignol, N. T. Thoung, and C. Helene, *Bioconj. Chem.*, **1**, 108 (1990).

105. B. L. Lee, K. R. Blake and P. S. Miller, *Nucleic Acids Res.*, **16**, 10681 (1988).

106. B. L. Lee, A. Murakami, K. R. Blake, S.-B. Lin, and P. S. Miller, *Biochem.*, **27**, 3197 (1988).

107. D. Praseuth, M. Chassignol, M. Takasugi, T. Le Doan, N. T. Thuong, and C. Helene, *J. Mol. Biol.*, **196**, 939 (1987).

108. C. Helene, *Br. J. Cancer*, **60**, 157 (1989).

109. J. M. Kean, A. Murakami, K. R. Blake, C. D. Cushman, and P. S. Miller, *Biochemistry*, **27**, 9113 (1988).

110. T. Saison-Behmoaras, B. Tocque, I. Rey, M. Chassignol, N. T. Thuong, and C. Helene, *Embo J.*, **10**, 1111 (1991).

111. B. C. F. Chu and L. E. Orgel, *Proc. Natl. Acad. Sci. USA*, **82**, 963 (1985).

112. A. S. Boutorin, V. V. Vlassov, S. A. Kazakov, I. V. Kutiavin, and M. A. Podyminogin, *FEBS Lett.*, **172**, 43 (1984).

113. J. S. Sun, J C. Francois, R. Lavery, T. Saison-Behmoaras, T. Montenay-Garestier, N. T. Thuong, and C. Helene, *Biochem.*, **27**, 6039 (1988).

114. C.-H. B. Chen, and D. S. Sigman, *Proc. Natl. Acad. Sci. USA*, **83**, 7147 (1986).

115. C. Helene, T. Le Doan, and N. T. Thuong, in *Photochemical Probes in Biochemistry*, P. E. Nielsen, Ed., Kluwer Academic Publishers, 1989, p. 219.

116. C. Helene and N. T. Thuong, in *Working Group on Molecular Mechanisms of Carcinogenic and Antitumor Activity*, C. Chagas adn B. Pullman, Eds., Pontificaiae Academiae Scientarium Scripta Varia, Vatican City, 1987, p. 205.

117. C. Helene and N. T. Thuong, *Genome*, **31**, 413 (1989).

118. T. R. Cech, *Science*, **236**, 1532 (1987).

119. J. A. McSwiggen and T. R. Cech, *Science*, **244**, 679 (1989).

120. D. Herschlag and T. R. Cech, *Nature*, **344**, 405 (1990).

121. D. Cook, et al., Unpublished data, 1992.

122. A. D. Ellington and J. W. Szostak, *Nature*, **355**, 850 (1992).

123. L. C. Bock, L. C. Griffin, J. A. Latham, E. H. Vermaas, and J J. Toole, *Nature*, **355**, 564 (1992).

124. C. Tuerk and L. Gold, *Science*, **249**, 505 (1990).

125. A. D. Ellington and J. W. Szostak, *Nature*, **346**, 818 (1990).

126. P. Dehua, H. D. Ulrich, and P. G. Schultz, *Science*, **253**, 1408 (1991).

127. G. D. Hoke, K. Draper, S. M. Freier, C. Gonzalez, V. B. Driver, M. C. Zounes, and D. J. Ecker, *Nucleic Acid Research*, **19**, 5743 (1991).

128. E. Wickstrom, *J. Biochem. Biophy. Meth.*, **13**, 97 (1986).

129. C. Cazenave, M. Cheurier, N. T. Thuong, and C. Helene, *Nucleic Acid Res.*, **15**, 10507 (1987).

130. A. Harel-Bellan, S. Durum, K. Muegge, A. K. Abbas and W. L. Farrar, *J. Exp. Med.*, **168**, 2309 (1988).

131. J. M. Campbell, T. A. Bacon, and E. Wickstrom, *J. Biochem. and Biophysical Methods*, **20**, 259 (1990).

132. J. S. Cohen, in *Design of Anti-AIDS Drugs*, De Clercq, Ed., Elsevier, 1990, p. 195.

133. M. Matsukura, K. Shinozuka, G. Zon, H. Mitsuya, M. Reitz, J. S. Cohen, and S. Broder, *Proc. Natl. Acad. Sci. USA*, **84**, 7706 (1987).

134. P. S. Miller, C. H. Agris, L. Aurelian, K. R. Blake, S. B. Lin, A. Murakami, M. P. Reddy, C. Smith, and P. O. P. Ts'o, in *Interrelationship Among Aging, Cancer and Differentiation*, B. Pullman et al., Eds., D. Reidel Publishing Co., Mass., 1985, p. 207.

135. P. S. Miller, C. H. Agris, K. R. Blake, A. Murakami, S. A. Spitz, P. M. Reddy, and P. O. P. Ts'o, in *Nucleic Acids: The Vectors of Life*, B. Pullman and J. Jortner, Eds., D. Deidel Publishing, Doredrecht, Holland, 1983, p. 521.

136. P. S. MIller, K. B. McParland, K. Jayaraman, and P. O. P. Ts'o, *Biochemistry*, **20**, 1874 (1981).

137. P. S. Miller and P. O. P. Ts'o, *Anti-Cancer Drug Design*, **2**, 117 (1987).

138. P. O. P. Ts'o, P. S. Miller, L. Aurelian, A. Murakami, C. Agris, K. R. Blake, S. B. Lin, B. L. Lee, and C. C. Smith, in *Biological Approaches to the Controlled Delivery of Drugs*, Annals of the New York Academy of Sciences, 1987, p. 507.

139. S. Agrawal and J Goodchild, *Tetrahedron lett.*, **28**, 3539 (1987).

140. K. L. Agrawal and F. Fiftina, *Nucleic Acids Res.*, **6**, 3009 (1979).

141. P. S. Miller, N. Dreon, S. M. Pulord, and K. B. McParland, *J. Biol. Chem.*, **255**, 9659 (1980).

142. M. Koziolkiewicz, B. Uznanski, W. J. Stec, and G. Zon, *Chem. Scripta*, **26**, 251 (1986).

143. P. S. Miller and P. O. P. Ts'o, *Ann. Reports Med. Chem.*, **23**, 295 (1988).

144. P. S. Miller, S. Chandrasegaran, D. L. Dow, S. M. Pulford, and L. S. Kan, *Biochemistry*, **21**, 5468 (1982).

145. T. A. Bacon, F. Morvan, B. Rayner, J. L. Imbach, and E. Wickstrom, *J. Biochem. Biophys. Methods* **16**, 311 (1988).

146. F. Morvan, B. Rayner, J. Imbach, S. Thenet, J. Bertrand, J. Paoletti, C. Malvy, and C. Paolett, *Nucleic Acids Res.* **15**, 3421 (1987).

147. F. Morvan, C. Genu, B. Rayner, and J.-L. Imbach, *Biochem. Biophys. Res. Comm.*, **172**, 537 (1990).

148. S. Thenet, F. Morvan, J. R. Bertrand, C. Gauthier, and C. Malvy, *Biochimie*, **70**, 1729 (1988).

149. B. S. Sproat, A. L. Lamond, B. Beijer, P. Neuner, and U. Rynder, *Proc. Natl. Acad. Sci. USA*, **87**, 3391 (1990).

150. C. J. Guinosso, G. D. Hoke, D. J. Ecker, C. K. Mirabelli, S. T. Crooke, and P. D. Cook, *Nucleosides & Nucleotides*, **10**, 259 (1991).

151. C. A. Stein, K. Mori, S. L. Loke, C. Subasinghe, K. Shinozuka, J. S. Cohen, and L. M. Neckers, *Gene*, **72**, 333 (1988).

152. P. Vespieren, A. W. C. A. Cornelissen, N. T. Thuong, C. Helene, and J. J. Toulme, *Gene*, **61**, 307 (1987).

153. J. J. Toulme, H. M. Krisch, N. Loreau, N. T. Thuong, and C. Helene, *Proc. Natl. Acad. Sci. USA*, **83**, 1227 (1986).

154. M. Lemaitre, C. Bisbal, B. Bayard and B. Lebleu, *Nucleosides Nucleotides*, **6**, 311 (1987).

155. J. P. Leonetti, B. Rayner, M. Lemaitre, C. Gagnor, P. G. Milhaud, J.-L. Imbach, and B. Lebleu, *Gene*, **72**, 323 (1988).

156. M. Manoharan, C. J. Guinosso, and P. D. Cook, *Tetrahedron Letters*, **32**, 7171 (1991).

157. K. Yamanal, Y. Nishijima, T. Ikeda, T. Gokota, H. Ozaki, H. Nakano, O. Sangen, and T. Shimidzu, *Bioconjugate Chem.*, **1**, 319 (1990).

158. K. Ramasamy, R. S. Springer, J. F. Martin, S. M. Freier, G. D. Hoke, T. W. Bruice, and P. D. Cook, *International Union of Biochemistry Conference on Nucleic Acid Therapeutics*, **82** (1991).

159. R. Casale and L. W. McLaughlin, *J. Amer. Chem. Soc.*, **112**, 5264 (1990).

160. O. L. Acevedo, G. D. Hoke, S. Freier, M.

Zounes, C. G. Guinosso, R. S. Springer, and P. D. Cook, *Intl. Union of Biochemistry Conference on Nucleic Acid Therapeutics*, 50 (1991).

161. Y. S. Sanghvi, G. D. Hoke, M. Zounes, H. Chan, O. Acevedo, D. J. Ecker, C. K. Mirabelli, S. T. Crooke, and P. D. Cook, *Nucleosides & Nucleotides*, **10**, 345 (1991).

162. R. M. Crooke, *Anti-Cancer Drug Design*, **6**, 609 (1991).

163. Y. Shoji, S. Akhtar, A. Periasamy, B. Herman, and R. L. Juliano, *Nucleic Acids Res.* **19**, 5543 (1991).

164. C. J. Marcus-Sekura, A. M. Woerner, K. Shinozuka, G. Zon, and G. V. Quinnan, Jr., *Nucleic Acids Res.*, **15**, 5749 (1987).

165. W. Gao, C. A. Stein, J. S. Cohe, G. E. Dutschman, and C.-Y. Cheng, *J. Biol. Chem.*, **2643**, 11521 (1989).

166. R. M. Crooke, in *Antisense Research and Applications*, S. T. Crooke and B. Lebleu, Eds., CRC Press, Boca Raton, Fla., 1993, p. 427.

167. C. F. Bennett, M.-Y. Chiang, H. Chan, J. Shoemaker, and C. K. Mirabelli, *Molecular Pharmacology*, **41**, 1023 (1992).

168. J. P. Leonetti, G. Degols, P. Milhaud, C. Gagnor, M. Lemaitre, and B. Lebleu, *Nucleosides Nucleotides*, **8**, 825 (1989).

169. J.-P. Leonetti, G. Degols, B. Lebleu, *Bioconj. Chem.*, **1**, 149 (1990).

170. R. G. Shea, J. C. Marsters, and N. Bischofberger, *Nucleic Acids Res.*, **18**, 3777 (1990).

171. A. V. Kabanov, S. V. Vinogradov, A. V. Ovcharenko, A. V. Krivonos, N. S. Melik-Nubarov, V. I. Kiselev, and E. S. Severin, *FEBS Lett.*, **259**, 327 (1990).

172. S. L. Loke, C. Stein, X. Zhang, M. Avigan, J. Cohen, and L. Neckers, *Curr. Top. Microbiol. Immunol.*, **141**, 282 (1988).

173. C. Bisbal, B. Bayard, M. Lemaitre, L. Leserman, and B. Lebleu, *Drugs of the Future*, **12** 793 (1987).

174. S. L. Loke, C. A. Stein, X. H. Zhang, K. Mori, M. Nakanishi, C. Subasinghe, J. S. Cohen, and L. M. Neckers, *Proc. Natl. Acad. Sci. USA*, **86**, 3474 (1989).

175. T.-L. Chem, P. S. MIller, P O. Ts'o, and O. M. Colvin, *Drug Metabolism and Diastribution*, **18**, 815 (1990).

176. P. Iversen, *Anti-Cancer Drug Design*, **6**, 531 (1991).

177. Y. S. Sanghvi, in *Antisense Research and Applications*, S. T. Crooke and B. Lebleu, Eds., CRC Press, Boca Raton, Fla, 1993, p. 273.

178. R. Heikkila, G. Schwab, R. Wickstrom, et al., *Nature*, **328**, 445 (1987).

179. C. H. Agris, K. R. Black, P. S. Miller, M. P. Reddy, and P. O. P. Ts'o, *Biochemistry*, **25**, 6268 (1986).

180. T. Ishikawa, F. Yoneda, et al. *Biorg. & Med. Chem. Letts.*, **1**, 523 (1991).

181. T. T. Nikiforov and B. A. Connolly, *Tet. Letts.*, **32**, 3851 (1991).

182. K. T. P. Lin, and D. M. Brown, *Nucleic Acids Res.*, **17**, 10373 (1989).

183. H. Inoue and E. Ohtsuka, *Nucleic Acids. Res.*, **13**, 7119 (1985).

184. Y. S. Sanghvi, G. D. Hoke, S. M. Freier, M. C. Zounes, C., Gonzalez, L. Cummins, H. Sasmor, and P. D. Cook, *Nucleic Acids Res.*, **21**, 3197 (1993).

185. L. Hagenberg, H. G. Gassen, and H. Matthaei, *Biochem. Biophy. Res. COmm.*, **50**, 1104 (1973).

186. B. S. Sproat, A. M. Irabarren, et al., *Nucleic Acids Res.*, **19**, 733 (1991).

187. F. H. Martin, M. M. Castro, et al., *Nucleic Acids. Res.*, **13**, 8927 (1985).

188. J. S. Koh and P. B. Dervan, *J. Am. Chem. Soc.*, **114**, 1470 (1992).

189. L. C. Griffin, L. L. Kiessling, P. A. Beal, P. Gillespie, and P. B. Dervan, *J. Am. Chem. Soc.*, **114**, 7976 (1992).

190. M. Manoharan, in *Antisense Research and Therapeutics*, S.T. Crooke and B. Lebleu, Eds., CRC Press, Inc., Boca Raton, Fla, 1993, p. 303.

191. G. D. Hoke, K. Draper, S. M. Freier, C. Gonzalez, V. B. Driver, M. C. Zounes, and D. J. Ecker, *Nucleic Acids Res.*, **19**, 5743 (1991).

192. B. P. Monia, E. A. Lesnik, C. Gonzalez, W. F. Lima, D. McGee, C. J. Guinosso, A. M. Kawasaki, P. D. Cook, and S. M. Freier, *J. Biol. Chem.*, **268**, 14514 (1993).

193. A. Boutorine, C. Huet, T. Saison, C. Helene and T. Le Doan, *Conf. on Nucleic Acid Therapeutics*, 60 (*abstract* 1991).

194. T. S. Sergeyev, T. S. Godovikova, and V. F. Zarytova, *FEBS Letts.*, **280**, 271 (1991).

195. K. Nagai and S. M. Hecht, *J. Biol. Chem.*, **266**, 23994 (1991).

196. Y. S. Sanghvi and P. D. Cook, in *Nucleosides and Nucleotides as Antitumor and Antiviral Agents*, C. K. Chu & D. C. Baker, Eds., Plenum Press, New York, 1993, p. 311.

197. P. E. Nielsen, M. Egholm, R. H. Berg, and O. Buchardt, in *Antisense Research and Application*, S. T. Crooke and B. Lebleu, Eds., CRC Press, Inc., Boca Raton, Fla., 1993, p. 363.

198. M. Egholm, O. Buchardt, P. E. Nielsen, and R. H. Berg, *J. Amer. Chem. Soc.*, **114**, 1895 (1992).

199. J. C. Hanvey, N. J. Peffer, J. E. Bisi, S. A. Thomson, R. Cadilla, J. A. Josey, D. J. Ricca, C. F. Hassman, M. A. Bonham, K. G. Au, S. G. Carter, D. A. Bruckenstein, A. L. Boyd, S. A.

Noble, and L. E. Babiss, *Science*, **258**, 1481 (1992).

200. J. S. Cohen, Ed., *Oligodeoxynucleotides. Antisense Inhibitors of Gene Expression.*, CRC Press, Inc., Boca Raton, Fla., 1989, 255 pp.

201. J. N. M. Mol, A. R. van der Krol, Eds., *Antisense Nucleic Acids adn Proteins. Fundamentals and Applications*, Marcell Dekker, New York, 1991, 231 pp.

202. L. Perlaky, Y. Saijo, R. K. Busch, C. F. Bennett, C. F. Mirabelli, S. T. Crooke, and H. Busch, *Anti-Cancer Drug Design*, **8**, 3 (1993).

203. M. Simons, E. R. Edelman, J.-L. DeKeyser, R. Langer, and R. D. Rosenberg, *Nature*, **359**, 67 (1992).

204. R. M. Burch and L. C. Mahan, *J. Clin. Invest.*, **88**, 1190 (1991).

205. I. Kitajima, T. Shinohara, J. Bilakovics, D. A. Brown, X. Xu, and M. Nerenberg, *Science*, **258**, 1792 (1992).

206. C. K. Mirabelli and S. T. Crooke, in *Antisense Research and Applications*, S. T. Crooke and B. Lebleu, Eds., CRC Press, Boca Raton, Fla., 1993, p. 7.

207. W. J. Stec, G. Zon, W. Egan, and B. Stec. *J. Am. Chem. Soc.*, **106**, 6077–6079 (1984).

208. K. G. Draper and V. B. Driver, *International Herpesvirus Workshop* (1991, *abstract*).

209. V. V. Vlassov, Meeting on "Oligodeoxynucleotides as Antisense Inhibitors of Gene Expression: Therapeutic Implications," June 18–21, 1989, Rockville, Md., (abstract).

210. P. S. Miller, C. H. Agris, L. Aurelian, K. R. Blake, A. Murakami, M. P. Reddy, S. A. Spitz, and P. O. P. Ts'o, *Biochimie*, **67**, 769–776 (1985).

211. G. Goodarzi, S. C. Gross, A. Tewari, and K. Watabe, *J. Gen. Virol.*, **71**, 3021–3025 (1990).

212. E. L. Wickstrom, T. A. Bacon, A. Gonzalez, G. H. Lyman, and E. Wickstrom, *In Vitro Cell Develop. Biol.*, **25**, 297–302 (1989).

213. A. M. Gewirtz and B. Calabretta, *Science*, **242**, 1303–1306 (1988).

214. J. C. Reed, M. Cuddy, S. Haldar, C. Croce, P. Nowell, D. Makover, and K. Bradley, Proc. Natl. Acad. Sci. USA, **87**, 3660–3664 (1990).

215. D. M. Tidd, P. Hawley, H. M. Warenius, and I. Gibson, *Anti-Cancer Drug Design*, **3**, 117–127 (1988).

216. J. W. Jaroszewski, O. Kaplan, J. L. Syi, M. Sehested, P. J. Faustino, P. J. and J. S. Cohen *Cancer Comm.*, **2**, 287–294 (1990).

217. D. Jaskulski, J. K. DeRiel, W. E. Mercer, B. Calabretta, and R. Baserga, *Science*, **240**, 1544–1546 (1989).

218. M. C. Brichenall-Roberts, L. A. Falk, C. Ferrer, and F. W. Ruscetti, *J. Cell. Biochem. Suppl.* **13 (Part C)**, 188 (1989, abstract).

219. L. C. Yeoman, Y. J. Daniels, and M. J. Lynch, Meeting on "Oligodeoxynucleotides as Antisense Inhibitors of Gene Expression: Therapeutic Implications," June 18–21, 1989, Rockville, Md., (abstract).

220. R. S. Morrison, *J. Biol. Chem.*, **266**, 728–734 (1991).

221. K. R. Blake, A. Murakami, and P. S. Miller, *Biochem.*, **24**, 6132–6138 (1985).

222. A. Caceres and K. S. Kosik, *Nature*, **343**, 461–463 (1990).

223. G. Tortora, T. Clair, and Y. S. Cho-Chung, *Proc. Natl. Acad. Sci. USA*, **87**, 705–708 (1990).

224. D. Bories, M.-C. Raynal, D. H. Solomon, Z. Darzynkiewicz, and Y. E. Cayre, *Cell*, **59**, 959–968 (1989).

225. M. A. Clark, L. E. Ozgur, T. M. Conway, J. Dispoto, S. T. Crooke, and J. S. Bomalaski, *Proc. Natl. Acad. Sci. USA*, **88**, 5418–5422 (1991).

226. J. A. M. Maier, P. Voulalas, D. Roeder, and T. Maciag, *Science*, **249**, 1570–1574 (1990).

227. J. Manson, T. Brown, and G. Duff, *Lymphokine Res.*, **9**, 35–42 (1990).

228. J. R. Florini and D. Z. Ewton, *J. Biol. Chem.*, **265**, 13435–13437 (1990).

229. H. Acha-Orbea, L. Scarpellino, S. Hertig, M. Dupuis and J. Tschopp, *EMBO Journal*, **9**, 3815–3819 (1990).

230. C. R. Brandt, L. M. Coakley, D. R. Graud, and K. G. Draper, *Assoc. Res. in Vision and Ophthalmology*, Tampa, Fla., (1991 abstract).

CHAPTER TWENTY-TWO

Carbohydrate-based Therapeutics

JOHN H. MUSSER
PÉTER FÜGEDI
MARK BRIAN ANDERSON

Glycomed, Inc.
Alameda, California, USA

CONTENTS

1 Introduction, 902
2 Carbohydrate-related Pharmaceuticals, 903
  2.1 Antibiotics, 904
  2.2 Nucleosides, 906
  2.3 Cardiac glycosides, 906
  2.4 Synthetic carbohydrate drugs, 907
3 Pharmacological Considerations, 907
  3.1 Absorption, 908
  3.2 Distribution, 908
  3.3 Metabolism, 908
  3.4 Excretion, 909
  3.5 Binding affinities, 909
4 New Techniques and Instrumentation, 909
  4.1 Instrumentation, 910
    4.1.1 Isolation and separation, 910
    4.1.2 Structure determination, 910
    4.1.3 Conformational studies, 911
  4.2 Synthesis, 912
    4.2.1 Chemical, 912
    4.2.2 Enzymatic, 915
    4.2.3 Glycomimetics, 917
    4.2.4 Carbohydrates as chiral synthons, 917
5 Glyconconjugates, 919
  5.1 Glycolipids, 919
  5.2 Proteoglycans, 922
  5.3 Glycoproteins, 925
6 Enzyme Inhibitors of Carbohydrate Biosynthesis and Catabolism, 926
  6.1 Glycosidase inhibitors, 926

Burger's Medicinal Chemistry and Drug Discovery,
Fifth Edition, Volume 1: Principles and Practice,
Edited by Manfred E. Wolff.
ISBN 0-471-57556-9 © 1995 John Wiley & Sons, Inc.

6.2 Glycosyltransferase inhibitors, 928

7 Immunomodulation, 929
  7.1 Antibacterial vaccines, 929
  7.2 Immunostimulants and adjuvants, 931
    7.2.1 Muramyl dipeptide and analogs, 931
    7.2.2 Cord factor and analogs, 932
    7.2.3 Lipid A and analogs, 933
    7.2.4 Antitumor polysaccharides, 934
    7.2.5 Glycolipid analogs, 934
    7.2.6 Saponins, 935
    7.2.7 Therafectin, 935

8 Carbohydrate-mediated Cell–Cell
  Interactions, 935
  8.1 Blood group carbohydrates, 935
  8.2 Selectin-mediated adhesion, 937
  8.3 Sperm–egg adhesion, 937
  8.4 Microorganism–cell interaction, 938
  8.5 Cancer metastasis, 938

9 Summary, 938

1 INTRODUCTION

Currently, there are few examples of therapeutics based on carbohydrates; however, by the 21st century research on carbohydrates will emerge as significant new approach to drug discovery. Historically, the pharmaceutical impact of this class of biomolecules has been underestimated. Carbohydrates were considered to function as merely energy storage or mechanical support polymers such as starch and cellulose, respectively. In addition, carbohydrates were widely found in significant concentration in plants but only sparingly found in localized areas of animal tissue. Furthermore, the lack of adequate research tools made the localization and functional characterization of these molecules difficult. Structural analysis requires not only the determination of the component monosaccharides and their sequences but identification of the anomeric configuration, the linkage position, and any additional substituents, such as acetyl, methyl, 1-carboxyethyl, sulfate, phosphate, etc. Synthesis problems derived from the multifunctional nature of the compounds, and the lack of methods for controlling the anomeric stereochemistry presented additional im-

pediments to progress. Finally, both carbohydrate chemists and biochemists have been isolated from mainstream drug discovery scientists. Thus all the above factors have historically combined to diminish the importance of carbohydrates as a source for drug discovery leads.

Research on carbohydrates, however, is undergoing considerable growth and saccharide-based structures are now serving as drug discovery leads (1). Indeed, this is the first edition of Burger's Medicinal Chemistry which contains a chapter dedicated solely to carbohydrate-based therapeutics (2). The reason for the rapid growth of carbohydrate structures serving as new leads is based on fundamental and interdependent cellular processes of recognition, regulation, and growth.

Carbohydrates are critical in the operation of fundamental biological processes of cellular recognition. Bacterial and viral infections are preceded by cell surface recognition events, and the response by the body's immune defense is initiated in part by C-type lectin interactions. When cellular regulatory mechanisms become faulty, as in autoimmune diseases or cancer, cell surface carbohydrates change in structure and composition. Indeed, egg–sperm recognition, which is required for propagation, may be mediated by carbohydrate–protein interactions. Deficiencies in carbohydrate synthesis and metabolism are also implicated in a series of genetic diseases.

With more knowledge accumulating on carbohydrate-containing complex molecules (3), it is clear that carbohydrates, just like proteins and nucleic acids, play an important role in recognition processes. Biologists are discovering that "the specificity of many natural polymers is written in terms of sugar residues, not of amino acids or nucleotides" (4). In the carbohydrate-containing complex molecules, the glycoconjugates, the carbohydrate is attached to proteins to form glycoproteins and proteoglycans, or to different types of lipids to form glycolipids. The glycoconjugates are typical components of cell membranes, cell walls and organelle membranes, with their oligosaccharide chains protruding. The exposed oligosaccharide chains play important roles in intercellular recognition processes, acting as receptors for proteins, enzymes, and viruses and serving as determinants of immunological specificity. In addition to molecule–molecule and cell–molecular interaction, glycoconjugates may act on a cell–cell level. For example, it is now thought, that E- and P-selectins embedded in endothelial cells bind with carbohydrate epitopes on certain inactive glycoprotein receptors or integrins expressed on circulating leukocytes, which in turn are activated and subsequently bind intercellular adhesion molecules (ICAMs) (5). The whole process thus is initiated by carbohydrate recognition and results in cell–cell adhesion and extravasation of leukocytes at a site of inflammation.

In parallel, chemists recognizing that carbohydrates are ideally suited as carriers of biological specificity as they are innately exquisite forms of concise informational packages. In comparison to polypeptides or oligonucleotides, carbohydrates have the potential for greater complexity on a unit basis. Two identical amino acids or nucleotides when joined together yield only one dipeptide or one dinucleotide, whereas when two identical monosaccharides are linked, 11 different disaccharides are possible, considering only the most frequently occurring pyranose forms (6). A recent calculation gave the number of isomeric linear hexasaccharides as nearly 200 billion, while the actual number of possible structures is astronomical, taking into account branched structures (7). Branching is a unique structural feature of carbohydrate polymers not found in the other basic biopolymers: proteins and nucleic acids. Besides this structurally built-in capability of carbohydrates to serve as specific information carriers, they are also well suited for this function biochemically. Because carbohydrates are not direct gene products, their biosynthesis is regulated on different posttranslational levels.

With the recognition that complex oligosaccharides and polysaccharides modulate important physiological processes, research on carbohydrates promises to be a major focus of drug discovery leads (8–10). This chapter starts with a discussion of carbohydrate-containing therapeutics already in use and then discusses fields that show promise for the future. Because the current progress in carbohydrate research is substantially the result of progress in analytical chemistry methods and synthetic techniques, a discussion of these topics is also included.

2 CARBOHYDRATE-RELATED PHARMACEUTICALS

Despite the neglect of saccharides in drug discovery, several carbohydrate or carbohydrate-containing compounds are already in use, although their discovery was generally not the result of understanding the biological role of carbohydrates. These include antibiotics, nucleoside antivirals and anticancer agents, and cardiac glycosides.

2.1 Antibiotics

Among the carbohydrate-containing therapeutics, antibiotics are definitely the most widely used. Numerous antibiotics contain carbohydrate moieties (11). The first representative was streptomycin (Fig. 22.1) isolated by Waksman and co-workers from *Streptomyces griseus* in 1944. Streptomycin is a member of the class of aminoglycoside antibiotics (12) that have an oligosaccharide-like structure and a terminal unit that is not a sugar but an aminocyclitol (streptidine, 2-deoxystreptamine, fortamine B). Several other classes of antibiotics contain carbohydrate units, including the anthracyclines, macrolides, glycopeptides, polyethers, lincosaminides, aurelic acids, and polyene antibiotics. The field has been extensively reviewed (13–16) and no attempt will be made to discuss these agents here except to comment on the structure and function of carbohydrate moieties.

No general rule as to the role of carbohydrates is found, but the sugars seem to be essential in conferring optimum activity to antibiotics. Synthetic modification of carbohydrate moiety constitutes an important tool to generate both an improved therapeutic index and an ability to avoid resistance. Carbohydrate-containing antibiotics often contain rare sugars of unique structures. Even the first representative of

the carbohydrate-containing antibiotics, streptomycin, contains unusual sugars: a branched-chain aldehydrofuranose L-streptose and an *N*-methyl-L-glucosamine. Further examples of sugars occurring typically in antibiotics include (*1*) the different isomers of 2,6-dideoxyhexoses, including D-olivose, which occurs in mithramycin (Fig. 22.2) (17), chromomycin, and olivomycin; (*2*) the branched-chain sugars represented by D-mycarose in mithramycin; and (*3*) 3-amino-2,3,6-trideoxyhexoses such as L-daunosamine, which is the carbohydrate component of adriamycin (Fig. 22.3). The synthesis of 2-deoxy-sugar–containing oligosaccharide components of antibiotics is the subject of a recent review (18).

Besides antibacterial, antiviral, and antitumor activities, carbohydrate-containing compounds are also found as antiparasitic agents. The avermectins are a family of naturally occurring macrocyclic lactonic glycosides (19), these compounds and the structurally related milbemycins (20–22) have significant antiparasitic activities (23). Ivermectin (22,23-dihydroavermectin B_1) (Fig. 22.4) (24, 25) are used as an anthelmintics mainly in animals but also in humans. A key feature of the avermectins is the oleandrosyloleandrose disaccharide unit at the C-13 position, which appears to contribute to antianthelmintic potency (26, 27).

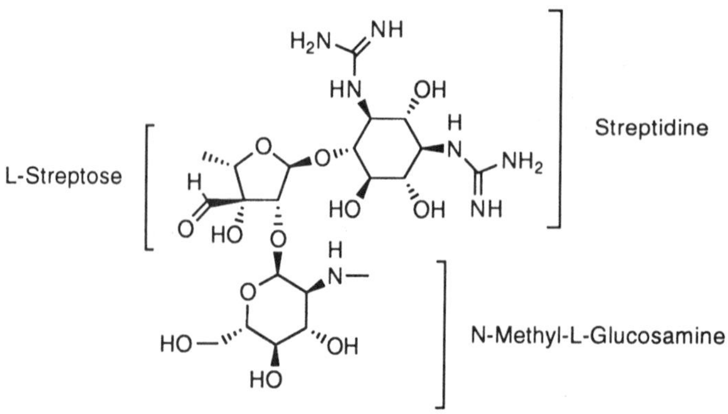

Fig. 22.1 Streptomycin.

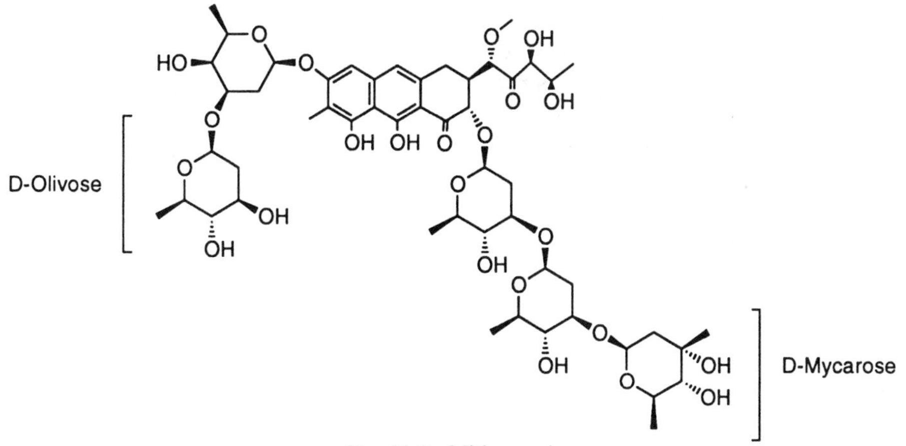

Fig. 22.2 Mithramycin.

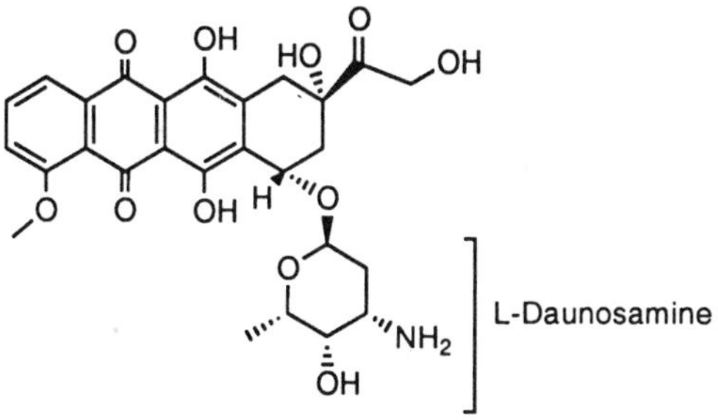

Fig. 22.3 Adriamycin.

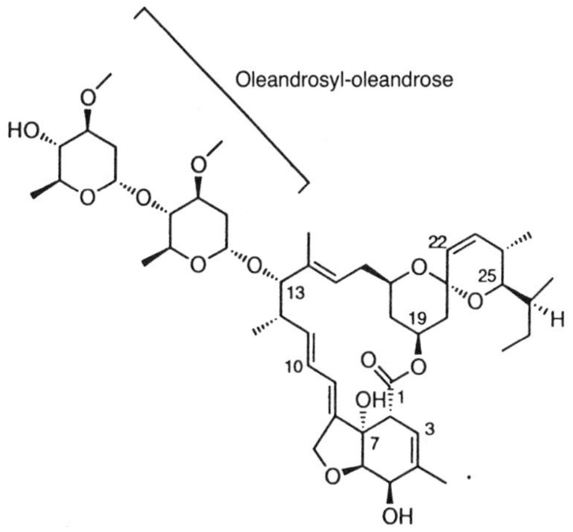

Fig. 22.4 Avermectin.

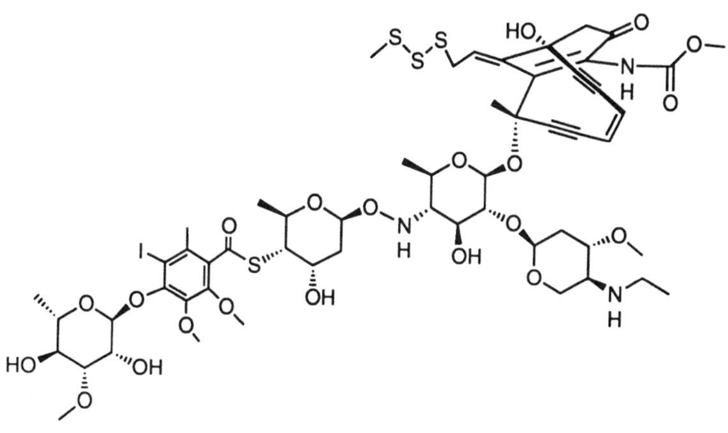

Fig. 22.5 Calicheamicin γ_1.

The long-term interest in antibiotics and the occurrence of rare sugars, combined with the complexity of the overall structures, serve as challenges and strong impetus for carbohydrate synthesis. This has resulted in the development of several semisynthetic antibiotics and the total synthesis of many highly complex structures. A current excellent example is the total synthesis calicheamicin γ_1 (28) (Fig. 22.5).

2.2 Nucleosides

Another large group of carbohydrate-containing therapeutics are the nucleoside analogs. In addition to the nucleosides that occur in nucleic acids, several others, including not only N- but C-glycosides, have been isolated from natural sources (29). These compounds have a wide range of biological activities, including antibacterial, antifungal, antiviral, and antitumor activities. In addition to the naturally occurring compounds, synthetic nucleoside and nucleotide analogs have also gained importance as antiviral and antitumor agents (30). Modifications of the appended carbohydrate moieties were extensively studied and have resulted in therapeutically useful compounds. For example, the anti-HIV drug AZT (Fig. 22.6) and the antiherpes drug acyclovir (Fig. 22.7) are useful repre-

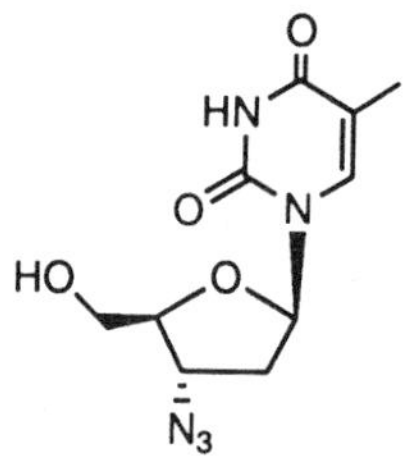

Fig. 22.6 AZT.

Fig. 22.7 Acyclovir.

sentative carbohydrate-based therapeutics. In addition to AZT, ddI (2',3'-dideoxyinosine) and ddC (2',3'-dideoxycytidine) are also approved drugs for the treatment of AIDS. AIDS-driven nucleoside chemistry has recently been reviewed (31).

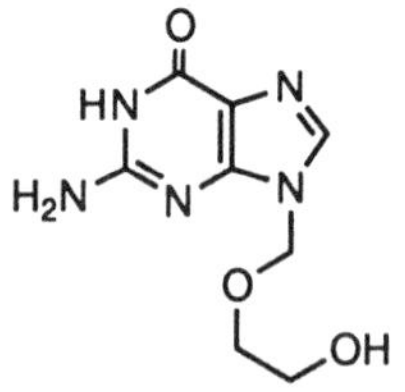

2.3 Cardiac Glycosides

In addition of compounds of microbial origin, carbohydrate-containing therapeutics also are isolated from plants. The cardiac glycosides digoxin and digitoxin (Fig. 22.8) are isolated from *Digitalis lanata*

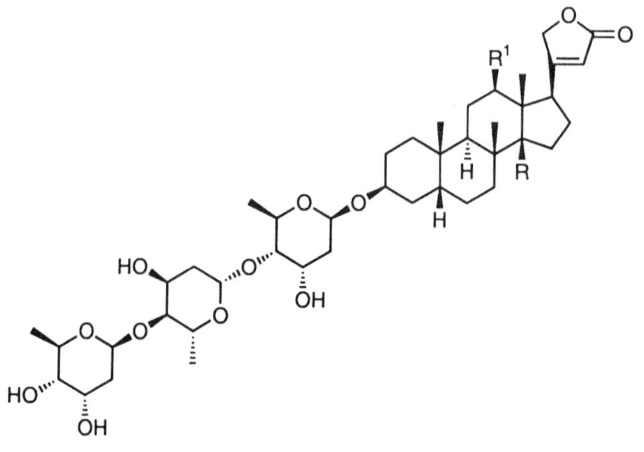

Fig. 22.8 Cardiac glycodise. Digoxin: R = OH, R^1 = OH; digitoxin: R = OH, R^1 = H.

and *D. purpurea* and are used in the treatment of heart arrhythmias, despite their narrow therapeutic index (32). These compounds cause a positive inotropic effect: an increase in the cardiac beat volume by enhancing contractility. Their mechanism of action seems to be associated with the inhibition of the transport enzyme sodium–potassium-ATPase (33). The structure–activity relationship (SAR) of cardiac glycosides is complex in that both the steroid and carbohydrate segments are implicated in binding (34, 35). However, the pharmacokinetics is significantly influenced by the saccharide portion. Present conformation (36) and synthetic (18) studies may form the basis of a future generation of drugs with improved therapeutic indices.

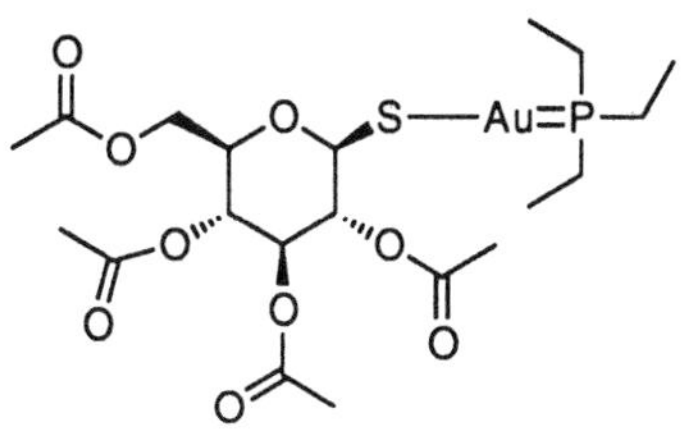

2.4 Synthetic Carbohydrate Drugs

In contrast to the above classes, there are a relatively small number of synthetic carbohydrate drugs. In many cases, the carbohydrate serves as a carrier of a known pharmacophore group. The carbohydrate carrier may modify an aspect of absorption, distribution, metabolism, or excretion of the drug. Examples of this type of therapeutic agent with a carbohydrate backbone include Degranol, Mannitol-Myleran, Zytostop, and Mylebromol (37). These carbohydrate-based cytostatics are biological alkylating agents employed as antineoplastic agents. Similar examples from another field include the nitrate esters of isosorbide. Isosorbide-5-nitrate and isosorbide dinitrate are established vasodilatory drugs.

Other examples of carbohydrate-based synthetic drugs take the form of metal complexes. The disease-modifying antirheumatic drug Auranofin (Fig. 22.9), is a gold-containing complex with peracetylated thioglucose (38). The basic aluminum salt of the fully sulfated derivative of saccharose, Sucralfate (Fig. 22.10), is used in ulcer treatment (39).

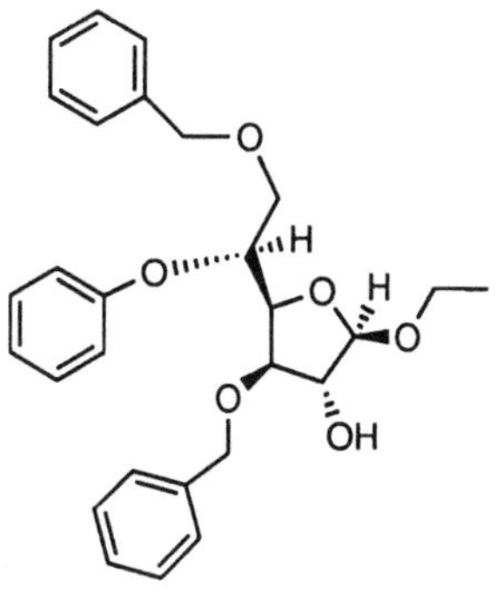

Fig. 22.9 Auranofin.

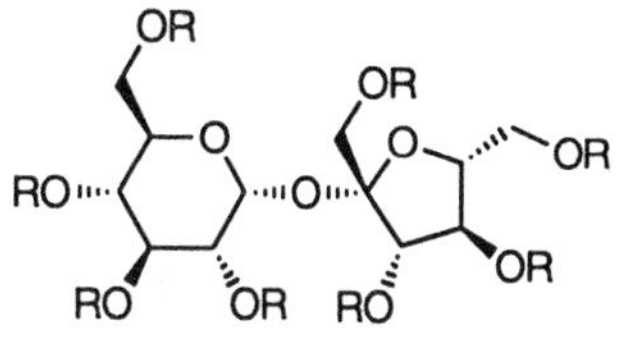

R = SO₃[Al₂(OH)₅]

Fig. 22.10 Sucralfate. R = SO$_3$[Al$_2$(OH)$_5$].

Fig. 22.11 Glyvenol.

In addition to acting as a modifier, carbohydrates can induce activity. For example, a simple benzylated D-glucose derivative, Glyvenol (Fig. 22.11), is used as an antiinflammatory drug (40–42). The approach of using carbohydrates as pharmacological modifiers of therapeutic agents has considerable potential, which at present is far from being fully exploited.

3 PHARMACOLOGICAL CONSIDERATIONS

Because the carbohydrate class of therapeutic agents is not mature, a concise

discussion of the pharmacological considerations is not possible at this time. However, an examination of the absorption,
distribution, metabolism, and excretion of
aminoglycosides, cardiac glycosides, and
heparin (43) may have value in the design
of new carbohydrate-based therapeutic
agents.

3.1 Absorption

The aminoglycosides are poorly absorbed
after ingestion or topical application and
thus are usually given intravenously or by
intramusculature injection. They are not
lipophilic and do not penetrate into cells or
cross the blood–brain barrier. In contrast,
cardiac glycosides contain a steroid nucleus
and, therefore, are more lipid soluble than
the aminoglycosides. Digoxin, the most
commonly used cardiac glycoside, is orally
active; however, another *Digitalis* preparation, ouabain, can only be given intravenously. The aglycons of cardiac glycosides,
termed genins, are shorter acting and less
potent than the glycosides. The attached
sugar molecules increase solubility in water
and tissue penetration. Like the aminoglycosides, heparin may be administered as
a constant intravenous infusion for symptomatic treatment of deep vein thrombosis
or by the subcutaneous route for prophylaxis. Note, however, there are recent
reports that heparin is absorbed by gastric
administration (44). Nevertheless, it is apparent that for carbohydrates to possess
oral activity, a certain degree of lipid solubility is required for absorption.

3.2 Distribution

Aminoglycosides distribute primarily into
the extracellular fluid space. Adipose tissue
is poorly penetrated, as would be expected
form a class of highly water-soluble compounds. The activity of aminoglycosides is

reduced at low pH and in the presence of
leukocytes, because of protein binding. In
contrast, there is a high volume of distribution of cardiac glycosides to organs,
which may be explained by greater lipid
solubility. Indeed, digoxin has a high affinity for heart muscle, where it is concentrated. High digoxin concentrations are
also attained in skeletal muscles, liver,
brain, and kidneys. Heparin concentrates
mainly within the vascular endothelia, and
because it does not cross the placenta, it is
the anticoagulant drug of choice for use
during pregnancy.

3.3 Metabolism

It is ironic when considering the nature of
this chapter that the primary metabolism of
drugs involves conjugation with polar
groups such as carbohydrates. Thus metabolism renders lipid-soluble substances
water-soluble and more readily excretable.
Because carbohydrate drugs are already
water-soluble, conjugation is not an important process in carbohydrate drug metabolism. Although conjugations almost
always result in inactivation for typical
drugs, this may not be a problem for
carbohydrate-based drugs. Nevertheless,
because of intrinsic water solubility, carbohydrate drugs are almost exclusively removed from circulation by the kidneys.
Carbohydrate drugs also appear to be resistant to significant metabolic transformation.

For example, aminoglycosides are quite
water soluble and are metabolically stable.
In patients with normal renal function, the
half-life of aminoglycosides is about 1.5 to
5.0 h (average $t_{1/2} = 3$ h). By comparison,
digoxin is also cleared by the kidneys, but
the serum half-life averages 1.6 days. In
general, the cardiac glycosides are not
highly metabolized and are excreted largely
unaltered. In contrast, the half-life of
heparin is approximately 1.5 h, and it is

inactivated by the liver. The relative long metabolic half-life for digoxin suggests that the aglycone may be responsible by inducing a certain degree of lipid solubility into an otherwise water-soluble trisaccharide.

3.4 Excretion

The aminoglycosides are urinary eliminated almost exclusively by glomerular filtration without any metabolism or active tubular secretion. Their binding to serum proteins is negligible. Likewise, digoxin is cleared by the kidneys via filtration at the glomerulus, but there is significant secretion by the tubules. Heparin appears to be mostly cleared by the reticuloendothelial system.

From the forgoing discussion it is clear that chemical lipid–water partitioning may be critical to the pharmacological behavior of carbohydrate drugs. Thus, in the design of new therapeutic agents based on carbohydrates, it may be appropriate to consider the synthesis of hydrocarbon or aromatic appendages to the parent carbohydrate to increase lipid solubility. A subsequent examination of octanol–water partition coefficients correlated with activity may then provide improved carbohydrate-based drug candidates.

3.5 Binding Affinities

A general criticism of carbohydrates as leads for drug discovery is their low receptor binding affinities, with dissociation constants of the enzyme–inhibitor complex (K_i) often in the millimolar range. It is clear that for cell–cell interactions, which involve several cooperative interaction sites, a univalent analog must be a significantly better ligand than the natural structure to compete as an inhibitor.

One way of making synthetic carbohydrates more avid is to prepare multivalent presentation constructs with identical carbohydrate groups attached. These constructs might mimic what is thought to occur in nature, in that each individual carbohydrate interaction contributes to the strength of the whole. For example, the binding between trivalent glycopeptide structures with defined geometry to the asialoglycoprotein receptor of rat hepatocytes is reported to increase the K_i by three orders of magnitude over the monovalent precursor (45). Also, it was shown that for the binding of influenza virus, for which sialic acid is the receptor, the glycoprotein equine 2-macroglobulin, which has multiple sialic acid–containing oligosaccharide chains, is 4,000,000-fold more potent as an inhibitor than the isolated oligosaccharide chains of the same glycoprotein (46). The importance of multivalency in this case is further supported by the results that copolymerized sialic acid derivatives give a three- to four-order-of-magnitude increase in binding constants over sialic acid monomers (47, 48). Although weak K_i's are frequently associated with carbohydrate–receptor interactions, there are exceptions with median effective concentrations (EC_{50}) in the nanomolar range (49).

4 NEW TECHNIQUES AND INSTRUMENTATION

Evolutionary advances in isolation and analytical instrumentation, structure determination, and conformational studies are greatly facilitating the discovery of potential therapeutics based on glycoconjugates and polysaccharides. The classical methods of structure determination such as acid hydrolysis, methylation analysis, and specific degradation methods (50) are still invaluable tools, but the pharmaceutical industry requires additional technical solutions to analysis and identification. For example, in the case of recombinant glycoproteins in pharmaceutical interest, for which not only structure elucidation but also lot-to-lot characterization are critical to pharmaceutical product development and quality control, a combination of analytical techniques is currently being used to characterize carbohydrates (51).

The following section is organized in two main parts: instrumentation, which deals with isolation and structure determination, and synthesis. Significant information is provided on the synthesis of carbohydrates, because the new techniques currently under development will play a critical role in the discovery of carbohydrate-based therapeutics. Note that in the carbohydrate biopolymer class, there is no corresponding paradigm for the recombinant DNA technology that currently exists for protein generation. In addition, unlike peptides and oligonucleotides, there are no automated synthesis methods for oligosaccharide generation.

4.1 Instrumentation

4.1.1 ISOLATION AND SEPARATION. Recent developments in chromatographic techniques of carbohydrates—including gas–liquid chromatography (GLC), high pressure liquid chromatography (HPLC), thin-layer chromatography (TLC), and supercritical fluid chromatography (SCFC)—facilitate isolation and analysis (52, 53). The technique of high-pH anion exchange (HPAE) chromatography, normally with pulsed amperometric detection (PAD), is capable of separating closely related oligosaccharides of glycoconjugates (54, 55) and permitting compositional monosaccharide analysis of hydrolized samples (56). The HPLC version of affinity chromatography, which uses lectins, carbohydrate-binding proteins of nonimmune origin, is based on specific interactions between the mobile and nonmobile phases, and is efficient in characterizing and separating oligosaccharides and glycopeptides, even those with similar sizes and charges (57). Electrophoretic

methods in combination with enzymatic degration and chemical modification show promise as sensitive methods of identification, sequencing, and oligosaccharide mapping (58–60). The high resolving power of capillary electrophoresis makes it a promising analytical technique for charged oligosaccharides (61).

4.1.2 STRUCTURE DETERMINATION. Evolutionary advances in analytical instrumentation are greatly facilitating the discovery of new oligosaccharides and polysaccharides, which may serve as new leads in the rational design of drugs. In addition, analytical techniques are providing insights into molecular interactions of carbohydrates with other biopolymer classes.

X-ray crystallographic data help clarify the atomic features of protein–carbohydrate interactions (62, 63). The importance of polar and nonpolar residues for carbohydrate recognition and affinity is becoming clearer with respect to hydrogen bonds, van der Waals contacts per sugar unit, and the involvement of water molecules. Apparently, most protein–carbohydrate complexes show stacking of aromatic residues of the protein against both sides of the sugar ring.

Another explanation for protein–carbohydrate interactions, one that has considerably more historical background and theoretical depth, is the hydrated polar gate principle (64, 65). According to this principle, there are large lipophilic domains that constitute the binding epitope on lectin surfaces, and adjacent to these lipid domains are key polar groups that serve to direct, orient, and most important, help strip the carbohydrate moiety of its hydration sphere. Indeed, crystallographic evidence indicates that with carbohydrate–lectin complexes, such as in the high affinity complex of L-arabinose and its transport protein, there are a considerable number of hydrogen bonds and van der Waals contacts that stabilize the interactions (66).

Obtaining high quality mass spectra of large oligo- and polysaccharide molecules by fast atom bombardment (FAB) is now routine (67). The new technique of electrospray mass spectrometry holds additional promise for carbohydrate structural elucidation. For example, in a study of a breast tumor–associated epitope of an *O*-linked mucin defined by a monoclonal antibody, the presence of *N*-glycolylneuraminic acid was confirmed by electrospray ionization (68). Posttranslational modifications of proteins often involve glycosylation and a degree of uncertainty as far as resulting structure. Use of electrospray ionization confirmed the presence of a single *O*-linked *N*-acetylglucosamine substitution of the lens crystalline A_2 subunit (69). The ionspray mass spectrometry technique has the capability to detect noncovalent receptor–ligand complexes. Indeed, enzyme–substrate and enzyme–product complexes of hen egg-white lysozyme and *N*-acetylglucosamine oligosaccharides are observed with the use of ion-spray mass spectrometry (70).

NMR spectroscopy continues to be an invaluable tool both for structural determination and conformational studies. Structural analysis is facilitated not only by multidimensional NMR techniques (71) but also by the building of carbohydrate NMR databases (72) and the creation of computer programs (73) capable of automatic structure determination based on the NMR spectra of the material.

Parallel to advances in instrumental techniques, progress in chemical methodologies also continues. New and improved methods of derivatization (52, 58, 74) facilitate separations, increase the sensitivity of detection and afford more reliably derivatized material for structural work. In structure elucidation methodologies, the reductive cleavage method (75) and the increasing use of enzymes are particularly noteworthy.

4.1.3 CONFORMATIONAL STUDIES. Information about the molecular shape is essential for understanding biological properties

and provides a major tool for drug design. The study of carbohydrate conformation (76, 77) requires the combined use of experimental techniques, such as NMR, and theoretical approaches, such as computational methods.

A major factor determining the conformation of carbohydrates is the anomeric effect (78), the tendency of electronegative substituents at the anomeric center to favor axial over the equatorial orientation. Although the anomeric effect has multiple origins and varied definitions (78–83), it is essentially thought of as a stereoelectronic phenomenon, in which the lone pair orbital of the ring oxygen in the carbohydrate ring interacts with the antibonding orbital of the polarized substituent's (C–X) bond to provide stabilization. The term *exo*-anomeric effect was introduced to describe the preferred rotamers of the aglycon around the glycosidic bond (78, 84, 85). Therefore, the *exo*-anomeric effect is critical in determining the overall shape of oligosaccharides. These effects also are crucial for understanding the reactivity and the stereochemical outcome of carbohydrate reactions.

Computational chemistry, a multidisciplinary field of research, is an important tool in the study of chemical and physical properties of carbohydrates (86). Computational chemistry is especially important in the study of conformation and the promise of computer-assisted drug design. *Ab initio* calculations are giving insight into the basic properties of these molecules, including monosaccharide conformation (87) and the anomeric effect (88–90). Semiempirical and especially molecular mechanics calculations can handle larger molecules and, therefore, are more practically oriented. A simplified force field, the hard sphere *exo*-anomeric (HSEA) effect (91, 92) is widely used, and during the past decade it has provided insight into the conformation of many biologically important oligosaccharides, including the blood group oligosaccharides (91, 93). More accurate parametrizations of the anomeric effect (94) and more precise hydrogen bonding (95) and solvent interaction terms are being used to generate better models (96). A different approach, molecular dynamics simulation, is gaining popularity and gives more insight into the fluctuations and transitions of molecules (97).

In carbohydrate chemistry, the majority of molecular modeling studies are focused on oligosaccharides. In some cases, glycoconjugates were also studied. However, with the advances in computer technology and computational methods additional reports on carbohydrate–receptor interactions will emerge.

Of all the experimental techniques used to study carbohydrate conformation in solution, NMR techniques are the most valuable, by far. Nuclear Overhauser enhancements (nOes) across the glycosidic bond (98) are easily obtainable, but the time-averaged nature of the nOes might result in virtual conformations with relatively low statistical weight and high nOes (99). Therefore, to get more conformational constraints, it is desirable to get nOes between other sites. Fine analysis of changes in chemical shifts due to the proximity of other groups and the determination of the $^3J_{^{13}C}$, ^1H coupling constants (100, 101) and spin-lattice relaxation rates (102) can give further support to the deduced conformation. It is interesting to note that *C*-glycosides have recently been shown to have similar conformational preferences to that of *O*-glycosides (103).

4.2 Synthesis

Compared with the synthesis of peptides and oligonucleotides, the synthesis of complex carbohydrate-containing molecules is far more difficult. The synthesis of large peptides and oligonucleotides is easily achieved by solution chemistry or automated techniques on solid support. In contrast, until quite recently, "syntheses of trisaccharides with various structural units and types of linkages were successful only in isolated cases" (104). There are no automated, solid-phase techniques available for carbohydrate synthesis. Only a small number of the higher oligomers are available by traditional methods (105–108). Although the use of enzymes has the potential to produce complex oligo- and polysaccharides, significant technical difficulties must be solved before they can be commonly used in carbohydrate drug discovery.

4.2.1 CHEMICAL. The two major problems for any carbohydrate synthesis are regioselectivity and stereoselectivity. Because of the multifunctional nature of the carbohydrate molecules, any unambiguous synthesis requires the use of protecting groups on hydroxyls or other functional groups not involved in the reaction. Persistent blocking groups are required for the functionalities that are not involved in the whole synthetic scheme, whereas temporary protecting groups are required on functionalities that must be manipulated at a later stage of the synthesis. Benzyl ethers are most commonly used as persistent blocking groups in combination with temporary acyl groups.

From the plethora of blocking groups currently available (109), the most valuable are the ones that can be introduced in a regioselective manner. A detailed discussion of protecting group strategies and manipulations is beyond the scope of this chapter, and the reader is encouraged to consult relevant handbooks (110) and the specific literature; nevertheless, a few protection methods that have proved to be of general value are mentioned here.

The normally higher reactivity of primary hydroxyls compared with secondary ones is exploited to give synthetically useful regioselective substitution at O-6 in hexopyranosides or at O-5 in pentofuranosides by using bulky groups such as trityl, *tert-*

butyldimethylsilyl, and *tert*-butyldiphenyl-silyl. Cyclic acetals, such as benzylidene and isopropylidene, are used to protect both the O-4 and O-6 positions in hexopyranosides and/or a vicinal axial–equatorial hydroxyl pair. The advantages of the benzylidene acetals are that they can be removed to liberate both hydroxyls and the acetal ring can be reductively cleaved in both directions regioselectively to generate a benzyl ether and one free hydroxyl (111, 112) (Fig. 22.12). These reactions are extended to derivatives of benzylidene acetals substituted either at the acetal carbon (113) or in the aromatic ring (114); the latter case provides derivatives that the substituted benzyl protecting group can be selectively removed in the presence of benzyl groups. The direction of the reductive cleavage on 1,3-dioxolane-type

benzylidene acetals depends on the stereochemistry of the acetal carbon. Thus it is possible to prepare either axial O-benzyl–equatorial hydroxyl or axial hydroxyl–equatorial O-benzyl derivatives (115) (see Fig. 22.12). Cyclic orthoester derivatives on *cis* axial–equatorial diols are also selectively opened to give the acyl derivative on the axial hydroxyl (116). In the case of 4,6-O-cyclic orthoesters, after an additional acyl migration step, the 6-O-acyl derivatives are obtained in good yields (117). An especially useful method for both selective acylation and alkylation is the regioselective enhancement of nucleophilicity via the dibutylstannylene or tributylstannyl alkoxides (118). The reaction normally gives substitution on an equatorial hydroxyl neighboring an axial one. An alternative for selective substitution is to use phase-

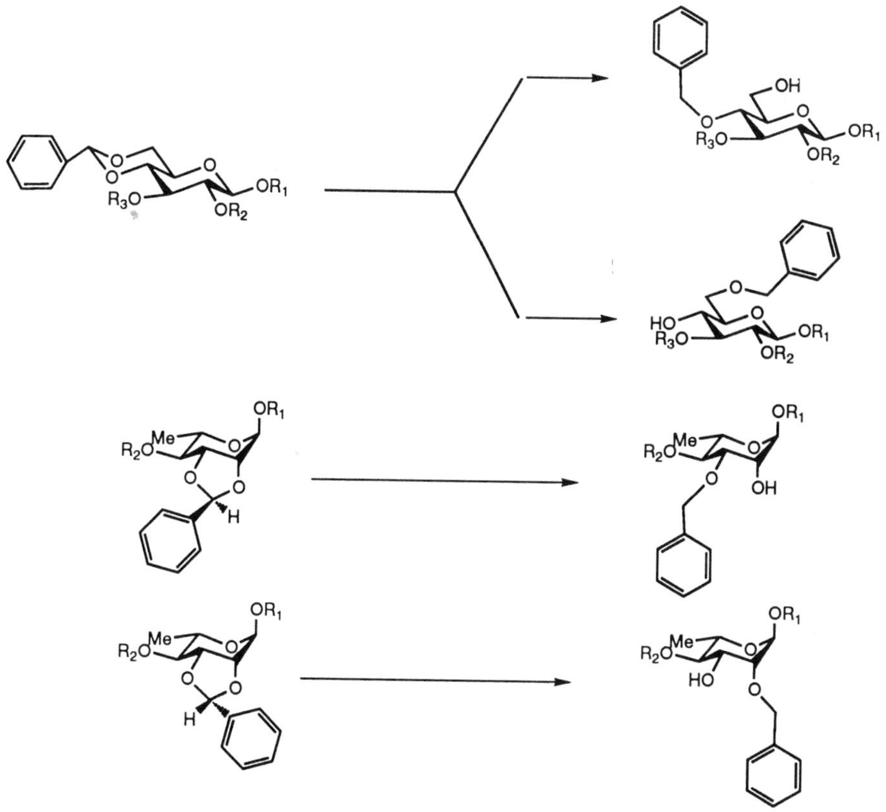

Fig. 22.12 Benzylidine openings.

transfer catalyzed reactions, for which the regioselectivity is governed by other factors (119).

Although the above reactions are generally applicable, depending on the structure of the particular carbohydrate, more efficient routes are often possible. Reviews on the synthesis of partially alkylated derivatives (120), regioselective substitution reactions (121), and selective deprotection methods (122) leading to partially substituted carbohydrate derivatives are useful guides.

In contrast to peptide or oligonucleotide synthesis, the reaction of the glycosidic linkage between carbohydrate monomers requires stereocontrol of the newly formed linkage. Glycosides that have a trans relationship of the C-1 and C-2 substituents are synthesized by taking advantage of neighboring group participation from the 2 position. With acyl-type protecting groups at C-2 the reaction proceeds via an acyloxonium cation intermediate that reacts with a nucleophile to give 1,2-trans stereochemistry in the product, whereas, the oxocarbonium ion is expected to give mixtures of the 1,2-cis and 1,2-trans products (Fig. 22.13). For the synthesis of 1,2-*cis* glycosides, a prerequisite is, therefore, the use of nonparticipating blocking groups at the 2

position. Using a nonparticipating substituent, however, does not necessarily result in the formation of 1,2-*cis* glycosides; the stereoselectivity depends in a complex manner on the reactivities of the glycosyl donor and acceptor, the strength of the promoter used for the reaction, the solvent, and the reaction temperature (104). Note that the reactivities of the glycosyl donors and acceptors are influenced by the protecting groups used, and in several cases, changing a single protecting group at a remote position may result in drastic changes in stereoselectivity and yields.

Significant progress is being made with glycosylation methodologies. In addition to traditional methods that use glycosyl bromides as glycosyl donors in Koenigs-Knorr type reactions (123), several new classes of glycosyl donors are in use. Glycosyl trichloroacetimidates (124) are especially efficacious and have the added advantage that they can be activated by Lewis acids, thereby avoiding the use of the expensive and toxic heavy-metal salts used in Koenigs-Knorr reactions. A disadvantage of both the glycosyl bromides and the trichloroacetimidates is the sensitivity of these groups at the anomeric position. Hardly any chemical manipulations can be made at other positions in their presence;

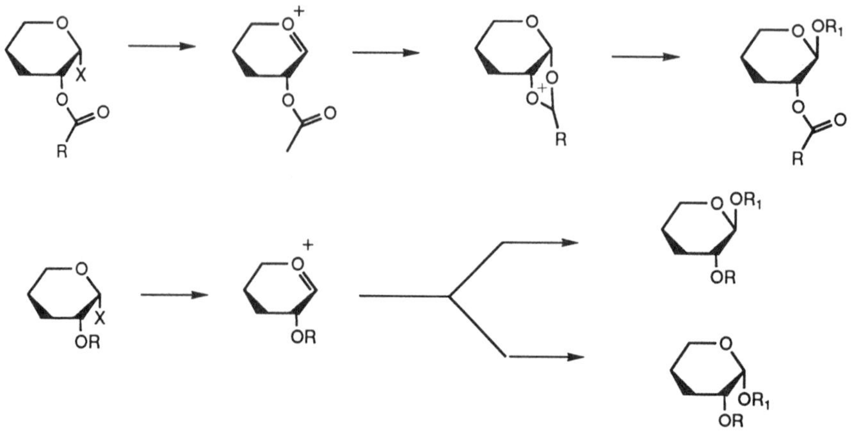

Fig. 22.13   *cis*- and *trans*-Glycosidations.

therefore, the anomeric hydroxyl must be protected by some other group first and then converted into the actual glycosylating species before glycosylation. Glycosyl fluorides (125), and especially thioglycosides (126), offer a solution to this problem. These not only are compatible with most of the common protecting group manipulations but also can serve as glycosyl acceptors. This is especially advantageous in block synthesis of larger molecules for which an oligosaccharide can be assembled on a thioglycoside and the block is used directly, without an additional activation step, as a glycosyl donor. Thioglycosides also have the flexibility of being easily converted into other types of glycosyl donors (bromides, fluorides) if required (127). Interestingly, some types of O-glycosides (pentenyl glycosides) can also be used to create new O-glycosidic bonds (128), and pentenyl glycosides have the same type of advantages as the above glycosyl donors. New methods of activation are also available for glycals (129), and the use of these glycosyl donors can be advantageous if further chemical manipulations at C-2 are required.

Because the C-2 substituent is of crucial importance to the outcome of glycosylation reactions, synthesis of glycosides of 2-deoxy- and 2-amino-2-deoxy-sugars have some special features. Syntheses of these classes of glycosides have been recently reviewed (18, 130). The synthesis of oligosaccharides and glycoconjugates of biological interest are summarized in several excellent reviews (131–137). The tremendous progress made in synthetic methodologies makes it possible to target large and structurally highly complex oligosaccharides, e.g., a regiocontrolled and stereocontrolled synthesis of a pentacosasaccharide (a 25-mer), the carbohydrate part of a glycosyl ceramide, was recently accomplished (138).

Despite significant achievements, the present status of oligosaccharide synthesis is still best summarized this way:

Although we have learned now how to synthesize oligosaccharides, it should be emphasized that each oligosaccharide synthesis remains an independent problem, whose resolution requires considerable systematic research and a good deal of know-how. There are no universal reaction conditions for oligosaccharide synthesis (104).

Thus it is understandable that early efforts for the solid-phase synthesis of oligosaccharides (139) did not result in practically useful procedures. Although promising advances in the chemistry of polymer-supported synthesis have been made (140, 141), the generality and usefulness of these methodologies remain to be seen before they can be applied to automated instrumentation.

4.2.2 ENZYMATIC. Enzymatic synthesis of carbohydrate-based therapeutics is an emerging technology (142–147). Currently, enzymatic synthesis is of limited pharmaceutic value. Nevertheless, an indication of the potential of using enzymes is in the carbohydrate field where the largest scale enzymatic transformations are used at present, i.e., the conversion of starch to glucose and glucose to high fructose corn syrup (142). Enzymatic synthesis of carbohydrates has the capability to solve both the regio- and stereoselectivity problems associated with carbohydrate synthesis.

For example, enzymatic syntheses is used in the preparation of monosaccharides and analogs using aldolases (144–146, 148). Enzymic synthesis for oligosaccharides (144–146, 149) avoids the protection and deprotection steps, and in principle, complete regio- and stereoselectivity can be ensured. With respect to the chiral nature of enzymes, the preparation of optically pure compounds from inexpensive racemic mixtures is possible, and with symmetrical starting materials, enzymes are able to differentiate between prochiral centers, giving products of high enantiomeric excess (145).

There are three strategies available for enzymic oligosaccharide synthesis: (*1*) the Leloir pathway, which uses the activated sugar nucleotides as glycosyl donors and glycosyl transferases and essentially follows the biochemical pathway by which oligosaccharides are synthesized; (*2*) glycosidases under conditions that reverse the normal reaction of enzymatic glycosidic hydrolyzation; and (*3*) enzymes that use glycosyl 1-phosphates as donors.

From the three possible routes, the Leloir pathway (Fig. 22.14) offers an ideal solution, and it has been successfully used for the synthesis of several prototypical oligosaccharides. Ideally, a transferase enzyme catalyzes the transfer of the glycosyl unit from a sugar nucleotide donor to the acceptor with complete stereo- and regioselectivity. Although several glycosyltransferases have been cloned (150), the practical basis of widely using this enzyme technology is still distant. It is estimated that more than 100 glycosyltransferases are required for the synthesis of known carbohydrate structures occurring on glycolipids and glycoproteins of mammals. Because in mammalian systems only eight sugar nucleotide donors are commonly found (UDP-Glc, UDP-Gal, UDP-

GlcNAc, UDP-GalNAc, UDP-GlcA, GDP-Man, GDP-Fuc, CMP-Neu5Ac), it may be speculated that a great deal of sequence homology could exist in glycosyltransferases. Despite a common domain structure, however, surprisingly few regions of homology have been found.

Although glycosyltransferases have great promise, there are several drawbacks at present concerning their use. One is their limited availability and the relatively large number of enzymes that must be cloned for the synthesis of a complex oligosaccharide. For example, in the biosynthesis of oligosaccharide chains of glycoproteins at least six GlcNAc-transferases are known, and all transfer the same monosaccharide (*N*-acetyl-D-glucosamine) to an identical acceptor (D-mannose), but each transfer occurs in different environment of the growing oligosaccharide chain. Another disadvantage is that glycosyltransferases require the use of a stoichiometric amount of the activated glycosyl donor. Progress has been made to generate most of the nucleoside phosphate sugars on a practical scale (151). Also routes for regenerating the nucleotide sugars *in situ* in the reaction mixtures are available (149); however, they require the use of additional enzymes. Therefore, a complete enzymatic synthesis of an oligosaccharide requires, in addition to the

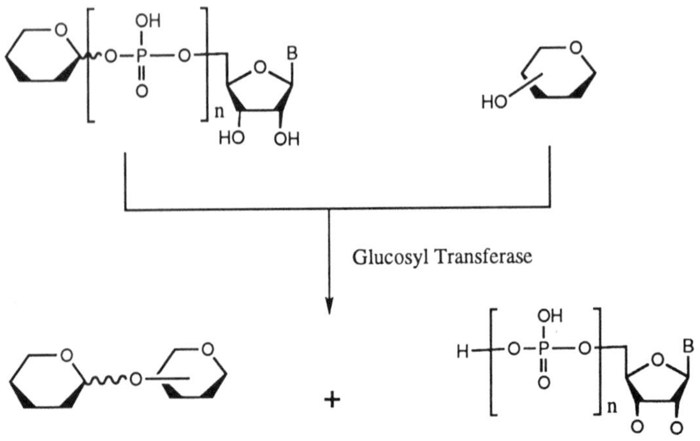

Fig. 22.14 Glucosyltransferase.

appropriate glycosyltransferases the use of enzymes (aldolases, oxidoreductases) to synthesize the rare sugars of the sequence, enzymes to generate and regenerate the nucleotide sugars, enzymes (phosphatases) to handle inhibition problems, and cofactors. In spite of the complexities, significant advances have been made, and in the future large-scale enzymatic synthesis of carbohydrates may be practical.

A significant technical advance that aids enzymatic synthesis of carbohydrate-based therapeutics is the use of immobilized enzymes (146). Since some glycosyltransferases tolerate substrate analogs, the synthesis of unnatural structures may be exploited with currently available enzymes (152). In the future, enzymatic synthesis may be aided by site-directed mutagenesis.

The use of glycosidase and transglycosidase enzymes for the synthesis of glycosyl bonds offers several advantages (153–156). A lot of glycosidases are readily available, and they do not require nucleotide sugars as glycosyl donors. On the other hand, glycosidases naturally catalyze the hydrolysis of the glycosidic bonds and not their formation, and the equilibrium lies in favor of the hydrolized products. Approaches used to run glycosidases in reverse are divided into thermodynamic and kinetic types. With the thermodynamic type, the equilibrium is shifted in the desired direction through a high concentration of the sugars, using organic cosolvents, high temperatures, and extraction methods. In the kinetic approach a derivative such as an aryl glycoside or a glycosyl fluoride is used as a donor, and the method takes advantage of the fact that glycosidases transfer glycosyl units not only to water but also onto other substrates. Since glycosidases have a stereospecific preference for the anomeric linkage, the stereoselective outcome of using glycosidases in reverse is generally excellent. Regioselectivity is difficult to predict, however. It seems to depend on a series of factors, including reaction conditions and the precise structure of the acceptor.

The major advantages of using glycosidases for enzymatic synthesis at present are low cost, relative simplicity, and the potential to create a series of related structures with ease. Nevertheless, targeting highly specific structures with glycosyltransferases may require an initial higher research investment, but this may be more rewarding in the long term. Although the chemical and enzymic syntheses of carbohydrate-based therapeutics appears to be at odds, a combination of the two may be especially valuable. A recent example of chemoenzymatic synthesis is the preparation of ganglioside G_{M3} (157).

4.2.3 GLYCOMIMETICS. In addition to the preparation of the naturally occurring carbohydrates, there are efforts devoted to the synthesis of compounds in which either the ring or the glycosidic oxygen is replaced by a carbon or heteroatom. These compounds include the carbasugars, in which the ring oxygen is replaced by carbon (158, 159), and C-glycosides, in which the glycosidic oxygen is replaced by carbon (160). Similarly, nitrogen, sulfur, selenium (161), and phosphorus (162) rings and linker variants (163) are possible. Finally, fluorine is often substituted for the hydroxyl groups, which maintains similar electronegativity but loses hydrogen donor ability (164). Synthesis of carbon, heteroatom, and fluorine carbohydrate variants may be thought of as first-generation glycomimetics.

4.2.4 CARBOHYDRATES AS CHIRAL SYNTHONS. On a chiral atom/cost basis carbohydrates are by far the least expensive starting material for enanteriomerically pure pharmaceuticals. This recognition combined with the developments in synthetic methodologies resulted in an upsurge in the synthesis of pharmaceutically important molecules. The current trend in the pharamaceutical industry is to shift from racemates to enantiomerically pure compounds. This shift gives added impetus to the use of carbohydrate-derived synthons in drug synthesis. Although it is beyond the scope of this Chapter to cover all the important developments in the use of carbohydrates as chiral synthons, it is sufficient to mention a few examples. Optically active compounds, such as muscarine analogues, (+)-biotine, prostaglandins, β-lactames, other antibiotics, and pheromones, can now be synthesized starting from carbohydrates. This topic is annually reviewed and is the subject of an excellent textbook (165, 166).

Advances made in chiral synthesis have allowed scientists to seek synthetic targets of much larger size and complexity than was commonly pursued in the past. Palytoxin (Fig. 22.15), a highly toxic princi-

ple isolated from *Palythoa toxica* contains not less than 64 stereocenters (167), and it is one of the largest and most complicated synthetically targeted molecules (168, 169). As a research tool, palytoxin is used to induce contraction and release of norepinephrine and prostaglandins in the aorta (170), to inhibit the action on Na^+/K^+-ATPase (171), to induce permeability changes in excitable membranes (172), and to contract vascular smooth muscles (173). Palytoxin can be viewed as *C*-glycosides core units, and efforts toward its total synthesis resulted in the total synthesis of palytoxin carboxylic acid and palytoxin amide (174). Palytoxin carboxylic acid is constructed from *C*-glycosides in a logical fashion. Further examples of chiral synthesis are the total syntheses of okadaic acid (175) (Fig. 22.16), a protein phosphatase inhibitor (176), and avermectin (177).

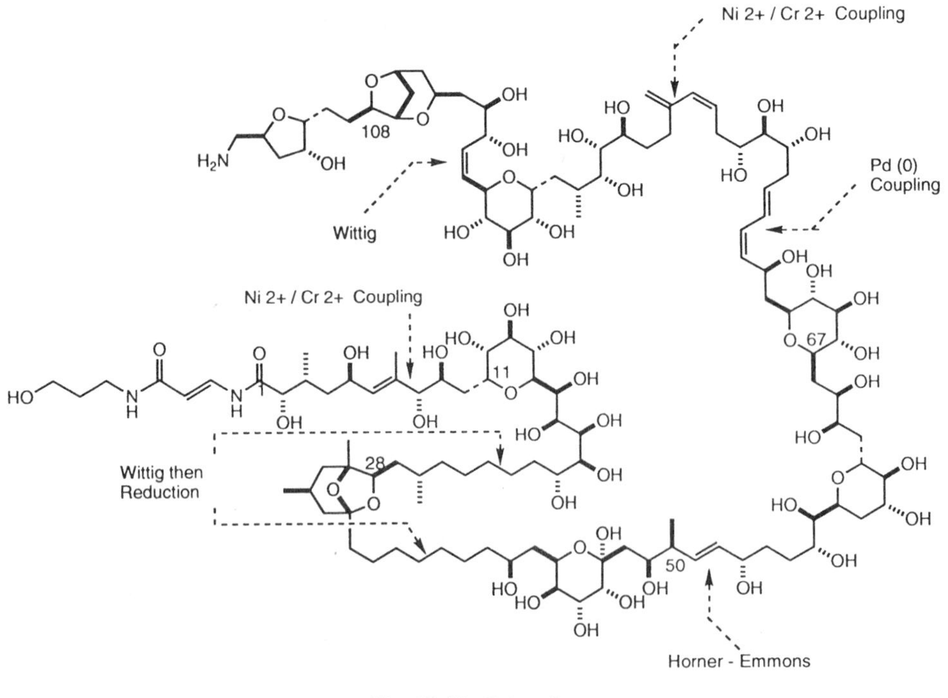

Fig. 22.15 Palytoxin.

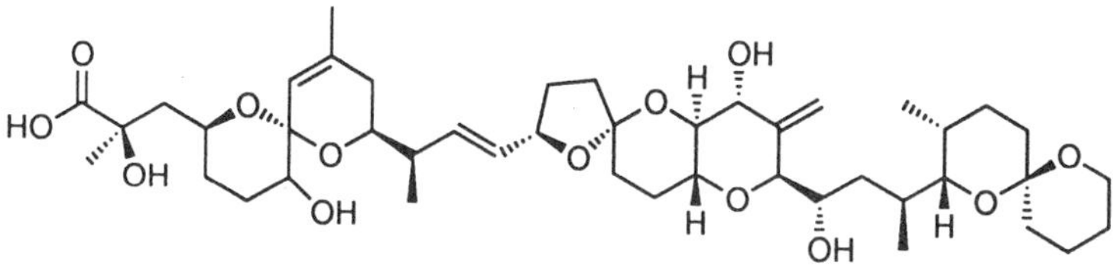

Fig. 22.16 Okadaic acid.

5 GLYCOCONJUGATES

Many carbohydrates of current interest are expressed as glycoconjugates (178). They are classified as glycolipids, proteoglycans, and glycoproteins and may either be anchored in the cell surface membrane, secreted as semisoluble substances, or deposited as insoluble substances. A brief description of each glycoconjugate follows.

5.1 Glycolipids

Although the carbohydrate portion of glycolipids imparts greater biological significance, these molecules are normally classified according to the structure of their lipid components. For example, glycolipids are subdivided into (1) glycosphingolipids; (2) glycerol-type glycolipids or glycosylated glycerols, which have fatty acid substituents on the glycerol; (3) ester-type glycolipids or esters of carbohydrates, which have fatty acids; (4) steryl glycosides or glycosylated derivatives of sterol; and (5) polyisoprenol-type glycolipids in which the sugar is normally linked via a phosphate bridge to the polyisoprenols (179). Recent additions to this list are the glycosylphosphatidyl-inositols (180), which serve as anchors for either proteins, oligosaccharides, or polysaccharides to cellular membranes through a covalent linkage. By far the most important among glycolipids are the glyco-sphingolipids.

In glycosphingolipids the carbohydrate is glycosidically linked to a long-chain 2-amino-1,3-diol, which is most commonly sphingosine (D-*erythro*-1,3-dihydroxy-2-amino-4,5-*trans*-octadecene) (Fig. 22.17) the amino group of sphingosine is normally substituted by a fatty acid, giving a structure known as ceramide (see Fig. 22.17). Glycosphingolipids containing sialic acid are called gangliosides. Glycosphingolipids are ubiquitous membrane components, and a large number of structures that differ in carbohydrate structure are known (181).

Glycolipids are well known as essential structural constituents of the cell membrane bilayers. However, recent results indicating dramatic changes in glycolipid composition observed during both ontogenesis and oncogenesis suggest roles for this class of compounds in extracellular communication (182). Indeed, glycolipids are critical in cellular interaction and differentiation. For example, the Lewis x (Le^x) (Fig. 22.18) is strongly expressed in early embryogenesis at the 8- to 32-cell stage (morula), and it disappears after compaction (183, 184). Interestingly there is evidence that cell–cell recognition in this case is not the result of the usual protein–carbohydrate interaction but to carbohydrate–carbohydrate interactions (185). Membrane glycosphingolipids are implicated in regulation of cell growth (contact inhibition), and changes of the cell cycle are manifested in glycosphingolipid synthesis (182). Oncogenic transformations produce tumor-distinctive glycolipids, some of which may be tumor-associated antigens or markers. Essentially, all human cancers exhibit an aberrant glycosylation pattern in

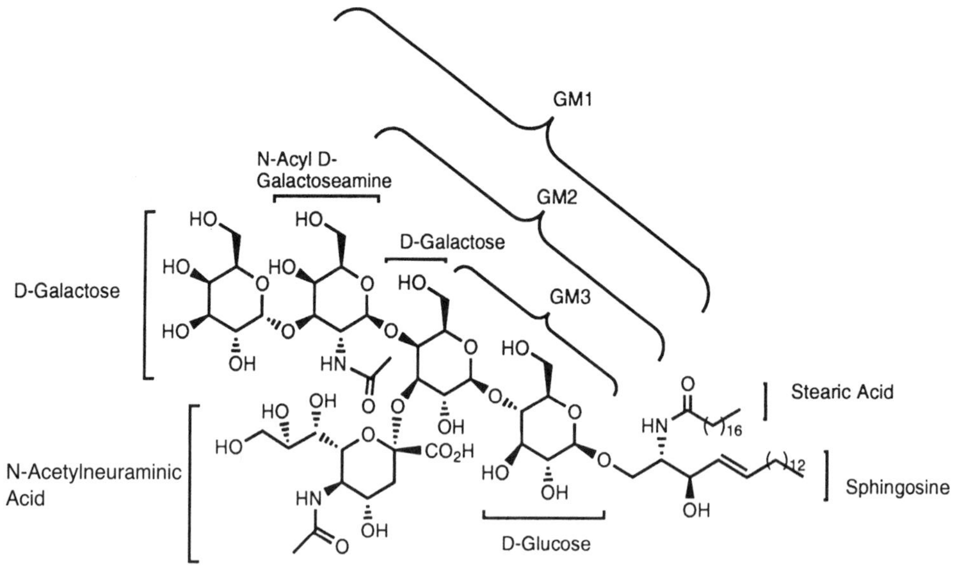

Fig. 22.17 Gangliosides: G_{M1}, G_{M2}, and G_{M3}.

their glycolipids (182–186) e.g., the structures Le^x, Le^a, Le^b, Le^y, sialyl Le^a, sialyl Le^x, and disialyl Le^a have all been characterized as tumor-associated antigens. It is important to note, however, that although these structures might be absent in their progenitor cell types they may be normal components of other cell types. Only a few tumor-associated antigens, such as the Forssman antigen, are known to be virtually absent in normal tissues. Glycolipids and glycoproteins share a lot of common tumor-

associated antigens that are expressed on both classes of glycoconjugates, though there are some antigens that occur exclusively in only one of these types of glycoconjugates (186).

Glycolipids also play a role in immune recognition. They can serve as cell surface antigens, including blood group antigens. Note that B- or T-cell response is also modulated by gangliosides (182). Finally, glycolipids also interact with a series of bioactive factors, including bacterial toxins

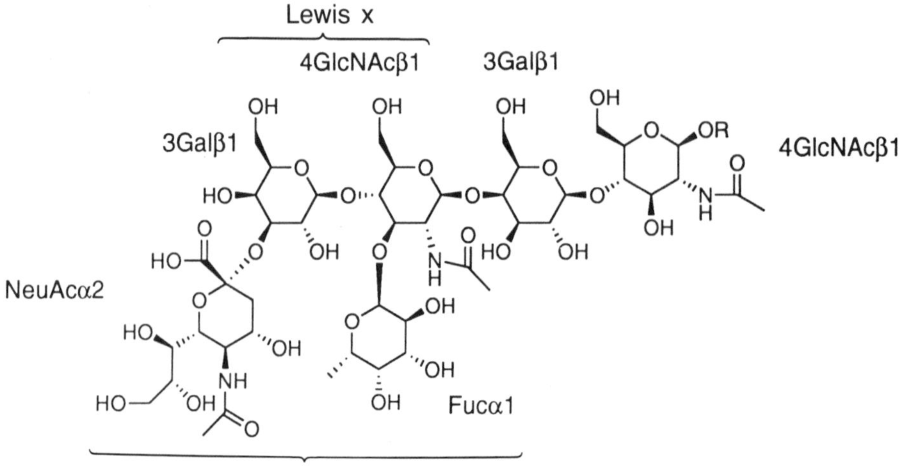

Fig. 22.18 Sialylated Lewis x hexasaccharide.

(187), glycoprotein hormones, and interferon (182).

A new dimension to the biological role of glycosphingolipids, which is different from extracellular communication, was recently added (188, 189). These compounds, or their catabolites, are modulating transmembrane signal transduction, suggesting a new function of being potential second mesengers. It has been shown that both protein kinase C and growth factor receptor–associated protein kinases are modulated by gangliosides or their breakdown products. G_{M3} was shown to inhibit epidermal growth factor–dependent tyrosine phosphorylation of the epidermal growth factor (EGF) receptor (190), the ganglioside 2,3-disialosyl-paragloboside inhibits insulin-dependent cell proliferation via effects on the tyrosine kinase activity of the receptor (191). G_{M1} seems to modulate cellular proliferation through a still undefined growth-signaling pathway (189). Similar effects are observed with breakdown products of glycosphingolipids. For example, sphingosine is a potent and specific inhibitor of protein kinase C (192), and the possibility of a sphingolipid cycle similar to that of the phosphoglycerolipid cycle is hypothesized (189), with implications in cell growth regulation. Indeed, a metabolite of glycosylsphingosines (N,N-dimethylsphingosine) acts as an enhancer for EGF receptor kinase and produces EGF-like activity (193). Studies on the metabolism and intracellular transport of glycosphingolipids (194) will give additional information on their biological role.

Gangliosides are found on the plasma membranes of vertebrate cells and are particularly concentrated in neural tissue. Over 100 gangliosides are known (195). Gangliosides may be of value for nerve growth and neural repair, although this is not universally accepted as their mechanisms of action remain elusive (196). Apparently, gangliosides act in a multifactorial fashion to modulate cAMP levels, protein kinases, and nerve growth factors.

In different animal models of brain damage, the monosialoganglioside G_{M1} appears to preserve the activity of the enzyme Na^+/K^+-ATPase, which is essential for membrane function (197) (see Fig. 22.17). In brain-damaged rats, functional improvement is noted with chronic G_{M1} administration (198). G_{M1} also decreases the neurotoxicity of excitatory amino acids such as glutamate (199, 200). Studies on the protection of glutamate-induced neuronal death with G_{M1} and the semisynthetic analogs LIG_{A4} (G_{M1} with N-acetyl-sphingosine), LIG_{A20} (G_{M1} with N-dichloroacetyl-sphingosine) and PK_{S3} (G_{M1} with D-erythro-1,3-dihydroxy-2-dichloroacetamido-4-trans-octadecene) indicate that analogs may be more potent than the parent compound (201). The order of potency for the protection is $G_{M1} < PK_{S3} < LIG_{A4} \leq LIG_{A20}$.

Clinical trials are under way with G_{M1} that could determine whether this agent can play a significant role in repairing nervous tissue damaged by stroke (197) or spinal injury (202). The treatment of hypoxic and ischemic brain damage (203), the relevance to neurosurgery (204), studies on the mechanism of action (205), the treatment of stroke (206), cellular proliferation and signal transduction pathways (189), and thyrotrophin-releasing hormone in peripheral neuromuscular diseases (207) are areas of recent reviews on gangliosides. However, the reader is cautioned about the utility of gangliosides in the treatment of nerve damage because of the uncertainty in mechanism of action and efficacy in humans and because of potential toxicity. Indeed, some have argued that ganglioside use in neurological diseases of humans should be suspended (208).

In addition to nerve damage indications, glycosphingolipids may have use in the diagnosis and treatment of cancer. There have been indications since the 1960s that sera of patients with cancer show elevated levels of tumor antigens and antibodies related to carbohydrate structures of glycolipids (209). Monoclonal antibodies directed against antigens associated with difficult to diagnose, early stage tumors, such as pancreatic cancer, can be of special value (201). Imaging of tumor locations is of great clinical importance, which can also be addressed by labeled antibodies against tumor-associated antigens (186).

Tumor-associated carbohydrate antigens can be the basis of different therapeutical strategies. Since specific glycolipid antigens are expressed by human cancer cells (186, 211), the use of antibody treatment may be appropriate. Thus gangliosides G_{G3}, G_{D3}, G_{D2}, and G_{M3} expressed by cancer cells in lymphoma and malignant melanoma are suitable targets for passive immunotherapy with monoclonal antibodies (186). A vaccine containing antibodies against the sialyl-Tn antigen (glycoprotein) (212) is in phase II clinical trials against breast cancer. An alternative strategy is active immunotherapy with vaccines (186, 213). Approaches to augmenting the IgG antibody response to melanoma ganglioside vaccines was recently reviewed (214). Gangliosides may play a direct role in immunomodulation, as there is now evidence for their role in T-cell activation (215). Another promising approach that uses monoclonal antibodies as magic bullets to carry therapeutically active agents to target cells has yet to show efficacy; however, this result may be due to technical difficulties and not failure of the basic approach (186).

Gangliosides also modulate copper ions concentrations and angiogenic capacity of adult tissues (216). Gangliosides have a direct effect on size of tumor vascular network and tumor growth rate or cell population. The angiogenic capacity of tumors and the role that prostaglandin E_1 plays as an angiogenesis factor, the relationship between acquisition of angiogenic capacity and neoplastic transformation of a cell population, the modification of tissue composition at the onset of angiogenesis,

and the behavior of copper ions and copper carriers in the course of the angiogenic response are influenced by gangliosides G_{M1} and G_{T1b} *in vivo*.

5.2 Proteoglycans

Proteoglycans are glycoconjugates composed of glycosaminoglycan (GAG) chains covalently bound to a protein core (217–220). The GAG chains are built up of long, linear sequences of alternating hexosamine (D-glucosamine of D-galactosamine) and hexuronic acid (D-glucuronic acid or L-iduronic acid) units that carry sulfate substituents at various positions. The special cases of hyaluronic acid, which occurs as a free GAG without a protein, and keratan sulfate, in which the hexuronic acid is replaced by the neutral sugar D-galactose, are also considered proteoglycans. Despite the regularity in the alternating sequence of the amino and uronic acid–type sugars, GAGs generally show substantial structural heterogeneity. Nevertheless, their simplest classification is based on their most typical monosaccharide constituents, e.g., hyaluronic acid (β-D-GlcA, β-D-GlcN), chondroitin 4- and 6-sulfates (β-D-GlcA, β-D-GalN), dermatan sulfate (α-L-IdoA, β-D-GalN), heparan sulfate and heparin (α-L-IdoA, α-D-GlcN), and keratan sulfate (β-D-Gal, β-D-GlcN). They occur intracellularly, at the cell surface, and in the intracellular matrix. Their biological functions are also varied, from their long-known contribution to the organization and physical properties of the extracellular matrix to more recently observed effects on various cellular processes, such as cell adhesion and proliferation.

Besides hyaluronan, which has been used in surgery because of its elastoviscous properties and effects on wound healing, heparin (221, 222) is by far the pharmaceutically most important glycosaminoglycan.

Heparin has been used clinically since 1937, because of its blood anticoagulant properties and its usefulness to treat thromboembolic disorders. Originally, it was introduced to prevent thrombosis in surgical patients, followed by its use for the treatment of deep venous thrombosis, and preventing complications following vascular surgery, myocardial infarction, and extracorporeal circulation. Although heparin is used as a drug for the treatment of thrombosis, bleeding complications narrow the range in which heparin can safely and efficaciously be administered.

Low molecular weight heparins (LMWHs) are under study to circumvent these problems (223–225). Commercial heparin preparations, depending on their source, normally have molecular weights in the 6,000 to 30,000 range, whereas LMWHs have molecular weights between 3,000 and 6,000. The mechanism of action of LMWHs is understood with respect to antithrombic therapy (226) (Fig. 22.19). Although LMWHs are uniform with respect to the inability to inactivate thrombin, an analysis of LMWHs in the prophylaxis of venous thrombosis revealed that antifactor Xa activity can vary significantly among different preparations with similar molecular weights (227). There are several LMWHs currently undergoing clinical trials for prophylaxis of thromboembolism and perioperative deep vein thrombosis in gen-

eral surgery. These LMWHs include Fragmin (228), Logiparin (229), Lomoparin (230), Enoxaparin (231), Fraxiparine (232), and RD heparin (233).

Although heparin has been used in the clinical setting for more than 50 yr, its mode of action is only now being understood. This understanding is leading efforts to develop low molecular weight synthetic compounds that have promise as drugs. With knowledge accumulating on the blood coagulation cascade and the understanding of the role of GAGs in self-regulation (234), the minimum antihrombin III (ATIII) binding sequence of heparin is narrowed down to a pentasaccharide (Fig. 22.20, R = H) (235, 236), and this hypothesis was confirmed by synthesis (237). This unique sequence occurs with low frequency in heparin chains and contains a D-glucosamine-2,3,6-tri-sulfate unit, previously not found in GAGs. SAR studies of ATIII pentasaccharide (Fig. 22.20, R = H) indicate that regiosulfation and carboxylate stereochemistry are critical for biological activity (238, 239). For example, an extra 3-O-sulfate group on the reducing sugar (ORG 31550; Fig. 22.20, R = OSO_3-Na^+) enhances the interaction with the protein (240), whereas an extra 3-O-sulfate on the glucuronate impedes binding to ATIII. ORG 31550 is in clinical studies. A molecular model to explain many of the aspects of the binding of the pentasaccharide se-

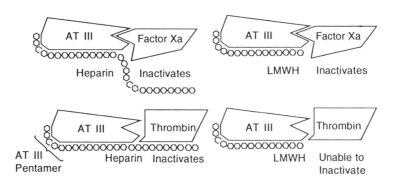

Fig. 22.19 Mechanism of clotting factor inactivation for heparin and LMWH.

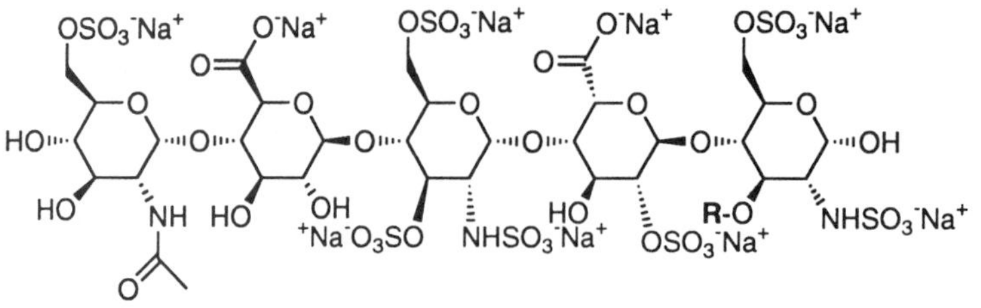

Fig. 22.20 Pentasaccharide sequences. (**1**) R = H; (**2**) R = OSO$_3^-$Na$^+$.

quence (Fig. 22.20, R = H) to ATIII is under development (241). Further SAR studies indicate that D-glucosamine-N-sulfates in the original structure can be replaced with glucose 2-O-sulfates and that nonsulfated hydroxyls can be retained O-alkylated (242), substantially reducing the number of necessary synthetic steps (238). The original synthesis of ATIII pentasaccharide required not less than 83 steps for the preparation of only the monosaccharide synthons (243). Taken together, it appears that these highly negatively charged oligosaccharides have specific requirements with respect to charge distribution and spatial orientation.

Besides its anticoagulant activity, heparin has antiviral activity, effects on smooth muscle cell proliferation, angiogenesis modulating activity, and effects on lipases activity. On the molecular level, heparin interacts with a large number of proteins, including growth factors (244), fibronectin (245) and von Willebrand factor (246). Theoretically, 17 different HexAαGlcN sequences may exist in the heparin chain, which results in millions of possible epitopes on the hexa-decasaccharide level that could interact with proteins. In a classical lock-and-key model, heparin can be viewed as "a bag of skeleton keys which fit many locks" (247). In addition to the ATIII sequence, the specific sequence responsible for the binding of heparin with basic fibroblast growth factor (bFGF) (248) was recently identified as a hexasaccharide (GM 1115) (Fig. 22.21).

Although there are additional interactions of heparin with individual proteins that may be caused by specific epitopes in the heparin structure, the possibility exists that some of the interactions of the highly negatively charged heparin and proteins are mostly electrostatic in nature. This forms the basis of another drug development strategy for heparin mimics: using highly charged synthetic molecules as possible heparin surrogates. Aprosulate (249, 250), a structurally simple tethered sulfatoid, is in clinical trials as a possible antithrombotic drug.

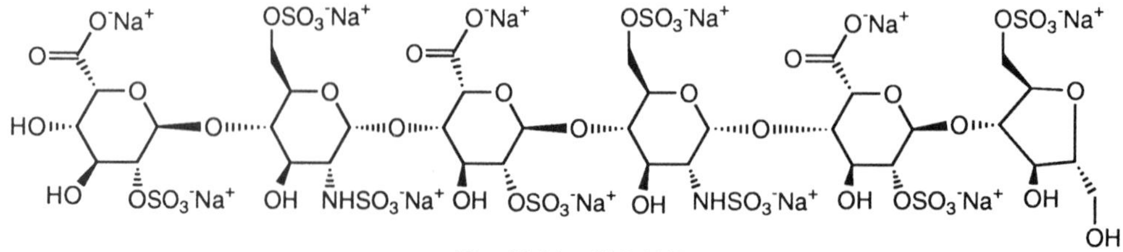

Fig. 22.21 GM 1115.

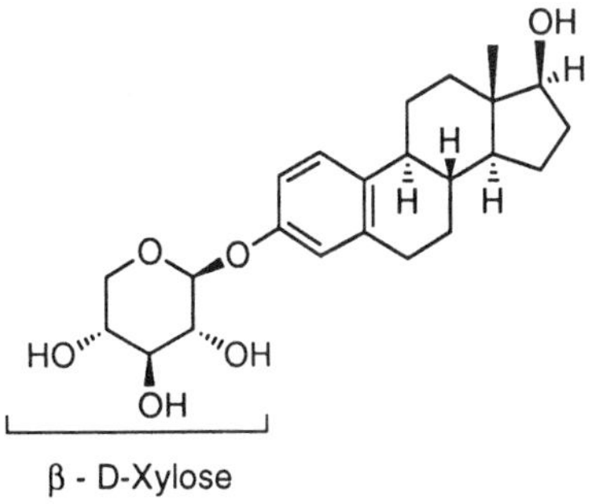

β - D-Xylose

Fig. 22.22 Estradiol-β-D-xyloside.

The GAG chains in typical proteogly-cans are attached to the hydroxyl group of a serine residue in the protein via a linkage region of the structure β-D-GlcpA-(1-3)-β-D-Galp-(1-3)-β-D-Galp-(1-4)-β-D-Xylp. In contrast to direct binding, a novel way to modulate GAG-related biological activities is to induce the endogenous synthesis of GAG oligosaccharide sequences. A series of lipophilic β-D-xylosides was synthesized to examine the structural requirements of the aglycone for GAG priming (251, 252). Of particular interest is estradiol β-D-xyloside, which primes heparin sulfate efficiently in a number of cell types, including CHO, BHK, BAE, and Balb/cs (Fig. 22.22). It is also known that β-glycoside derivatives of 5-thio-β-D-xylopyranosides have increased activity compared with their oxygen analogs (253).

5.3 Glycoproteins

Carbohydrates are attached to mammalian proteins primarily at hydroxyl groups of serines or threonines as O-glycosides or at amido groups of asparagines as N-glycosides (254). The N-linked oligosaccharide chains have a common pentasaccharide core attached to the asparagine in a Asn-X-Ser/Thr sequence (255). This is the result of a common mechanism in biosynthesis in which a branched (Glc)3(Man)9(GlcNAc)2

tetradecasacchride is assembled first, linked by a high energy pyrophosphate bond to the carrier lipid, dolichol. Transfer from the lipid to the protein is followed by "trimming" with specific glucosidases and mannosidases, and the oligosaccharide chain is further modified by stepwise addition of individual sugar units with specific glycosyltransferases. The resulting oligosaccharide chains are classified as high mannose type, hybrid type, or complex type, depending on the extent to which they were processed in the biosynthetic scheme. O-linked carbohydrate chains most commonly have an α-D-GalNAc unit linked to the hydroxyl group of serine or threonine, though other less common types of linkages are also known (256). In contrast to the N-linked glycan chains, no consensus sequence specifying the O-glycosylation sites is known (257). The major source of diversity in both the N- and O-linked oligosaccharide chains of glycoproteins results from variations at the nonreducing terminal, although glycolipids and glycoproteins share a lot of common sequences. The carbohydrate groups on natural glycoproteins confer important physical properties (such as conformational stability, protease resistance, charge and water-binding capacity) and have essentially the same role in the "social life" of cells as the oligosaccharide chains of glycolipids.

Glycoproteins generally show significant microheterogeneity; a potential glycosylation site can carry different oligosaccharide chains or no carbohydrate at all, resulting in different glycoforms of the protein (258). Factors that determine the actual oligosaccharide structure on a potential glycosylation site of a protein are at present poorly understood.

The glycosylation pattern of a protein or glycoform can affect a protein-based drug's potency and determine its target tissue. Indeed, lack of proper glycosylation by microorganisms has mandated the use of mammalian cells in production, instead of simpler bacterial fermentations. Thus carbohydrate research may affect second-generation protein products, improving their efficacy and possibly reducing dosage levels and side effects. Redesigned glycosylation patterns may also provide glycoproteins that will target specific tissues, have longer half-lives, or be more stable or soluble. Many protein-based therapeutics either fail to function or cause immune reactions when not properly glycosylated. For recombinant glycoproteins used as therapeutics, the preparation of the proper glycoform can be a critical issue. Erythropoietin (EPO), which is used in the treatment of anemia caused by renal failure has one O-linked and three N-linked glycosylation sites. Removal of the terminal sialic acid results in loss of *in vivo* activity and rapid clearance from circulation (259). Different glycoforms of tissue-type plasminogen activator (t-PA), which is used to dissolve blood clots following heart attacks and strokes, also have differences in their biological activities. Type 2 t-PA, which has two N-linked glycan chains, is two to three times more active in fibrin-dependent plasminogen activation than type 1 t-PA, which has three N-linked glycan chains (260). Researchers are learning about transport systems in biological systems in regard to absorption, distribution, and metabolism of drugs. For example, significant improvement is observed with peptide renin inhibitors when they are synthetically converted into glycopeptides (261).

With respect to regulatory and proprietary issues, protein glycoforms are becoming part of the strategy for patent applications and drug development. Both regulatory agencies and industry are concerned with carbohydrate characterization, because it effects protein drug efficacy in terms of pharmacokinetics and tissue distribution, safety as it relates to immune reactions, and innovation as it pertains to patent strategy (262).

6 ENZYME INHIBITORS OF CARBOHYDRATE BIOSYNTHESIS AND CATABOLISM

Inhibition of enzymes associated with an important physiological and/or pathological reaction is a classical approach in drug design. From the large variety of different types of enzymes involved in carbohydrate anabolism and catabolism—aldolases, transaldolases, transketolases, phosphorylases, kinases, phosphatases, isomerases, oxidoreductases, nucleotidyltransferes, glycosyltransferases, and glycosidases—nucleotidyltransferases, glycosyltransferases, and glycosidases are most directly connected to the biosynthesis and metabolism of complex carbohydrates.

6.1 Glycosidase Inhibitors

Glycosidases, or glycosyl hydrolases, catalyze the hydrolytic cleavage of glycosidic bonds. In the digestive system, they perform the degradation of poly- and oligosaccharides into absorbable forms, whereas other glycosidases play a role in the processing or trimming the oligosaccharides of the N-linked chains in glycoproteins. Inhibition of glycosidases (263) has received the preponderance of attention from the research community.

Glycosidases in the intestinal system (e.g., the different amylases, maltase, and sucrase) perform the degradation of polysaccharides from food such as starch. Their oligosaccharide degradation products are then converted into absorbable D-glucose, which in turn is introduced into secondary metabolism. The pseudotetrasaccharide Acarbose (Fig. 22.23) is produced by strains of *Actinomycetales* and is a competitive inhibitor of intestinal α-glucosidases, such as glucoamylase and sucrase (264, 265). Administration of Acarbose delays the digestion of sucrose and complex carbohy-

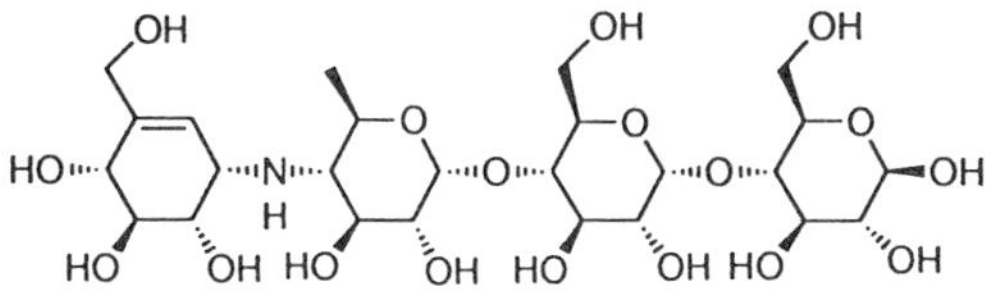

Fig. 22.23 Acarabose.

Fig. 22.25 Swainsonine.

drates, thus retarding the absorption of glucose and fructose and reducing postprandial hyperglycemia. Acarbose also inhibits hyperinsulinemia. It is the first representative of a new class of oral antidiabetic drugs: α- and β-glucosidase inhibitors (266, 267). A series of homologues of Acarbose is known, the members at which differ in the number of the D-glucose units at the reducing and nonreducing ends. Other structurally related compounds (trestatins, adiposins, and oligostatins) are also known (264, 265). SAR studies on the natural and synthetic compounds show that the critical element for the α-glucosidase inhibitory activity is the pseudodisaccharide (acarviosine) built up from an unsaturated cyclitol and the neighboring 4-amino-4,6-dideoxy-D-glucose unit (268–271). The secondary amino group of acarviosine is thought to bind to a carboxyl group in the active center of the enzymes, thereby preventing the protonation of the interglycosidic oxygen of the substrate and thus hydrolysis. The inhibitory potency of acarbose against the different intestinal α-glycosidases decreases in the following order: glucoamylase > sucrase > maltase > isomaltase. It has about 15,000 times higher affinity for sucrase than the enzyme's natural substrate, sucrose. Homologues of acar-

bose with more D-glucose units have less activity against sucrase but higher inhibitory activity against amylase. The pharmacodynamic and pharmacokinetic properties of acarbose and its therapeutic potential have been reviewed (267).

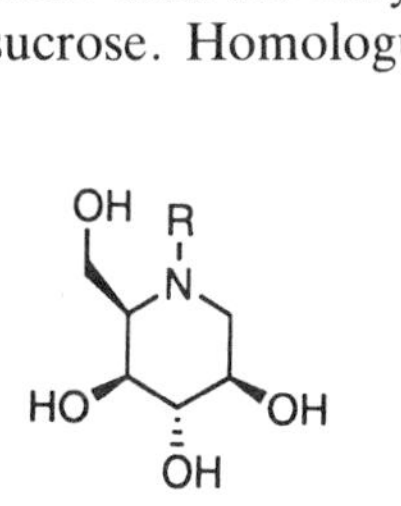

A family of azasugar glycosidase inhibitors from natural sources are of interest because of their unique structures and because of their therapeutical potential as anticancer and anti-HIV agents (272). The archetypal molecule deoxynojirimycin (Fig. 22.24) is isolated from *Streptomyces* (273). Related compounds that have nitrogen—e.g., polyhydroxylated piperidines, pyrrolidines, indolizidines such as swainsonine (Fig. 22.25) and castanospermine (see Fig. 22.26), and pyrrolizidines—are isolated from other natural sources. A large number of deoxynojirimycin and castanospermine analogues have been synthesized (274). In addition, different stereoisomers and substituted derivatives of these compounds as well as the structurally somewhat different aminocyclopentitol derivatives (e.g., mannostatin) have been extensively studied as potentially specific inhibitors of particular glycosidases (263, 274). The primary importance of this class of enzyme inhibitors (besides the effect of inhibiting enzymes in intestinal digestion) is due to its inhibitory effects in the posttranslational trimming process of *N*-linked glycan chains of glycoproteins (275–277). Since processed oligo-

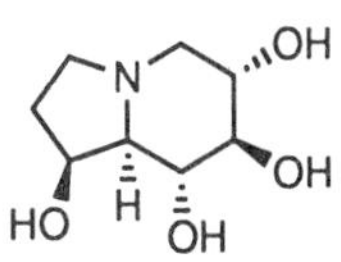

Fig. 22.24 Deoxynojirimycin (R = H) and *N*-butyldeoxynojirimycin (R = Bu).

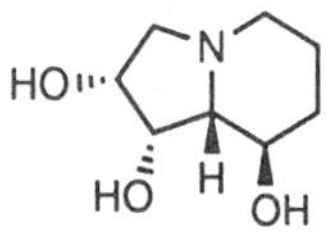

Fig. 22.26 Castanospermine.

saccharides are altered in cancer, a potential therapeutic strategy for cancer is the use of glycosidase inhibitors to prevent the synthesis of aberrant N-linked glycan chain structures. Castanospermine, an inhibitor of glucosidase I, is effective in reducing the growth of v-*fms* transformed rat cells in nude mice *in vivo* (278). There is evidence that swainsonine also acts as an immunomodulator to augment natural killer cell activity (279). Alteration of the glycan structure on viral glycoproteins might affect the infectivity of the viruses. This appears to be the case with inhibitors of α-glucosidase I and II and HIV. Deoxynojirimycin and castanospermine also reduce HIV infectivity and replication (280, 281). Some substituted derivatives—N-butyl-deoxynorjirimycin (see Fig. 22.24) (282) and 6-O-butyryl-castanospermine (283)—are more potent than their parent compounds and N-butyl-deoxynojirimycin is in clinical trials as an anti-HIV drug.

6.2 Glycosyltransferase inhibitors

Glycosyltransferases have the ability to transfer specifically glycosyl residues from sugar nucleotides to hydroxyl groups of acceptor oligosaccharides. In some cases, glycosyltransferases can transfer phosphate-linked lipid derivatives to acceptor groups. Specific inhibition of a given glycosyltransferase results in decreased expression of its product. Inhibition of the synthesis of the activated form of some sugars is an alternative stragey in drug discovery, which may have similar consequences to that of inhibiting glycosyltransferases. Inhibition of glycosyltransferases is of special importance in the modulation of O-linked oligosaccharides of glycoproteins or glycolipids, for which there is no trimming process in the biosynthesis.

Compared with the inhibition of glycosidases, the field of glycosyltransferase inhibitors is less well developed. The antibiotic tunicamycin, isolated from *Strep-*

tomyces (284) is the best example with $K_i = 50$ nM (Fig. 22.27). It inhibits the first step of the synthesis of asparagine-linked glycan chains, the transfer of GlcNAc-1-P from UDP-GlcNAc to the lipid acceptor dolichyl-P to form dolichyl-PP-GlcNAc.

Finding inhibitors of glycosyltransferases that catalyze a growing glycan chain has been less successful than that of the glycosidase inhibitors. Nevertheless, a number of deoxygenated oligosaccharide acceptor analogs are known as specific inhibitors of glycosyltransferases (285). For example, 2-deoxy-Gal-β-[1-3]-GlcNAl-β-[1-x]-C$_8$ ester (Fig. 22.28) inhibits α-(1-2)-fucosyltransferase isolated from pig submaxillary with a K_i of 0.8 mM, and a related analog inhibited β(1-6)-N-acetylglucosaminyltransferase V isolated from hamster kidney with a K_i of 0.063 mM. Both inhibitors are competitive. Synthesis of bisubstrate analogs, thought to better mimic the transition state, is an alternative approach. A bisubstrate analog competitively inhibited α(1-2)-fucosyltransferase with a K_i in the micromolar range (286), but compounds of this type require elaborate synthesis.

Rational design of glycosyltransferase inhibitors at present is limited by the fact that there is no clear mechanism for these enzymes. With the growing number of

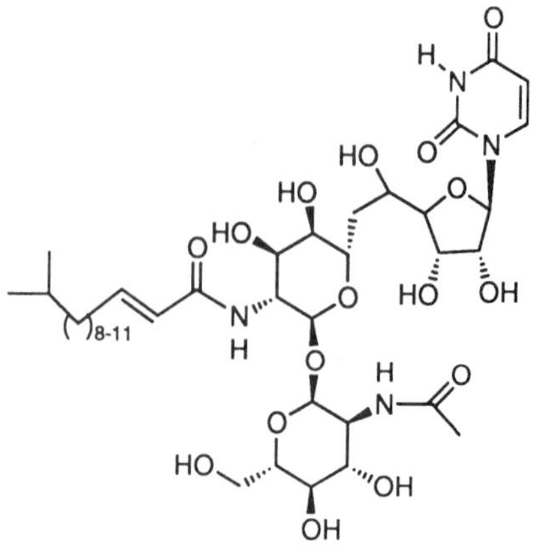

Fig. 22.27 Tunicamycin.

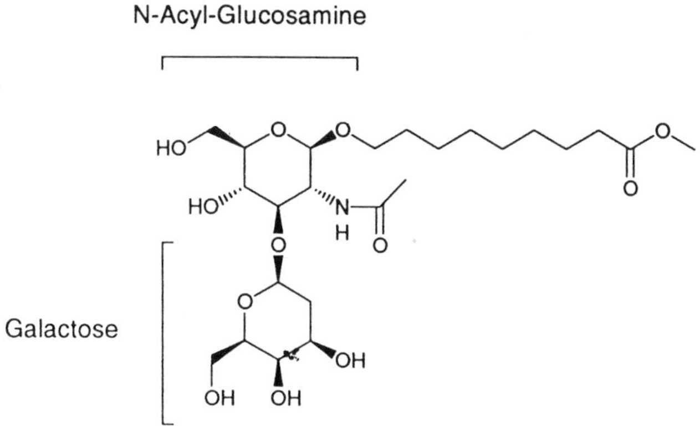

N-Acyl-Glucosamine

Galactose

Fig. 22.28 (3) 2-Deoxy-Gal-β-1,3-GlcNac-β-1,X-C$_8$ ester.

cloned enzymes and the possibility of obtaining an X-ray structure, a deeper insight into the mechanism might result in a breakthrough glycosyltransferase inhibitor.

Another possible approach to down regulate glycosylation is to inhibit the nucleotidyltransferases that synthesize the activated forms of monosaccharides. The eight-carbon sugar 3-deoxy-D-*manno*-2-octulosonic acid (Kdo) is a constituent of the lipopolysaccharides (LPS) of Gram-negative bacteria (287). It occurs in the inner-core region of the LPS, serving as a bridge between lipid A and *O*-specific side chain. The synthesis of the activated form of Kdo (CMP-Kdo) from β-Kdo and CTP catalyzed by the enzyme CMP-Kdo synthetase is thought to be the rate-limiting step in LPS biosynthesis (288). Since bacteria that lack the core region are nonvirulent, inhibitors of CMP-Kdo synthetase are potentially useful as antibacterial agents (289). A large number of Kdo analogues have been synthesized (290, 291), and many of them are active *in vitro*. Their use, however, is hampered by their inability to cross the cytoplasmic membrane.

7 IMMUNOMODULATION

Modulation of the immune system by either stimulation or suppression is an important

pharmacological target for carbohydrate-based therapeutics. Specific stimulation of the immune system or enhancement of the immune response against a given structure is the aim of vaccinations. The problem of attempting immunization with weakly immunogenic compounds, such as subunit vaccines and carbohydrate vaccines, requires the use of adjuvants to enhance the specific immune response to antigens. Nonspecific stimulation, which is a general enhancement of the immune response, might be advantageous in other situations. For example, infection in major surgery, cancer, and AIDS the patient could benefit from the nonspecific stimulation of the immune system. Reviews on immunomodulation indicate a number of agents that are carbohydrates (292–296).

7.1 Antibacterial Vaccines

The recognition that specific polysaccharides of the bacterial cell surface are antigenic is mostly due to the pioneering work of Avery and Heidelberger (297, 298). They showed that a polysaccharide from *Pneumococcus* elicited an immune reaction that demonstrated, for the first time, that a material other than a protein can be antigenic (297). Since the original findings were on the *Pneumococci* and pneumoccocal pneumonia then had an extremely high mortality rate, the prevention of bacterial infections by using bacterial polysaccharide vaccines was given priority over other aproaches. For example, a multivalent vaccine from early work, licensed in 1945 for the Squibb Co., provided 100% efficacy in prevention pneumonia in army recruits. However, this critical stage in the development of carbohydrate-based antibacterial vaccines coincided with the discovery of antibiotics, which overshadowed the early promise of polysaccharide vaccines. Nevertheless, researchers continued their studies on the structure, immunology, and potential uses of bacterial polysaccharides for diagnosis or prevention of bacterial infection (299–302). In an age of potent analytical tools, it is interesting that immunodominant structures of many bacterial polysaccharides were originally determined by total synthesis (303).

Despite the success of antibiotics, pneumococcal pneumonia still occurs with the same frequency and mortality rate as in the preantibiotic era. Moreover, epidemics of meningitis continue not only in Third World countries but also in Scandinavia, and in the United States, bacterial meningitis is still the leading cause of acquired mental retardation (299, 304). Government programs, such as the attempt to eradicate brucellosis in veterinary medicine in Canada, continue to renew interest in carbohydrate-based vaccines. Indeed polysaccharide vaccines may be among the safest in use, because millions of individuals have been injected with these agents without a recorded fatality or serious morbidity (299).

Depending on type, bacteria express different carbohydrate antigens on their cell surfaces, including the *O*-specific side chains of lipopolysaccharides and capsular polysaccharides. Both types consist of repeating oligosaccharide units, ranging in size from di- to hexasaccharides, and are the primary candidates for vaccine genera-

tion. Target infections are determined by their clinical importance, the existence of meaningful epidemiological studies, and the identification of stable polysaccharide antigens. The most important bacterial strains targeted at present are *Streptococcus pneumonia*, *Neisseria meningitidis*, and *Haemophilus influenza*. Other possible candidates include group B *streptococci*, *Klebsiella*, *Pseudomonas aeruginosa*, and *E. coli*. Since bacteria have several immunotypes, most cases have a multivalent vaccine directed against the important serotypes. For example, a multivalent vaccine, including more than 20 serotypes based on the prevalence of types isolated in the United States, and Europe, is used against *S. pneumonia* (302, 305).

A tetravalent vaccine against *N. meningitidis*—the bacterium that causes severe meningococcal disease, especially in the so-called meningitis belt of sub-Sahara Africa—includes serogroups A, C, Y, and W135 and is now available in the United States (306). Development of a vaccine against serotype B, however, remains elusive (307), because the capsular polysaccharide mimics structures normally occuring in mammals. Therefore, other approaches that do not use capsular polysaccharides, including the use of lipopolysaccharides in combination with outer membrane proteins (308, 309), are under investigation.

A problem in immunization with pure polysaccharides is that the vaccines tend to be T-cell–independent antigens and no immunological memory is formed, making effective vaccination of immunologically naive subjects (young children) especially difficult. A possible solution is demonstrated with the development of vaccines against *H. influenzae* type b, which is the leading cause of meningitis in children under the age of 5. A pure polysaccharide vaccine is effective in children older than 24 months (310). An important way to enhance the immunogenecity of pure polysaccharides (311) is to conjugate them to protein carriers (312), which converts them to thymus-dependent antigens. Several vaccines consisting of the *H. influenzae* type b polysaccharide conjugated to proteins—such as diphtheria toxoid CRM 197 (a nontoxic mutant diphtheria toxin) and an outer membrane protein complex (OMPC) of *N. meningitidis*—are now available; these vaccines are for infants as young as 2 months old (310).

Currently used vaccines are bacterial polysaccharides or the corresponding protein conjugates. Because of the extensive synthetic work on bacterial oligosaccharides, however, their is potential for synthetic vaccine development. Chemical synthesis of different size oligomers of the repeating units helps to determine the minimum size of the carbohydrate portion required for an efficient vaccine and indicates that fully synthetic structures can substitute for bacterial isolates (313, 314).

Since most bacterial strains express different capsular and/or lipopolysaccharide structures, which results in the generation of different serotypes, the use of multivalent vaccines is required. There may be alternative approaches, however. The core region connecting the lipid A part with the structurally divergent *O*-specific side chains of the lipopolysaccharides of *Enterobacteriae* has a rather conservative structure. This raises the possibility that, theoretically, a vaccine based on the core structure might give protection against a broad range of bacteria. Indeed, oligosaccharide fragments of the inner and outer core are the subjects of intensive synthetic and immunological studies.

7.2 Immunostimulants and Adjuvants

Although the physicochemical properties and the mode of administration are critical to achieve adjuvant activity (315–318), a discussion based on structural types might be more useful with immunostimulants and adjuvants.

7.2.1 MURAMYL DIPEPTIDE AND ANALOGUES. Microbial invaders that can stimulate the host's defense system are expected on evolutionary grounds. Water-in-oil emulsions of killed mycobacteria (Freund's complete adjuvant) are known to stimulate the immune system, and analyses of these preparations have revealed the structures responsible for this effect. The minimum structural fragment of the cell wall peptidoglycan of *Mycobacterium tuberculosis* that has immunostimulant activity is *N*-acetylmuramyl - L - alanyl - D - isoglutamine, or muramyl dipeptide (MDP) (319) (Fig. 22.29).

MDP has several biological activities: (*1*) when given without an antigen, it stimulates nonspecific resistance against bacterial, viral, and parasite infections and against tumors and (*2*) when given with an antigen, it has adjuvant activity, stimulates the immune response against the antigen, and induces delayed-type hypersensitivity. It also has somnogenic activity. MDP has a set of pharmacologically undesired effects, however, such as pyrogenicity and induction of arthritis.

The underlying biological mechanism for these effects is highly complex and not completely understood (316, 320). Several cell types of the immune system, both macrophages and B-cells are involved, although T-cells are also stimulated by MDP. The influence of MDP on macrophages

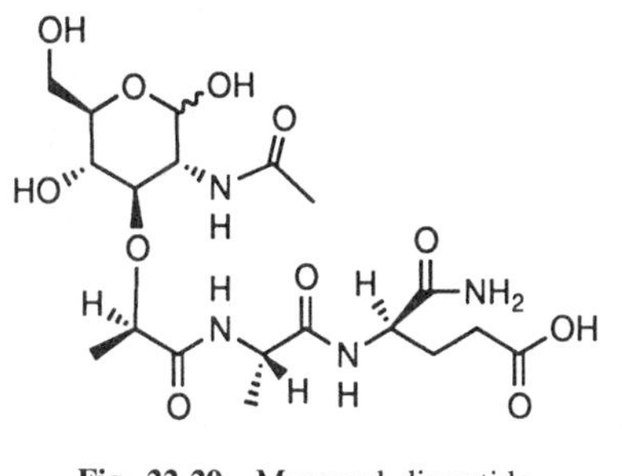

Fig. 22.29 Muramyl dipeptide.

results in the production of interleukin-1 (IL-1), which is one factor in explaining the observed immune enhancement. Stimulation of IL-1 production can also explain some of the undesired effects.

Since MDP is not acceptable for human use, the target in MDP drug design is to maintain the activity of the enhancement of B-cell function, resulting in the production of polyclonal antibodies, and to eliminate the undesired effects. The structure of MDP was confirmed by chemical synthesis (321), and because several hundred MDP derivatives were prepared, detailed SAR data are now available (322, 323).

For example, the cyclic pyranosidic structure is essential for activity; however, the anomeric hydroxyl group can be eliminated or replaced by a thiol residue. The α- and β-glycosides are also active. The primary hydroxyl group at C-6 can be replaced with an amino or acylamido function. Lipophilic 6-O-acyl derivatives are poor adjuvants for humoral reponse relative to MDP, but they induce cellular response and increase nonspecific resistance. The acetyl group at the C-2 amino function can be replaced by other acyl groups. The side chain methyl group of the lactyl residue is not essential; replacement of this group by hydrogen (nor-MDP), however, results in reduction of side effects. Similarly, the methyl group of the alanyl residue is not essential. The substituion at this position, however, must retain the L-configuration. Furthermore, the D-configuration of the terminal glutamyl residue is important because the aspartyl analogue is inactive, although the carboxyls can be free acids, esters, or primary amides. Extension of the peptide moiety by a stearoyl-L-lysine residue significantly enhances activity. The addition of a second glucosamine residue at C-4 of nor-MDP and substitution of the alanyl by an γ-aminobutyryl residue increases the adjuvant activity and reduces pyrogenicity. Some analogs are reported to be devoid of the

pyrogenic effect. It should be mentioned, however, that the diverse biological activities of MDP and its analogs create problems in SAR analysis.

Of the large number of MDP analogs synthesized thus far, Murabutide and Muramethide are considered the best drug candidates. Murabutide is as effective as MDP as an adjuvant, but it has nonspecific immunostimulant activity. Murabutide is nonpyrogenic and is devoid of other unwanted biological properties of MDP. Murabutide has undergone clinical trials as a vaccine adjuvant (324) and is also in clinical trials as an immunostimulant for cancer patients (292). Another MDP analog, Romurtide is licensed in Japan to induce bone marrow recovery in connection with cancer chemotherapy (325).

7.2.2 CORD FACTOR AND ANALOGS. Another class of immunostimulant compounds isolated from mycobacteria are the cord factors, ester derivatives of trehalose with long-chain fatty acids (296, 316, 317, 323). The 6,6'-O-dimycolate of α,α-trehalose, or trehalose dimycolate (TDM), was originally isolated from *Mycobacterum tuberculosis* (Fig. 22.30). (Mycolic acids are long-chain α-branched β-hydroxy acids of chain length C85–C90.) Related compounds with shorter-chain fatty acids (C28–C36) also are isolated from *Corynebactrium* and *Nocardia*. The immunostimulant properties, including adjuvant, antibacterial, antitumor,

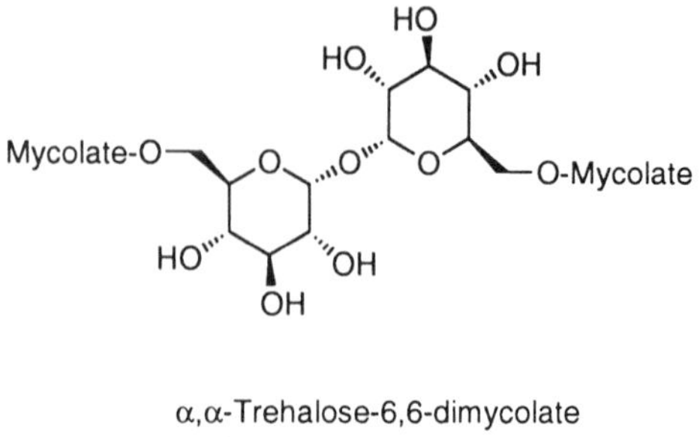

α,α-Trehalose-6,6-dimycolate

Fig. 22.30 Trehalose 6,6-dimycolate.

and antiparasitic activities, are well studied (326–328). Synthetic studies on producing cord factor analogs are aimed to reduce the toxicity and granuloma-forming activity of TDM. One approach of SAR studies is focused on the use of shorter-chain esters or cutting the molecule in half (329). The 6-*O*-mycoloyl ester 1-deoxy-*N*-acetyl-D-glucosamine, is devoid of toxicity but is a potent macrophage activator (330). In another approach, the ester functionalities are regioinverted (331, 332), and the corresponding uronic acid esters are termed "mirror" pseudocord factors.

7.2.3 LIPID A AND ANALOGS. Another class of bacteria-derived compounds are the lipopolysaccharide (LPS) endotoxins of Gram-negative bacteria, which have potent effects on the immune system, especially B-lymphocytes and macrophages (292). After the general architecture of LPS was described (333, 334), it became clear that the lipid A portion of LPS is reponsible for the observed endotoxicity (335). As with MDP and cord factor, however, lipid A itself is unsuitable for use in humans and

animals, as it has a series of undesired effects; the most notable are extreme toxicity and pyrogenicity. Detoxified forms of lipid A provide chemically defined safe forms for preclinical testing as immunotherapeutics. The gross chemical structure of lipid A was established in the 1970s (335), and several synthetic analogues were synthesized and tested (334). Details of the structure had to be revised in 1983, and the structure of lipid A from *E. coli* is now firmly established and has been confirmed by synthesis (337) (Fig. 22.31). Lipid A's of other bacterial strains, such as *Salmonella minnesota*, show minor differences in the fatty acid chain lengths.

During the course of purification and characterization of lipid A, several related structures, such as lipid X and lipid Y, were isolated (338). A derivative lacking the phosphate on the reducing end (monophosphoryl lipid A, or MPL) shows substantially reduced pyrogenicity and lethality while retaining the full immunostimulant and adjuvant properties (339, 340). MPL is described as the "long sought after utilitarian immunotherapeutic form of endotox-

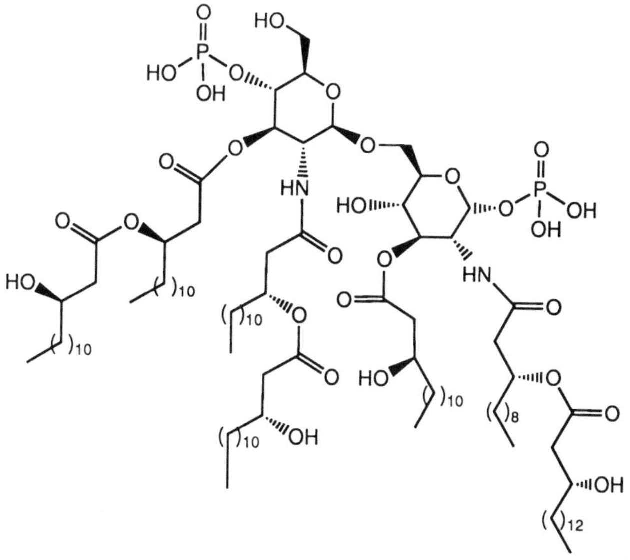

Fig. 22.31 Lipid A.

in." Early clinical trial data for remission of melanoma by treatment with MPL are reported (341).

Synthetic studies on lipid A components, in addition to proving the structures of the natural products, provide important SAR information. In retaining the immuno-stimulant activity but eliminating the unde-sired side effects, analogs of the nonreduc-ing end monosaccharide turned out to be especially valuable. A wide variety of fatty acid–substituted 4-O-phosphono-D-glucosamine derivatives, including GLA-60 (342) were prepared; GLA-60 shows strong immunostimulatory activity but no pyro-genicity. SAR studies indicate that the number, position, and chain length of the actyl groups are critical for biological activi-ty. Best results are obtained with com-pounds that have a total of three acyl groups, one in the form of acyloxyacyl and the third one with a free OH on a 3-hydroxy fatty acid (343). The chain length and configuration of C-3 of the fatty acid also affects biological activity (344). Re-placement of the O-3 acyloxy residue with a long-chain alkyl ether group gave inactive compounds (345), but using a C-2–branch-ed 2-alkyl–fatty acid instead of the 3-acyloxyacyl group retained activity (346). Some 1-deoxy derivatives are active (347); fluorinated analogs, however, are essential-ly inactive (348).

In another approach, conjugates of two immunologically active components of bac-terial cell walls—lipid A and muramyl dipeptide analogs, with an oligosuccinyl-type spacer were prepared. They have activity equivalent to MDP in inducing delayed-type hypersensitivity (349).

7.2.4 ANTITUMOR POLYSACCHARIDES. Stim-ulation of nonspecific host defense is ob-served with a number of polysaccharides of diverse origins, including bacteria, fungi, yeast, and plants. Their potential in an-titumor therapy merits a brief discussion (350, 351).

Most of the antitumor polysaccharides are D-glucans. A characteristic example of a β-D-glucan is lentinan (352), a high molecular weight β-(1-3)-glucan with β-(1-6) branching. This polysaccharide is ex-tracted from the edible mushroom Lentinus edodes (Berk.) Sing. Lentinan is believed sequentially to enhance IL-1 production, T-cell function, and natural killer (NK) cell activity. No direct effect on phagocytosis or interferon production is involved. Lentinan is licensed in Japan and is in clinical trials in the United States.

Active homo- and heteropolysaccharides combine with structural diversity and com-plexity of these classes to make SAR studies of saccharide-based antitumor espe-cially difficult. A prerequisite for biological activity is that the compounds should not be quickly hydrolyzed by humoral glycosid-ases. In general, polysaccharides with a linear backbone without excessively long branches are the most active. β-D-Glucans that have mostly (1-3) linkages are more potent than β-(1-6)-glucans, whereas poly-saccharides with (1-4) linkages are less potent. The importance of highly ordered three-dimensional structures (triple helices) appear to be required for the activity (353), but recent data do not support this hypoth-esis (354, 355). A series of different chemi-cally modified derivatives of the native polysaccharides, consisting mostly of charged and glycosylated derivatives, are currently under evaluation as possible an-titumor agents.

7.2.5 GLYCOLIPID ANALOGS. Glycolipid analogues that show promise as potential adjuvants are N-alkylglycosyl amides of long-chain fatty acids (356). These are structurally related to naturally occurring glycolipids: glycosphingolipids and gly-coglycerolipids. Compounds of this class produce a dose-dependent increase in the formation of antibodies. Alone they have no mitogenic activity, their effect is in-dependent of T-lymphocytes, and the for-

mation of antibodies is detectable only in combintion with the antigen stimulus on B-lymphocytes. Modifications in the sugar residue, the lipophilic group, and the branching region have been reported. Among the sugar residues studied, β-D-glucopyranosyl and 2-(N-acyl)amino-2-de-oxy-β-D-glucopyranosyl have the highest activity. The alkyl chain must be at least 12 carbon atoms long, and the amide group appears to be essential. Interestingly, glycosylamido derivatives of MDP are inactive. From the compounds studied, N-(2-deoxy-L-leucylamino-β-D-glucopyranosyl)-N-octadecyldodecanamide acetate (BAY R 1005) is in development.

7.2.6 SAPONINS. Several saponins, terpenoid or steroid glycosides of oligosaccharides with surfactant properties, show different adjuvant activity (357). Extracts of the bark of the South American tree *Quillaja saponaria* Molina, that contain a mixture of triterpenoid saponins have strong immunoadjuvant effects (358). They also lower plasma cholesterol levels. Despite the potential use of *Quillaja* saponins as adjuvants, their application has been limited because of undesirable side effects, including toxicity and hemolytic activity. Some partially purified fractions, Quil A and Quillayanin, are valuable as vaccine adjuvant, e.g., against foot-and-mouth disease (359). Specially formulated particles, complexes of Quil A with membrane proteins, induce serum antibody titers about 10-fold higher than immunization with protein micelles alone (360). Components of *Quillaja* saponins, purified to homogeneity (361, 362) reveal that there is no correlation between hemolytic activity, lethality, and adjuvant activity. One fraction QS21 (Stimulon), is undergoing clinical testing as an adjuvant in several therapeutic areas. For example, human trials against malignant melanoma have started, and it is given with synthetically engineered vaccines against malaria. It is also under study as an

Fig. 22.32   Therafectin.

adjuvant in a cytomegalovirus vaccine and for use as a potential veterinary vaccines.

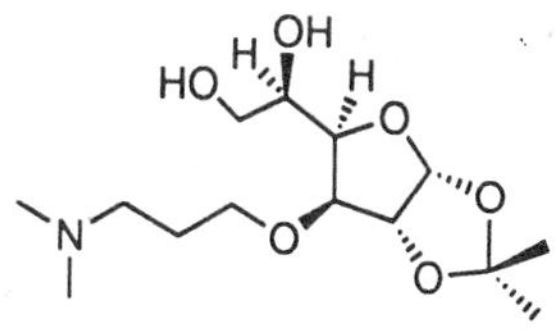

7.2.7 THERAFECTIN. Therafectin, a structurally simple synthetic D-glucose derivative, has stimulatory effects on immune cells and does not interfere with vital cell functions (Fig. 22.32). It protects mice from infection with herpesvirus, influenza virus, and *Candida* and prolongs the life span of mice inoculated with B16 melanoma. It is promised as a potent macrophage activator in patients with rheumatoid arthritis and AIDS needs to be further demonstrated (363). Therafectin has gone through phase III clinical trials for the treatment of rheumatoid arthritis but has not been approved by the U.S. FDA.

8 CARBOHYDRATE-MEDIATED CELL–CELL INTERACTIONS

Cell surface glycoconjugates may act as cell–cell recognition molecules via specific binding between carbohydrates on one cell and protein receptors on an opposing cell, specific interactions directly between carbohydrates on opposing cells, or indirectly via intermediate molecules, such as, antibodies (364). In the area of cell surface glycoconjugates, one finds the blood group antigens. Blood groups are genetically regulated carbohydrate antigens found on cell surfaces (365).

8.1 Blood Group Carbohydrates

In red blood cells (erythrocytes), the carbohydrate side chains can determine the blood group specificity and antigenicity. The major red cell antigens are called the ABO antigens, and different individuals carry either the A antigen, the B antigen, both (group AB), or the H antigen (group O). The existence of these strong antigenic differences means that, with certain exceptions, it is only possible to transfuse blood between individuals of the same blood group. Individuals with AB blood can accept blood of any ABO type, because they lack antibodies for A and B antigens. Individuals with O blood are universal blood donors because they do not have A and B antigens.

Although the ABO blood group is not under direct genetic control, enzymes that control its biosynthesis are gene products (366). The ABO enzymes catalyze the attachment of sugar residues to already existing oligosaccharide chains common to many cell types. For example, individuals with the A allele produce 2-acetamido-D-galactosyltransferase, and individuals with the B allel produce D-galactosyltransferase, resulting in the biosynthesis of the A and B tetrasaccharide determinants, respectively. Those individuals who have both alleles express both transferases, and those individuals with neither produce no A- or B-applicable transferases. It is interesting to note that there is only a four amino acid residue difference between A and B transferases, and that a single-base deletion is found in the O allele (367).

The ABO antigen determinants have been investigated (93, 368), and the conformation of the blood group determinant was studied by hard-sphere/exoanomeric calculations, 1H NMR, nOe, and T1 experiments (91). There are additional studies on the binding of the ABO blood group antigens (93, 369–371).

A complication of the ABO determinants involves the structural backbone (Fig. 22.33). Type I and II determinants

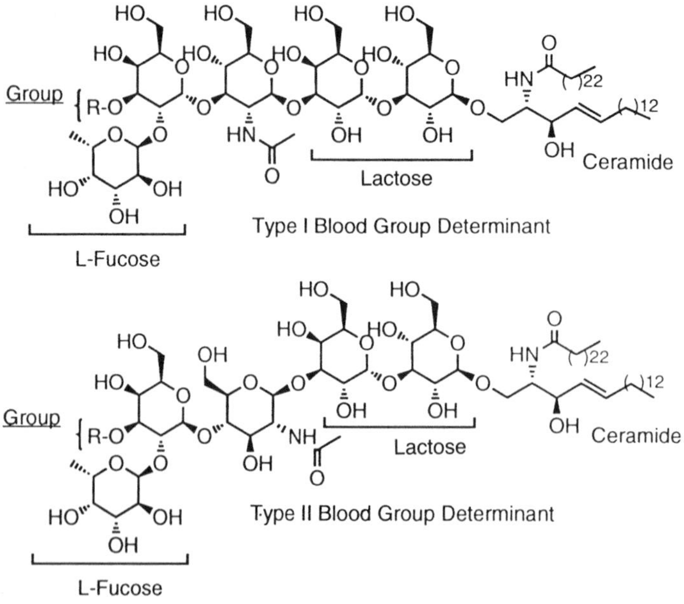

Fig. 22.33 Blood group determinants. Group A: R = α-D-N-acetylaminogalactosyl; group B: R = α-D-galactosyl; group O: R = H.

differ in the galactosyl–glucosamine linkage of the core trisaccharide. For example, in type I determinants, the internal galactosyl moiety is bound to the three position of the glucosamine, whereas, in type II, the internal galactosyl moiety is bound to the four position of the glucosamine. Currently, there appears to be no biological impact of type I versus type II backbone with respect to blood group specificity and antigenicity. Nevertheless, differences may be noted in the emerging field of selectin-mediated adhesion and the structurally related Lewis determinants.

8.2 Selectin-mediated Adhesion

Adhesion of cells in the immune system is clinically important when considering such indications as cancer; microbial infection; and inflammatory, allergic, and autoimmune diseases. Lectins are simply carbohydrate-binding proteins. The structure of the calcium-dependent (C-type) lectin domain from a rat mannose-binding protein was determined by X-ray crystallography, employing multiwavelength anomalous dispersion phasing (372). These results are significant, since the structure may be used to gain insight into other carbohydrate-binding proteins such as the selectins.

The selectins are a family of glycoproteins that are implicated in the adhesion of leukocytes to platelets or vascular endothelium (373). Adhesion is an early step in leukocyte extravasation, whose sequelae includes thrombosis, recirculation, and inflammation. An excellent review on leukocyte adhesion in inflammation and the immune system was recently published (374). Three protein receptors, E-, L- and P-selectins are assigned to the selectin family based on their cDNA sequences. Each contains a domain similar to C-type lectins, an epidermal growth factor-like domain, and several complement binding protein-like domains (375). An intense effort is ongoing to define the native carbohydrate ligands for each selectin receptor. In the case of E-selectin (ELAM-1, LECAM-2) several laboratories have described the ligands from myeloid cells as the sialyl Lewis x (sLe^x) epitope (376). Current information suggests that sLe^x is also a carbohydrate ligand for P-selectin (GMP-140, LECAM-3) (377) and L-selectin (LECAM-1) (378). Other ligands for the selectins have been partially identified. For example, a sulfated 50 kD glycoprotein that contains both sialic acid and fucose is reported to be a ligand for the L-selectin receptor (379). Finally, there are data that suggest that the heterogeneous 3-O-sulfated galactosylceramides, referred to as sulfatides, bind to both the L-selectin (380) and P-selectin (381) receptors. However, this binding does not appear to be calcium dependent.

A synthetic peptide, CQNRYTDLVAIQNKNE, inhibits neutrophil binding to P-selectin (382). This protein was designed based on an epitope that spans residues 19 to 34 to the P-selectin domain and is recognized by a blocking monoclonal antibody. Although neutrophil recognition is thought to require a calcium-induced conformational change in the lectin domain of GMP-140, this result indicates that a small polypeptide may be used to block this interaction.

8.3 Sperm–Egg Adhesion

Evidence is accumulating that mammalian sperm cells in general express proteins that interact specifically with saccharide receptors on eggs. For example, a 56 kD mouse sperm cell surface protein (ZP3) that specifically binds to the oligosaccharide part of a glycoprotein on unfertilized mouse eggs is similar in size to lectin-like receptors on sperm of other animal species (383). Indeed, attachment of mouse blastocysts to endometrial cells is inhibited by a distinct pentasaccharide. Thus new possibilities for contraception may be possible by modulating fertilization processes that are based on protein–carbohydrate interactions.

8.4 Microorganism–Cell Interaction

Carbohydrates are critical in the initiation of bacterial and viral infections. It is well established that bacterial lectins play a significant role in host cell recognition, adherence, and initiation of infection (384). For example the α-mannosides inhibits *E. coli* adherence to epithelial cells and is 10-fold more potent than naturally occurring oligosaccharides and 1000-fold more potent than α-methyl mannoside. This demonstrates that mannoside derivatives can specifically inhibit bacterial infections, at least in rodent experimental models. Both glycoproteins and glycolipids contain terminal sialic acids, which bind influenza virus *in vitro* (46). Another factor is multivalent binding via the viral hemagglutinins, which are trimeric in the viral envelope and bind most avidly to multiple optimally spaced carbohydrate determinants. In addition to influenza, several other viruses are reported to bind to glycoconjugates, including rabies virus, Sendai virus, Newcastle disease virus, and retroviruses (385).

8.5 Cancer Metastasis

There is strong evidence that specific cell surface carbohydrates expressed on colonic, pancreatic, and other tumors are involved in metastasis (386). Colonic and pancreatic tumors exhibit high levels of sLe^x as they progress through metastatic stages of malignancy; human urinary bladder carcinoma metastatic potential is correlated with expression of sLe^x; and a large proportion of stomach intramucosal carcinomas, gastric adenomas, and goblet cells of intestinal metaplasia exhibit sLe^x (387).

Indeed, the primary adhesion event for circulating metastatic cells may use the same identical adhesive system as that for lymphocytes. Thus a carbohydrate lead may be of value in prophylactic therapy after primary tumors are discovered and during and after surgery when metastatic-potentiated cells may be dislodged into the circulation.

9 SUMMARY

Carbohydrate-containing biomolecules are found on all cell surfaces, and because of their inherent strucural diversity, many oligosaccharides are information carriers and recognition molecules. It is now clear that carbohydrates are critical in the operation of fundamental biological processes of cellular recognition and that the specific interaction of many biopolymers is mediated by complex carbohydrates, not by proteins or by oligonucleotides. Carbohydrate groups provide signals for protein or lectin targeting and cell–cell interactions and serve as receptors for binding toxins, viruses, and hormones. They control vital events in fertilization and early development, regulate many critical immune system recognition events, and target aging cells for destruction.

Because carbohydrates have the highest potential for complexity on a unit basis compared with amino acids, nucleosides, and lipids, they are the ideal carriers of biological specificity. Nature appears to have taken full advantage of these innately exquisite forms of concise informational packages, and only recently have we been able employ this information in the design of carbohydrate-containing therapeutics.

Current progress in carbohydrate research is primarily the result of progress in analytical chemistry methods and synthetic techniques. As noted earlier, the carbohydrate biopolymer class has no corresponding recombinant DNA technology paradigm as exists for protein generation. In carbohydrate chemistry, the significant progress in chemical analysis—such as mass spectrometry (which employs electrospray techniques) and NMR (which uses nOe)—has served as a technological substitute for biological-based characterizations used with the protein or nucleoside biopolymer classes. In addition, unlike peptides and oligonucleotides, there are no automated synthesis methods for oligosaccharide generation. The significant information now available on carbohydrate synthesis will play a critical role in the discovery of carbohydrate-based therapeutics. Since enzymatic carbohydrate chemistry has the capability to solve both regio- and stereoselectivity problems associated with carbohydrate synthesis, it is expected that enzymes will play larger role in the production of carbohydrate-based therapeutics in the future.

Despite the neglect of saccharides in drug discovery, several carbohydrate-containing drug classes (including antibiotics, nucleoside antivirals and anticancer agents, and cardiac glycosides) are in use. An examination of the absorption, distribution, metabolism, and excretion of these agents indicate that, in the design of new therapeutic agents based on carbohydrates, it may be appropriate to consider the synthesis of hydrocarbon or aromatic appendages to the parent carbohydrate to increase lipid solubility. It is also suggested that glycomimetics may be more readily accessible than peptidomimetics. Furthermore, the approach of using carbohydrates as pharmacological modifiers of therapeutic agents has considerable potential, which at present is far from being fully exploited. Finally, carbohydrates can alter drug pharmacokinetics and efficacy.

Taken together, knowledge of oligosaccharide synthesis, structure, and function can serve the medicinal chemist well in the design of new therapeutic agents based on carbohydrates (9).

REFERENCES

1. J. H. Musser in J. A. Bristol, ed., *Annual Report of Medicinal Chemistry*, Vol. 27, New York, Academic Press, 1992, p. 301.

2. M. A. Wolff, ed., *Burger's Medicinal Chemistry*, 4th ed., John Wiley & Sons, Inc., New York, 1979.

3. N. Sharon, *Complex Carbohydrates. Their Chemistry, Biosynthesis, and Functions*, Addison-Wesley, Publishing Co., Inc., Reading, Mass., 1975.

4. Ref. 3, p. 26.

5. P. Kotovuori, E. Tontti, R. Pigott, M. Shepherd, M. Kiso, A. Hasegawa, R. Renkonnen, P. Nortamo, D. C. Altieri, and C. G. Gahmberg, *Glycobiol.*, **3**, 131 (1993).

6. Ref. 3, p. 7.

7. R. A. Laine, personnel communication.

8. J. H. Musser in C. G. Wermuth, ed., IUPAC *Monograph Medicinal Chemistry for the 21st Century*, Blackwell Scientific, Oxford, UK, 1992, p. 25.

9. R. L. Schnaar, *Adv. Pharmacol.*, **23**, 35 (1992).

10. K.-A. Karlsson, *Trends Pharm. Sci.*, **12**, 265 (1991).

11. A. K. Mallams in J. F. Kennedy, ed., *Carbohydrate Chemistry*, Oxford University Press, Oxford, UK, 1988, p. 73.

12. S. Umezawa, *Adv. Carbohydr. Chem. Biochem.*, **30**, 111 (1974).

13. U. Hollstein in Ref. 2, p. 173.

14. G. Lukacs, ed., *Recent Progress in the Chemical Synthesis of Antibiotics and Related Microbial Products*, Springer-Verlag, New York, 1993.

15. E. F. Gale, E. Cundliffe, P. E. Reynolds, M. H. Richmond, and M. J. Waring, *The Molecular Basis of Antibiotic Action*, 2nd ed., John Wiley & Sons, Inc., New York, 1981.

16. L. P. Garrod, H. P. Lambert, and F. O'Grady, *Antibiotic and Chemotherapy*, 5th ed., Chirchill Livingston, Edinburgh, UK, 1981.

17. J. Thiem and B. Meyer, *Tetrahedron*, **37**, 551 (1981).

18. J. Thiem and W. Klaffke, *Topics Curr. Chem.*, **154**, 285 (1990).

19. R. W. Burg, B. M. Miller, E. E. Baker, J. Birnbaum, S. A. Currie, R. Hartman, Y.-L. Kong, R. L. Monaghan, G. Olson, I. Putter, J. B. Tunac, H. Wallick, E. O. Stapley, R. Oiwa, and S. Omura, *Antimicrob. Agents Chemother.*, **15**, 361 (1979).

20. Y. Takiguchi, H. Mishima, M. Okuda, M. Terao, A. Aoki, and R. Fukuda, *J. Antibiotics*, **33**, 1120 (1980).

21. H. G. Davies and R. H. Green, *Chem. Soc. Rev.*, **20**, 211 (1991).

22. H. G. Davies and R. H. Green, *Chem. Soc. Rev.*, **20**, 271 (1991).

23. M. H. Fisher and H. Mrozik, *Annu. Rev. Pharmacol. Toxicol.*, **32**, 537 (1992).

24. W. C. Campbell, M. H. Fisher, E. O. Stapley, G. Albers-Schönberg, and T. A. Jacob, *Science*, **221**, 823 (1983).

25. K. L. Goa, D. McTavish, and S. P. Clissold, *Drugs*, **42**, 640 (1991).

26. H. Mrozik, B. O. Linn, P. Eskola, A. Lusi, A. Matzuk, F. A. Preiser, D. A. Ostlind, J. M. Schaeffer, and M. H. Fisher, *J. Med. Chem.*, **32**, 375 (1989), and references therein.

27. H. G. Davies and R. H. Green, *Natural Product Rep.*, **3**, 87 (1986).

28. K. C. Nicolaou, C. W. Hummel, E. N. Pitsinos, M. Nakada, A. L. Smith, K. Shibayama, and H. Saimoto, *J. Am. Chem. Soc.*, **114**, 10082 (1992).

29. J. A. Secrist III in J. F. Kennedy, ed., *Carbohydrate Chemistry*, Oxford University Press, Oxford, UK, 1988, p. 134.

30. J. C. Martin, ed., *Nucleotide Analogues as Antiviral Agents*, ACS Symposium Series, **401**, American Chemical Society, Washington, D.C., 1989.

31. D. M. Huryn and M. Okabe, *Chem. Rev.*, **92**, 1745 (1992).

32. S. Smith, *J. Chem. Soc.*, 508 (1930).

33. K. R. H. Repke and W. Schönfeld, *Trends Pharmacol. Sci.*, **5**, 393 (1984).

34. W. Schönfeld, R. Schönfeld, K. H. Menke, J. Weiland, and K. R. H. Repke, *Biochem. Pharmacol.*, **35**, 3221 (1986).

35. H. Rathore, A. H. L. From, K. Ahmed, and D. S. Fullerton, *J. Med. Chem.*, **29**, 1945 (1986).

36. A. E. Aulabough, R. C. Crouch, G. E. Martin, A. Ragouzeous, J. P. Shockcor, T. D. Spitzer, R. D. Farrant, B. D. Hudson, and J. C. Lindon, *Carbohydr. Res.*, **230**, 201 (1992).

37. L. Varga and J. Kuszmann, *Magy. Kemikusok Lapja*, 373 (1972).

38. D. T. Walz in M. E. Goldberg, ed., *Pharmacological and Biochemical Properties of Drug Substances*, Vol. 2, American Pharmaceutical Association, Washington, D.C., 1979, p. 400.

39. R. N. Brogden, R. C. Heal, T. M. Speight, and G. S. Avery, *Drugs*, **27**, 194 (1984).

40. G. Huber and A. Rossi, *Helv. Chim. Acta*, **51**, 1185 (1968).

41. R. Jaques, G. Huber, L. Neipp, A. Rossi, B. Schär, and R. Meier, *Experientia*, **23**, 149 (1967).

42. L. Reisterer and R. Jaques, *Experientia*, **24**, 581 (1968).

43. R. J. Kandrotas, *Clin. Pharmacokinet.*, **22**, 359 (1992).

44. L. B. Jaques, L. M. Hiebert, and S. M. Wice, *J. Lab. Clin. Med.*, **117**, 122 (1991).

45. K. G. Rice, O. A. Weisz, T. Barthel, R. T. Lee, and Y. C. Lee, *J. Biol. Chem.*, **265**, 18429 (1990).

46. T. J. Pritchett and J. C. Paulson, *J. Biol. Chem.*, **264**, 9850 (1989).

47. M. N. Matrosovich, L. V. Mochalova, V. P. Marinina, N. E. Byramova, and N. V. Bovin, *FEBS Lett.*, **272**, 209 (1990).

48. A. Spaltenstein and G. M. Whitesides, *J. Am. Chem. Soc.*, **113**, 686 (1991).

49. J.-J. Cheong, W. Birberg, P. Fügedi, Å. Pilotti, P. J. Garegg, N. Hong, T. Ogawa, and M. G. Hahn, *Plant Cell.*, **3**, 127 (1991).

50. B. Lindberg, J. Lönngren, and S. Svensson, *Adv. Carbohydr. Chem. Biochem.*, **31**, 185 (1975).

51. M. W. Spellman, *Anal. Biochem.*, **62**, 1714 (1990).

52. S. C. Churms, *J. Chromatogr.*, **500**, 555 (1990).

53. K. B. Hicks, *Adv. Carbohydr. Chem. Biochem.*, **46**, 17 (1988).

54. Y. C. Lee, *Anal. Biochem.*, **189**, 151 (1990).

55. R. R. Townsend, M. R. Hardy, and Y. C. Lee, *Meth. Enzymol.*, **179**, 65 (1989).

56. M. R. Hardy, *Meth. Enzymol.*, **179**, 76 (1989).

57. E. D. Green and J. U. Baenzinger, *Trends Biochem. Sci.*, **14**, 168 (1989).

58. P. Jackson, *Biochem. Soc. Trans.*, **21**, 121 (1993).

59. P. Jackson, *Biochem. J.*, **270**, 705 (1990).

60. K. B. Lee, A. Al-Hakim, D. Loganathan, and R. J. Linhardt, *Carbohydr. Res.*, **214**, 155 (1991).

61. S. L. Carney and D. J. Osborne, *Anal. Biochem.*, **195**, 132 (1991).

62. N. K. Vyas, *Curr. Opin. Struct. Biol.*, **1**, 732 (1991).

63. N. Sharon and H. Lis, *Chem. Brit.*, 679 (1990).

64. R. U. Lemieux, A. P. Venot, U. Spohr, P. Bird, G. Mandal, N. Morishima, O. Hindsgaul, and D. R. Bundle, *Can. J. Chem.*, **63**, 2664 (1985).

65. R. U. Lemieux in *Proceedings of the Seventh International Symposium on Medical Chemistry*, Vol. 1, Uppsala, Sweden, 1984, p. 329.

66. F. A. Quiocho, *Ann. Rev. Biochem.*, **55**, 287 (1986).

67. A. Dell, *Adv. Carbohydr. Chem. Biochem.*, **45**, 19 (1987).

68. P. L. Devine, B. A. Clark, G. W. Birrell, G. T. Layton, B. G. Ward, P. F. Alewood, and I. F. C. McKenzie, *Cancer Res.*, **51**, 5826 (1991).

69. E. P. Roquemore, A. Dell, H. R. Morris, M. Panico, A. J. Reason, L.-A. Savoy, G. J. Wistow, J. S. Zigler Jr., B. J. Earles, and G. W. Hart, *J. Biol. Chem.*, **267**, 555 (1992).

70. B. Ganem, Y.-T. Li, and J. D. Henion, *J. Am. Chem. Soc.*, **113**, 7818 (1991).

71. J. Dabrowski, *Meth. Enzymol.*, **179**, 122 (1989).

72. J. A. van Kuik, K. Hård, and J. F. G. Vliegenthart, *Carbohydr. Res.*, **235**, 53 (1992).

73. P.-E. Jansson, L. Kenne, and G. Widmalm, *J. Chem. Info. Comput. Sci.*, **31**, 508 (1991).

74. I. Ciucanu and F. Kerek, *Carbohydr. Res.*, **131**, 209 (1984).

75. J.-G. Jun and G. R. Gray, *Carbohydr. Res.*, **163**, 247 (1987).

76. J. F. Stoddart, *Stereochemistry of Carbohydrates*, Wiley-Interscience, New York, 1971.

77. B. Meyer, *Topics Curr. Chem.*, **154**, 141 (1990).

78. R. U. Lemieux and S. Koto, *Tetrahedron*, **30**, 1933 (1974).

79. I. Tvaroska and T. Bleha, *Adv. Carbohydr. Chem. Biochem.*, **47**, 45 (1989).

80. W. A. Szarek and D. Horton, eds., *The Anomeric Effect, Origin and Consequences*, ACS Symposium Series, **87**, American Chemical Society, Washington, D.C., 1979.

81. P. Deslongchamps, *Stereoelectronic Effects in Organic Chemistry*, Pergamon Press, Oxford, UK, 1983.

82. A. J. Kirby, *The Anomeric Effect and Related Stereoelecronic Effects at Oxygen*, Springer-Verlag, Berlin, 1983.

83. V. G. S. Box, *Heterocycles*, **31**, 1157 (1990).

84. R. U. Lemieux, A. A. Pavia, J. C. Martin, and K. A. Watanabe, *Can. J. Chem.*, **47**, 4427 (1969).

85. R. U. Lemieux, S. Koto, and D. Voisin in Ref. 80, p. 17.

86. A. D. French and J. W. Brady, eds., *Computer Modeling of Carbohydrate Molecules*, ACS Symposium Series, **430**, American Chemical Society, Washington, D.C., 1990.

87. E. C. Garrett and A. S. Serianni in Ref. 86, p. 91.

88. S. Wolfe, M.-H. Whangbo, and D. J. Mitchell, *Carbohydr. Res.*, **69**, 1 (1979).

89. G. A. Jeffrey and J. H. Yates, *Carbohydr. Res.*, **96**, 205 (1981).

90. G. A. Jeffrey, J. A. Pople, J. S. Binkley, and S. Vishveshwara, *J. Am. Chem. Soc.*, **100**, 373 (1978).

91. R. U. Lemieux, K. Bock, L. T. J. Delbaere, S. Koto, and V. S. Rao, *Can. J. Chem.*, **58**, 631 (1980).

92. H. Thogersen, R. U. Lemieux, K. Bock, and B. Meyer, *Can. J. Chem.*, **60**, 44 (1982).

93. R. U. Lemieux, *Chem. Soc. Rev.*, **7**, 423 (1978).

94. S. W. Homans, *Biochemistry*, **29**, 9110 (1990).

95. G. A. Jeffrey, in Ref. 86, p. 20.

96. I. Tvaroska and T. Kozar, *Chem. Papers*, **41**, 501 (1987).

97. J. W. Brady, *Curr. Opin. Struct. Biol.*, **1**, 711 (1991).

98. K. Bock, *Pure Appl. Chem.*, **55**, 605 (1983).

99. D. A. Cumming and J. P. Carver, *Biochemistry*, **26**, 6664 (1987).

100. D. Y. Gagnaire, R. Nardin, F. R. Taravel, and M. R. Vignon, *Nouv. J. Chim.*, **1**, 423 (1977).

101. G. K. Hamer, F. Balza, N. Cyr, and A. S. Perlin, *Can. J. Chem.*, **56**, 3109 (1978).

102. P. Dais and A. S. Perlin, *Adv. Carbohydr. Chem. Biochem.*, **45**, 125 (1987).

103. T.-C. Wu, P. G. Goekjian, and Y. Kishi, *J. Org. Chem.*, **52**, 4819 (1987).

104. H. Paulsen, *Angew. Chem. Int. Ed. Engl.*, **21**, 155 (1982).

105. A. F. Bochkov and G. E. Zaikov, *Chemistry of the O-glycosidic Bond: Formation and Cleavage*, Pergamon Press, Oxford, UK, 1979.

106. A. Lipták, P. Fügedi, and Z. Szurmai, *Handbook of Oligosaccharides*, Vol. 1, CRC Press, Boca Raton, Fla., 1990.

107. A. Lipták, Z. Szurmai, P. Fügedi, and J. Harangi, *Handbook of Oligosaccharides*, Vol. 2, CRC Press, Boca Raton, Fla., 1991.

108. A. Lipták. Z. Szurmai, P. Fügedi, and J. Harangi, *Handbook of Oligosaccharides*, Vol. 3, CRC Press, Boca Raton, Fla., 1991.

109. T. W. Green, and P. G. M. Wuts, *Protective Groups in Organic Synthesis*, John Wiley & Sons, Inc., New York, 1991.

110. R. L. Whistler and J. M. BeMiller, eds., *Methods in Carbohydrate Chemistry*, Vols. 1–8, Academic Press, New York, 1962–1980.

111. P. Fügedi, A. Lipták, P. Nánási, and J. Szejtli, *Carbohydr. Res.*, **104**, 55 (1982) and references therein.

112. P. J. Garegg and H. Hultberg, *Carbohydr. Res.*, **93**, c10 (1981).

113. A. Lipták and P. Fügedi, *Angew. Chem. Int. Ed. Engl.*, **22**, 255 (1983).

114. R. Johansson and B. Samuelsson, *J. Chem. Soc., Perkin Trans. 1*, 2371 (1984).

115. A. Lipták, P. Fügedi, and P. Nánási, *Carbohydr. Res.*, **51**, c19 (1976).

116. R. U. Lemieux and H. Driguez, *J. Am. Chem. Soc.*, **97**, 4069 (1975).

117. S. Oscarsson and M. Szönyi, *J. Carbohydr. Chem.*, **8**, 663 (1989).

118. S. David and S. Hanessian, *Tetrahedron*, **41**, 643 (1985).

119. P. J. Garegg, T. Iversen and S. Oscarson, *Carbohydr. Res.*, **50**, c12 (1976).

120. J. Stanek, Jr., *Topics Curr. Chem.*, **154**, 209 (1990).

121. A. H. Haines, *Adv. Carbohydr. Chem. Biochem.*, **33**, 11 (1976).

122. A. H. Haines, *Adv. Carbohydr. Chem. Biochem.*, **39**, 13 (1981).

123. K. Igarashi, *Adv. Carbohydr. Chem. Biochem.*, **34**, 243 (1977).

124. R. R. Schmidt, *Angew. Chem. Int. Ed. Engl.*, **25**, 212 (1986).

125. T. Mukaiyama, Y. Murai, and S. Shoda, *Chem. Lett.*, 431 (1981).

126. P. Fügedi, P. J. Garegg, H. Lönn, and T. Norberg, *Glycoconjugate J.*, **4**, 97 (1987).

127. K. C. Nicolaou, R. E. Dolle, and D. P. Papahatjis, *J. Am. Chem. Soc.*, **106**, 4189 (1984).

128. B. Fraser-Reid, U. E. Udodong, Z. F. Wu, H. Ottoson, J. R. Merritt, C. S. Rao, C. Roberts, and R. Madsen, *Synlett.*, 927 (1992).

129. R. L. Halcomb and S. J. Danishefsky, *J. Am. Chem. Soc.*, **111**, 6661 (1989).

130. J. Banoub, P. Boullanger, and D. Lafont, *Chem. Rev.*, **92**, 1167 (1992).

131. H. Kunz, *Angew. Chem. Int. Ed. Engl.*, **26**, 294 (1987).

132. R. R. Schmidt, *Pure Appl. Chem.*, **61**, 1257 (1989).

133. H. Paulsen, *Angew. Chem. Int. Ed. Engl.*, **29**, 823 (1990).

134. J. Gigg and R. Gigg, *Topics Curr. Chem.*, **154**, 77 (1990).

135. K.-H. Jung and R. R. Schmidt, *Curr. Opin. Struct. Biol.*, **1**, 721 (1991).

136. K. C. Nicolaou, *Chemtracts-Org. Chem.*, **4**, 181 (1991).

137. P. Sinaÿ, *Pure Appl. Chem.*, **63**, 519 (1991).

138. Y. Matsuzaki, Y. Ito, Y. Nakahara, and T. Ogawa, *Tetrahedron Lett.*, **34**, 1061 (1993).

139. J. M. Frechét and C. Schuerch, *J. Am. Chem. Soc.*, **94**, 604 (1972).

140. S. P. Douglas, D. M. Whitfield, and J. J. Krepinsky, *J. Am. Chem. Soc.*, **113**, 5095 (1991).

141. S. J. Danishefsky, K. F. McKlure, J. T. Randolph, and R. B. Rugerri, *Science*, **260**, 1307 (1993).

142. A. Akiyama, M. Bednarski, M.-J. Kim, E. S. Simon, H. Waldmann, and G. M. Whitesides, *Chemtech.*, 627 (1988).

143. C.-H. Wong, *Science*, **244**, 1145 (1989).

144. E. J. Toone, E. S. Simon, M. D. Bednarski, and G. M. Whitesides, *Tetrahedron*, **45**, 5365 (1989).

145. D. G. Drueckhammer, W. J. Hennen, R. L. Pederson, C. F. Barbas, C. M. Gautheron, T. Krach, and C.-H. Wong, *Synthesis*, 499 (1991).

146. S. David, C. Augé, and C. Gautheron, *Adv. Carbohydr. Chem. Biochem.*, **49**, 175 (1991).

147. M. D. Bednarski and E. S. Simon, eds., *Enzymes in Carbohydrate Synthesis*, ACS Symposium Series, **466**, American Chemical Society, Washington, D.C., 1991.

148. C.-H. Wong in Ref. 147, p. 23.

149. Y. Ichikawa, G. C. Look, and C.-H. Wong, *Anal. Biochem.*, **202**, 215 (1992).

150. J. C. Paulson and K. J. Colley, *J. Biol. Chem.*, **264**, 17615 (1989).

151. J. E. Heidlas, K. W. Williams, and G. M. Whitesides, *Acc. Chem. Res.*, **25**, 307 (1992).

152. O. Hindsgaul, K. J. Kaur, U. B. Gokhale, G. Srivastava, G. Alton, and M. Palcic in Ref. 147, p. 38.

153. K. G. I. Nilsson, *Trends Biotecnol.*, **6**, 256 (1988).

154. K. G. I. Nilsson in Ref. 147, p. 51.

155. G. L. Cote and B. Y. Tao, *Glycoconjugate J.*, **7**, 145 (1990).

156. M. L. Sinnott, *Chem. Rev.*, **90**, 1171 (1990).

157. Y. Ito and J. C. Paulson, *J. Am. Chem. Soc.*, **115**, 1603 (1993).

158. T. Suami, *Topics Curr. Chem.*, **154**, 257 (1990).

159. T. Suami and S. Ogawa, *Adv. Carbohydr. Chem. Biochem.*, **48**, 21 (1990).

160. M. H. D. Postema, *Tetrahedron*, **48**, 8545 (1992).

161. H. Paulsen and K. Todt, *Adv. Carbohydr. Chem. Biochem.*, **23**, 115 (1968).

162. H. Yamamoto and S. Inokawa, *Adv. Carbohydr. chem. Biochem.*, **42**, 135 (1984).

163. M. Blanc-Muesser, L. Vigne, H. Driguez, J. Lehmann, J. Steck, and K. Urbahns, *Carbohydr. Res.*, **224**, 59 (1992).

164. T. Tsuchiya, *Adv. Carbohydr. Chem. Biochem.*, **48**, 91 (1990).

165. *Specialist Periodical Reports, Carbohydrate Chemistry*, Royal Society of Chemistry, Cambridge, UK.

166. S. Hanessian, *Total Synthesis of Natural Products—The Chiron Approach*, Pergamon Press, Oxford, UK, 1983.

167. Y. Kishi, *Pure Appl. Chem.*, **61**, 313 (1989).

168. D. Uemura, K. Ueda, Y. Hirata, H. Naoki, and T. Iwashita, *Tetrahedron Lett.*, **22**, 2781 (1981).

169. J. K. Cha, W. J. Christ, J. M. Finan, H. Fujioka, Y. Kishi, L. L. Klein, S. S. Ko, J. Leder, W. W. McWhorter Jr., K.-P. Pfaff, M. Yonaga, D. Uemura, and Y. Hirata, *J. Am. Chem. Soc.*, **104**, 7369 (1982).

170. H. Nagase and H. Karaki, *J. Pharmacol. Exp. Ther.*, **242**, 1120 (1987).

171. E. Habermann, *Toxicon.*, **27**, 1171 (1989).

172. L. Lauffer, S. Stengelin, L. Béress, and F. Hucho, *Biochim. Biophys. Acta.*, **818**, 55 (1985).

173. H. Ozaki and co-workers, *Jpn. J. Pharmacol.*, **33**, 1155 (1983).

174. R. W. Armstrong, J. M. Beau, S. H. Cheon, W. J. Christ, H. Fujioka, W.-H. Ham, L. D. Hawkins, H. Jin, S. H. Kang, Y. Kishi, M. J. Martinelli, W. W. McWhorter Jr., M. Mizuno, M. Nakata, A. E. Stutz, F. X. Talamas, M. Taniguchi, J. A. Tino, K. Ueda, J. Uenishi, J. B. White, and M. Yonaga, *J. Am. Chem. Soc.*, **111**, 7530 (1989).

175. M. Isobe, Y. Ichikawa, D.-L. Bai, H. Masaki, and T. Goto, *Tetrahedron*, **43**, 4767 (1987).

176. C. Bialojan and A. Takai, *Biochem. J.*, **256**, 283 (1988).

177. S. J. Danishefsky, D. M. Armistead, F. E. Wincott, H. G. Selnick, and R. Hungate, *J. Am. Chem. Soc.*, **109**, 8117 (1987).

178. M. I. Horowitz and W. Pigman, *The Glycoconjugates*, Vols. 1–4, Academic Press, New York, 1977–1982.

179. I. M. Morrison in Ref. 11, p. 196.

180. J. R. Thomas, R. A. Dwek, and T. W. Rademacher, *Biochemistry*, **29**, 5413 (1990).

181. C. M. Stults, C. C. Sweeley, and B. A. Macher, *Meth. Enzymol.*, **179**, 167 (1989).

182. S. Hakomori, *Ann. Rev. Biochem.*, **50**, 733 (1981).

183. T. Feizi, *Nature*, **314**, 53 (1985).

184. T. Feizi and R. A. Childs, *Trends Biochem. Sci.*, 24 (1985).

185. I. Eggens, B. Fenderson, T. Toyokuni, B. Dean, M. Stroud, and S. Hakomori, *J. Biol. Chem.*, **264**, 9476 (1989).

186. S. Hakomori, *Adv. Cancer Res.*, **52**, 257 (1989).

187. K.-A. Karlsson, *Ann. Rev. Biochem.*, **58**, 309 (1989).

188. S. Hakomori, *J. Biol. Chem.*, **265**, 18713 (1990).

189. A. Olivera and S. Spiegel, *Glycoconjugate J.*, **9**, 110 (1992).

190. E. G. Bremmer, J. Schlessinger, and S. Hakomori, *J. Biol. Chem.*, **261**, 2434 (1986).

191. H. Nojiri, M. Stroud, and S. Hakomori, *J. Biol. Chem.*, **266**, 4531 (1991).

192. Y. A. Hannun and R. M. Bell, *Science*, **243**, 500 (1989).

193. Y. Igarashi, K. Kitamura, T. Toyokuni, B. Dean, B. Fenderson, T. Ogawa, and S. Hakomori, *J. Biol. Chem.*, **265**, 5385 (1990).

194. G. Schwarzmann and K. Sandhoff, *Biochemistry*, **29**, 10865 (1990).

195. R. A. Dwek, *Glycoconjugate J.*, **9**, 109 (1992).

196. A. C. Cuello, *Adv. Pharmacol.*, **21**, 1 (1990).

197. D. B. Jack, *Drug News Prosp.*, **3**, 292 (1990).

198. D. G. Stein, *Acta Neurobiol. Exp.*, **50**, 405 (1990).

199. A. Guidotti, H. Manev, M. Favaron, G. Brooker, and E. Costa, *Adv. Exp. Med. Biol.*, **268**, 135 (1990).

200. F. M. Vaccarino, *Psychopharmacol. Bull.*, **24**, 403 (1988).

201. H. Manev, M. Favaron, S. Vicini, A. Guidotti, and E. Costa, *Pharmacology*, **252**, 419 (1990).

202. G. Gutfeld, *Prevention*, **43**, 16 (1991).

203. G. Rotondo, G. Maniero, and G. Toffano, *Aviat. Space Environ. Med.*, **61**, 162 (1990).

204. F. A. Rodden, H. Wiegandt, and B. L. Bauer, *J. Neurosurg.*, **74**, 606 (1991).

205. R. W. Ledeen, G. Wu, M. S. Cannella, Oderfeld, B. Nowak, and A. C. Cuello, *Acta Neurobiol. Exp.*, **50**, 439 (1990).

206. S. Braune, *Drugs Aging*, **1**, 57 (1991).

207. W. G. Bradley, *Muscle Nerve*, **13**, 833 (1990).

208. P. O. Behan and B. A. G. Haniffah, *Br. Med. J.*, **305**, 1309 (1992).

209. C. Tal, T. Dishon, and J. Gross, *Br. J. Cancer.*, **18**, 111 (1964).

210. C. Haglund, P. J. Roberts, P. Kuusela, T. M. Scheinin, O. Mäkelä, and H. Jalanko, *Br. J. Cancer.*, **53**, 197 (1986).

211. G. Ritter and P. O. Livingston, *Semin. Cancer Biol.*, **2**, 401 (1991).

212. B. M. Longenecker, M. Reddish, R. Koganty, G. D. MacLean, *Ann. N. Y. Acad. Sci.*, **690**, 276 (1993).

213. P. Hersey, *Cancer Treat. Res.*, **54**, 137 (1991).

214. P. O. Livingston, *Cancer Weekly*, **1**, 17 (1993).

215. H. Yuasa, D.-A. Scheinberg, and A.-N. Houghton, *Tissue Antigens*, **36**, 47 (1990).

216. P. M. Gullino, M. Ziche, and G. Alessandri, *Cancer Metastasis Rev.*, **9**, 239 (1990).

217. L. Kjellen and U. Lindahl, *Ann. Rev. Biochem.*, **60**, 443 (1991).

218. M. Höök, L. Kjellèn, S. Johansson, and J. Robinson, *Ann. Rev. Biochem.*, **53**, 847 (1984).

219. V. C. Hascall in V. Ginsburg and P. Robbins, eds., *Biology of Carbohydrates*, Vol. 1, John Wiley & Sons, Inc., New York, 1981, p. 1.

220. H. E. Conrad, *Ann. N. Y. Acad. Sci.*, **556**, 18 (1989).

221. D. A. Lane and U. Lindahl, eds., *Heparin, Chemical and Biological Properties*, *Clinical Applications*, CRC Press, Inc., Boca Raton, Fla., 1989.

222. B. Casu, *Adv. Carbohydr. Chem. Biochem.*, **43**, 51 (1985).

223. J. Harenberg, *Semin. Throm. Hemostasis*, **16**, 12 (1990).

224. E. Holmer in Ref. 221, p. 575.

225. C. E. Donayre, K. Ouriel, R. Y. Rhee, and C. K. Shortell, *J. Vascular Surgery*, **15**, 675 (1982).

226. F. A. Ofosu and T. W. Barrowcliffe in J. Hirsh, ed., *Antithrombic Therapy, Bailliere's Clinical Haematology*, Vol. 3, Bailliere Tindall, London, 1991, p. 505.

227. F. R. Rosendaal, M. T. Nurmohamed, H. R. Buller, E. Dekker, J. P. Vandenbrouche, and E. Briet, *Thromb. Haemost.*, **65**, 927, (1991).

228. P. Hartle, P. Brucke, E. Dienstl, and H. Vinazzer, *Thromb. Res.*, **57**, 577 (1990).

229. A. Leizorovicz, H. Picolet, J. C. Peyrieux, and J. P. Borssel, *Br. J. Surg.*, **78**, 412 (1991).

230. J. Leclerc, W. Geerts, L. Desjardins, F. Jobin, F. Delorme, and J. Bourgouin, *Thromb. Haemost.*, **65**, 753, (1991).

231. M. N. Levine, J. Hirsh, M. Gent, A. G. Turpie, J. Leclerc, P. J. Powers, and R. M. Jay, *Ann. Intern. Med.*, **114**, 545 (1991).

232. P. F. Leyvraz, F. Bachman, J. Hoek, H. R. Bueller, M. Postel, M. Samama, and M. D. Vandenbroek, *Br. Med. J.*, **303**, 543 (1991).

233. J. Heit, C. Kessler, E. Mammen, H. Kwaan, J. Neemah, V. Cabanas, A. Trowbridge, and B. Davidson, *Blood*, **79**, (1992).

234. M.-C. Bourin and U. Lindahl, *Biochem. J.*, **289**, 313 (1993).

235. L. Thunberg, G. Bäckström, and U. Lindahl, *Carbohydr. Res.*, **100**, 393 (1982).

236. J. Choay, J. C. Lormeau, M. Petitou, P. Sinaÿ, and J. Fareed, *Ann. N. Y. Acad. Sci.*, **370**, 644 (1981).

237. P. Sinaÿ, J.-C. Jacquinet, M. Petitou, P. Duchaussoy, I. Lederman, J. Choay, and G. Torri, *Carbohydr. Res.*, **132**, C5 (1984).

238. M. Petitou and C. A. A. van Boeckel, *Progr. Chem. Org. Natural Products*, **60**, 143 (1992).

239. C. A. A. van Boeckel, P. D. J. Grootenhuis, and C. A. G. Haasnoot, *Trends Pharm. Sci.*, **12**, 241 (1991).

240. C. A. A. van Boeckel, T. Beetz, and S. F. van Aelst, *Tetrahedron Lett.*, **29**, 803 (1988).

241. P. D. J. Grootenhuis and C. A. A. A. van Boeckel, *J. Am. Chem. Soc.*, **113**, 2743 (1991).

242. J. Basten, G. Jaurand, B. Olde-Hanter, P. Duchuassoy, M. Petitou, and C. A. A. van Boeckel, *Bioorg. Med. Chem. Lett.*, **2**, 905 (1992).

243. J. Choay, *Ann. N. Y. Acad. Sci.*, **556**, 61 (1989).

244. W. H. Brugess and T. Maciag, *Ann. Rev. Biochem.*, **58**, 575 (1989).

245. J. Pawes and N. Pavak, *Thromb. Haemost.*, **65**, 829 (1991).

246. M. Sobel, P. M. McNeil, P. L. Carlson, J. C. Kermode, B. Adelman, R. Conroy, and D. Marques, *J. Clin. Invest.*, **87**, 1787 (1991).

247. L. B. Jacques, *Trends Pharmacol. Sci.*, **3**, 289 (1982).

248. D. J. Tyrell, M. Isihara, N. Rao, A. Horne, M. C. Kiefer, G. B. Stauber, L. H. Lam, and R. J. Stack, *J. Biol. Chem.*, **268**, 4684 (1993).

249. R. J. Klauser, R. W. Raake, E. Meinetsberger, and P. Zeiller, *J. Pharm. Exp. Therapeut.*, **259**, 8 (1991).

250. A. Sugidachi, F. Asai, and H. Koike, *Thrombosis Res.*, **69**, 71 (1993).

251. F. L. Lugemwa and J. D. Esko, *J. Biol. Chem.*, **266**, 6674, (1991).

252. F. Bellamy, D. Horton, J. Millet, F. Picart, S. Samreth, and J. B. Chazan, *J. Med. Chem.*, **36**, 898 (1993).

253. V. Barberousse, F. Bellamy, J. Millet, P. Renaut, and S. Samreth, paper presented at the Seventh European Carbohydrate Symposium, Cracow, Poland, August 22–27, 1993.

254. J. C. Paulson, *Trends Biochem. Sci.*, **14**, 272 (1989).

255. R. Kornfeld and S. Kornfeld, *Ann. Rev. Biochem.*, **54**, 631 (1985).

256. C.-R. Torres and G. W. Hart, *J. Biol. Chem.*, **259**, 3308 (1984).

257. N. Jentoft, *Trends Biochem. Sci.*, **15**, 291 (1990).

258. T. W. Rademacher, R. B. Parekh, and R. A. Dwek, *Ann. Rev. Biochem.*, **57**, 785 (1988).

259. K. Yamaguchi, K. Akai, G. Kawanishi, M. Ueda, S. Masuda, and R. Sasaki, *J. Biol. Chem.*, **266**, 20434 (1991).

260. A. J. Wittwer, S. C. Howard, L. S. Carr, N. K. Harakas, J. Feder, R. B. Parekh, P. M. Rudd, R. A. Dwek, and T. W. Rademacher, *Biochemistry*, **28**, 7662 (1989).

261. J. F. Fisher, A. W. Harrison, G. L. Bundy, K. F. Wilkinson, B. D. Rusht, and M. J. Ruwart, *J. Am. Chem. Soc.*, **34**, 3140 (1991).

262. P. Knight, *Biotechnology*, **7**, 35 (1989).

263. G. Legler, *Adv. Carbohydr. Chem. Biochem.*, **48**, 319 (1990).

264. D. D. Schmidt, W. Frommer, B. Junge, L. Müller, W. Wingender, E. Truscheit, and D. Schäfer, *Naturwissenschaften*, **64**, 535 (1977).

265. E. Truscheit, W. Frommer, B. Junge, L. Müller, D. D. Schmidt, and W. Wingender, *Angew. Chem. Int. Ed. Engl.*, **20**, 744 (1981).

266. E. Truscheit, I. Hillebrand, B. Junge, L. Müller, W. Puls, and D. Schmidt, *Progr. Clin. Biochem. Med.*, **7**, 17 (1988).

267. S. P. Clissold and C. Edwards, *Drugs*, **35**, 214 (1988).

268. S. Ogawa and Y. Shibata, *J. Chem. Soc. Chem. Commun.*, 605 (1988).

269. M. Hayashida, N. Sakairi, H. Kuzuhara, and M. Yajima, *Carbohydr. Res.*, **194**, 233 (1989).

270. S. Ogawa, Y. Shibata, Y. Kosuge, K. Yasuda, T. Mizukoshi, and C. Uchida, *J. Chem. Soc. Chem. Commun.*, 1387 (1990).

271. Y. Shibata, Y. Kosuge, T. Mizukoshi, and S. Ogawa, *Carbohydr. Res.*, **228**, 377 (1992).

272. Y. Yoshikuni, *Trends Glycosci. Glycotech.*, **3**, 184 (1991).

273. N. Ishida, K. Kumagai, T. Niida, T. Tsuruoka, and H. Yumato, *J. Antibiot.*, **20**, 66 (1967).

274. B. Winchester and G. W. J. Fleet, *Glycobiology*, **2**, 199 (1992).

275. U. Fuhrmann, E. Bause, and H. Ploegh, *Biochim. Biophys. Acta*, **825**, 95 (1985).

276. A. D. Elbein, *Ann. Rev. Biochem.*, **56**, 497 (1987).

277. W. McDowell and R. T. Schwarz, *Biochimie*, **70**, 1535 (1988).

278. G. K. Ostrander, N. K. Scribner, and L. R. Rohrschneider, *Cancer Res.*, **48**, 1091 (1988).

279. M. J. Humphries, K. Matsumoto, S. L. White, R. J. Molyneux, and K. Olden, *Cancer Res.*, **48**, 1410 (1988).

280. R. A. Gruters, J. J. Neefjes, M. Tersmette, R. E. Y. de Goede, A. Tulp, H. G. Huisman, F. Miedema, and H. L. Ploegh, *Nature*, **330**, 74 (1987).

281. B. D. Walker, M. Kowalski, W. C. Goh, K. Kozarsky, M. Krieger, C. Rosen, L. Rohrschneider, W. A. Hasseltine, and J. Sodroski, *Proc. Natl. Acad. Sci. U. S. A.*, **84**, 8120 (1987).

282. A. Karpas, G. W. J. Fleet, R. A. Dwek, S. Petursson, S. K. Namgoong, N. G. Ramsden, G. S. Jacob, and T. W. Rademacher, *Proc. Natl. Acad. Sci. U. S. A.*, **85**, 9229 (1988).

283. P. S. Sunkara, D. L. Taylor, M. S. Kang, T. L. Bowlin, P. S. Liu, A. S. Tyms, and A. Sjoerdsma, *Lancet*, 1206 (1989).

284. A. Takatsuki, K. Arima, and G. Tamura, *J. Antibiot.*, **24**, 215 (1971).

285. O. Hindsgaul, K. J. Kaur, G. Srivastava, M. Blaszczyk-Thurin, S. C. Crawley, L. D. Heerze, and M. M. Palcic, *J. Biol. Chem.*, **266**, 17858 (1991).

286. M. M. Palcic, L. D. Heerze, O. P. Srivastava, and O. Hindsgaul, *J. Biol. Chem.*, **264**, 17174 (1989).

287. F. M. Unger, *Adv. Carbohydr. Chem. Biochem.*, **38**, 323 (1981).

288. P. H. Ray, C. D. Benedict, and H. Grasmuk, *J. Bacteriol.*, **145**, 1273 (1981).

289. S. M. Hammond, A. Claesson, A. M. Jansson, L.-G. Larsson, B. G. Pring, C. M. Town, and B. Ekström, *Nature*, **327**, 730 (1987).

290. A. Claesson, K. Luthman, K. Gustafsson, and G. Bondesson, *Biochem. Biophys. Res. Commun.*, **143**, 1063 (1987).

291. F. O. Andersson, B. Classon, and B. Samuelsson, *J. Org. Chem.*, **55**, 4699 (1990).

292. J. W. Hadden, *Trends Pharm. Sci.*, **14**, 169 (1993).

293. V. Ruszala-Mallon, Y.-I. Lin, F. E. Durr, and B. S. Wang, *Int. J. Immunopharmac.*, **10**, 497 (1988).

294. J. P. Devlin and K. D. Hargrave, *Tetrahedron*, **45**, 4327 (1989).

295. A. S. Fauci, S. A. Rosenberg, S. A. Sherwin, C. A. Dinarello, D. L. Longo, and H. C. Lane, *Ann. Intern. Med.*, **106**, 421 (1987).

296. P. Dukor, L. Tarcsay, and G. Baschang, *Ann. Rep. Med. Chem.*, **14**, 146 (1979).

297. Ref. 3, p. 27.

298. M. Heidelberger and O. T. Avery, *J. Exp. Med.*, **38**, 73 (1923).

299. J. B. Robbins, *Immunochem.*, **15**, 839 (1978).

300. C. T. Bishop and H. J. Jennings in G. O. Aspinall, ed., *The Polysaccharides*, Vol. 1, Academic Press, New York, 1982, p. 291.

301. H. J. Jennings, *Adv. Carbohydr. Chem. Biochem.*, **41**, 155 (1983).

302. C.-J. Lee, *Molecular Immunol.*, **24**, 1005 (1987).

303. D. R. Bundle, *Top Curr. Chem.*, **154**, 1 (1990).

304. R. Austrian, *J. Infect. Dis.*, **131**, 474 (1975).

305. D. M. Jones, *J. Antimicrob. Chemother.*, **31** (Suppl. B), 93 (1993).

306. C. E. Frasch in A. Mizrahi, ed., *Bacterial Vaccines*, John Wiley-Liss, New York, 1990, p. 123.

307. D. M. Jones, *J. Med. Microbiol.*, **38**, 77 (1993).

308. J. T. Poolman in Ref. 306, p. 57.

309. A. F. M. Verheul, H. Snippe, and J. T. Poolman, *Microbiol. Rev.*, **57**, 34 (1993).

310. M. Santosham, *Vaccine*, **11** (Suppl. 1), S52–S57 (1993).

311. W. F. Goebel and O. T. Avery, *J. Exp. Med.*, **54**, 431 (1931).

312. W. E. Dick Jr. and M. Beurret in J. M. Cruse and R. E. Lewis Jr., eds., *Conjugate Vaccines*, S. Karger Verlag, Basel, Switzerland, 1989, p. 48.

313. S. Nilsson, M. Bengtsson, and T. Norberg, *J. Carbohydr. Chem.*, **11**, 265 (1992).

314. C. C. A. M. Peeters, D. Evenberg, P. Hoogerhout, H. Käyhty, L. Saarinen, C. A. A. van Boeckel, G. A. van der Marel, J. H. van Boom, and J. T. Poolman, *Infect. Immun.*, **60**, 1826 (1992).

315. F. M. Audibert and L. D. Lise, *Trends Pharmacol. Sci.*, **14**, 174 (1993).

316. R. K. Gupta, E. H. Relyveld, E. B. Lindblad, B. Bizzini, S. Ben-Efraim, and C. K. Gupta, *Vaccine*, **11**, 293 (1993).

317. L. F. Woodard in Ref. 306, p. 281.

318. H. S. Warren and L. A. Chedid, *CRC Crit. Rev. Immunol.*, **8**, 83 (1988).

319. F. Ellouz, A. Adam, R. Ciorbaru, and E. Lederer, *Biochem. Biophys. Res. Commun.*, **59**, 1317 (1974).

320. D. E. S. Stewart-Tull, *Ann. Rev. Microbiol.*, **34**, 311 (1980).

321. C. Merser, P. Sinaÿ, and A. Adam, *Biochem. Biophys. Res. Commun.*, **66**, 1316 (1975).

322. P. Lefrancier and E. Lederer, *Pure Appl. Chem.*, **59**, 449 (1987).

323. E. Lederer, *J. Med. Chem.*, **23**, 819 (1980).

324. E. Telzak, S. M. Wolff, C. A. Dinarello, T. Conlon, A. El Kholy, G. M. Bahr, J. P. Choay, A. Morin, and L. Chedid, *J. Infect. Dis.*, **153**, 628 (1986).

325. I. Azuma, *Int. J. Immunopharmacol.*, **14**, 487 (1992).

326. A. Bekierkunst, I. S. Levij, E. Yarkoni, E. Vilkas, A. Adam, and E. Lederer, *J. Bacteriol.*, **100**, 95 (1969).

327. G. Lemiare, J. P. Tenu, and J.-F. Petit, *Medic. Res. Rev.*, **6**, 243 (1986).

328. N. Rastogi and H. L. David, *Biochimie*, **70**, 1101 (1988).

329. F. Numata, H. Ishida, K. Nishimura, I. Sekikawa, and I. Azuma, *J. Carbohydr. Chem.*, **5**, 127 (1986).

330. T. Sakurai, I. Saiki, H. Ishida, K. Takeda, and I. Azuma, *Vaccine*, **7**, 269 (1989).

331. M. B. Goren and K.-S. Jiang, *Chem. Phys. Lipids*, **25**, 209 (1979).

332. H. H. Baer and R. L. Breton, *Carbohydr. Res.*, **209**, 181 (1990).

333. O. Westphal and O. Lüderitz, *Angew. Chem.*, **66**, 407 (1954).

334. L. Anderson and F. M. Unger, eds., *Bacterial Lipopolysaccharides. Structure, Synthesis, and Biological Activities*, ACS Symposium Series, **231**, American Chemical Society, Washington, D.C., 1983.

335. O. Lüderitz, C. Galanos, V. Lehmann, H. Mayer, E. T. Rietschel, and J. Weckesser, *Naturwissenschaften*, **65**, 578 (1978).

336. M. Imoto, S. Kusumoto, T. Shiba, H. Naoki, T. Iwashita, E. T. Rietschel, H.-W. Wollenweber, C. Galanos, and O. Lüderitz, *Tetrahedron Lett.*, **24**, 4017 (1983).

337. M. Imoto, H. Yoshimura, N. Sakaguchi, S. Kusumoto, and T. Shiba, *Tetrahedron Lett.*, **26**, 1545 (1985).

338. M. Nishijima, F. Amano, Y. Akamatsu, K. Akagawa, T. Tokunaga, and C. R. H. Raetz, *Proc. Natl. Acad. Sci. U. S. A.*, **82**, 282 (1985).

339. N. Qureshi, P. Mascagni, E. Ribi, and K. Takayama, *J. Biol. Chem.*, **260**, 5271 (1985).

340. K. Takayama, N. Qureshi, E. Ribi, and J. L. Cantrell, *Rev. Infect. Dis.*, **6**, 439 (1984).

341. J. A. Rudbach, J. L. Cantrell, J. T. Ulrich, and M. S. Mitchell, *Adv. Exp. Med. Biol.*, **256**, 665 (1990).

342. M. Kiso, S. Tanaka, M. Fujita, Y. Fujishima, Y. Ogawa, H. Ishida, and A. Hasegawa, *Carbohydr. Res.*, **162**, 127 (1987).

343. Y. Kumazawa, M. Nakatsuka, H. Takimoto, T. Furuya, T. Nagumo, A. Yamamoto, J. Y. Homma, K. Inada, M. Yoshida, M. Kiso, and A. Hasegawa, *Infect. Immun.*, **56**, 149 (1988).

344. Y. Ogawa, Y. Fujishima, H. Ishida, M. Kiso, and A. Hasegawa, *Carbohydr. Res.*, **197**, 281 (1990).

345. M. Shiozaki, Y. Kobayashi, N. Ishida, M. Arai, T. Hiraoka, M. Nishijima, S. Kuge, T. Otsuka, and Y. Akamatsu, *Carbohydr. Res.*, **222**, 57 (1991).

346. Y. Ogawa, Y. Fujishima, H. Ishida, M. Kiso, and A. Hasegawa, *Carbohydr. Res.*, **220**, 155 (1991).

347. Y. Kumazawa, S. Ikeda, H. Takimoto, C. Nishimura, M. Nakatsuka, J. Y. Homma, A. Yamamoto, M. Kiso, and A. Hasegawa, *Eur. J. Immunol.*, **17**, 663 (1987).

348. Y. Kobayashi, N. Ishida, M. Arai, M. Shiozaki, T. Hiraoka, M. Nishijima, S. Kuge, T. Otsuka, and Y. Akamatsu, *Carbohydr. Res.*, **222**, 83 (1991).

349. A. Hasegawa, E. Seki, Y. Fujishima, K. Kigawa, M. Kiso, H. Ishida, and I. Azuma, *J. Carbohydr. Chem.*, **5**, 371 (1986).

350. R. L. Whistler, A. A. Bushway, P. P. Singh, W. Nakahara, and R. Tokuzen, *Adv. Carbohydr. Chem. Biochem.*, **32**, 235 (1976).

351. H. Furue, *Drugs Today*, **23**, 335 (1987).

352. Y. Y. Maeda and G. Chihara, *Nature*, **229**, 634 (1971).

353. H. Saito, T. Ohki, and T. Sasaki, *Carbohydr. Res.*, **74**, 227 (1979).

354. Y. Y. Maeda, S. T. Watanabe, C. Chihara, and M. Rokutanda, *Cancer Res.*, **48**, 671 (1988).

355. S. Demleitner, J. Kraus, and G. Franz, *Carbohydr. Res.*, **226**, 247 (1992).

356. O. Lockhoff, *Angew. Chem. Int. Ed. Engl.* **30**, 1611 (1991).

357. R. G. Espinet, *Gac. Vet. (B. Aires)*, **13**, 268 (1951).

358. R. Richou, P. Lallouette, and H. Richou, *Rev. Immunol. Ther. Antimicrob.*, **33**, 155 (1969).

359. K. Dalsgaard, *Arch. ges. Virusforsch.*, **44**, 243 (1974).

360. B. Morein, B. Sundquist, S. Höglund, K. Dalsgaard, and A. Osterhaus, *Nature*, **308**, 457 (1984).

361. R. Higuchi, Y. Tokimitsu, and T. Komori, *Phytochemistry*, **27**, 1165 (1988).

362. C. R. Kensil, U. Patel, M. Lennick, D. Marciani, *J. Immunol.*, **146**, 431 (1991).

363. J. M. Goldsmith, J. Huprikar, S. J. Y. Wu, and J. P. Phair, *J. Immunopharmacol.*, **8**, 1 (1986).

364. N. Kojima, and S. Hakomori, *J. Biol. Chem.*, **264**, 20159 (1989).

365. T. Feizi, *Trends Biochem. Sci.*, **15**, 330 (1990).

366. W. M. Watkins, *Adv. Hum. Genet.*, **10**, 1 (1980).

367. F. Yamamoto, H. Clausen, T. White, J. Marken, S. Hakomori, *Nature* **345**, 229 (1990).

368. R. U. Lemieux, in K. J. Laidler, ed., *Frontiers of Chemistry*, Pergamon Press, New York, 1982.

369. E. F. Hounsell, *Chem. Soc. Rev.*, **16**, 161 (1987).

370. W. M. Watkins, *Biochem. Soc. Symp.*, **40**, 125 (1974).

371. Z.-Y. Yan, B. N. N. Rao, and C. A. Bush, *J. Am. Chem. Soc.*, **109**, 763 (1987).

372. W. I. Weis, R. Kahn, R. Fourme, K. Drickamer, and W. A. Hendrickson, *Science*, **254**, 1608 (1991).

373. L. Osborn, *Cell*, **62**, 3 (1990).

374. T. A. Springer, *Nature*, **346**, 425 (1990).

375. L. Lasky, *Cell*, **56**, 1045 (1989).

376. B. K. Brandley, S. J. Sweidler, and P. W. Robbins, *Cell*, **63** (1990)

377. M. J. Pauley, M. L. Phillips, E. Warner, E. Nudleman, A. K. Singhal, S. I. Hakomori, and J. C. Paulsen, *Proc. Natl. Acad. Sci. U. S. A.*, **88**, 6224 (1991).

378. C. Foxall, S. R. Watson, D. Dowberko, C. Fennie, L. A. Lasky, M. Kiso, A. Hasegawa, D. Asa, and B. K. Brandley, *J. Biol. Chem.*, **117**, 895 (1992).

379. Y. Imai, M. S. Singer, C. Fennie, L. A. Lasky, and S. D. Rosen, *J. Cell Biol.*, **113**, 1213 (1991).

380. Y. Imai, D. D. True, M. S. Singer, and S. D. Rosen, *J. Cell Biol.*, **111**, 1225 (1990).

381. A. Aruffo, W. Kolanus, G. Walz, P. Fredman, and B. Seed, *Cell*, **67**, 35 (1991).

382. J. G. Geng, K. L. Moore, A. E. Johnson, and R. P. McEver, *J. Biol. Chem.*, **266**, 33 (1991).

383. J. D. Bleil and P. M. Wassarman, *Proc. Natl. Acad. Sci. U. S. A.*, **87**, 5563 (1990).

384. I. Ofek and N. Sharon, *Curr. Topics Microbiol. Immunol.*, **151**, 91 (1990).

385. R. E. Willoughby, R. H. Yolken, and R. L. Schnaar, *J. Virol.*, **64**, 4830 (1990).

386. T. Imura, Y. Matsushita, S. D. Hoff, T. Yamori, S. Nakamori, M. L. Frazier, G. G. Giacco, K. R. Cleary, and D. M. Ota, *Semin. Cancer Biol.*, **2**, 129 (1991).

387. T. Matsusako, H. Muramatsu, T. Shirahama, T. Muramatu, and Y. Ohi, *Biochem. Biophys. Res. Commun.*, **181**, 1218 (1991).

CHAPTER TWENTY-THREE

Metabolic Considerations in Prodrug Design

L. P. BALANT

Clinical Research Unit,
Psychiatric University Institutions of Geneva
Geneva, Switzerland

E. DOELKER

School of Pharmacy,
University of Geneva, Switzerland

CONTENTS

1 Introduction, 950
  1.1 The pharmacokinetic point of view, 951
  1.2 The pharmaceutical point of view, 952
  1.3 The regulatory point of view, 952
2 Chemical Bond, 953
  2.1 Esters, 954
  2.2 Mannich bases, 956
  2.3 Macromolecular prodrugs, 956
  2.4 Prodrug derivatives of peptides, 958
  2.5 Peptide esters of drugs, 958
  2.6 Amine Prodrugs, 959
  2.7 Lipidic peptides, 959
  2.8 Chemical hydrolysis, 959
3 Gastrointestinal Absorption, 960
  3.1 Improvement of gastrointestinal
    tolerance, 960
  3.2 Increase in systemic availability, 960
  3.3 Sustained release prodrug systems, 962
  3.4 Improvement of taste, 964
  3.5 Diminishing gastrointestinal absorption, 964
4 Parenteral Administration, 964
  4.1 Increased aqueous solubility, 964
  4.2 Improvement in the shelf life of
    parenterals, 965
5 Distribution, 966
  5.1 Tissue targeting, 966

Burger's Medicinal Chemistry and Drug Discovery,
Fifth Edition, Volume 1: Principles and Practice,
Edited by Manfred E. Wolff.
ISBN 0-471-57556-9 © 1995 John Wiley & Sons, Inc.

5.2 Activation at the site of action, 966
5.3 Reversible and irreversible conversion, 967
5.4 The double prodrug concept for drug targeting, 968

6 Transdermal Absorption, 968

7 Ocular Absorption, 969
   7.1 Some typical examples, 969
   7.2 Ocular "pharmacokinetics", 971

8 Pharmacokinetic and Biopharmaceutical Aspects, 971
   8.1 Compartmental approach, 971
   8.2 Clearance approach, 972
   8.3 Study design for kinetic studies in humans, 973
   8.4 Bioavailability assessment, 973
   8.5 Comparison of animal and human data, 974
   8.6 Validity of classical pharmacokinetic concepts for prodrug design, 975

9 Some Considerations for Prodrug Design, 975
   9.1 Rationale of prodrug design, 975
   9.2 Practical considerations, 976

10 Conclusions, 976

1 INTRODUCTION

The term prodrug was first introduced by Albert in 1958 (1) to describe compounds which undergo biotransformation prior to exhibiting their pharmacological effects. Since then, many papers have been published on this subject (2–8). Basically, prodrug design comprises an area of drug research that is concerned with the optimization of drug delivery. This may be "systemic delivery" after oral or topical administration or "delivery to the site of action," independently of the route of administration. The rationale for prodrug design is that a molecule with optimal structural configuration and physicochemical properties for eliciting the desired pharmacological action and the expected therapeutic effect does not necessarily possess the best molecular form and properties for its delivery at the receptor sites. By attachment of a promoiety to the active moiety, a prodrug is formed that is designed to overcome the barrier that hinders the optimal use of the active principle (9). Usually, the use of the term prodrug implies a covalent

link between an "active moiety" and a "carrier moiety," but some authors also use this term to characterize some form of salts of the active principle. In this chapter, only covalently bound moieties will be considered.

Prodrugs also occur in the organism. As an example of an endogenous prodrug, proinsulin is synthesized in the pancreas to be released as its active moiety insulin and an inactive propeptide. To some extent the bioactivation of neurotransmitters could also be termed prodrug design by nature and there are many other examples in the realm of mammalian endogenous compounds. Prodrugs derived from plant sources also exist. As an example, codeine activation to morphine is essential for its analgesic effect (Section 5.2).

Finally, prodrugs were first synthesized before the concept was introduced by Albert. As an example, heroin is to some extent an "accidental" prodrug. As a matter of fact, morphine crosses the blood-brain carrier relatively slowly. Diacetylmorphine (heroin) has a greater lipid solubility, and thus transfers into the brain where hydrolysis converts heroin to morphine. The latter is ultimately responsible for the pharmacological effect (10). This is a good example of a prodrug which has found unintended use outside the field of medicine, although it has also been used to treat chronic pain.

The present chapter concentrates on prodrugs designed by pharmaceutical chemists to overcome pharmaceutical or pharmacokinetic (essentially metabolic) problems encountered with active principles. Although the chapter does not consider the chemical methods used to synthesize prodrugs, the reader more specifically interested in chemical synthesis can find relevant bibliography in references presented in the following paragraphs. The investigations presented in this chapter have been selected, not because they lead to a commercialized drug product, but in order to illustrate the types of problems pharmaceutical chemists have tried to solve, and the metabolic, kinetic or pharmaceutic rationale behind these attempts. Although very little published information is available on pharmacokinetic methods useful in the study of prodrugs and on regulatory requirements needed for prodrug development, the authors have tried to develop some general ideas which might be useful in this regard.

1.1 The Pharmacokinetic Point of View

A prerequisite for the design of safe drugs is knowledge about the various metabolic reactions that xenobiotics and endogenous compounds undergo in the organism. Since pharmacological activity depends on molecular structure, the medicinal chemist is restricted in the choice of functional groups for the design of new drugs. Often he or she encounters a situation where a structure has adequate pharmacological activity, but has an inadequate pharmacokinetic profile (i.e., absorption, distribution, me-

tabolism and excretion). This is because the compounds synthesized by the medicinal chemist are usually screened on the basis of *in vitro* testing and because pharmacology and pharmacokinetic departments in the pharmaceutical industry often do not collaborate at the early stage of drug development. It is only later, when the new compound is tested in animals or in humans that pharmacokinetic disadvantages become obvious. In many cases the compound is discarded, but in some instances pharmaceutics can help solve the problem if drug behavior in the gastrointestinal tract is involved, or if the elimination half life is too short. In the first case, innovative pharmaceutical formulations or new routes of administration can be devised. In the second case, slow release formulations may help overcome the problem.

More difficult is the situation where a drug should be available as a solution but its solubility is too low to allow easy parenteral or ocular administration. In such cases the prodrug approach may be appropriate, as discussed briefly below (Section 4.1). The same applies to the improvement in the half-life of unstable parenterals (Section 4.2). Similarly, gastrointestinal membrane or transdermal passage, as well as hepatic first-pass metabolism, are difficult to change by pharmaceutical approaches, being inherent in the molecular structure of the active moiety. In order to improve the pharmacokinetic properties of a molecule displaying such problems, one must modify its chemical structure. This can be done by the design of a prodrug or by the synthesis of an analogue with improved pharmacokinetic properties. The latter case falls outside the scope of the present review. Accordingly, the following paragraphs will be mainly concerned with prodrugs.

Even if, according to the accepted definition, the couple "prodrug-and-its-active-derivative" should not be considered as the pair "parent-compound-and-metabolite," from a pharmacokinetic point of view the two entities are strictly identical. Accordingly, the equations used for the determination of the kinetics of metabolites (active or nor) are to be used (11–14). The basic equations will be presented below. As for metabolite kinetics, a clear appreciation of the pharmacokinetics of a substance generated *in vivo* is only possible if the fraction of metabolite formed from its precursor is known. In most cases, prodrug design tends to produce substances which are totally bioactivated by one chemical route. This is, however, not necessarily the case, and adequate provision must be made for such deviations from the ideal case when planning and interpreting the results in pharmacokinetic and relative bioavailability investigations.

1.2 The Pharmaceutical Point of View

From a pharmaceutical point of view, prodrugs can be defined as precursors of active principles that can be utilized to modify a variety of both pharmaceutical and biological properties, including, as discussed above, modification of the pharmacokinetics of the drug *in vivo* to improve absorption, distribution, metabolism, and excretion. This may lead to improvement of bioavailability by increased aqueous solubility, increase of drug product stability, enhancement of patient acceptance and compliance by minimizing taste and odor problems, elimination of pain on injection, and decrease of gastrointestinal irritation. It is usually accepted that a prodrug should not possess any relevant pharmacological activity. In this context the term prodrug is used essentially when chemical modifications are deliberately introduced to improve an unsatisfactory situation encountered when the active compounds are administered per se. The classical example is the synthesis in 1899 of aspirin in an attempt to improve therapy with salicylic acid.

This chapter deals essentially with enhancement of gastrointestinal availability of drugs through prodrug administration, but some other aspects of the prodrug concept are also discussed briefly.

1.3 The Regulatory Point of View

Presently there is no clear opinion about the requirements for the development of a prodrug. In general, regulatory agencies are reluctant to register this type of product. Of particular concern is the fact that toxicological studies might not be relevant for human use of the drug because of differences in the rate and/or extent of formation of the active moiety.

This problem was raised by Aungst et al. in 1987 (15) concerning the extrapolation of data from animal models to humans. Discussing the results of their pharmacokinetic studies of nalbuphine prodrugs, a narcotic agonist/antagonist, they stated: "Animal models should be similar to humans in regard to: (i) nalbuphine disposition (bioavailability) after oral dosing; and (ii) prodrug hydrolysis rates." It is evident that due to great interspecies variability in xenobiotic metabolism (well known from a toxicological point of view) this goal is quite difficult to achieve. Accordingly, animal experiments should be analyzed with caution, and confirmatory experiments in humans must be performed. It could even be argued that for some active principles it would be wiser to conduct all experiments in humans. As an example of inter-species differences, it was found (16) that the pivaloyloxyethyl ester of methyldopa was essentially hydrolyzed presystematically to pivalic acid and methyldopa, while the succinimidoetinyl derivative was readily hydrolyzed in the rat, but not in the dog. Similarly, it was found that for dyphylline prodrugs the relative rates of active moiety release were

1.3 to 13 times faster in rabbit plasma than human plasma (17).

Nomenclature is also a subject of confusion, although of much lesser importance than the metabolic aspects discussed in the previous paragraph. As examples of potential confusion, some terms used in Europe will briefly be discussed. A similar confrontation of definitions could also be made for other countries. The nomenclature adopted in 1965 (18) by the European communities presents no problem for prodrugs:

- *Proprietary medicinal product*: Any ready-prepared medicinal product placed on the market under a special name and in a special pack.
- *Medicinal product*: Any substance or combination of substances presented for treating or preventing disease in human beings or animals.
- *Substance*: Any matter irrespective of origin which may be human, animal, vegetable, chemical.

In its Notice on "Studies of Prolonged-Action Forms in Man" dated 1987 (19), the EC introduces the term of "*active principle*" presented in "pharmaceutical forms." This concept may apply to prodrugs, but only indirectly since the substance contained as such in the pharmaceutical form is not exactly the active principle. Similarly, in the Council recommendation of 1987 on Investigation on Bioavailability (20), the terms "*active drug ingredient or therapeutic moiety*" of a drug are used to define the chemical species which should be measured. Finally, in a newer definition of bioavailability, the term "*active substance*" is used (21).

In most situations, the terminology can be adapted to the characterization of the pharmacokinetics of prodrugs. Some authors use the terminology of a "prodrug" being bioactivated to the "drug" or even to the "parent drug," which is a rather misleading nomenclature. In order to avoid confusion with the term "drug product" which is often used to describe the "pharmaceutical form," the term "prodrug" and "active moiety" will generally be used in the present review. There are, however, situations in which great care must be taken to analyze the potential consequences of imprecise definitions of these concepts. Paragraph 8.4. on bioavailability assessment of prodrugs is a good example of such potential problems.

Finally, there is one type of prodrug that may create potential problems at the regulatory level, and it is represented by all prodrugs aiming at a prolongation of the duration of action of an active substance. As an example, it is not totally clear from the available guidelines how a prodrug administered intravenously as a solution with prolonged release properties should be compared to the "drug" given by the same route of administration. In these cases, it is hoped that scientific common sense will prevail over strict adherence to guidelines that were not written with such particular cases in mind.

2 CHEMICAL BOND

Prodrug design and synthesis is an important field of pharmaceutical chemistry. This chapter will, however, be centered around pharmaceutical aspects of prodrugs. From a pharmacokinetic point of view it is important to understand the nature of the chemical bond linking the active moiety to its "carrier moiety," and the nature of the "carrier moiety." Knowledge of the nature of the chemical bond may help to explain the nature of the biotransformation process and its location in specific tissues or cells. The study of the fate in the body of the "carrier" moiety is particularly important from a safety point of view and should be investigated just as thoroughly as the active moiety. Clearly, in some cases, such as the esters of methanol or ethanol, the fate of the released "carrier moiety" is well known, and no extra study is needed during drug development. In other cases, additional pharmacokinetic investigations may be necessary.

A basic requirement for prodrug design is naturally the adequate reconversion of the prodrug to the active moiety *in vivo*. This prodrug-drug conversion may take place before absorption (e.g., in the gastrointestinal system), during absorption (e.g., in the gastrointestinal wall or in the skin), after absorption, or at the specific site of drug action. The prodrug being usually inactive, it is important that the conversion be essentially complete because intact prodrug represents unavailable drug. However, the rate of conversion depends on the specific goal of prodrug design. As two opposite examples, a prodrug designed to overcome low solubility for an intravenous formulation should be converted very rapidly to the active moiety following injection. Conversely, if the objective of the prodrug is to produce a sustained drug action through rate-limiting conversion, the rate of conversion should not be too fast. Depot neuroleptics designed for once a month intramuscular administration are an interesting case. As discussed in Section 3.3, the rate limiting steps is their diffusion from the oily depot to the blood stream, the conversion in plasma to the active moiety being very fast, as for most ester prodrugs.

This clearly indicates that the nature of the bond between the carrier and the active moiety plays a major role in prodrug design and that pharmacokinetic considerations are of uttermost importance in this context. In the following sections, some typical kinds of chemical bonds will be discussed. It is not intended here to present an overview on this subject, but only to give some examples of how chemistry and pharmacokinetics interact in the field of prodrugs.

For a more detailed review of xenobiotic conversion in the body, see chapter six (22), and a review by the late H. Bundgaard (9), who has been so active in this field and whose work inspired parts of this chapter.

In any case, the necessary conversion or activation of prodrugs in the body can take place by a variety of chemical or enzymatic reactions which, as stated before, must be selected in order to achieve optimal conversion site and rate. There are, however, some limitations to this choice since the active moiety must have adequate chemically functional groups for the attachment of the carrier moiety. The most common prodrugs are those requiring a hydrolytic cleavage mediated by enzymatic catalysis, but reductive and oxidative reactions have also been used for the *in vivo* regeneration of the active moiety. Besides usage of the various enzyme systems of the body to carry out the necessary activation of prodrugs, the buffered and relatively constant value of the physiological pH may be useful in triggering the release of a drug from a prodrug. In these cases, the prodrugs are characterized by a high degree of chemical lability at pH 7.4, while preferably exhibiting a higher stability at other pH values.

2.1 Esters

As stated above, the rational design of biologically reversible drug derivatives is based on the ability of the host tissue to regenerate the active moiety. This is frequently accomplished through the mediation of an enzyme system. Enzymes considered important to orally administered prodrugs are found in the gut wall, liver and blood. In addition, enzyme systems present in the gut microflora may be important in metabolizing the prodrug before it reaches the intestinal cells (23). Due to the wide variety of esterases present in the target tissues for oral prodrug-regeneration, it is not surprising that esters are the most numerous prodrugs designed when gastrointestinal absorption is considered. The consequence, however, of this multiplicity of esterases is that prodrug stability or instability must not only be tested in plasma, but also in the presence of gut, liver or brain esterases, as shown for example in a study of a series of prodrug esters, including various acylated acetaminophen and acetylaminobenzoate compounds (24).

By appropriate esterification of molecules containing a hydroxyl or carboxyl groups, it is possible to obtain derivatives with almost any desirable hydro- or lipophilicity as well as *in vivo* lability. Some aliphatic or aromatic esters are not sufficiently labile *in vivo* to ensure an adequate rate and extent of prodrug conversion. For example, simple alkyl or aryl esters of penicillins are not hydrolyzed to the active free penicillin acid *in vivo* and therefore have no therapeutic potential. The reason is to be found in the highly sterically hindered environment about the carboxyl group in the penicillin molecule which makes enzymatic attack very difficult. This shortcoming can be overcome by preparing a double ester type in which the terminal ester grouping is less sterically hindered. The first step in the hydrolysis of such an ester is enzymatic cleavage of the terminal ester bond with formation of a highly unstable hydroxymethyl ester which rapidly dissociates to the acidic drug. This approach has been successfully used in pivampicillin (**1**) to improve the oral bioavail-

ability of ampicillin (Section 3.2.). Other approaches used to overcome this problem are based on the use of carrier moieties which give highly labile esters. For example, glycolamide esters have been synthesized in this context (25).

Chloramphenicol prepared as its palmitate ester is an interesting study example with respect to polymorphism. This ester, synthesized to avoid the bitterness of the active moiety (see below), exists as four polymorphs, three crystalline forms and an amorphous one. Polymorphs A and B have been found in commercial preparations, but only form B leads to satisfactory blood levels. This effect was first attributed to the lower solubility of the "inactive" form A (26), but it was later proved that the higher susceptibility of form B to esterases was, in fact, involved (27).

In some cases, such as that of terbutaline (28), it was observed that improved absorption of the diester ibuterol was accompanied by shorter effect duration and a slightly increased extent of first-pass metabolism. Other prodrugs were thus synthesized in an attempt to improve resistance to first-pass hydrolysis. Preliminary results with bambuterol (**2**), an *N*-isostere of

(2)

ibuterol, displayed improved hydrolytic stability. This might result from the introduction of the nitrogen atom reducing the reactivity of the acyl function, and/or dimethycarbamate being a cholinesterase inhibitor, bambuterol hydrolysis could be partially inhibited because of reversible inhibition of the esterases responsible for its own degradation.

(1)

2.2 Mannich Bases

Mannich base prodrugs are said to enhance the delivery of their parent drugs through the skin because of enhanced water solubility, as well as enhanced lipid solubility. Those more polar prodrugs are also more effective in improving topical delivery than prodrugs that have been designed to incorporate only lipid solubilizing groups into the structure of the parent drug (29). Mannich base prodrugs are regenerated by chemical hydrolysis (Section 2.8) without enzymatic catalysis (30). Various other chemical approaches can be used in order to achieve increased skin permeability by enhancing both water solubility and lipid solubility (31).

2.3 Macromolecular Prodrugs

Proteins (such as antibodies and lipoproteins), liposomes, synthetic polymers or polysaccharides (such as dextran and insulin) are various types of macromolecules used as drug delivery systems. Polymers are used extensively in these systems, including nanoparticles, microcapsules, laminates, matrices and microporous powders. In all these delivery systems, the drug is merely dispersed or incorporated into the system without the formation of a covalent bond between the drug and the polymer. The present chapter will discuss only those polymeric drugs in which an active moiety is covalently bound to a polymeric backbone. As a complement, a recent review of drug–polymer conjugates as a potential for improved chemotherapy is available (32) and contains extensive bibliography. It must also be mentioned that some pharmaceutical chemists have combined a prodrug with another drug delivery system, such as liposomes or polymer conjugates as exemplified for 5-fluoro-2′-deoxyuridine (33).

Although the terms macromolecular prodrug or polymeric prodrug systems are

recent, the interest in the temporary covalent binding of pharmacologically active compounds to macromolecules for sustained release has been recognized for many years as a potential method for controlled drug delivery and has received increasing attention (34).

As discussed below, as early as 1975 Ringsdorf (35) drew attention to the need for tailor-made macromolecular prodrugs with a view to attaching a homing device or directing units, solubilizing units, and using a biostable or biodegradable backbone. Besides monoclonal antibodies used in conjunction with anticancer drugs, other macromolecules, such as polyvinylic or polyacrylic, polysaccharidic, and poly(α-amino acid) backbones, have been mostly used. Theoretically, the main advantage of synthetic polymers over naturally occurring macromolecules is that they can be tailored to meed individual requirements.

As typical examples, one may mention dextran, soluble starch or hydroxyethyl starch-based ester-prodrugs of naproxen (36, 37), or dextran based prodrugs of mitomycin C (38, 39). Other polysaccharides have been tested for their usefulness as transport groups for therapeutic agents, such as starch for acetyl salicylic acid (40, 41), inulin for procainamide (42, 43), agarose for mitomycin (44) or for adriamycin (45), soluble starch for nicotonic acid (46) or for salicylate (47), cellulose for insulin (48), and hydroxypropyl cellulose for estrone and testosterone (49, 50). However, clinical experience with such prodrugs is still too limited for an adequate judgment on this aspect of macromolecular prodrugs.

Many other polymers have been tested as backbones for prodrugs. As examples, one may list poly-L-(glutamic acid) for clonidine controlled release (51), hyaluronic acid for hydrocortisone and derivatives (52–54), or the synthetic polyanionic polymer Pyran for the antitumor, antibacterial and antiviral agent muramyl dipeptide (55). Hyaluronic acid and Pyran are interesting in the sense that they add a new dimension to the macromolecular prodrug approach. Hyaluronic acid is believed to be potentially useful for the control of infection or inflammation in the eye following surgery and to promote wound healing; its use as a prodrug backbone could also transform it into an active ingredient in some indications (55). Similarly, Pyran has an effect on the immune system and it has been postulated that, combined with specific active principles, it could also play an active role in the effects of the drug (55). In these two cases, the prodrug would give rise to two active moieties with possibly complementary therapeutic activities. Other polymers have also been tested as exemplified by fluorouracil derivatives of organosilicon (56) or polyacrylates (57).

Recently, drug-antibody conjugates have become realities in the context of drug transport, drug targeting, and cancer therapy. An aspect of macromolecular prodrug synthesis that seems still to present a technical problem is the development of selective antitumor drug-protein conjugates with a covalent and reversible linkage for stability in biological fluids, together with adequate release at the site of action. As a matter of fact, a major problem is the rapid clearance of such complexes from the blood stream because they are frequently recognized as foreign materials by cells of the recituloendothelial system.

From a theoretical point of view, Ringsdorf (35) proposed a model for macromolecular prodrugs. The backbone must contain three essential units:

- A device for controlling the physicochemical properties of the entire macromolecule, which mainly controls the hydrophilic–lipophilic balance, the electronic charge, and the solubility of the system.
- The active moiety which must be covalently bound to the polymer and must remain attached to it until the macromolecule reaches the desired site of action. The active molecule must be detached from the parent polymer at the site of action, the release taking place by hydrolysis or by specific enzymatic cleavage of the drug–polymer bond. In many cases, the active moiety is attached to the polymer through a spacer molecule which is an amino acid or other simple molecule. The choice of the spacer molecule is of crucial importance for the generation of adequate releasing characteristics.
- The "homing device" which should guide the entire drug polymer conjugates to the target tissue. Presently, antibodies are mainly used for this purpose, but other approaches are possible. For example, since a variety of cell systems are known to possess cell surface lectins with well defined sugar specificity, glucosylated polymers could be of interest as potential cell specific homing devices.

The choice of an active moiety for use in this type of systems is based on three criteria (58):

- Only potent substances can be used because there is a restriction on the amount of drug that can be administered.
- The active moiety must have a functional group by which it can bind with the polymer backbone directly or by means of a spacer molecule.
- The active substance must be sufficiently stable and should not be excreted in its conjugate form until it is released at the desired site.

As can be seen from this list of criteria, macromolecular prodrugs represent a true challenge for the pharmaceutical chemist in particular because very little is known about the behavior of xenobiotic macromolecules in the human body. Not only are the pharmacokinetic properties of such substances not well investigated, but their potential to provoke immunological reactions represents an additional difficulty. Such properties depend not only on the type of polymer, but also on its size. This introduces an additional pharmacokinetic variable. As an example, small peptides tend to be easily taken up by the hepatocytes; larger molecules are filtered by the glomerulus and taken up by the tubular cells where they are catabolyzed; still larger molecules, although filtered, are not taken up in the tubules, whereas moderately large molecules are not filtered at all. As a consequence, it is probable that much more basic research on the kinetics of these compounds is needed before the pharmaceutical chemists can select on scientifically sound bases the most adequate "backbone" molecule.

2.4 Prodrug Derivatives of Peptides

A major obstacle to the application of peptides as clinically useful drugs is their poor delivery characteristics. Most peptides are rapidly metabolized by proteolysis at most routes of administration and they possess short biological half-lives due to rapid metabolism (59, 60). In addition, they are generally non-lipophilic compounds showing poor biomembrane penetration characteristics which lead to poor absorption and low availability at their potential site of action. A possible approach to solve these delivery problems may be derivatization of the bioactive peptide to produce prodrugs or transport forms which possess enhanced physicochemical properties (9). Thus derivatization may, on one hand, protect small peptides against degradation by enzymes present at the mucosal barrier, and, on the other hand, render hydrophilic peptides more lipophilic and hence facilitate their absorption (61). Such an approach has, for example, been

proposed for thyrotropin-releasing hormone (THR) (3), a hypothalamic tripep-

(3)

tide that regulates the synthesis and secretion of thyrotropin from the anterior pituatary gland. THR is a potential drug for the management of neurological disorders. Its clinical use is greatly hampered by its rapid metabolism leading, after parenteral administration, to a half-life of a few minutes. Moreover, its very low lipophilicity limits its ability to penetrate the blood-brain barrier. The prodrug approach has been tested and found potentially useful to improve the pharmacokinetic characteristics of THR (62, 63), in particular in protecting it against cleavage by carboxypeptidase A. The same approach has been used to protect peptides against degradation by another pancreatic proteolytic enzyme, α-chymotrypsin (64).

Another area of considerable interest is the use of the prodrug concept for better kinetic properties of angiotensin converting-enzyme inhibitors (Section 3.2) or fibrinolytic enzymes (65).

2.5 Peptide Esters of Drugs

In the preceding section *prodrugs of peptides* were considered. They should not be confused with *peptide esters of drugs*. In the latter case, one forms α-amino acid or related short-chained aliphatic amino esters, for example, as a useful means of increasing the aqueous solubility of drugs containing a hydroxyl group, e.g., with the aim of developing improved preparations for parenteral administration (66, 67). Ideally, such prodrugs should possess high water solubility at the pH of optimum stability and sufficient stability in aqueous solution to allow long-term storage (>2 years) of ready-to-use solutions, and yet they should be converted quantitatively and rapidly *in vivo* to the active moiety. Considering these desirable properties of the prodrugs, the use of α-amino acids or related esters is not without problems. Although they are generally readily hydrolyzed by plasma enzymes (68, 69), they exhibit poor stability in aqueous solutions as exemplified with esters of metronidazole (69, 70), acyclovir (71), corticosteroids (72, 73), and paracetamol (74, 75). One of the solutions to overcome such problems is the use of adequately selected spacer groups (Section 4.1).

2.6 Amine Prodrugs

The presence of a primary amine group in a drug can affect its physico-chemical and biological properties in different ways (76). For example, drugs containing a primary amine group can undergo intra- or intermolecular aminolysis reactions leading to reactive and/or potentially toxic products. When the primary amine group is present in a molecule with another ionizable functionality, such as a carboxylic acid group, the molecule can display poor aqueous solubility and liposolubility due to the zwitterionic nature of the molecule in the physiological pH range, thereby potentially limiting its dissolution rate and/or its passive permeability. This is exemplified by the fact that after oral administration, the systemic availability of many peptides is low, in part also because of their enzymatic lability (see Section 2.4).

In addition, the terminal free amino acid groups are recognition sites for proteolytic enzymes, such as aminopeptidase and trypsin, present in the gastrointestinal tract lumen, the brush border region and the cytosol of the intestinal mucosa cells. For all these reasons the prodrug approach has been advocated (76, 77) for the improvement of the *in vivo* behavior of active principles containing primary amine groups. However, many attempts to impart "ester characteristics" (see Section 2.1) to amines have met with limited success, and other approaches, such as the synthesis of pro-prodrugs for amide prodrugs, have been described (77). The pro-prodrug, for example, is designed to be stable chemically, and is biologically converted to a prodrug. The latter is then chemically activated to the active amine group containing substance. If the rate of the chemical reaction is sufficiently rapid, the biological reaction will become the rate-determining process in the overall activation. A derivative with these qualities has been said to possess an "enzymatic trigger" (78).

2.7 Lipidic Peptides

The α-amino acids with long hydrocarbon side chains, the so-called lipidic amino acids and their homo-oligomers, the lipidic peptides, represent a class of compounds which combine structure features of lipids with those of amino acids. Several uses of lipidic amino acids and peptides have been proposed. Of particular interest is their potential use as a drug delivery system (79). The lipidic amino acids and peptides could be covalently conjugated to or incorporated into poorly absorbed peptides and drugs, to enhance the passage of the pharmacologically active compounds across biological membranes. Because of their bifunctional nature, the lipidic amino acids and peptides have the capacity to be chemically conjugated to drugs with a wide variety of functional groups. The linkage between drug and lipidic unit may either be biologically stable (i.e., a new drug is formed) or possess biological or chemical instability (i.e., the conjugate is a prodrug). In either case, the resulting conjugates would be expected to possess a high degree of membranelike character which may be sufficient to facilitate their passage across membranes. The long alkyl side chains may also have the additional effect of protecting a labile parent drug from enzymatic attack, thereby enhancing metabolic stability.

2.8 Chemical Hydrolysis

A serious drawback of prodrugs requiring chemical (i.e., non-enzymatic) release of the active moiety is the inherent lability of these compounds, raising some stability-formulation problems at least in cases of solution preparations. Such problems may sometimes be overcome by using an approach involving pro-prodrugs or double prodrugs, where use is made of an enzymatic release mechanism prior to the spontaneous chemical reaction. It is then possible to overcome the stability problem of the prodrug.

3 GASTROINTESTINAL ABSORPTION

3.1 Improvement of Gastrointestinal Tolerance

The gastrointestinal lesions produced by the acid nonsteroidal anti-inflammatory agents are generally believed to be caused by two different mechanisms: a direct contact mechanism on the gastrointestinal mucosa and a generalized systemic action appearing after absorption, which can be demonstrated following intravenous administration. The relative importance of these mechanisms may vary from drug to drug. Acetylsalicylic acid and most newer NSAI drugs are carboxylic acids. Tempor-

ary masking of the acid function has been proposed as a promising means of reducing gastrointestinal toxicity resulting from the direct mucosal contact mechanism (80–87).

Several attempts have been made to develop bioreversible derivatives of acetylsalicylic acid (88–90). They nicely illustrate the potential problems encountered with prodrugs of prodrugs. A major difficulty in the design of aspirin prodrugs is the great enzymatic lability of the acetyl ester in aspirin derivatized at its carboxyl group. Therefore, a prerequisite for any true aspirin prodrug is for the masking group to cleave faster than the acetyl ester moiety. Otherwise, the derivatives will behave as prodrugs of salicylic acid.

3.2 Increase in Systemic Availability

Until recently it seemed that the most fruitful area of derivatization was the improvement of passive drug absorption through epithelial tissue. Accordingly, an immense number of prodrugs featuring the addition of a hydrophobic group have been prepared in order to improve their gastrointestinal absorption. As early as 1975, Sinkula and Yalkowsky (23) listed a number of drug derivatives utilized as modifiers of absorption, and the list has steadily increased since then. It is in the field of poorly absorbed penicillin derivatives that the most successful prodrugs have been produced and commercialized. They include esters (Section 2.1) of ampicillin (e.g., bacampicillin, pivampicillin (1) and talampicillin), mecillinam (pivmecillinam), and carbenicillin (carfecillin: for urinary tract infections only). As an example, plasma concentrations of ampicillin attained with these esters are systematically higher than those seen after oral ampicillin (91–93). Other antibiotics for which the prodrug approach has been tested include cefotiam (94) and erythromycin (95).

Furosemide (4) provides an interesting

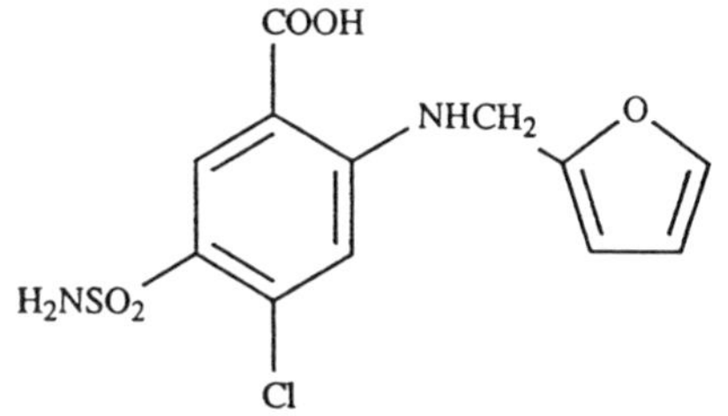

(4)

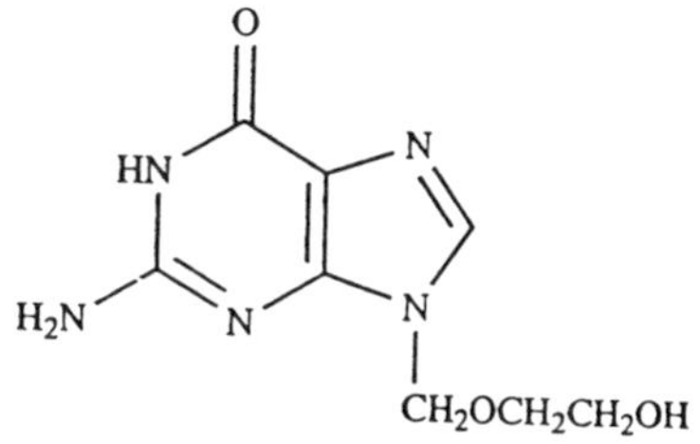

(5)

example of the use of the prodrug concept for a substance presenting biopharmaceutical problems (96). This loop diuretic is only incompletely (40–60%) absorbed following oral administration (97) and, in addition, the systemic availability (both in terms of rate and extent of absorption) shows a high degree of inter- and intra-individual variability. Various possible reasons for the relatively low systemic availability have been considered, such as acid-catalyzed degradation of the drug in the stomach, first-pass metabolism in the gut wall or in the liver, dissolution limited absorption, and site-limited or site-specific absorption, but no firm explanation has been given (97). Data obtained in rats appear to indicate that the occurrence of a site-related absorption from the stomach or the upper part of the gastrointestinal tract is the most likely explanation for the incomplete and variable absorption pattern of furosemide. On the other hand, because of the short duration of the diuretic effect of conventional furosemide tablets or capsules, various slow-release preparations have been developed. A disadvantage of these preparations is, however, that their relative bioavailability is reduced to about 50% as compared to conventional tablets. This is why the prodrug approach has been proposed (96) in order to improve the oral bioavailability characteristics of furosemide drug products.

Acyclovir (5) is an interesting example of prodrug or pro-prodrug design for improved gastrointestinal absorption. This antiherpetic agent exhibits great selectivity in its antiviral action through conversion to the active triphosphorylated species by virtue of virus-specific thymidine kinase (98, 99). Acyclovir is thus a prodrug exhibiting site-specific conversion to the active moiety (Section 5.2). It suffers, however, from poor oral systemic availability, only 15–20% of an oral dose being absorbed in humans (100, 101). This can most likely be ascribed to the poor water-solubility and low lipophilicity of the compound. Deoxyacyclovir (desiclovir) has been found to be a promising prodrug with improved oral absorption (102). The compound is 18 times more water-soluble than acyclovir and is also more lipophilic. Its systemic availability is about 75% in healthy humans (103). From a formal point of view, deoxyacyclovir is a pro-prodrug (Section 5.4).

Prodrug design has also been successful in the area of angiotensin, converting enzyme inhibitors, enalapril (6) being an ester prodrug of enaprilate (7) which has not

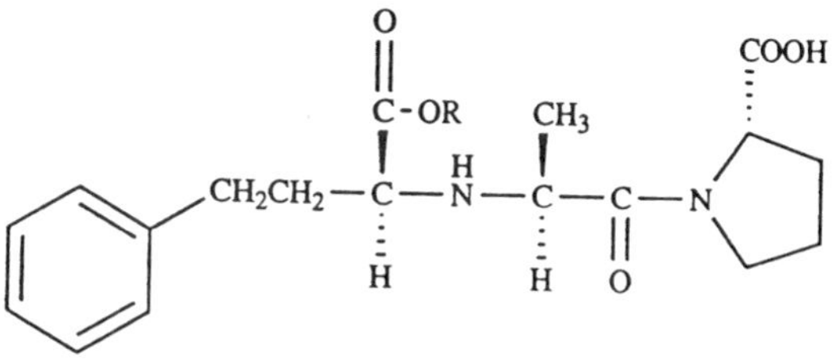

(6)   R = C$_2$H$_5$
(7)   R = H

been developed as such, but immediately commercialized as its prodrug. Enalaprilate binds tightly to the angiotensin-converting enzyme, yet is transported with low efficacy by the peptide carrier in the gastrointestinal tract. The prodrug enalapril has a higher apparent affinity for the carrier. This indicates that the reason for good oral absorption of enalapril is that it makes enalaprilate more peptide-like, rather than more nonpolar (104). Dicarboxylic acid ACE inhibitors in development or commercialized based on esterification of the same carboxyl group include perindoprilate, ramiprilate, cilazaprilate and benazeprilate.

Mixed triglycerides formed by coupling of drugs to diglycerides exhibit physicochemical properties (105) and absorption characteristics (106) similar to those of natural triglycerides, resulting in a different pharmacokinetic and/or pharmacodynamic profile compared to that of the unmodified drug. Such an approach has been used in order to improve the oral systemic availability of phenytoin (107).

The concept of bioreversible chemical modification has been proposed in order to diminish the gastrointestinal and/or hepatic first-pass metabolism of drugs with high extraction ratios. This approach has been tried for a number of drugs such as methyldopa (16, 108, 109), dopamine (110), etilefrine (111), L-dopa (112), terbutaline (113), salicylamide (114), 5-fluorouracil (115-117), progesterone (118), β-estradiol (119), naltrexone (120, 121), N-acetylcysteine (122), and peptides (123).

For some prodrugs a specific problem may arise if presystemic isomerization to an inactive compound occurs. As an example, ester prodrugs of the delta-3-isomers of cephalosporins may isomerize to the microbiologically inactive delta-2-isomer (124), and it is important for clinical effectiveness that, after reaching the blood, hydrolysis of the ester group proceeds much more rapidly than isomerization of the delta-3 double bond.

Another interesting approach is the utilization of peptide carrier systems to improve intestinal absorption (125). The concept is based on the relatively recent finding that the intestinal mucosal cell peptide transporter has a relatively broad specificity. These findings suggest that this transporter could serve for polar prodrugs and analogues of di- and tripeptides. The general scheme is that a polar drug with a low membrane permeability is converted into a prodrug that is transported via the peptide carrier into the mucosal cell. This prodrug may still be very polar since what is required is the correct structural features for the peptide carrier-mediated transport. The prodrug can still possess a high aqueous solubility in the gastrointestinal lumen. Following membrane transport, the prodrug is subsequently hydrolyzed by a mucosal cell cytosolic enzyme.

3.3 Sustained Release Prodrug Systems

Sustained release products have become one of the major areas of pharmaceutical research. However, some sustained release preparations available on the market for many years are in fact derived from prodrug design. The prodrug approach has been applied, for example, for depot neuroleptics. Esterification of the active substance with decanoic acid yields a very lipophilic prodrug which is dissolved in Viscoleo. Intramuscular injection creates an oily depot from which the prodrug slowly diffuses into the systemic circulation where esterases quickly release the active substances. These depot forms allow the drug to be given only once or twice a month. It is thus not a slow bioactivation of the therapeutic moiety that is involved in the present case, but a slow release from an oily depot. The synthesis of the esterified precursor of neuroleptics permitted a new approach to long term treatment of schizophrenia. Compounds available in depot prodrug formulations include haloperidol, fluphenazine (**8**), flupenthioxol and zu-clopentixol (126, 127). It must, however, be stressed that prodrug design alone was not sufficient for depot neuroleptics. A specific solvent (a vegetable oil) and a specific route of administration (in-tramuscular) had to be combined with the prodrug concept since the release of the active moiety from the decanoate esters (**9**)

(**8**)   R = H

(**9**)   R = C$_9$H$_{19}$CO⁻

is almost instantaneous when the prodrug reaches the systemic circulation. These examples are excellent illustrations of successful prodrugs which have had a major impact on therapy by the modification of pharmacokinetic and biopharmaceutic characteristics of well established agents. Due to the lability of ester bonds in biological fluids, ester prodrugs are usually not designed (with the exceptions mentioned above) for sustained release systems, although such an approach has been tried with zidovudine in an attempt to reduce side effects in the treatment of AIDS (128).

Other slow release systems have been devised on the basis of prodrug design. They rely more specifically on the slow delivery of the active moiety from a prodrug to which it is covalently bound. As an example, a catechol monester of L-dopa has been shown, in rats, to exhibit longer duration of plasma L-dopa concentrations as evaluated from "mean residence time" (129). Similarly, carbamate prodrugs have been used for a dopamine agonist early in

drug development (130). Classically, sustained release systems using polymer matrices rely on release of the drug by either diffusion through the matrix, erosion of the matrix, or a combination of both. The prodrug concept can also be applied for such systems, for example by covalently binding the drug to a biodegradable polymer. This approach has been tested for naltrexone (131) and prazosin (132), but these prodrugs are not intended for oral administration. In these systems, two physicochemical processes may influence drug release. First, drug is released from the backbone polymer by hydrolysis (enzyme and/or acid-base catalyzed). Second, free drug diffuses through the polymer matrix. If the rate of hydrolysis is lower than the rate of diffusion, it will govern the release rate. The fact that this rate limiting process occurs at the boundary between unaffected nonswollen and previously swollen, degraded, or permeated material implies particular pharmaceutical designs (see also Section 2.3).

Another procedure that has been followed is synthesizing a monomer with the active substance, and then polymerizing this new molecule. Chloramphenicol has thus been attached to a methacrylic derivative by an acetal function, and then copolymerized with 2-hydroxyethyl-methacrylate (133). The copolymer can then, in addition, be dispersed into a biocompatible nondegradable polymer, such as Eudragit, playing the role of a polymer matrix (134).

Ion-exchange systems have found many medicinal applications. As a controlled-release system, ion-exchange resins offer the benefit that release of a complexed drug is initiated by an influx of competing ions from the gastrointestinal tract. However, in general, release rates from unmodified resins are too great for adequate control of delivery, and diffusional barriers to delay drug egress are employed in some preparations. Homologous series of *O-n*-acyl propanolol prodrugs have been used to study the influence of physicochemical properties of the drug on its release from resinates (135, 136).

3.4 Improvement of Taste

Although not directly related to the physiological process of absorption, it may happen that oral drugs with a markedly bitter taste may lead to poor compliance if administered as a solution, a syrup or an elixir. The prodrug approach has been used in this context for chloramphenicol, clindamycin or metronidazole (6). 3-Hydroxymorphinan opioid analgesics or antagonists are good examples of the potential of prodrug design because of their low oral bioavailability due to high first-pass metabolism and bitter taste (137). Oral administration is limited for most of these compounds and systemic availability can be substantially improved by sublingual dosing. However, discomfort due to bitter taste is a common complaint from patients administered morphine or similar compounds buccally. Many prodrugs of these analgesics or their antagonists do not taste bitter and may represent an attractive alternative to injections when the oral route is not adequate due to low systemic availability.

3.5 Diminishing Gastrointestinal Absorption

Colon-specific drug delivery has potential in the treatment of a variety of colonic diseases (e.g., colitis, colon cancer, radiation-induced colitis, and irritable bowel syndrom). The overall concept is to deliver an active ingredient as a prodrug having the ability to remain unabsorbed in the upper gastrointestinal tract, and subsequently to release active substance, for example, by the action of bacterial glycosidases in the large intestine. Such an approach has been attempted for steroidal anti-inflammatory drugs, such as dexamethasone (138, 139). This type of prodrug is interesting from a pharmacokinetic point of view since diminished systemic availability must be shown together with an increased local availability as compared to the active moiety administered per se. Thus specific colon delivery (140) and stability in various location of the gastrointestinal tract (141) should be tested. Animal and *in vitro* models for such studies include "conventional," colitic and germfree rats (140, 141), or the guinea pig (142) as used for the study of dexamethasone β-D-glucosides or β-D-glucuronides. *In vitro* models are also used to investigate colonic membrane transfer. They include different intestinal preparations and monolayer cultures. These cell cultures can express a variety of the characteristic morphological, cytochemical and transport features found in the intestinal enterocytes.

4 PARENTERAL ADMINISTRATION

Although it is not common to prepare prodrugs for parenteral administration, some situations may occur in which this might be useful in increasing the amount of active moiety that will reach the systemic circulation.

4.1 Increased Aqueous Solubility

Examples in which increased "pharmaceutical availability" is important include glucocorticoids (such as dexamethasone (**10**) or methylprednisolone) used at high doses for emergency treatment of shock or other life threatening situations. As their water solubility is very low, these drugs are generally administered in the form of water-soluble esters as hemisuccinates and phosphates (**11**) (143–145). A similar approach has been used for allopurinol (146)

(10) R = H

(11) R = $\begin{array}{c} O \\ \| \\ P - ONa \\ | \\ ONa \end{array}$

and acyclovir (147) in order to make them suitable for parental or rectal administration as a solution. However, as simple as parenteral administration may seem compared to oral administration, the situation is often more complicated than expected. As an example, fetindomide is a potential prodrug of mitindomide, an antitumor agent with poor solubility in water and in most pharmaceutically acceptable solvents (148). The prodrug was designed so that mitindomide would be released *in vivo* by the loss of two molecules of phenylalanine and formaldehyde. It was observed that *in vitro* formaldehyde exerts a catalytic effect on fetindomide hydrolysis (148). This study shows that the choice of a spacer group (in this case formaldehyde) is not always without important practical consequences. Another potential problem described for chloramphenicol sodium succinate, is incomplete hydrolysis leading to a "systemic availability" that is less than expected (149, 150).

Spacer groups play an important role for the design of peptide esters with adequate solubility and stability (Section 2.5). Spacer groups are also important for other types of prodrugs designed to increase water solubility. Dextran-linked water-soluble prod-

rug esters of metronidazole (151) are a good example of the importance of the spacer. The antitrichomal activity measured *in vitro* on *Trichomonas vaginalis* seemed to be correlated with the release rate of the active moiety, metronidazole, and with the hydrophobicity of the spacer. Metronidazole ester-prodrugs have also been designed for formulating a parenteral solution to be administered by a single injection instead of repeated infusions. This form should be useful for rapid onset of action in the treatment of anaerobic bacteria (152).

4.2 Improvement in the Shelf Life of Parenterals

For a prodrug, the true utilization time has been defined (153) as the time during which the total concentration of prodrug and drug equals or exceeds 90% of the original prodrug concentration. It has consequently been argued that the storage of active ingredients in solutions as prodrugs might produce advantages (154). If it is assumed that a solution of the parent drug is useful until its concentration decreases to 90% of its initial value ($t_{90\%}$), a prodrug utilization time can be defined as the time during which administration of the prodrug provides a bioavailable dose of drug equal to or better than the parent drug at $t_{90\%}$. Under optimal conditions, $t_{90\%}$ of the prodrug might be rather longer than $t_{90\%}$ for the active moiety stored as such. Caution must, however, be used since this concept is valid only if the prodrug degrades to the active principle and if the given definition is considered valid for the drug product under scrutiny.

A problem arises when a prodrug in solution prematurely converts to the drug via chemical hydrolysis during storage and simultaneously to an inactive product via a degradation pathway similar to that of the parent drug. For example, hydrolysis of ester prodrugs of penicillins may yield the corresponding penicillins, while simultaneously forming inactive β-lactam degradation products.

5 DISTRIBUTION

5.1 Tissue Targeting

An interesting approach of specific drug delivery to the liver has been attempted with glutathione as a dextran conjugate for the potential treatment of hepatic poisoning (155). This prodrug was developed with the aim of overcoming both the poor hepatic uptake of glutathione and its rapid renal degradation into constituent amino acids. Similarly, the cholesterol-lowering agents lovostatin and simvastatin are prodrugs showing a liver-specific uptake and bioactivation following oral administration (156, 157).

Tissue targeting may also be directed at tumors using monoclonal antibodies, as briefly mentioned above. Finally, brain targeting can also be attempted with the prodrug approach as exemplified by estradiol using a redox-based chemical delivery system (158).

It is possible that for such types of drugs, new pharmacokinetic approaches would have to be derived in order to correctly describe their behavior in the body, in particular if one is interested to evaluate the degree of tissue targeting.

5.2 Activation at the Site of Action

Several examples of prodrugs are found in the purine and pyrimidine analogs which substitute for natural nucleotides and inhibit nucleic acid formation. For example, 5-fluorouracil is essentially harmless to mammalian host and tumor cells. Upon administration, the drug is subject to one of two opposing metabolic fates. Inactivation and elimination are accomplished by catabolism

(about 80% of the dose) and by urinary excretion of unchanged drug (about 5–20%). On the other hand, cytotoxicity in host and tumor cells only occurs following anabolism in actively proliferating cells. Due to a marked first-pass metabolism, oral administration leads to highly variable systemic availability and is thus an unsuitable and unreliable mode of therapy. It seems thus possible to improve oral delivery of this drug using the prodrug approach (115, 117). As a matter of fact, 5'-deoxy-5-fluorouridine is a sugar derivative presently in clinical trials for the oral route. It is a pro-prodrug if 5-fluorouracil is considered a prodrug. The pro-prodrug has a half-life of about 10 to 30 minutes in patients and is transformed mostly into 5-fluorouracil. It is possible that the therapeutic index of 5-fluorouracil might be increased by the prodrug approach. It seems that doxifluridine is selectively activated to 5-fluorouracil in sensitive tumor cells as opposed to bone-marrow cells (159). Should this be conclusively demonstrated, it would be an interesting example of increased target organ availability due to prodrug derivatization. The kinetics of 5-fluorouracil and its metabolites are essentially non-linear. Therefore it is extremely difficult to build models that would correctly describe the cascade of non-linear transformations that are observed, starting from drug absorption to its transformation into the active moiety.

The case of the antiherpes agent acyclovir has been discussed previously (Section 3.2). This is also a prodrug with site-specific activation. A similar situation has been exploited in cancer chemotherapy because of the increased secretion of the plasminogen activator urokinase by various tumors and metastases as compared to normal cells. This may be used for the synthesis of urokinase-labile prodrugs of anticancer agents. In this case the transport or promoiety must be carefully selected so that the active moiety is specifically released by urokinase at an appropriate rate.

In addition the chemical properties of the active moiety per se must be such as to affect adequately the susceptibility of the carrier-active substance bond to be cleaved by the enzyme (160), because if chemical properties of the active moiety are such as to render the prodrug resistant to urokinase action, the rate and extent of delivery in the target cell may then be inappropriate for adequate cancer therapy.

Omeprazole (**12**), a potent anti-ulcer

(12)

agent, is an effective inhibitor of gastric acid secretion, as it is an inhibitor of the gastric H^+,K^+-ATPase (unlike acid secretion inhibitors such as cimetidine). The enzyme H^+,K^+-ATPase is responsible for gastric acid production and is located in the secretory membranes of the parietal cells. Omeprazole itself is not an active inhibitor of this enzyme, but is transformed within the acid compartments of the parietal cell into the active inhibitor, close to the enzyme.

Orally administered amines do not cross the blood-brain barrier, but neutral amino acids such as α-methyldopa are transported into the brain by a specific carrier system. α-Methyldopa is subsequently concentrated in neuronal cells where it becomes a substrate in the catecholamine biosynthesis and is transformed into α-methylnoradrenaline (161).

Codeine activation to morphine by demethylation is controlled by the activity of the polymorphic cytochrome CYP2D6 (162). The clinical relevance of this observation derives from the fact that about

10% of Caucasians lack this metabolic pathway. Since poor metabolizers cannot activate this widely used drug, for them codeine is an ineffective analgesic (163). A similar observation has been made for the metabolic activation of hydrocodone to hydromorphone (164).

These substances metabolized within the central nervous system illustrate well one of the difficulties that may be encountered with prodrug kinetics. The prodrug may follow an ADME pattern perfectly well described by its systemic availability, volume of distribution, hepatic and renal clearances, but still have a pharmacological effect of which the dependency on blood kinetics is only indirect. This is particularly true if the drug must diffuse through the blood–brain barrier, and is then metabolized by enzyme systems different from those found in the liver.

5.3 Reversible and Irreversible Conversion

The natural conversion of an inactive stereo-isomer to an active one is another case in which no *a priori* intention existed when the compound was synthesized. Ibuprofen is a good example. From a pharmacokinetic point of view, one may consider that the reversibly formed metabolite represents a compartment for the parent compound, and adequate provision must be taken when analyzing this type of data.

Sulindac (**13**) is an interesting case of reversible metabolism to an active derivative by reduction to a sulfide. It is also metabolized irreversibly to an inactive sulfone (165, 166). *In vitro* anti-inflammatory test systems considered relevant to *in vivo* efficacy and correlations between drug concentration and biological effect ex vivo suggest that sulindac is a prodrug. Re-oxidation of the sulfide to the parent form occurs before elimination, but the sulfide has a long half-life and prolonged duration of action. There is strong evidence that

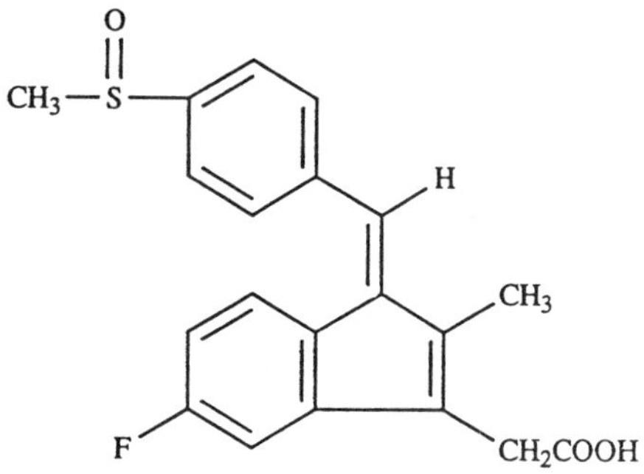

(13)

both liver (167) and gut flora (168) contribute to sulfide generation.

Although many alkylating agents are administered in the active form, cyclophosphamide (**14**) is a prodrug activated in the

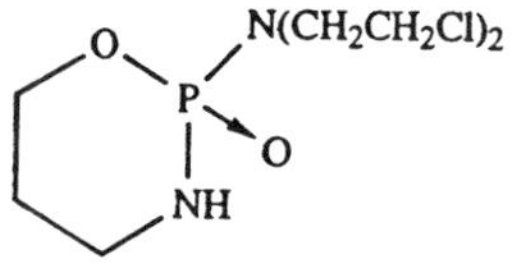

(14)

liver. Initial conversion is to 4-hydroxy-cyclophosphamide, which is in spontaneous equilibrium with its tautomeric form, aldophosphamide. These function as inactive "transport" molecules (169). Subsequent spontaneous elimination of acrolein from aldophosphamide generates the active moiety, phosphoramide mustard.

It is evident that modelling of such compounds is difficult, and that great care must be taken not to generate models that have too many degrees of freedom or that cannot be solved in a univocal way.

5.4 The Double Prodrug Concept for Drug Targeting

Drug targeting may present particular problems that cannot be solved by a "sim-

ple" prodrug design (i.e., one transport plus one active moiety). For example, a prodrug designed to promote site specific delivery through a target-specific cleavage mechanism (e.g., due to a specific enzyme activity) may not be successful if it is not able to reach the target tissue. For optimal activity, both conditions should be fulfilled at the same time. A promising solution to this problem is the double prodrug concept (78). Drug targeting may be achieved by preparing a prodrug form with good properties for transport of a prodrug which exhibits a site-specific bioactivation. Pilocarpine is a good example of an active moiety for which the double prodrug approach may be useful to overcome unfavorable pharmacokinetic properties (Section 7.1). Acyclovir is another example for which the double prodrug design might be useful (Section 3.2).

6 TRANSDERMAL ABSORPTION

Metabolism of drugs by the skin is gaining interest due to its pharmacokinetic, pharmacological, therapeutic, and toxicological implications. The metabolic capacity of the skin can be exploited in the field of dermal drug delivery through the use of prodrugs (170). The prodrug approach in dermal drug delivery must clearly separate optimization of systemic delivery from delivery to the dermis for the treatment of skin diseases. The physicochemical attributes needed to reach these two objectives are clearly different.

The prodrug approach in dermal drug delivery has been the subject of numerous investigations, and various drugs have been considered, such as vidarabine (171), aspirin (172), theophylline (29, 173, 174), purine analogs (175-178), 5-fluorouracil (173–175), indomethacin (179–181), dithranol (182), lonapalene (183), mitomycin C (184, 185), metronidazole (186, 187), 5-fluorocytosine (188), nicorandil (189) or zidovudine (190, 191). These investigations have shown that although the effect is generally relatively small, drug derivatives can be made to permeate the skin more readily than the parent compound. However, guidelines for enabling optimal dermal delivery by use of the prodrug approach are still lacking. Few reports on prodrugs have dealt with derivatives consisting of homologous series (192), and few systematic evaluations of their physico-chemical properties relevant for penetration of human skin have been published (193). Nevertheless, recent reviews of prodrug design for topical application are available (194, 195).

7 OCULAR ABSORPTION

A major challenge in ocular therapeutics is improving the poor local availability of topically applied ophtalmic drugs (196). Such low availability, often less than 10% of the applied dose, is largely due to precorneal processes that rapidly remove drugs from their absorption site and to the existence of the corneal structure designed to restrict passage of xenobiotics (197). During the past two decades, considerable effort has been devoted to prolonging precorneal drug retention through vehicle manipulations (viscosity, polymeric inserts) with the hope of enhancing ocular availability. Thus far, it seems that such methods have only resulted in moderate success. This is probably due to the modest improvement in ocular drug availability as exemplified by viscous solutions and by the lack of patient acceptance as exemplified by inserts (196).

As stated by Lee (196), once the mechanisms have been better understood, by which topically applied drugs are ocularly absorbed, it would become possible to attempt other approaches to enhance corneal drug permeability:

- Modification of the *integrity of the corneal epithelium* transiently by using penetration enhancers.
- Modification of the *physico-chemical characteristics of the drug product* through ion pair formation.
- Modification of the *physico-chemical characteristics of the active principle* by product derivatization.

However, thus far, only the prodrug approach seems to have met objectives allowing commercialization of such ophtalmic products.

7.1 Some Typical Examples

Prodrugs have been designed to improve corneal absorption. This approach has been applied with epinephrine (198–202), terbutaline (203), various prostaglandins (204), phenylephrine (205–207) and pilocarpine (208–213). For some pilocarpine derivatives, the double prodrug approach has been used in order to improve eye irritation and poor water solubility (212, 213) (Section 5.4).

As discussed by Bundgaard (9), the latter drug is an interesting example of the potential of the double prodrug approach since it presents significant delivery problems. Its ocular availability is low, the elimination of the drug from its site of action in the eye is fast, resulting in a short duration of action. Furthermore, undesirable side effects, such as myopia and miosis, frequently occur as a result of non corneal absorption or transient peaks of high drug concentration in the eye. To be useful, a potential prodrug should exhibit a higher lipophilicity than pilocarpine in order to enable efficient penetration through the corneal membrane. It should possess sufficient aqueous solubility and stability for formulation as eyedrops, it should be converted to the active parent drug within the cornea or once the corneal barrier has been passed, and it should lead to controlled release and hence prolonged duration of action of pilocarpine. Various diesters of pilocarpic acid (15) have been

(15)

shown to possess these desirable attributes (208–210). The compounds are highly stable in aqueous solution at pH 5–6, but readily converted quantitatively to pilocarpine (16) in the eye through a sequential

(16)

process involving enzymatic hydrolysis, followed by spontaneous ring-closure of the intermediate pilocarpic acid monoesters. The latter derivatives were originally developed as prodrug forms, but they suffered from limited stability in aqueous solutions. This stability problem was solved by forming double prodrug pilocarpic acid esters. Because of their blocked hydroxyl group, these compounds are unable to undergo cyclization to pilocarpine in the absence of hydrolytic enzymes.

β-Adrenergic receptor blockers are widely used in the treatment of glaucoma. Their therapeutic usefulness may be limited by a relatively high incidence of cardiovascular and respiratory side effects. These arise as a result of absorption of the topically applied drug into the systemic

circulation, and are essentially the same as those seen with oral drug administration. A potentially useful approach for decrease in the systemic absorption of topically applied β-adrenergic receptor blockers, thereby diminishing their adverse effects, may be the development of prodrugs with improved corneal absorption characteristics (214, 215). This approach has been variably successful with nadolol (216, 217), propanolol (218) and timolol (219–226).

Timolol has been particularly well studied in the context of prodrug design for a reduction of systemic availability of ocularly applied xenobiotics (196). This aim is achieved by either reducing the instilled dose in proportion to the degree of enhancement in corneal drug absorption (221, 222), or by increasing the lipophilicity of the prodrugs, thereby impeding their absorption into the systemic circulation without negatively affecting their ocular absorption (215). The basis for the second method is the differential lipophilic characteristics of the membranes responsible for ocular absorption (cornea) and systemic absorption (conjunctival and nasal mucosa). Both methods have been found to be feasible in the case of timolol. It has thus been shown that it is possible to design prodrugs that are poorly absorbed into the blood stream and yet well absorbed into the eye.

An even more extreme situation is found with carbonic anhydrase inhibitors, such as acetazolamide, ethoxyzolamide and methazolamide, which are useful for the treatment of glaucoma. Due to their limited aqueous solubility or unfavorable lipophilicity, they are not active when given topically to the eye and must be given orally or parenterally. Systemic side effects severely limit this mode of therapy and consequently, great activities are presently under way to find a new carbonic anhydrase inhibitor readily penetrating the cornea, or to prepare a prodrug with adequate water solubility and lipophilicity combined with the ability to be reconverted to the parent sulfonamide following a corneal passage (227–229).

As stated by Lee (196), although prodrugs hold great promise in improving ocular delivery, they have yet to be considered routinely for improving the physicochemical characteristics of potent active principles originally developed for systemic use because in many cases such active substances show inacceptable side effects when they reach the systemic circulation after ocular application. The key of a new approach would be to take advantage of the ability of prodrugs to enhance the ocular potency of a drug candidate originally designed for systemic use, but which has been, in a second step, deliberately chosen for ophtalmology because of its lack of systemic potency. This would be an attempt to achieve relative "oculoselectivity." Therefore, the salient feature of the proposed approach is to select a less potent drug candidate so as to minimize the incidence of systemic side effects and then to offset this loss in potency by enhancing its ocular absorption using prodrug design.

7.2 Ocular "Pharmacokinetics"

For all routes of administration, the absorption, distribution and elimination kinetics are important for obtaining the desired therapeutic effect. For drugs expected to act in the eye after ocular absorption pharmacokinetic parameters are difficult to obtain in animals and humans. Accordingly, it has been proposed to rely essentially on pharmacodynamic measurements using a specific biological response after topical administration (230, 231). For example, the apparent absorption and elimination kinetics in the human iris have been estimated for several commonly used drugs, such as tropicamide (232, 233), pilocarpine (233, 234), homatropine (235) and penhylephrine (236, 237), using the

measurement of pupil-response versus time profiles. Such an approach is based on the assumption that the extent of the mydriasis is an instantaneous response to the quantity of the active principle residing in the biophase (iris dilator muscle) so that the time course of the pupil response directly reflects the change of the drug in the iris.

As reported by Chien and Schoenwald (231), for phenylephrine, a drug used during cataract surgery and ophtalmoscopic examination, the situation may be more complicated. As a matter of fact, a rebound miosis can be observed in some patients (238–240). A subsequent instillation of phenylephrine in these patients may then result in a reduction of mydriasis, suggesting that mydriatic tolerance may develop in the iris muscle. As a consequence, mydriasis measurement may not accurately reflect the pharmacokinetic behavior of the active principle. To test this hypothesis the authors (231) compared pharmacokinetic and pharmacodynamic parameters obtained in the rabbit eye after topical instillation of phenylephrine and one of its prodrugs. The study showed indeed that the kinetic parameters of phenylephrine estimated from its mydriasis profile did not accurately reflect the kinetics of drug distribution in the iris. These parameters also varied with the instillation of phenylephrine solution or prodrug suspensions. Such results clearly indicate that the study of the local kinetics of a drug or a prodrug after topical administration is a quite difficult task and that dynamic results obtained in humans should be extrapolated with care if pharmacokinetic deductions are made from this type of data.

8 PHARMACOKINETIC AND BIOPHARMACEUTICAL ASPECTS

8.1 Compartmental Approach

If one considers the one-compartment open body model with first-order input and output, the concentration-time curve for the parent compound can be described by the Bateman function. For most drugs the absorption rate constant is significantly larger than the elimination rate constant. As a consequence, the shape of the concentration versus time curve will, after some time, depend only on the elimination rate constant. During the postabsorptive phase, it will therefore be possible to estimate the "apparent half-life of elimination", which is related to the first-order elimination rate constant. On the other hand, if elimination is faster than absorption, the rate constant obtained from the slope of the terminal portion of the curve will be the absorption rate constant and not the elimination rate constant. This is called a flip-flop situation, and may be observed with drugs that are very rapidly eliminated or with dosage forms that slowly release the drug in an apparent first-order fashion.

The pharmacokinetic properties of metabolites are particularly interesting in this respect. At one time it was generally assumed that metabolite elimination was faster than formation because metabolites were considered to be more easily eliminated from the body than the parent compound. This assumption may be true when polar compounds, such as glucuronides, sulfates, or glycine conjugates, are the major biotransformation products, but need not be true when drugs are, for example, acetylated or hydroxylated. Nevertheless, a basic difference usually exists between parent drug and metabolite kinetics: for metabolites, elimination is normally faster than formation, whereas for most drugs elimination is slower than gastrointestinal absorption. The consequence of this reversal is that metabolites often show flip-flop kinetics.

For prodrugs, the situation is basically different since, in most cases, the chemical bond between transport moiety and active moiety is designed as labile in order to avoid, for example, urinary elimination of

the prodrug which would diminish the amount of active compound available at the site of action. However, this is not an inviolated rule, in particular if prodrug design is used to provide "slow formation" of the active moiety.

The pharmacokinetic models used to describe prodrug and active moiety kinetics are similar to those used for metabolites (11). It may thus often be difficult to calculate individual rate constants, when prodrug transformation occurs both on first-pass and after reaching the systemic circulation. Even if complicated models are of little probable help for data analysis, they may be useful to determine the relative influence of the different rate constants on the behavior of the prodrug and the active moiety. For example, comparing simulated data obtained with different models may allow to evaluate the impact of prodrug excretion on the AUC of the active moiety in function of the prodrug transformation rate.

8.2 Clearance Approach

The clearance concept can successfully be applied to analyze metabolite kinetics in blood (13). It can, by analogy, be used for the kinetics of the active moiety after prodrug administration. As with the compartmental approach, care must be taken when prodrug transformation occurs during first-pass and/or prodrug excretion is important after it reaches the systemic circulation. Here again, some differences with metabolite kinetics occur in function of two different aspects:

1. Metabolite kinetics of classical drugs are not always studied after their administration to man, whereas the active moiety of a prodrug should always be well investigated from a pharmacokinetic point of view. This means that the basic pharmacokinetic parameters (11)

are estimated, and that they can be used to extract relevant information when the prodrug is administered.

2. Metabolite formation is usually the rate limiting step, whereas this is not the case for the active moiety of a prodrug.

It must be stated that these two considerations also hold for the compartmental approach, although in the latter case, the danger of calculating artifactual parameters is more critical.

8.3 Study Design for Kinetic Studies in Humans

Ideally, the kinetics of the prodrug and the active moiety should be studied in the same patients or healthy volunteers. It is not possible to provide generally valid guidelines for study design since, as described in the previous paragraphs, many factors may influence the analysis of the data, and consequently the way in which data must be collected. For example, it is certainly very different to study a prodrug such as bacampicillin with a very fast release of ampicillin after oral administration, or the decanoic ester of haloperidol given intramuscularly as a depot preparation in an oily vehicle.

Planning pharmacokinetic studies for topically applied prodrugs is even more problematic, and it must be realized that even kinetic studies of topically applied drugs (i.e., dermal, ocular, rectal, etc.) are not yet clearly delineated. In particular, analytical sensitivity often represents a major obstacle for the conduct of properly designed pharmacokinetic investigations (11).

Finally, it must be remembered that a prodrug intended for oral administration may show perfectly adequate release performances under normal conditions, but be unreliable (i.e., not transformed to the

active moiety) in liver disease. This may be seen if regeneration occurs enzymatically in the liver. The prodrug should, accordingly, be tested in this pathological situation before marketing.

8.4 Bioavailability Assessment

The concept of bioavailability was developed in the early 1960s, when it was realized that the same active drug ingredient, in the same dose but formulated in different pharmaceutical products, might not have the same therapeutic and/or toxicological properties, even if the two formulations were administered according to the same dosage regimen. Since that time, numerous efforts have been made to establish definitions and guidelines for experimental protocols, specifications of analytical methods, calculations of target pharmacokinetic parameters, statistical procedures and clinical relevance of bioavailability studies. Over the years it has become evident that there are some active substances or particular situations to which the definitions are only partly applicable. A workshop was organized in 1989 to highlight some of those cases and to discuss the applicability of the current definitions, with special reference to their use in drug registration documents. A positon paper presented the conclusions and consensus reached by participants from Academia, the Pharmaceutical Industry and Regulatory Authorities in a number of countries (241).

It was recognized that currently available and recognized definitions of bioavailability based on the concept of "active drug ingredient" or "therapeutic moiety," render it mandatory to consider measurement of pharmacologically active metabolites. In this context two cases were considered:

- An active drug ingredient is metabolized to active metabolites.

● An inactive pro-drug is biotransformed to active metabolites.

In the latter situation, two typical cases were discussed.

Case A: When a prodrug is pharmacologically inactive and is subject to an important pre-systemic transformation to the active moiety, it is correct to administer the active moiety by the intravenous route as the reference pharmaceutical form, as long as its behavior (CL, V_d) is identical for both modes of administration. The ratio of dose-normalized AUCs after oral and intravenous administration is the absolute bioavailability of the active moiety. This is, for example, the procedure that was used with ampicillin and its prodrugs bacampicillin and pivampicillin (93).

Case B: When a prodrug is pharmacologically inactive, subject to important pre-systemic and/or systemic biotransformation to the active moiety, and intended for both oral and intravenous administration, two practical situations may occur: the active moeity is available for parenteral administration or the active moiety cannot be administered intravenously to humans for practical, safety or ethical reasons.

In the first situation, the procedure described in Case A is applicable. In the second situation, it is necessary to administer the parent prodrug compound intravenously as the reference compound. The ratio of the dose-normalized AUCs of the parent prodrug indicates its absolute bioavailability; this parameter is often close to zero and of limited clinical relevance because by definition the prodrug is not active. The absolute bioavailability of the active moiety cannot usually be calculated, unless it is demonstrated that the prodrug is entirely biotransformed to the active moiety, or if the amount of parent drug transformed to other metabolites can be calculated for both routes of administration. Even if the absolute bioavailability of the active metabolite cannot be calculated in the strict sense

of pharmacokinetic definitions, clinically relevant conclusions about the behavior of the active moiety after i.v. and p.o. administration may nevertheless be obtained from analysis of its concentration- time curves. For example, if these curves are similar (AUC, t_{max}, C_{max}) after both modes of administration, it is probable that therapeutic effects will be similar. In addition, if AUCs are equivalent, it can be stated that equivalent amounts of the active moiety are made available to the body following i.v. and p.o. administration (241).

8.5 Comparison of Animal and Human Data

As briefly discussed in Section 1.3, it is often difficult to compare pharmacokinetic data of prodrugs obtained in animals and humans. A basic problem is raised by the fact that the enzymatic systems responsible for the bioactivation of the prodrug are not identical in different mammal species including man. Another, complicating factor is when the metabolism of the active moiety also differs in different animals. As an example, methylprednisolone showed nonlinear kinetics in the rat (145), but linear kinetics in humans (144). It then becomes very difficult to analyse the respective advantages of different prodrugs tested in different animal species. Great care should thus be laid on proper and complete study design to allow for such comparisons, as showed for example with a series of ester prodrugs of valproic acid (242) in dogs, of 5-fluorouracil prodrugs in the intestine of rabbits (243) or diacid angiotensin- converting enzyme inhibitors (244).

In view of these difficulties, it should be envisaged to test prodrug approaches at a very early stage of drug development if particular pharmacokinetic problems of specially interesting active moieties are detected. If liver metabolic activities are involved it might be useful to consider the use of liver microsome preparations as shown for new dopaminergic compounds (245), and to include human microsomes in order to gain some insight into the situation potentially encountered in humans.

8.6 Validity of Classical Pharmacokinetic Concepts for Prodrug Design

As seen in the previous paragraphs, classical pharmacokinetic concepts can be used for the study of prodrugs despite the fact that they have essentially been derived from theoretical considerations related to the situation where the parent compound is the active moiety. As for metabolite kinetics, difficulties arise when the prodrug is not totally biotransformed to the "drug." There is one situation, however, in which it is questionable whether these concepts are fully appropriate, namely drug targeting. For example, if a prodrug is very specifically targeted to one type of cells or to one organ system, it might be necessary to define a "targeting index" to describe distribution of the prodrug and the active moiety, since a concept such as the apparent volume of distribution might only poorly describe the distribution properties of the therapeutic agent. The same restriction may apply to the concepts of systemic availability, systemic clearance and apparent half-life of elimination. This does not mean that classical pharmacokinetic concepts would become invalid because they are robust and well validated, but that some creativity is probably necessary in order to improve the descriptive power of pharmacokinetics in order to allow comparisons of "drug" and prodrug or between prodrugs. Similar considerations also apply to the concepts basic to biopharmaceutic evaluations. If the necessity to define new pharmacokinetic parameters for the description of targeted prodrugs is accepted, it will be of utmost importance to define only concepts that can be quantified based

on experimental data. It is possible that development of imaging techniques such as PET- or NMR-scan will give an impetus to these foreseeable developments in pharmacokinetics.

A problem requiring special attention is the stereoselective *in vivo* activation of prodrugs derived from racemic mixtures, as exemplified by the stereoselective hydrolysis of *O*-acetyl-propanolol (246), for which it was also found that the selectivity of plasma enzyme urase differs from that of liver and intestine enzymes.

9 SOME CONSIDERATIONS FOR PRODRUG DESIGN

9.1 Rationale of Prodrug Design

The design of prodrugs in a rational manner requires, as stated by Bundgaard (9), that the underlying causes which necessitate or stimulate the use of the prodrug approach be defined and clearly understood. It may then be possible to identify the means by which the difficulties can be overcome. The rational design of the prodrug can thus be divided into three basic steps:

- Identification of the drug delivery problem.
- Identification of the physicochemical properties required for optimal delivery.
- Selection of a prodrug derivative that has the proper physicochemical properties and that will be cleaved in the desired biological compartment.

In this context it must be accepted that a very close collaboration is needed between the pharmaceutical chemists active in drug synthesis and those working in the area of xenobiotic metabolism. This is particularly important if more targeted prodrugs are designed in function of enzymes available at the right place, in the right amount and with the right prodrug specificity.

9.2 Practical Considerations

In the rational design and synthesis of prodrugs, several factors should be considered before starting the development of a new compound intended for large-scale production (247):

- The chemical intermediates or modifiers should be available in a high state of purity at reasonable cost.
- Complicated synthetic schemes should be avoided and purification steps should be efficient without markedly increasing production costs. The production should be easy to scale-up from the bench mark to industrial production.
- The prodrug should be stable in bulk form. This is of particular importance for substances like esters, which are likely to be degraded in the presence of even trace amounts of moisture.
- The *in vivo* lability should be efficient to permit release of the active moiety at a rate adequate to ensure its therapeutic activity. Regeneration can be either chemical (pH effects) and/or enzymatic.
- The prodrug and the "carrier moiety" should be nontoxic. Relatively "safe" moieties include amino acids, short to medium length alkyl esters, and some of the macromolecules described previously.
- The pharmacokinetics of the active moiety should be well documented before starting prodrug synthesis, and, at a later stage, prodrug kinetics should be thoroughly investigated in man.
- The biopharmaceutical consequences for prodrug formulations should be carefully evaluated.
- Last but not least, the prodrug should present some clinically relevant advantages over the active principle administered directly. In this context, it must be remembered that modification of one pharmacokinetic property frequently alters other properties of the drug molecule and caution must thus be exercised when embarking on a program of this nature.

10 CONCLUSIONS

Although prodrug design started more than 30 years ago and many reviews have been written on this subject, very little information is available in official guidelines or pharmacokinetic textbooks on the regulatory requirements or data analysis for this type of compounds. This chapter is an attempt to gather and confront available information on the subject.

Some basic problems have, however, been left untouched. For example, the difficulty of extrapolating data from animal to humans encountered during toxicokinetic and toxicologic studies with drugs is amplified with prodrugs since not only metabolism of the active moiety might differ, but also its availability from the prodrug. As a matter of fact, there is presently no published rationale for the conduct of animal and human pharmacokinetic programs during prodrug research and development.

The authors concluded a review on prodrugs (7), quoting the question asked in 1985 (248) by Stella et al.: "Do prodrugs have advantages in clinical practice?" The opinion was the following: "Today, the answer is certainly YES in some particular cases, but for many drugs this aspect of drug design has received no clear and satisfactory solution. The main reason for this situation is that most prodrugs have been synthesized starting from valuable and well-known drugs. As a consequence, the potential advantage of the new chemical entity over its "seasoned precursor" has often been only marginal. It is thus important that in the future, drug design of new chemical entities should incorporate "delivery and/or targeting components" from the earliest stages of research and development. This strategy might help substances too toxic, or unable to show adequate pharmacologic effects in their basal form to go through primary and secondary screening, before successfully reaching human testing. It is evident that if such an approach were to become an integral part of basic drug design and not just a hindsighted attempt to solve problems associated with older drugs, it would also be necessary to develop new biopharmaceutical and pharmacokinetic approaches to tackle the new challenges." After five years, the authors still believe that this is a valid statement.

After this chapter, which focused more on pharmacokinetic aspects than on chemical synthesis, we can conclude that, indeed, additional thinking on new ways to approach the toxicokinetic and the clinical pharmacokinetics of prodrugs and their active moiety is of paramount importance if prodrug design is to remain (or to become?) an important part for research and development of new therapeutic agents. In parallel, great efforts must be undertaken in order to better understand the molecular basis of xenobiotic metabolism. It should then be easier to synthesize compounds which would show the most appropriate physicochemical characteristics.

REFERENCES

1. A. Albert, *Nature*, **182**, 421 (1958).

2. T. Higuchi and V. Stella, *Pro-drugs as Novel Drug Delivery Systems*, American Chemical Society, Washington DC, 1975.

3. E. B. Roche, *American Pharmaceutical Association/Academy of Pharmaceutical Sciences*, Symposium, Washington D.C., 1977.

4. L. Å. Svensson, *Pharm. Weekblad*, **122**, 245 (1985).

5. W. I. Higuchi, A. Kusai, J. L. Fox, N. A. Gordon, N. F. H. Ho, C. C. Hsu, D. C. Baker, and W. M. Shannon, in T. J. Roseman and S. Z. Mansdorf, Eds., *Controlled Release Delivery Systems*, Marcel Dekker, New York, 1983, p. 43.

6. D. G. Waller and C. F. George, *Brit. J. Clin. Pharmacol.*, **28**, 497 (1989).

7. L. P. Balant, E. Doelker, and P. Buri, *Europ. J. Drug. Metab. Pharmacokin.*, **15**, 143 (1990).

8. L. P. Balant, E. Doelker, and P. Buri in A. Rescigno and A. K. Thakur, Eds., *New Trends in Pharmacokinetics*, Plenum Press, New York, 1991, p. 281.

9. H. Bundgard, *Drugs of the Future*, **16**, 443 (1991).

10. C. E. Inturrisi, B. M. Mitchell, K. M. Foley, M. Schulz, S. Seung-Uon, and R. W. Houde, *New Engl. J. Med.* **310**, 1213 (1984).

11. L. P. Balant and J. McAinsh in P. Jenner and B. Testa, Eds., *Concepts in Drug Metabolism*, Marcel Dekker, New York, Part A, 1980, p. 311.

12. M. Gibaldi and D. Perrier, *Pharmacokinetics*, 2nd ed., Marcel Dekker, New York, 1982, 494 pp.

13. M. Rowland and T. N. Tozer, *Clinical Pharmacokinetics*, 2nd ed., Lea & Febiger, Philadelphia, 1989, 546 pp.

14. L. Benet in M. E. Wolff Ed., *Burger's Medicinal Chemistry and Drug Discovery*, 5th ed., John Wiley & Sons, Inc., New York, Vol. 1, Chapter 5.

15. B. J. Aungst, M. J. Myers, E. G. Shami and E. Shefter, *Int. J. Pharm.* **38**, 199 (1987).

16. S. Vickers, C. A. H. Duncan, H. G. Ramjit, M. R. Dobrinska, C. T. Dollery, H. J. Gomez, H. L. Leidy, and W. C. Vincek, *Drug Metab. Dispos.*, **12**, 242 (1984).

17. H. P. Huang and J. W. Ayres, *J. Pharm. Sci.* **77**, 104 (1988).

18. Council directive 65/65/EEC, *Official J. Europ. Comm.*, **22**, 2, (1965).

19. Note for Guidance, *Commission of the European Communities* (III/1962/87) (1987).

20. Council Recommendation 87/176/EEC, *Official J. Europ. Comm.*, L 73 (1987).

21. Note for Guidance, *Commission of the European Communities* (III/54/89) (1991).

22. B. Testa in M. E. Wolff Ed., *Burger's Medicinal Chemistry and Drug Discovery*, 5th Ed., John Wiley & Sons, New York, Chapt. 6.

23. A. A. Sinkula and S. H. Yalkowsky, *J. Pharm. Sci.*, **64**, 181 (1975).

24. H. Seki, T. Kawaguchi and T. Higuchi, *J. Pharm. Sci.*, **77**, 855 (1988).

25. N. M. Nielsen and H. Bundgaard, *J. Pharm. Sci.*, **77**, 285 (1988).

26. A. Aguiar and J. E. Zelmer, *J. Pharm. Sci.*, **58**, 983 (1969).

27. A-. Burger, *Sci. Pharm.*, **45**, 269 (1977).

28. O. A. T. Olsson and L. A. Svensson, *Pharm. Res.*, **1**, 19 (1984).

29. K. B. Sloan and N. Bodor, *Int. J. Pharm.*, **12**, 299 (1982).

30. M. Johansen and H. Bundgaard, *Arch. Pharm. Chem. Sci.*, **9**, 40 (1981).

31. K. G. Siver and K. B. Sloan, *J. Pharm. Sci.*, **79**, 66 (1990).

32. R. Duncan, *Anti-Cancer Drugs*, **3**, 175 (1992).

33. T. Kawaguchi, A. Tsugane, K. Higashide, H. Endoh et al., *J. Pharm. Sci.*, **81**, 508 (1992).

34. M. Vert, *Polyvalent Polymeric Drug Carriers, Critical Reviews in Therapeutic Drug Carrier Systems*, Vol. 2, CRC Press, Boca Raton, Fla., 1986, pp. 292, 327.

35. H. Ringsdorf, *J. Polym. Sci. Polym. Symp.*, **51**, 135 (1975).

36. E. Harboe, C. larsen, M. Johansen, and h. P. Olesen, *Int. J. Pharmac.*, **53**, 157, (1989).

37. C. Larsen, *Int. J. Pharm.*, **51**, 223 (1989).

38. K. Sato, K. Itakura, K. Nishida, Y. Takaura, M. Hashida, and H. Sezaki, *J. Pharm. Sci.*, **78**, 11 (1989).

39. T. Fujita, Y. Yasuda, Y. Takakura, M. Hashida, and H. Sezaki, *J. Contr. Rel.*, **11**, 149 (1990).

40. K. Kratzl and E. Kaufmann, *Monatschr. Chem.*, **92**, 371 (1961).

41. K. Kratzl, E. Kaufmann, O. Kraupp, and H. Stormann, *Monatschr. Chem.*, **92**, 378 (1961).

42. J. P. Remon, R. Duncan, and E. Schacht, *J. Control. Rel.* **1**, 47 (1984).

43. E. Schacht, E. Ruys, J. Vermeersch, and J. P. Remon, *J. Control. Rel.*, **1**, 33 (1984).

44. T. Kojima, M. Hashida, S. Muranishi, and H. Sezaki, *Chem. Pharm. Bull.* **26**, 1818 (1978).

45. T. R. Tritton, G. Yee and L. B. Wingaard, *Fed. Proc.*, **42**, 284 (1983).

46. L. Puglisi, V. Caruso, R. Paoletti, P. Ferruti, and M. C. Tanzi, *Pharmacol. Res. Commun.*, **8**, 379 (1976).

47. A. Havron, B. Z. Weiner, and A. Zilkha, *J. Med. Chem.*, **17**, 770 (1974).

48. M. Singh, P. Vasudevan, T. J. M. Sinha, A. R. Ray, M. M. Misro, and K. Guha, *J. Biomed. Mater. Res.*, **15**, 655 (1981).

49. S. Yolles, J. F. Morton and M. F. Sartori, *J. Polym. Sci. Polym. Chem. Ed.*, **17**, 4111 (1979).

50. S. Yolles, *J. Parenter. Drug Assoc.*, **32**, 188 (1987).

51. X. Li, N. W. Adams, D. B. Bennet, and S. W. Kim, *Proceed. Intern. Symp. Control. Rel. Bioact. Mater.*, **17**, 244 (1990).

52. H. N. Joshi, V. J. Stella, and E. M. Topp, *Proceed. Intern. Symp. Control. Rel. Bioact. Mater.*, **17**, 244 (1990).

53. L. Goei, E. Topp, V. Stella, et al. in R. M. Ottenbrite and E. Chiellini Eds., *Polymers in Medicine – Biomedical and Pharmaceutical Applications*, Technomic Publishing Co., Lancaster, Pa., 1992, p. 85.

54. L. Goei, *Ibid.*, p. 93. Eds., *Polymers in Medicine – Biomedical and Pharmaceutical Applications*, Technomic Publishing Co., Pa. 1992, p. 93.

55. T. M. T. Turk, S. Webb and R. M. Ottenbrite in R. M. Ottenbrite and E. Chiellini Eds., *Polymers in Medicine – Biomedical and Pharmaceutical Applications*, Technomin Publishing Co., Lancaster, Pa., 1992, p. 167.

56. T. Ouchi, K. Hagita, M. Kwashima, T. Inoi, and T. Tashiro, *J. Contr. Rel.*, **8**, 141 (1988).

57. T. Ouchi, H. Fujie, S. Jokei, Y. Sakamoto, H. Chikashita, T. Inoi, and O. Vogl, *J. Polym. Sci., Polym. Chem. Ed.*, **24**, 2059 (1986).

58. N. N. Joshi, *Pharm. Technol.*, **12**, 118 (1988).

59. M. J. Humphreys and P. S. Ringrose, *Drug Metab. Rev.*, **17**, 283 (1986).

60. V. H. L. Lee and A. Yamamoto, *Adv. Drug Deliv. Rev.*, **4**, 171 (1990).

61. H. Bundgaard in S. S. Davis, L. Illum and E. Tomlinson Eds., *Delivery Systems for Peptide Drugs*, Plenum Press, New York, 1986, p. 49.

62. H. Bundgaard and J. Møss, *Pharm. Res.*, **7**, 885 (1990).

63. J. Møss and H. Bundgaard, *Int. J. Pharm.*, **74**, 67 (1991).

64. A. H. Kahns and H. Bundgaard, *Pharm. Res.*, **8**, 1533 (1991).

65. F. Markwardt, *Pharmazie*, **8**, 521 (1989).

66. H. Bundgaard, *Design of Prodrugs: Bioreversible Derivatives for Various Functional Groups and Chemical Entities*, Elsevier, Amsterdam, New York, 1985, pp. 1, 92.

67. E. Jensen and H. Bundgaard, *Internat. J. Pharm.*, **71**, 117 (1991).

68. H. Bundgaard, C. Larsen, and P. Thorbek, *Int. J. Pharm.*, **18**, 67 (1984).

69. H. Bundgaard, C. Larsen, and E. Arnold, *Int. J. Pharm.*, **18**, 79 (1984).

70. M. J. Cho and L. C. Haynes, *J. Pharm. Sci.*, **74**, 883 (1985).

71. L. Colla, E. De Clercq, R. Busson, and H. Vanderhaeghe, *J. Med. Chem.*, **26**, 602 (1983).

72. M. Kawamura, R. Yamamoto, and S. Fujisawa, *J. Pharm. Soc. Jap.*, **91**, 863 (1971).

73. K. Johnson, G. L. Amidon, and S. Pogany, *J. Pharm. Sci.*, **74**, 87 (1985).

74. E. Jensen, E. Falch, and H. Bundgaard, *Acta Pharm. Nord.*, **3**, 31 (1991).

75. I. M. Kovach, I. H. Pitman, and T. Higuchi, *J. Pharm. Sci.*, **70**, 881 (1981).

76. V. H. Naringrekar and V. J. Stella, *J. Pharm. Sci.*, **79**, 138 (1990).

77. K. L. Amsberry, A. E. Gerstenberger, and R. T. Borchardt, *Pharm. Res.*, **8**, 455 (1991).

78. H. Bundgaard, *Adv. Drug Del. Rev.*, **3**, 39 (1989).

79. I. Toth, R. A. Hughes, M. R. Munday, C. A. Murphy, P. Mascagni, and W. A. Gibbons, *Int. J. Pharm.*, **68**, 191 (1991).

80. V. Cioli, S. Putzolu, V. Rossi, and C. Corradino, *Toxicol. Appl. Pharmacol.*, **54**, 332 (1980).

81. H. Bundgaard and N. M. Nielsen, *Int. J. Pharm.*, **43**, 101 (1988).

82. F. J. Perisco, J. F. Pritchard, M. C. Fisher, K. Yorgey, S. Wong, and J. Carson, *J. Pharmacol. Exp. Ther.*, **247**, 889 (1988).

83. L. Gu, J. Dunn and C. Dvorak, *Drug Dev. Ind. Pharm.*, **15**, 209 (1989).

84. A. H. Kahns, P. B. Jensen, N. Mork, and H. Bundgaard, *Acta Pharm. Nord.*, **1**, 327 (1989).

85. M. C. Venuti, J. M. Young, P. J. Maloney, D. Johnson, and K. McGreevy, *Pharm. Res.*, **6**, 867 (1989).

86. V. R. Shanbhag, A. M. Crider, R. D. Gokhale, A. Harpalani, and R. M. Dick, *J. Pharm. Sci.*, **81**, 149 (1992).

87. V. K. Tammara, M. M. Narurkar, A. M. Crider, and M. A. Khan, *Pharm. Res.*, **10**, 1191 (1993).

88. H. Bundgaard, N. M. Nielsen, and A. Buur, *Int. J. Pharm.* **44**, 151 (1988).

89. M. Hundewadt and A. Senning, *J. Pharm. Sci.*, **80**, 545 (1991).

90. H. Tsunematsu, E. Ishida, S. Yoshida, and M. Yamamoto, *Int. J. Pharm.*, **68**, 77 (1991).

91. D. A. Leight, D. S. Reeves, K. Simmons, A. L. Thomas, and P. J. Wilkinson, *Brit. Med. J.*, **1**, 1378 (1976).

92. M. Rozencweig, M. Staquet, and J. Klastersky, *Clin. Pharmacol. Ther.*, **19**, 592 (1976).

93. M. Ehrnebo, S. O. Nilsson, and L. O. Boreus, *J. Pharmacokin. Biopharm.*, **7**, 429 (1979).

94. Y. Yoshimura, N. Hamaguchi, and T. Yashiki, *Int. J. Pharm.*, **38**, 179 (1987).

95. M. Marvola, S. Nykänen, and M. Nokelainen, *Pharm. Res.*, **8**, 1056 (1991).

96. N. Mørk, H. Bundgaard, M. Shalmi, and S. Christensen, *Int. J. Pharm.*, **60**, 163 (1990).

97. M. Hammarlund-Udenaes and L. Z. Benet, *J. Pharmacokinet. Biopharm.*, **17**, 1 (1989).

98. G. B. Elion, P. A. Furman, J. A. Fyfe, P. De Miranda, L. Beauchamp and H. J. Schaeffer, *Proc. Natl. Sci. USA*, **74**, 5716 (1977).

99. H. J. Schaeffer, L. Beauchamp, P. De Miranda, G. B. Elion, D. J. Bauer, and P. Collins, *Nature*, **272**, 583 (1978).

100. R. B. Van Dyke, J. D. Connor, C. Wyborny, M. Hintz and R. E. Keeney, *Amer. J. Med.*, **73(1A)**, 172 (1982).

101. P. De Miranda and M. R. Blum, *J. Antimicrob. Chemother.*, **12 (Suppl. B)**, 29 (1983).

102. T. A. Krenitsky, W. W. Hall, P. De Miranda, L. M. Beauchamp. H. J. Schaeffer, and P. D. Whiteman, *Proc. Natl. Acad. Sci. USA*, **81**, 3209 (1984).

103. B. G. Petty, R. J. Whitley, S. Liao, H. C. Krasny, L. E. Rocco, L. G. Davis, and P. S. Lietman, *Antimicrob. Agents Chemother.*, **31**, 1317 (1987).

104. D. I. Friedman and G. L. Amidon, *Pharm. Res.*, **6**, 1043 (1989).

105. J. R. Deverre, A. Gulik, Y. Letourneux, P. Courvreur, and J. P. Benoit, *Chem. Phys. Lipids*, **59**, 75 (1991).

106. A. Garzon-Aburbeh, J. H. Poupaert, M. Claesen, and P. Dumont, *J. Med. Chem.*, **29**, 687 (1986).

107. G. K. E. Scriba, *Pharm. Res.*, **10**, 1181 (1993).

108. S. Vickers, C. A. Duncan, S. D. White, G. O. Breault, R. B. Royds, P. J. De Schepper, and K. F. Tempero, *Drug Metab. Dispos.*, **6**, 646 (1978).

109. M. R. Dobrinska, W. Kukovetz, E. Beubler, H. L. Leidy, H. J. Gomez, J. Demetriades, and J. A. Bolognese, *J. Pharmacokin. Biopharm.*, **10**, 587 (1982).

110. K. Murata, K. Noda, K. Kohno, and M. Samejima, *J. Pharm., Sci.*, **78**, 812 (1989).

111. J. Wagner, H. Grill, and D. Henschler, *J. Pharm. Sci.*, **69**, 1423 (1980).

112. N. Bodor, K. B. Sloan, T. Higuchi, and K. Sasahara, *J. Med. Chem.*, **20**, 1435 (1977).

113. Y. Hörnblad, E. Ripe, P. O. Magnusson, and K. Tegnes, *Eur. J. Clin. Pharmacol.*, **10**, 9 (1976).

114. M. D'Souza, R. Venkataramanan, A. D'Mello, and P. Niphadkar, *Int. J. Pharm.*, **31**, 165 (1986).

115. A. Buur and H. Bundgaard, *J. Pharm. Sci.*, **75**, 522 (1986).

116. H. Sasaki, T. Takahashi, J. Nakamura, J.

Konishi, and J. Shibasaki, *J. Pharm. Sci.*, **75**, 676 (1986).

117. A. Buur and H. Bundgaard, *Int. J. Pharm.*, **36**, 41 (1987).

118. K. Basu, D. O. Kildsig, and A. K. Mitra, *Int. J. Pharm.*, **47**, 195 (1988).

119. M. A. Hussain, B. J. Aungst and E. Shefter, *Pharm. Res.*, **5**, 44 (1988).

120. M. A. Hussain, C. A. Koval, M. J. Myers, E. G. Shami, and E. Shefter, J. Pharm. Sci., **76**, 356 (1987).

121. M. A. Hussain and E. Shefter, Pharm. Res., **5**, 113 (1988).

122. A. H. Kahns and H. Bundgaard, *Int. J. Pharm.*, **62**, 193 (1990).

123. A. Buur and H. Bundgaard, *Int. J. Pharm.*, **46**, 159 (1988).

124. A. N. Saab, L. W. Ditter, and A. A. Hussain, *J. Pharm. Sci.*, **77**, 906 (1988).

125. J. P. F. Bai, M. Hu, P. Subramanian, H. I. Mosbert, and G. L. Amidon, *J. Pharm. Sci.*, **81**, 113 (1992).

126. A. E. Balant-Gorgia and L. P. Balant, *Clin. Pharmacokin.*, **13**, 65 (1987).

127. A. E. Balant-Gorgia, L. P. Balant, and A. Andreoli, *Clin. Pharmacokin.*, **25**, 217 (1993).

128. T. Kawaguchi, K. Ishikawa, T. Seki, and K. Juni, *J. Pharm. Sci.*, **79**, 531 (1990).

129. M. Ihara, Y. Tsuchiya, Y. Sawasaki, A. Hisaka, H. Takehana, K. Tomimoto, and M. Yano, *J. Pharm. Sci.*, **78**, 525 (1989).

130. I. Den Daas, P. De Boer, P. G. Tepper, H. Rollema, and A. S. Horn, *J. Pharm. Pharmacol.*, **43**, 11 (1991).

131. N. Negishi, D. B. Bennett, C. S. Cho, S. Y. Jeong, W. A. R. Van Heeswijk, J. Feijen, and S. W. Kim, *Pharm. Res.*, **4**, 305 (1987).

132. X. Li, N. W. Adams, D. B. Bennet, J. Feijen, and S. W. Kim, *Pharm. Res.*, **8**, 527 (1991).

133. J. C. Meslard, L. Yean, F. Subira, and J. P. Vairon, *Makromol. Chem.*, **187**, 787 (1986).

134. N. Chafi, J. P. Montheard, and J. M. Vergnaud, *Int. J. Pharm.*, **45**, 229 (1988).

135. W. J. Irwin and K. A. Belaid, *Int. J. Pharm.*, **46**, 57 (1988).

136. W. J. Irwin and K. A. Belaid, *Int. J. Pharm.*, **48**, 159 (1988).

137. M. A. Hussain, B. J. Aungst, C. A. Koval, and E. Shefter, *Pharm. Res.*, **5**, 615 (1988).

138. D. R. Friend, S. Phillips, A. McLeod, and T. N. Tozer, *J. Pharm. Pharmacol.*, **43**, 353 (1991).

139. B. Haeberlin and D. R. Friend, *Proceed. Intern. Symp. Control. Rel. Bioact. Mater.*, **19**, 287 (1992).

140. B. Haeberlin, L. Empey, R. Fedorak, H. Nolen III, and D. R. Friend, *Proceed. Intern. Symp. Control. Rel. Bioact. Mater.*, **20**, 174 (1993).

141. B. Haeberlin, H. Nolen III, W. Rubas, and D. R. Friend, *Proceed. Intern. Symp. Control. Rel. Bioact. Mater.*, **20**, 172 (1993).

142. D. R. Friend, S. Phillips, A. McLeod, and T. N. Tozer, *Proceed. Intern. Symp. Control. Rel. Bioact. Mater.*, **18**, 564 (1991).

143. P. Rohdewald, H. Möllmann, J. Barth, J. Rehder, and H. Derendorf, *Biopharm. Drug Disp.*, **8**, 205 (1987).

144. H. Möllmann, P. Rohdewald, J. Barth, M. Verho, and H. Derendorf, *Biopharm. Drug Disp.*, **10**, 453 (1989).

145. A. N. Kong and W. J. Jusko, *J. Pharm. Sci.*, **80**, 409 (1991).

146. H. Bundgaard, E. Jensen, E. Falch, and S. B. Pedersen, *Int. J. Pharm.*, **64**, 75 (1990).

147. H. Bundgaard, E. Jensen, and E. Falch, *Pharm. Res.*, **8**, 1087 (1991).

148. F. Sendo, C. Riley, and V. J. Stella, *Int. J. Pharm.*, **45**, 207 (1988).

149. M. C. Nahata and D. A. Powell, *Clin. Pharmacol. Ther.*, **30**, 368 (1981).

150. J. T. Burke, W. A. Wargin, R. J. Sheretz, K. L. Sanders, M. R. Blum, and F. A. Sarubbi, *J. Pharmacokin. Biopharm.*, **6**, 601 (1982).

151. H. Vermeersch, J. P. Remon, D. Permentier, and E. Schacht, *Int. J. Pharm.*, **60**, 253 (1990).

152. E. Jensen, H. Bundgaard and E. Falch, *Int. J. Pharm.*, **58**, 143 (1990).

153. M. A. Schwartz and W. L. Hayton, *J. Pharm. Sci.*, **61**, 906 (1972).

154. N. A. T. Nguyen, L. M. Mortada, and R. E. Notari, *Pharm. Res.*, **5**, 288 (1988).

155. Y. Kaneo, T. Tanaka, Y. Fujihara, H. Mori, and S. Iguchi, *Int. J. Pharm.*, **44**, 265 (1988).

156. D. E. Duggan, I. W. Chen, W. F. Bayne, R. A. Halpin, C. A. Duncan, M. S. Schwartz, R. J. Stubbs, and S. Vickers, *Drug Metab. Disp.*, **17**, 166 (1989).

157. S. Vickers, C. A. Duncan, I. W. Chen, A. Rosegay and D. E. Duggan, *Drug Metab. Disp.*, **18**, 138 (1990).

158. M. H. Rahimy, J. W. Simpkins, and N. Bodor, *Pharm. Res.*, **7**, 1061 (1990).

159. L. J. Schaaf, B. R. Dobbs, I. R. Edwards and D. G. Perrier, *Eur. J. Clin. Pharmacol.*, **34**, 439 (1988).

160. P. Kurtzhals and C. Larsen, *Acta Pharm. Nord.*, **1**, 269 (1989).

161. W. M. Pardridge, *Physiol. Rev.*, **63**, 1481 (1983).

162. P. Dayer, J. Desmeules, T. Leemann, and R.

Striberni, *Biochem. Biophys. Res. Commun.*, **152**, 411 (1988).

163. J. Desmeules, P. Dayer, M. P. Gascon, and M. Magistris, *Clin. Pharmacol.*, **45**, 122 (1989).

164. S. V. Otton, M. Schadel, S. W. Cheung, H. L. Kaplan, U. E. Busto, and E. M. Sellers, *Clin. Pharmacol. Ther.*, **54**, 463 (1993).

165. D. E. Duggan, L. E. Hare, C. A. Ditzler, B. W. Lei, and K. C. Kwan, *Clin. Pharmacol. Ther.*, **21**, 326 (1977).

166. D. E. Duggan, K. F. Hooke, R. M. Noll, H. B. Hucker, and C. G. Van Arman, *Biochem. Pharmacol.*, **27**, 2311 (1978).

167. K. Tatsumi, S. Kitimura, and S. Yanada, *Biochem. Biophys. Acta.*, **747**, 86 (1983).

168. H. A. Strong, N. J. Warner, A. G. Renwick, and C. F. George, *Clin. Pharmacol. Ther.*, **38**, 387 (1985).

169. M. Colvin, R. B. Brundrett, M. N. N. Kan, I. Jardine, and C. Feneslau, *Cancer Res.*, **36**, 1121 (1976).

170. S. Y. Chan and A. Li Wan Po, *Int. J. Pharm.*, **55**, 1 (1989).

171. C. D. Yu, J. L. Fox, N. F. H. Ho, and W. I. Higuchi, *J. Pharm. Sci.*, **68**, 1341 (1979).

172. T. Loftsson and N. Bodor, *J. Pharm. Sci.*, **70**, 750 (1981).

173. K. B. Sloan, S. A. M. Koch, and K. G. Silver, *Int. J. Pharm.*, **21**, 251 (1984).

174. K. B. Sloan, E. F. Sherertz, and R. G. McTiernan, *Int. J. Pharm.*, **44**, 87 (1988).

175. B. Møllgaard, A. Hoelgaard, and H. Bundgaard, *Int. J. Pharm.*, **12**, 153 (1982).

176. K. B. Sloan, M. Hashida, J. Alexander, B. Bodor, and T. Higuchi, *J. Pharm. Sci.*, **72**, 372 (1983).

177. K. G. Siver and K. B. Sloan, *Int. J. Pharm.*, **48**, 195 (1988).

178. A. N. Saab, K. B. Sloan, H. D. Beall, and R. Villanueva, *J. Pharm. Sci.*, **79**, 1099 (1990).

179. K. B. Sloan, S. Selk, J. Haslam, L. Caldwell, and R. Shaffer, *J. Pharm. Sci.*, **73**, 1734 (1984).

180. K. B. Sloan, *Adv. Drug Del. Rev.*, **3**, 67 (1989).

181. F. P. Bonina, L. Montenegro, P. De Capraris, E. Bousquet, and S. Tirendi, *Int. J. Pharm.*, **77**, 21 (1991).

182. W. Wiegrebe, A. Retzow, E. Plumier, N. Ersoy, A. Garbe, H. P. Faro, and R. Kunert, *Arzneim. Forsch.*, **34**, 48 (1984).

183. M. F. Powell, A. Magill, A. R. Becker, R. A. Kenley, S. Chen, and G. C. Visor, *Int. J. Pharm.*, **44**, 225 (1988).

184. M. Hashida, E. Mukai, T. Kimura, and H. Sezaki, *J. Pharm. Pharmacol.*, **37**, 542 (1985).

185. E. Mukai, K. Arase, M. Hashida, and H. Sezaki, *Int. J. Pharm.*, **25**, 95 (1985).

186. H. Bundgaard, A. Hoelgaard, and B. Mollgaard, *Int. J. Pharm.*, **15**, 285 (1983).

187. M. Johansen, B. Mollgaard, P. K. Wotton, C. Larsen, and A. Hoelgaard, *Int. J. Pharm.*, **32**, 199 (1986).

188. S. A. M. Koch and K. B. Sloan, *Int. J. Pharm.*, **35**, 243 (1987).

189. K. Sato, K. Sugibayashi, and Y. Morimoto, *Int. J. Pharm.*, **43**, 31 (1988).

190. T. Seki, T. Kawaguchi, and K. Juni, *Pharm. Res.*, **7**, 948 (1990).

191. T. Seki, T. Kawaguchi, K. Juni, K. Sugibayashi, and Y. Morimoto, *Proceed. Intern. Symp. Control. Rel. Bioact. Mater.*, **18**, 513 (1991).

192. R. P. Waranis and K. B. Sloan, *J. Pharm. Sci.*, **77**, 210 (1988).

193. D. A. W. Bucks, *Pharm. Res.*, **1**, 148 (1984).

194. V. H. L. Lee and V. H. K. Li, *Adv. Drug Deliv. Rev.*, **3**, 1 (1989).

195. K. B. Sloan, Ed., *Prodrugs – Topical and Ocular Drug Delivery*, Marcel Dekker, New York, 1992.

196. V. H. L. Lee, *J. Contr. Rel.*, **11**, 79 (1990).

197. V. H. L. Lee and J. R. Robinson, *J. Ocular Pharmacol.*, **2**, 67 (1986).

198. A. I. Mandell, F. Stenz, and A. E. Kitabchi, *Ophthalmology*, **85**, 268 (1978).

199. D. A. McLure, T. Higuchi, and V. J. Stella, Eds., in *Pro-drugs as Novel Drug Delivery Systems*, American Chemical Society, Washington, D.C., 1975, p. 224.

200. M. A. Hussain and J. E. Truelove, *J. Pharm. Sci.*, **65**, 1510 (1976).

201. N. Bodor and G. Visor, *Exp. Eye Res.*, **38**, 621 (1984).

202. N. Bodor and G. Visor, *Pharm. Res.*, **1**, 168 (1984).

203. T. L. Phipps, D. E. Potter, and J. M. Rowland, *J. Ocular Pharmacol.*, **2**, 225 (1986).

204. L. Z. Bito, *Exp. Eye Res.*, **38**, 181 (1984).

205. D. S. Chien and R. D. Schoenwald, *Biopharm. Drug Dispos.*, **7**, 453 (1986).

206. R. D. Schoenwald, J. C. Folk, V. Kumar, and J. G. Pier, *J. Ocular Pharmacol.*, **3**, 333 (1987).

207. R. D. Schoenwald and D. S. Chien, *Biopharm. Drug Dispos.*, **9**, 527 (1988).

208. H. Bundgaard, E. Falch, C. Larsen, G. L. Mosher, and T. J. Mikkelson, *J. Med. Chem.*, **28**, 979 (1985).

209. H. Bundgaard, E. Falch, C. Larsen, and T. J. Mikkelson, *J. Pharm. Sci.*, **75**, 36 (1986).

210. H. Bundgaard, E. Falch, C. Larsen, G. L.

Mosher, and T. J. Mikkelson, *J. Pharm. Sci.*, **75**, 775 (1986).

211. G. L. Mosher, H. Bundgaard, E. Falch, C. Larsen, and T. J. Mikkelson, *Int. J. Pharm.*, **39**, 113 (1987).

212. T. Järvinen, P. Suhonen, S. Auriola, J. Vepsäläinen, A. Urtti, and P. Peura, *Int. J. Pharm.*, **75**, 249 (1991).

213. P. Suhonen, T. Järvinen, P. Rytkönen, P. Peura, and A. Urtti, *Pharm. Res.*, **8**, 1539 (1991).

214. H. Bundgaard, A. Buur, S. C. Chang, and V. H. L. Lee, *Int. J. Pharm.*, **33**, 15 (1986).

215. H. Sasaki, D. S. Chien and V. H. L. Lee, *Pharm. Res.*, **Suppl.**, **5**, S98 (1988).

216. E. Duzman, C. C. Chen, J. Anderson, M. Blumenthal, and H. Twizer, *Arch. Ophthalmol.*, **100**, 1916 (1982).

217. E. Duzman, N. Rosen, and M. Lazar, *Br. J. Ophthalmol.*, **67**, 668 (1983).

218. A. Buur, H. Bundgaard, and V. H. L. Lee, *Int. J. Pharm.*, **42**, 51 (1988).

219. S. C. Chang, H. Bundgaard, A. Buur, and V. H. L. Lee, *Invest. Ophthalmol. Vis. Sci.*, **28**, 487 (1987).

220. H. Bundgaard, A. Buur, S. C. Chang, and V. H. L. Lee, *Int. J. Pharm.*, **46**, 77 (1988).

221. S. C. Chang, H. Bundgaard, A. Buur, and V. H. L. Lee, *Invest. Ophthalmol. Vis. Sci.*, **29**, 626 (1988).

222. S. C. Chang, D. S. Chien, H. Bundgaard, and V. H. L. Lee, *Exp. Eye Res.*, **46**, 59 (1988).

223. D. E. Potter, D. J. Sumate, H. Bundgaard, and V. H. L. Lee, *Curr. Eye Res.*, **7**, 755 (1988).

224. H. Sasaki, D. S. Chien, K. Lew, H. Bundgaard, and V. H. L. Lee, *Invest. Ophthalmol. Vis. Sci.* **Suppl.**, **29**, 83 (1988).

225. H. Sasaki, D. S. Chien, H. Bundgaard, and V. H. L. Lee, *Pharm. Res.*, **Suppl.**, **5**, S164 (1988).

226. D. S. Chien, H. Sasaki, H. Bundgaard, A. Buur, and V. H. L. Lee., *Pharm. Res.*, **8**, 728 (1991).

227. A. Bar-Ilan, N. I. Pessah, and T. H. Maren, *J. Ocular Pharmacol.*, **2**, 109 (1986).

228. J. D. Larsen, H. Bundgaard, and V. H. L. Lee, *Int. J. Pharm.*, **47**, 103 (1988).

229. J. D. Larsen, and H. Bundgaard, *Int. J. Pharm.*, **51**, 27 (1989).

230. D. M. Maurice and S. Mishima, in M. L. Sears Ed., *Pharmacology of the Eye*, Springer-Verlag, New York, 1984, p. 19.

231. D. S. Chien and R. D. Schoenwald, *Pharm. Res.*, **7**, 476 (1990).

232. V. F. Smolen and R. D. Schoenwald, *J. Pharm. Sci.*, **63**, 1582 (1974).

233. S. Yoshida and S. Mishima, *Jap. J. Ophthalmol.*, **19**, 121 (1975).

234. M. Sugaya and S. Nagataki, *Jap. J. Ophthalmol.*, **22**, 127 (1978).

235. H. D. Gambill, K. N. Ogle, and T. P. Kearns, *Arch. Ophthalmol.* **77**, 740 (1967).

236. S. Mishima, *Invest. Ophthalmol. Vis. Sci.*, **21**, 504 (1981).

237. S. Matsumoto, T. Tsuru, M. Araie, and Y. Komuro, *Jap. J. Ophthalmol.*, **26**, 338 (1982).

238. Y. Mitsui and Y. Takagi, *Arch. Ophthalmol.*, **65**, 626 (1961).

239. N. J. Haddad, N. J. Moyer, and F. C. Riley, Jr. *Am. J. Ophthalmol.*, **70**, 729 (1970).

240. S. M. Meyer and F. T. Fraunfelder, *Ophthalmology*, **87**, 1177 (1980).

241. L. P. Balant, L. Z. Benet, H. Blune et al., *Eur. J. Clin. Pharmacol.*, **40**, 123 (1991).

242. S. Hadad, T. B. Vree, E. Van Der Kleijn, and M. Bialer, *J. Pharm. Sci.*, **81**, 1047 (1992).

243. A. Buur, A. Yamamoto, and V. H. L. Lee, *J. Contr. Rel.*, **14**, 43 (1990).

244. J. D. Stuhler, H. Cheng, and B. R. Dorrbecker, *J. Pharm. Sci.*, **81**, 1071 (1992).

245. K. T. Hansen, P. Faarup, and H. Bundgaard, *J. Pharm. Sci.*, **80**, 793 (1991).

246. K. Takahashi, S. Tamagawa, J. Haginaka, H. Yasuda, T. Katagi, and N. Mizuno, *J. Pharm. Sci.*, **81**, 226 (1992).

247. A. A. Sinkula, *Pro-drugs as Novel Drug Delivery Systems*, ACS Symposium Series, *Application of the pro-drug approach to antibiotics*, American Chemical Society, 1975, pp. 116, 153.

248. V. J. Stella, W. N. A. Charman, and V. H. Naringrekar, *Drugs*, **29**, 445 (1985).

CHAPTER TWENTY-FOUR

Natural Products as Leads for New Pharmaceuticals

A. D. BUSS

Department of Natural Products,
Glaxo Research and Development Ltd.,
Middlesex, England

R. D. WAIGH

Department of Pharmaceutical Sciences,
Royal College,
University of Strathclyde,
Glasgow, Scotland

Burger's Medicinal Chemistry and Drug Discovery,
Fifth Edition, Volume 1: Principles and Practice,
Edited by Manfred E. Wolff.
ISBN 0-471-57556-9 © 1995 John Wiley & Sons, Inc.

CONTENTS

1 Introduction, 984
2 Drugs Affecting The Central Nervous
   System, 986
   2.1 Morphine alkaloids, 986
   2.2 Cannabinoids, 988
   2.3 Asperlicin, 989
3 Neuromuscular Blocking Drugs, 992
   3.1 Curare, decamethonium and atracurium, 992
4 Anticancer Drugs, 995
   4.1 Catharanthus (vinca) alkaloids, 995
   4.2 Taxol and taxotere, 996
   4.3 Podophyllotoxin, etoposide and
       teniposide, 1000
5 Antibiotics, 1003
   5.1 The β-lactams, 1003
   5.2 Erythromycin macrolides, 1009
   5.3 Echinocandins, 1012
6 Cardiovascular Drugs, 1014
   6.1 Lovastatin, simvastatin and pravastatin, 1014
   6.2 Teprotide and captopril, 1016
   6.3 Dicoumarol and warfarin, 1016
7 Antiasthma Drugs, 1017
   7.1 Khellin and sodium cromoglycate, 1017

7.2 Ephedrine, isoprenaline and salbutamol, 1020
8 Antiparasitic Drugs,   1021
    8.1 Artemisinin, artemether and arteether, 1021
    8.2 Quinine, chloroquine and mefloquine, 1023
    8.3 Avermectins and milbemycins, 1027
9 Conclusion,   1028

1 INTRODUCTION

The use of plants for medicinal purposes dates back thousands of years and even chimpanzees have been known to chew certain leaves only when suffering from gastro-intestinal disturbances (1). Natural products once served as the only source of medicines for mankind. Well known ancient herbal remedies include opium from which morphine and codeine are obtained, the belladona alkaloids, for example atropine used as a mydriatic, and the digitalis glycosides used as cardiac stimulants. In more recent times microbial metabolites have been utilized in medicine, for example, the naturally occurring fungal metabolites cyclosporin and lovastatin, are major drugs which are produced by fermentation and used for immunosuppression and to treat hypocholesterolemia, respectively. However, natural products have also been utilized as chemical models or templates for the design and synthesis of many other important drugs. Another opium alkaloid, papaverine, was used in this way and led to the synthesis of the open-chain analog, varapamil, which is used to treat cardiovascular disease and hypertension. Aspirin, of which some 25 million kilograms is produced annually, is derived from salicin, a secondary metabolite produced by the willow tree. The plant steroids diosgenin and hecogenin remain key precursors for the synthesis of many modern contraceptive drugs and other useful pharmaceuticals; including betamethasone for the treatment of eczema and psoriasis and beclomethasone for treating asthma. The abundance of plant and microbial secondary

metabolites and their value in medicine are undisputed, but one question that remains unanswered concerns the reasons for this abundance of complex chemical substances.

In the past, the production of alkaloids by the opium poppy (*Papaver somniferum*) was a mystery, considered by some to be a gift from a beneficient deity. Others assumed that the apparently useless secondary metabolites were simply waste products. Another view is that these compounds have a role in protecting the otherwise defenceless, stationary plant from attack by mammals, insects, fungi, bacteria, and viruses. Taking morphine as an example of a secondary metabolite whose value to the plant is not entirely obvious, it is instructive to consider the biosynthetic origin. From essential amino acids that have a role in primary metabolism, eight steps are required to reach (*R*)-reticuline (**1**), a typical 1-benzylisoquinoline which can act as a precursor for several alkaloids (eq. 24.1). To get to morphine however, first requires salutaridine synthase (2) which is highly substrate specific. The reaction is an example of oxidative coupling catalysed by a microsomal cytochrome P-450 enzyme and is regio- and stereoselective. Five more steps follow from salutaridine (**2**) to arrive at morphine (**3**), which is a major product. The presence of morphine in the tissues of *Papaver somniferum* must confer a selectional advantage on the plant (3): it is neither a waste product nor an irrelevance, genetic code is required for each of the many enzymes involved in the biosynthesis, valuable amino acids are utilized in forming the enzymes, and a relatively scarce nutrient (nitrogen) is locked up in the compounds produced. It would take only one mutation to destroy the plant's ability to synthesize morphine, liberating nutrient forms of nitrogen and other metabolites. If the morphine did not continue to have value for the plant, mutants would have arisen with the advantage of not having a drain on its metabolic resources.

We can only guess at the ecological functions of morphine. Perhaps a mammalian herbivore which consumed too many poppies would become drowsy and itself fall prey to another predator. But, what benefit do mammals gain from producing morphine? It is an amazing fact that mammals are also capable of producing morphine-type metabolites. Not only has morphine and it congeners been found

in mammalian tissue, but a highly regio- and stereoselective cytochrome P-450 enzyme has been discovered in pig's liver which is also responsible for the oxidative coupling of (R)-reticuline to salutaridine and thus the formation of the morphine-type metabolites in mammals (4). Whatever their natural protective functions, natural products are a rich source of biologically active compounds which have arisen as the result of natural selection, over perhaps three hundred million years. The challenge to the medicinal chemist is to exploit this unique chemical diversity. The following account illustrates how natural products have been used, often as "lead compounds", or templates for the development of useful medicines.

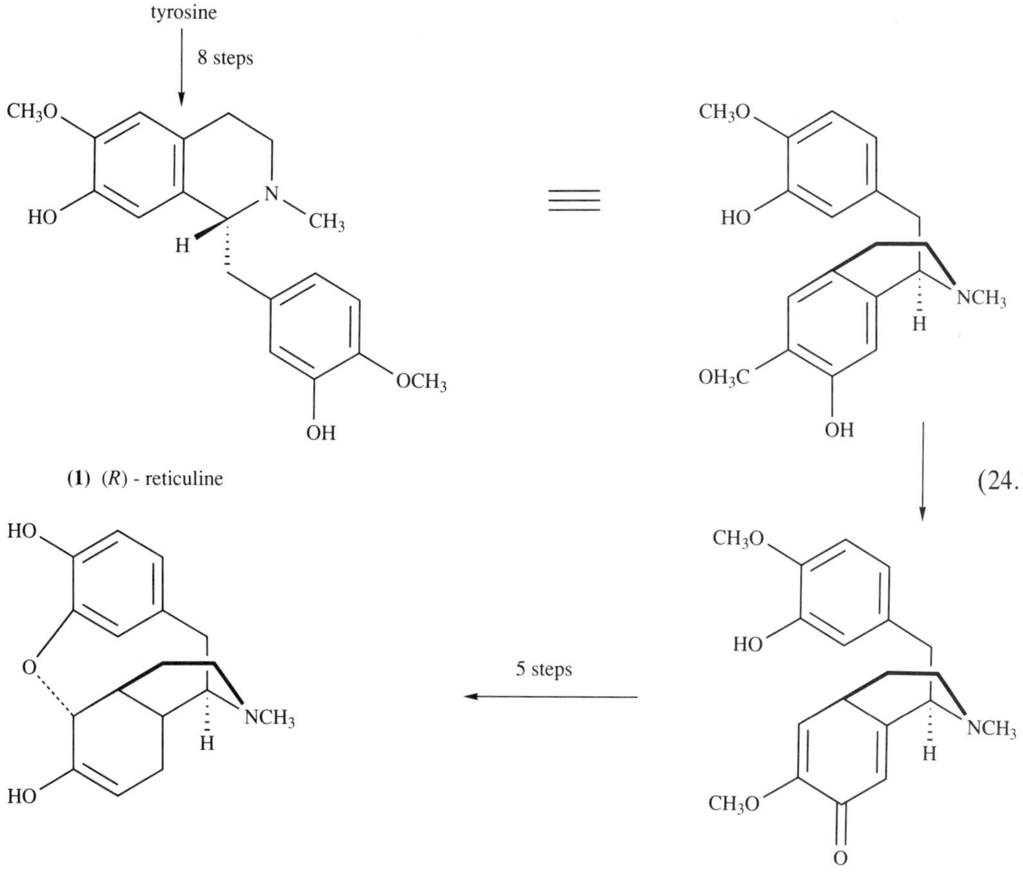

(1) (R) - reticuline

(3) morphine

(2) salutaridine

(24.1)

2 DRUGS AFFECTING THE CENTRAL NERVOUS SYSTEM

2.1 Morphine Alkaloids

The history of the opium alkaloids is too well known to warrant repetition here, but the analgesics based on morphine (3) are too important to be left out of an account of natural products as leads. We shall, therefore, summarize the clinically more important developments which have occurred since the isolation of morphine in 1803. Codeine (4) continues to be used widely for the treatment of moderate pain and although present in the opium poppy (*Papaver somniferum*), it is normally synthesized in higher yield from morphine (5).

Other than codeine, the earliest significant semisynthetic derivative of morphine is the diacetate, heroin (5), which is still widely used in terminal cancer where its addictiveness is irrelevant. Acetylation masks the polar hydroxy groups, so that penetration into the CNS is enhanced: hydrolysis then occurs to liberate the phenolic hydroxyl, giving an active analgesic, and ultimately regenerates morphine (6). Heroin was, therefore, one of the first prodrugs.

Modifications to the C-ring of morphine are legion, but none of the derivatives are free from addictive liability, though many have been used clinically. *N*-Demethylation and re-alkylation gives more interesting analogs, notably *N*-allylnormorphine, nalorphine (6), which is a morphine antagonist (7). Further modification leads to naloxone (7), which unlike nalorphine has very little agonist activity (8) and has retained a place in therapy for treatment of opiate-induced respiratory depression. Naloxone will also precipitate withdrawal symptoms in opiate addicts, thereby facilitating diagnosis.

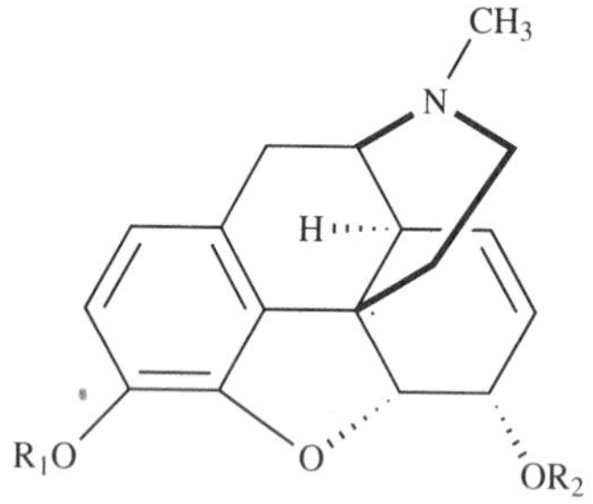

(3) morphine $R_1 = R_2 = H$

(4) codeine $R_1 = CH_3$, $R_2 = H$

(5) heroin $R_1 = R_2 = COCH_3$

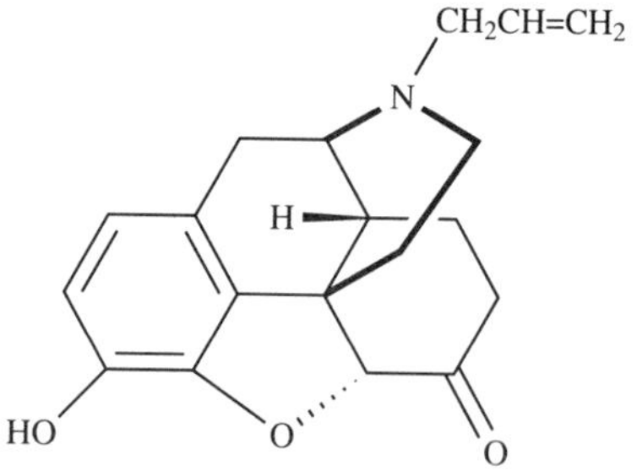

(7) naloxone

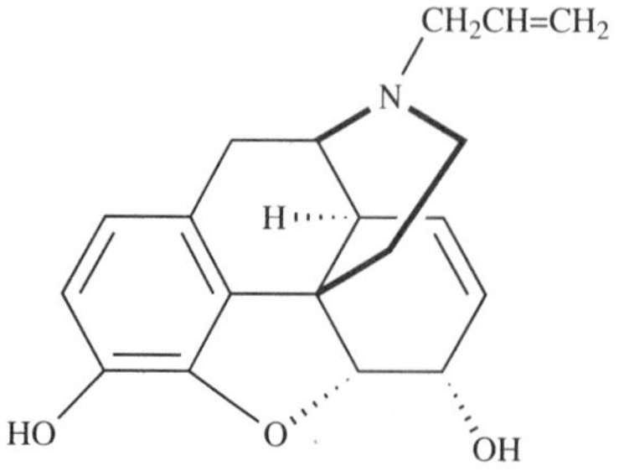

(6) nalorphine

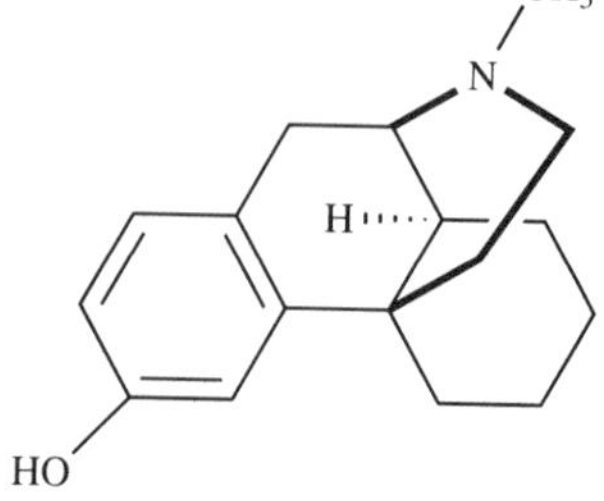

(8)

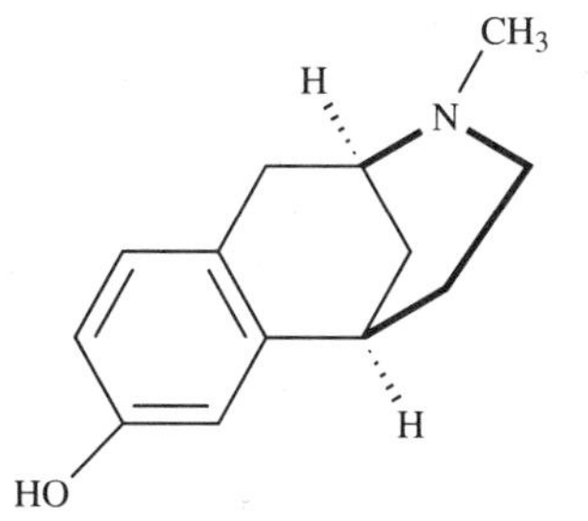

(9)

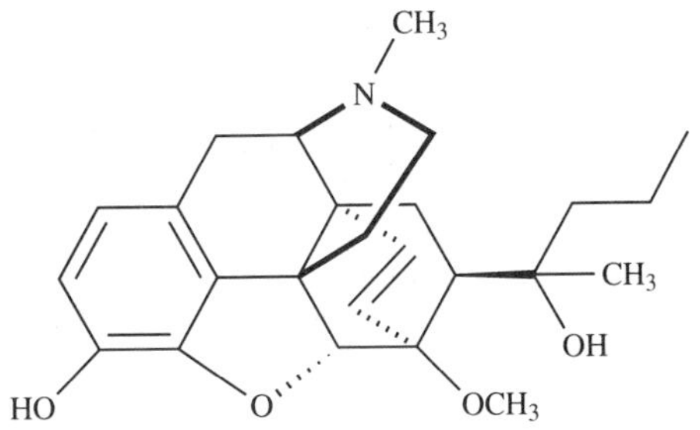

(11)

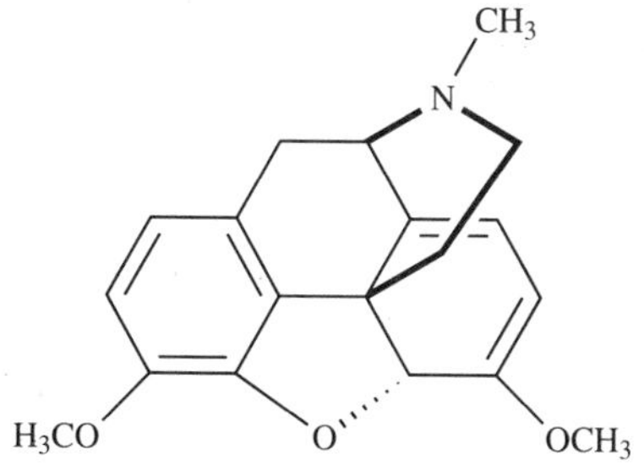

(10) thebaine

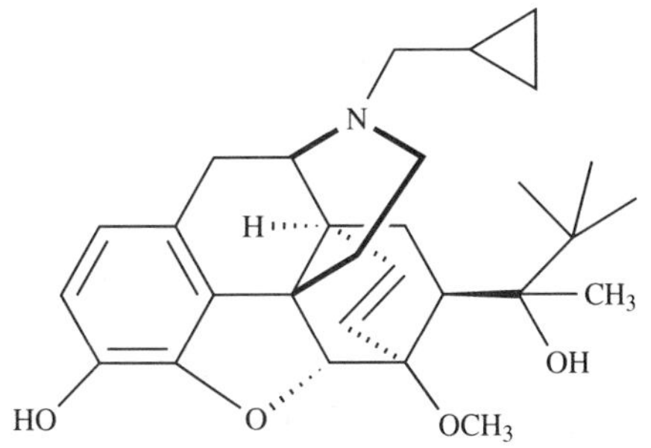

(12) buprenorphine

Total synthesis of morphine is difficult, but analogs lacking the dihydrofuran ring are accessible (9) from 1-benzylisoquinolines, in analogy with the biosynthesis of morphine, to give the morphinans (8). The system may be simplified even further (10) to given the benzomorphans (9), but neither these nor the morphinans have provided the long-sought analgesic without addictive properties.

A semisynthetic route to morphine analogs was found (11) from thebaine (10) using Diels-Alder reactions in the C-ring. Adducts such as (11) have the distinction of enormous potency (12), sufficient to immobilize rhinoceroses at moderate dose levels! Unfortunately, the addictive liability runs parallel to the increase in analgesic potency, a tendency which was partly overcome (13) in the analog buprenorphine (12).

All this work was carried out in ignorance of the nature of the natural transmitter(s), which proved, subsequently, to be the peptides known as endorphins and their pentapeptide fragments, the enkephalins (14). It is perhaps significant that vastly improved understanding of the biochemical basis for analgesia and the characterisation of a family of related receptors (15), known as δ, κ, and μ, has so far failed to yield any better drugs for the treatment of pain.

A series of analgesics which were discovered initially in an attempt to obtain smooth muscle relaxants based on another natural product, atropine (13), started with the observation that meperidine (pethidine) (14) unexpectedly produced a reaction in mice known as "Straub tail", normally characteristic of the morphine series (16). Pethidine (14) itself is still used widely in childbirth in the belief that there is a lower incidence of respiratory depression in the foetus. The realization that 4-phenyl-piperidines, which are not obvious structural analogs of morphine, could give rise to useful analgesic effects, led to the synthesis of many thousands of derivatives (17), many with far greater potency than pethidine (14). Unfortunately, as potency increases so do addiction liability and respiratory depression.

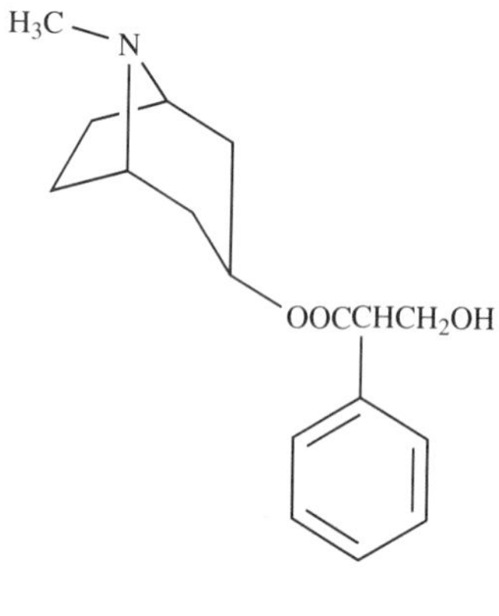

(13) atropine

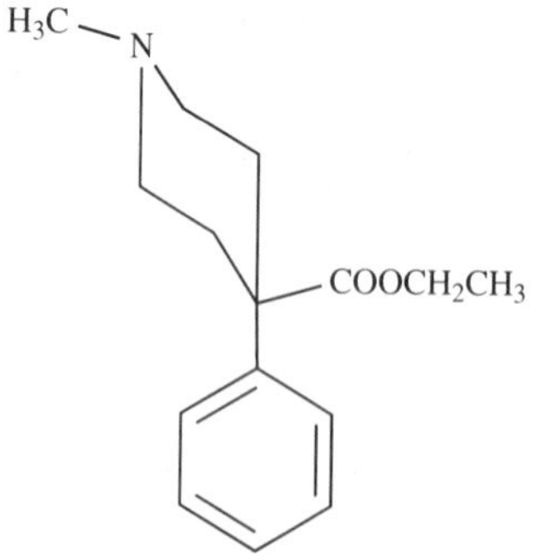

(14) pethidine

2.2 Cannabinoids

The plant *Cannabis sativa* has been used by humans for thousands of years, both for the effects when ingested and for making rope from the fibers in the stem. The major constituent of pharmacological interest is Δ_9-cannabinol (15) (THC) which has a multiplicity of actions. In animals the effects include sedation and apparent hallucinations (18), which are similar to the major effects in the CNS in humans. There are also cardiovascular effects, notably tachycardia and postural hypotension, which can be separated from the CNS action, as in the synthetic analog $\Delta_{6a,10a}$-dimethylheptyl-THC (16), which has minimal CNS activity (19).

Given the widespread illicit use of *C. sativa*, it was perhaps inevitable that eventually one or two cancer patients receiving chemotherapy would dose themselves with their own sedative in the form of marijuana. An unexpected blessing from this uncontrolled combination was a reduction in the nausea experienced during chemotherapy. A variety of anticancer agents cause severe nausea and vomiting, including nitrogen mustard, adriamycin, 5-azacytidine, cyclophosphamide and methotrexate: the unique situation arose in which the remedy was discovered by the patients themselves (20). Although it has been suggested that smoking reefers is the ideal route of administration, giving rapid absorption and close control of the effects, this peculiarly human form of self-abuse is unlikely to be recommended to those who are unaccustomed to it. In the event, when the physicians in charge were made aware of their patients' discovery, they devised a controlled clinical trial in which measured doses of THC were dissolved in sesame oil and administered in gelatin capsules. A placebo was similarly prepared for use in a randomised, double-blind, cross-over experiment (20). The results left no doubt that a majority of patients benefited from THC pretreatment, even those who had previously been refractory to the effects of the standard anti-emetics such as prochlorperazine. There remained the problem of tachycardia associated with THC treatment.

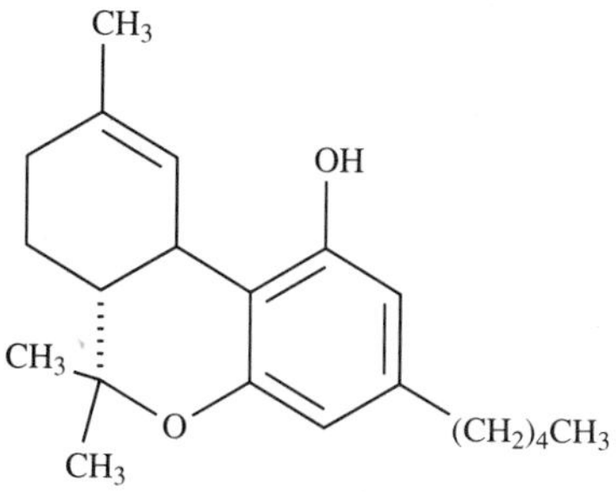

(15) THC

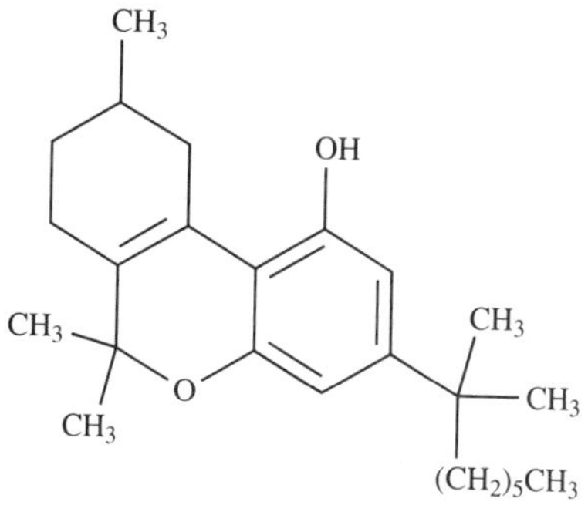

(16)

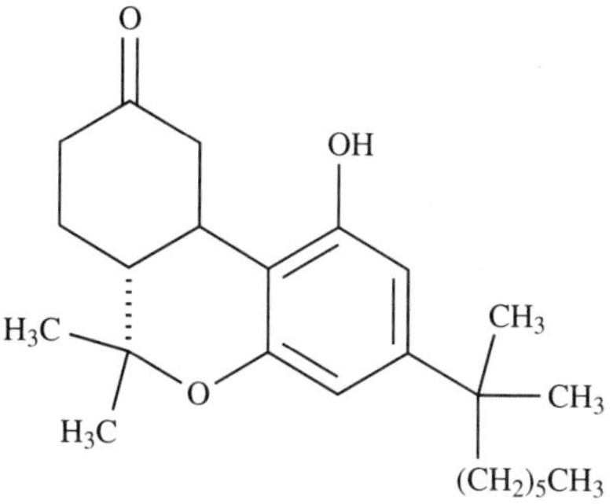

(17) nabilone

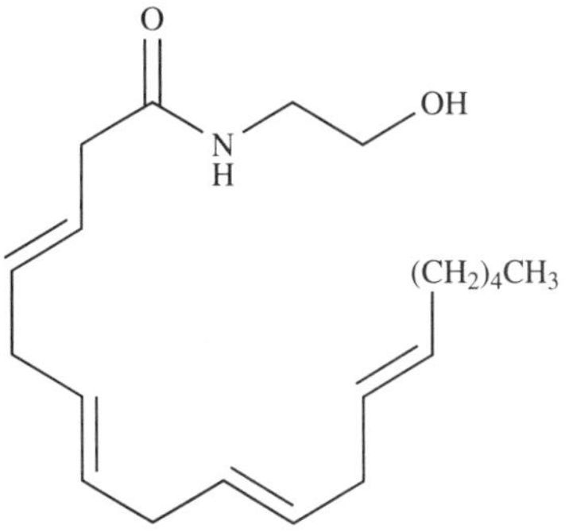

(18) anandamide

The multiplicity of effects of THC have led to the synthesis of large numbers of analogs (21), particularly in the hope of finding nonmorphine-like analgesics without addictiveness and without the other CNS effects of THC. The general impression is that the synthetic modifications are fairly random and have so far failed to provide an analgesic of clinical value. However, the analog (17) known as nabilone had been shown to possess less effect on the cardiovascular system than THC, while retaining the mixture of CNS actions, including analgesic, anti-anxiety and antipsychotic properties (22). When tested as an anti-emetic, nabilone proved to be superior to THC (23) and was approved subsequently for marketing. The first ten years of clinical experience has been reviewed (24).

More recently, an endogenous ligand for the 'THC receptor' has been identified as the long-chain ethanolamine derivative (18) known as anandamide (25). There is little obvious structural similarity between THC and anandamide, opening up new areas for research into analogs of the latter which may achieve the ultimate goal of separation of all the mixed effects of THC. Without THC, however, nobody would have looked for the endogenous ligand.

2.3 Asperlicin

Cholecystokinin (CCK) is a peptide hormone, present in the gut and CNS; it is one of the most abundant peptides in the brain (26, 27). The whole peptide is composed of

33 amino acids, but the C-terminal octapeptide H-Asp-Tyr(SO_3H)-Met-Gly-Trp-Met-Asp-Phe-NH_2 possesses the full range of activities, sufficient for it to be classed as a neurotransmitter (28). Specific, high-affinity binding sites have been found on mammalian CNS cell membranes and in other organs such as pancreas, gall-bladder, and colon (29). The latter have been classed as CCK-A receptors, but the majority of CNS receptors are classed as CCK-B, based on affinity differences for various agonists and antagonists (30). To confuse the issue slightly, the gastrin receptor in the stomach appears to be closely related to the CCK-B receptor (31) and is stimulated by the C-terminal tetrapeptide of CCK.

The effects of CCK on intestinal smooth muscle and pancreas are easy to demonstrate pharmacologically, unlike the role in the CNS which is a matter for conjecture. It was assumed that the CNS activity must be significant, given the abundance of the peptide in the brain, and that the discovery of antagonists might lead to new drug treatments, as yet unspecified (32). There were three ways in which the discovery of antagonists was undertaken. A group at Parke-Davis set out to mimic the natural octapeptide using the peptoid approach to arrive at stable analogs with oral bioavailability. In this they have been successful, producing potent and selective dipeptoid CCK-B antagonists which have interesting anxiolytic activity (33). However, these dipeptoids are not an appropriate subject for this chapter. In contrast, a group at Lilly used a routine screening program to identify CCK antagonists, resulting in a series of 4,5-diphenylpyrazolidinones which were developed to give potent CCK-B receptor antagonists able to discriminate between CCK-B and gastrin receptors (26). Again, it is not appropriate to discuss the work further in this context.

An alternative approach was to go searching in microbial broths, using an assay technique with radioreceptors as bait.

Perhaps surprisingly, this technique produced asperlicin (19), the first potent, competitive and selective CCK-A antagonist, from a culture medium of *Aspergillus alliaceus* (34). Subsequently, two Streptomyces antibiotics, anthramycin and virginiamycin M_1, were identified as having CCK antagonist properties (26). For the present purpose we shall confine ourselves to a discussion of the development of asperlicin.

Asperlicin is moderately potent, poorly soluble in water and not bioavailable by the oral route (35). When discovered it was also, with morphine, one of the very few non-peptides with affinity for a peptide receptor (peptoids are discounted in this assessment). It was an interesting target for synthetic modification, particularly viewed as a benzodiazepine derivative with potential CNS activity.

Based on the benzodiazepine nucleus, and an overt mimic of diazepam, one of the first successful synthetic analogs was L-364,286 (20) which had potency on CCK-A receptors similar to that of asperlicin. Further development along this line gave analogs with improved solubility in water and better oral bioavailability, but did not improve receptor affinity. To accomplish the latter required a move to 3-aminobenzazepines, specifically as their amides: the 2-indolyl derivative L-364,718, also known as MK-329 (21), is 5 orders of magnitude more potent at CCK-A receptors than asperlicin (36). MK-329 is also selective, has a long duration of action *in vivo* and may be given orally; it is being evaluated clinically, but so far with little excitement. Even so, MK-329 is the most potent and selective CCK-A antagonist currently available and it is a valuable pharmacological tool.

Modification of the 3-amide to give a urea linkage as in (22) led to a reduction in CCK-A receptor affinity. Importantly, discrimination between CCK-A and CCK-B receptors by (22) is governed by the stereo-

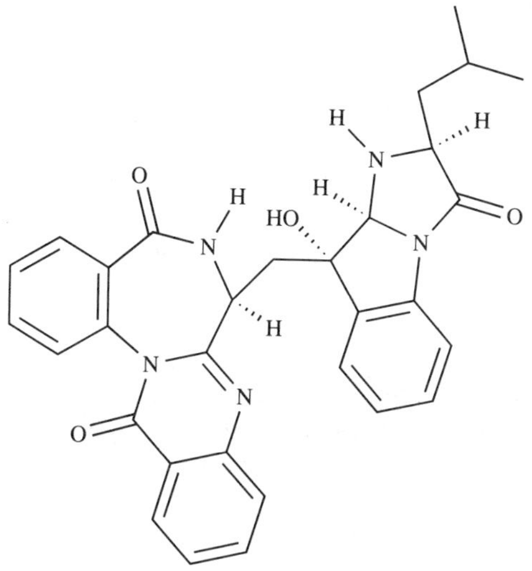

(**19**) asperlicin

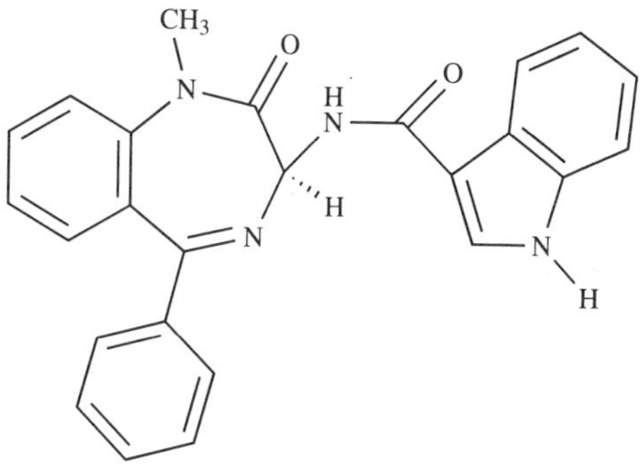

(**21**)

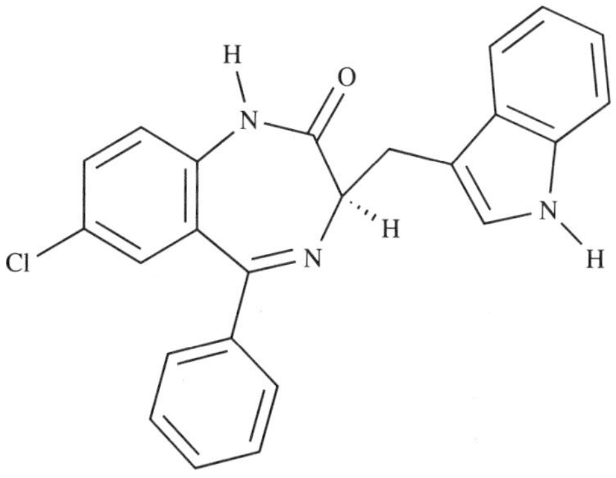

(**20**)

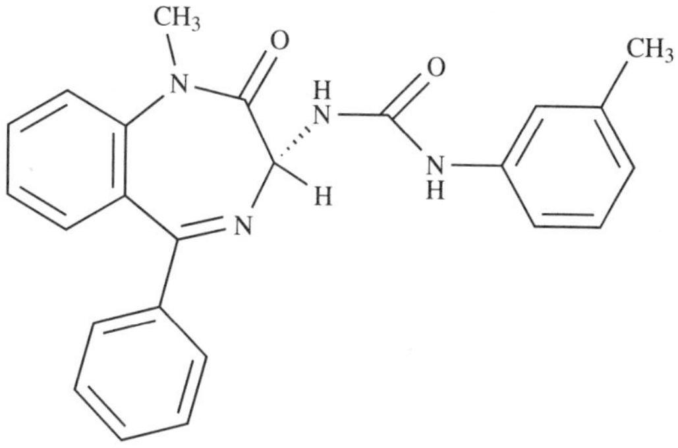

(**22**)

displays anxiolytic properties (26). It is undergoing phase 1 clinical trials.

An aspect of this research program which has stimulated some philosophical discussion concerns the dissimilarity between the nonpeptide ligands and the endogenous neurotransmitter. Both this aspect and the apparent versatility of benzodiazepine-derived molecules to bind

chemistry at C3, the (S)-enantiomer showing greater affinity for CCK-A receptors. The (R)-enantiomer prefers CCK-B receptors and has been shown to possess an attractive combination of biological effects. Known as L-365,260, the compound antagonizes gastrin-stimulated acid secretion in animal models and, among other CNS effects, induces analgesia in primates and selectively to a variety of functionally distinct receptors are explored in some depth by Evans et al. (32, 35, 36).

3 NEUROMUSCULAR BLOCKING DRUGS

3.1 Curare, Decamethonium, and Atracurium

The development and use of muscle relaxants, to allow a reduction in the level of anaesthesia during surgery, follows entirely from studies of South American arrow poisons (37) and particularly from the isolation by King (38) of pure D-tubocurarine (23) in the 1930s, from tube curare. Another of the South American blowpipe poisons, calabash curare, was used for similar purposes and developed (39, 40) to give alcuronium (24) from the alkaloid C-toxiferine I (25). Both types of curare paralyze skeletal muscle by a similar mechanism, antagonizing the effect of acetylcholine at the neuromuscular junction (41).

The muscle-paralyzing curare alkaloids are quaternary salts which are not absorbed when taken orally. For surgical procedures they must be administered by intravenous injection, which results in onset of paralysis in at most a few minutes: anaesthesia is normally induced prior to administration of the muscle relaxant (37), which is followed by artificial respiration. Although the neuromuscular blocking agents are potentially lethal when administered alone, in the environment of an operating theatre they are truly life-saving drugs which have made a major impact on survival rates during surgery.

At the time of King's work in the 1930s there were no spectroscopic aids to structure elucidation and it is not surprising that he made a small error in the structure assigned to D-tubocurarine, believing it to have two quaternary nitrogens, a mistake

which was not corrected (42) until 1970. The methylation product of D-tubocurarine, known as metocurine (26) is a more potent muscle relaxant. It was known for a long time as dimethyltubocurarine owing to the error in the structure allocated to compound (23). King's error, in assigning a bisquaternary structure to a molecule with one quaternary and one protonated tertiary nitrogen, led to a large number of highly active synthetic bisquaternaries. The simplest of these was decamethonium (27), being nothing more than two trimethylammonium end-groups connected with a decamethylene chain. As one of a series with different chain lengths (43), decamethonium became the prototype for many more complex structures with ten atoms between the quarternary centers, which appeared to be optimal for binding to the acetylcholine receptor at the neuromuscular junction.

Unlike tubocurarine, decamethonium depolarizes the muscle end-plate, rendering the membrane insensitive to acetylcholine (41). The action of tubocurarine is competitive and can be overcome with increased concentrations of acetylcholine, brought about by administration of an anticholinesterase: the latter is thus an antidote to tubocurarine, but not to decamethonium. Despite the lack of an antidote, decamethonium was used very widely for over two decades. One of its disadvantages is an overlong duration of action, during which time the patient has to be maintained on artificial respiration, because the muscle of the diaphragm is also susceptible to the actions of the drug. An early and highly successful attempt (44) to shorten the action of decamethonium gave suxamethonium (28), a diester formed between succinic acid and two molecules of choline.

Tubocurarine suffers from cardiovascular side-effects induced by direct interactions with ganglionic acetylcholine receptors and from stimulation of histamine

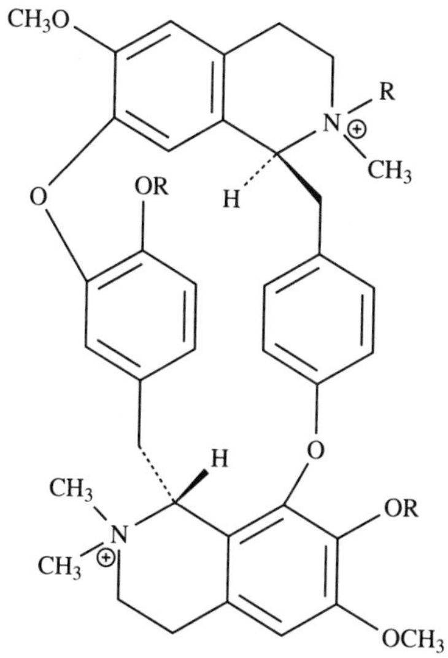

(23) tubocurarine R = H

(26) metocurine R = CH$_3$

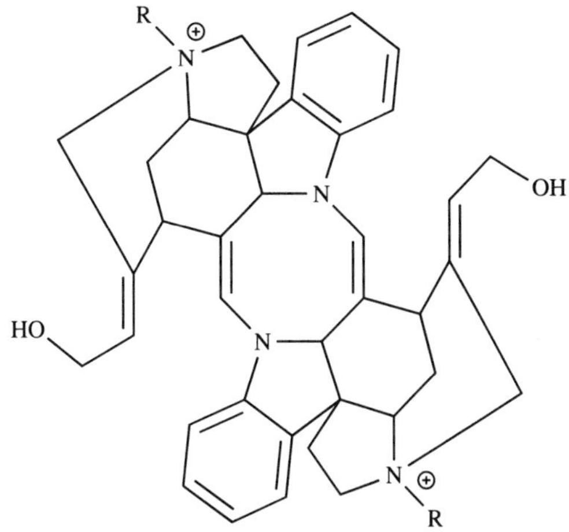

(24) R = CH$_3$ C-toxifermine I

(25) R = CH$_2$CH=CH$_2$ alcuronium

release, so analogs have been well worth pursuing. The macrocyclic structure of tubocurarine is a difficult synthetic target, but fortunately ring-opened analogs, such as laudexium (29), have high potency and relatively few side-effects (45). The main problem with (29) is the duration of action,

which at about 40 minutes is too long for many operations. Two approaches have been used to shorten the duration of action. The concept of pH-controlled Hofmann elimination was employed successfully (46) in the design of atracurium (30), which in clinical use (47) has the big

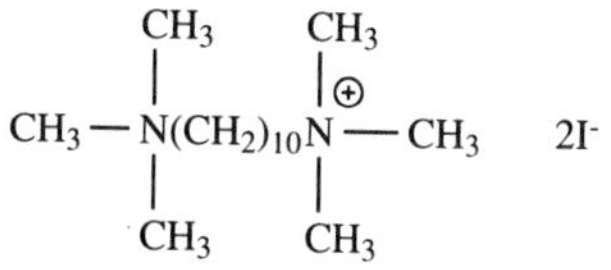

(27) decamethonium

2 Cl$^-$

(28) suxamethonium

2I$^\ominus$

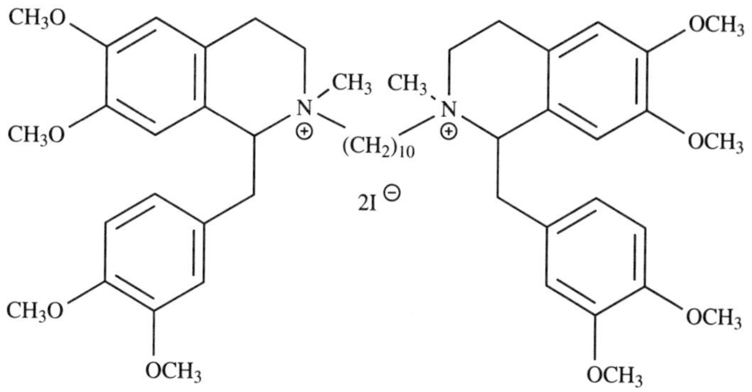

(29) laudexium

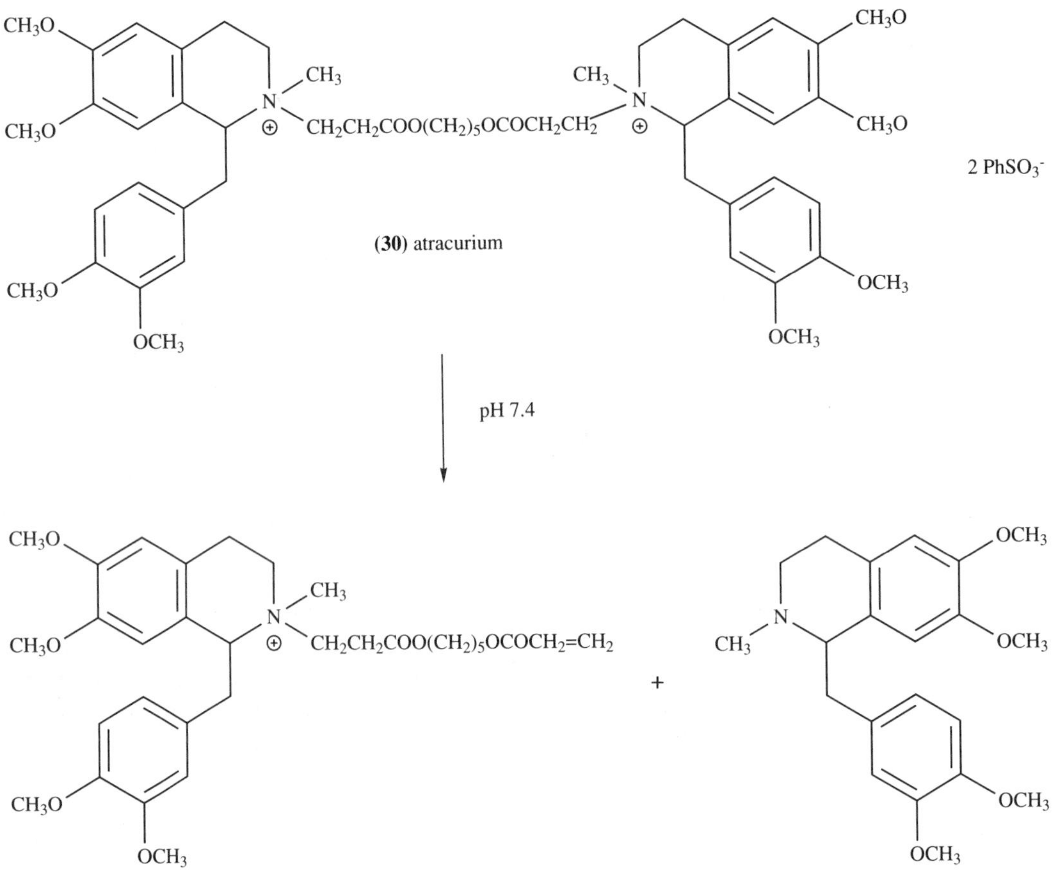

(30) atracurium

2 PhSO$_3^-$

pH 7.4

+

advantage that the drug disappears at a constant rate (eq. 24.2), irrespective of liver or kidney function. Some ester hydrolysis contributes to the destruction of atracurium *in vivo*, as might be expected. A slightly later development (48) centred on an empirical search for structures which would undergo ester hydrolysis more rapidly, resulting in mivacurium (31), which has a slightly shorter duration of action than atracurium, the latter being about 15–20 minutes.

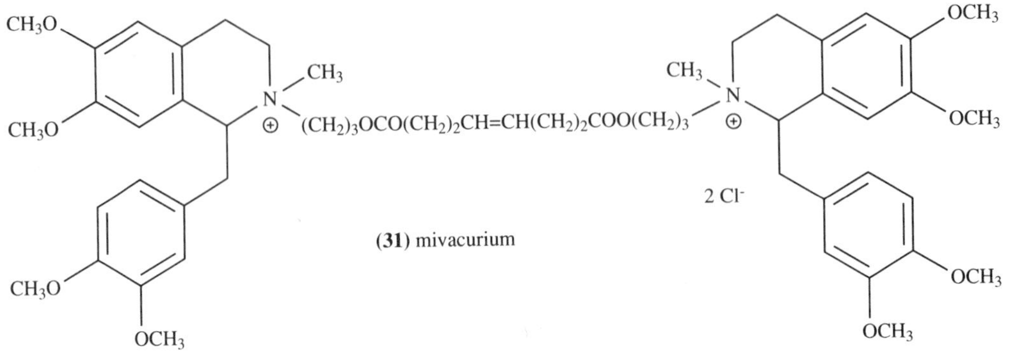

(31) mivacurium

2 Cl$^-$

4 ANTICANCER DRUGS

4.1 Catharanthus (Vinca) Alkaloids

In 1949 Canadian researchers at the University of Western Ontario began investigating the medicinal properties of the rosy periwinkle (*Catharanthus roseus*), a plant that had been used for many years to treat diabetes mellitus in the West Indies. Despite finding that the plant extract when given orally had no effect on blood sugar levels in rats or rabbits, the researchers noted that when given intravenously, the extract caused the animals to succumb to bacterial infection and die. This curious observation prompted further studies which showed that the plant extract reduced levels of white blood cells, caused granulocytopenia and bone marrow damage; toxic effects encountered with many antitumor drugs (49). These findings led the Canadian group to isolate an alkaloid fraction with potent cytotoxic activity. The active principle was eventually purified and became known as vinblastine (**32**), a dimeric indole-dihydroindole alkaloid.

Concurrently, researchers at the Lilly Research Laboratories had been investigating extracts of *C. roseus* and they too had detected cytotoxic activity, specifically against acute lymphocytic leukemia (50, 51). The U.S. group isolated several alkaloids, including vinblastine and another closely related alkaloid, vincristine (**33**).

Although many other alkaloids have been isolated from *C. roseus*, only vinblastine and vincristine have been developed for clinical use. The antiproliferative activity of the two compounds is related to their specific interaction with tubulin; preventing assembly of tubulin into microtubules and arresting cell division (52). However, despite this apparent identical mechanism of action an their clear chemical similarities, vinblastine and vincristine display very different clinical effects. Vinblastine, for example, is used to treat Hodgkin's disease and metastatic testicular tumors, whereas vincristine is used mainly in combination with other anticancer drugs for the treatment of acute lymphocytic leukemia in children. Toxicity profiles are also different, vinblastine causing bone-marrow depression, whereas peripheral neuropathy often proves to be dose-limiting in vincristine therapy.

Lilley introduced vinblastine and vincristine into the clinic in 1960 and 1963 respectively, but this did not preclude the search for improved derivatives. A chemical modification program aimed at improving antitumor activity and reducing toxicity was initiated in 1972 (53). Concern about the neurotoxicity displayed by vincristine, its chemical instability and low natural abundance (0.03 g/kg dried plant material), led to vinblastine being chosen as a template for semisynthetic modification. Selective ammonolysis of the ester function at C-3 and hydrolysis of the adjacent acetyl group yielded the desacetyl vinblastine amide, vindesine (**34**) (eq. 24.3). Better yields of vindesine were obtained from the hydrazide (**35**) on treatment with nitrous acid and reacting the resultant azide (**36**) with ammonia. The azide (**36**) proved to be a useful intermediate for the preparation of a range of substituted amides, but vindesine proved to be the derivative of choice with significant differences in the spectrum of antitumor activity and toxicity compared to the naturally occurring alkaloids. Phase I clinical trials commenced in 1977 and vindesine has been used for the treatment of non-small cell lung cancer, lymphoblastic leukemia, and non-Hodgkin's lymphomas. In combination with cisplatin, vindesine ranks among the foremost treatments for non-small cell lung cancer with respect to response rate and survival (54). Back in the 1950s, the U.S. researchers could not have guessed that thirty years on, the demand for Catharanthus alkaloids would necessitate the processing of around 8,000 kg of plant material per year (55)!

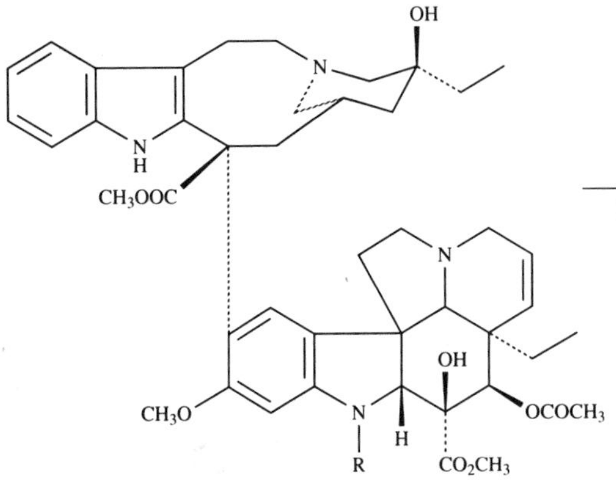

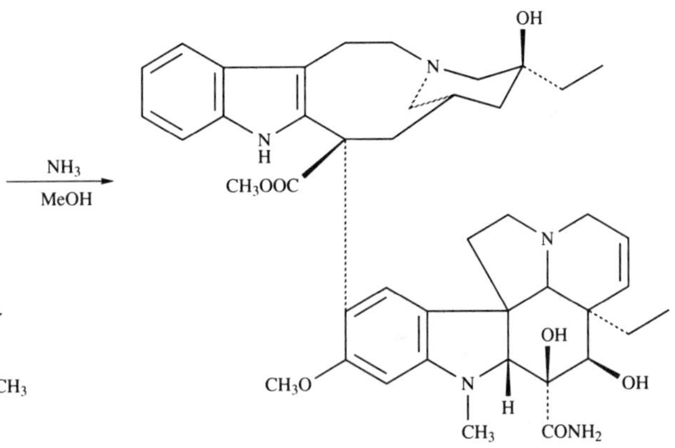

(32) vinblastine R = CH₃

(33) vincristine R = CHO

(34) vindesine

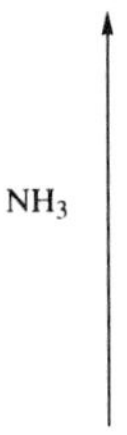

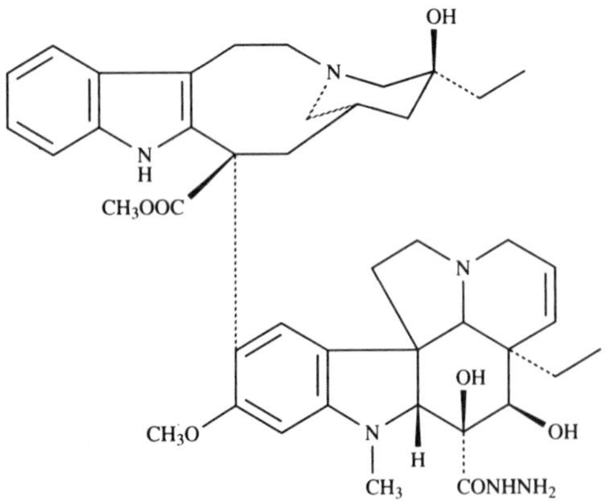

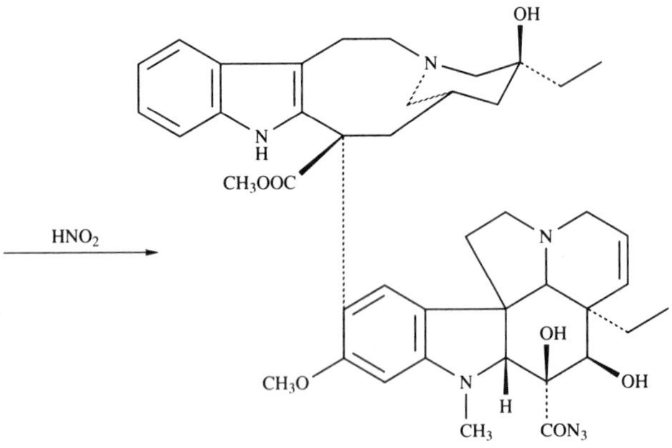

(35)

(36)

4.2 Taxol and Taxotere

Regarded as the tree of death by the Greeks and used to prepare arrow poison by the Celts, the yew tree has been associ-

ated with death and poisoning for centuries (56, 57). The English yew, *Taxus baccata*, was used to make funeral wreaths and it was believed that one could die by merely standing beneath the boughs of the tree.

Yew certainly contains highly toxic metabolites and their potency and fast duration of action has often made extracts of yew the poison of choice for numerous murders and suicide attempts. It is, therefore, ironical that extracts from the Pacific yew, *T. brevifolia*, after being tested in the National Cancer Institute's (NCI) screening program during the 1960s, yielded what has since been described (58) as the most exciting anticancer compound discovered in the last 20 years, namely taxol (**37**) (paclitaxel).

The initial isolation and characterization of taxol proved particularly difficult because of (a) its very low natural abundance in *T. brevifolia* bark (although this was the best known source, the isolated yield was only 0.02%, equivalent to 650 mg per tree), (b) the poor analytical data

obtained from the purified compound, and (c) the failure of taxol to given crystals which were suitable for x-ray analysis (59). The structure of taxol was published in 1971 (60), but further biological testing continued to be troubled by difficulties. The compound showed only modest *in vivo* activity in various leukemia assays which was no better than that displayed by a number of other new compounds at the time. In addition to the limited supplies of taxol (the complexity of the molecule precluded chemical synthesis), the compound was very poorly soluble in water which made formulation difficult. However, various new assays were developed in the 1970s, including the murine B16 melanoma model, in which taxol showed very good activity, and another boost came with Hor-

(**37**) taxol

(**38**) R = COCH₃ baccatin III

(**39**) R = H 10-desacetylbaccatin III

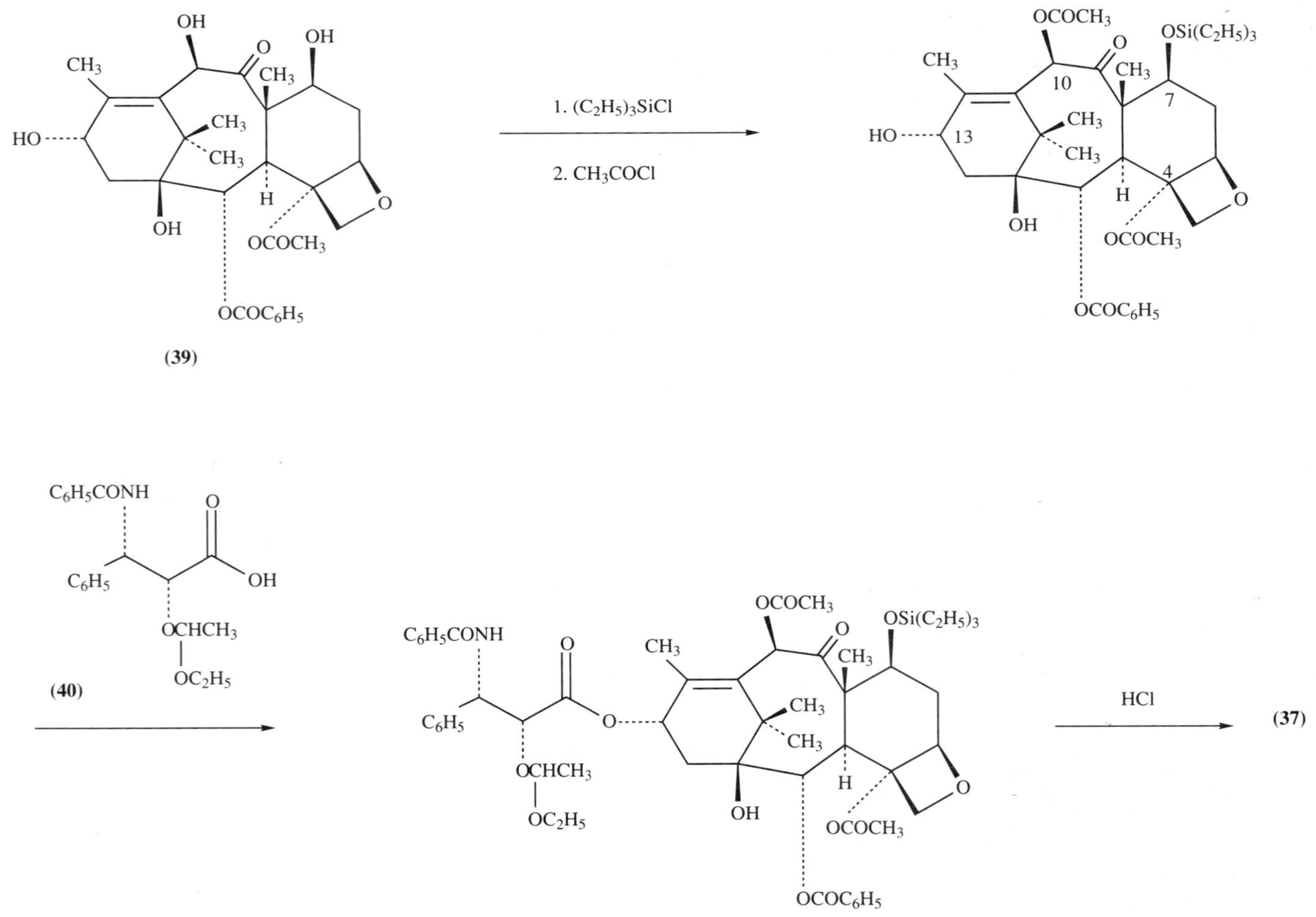

1. $(C_2H_5)_3SiCl$
2. CH_3COCl

(39)

(40)

HCl

(37)

witz et al. (61) discovered that the compound prevented cell division by a unique mode of action. In contrast to the antimitotic vinblastine and podophyllotoxin analogs (q.v.), which prevent microtubule assembly, taxol inhibits cell division by promoting assembly of stable microtubule bundles which leads to cell death.

Phase I clinical trials were initiated in 1983, but these were to proceed at a slow and tortuous pace and proved all but disastrous when the high levels of oil-based adjuvant used to formulate taxol caused severe allergic reactions in many volunteers. Undaunted by the formulation problem and spurred on by taxol's novel mechanism of action, clinicians were able eventually to minimize the allergic events and demonstrate useful activity. Phase II clinical trials began in 1985 despite continuing supply problems, and four years later the program received a significant boost when McGuire et al. (62) reported good responses from patients suffering from refractory ovarian cancer, a disease which kills some 12,500 women a year in the USA alone.

In 1991, Bristol-Myers Squibb in conjunction with the NCI agreed to manage the supplies of taxol and were granted a licence to develop the compound further. The following year the US Federal Drug Administration approved taxol for the treatment of ovarian cancer in patients unresponsive to standard treatments and in December 1993 approval was given for the treatment of metastatic breast cancer.

The sourcing of taxol from *T. brevifolia* was a major problem (63) because to treat just the groups of patients suffering ovarian cancer in the US would require about 25 kg of compound per year, necessitating the felling of some 38,000 trees (58)! Although the Pacific yew is not a rare tree, it is extremely slow growing and such harvesting could not be sustained indefinitely. It has been estimated that there are enough trees available to maintain a supply of taxol

for only the next 2–7 years (64). The isolation of taxol from other *Taxus* species has been investigated at length and reasonable quantities have been obtained from the needles of several species including *T. baccata*. Using the needles may help alleviate the supply problem because they can be harvested without damaging the tree, however, the needles contain much higher quantities of several biosynthetic precursors of taxol and two of these, baccatin III (**38**) and 10-desacetylbaccatin III (**39**) have been used to prepare taxol semisynthetically. One approach, developed by Potier et al. (65) involved acylation of the sterically hindered C-13 position of baccatin III with cinnamic acid and subsequent double bond functionalization via hydroxyamination to give taxol together with various regio- and stereoisomers. A better approach involved protection of 10-desacetylbaccatin III as the triethylsilyl ether (e.g. 24.4), followed by direct acylation with the phenylisoserine derivative (**40**), giving taxol in 38% overall yield (66). Further improvements were made using less sterically demanding acylating reagents, for example acylation with the β-lactam (**41**) gave taxol in up to 90% yield (67) and this may be the preferred method for commercial production in future.

These semisynthetic approaches also provide access to analogs with potential advantages over taxol itself. Structure–activity studies have shown that although the oxetane ring appears to be essential for activity, wide variation in the nature and stereochemistry of the C-13 ester sidechain can be tolerated. Thus, the *N-t-*(butoxycarbonyl) derivative, taxotere (**42**) (docetaxel), which appears to be more potent than taxol (68) and has better solubility characteristics, is being developed by Rhône-Poulenc Rorer and has entered Phase II clinical trials for the treatment of ovarian, breast, colon, and lung cancer.

Various "protaxols", designed to release taxol *in situ* under physiological conditions,

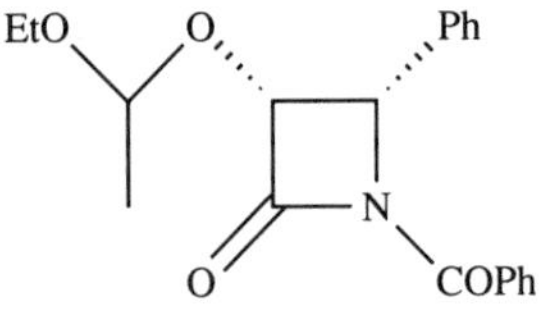

(41)

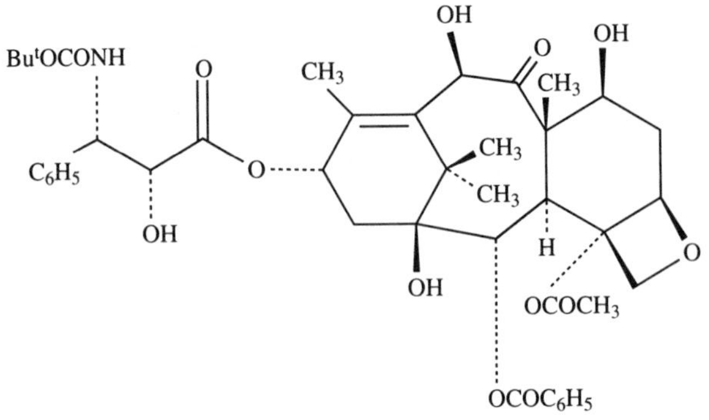

(42) taxotere

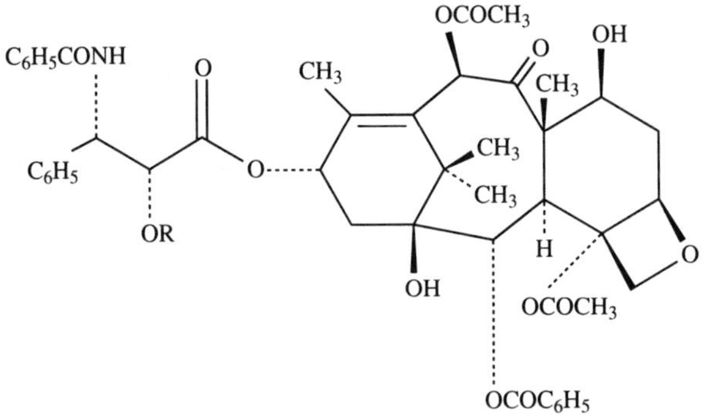

(43) R =

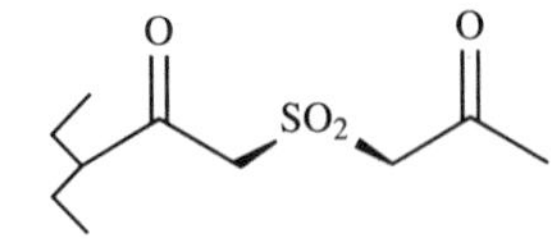

have been prepared by acylating the C-2′ hydroxyl group. Recently, Nicolaou et al. (69) reported the synthesis of the sulfone **(43)** which is soluble and stable in aqueous media, but is able to release taxol rapidly in human blood plasma.

Plant tissue culture (58), microbial fermentation (70), and total synthesis (71, 72) provide other possibilities for the production of taxol and its derivatives, although it is far from certain whether any of them will be commercially viable.

4.3 Podophyllotoxin, Etoposide, and Teniposide

The development of the natural constituents of Podophyllum into effective semi-synthetic and ultimately, totally synthetic compounds for the treatment of various kinds of cancer provides one of the most sustained and intriguing stories of drug discovery (73, 74). The story has all the classic ingredients, starting with observation and reasoning, extending through chance into new areas and characterized throughout by persistence and determination, particularly when biological activity had to be traced to very minor constituents in the crude plant extract.

Podophyllum peltatum (may apple, or American mandrake) and *P. emodi* are respectively American and Himalayan plants, widely separated geographically but used in both places as cathartics in folk medicine (75). An alcoholic extract of the rhizome known as podophyllin was included in many pharmacopoeias for its gastrointestinal effects; it was included in the U.S.P., for example, from 1820 to 1942. At about this time the beneficial effect of podophyllin, applied topically to benign tumors known as condylomata acuminata, was demonstrated clinically (76). This usage was not inspirational, since there are records of topical application in the treatment of cancer by the Penobscot Indians of Maine and subsequently, by various medical practitioners in the United States from the 19th century (77). The crude resinous podophyllin is an irritant, unpleasant mixture unsuited to systemic administration.

The first chemical constituent was isolated from podophyllin in 1880 and named podophyllotoxin (78). A structure was proposed in 1932 and after some fine tuning (79) was shown to be the lignan (44). As might be expected, the crude resin contains a variety of chemical types, including the flavonols quercetin and kaempferol (80). While these other constituents undoubtedly have biological activity, it is the lignans which have received most attention and to which we shall devote the remainder of this section.

Chemists at Sandoz in the early 1950s reasoned that crude podophyllin might contain lignan glycosides with anticancer activity which might be more water-soluble and less toxic than podophyllotoxin (73). The reasoning for the latter is not entirely clear, but in the event they proved to be correct in both respects. Careful isolation gave podophyllotoxin β-D-glucopyranoside (45), its 4′-desmethyl analog (46) and some less important lignans lacking the B-ring hydroxy group (81–83). Unfortunately, the sugar derivatives were less active as inhibitors of cell proliferation than the aglycones, as well as less toxic, however, as expected they were much more water soluble (73). While continuing work to isolate more natural lignans, a substantial program of structural modification of the known compounds was undertaken with a view to protecting the glucosides from hydrolytic enzymes and also to improve cellular uptake. Most of these changes were ineffective: the per-acylated derivatives, for example, were insoluble in water and had inferior cytostatic effects (84).

Condensation of the glucosides with a variety of aldehydes was more useful, in that not all the hydroxy groups were blocked. Despite this, water solubility was a problem with the podophyllotoxin derivatives (47). Gastrointestinal absorption was greatly improved, however, as was chemi-

(44) podophyllotoxin

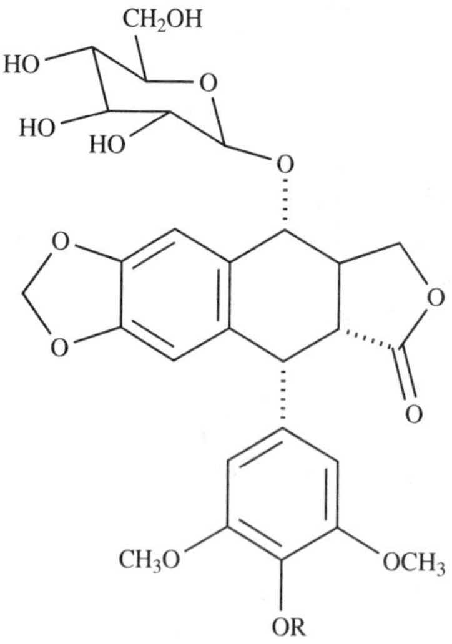

(45) R = CH$_3$

(46) R = H

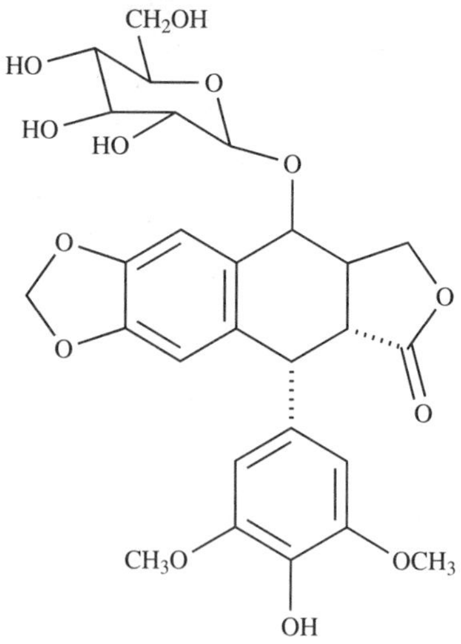

(50)

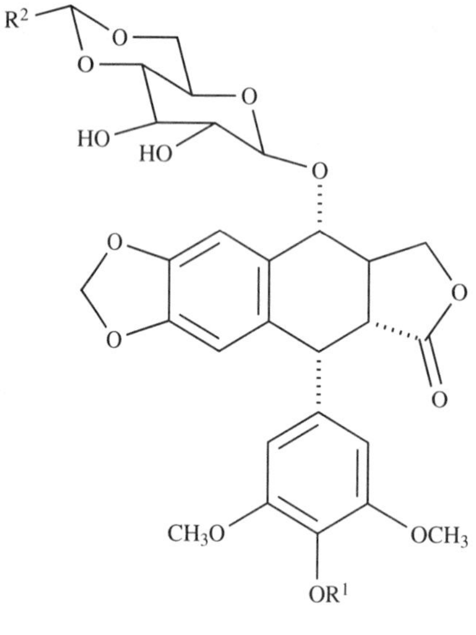

(47) R^1 = H,CH$_3$ R^2 = various alkyl, aryl

(48) R^1 = CH$_3$ R^2 = C$_6$H$_5$

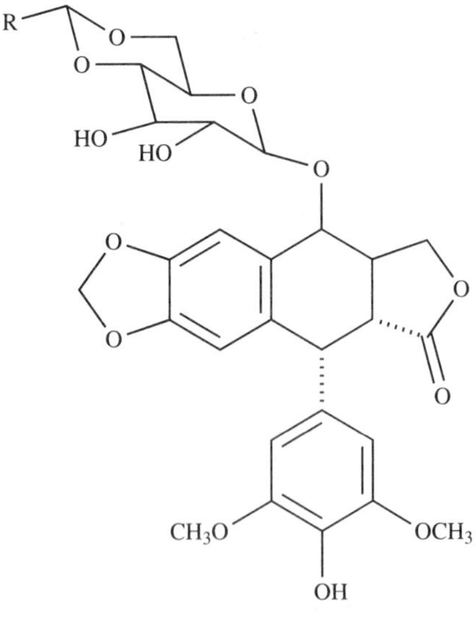

(49) R = C$_6$H$_5$

(51) R =

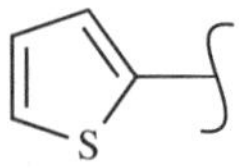

(teniposide)

(52) R = CH$_3$ (etoposide)

cal stability (85), and positive effects were observed in a few cancer patients with the benzylidene derivative (**48**). It was at this point that luck played a hand, backed up by a good deal of determination. A crude podophyllin fraction, which was simpler and cheaper to prepare than pure podophyllin glucoside, was also treated with benzaldehyde to give a mixture of benzylidene derivatives, about 80% of which was compound (**48**). The crude product was found to be more potent than compound (**48**) and subsequently to possess a different mode of action from the lead compounds: rather than arresting cells in metaphase, cells were prevented from entering mitosis altogether (86). The crude mixture was marketed for cancer treatment as Proresid^R.

Improved biological assay methods (87) indicated the presence of an unknown, highly active constituent of Proresid^R. For example, Proresid^R prolonged the life of mice inoculated with L1210 leukemia cells (74), an effect which was not observed with the known major constituent. In the early 1960s, chromatographic and spectroscopic techniques were not as highly developed as they are now and more than two years work was required to isolate and identify the unknown component of the mixture, which proved to be the 4′-desmethoxy-1-epi analog (**49**) of the podophyllotoxin glucoside adduct (73). Present only in very small amounts in the derivatised extract, it was necessary to devise a synthesis from readily available materials. It was fortunate that the desired 1β configuration was readily secured from 1α-hydroxy-4′-desmethylpodophyllotoxin, itself obtained by selective demethylation of podophyllotoxin: the remainder of the synthesis would now be considered fairly routine (88).

Given a large supply of the key intermediate (**50**) it was straightforward to prepare a number of aldehyde derivatives, resulting in analogs with up to a 1000-fold increase in potency (89). The selected adducts were those prepared from thiophen-2-aldehyde, giving teniposide (**51**), and from acetaldehyde, giving etoposide (**52**). Both drugs are of value in the treatment of small-cell lung cancer, testicular cancer, lymphomas and leukemias. The thiophene derivative is also of use in the treatment of brain tumors (74).

The natural products, podophyllotoxin and its congeners, are 'spindle poisons' which inhibit cell proliferation by binding to tubulin and preventing formation of microtubules (86). Presumably this effect is sufficient to account for the success of podophyllin in the treatment of condylomata acuminata, although the crude extract contains many other candidates for a contribution to the biological activity. As has been described, a very minor component of the natural mixture, missing the 4′ hydroxy group, having the 1β- instead of the 1α-hydroxy configuration and with this hydroxy group conjugated with β-D-glucose, must be treated with an aldehyde to produce the highly active and most important derivatives. These derivatives do not bind to tubulin, but have been shown to be inhibitors of topoisomerase II, which may account for most of the observed biological effects, including DNA strand breaks, which lead to anticancer activity (90).

5 ANTIBIOTICS

5.1 The β-Lactams

In 1929, Alexander Fleming published the results of his chance finding that a Penicillium mould caused lysis of staphylococcal colonies on an agar plate (91). He also showed that the culture filtrate, named penicillin, possessed activity against important pathogens including Gram-positive bacteria and Gram-negative cocci. However, it was not until 1940 that the true

therapeutic efficacy of penicillin was revealed, when Chain et al. (92) successfully
tested the material in mice which had been
previously infected with a lethal dose of
streptococci. Several years later the precise
chemical structure of the main active component, benzylpenicillin (53), was determined and efforts to synthesize the compound were initiated (93). Benzylpencillin
proved to be an elusive target due to the
instability of the β-lactam ring: it was
unstable under acid conditions and was
deactivated by β-lactamase enzymes produced by various Gram-positive and Gram-
negative bacteria.

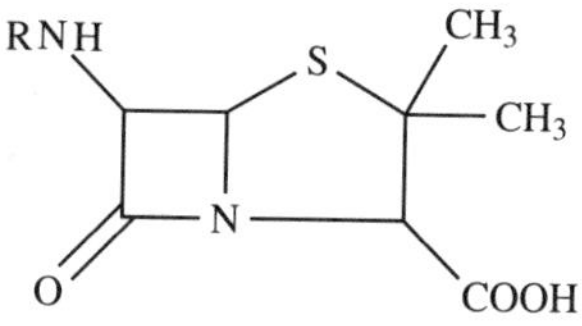

The discovery that the fused β-lactam
nucleus, 6-aminopenicillanic acid (6-APA)
(54), could be obtained from cultures of
Penicillium chrysogenum led to the preparation of new, semisynthetic derivatives
with improved stability to gastric acid and
β-lactamases, and with activity against a
wider range of pathogenic organisms (94).
Sheehan (95) showed that compound (54)
would react readily with acid chlorides to
form new penicillin derivatives with novel
substituents at the 6-position. Methicillin
(55), with a sterically demanding 2,6-di-
methoxybenzamide sidechain, was the first
semisynthetic penicillin to show resistance
to staphylococcal β-lactamases, but the
compound was still acid labile. Ampicillin
(56) has an α-aminophenylacetimido side-
chain and displays good activity against
Gram-negative organisms, it is stable to
acid and thus, can be administered orally
although it is susceptible to degradation by
β-lactamases. Amoxycillin (57) differs
from ampicillin by the addition of a single
hydroxy group, but the compound is better
absorbed by the gastrointestinal tract.

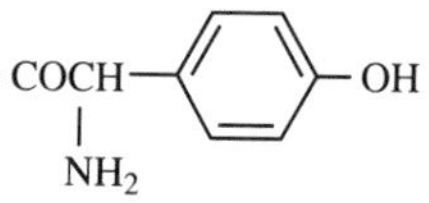

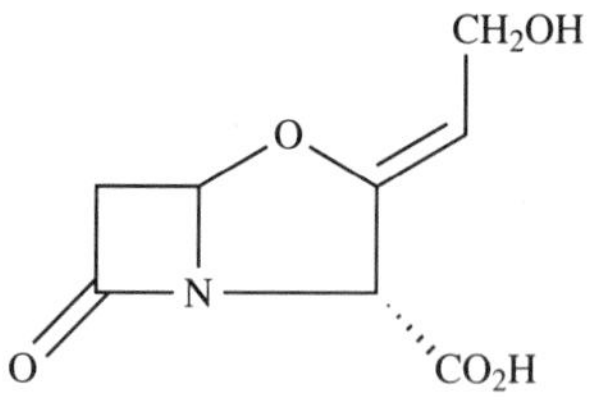

Clavulanic acid (58), isolated from
Streptomyces clavuligerus, is similar in
structure to the penicillins, except oxygen
replaces sulfur in the five-membered ring
(96). Clavulanic acid has weak antibacterial
activity, but is a potent inhibitor of β-
lactamases (97). A mixture of clavulanic

(53) benzylpenicillin   R = COCH₂Ph

(54) 6 - APA   R = H

(55) methicillin   R = CO—(2,6-dimethoxyphenyl)

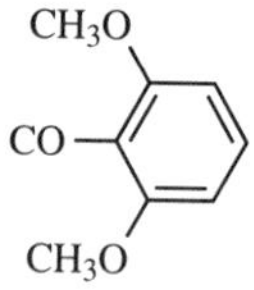

(56) ampicillin   R = COCHPh
                          |
                          NH₂

(57) amoxycillin   R = COCH—(4-hydroxyphenyl)—OH
                            |
                            NH₂

(58) clavulanic acid

acid and the β-lactamase-sensitive amoxycillin was introduced in 1981 as Augmentin and has proved to be an effective
combination used to combat β-lactamase-
producing bacteria (98). In 1991, ten years
after its launch, Augmentin became the
second best selling antibacterial worldwide.

The clinical introduction of the penicillin
group of antibiotics prompted an intensive
search for novel antibiotic-producing or-

ganisms and Selman Waksman demonstrated the value of actinomycetes in this role, discovering the aminoglycoside streptomycin (**59**) from *Streptomyces griseus* in 1943 (99). Pharmaceutical companies also embarked on large programs of screening soil samples for antibiotic-producing microorganisms (100). Chloroamphenicol (**60**) was isolated from *Streptomyces venezuelae* in 1948 and other clinically important antibiotics followed: chlortetracycline (**61**), neomycin (**62**), oxytetacyclin (**63**), erythromycin (**64**), oleandomycin (**65**), kanamycin (**66**) and rifamycin (**67**).

In 1948, Giuseppe Brotzu isolated the fungus *Cephalosporium acremonium* from a water sample collected off the coast of Sardinia. The culture showed significant antimicrobial activity, but Brotzu could not interest the Italian authorities in his discovery. He then turned to a friend in England for help, who arranged for Howard Florey at Oxford to receive a sample of the

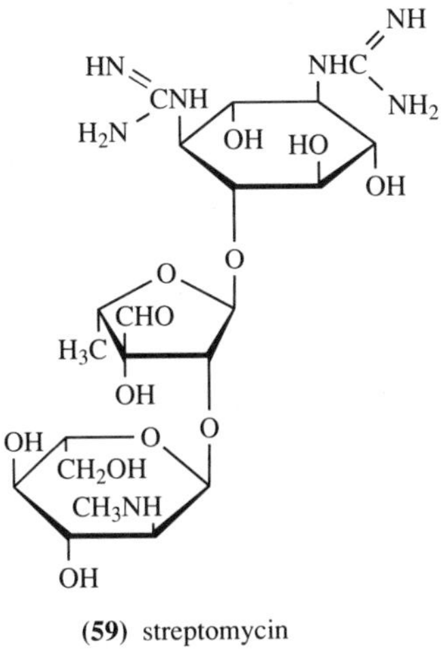

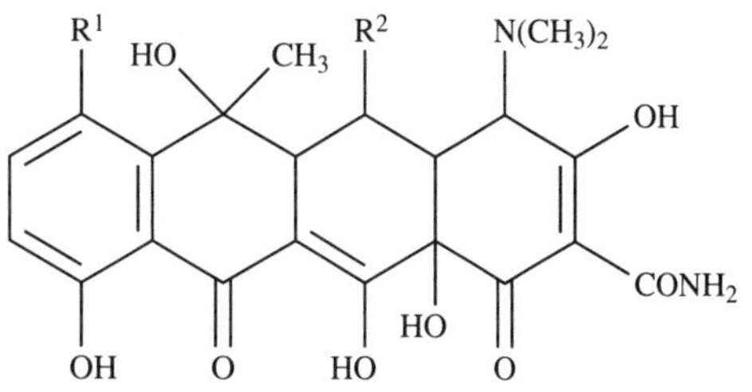

(**61**) chlortetracycline, R^1 = -Cl, R^2 = -H

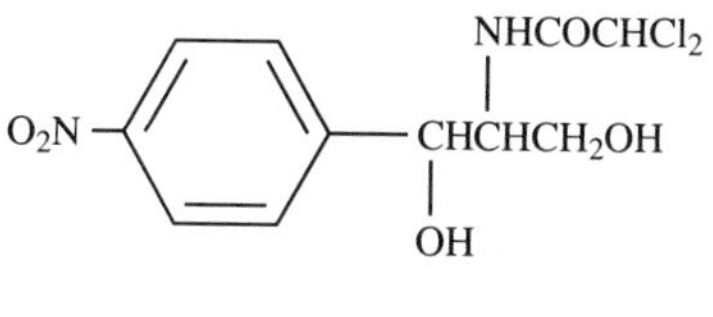

(**63**) oxytetracycline, R^1 = -H, R^2 = -OH

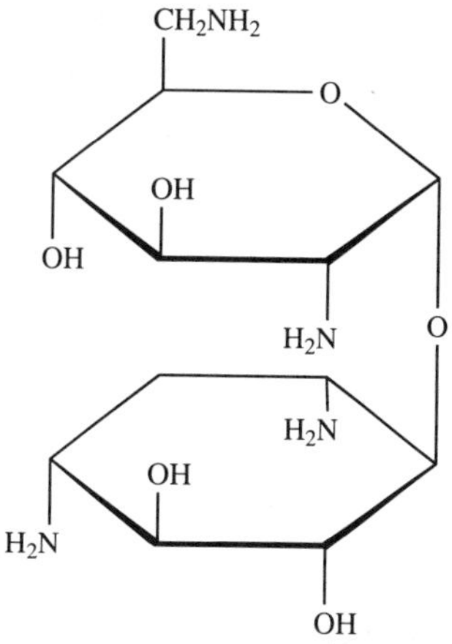

(**62**) neomycin

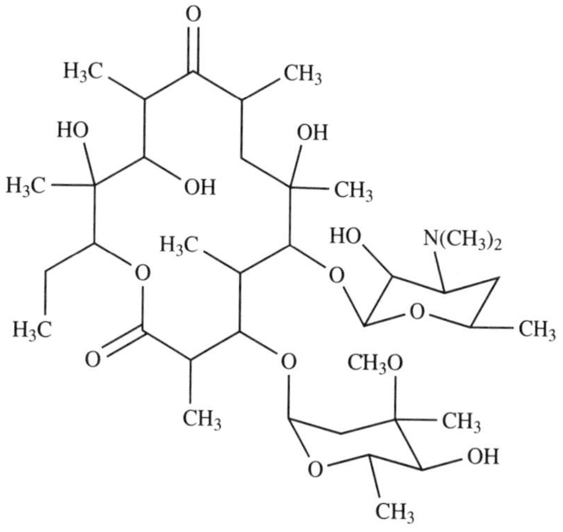

(**59**) streptomycin

(**60**) chloramphenicol

(**64**) erythromycin

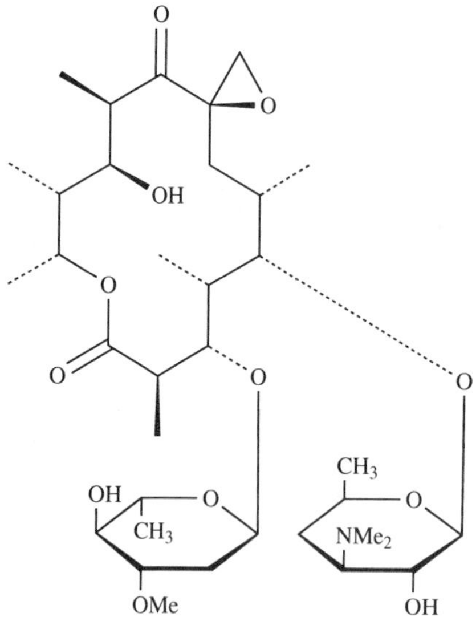

(65) oleandomycin

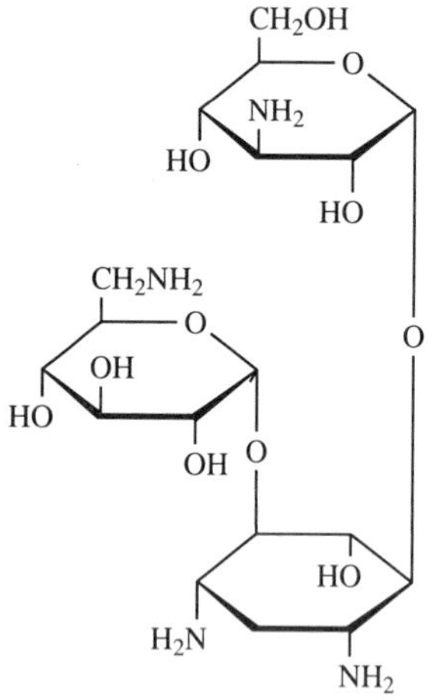

(66) kanamycin

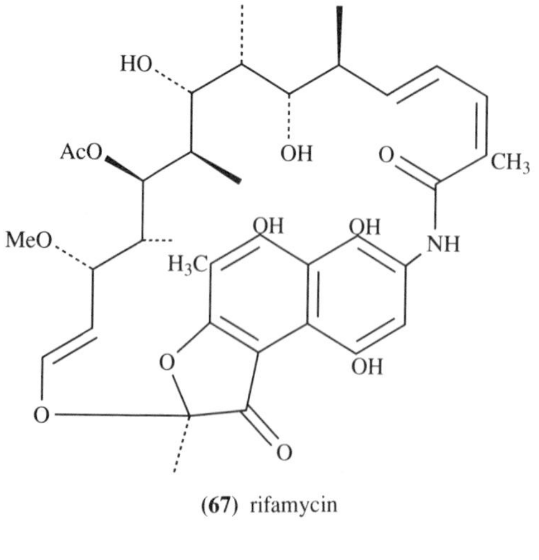

(67) rifamycin

producing culture. Eventually, an antibacterial substance was isolated and named cephalosporin C (**68**) (101). The compound, which had a similar structure to the penicillins, except it had a dihydrothiazine ring fused to the β-lactam core, showed good resistance to β-lactamases and was less toxic then benzylpenicillin. However, plans to market the compound were terminated with the introduction of methicillin (*supra vide*).

The discovery that the basic structural building block of cephalosporin C, namely 7-aminocephalosporanic acid (7-ACA) (**69**), could be synthesized led to the preparation of numerous cephalosporin derivatives in a similar way to the synthesis of penicillins from 6-aminopenicillanic acid (102, 103). Modification of the substituent at the 7-position, while retaining the 3-acetoxymethyl group, gave cephalothin (**70**), cephacetrile (**71**) and cephapirin (**72**), so-called "first generation" cephalosporins

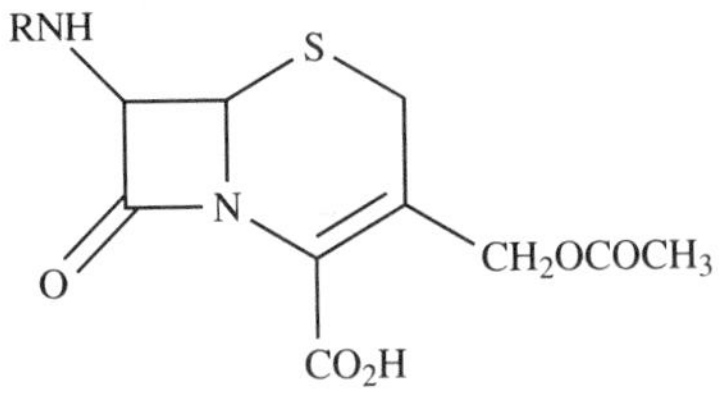

(**68**) cephalosporin C　　R = COCH₂CH₂CH₂CHNH₂

(**69**) 7-ACA　　R = H

(**70**) cephalothin　　R = COCH₂

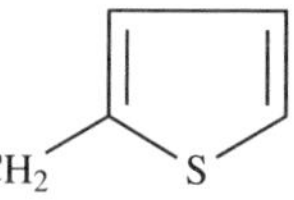

(**71**) cephacetrile　　R = COCH₂CN

(**72**) cephapirin　　R = COCH₂S

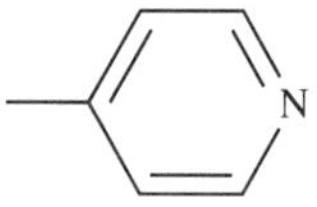

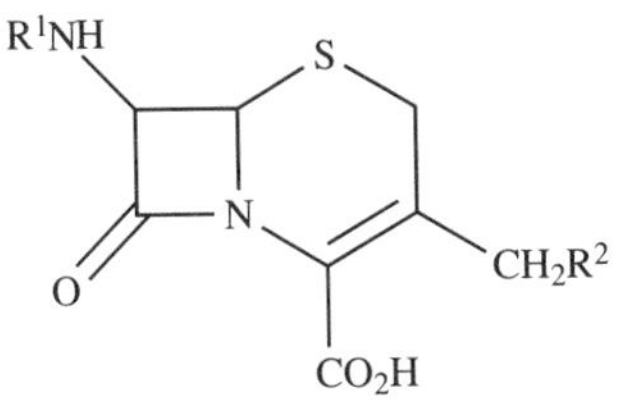

R^{1}NH

(73) cephaloridine   R^1 = COCH$_2$

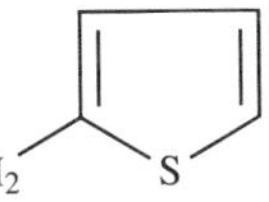

R^2 =

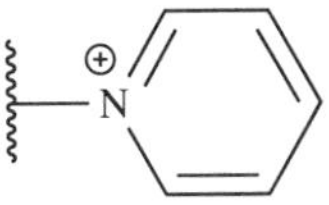

(74) cephaloglycin   R^1 = COCHPh

R^2 = OCOCH$_3$

(75) cephalexin   R^1 = COCHPh

R^2 = H

(76) cefadroxil   R^1 = COCH

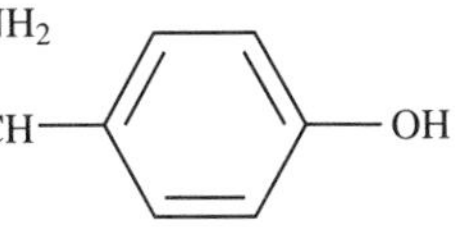

R^2 = H

(77) cephradine   R^1 = COCH

R^2 = H

CH$_2$R^2

CO$_2$H

R^{1}NH

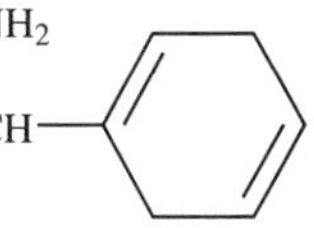

R^2

CO$_2$H

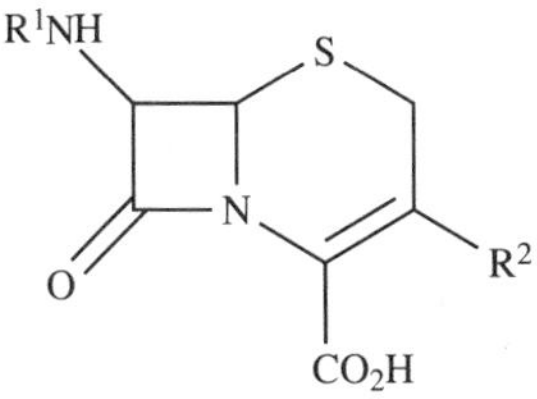

(78) cefaclor   R^1 = COCHPh   R^2 = Cl

(79) cephamandole   R^1 = COCHPh   R^2 = CH$_2$S

   CH$_3$

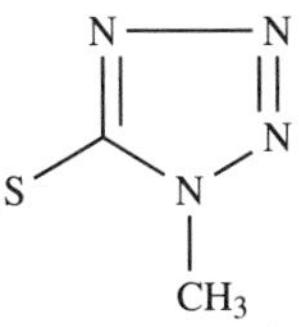

(80) cefuroxime   R^1 = COC   R^2 = CH$_2$OCONH$_2$

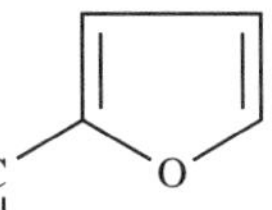

NOCH$_3$

(81) ceftazidime $R^1 = COC$ ... NH_2 $R^2 = CH_2-N^{\oplus}$ (pyridinium)

$OC(CH_3)_2$
CO_2H

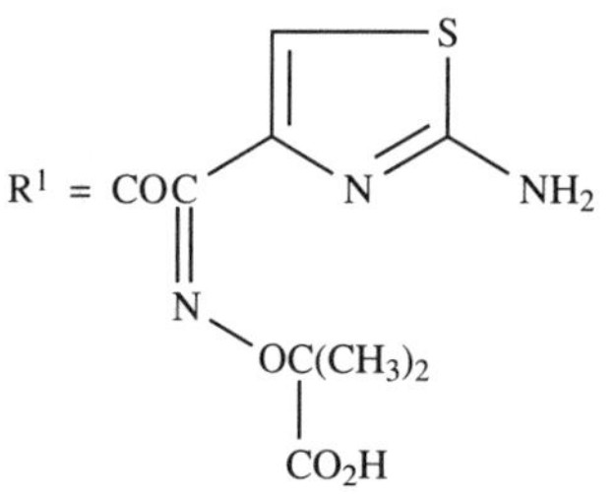

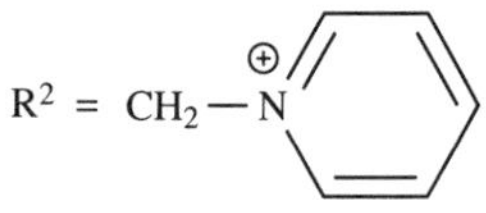

(82) ceftizoxime 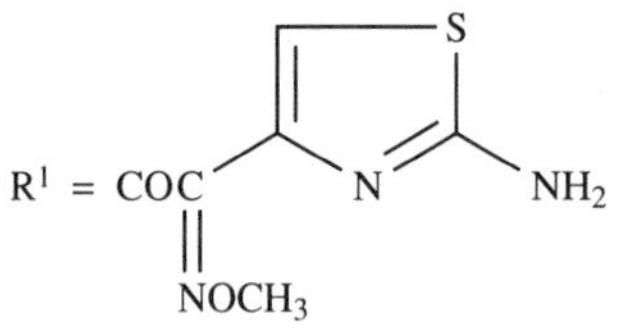 $R^1 = COC$ ... NH_2 $R^2 = H$

$NOCH_3$

(83) ceftriaxone $R^1 = COC$ ... NH_2 $R^2 = CH_2S$ (triazinyl)

$NOCH_3$

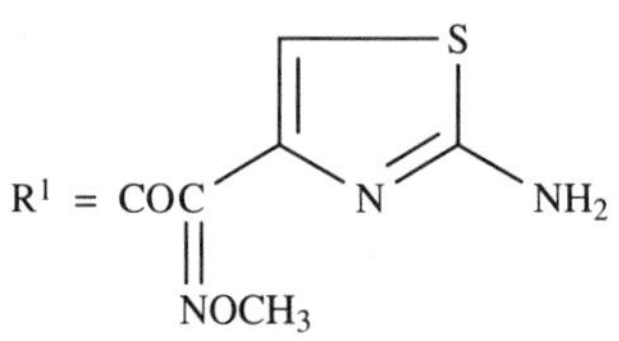

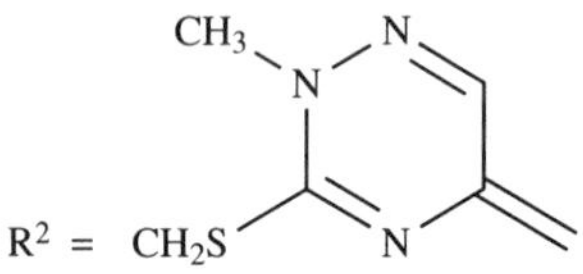

with good activity against Gram-positive bacteria, although the acetyl ester was susceptible to degradation by esterases and thus, limited the duration of action. Replacement of the acetoxy group by other substituents rendered the products less prone to esterase attack. For example, the pyridinium derivative, cephaloridine (73), has a longer duration of action than cephalothin.

The first orally active cephalosporin was cephaloglycin (74), which possessed a phenylglycine substituent in the C-7 sidechain, although the labile 3-acetoxymethyl group was retained. Replacing the acetoxy group with a proton or chlorine, for example cephalexin (75), cefadroxil (76), cephradine (77) and cefaclor (78), extended the duration of action of these orally active products. Cefaclor has been classified as a "second generation" cephalosporin because it has a wider spectrum of activity which includes Gram-negative bacteria such as

Haemophilus influenzae. Cephamandole (79) and cefuroxime (80) are parenterally administered cephalosporins with similar activities against clinically important Gram-negative bacteria and are also resistant to many types of β-lactamases.

The newer "third generation" cephalosporins, including ceftazidime (81), ceftizoxime (82) and ceftriaxone (83), which all contain an α-aminothiazolyl group in the C-7 sidechain, have been developed for treating specific pathogens such as *Pseudomonas aeruginosa.*

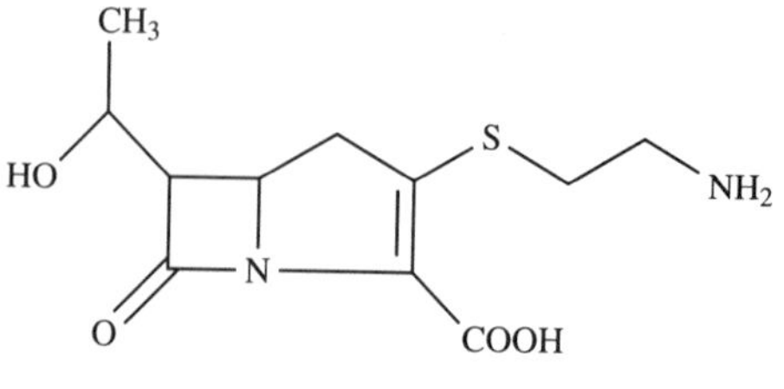

(84) thienamycin

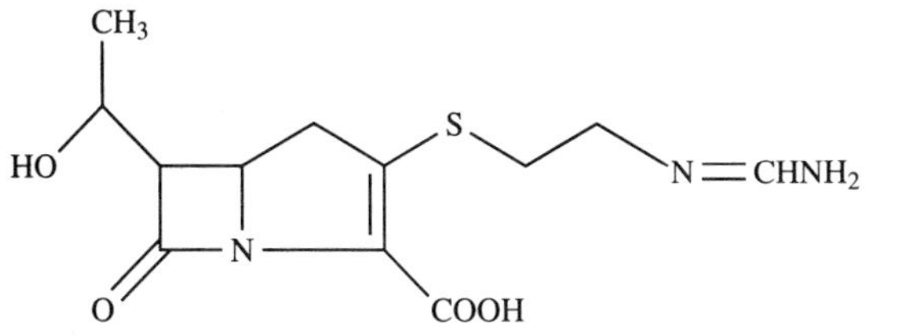

(85) imipenem

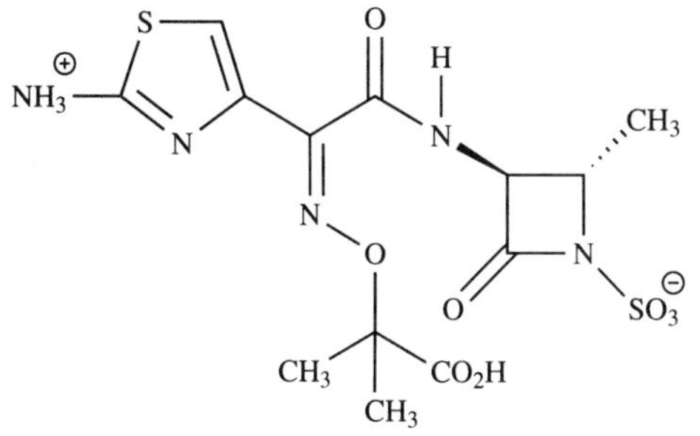

(86) azetreonam

a sidechain component common to the third generation cephalosporins (*supra vide*), showed specific activity against Gram-negative aerobic bacteria, including *Pseudomonas* spp., and was stable to most types of β-lactamases. The compound, aztreonam (**86**), became the first commercially available monobactam and showed a similar mode of action to the other β-lactam antibiotics by blocking bacterial cell wall synthesis (109).

5.2 Erythromycin Macrolides

Erythromycin (**87**) was isolated, in 1952, from a strain of *Saccharopolyspora erythraea* (formerly *Streptomyces erythreus*). As a broad-spectrum antibiotic erythromycin has proved invaluable for the treatment of bacterial infections in patients with β-lactam hypersensitivity and is also the drug of choice in the treatment of infections caused by species of *Legionella*, *Mycoplasma*, *Campylobacter* and *Bordetella* (110). It is surprising that in the forty years since the first clinical trials of erythromycin, few alternative or competing macrolides have surfaced.

Although safe and effective, erythromycin is not a perfect antibacterial. The presence of hydroxy groups suitably disposed with respect to the keto function at C9 leads to the formation of a tautomeric mixture of hemiketals which has only recently been characterized (111). The 6,9-hemiketal (**88**) may be dehydrated in stomach acid to give the inactive Δ_8 analog (**89**) which may undergo further ring closure to give the 9,12-tetrahydrofuran (**90**) which is also inactive (112) (eq. 24.5). The Δ_8 derivative (**89**) may be responsible for some gastrointestinal disturbance (113). To avoid these problems by increasing the stability to acid, the 2′-stearate, estolate and ethylsuccinate esters have been prepared (114), but even when the tablets are enteric-coated the bioavailability is erratic

Thienamycin (**84**), isolated from *Streptomyces cattleya* in 1976, represented a new class of β-lactam antibiotics produced by bacteria where the sulfur of the penicillin nucleus was replaced by a methylene group (104). An *N*-formylimidoyl derivative, imipenem (**85**), was the first example from this new class of carbapenem antibiotics to become available for clinical use (105). Imipenem has a very broad spectrum of activity against most Gram-positive and Gram-negative aerobic and anaerobic bacteria.

Screening bacteria such as *Pseudomonas acidophila* and *Chromobacterium violacium* for production of β-lactam antibiotics resulted in the discovery of naturally occurring monobactams which had moderate antimicrobial activity (106–108). Side-chain variations, as developed for the penicillins and cephalosporins, led to compounds with improved activity against both Gram-positive and Gram-negative bacteria. A derivative containing the α-aminothiazoyl group,

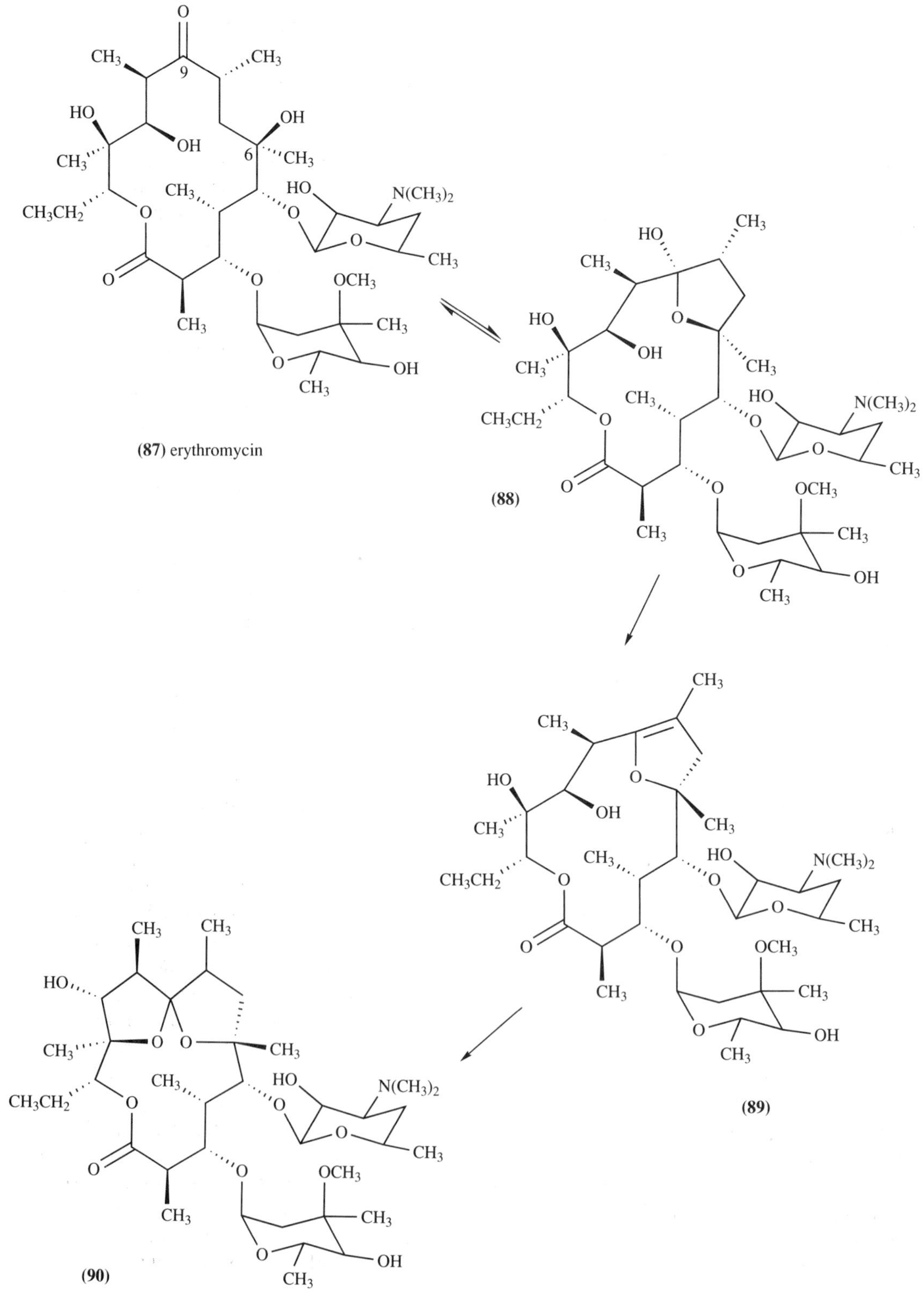

(87) erythromycin

(88)

(89)

(90)

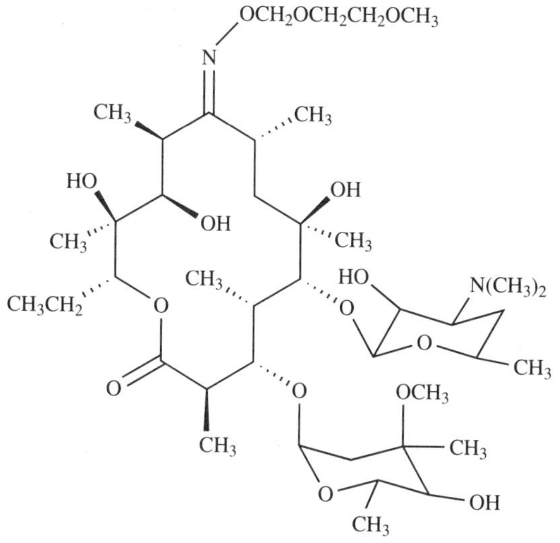

(91) roxithromycin

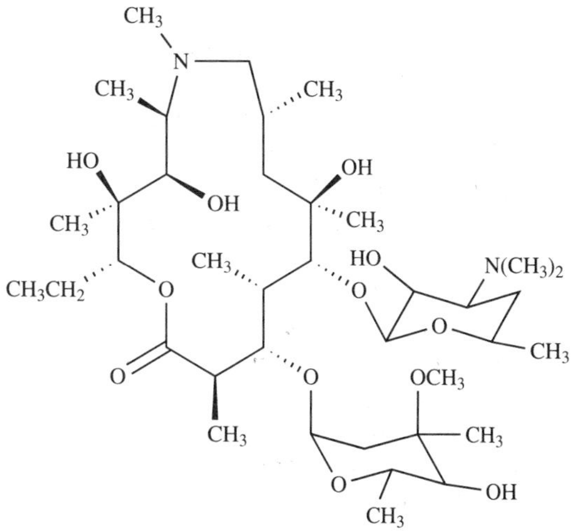

(93) azithromycin

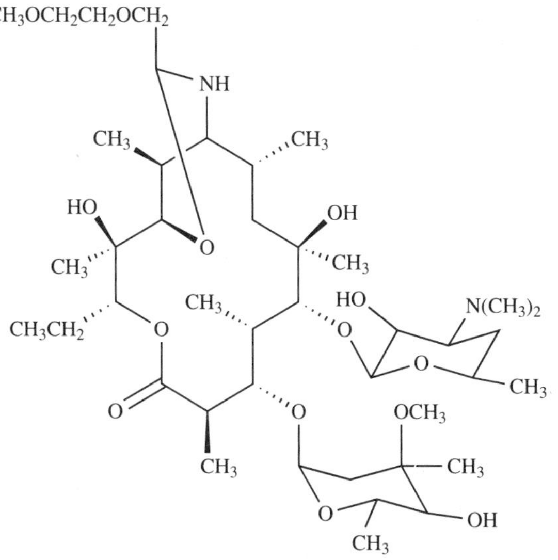

(92) dithromycin

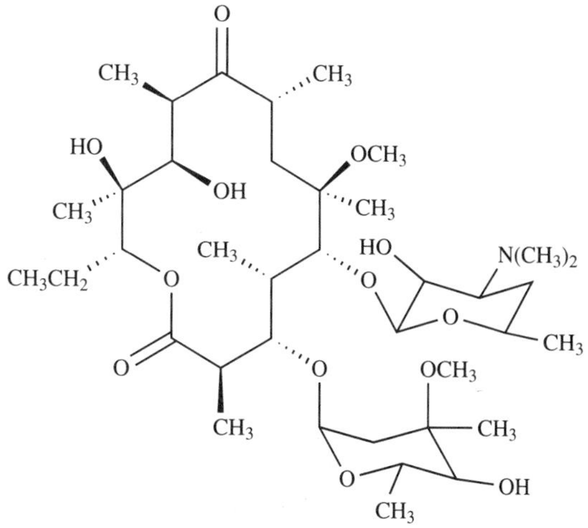

(94) clarithromycin

and relatively frequent dosing is required (110).

An understanding of the acid-catalyzed decomposition of erythromycin has led to a variety of very promising semisynthetic derivatives with improved oral bioavailability (115). The earliest of these was roxithromycin (91), which as a derivative of the oxime formed from the 9-ketone is less susceptible to acid-catalysed ring closure. Reductive amination of the 9-keto function gives erythromycylamine, which reacts with (2-methoxyethoxy)acetaldehyde (116) to give dirithromycin (92). Beckmann rearrangement of the 9-oxime followed by reduction and methylation (117) gives azithromycin (**93**) which shows good activity against Gram-negative bacteria, including *Haemophilus influenzae*. An alternative for prevention of cyclization between the 9-keto and 6-hydroxy is to mask the 6-hydroxy group. If the 6-hydroxy is methylated (118) the result is clarithromycin (**94**), which like (**91**), (**92**), and (**93**) has an improved pharmacokinetic profile compared to the parent molecule. Both azithromycin and clarithromycin have been approved for the treatment of various bacterial infections.

5.3 Echinocandins

The fungal metabolite echinocandin B (**95**) is one of the lipopeptides, in which a cyclic hexapeptide is combined with a long-chain fatty acid. Echinocandin B inhibits β-1,3-glucan synthesis and as a result has anti-Candida and anti-*Pneumocystis carinii* activity (119). As a group, the echinocandins are not orally bioavailable and are not very water-soluble (120) despite the hydrogen-bonding ability of the polyhydroxylated hexapeptide.

Synthesis of the cyclic hexapeptide is unattractive for the purpose of securing analogs with improved biological activity, owing to the unusual nature of the amino acids used and the complex stereochemistry generated by the high degree of hydroxylation. However, echinocandin B can be produced efficiently by fermentation of a culture of *Aspergillus nidulans* and then de-acylated by fermentation with *Actinoplanes utahensis* (121). The free amino group thus exposed can be derivatized with a number of active esters. Synthesis of the amide from 4-octylbenzoic acid gives

(**95**) echinocandin B, R = linoleyl

(**96**) cilofungin, R = —⟨benzene ring⟩—O(CH$_2$)$_7$CH$_3$

cilofungin (**96**), which has specifically high potency against *Candida albicans* and some other Candida species (121).

For systemic use cilofungin must be given intravenously and appears to be well tolerated. Given orally, the drug will eliminate Candida from the gastrointestinal tract (121).

An alternative approach in this chemical series starts with the echinocandin L-688, 786 (**97**), which differs from echinocandin B in the long-chain fatty acid and in some details in the hexapeptide (120). In this case the semisynthetic modification involves derivatization of the phenolic hydroxy group of the homotyrosine residue to

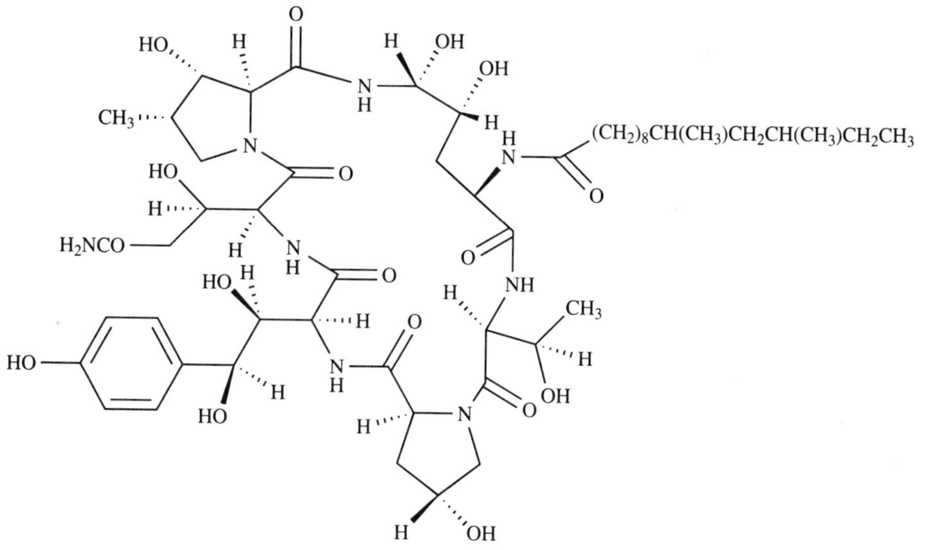

(**97**)

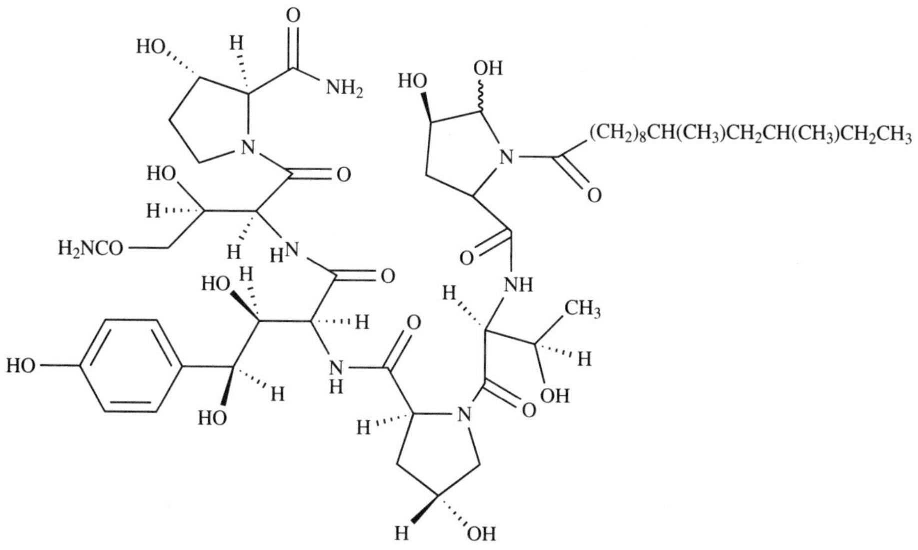

(**98**)

(99)

give enzymatically labile phosphate, carbamate, carbonate, or ester links. The derivatization step uses base catalysis, which carries the complication that the hydroxylated ornithine sidechain linked to one of the proline residues is a proaldehyde which is unstable in base, with irreversible ring-opening to give (**98**). Success depends on the use of solid LiOH.H$_2$O in dimethylformamide, which owing to limited solubility does not generate a strongly basic solution in the presence of excess derivatizing agent. The flexibility thus engendered in prodrug design allowed the synthesis of nine potential antimicrobial agents, of which the phosphate ester L-693, 989 (**99**) has been selected for potential development in the treatment of *P. carinii* infections and candidiasis.

6 CARDIOVASCULAR DRUGS

6.1 Lovastatin, Simvastatin, and Pravastatin

One of the most significant natural product discoveries in the last twenty years has been a fungal secondary metabolite called lovastatin (**100**). Heralded as a major breakthrough in the treatment of coronary heart disease (122), lovastatin was introduced onto the market by Merck in 1987 for the treatment of hypercholesterolemia, a condition marked by elevated levels of cholesterol in the blood.

Lovastatin works by inhibiting 3-hydroxy-3-methylglutaryl coenzyme A (HMG-CoA) reductase, a key rate-limiting enzyme in the cholesterol biosynthetic pathway. However, the first specific inhibitors of this enzyme were discovered several years earlier by Endo et al. at Sankyo (123). The compounds, which are structurally related to lovastatin, were isolated from *Penicillium citrinum* and shown to block cholesterol synthesis in rats and lower cholesterol levels in the blood. Development of the most active compound, designated ML-236B (**101**), is believed to have been curtailed due to toxicity problems (124).

Brown et al. at Beechams also reported the isolation of (**101**), but as a metabolite from *Penicillium brevicompactum* (125). The group, naming the compound compactin, reported its antifungal activity but failed to reveal its mode of action as an inhibitor of HMG-CoA reductase.

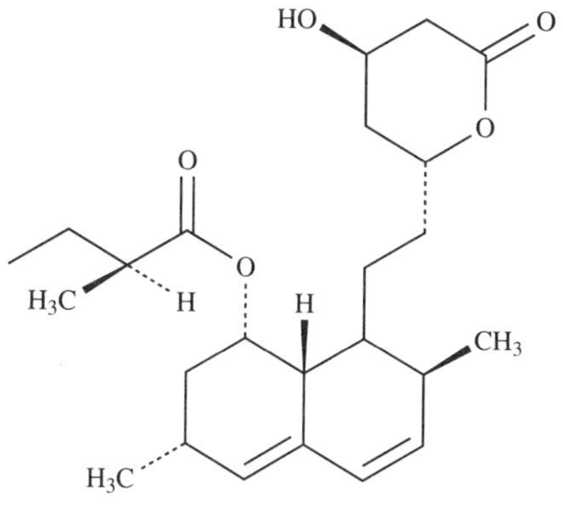

(100) lovastatin

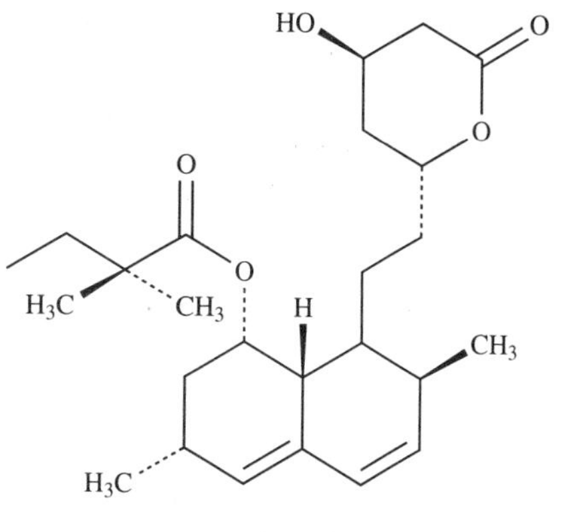

(102) simvastatin

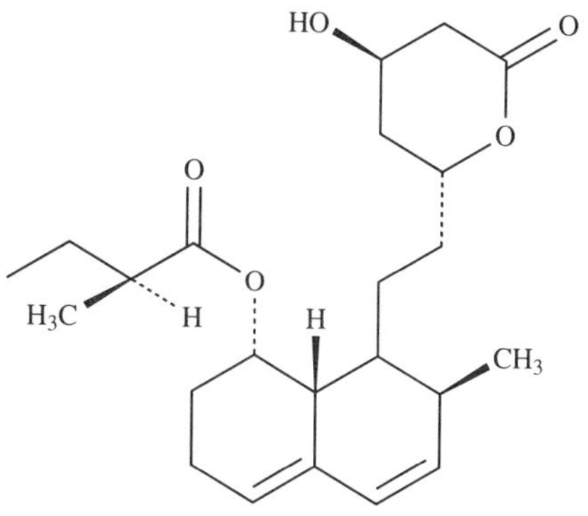

(101) compactin

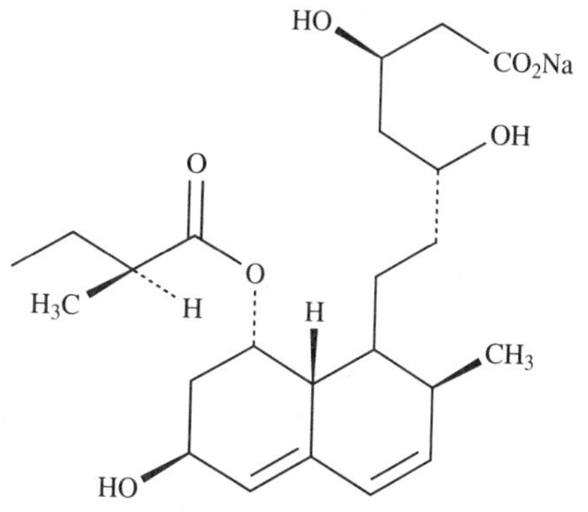

(103) pravastatin

The search for naturally occurring inhibitors of HMG-CoA reductase gained pace and after spending several years developing appropriate screens, Merck found during only the second week of testing a culture of *Aspergillus terreus* which displayed interesting inhibitory activity (126). In February 1979 the active component, lovastatin (mevinolin), was isolated and characterized (127), and in November the following year Merck were granted patent protection in the United States. Although lovastatin proved to be identical to monocolin K, a metabolite isolated earlier from *Monasus ruber* (128), the chemical structure of the latter compound had not been reported, whereas Merck filed for patent

protection giving complete structural details for lovastatin.

The discovery of compactin and lovastatin prompted efforts to develop derivatives with improved biological properties (129, 130). Modification of the methylbutyryl sidechain of lovastatin led to a series of new ester derivatives with varying potency and, in particular, introduction of an additional methyl group α to the carbonyl gave a compound with 2.5 times the intrinsic enzyme activity of lovastatin (131). The new derivative, named simvastatin (**102**), was the second HMG-CoA reductase inhibitor to be marketed by Merck and a third compound, pravastatin (**103**), has been launched by Sankyo and Squibb.

Pravastatin is the 6-hydroxy open hydroxy-acid derivative of compactin and was first identified as a urinary metabolite in dogs. Pravastatin is produced by microbial biotransformation of compactin.

6.2 Teprotide and Captopril

While studying the physiological effects of snake poisoning, Ferreira (132) discovered that specific components in the venom of the pit viper *Bothrops jararaca* inhibited degradation of the peptide bradykinin and potentiated its hypotensive action. The "potentiating factors" proved to be a family of peptides that worked by inhibiting the dipeptidyl carboxypeptidase, angiotensin converting enzyme (ACE) (133, 134). In addition to catalysing the degradation of bradykinin, ACE also catalyzes the conversion of human prohormone, angiotensin I, to the potent vasoconstrictor octapeptide, angiotensin II. However, the significance of ACE in the pathogenesis of hypertension was not fully appreciated until the 1970s after Ondetti et al. (135) had first isolated and then synthesized the naturally occurring nonapeptide, teprotide (**104**). The compound proved to a specific potent inhibitor of ACE and showed excellent antihypertensive properties in clinical trials, although its use was limited by the lack of oral activity.

The discovery of teprotide led to a search for new, specific, orally active ACE inhibitors. Ondetti et al. (135) proposed a hypothetical model of the active site of ACE, based on analogy with pancreatic carboxypeptidase A, and used it to predict and design compounds that would occupy the carboxy-terminal binding site of the enzyme. Carboxyalkanoyl and mercaptoalkanoyl derivatives of proline were found to act as potent, specific inhibitors of ACE and 2-D-methyl-3-mercaptopropanoyl-L-proline (**105**) (captopril) was developed and launched in 1981 as an orally active

Pyr-Trp-Pro-Arg-Pro-Gln-Ile-Pro-Pro

(104) teprotide

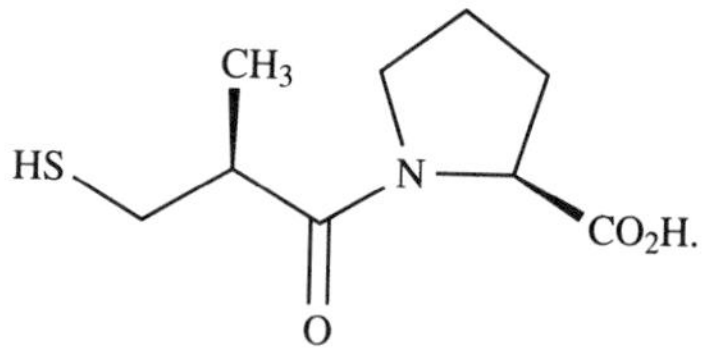

(105) captopril

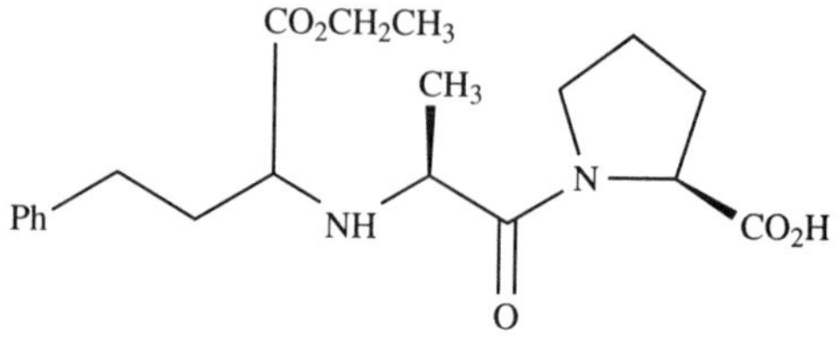

(106) enalapril

treatment for patients with severe, or advanced hypertension. Captopril, modeled on the biologically active peptides found in the venom of the pit viper, made an important contribution to the understanding of hypertension and paved the way for other ACE inhibitors, such as enalapril (**106**), which have had a major impact on the treatment of cardiovascular disease (136).

6.3 Dicoumarol and Warfarin

Sweet clover has a long history of medicinal use, often as an antiflammatory or analgesic preparation in the form of ointments and poultices. *Melilotus officinalis* (yellow sweet clover, or ribbed melilot) was reputed to have been a favorite herbal treatment used by King Henry VIII of England and the plant is still referred to as King's Clover in some publications (137).

The plant flourishes on poor soil and was cultivated extensively in Europe for cattle fodder and for soil improvement. In the early 1920s *M. officinalis* was planted on the prairies of North Dakota and Alberta, Canada, but with disastrous consequences. Soon cattle and sheep throughout these regions began literally bleeding to death. The mysterious hemorrhagic disease was traced to clover fodder which had not been stored properly and had become "spoiled", or moldy. However, the insolubility of the anticoagulant component and the difficulty of assaying extracts for biological activity made the task of isolating the active principle intractable (138). It took almost 20 years before the compound was identified as 3,3′-methylenebis(4-hydroxycoumarin) (**107**), an oxidative degradation metabolite of coumarin (**108**), itself a common component of *Melilotus* sp. Soon after the compound had been identified, trials were initiated which confirmed the oral anticoagulant activity in humans and in 1942 it was marketed under the name dicoumarol (**139**). The compound had a slow, erratic onset of action and efforts were initiated to prepare synthetic analogs which acted faster and had longer duration of action. A 4-hydroxycoumarin residue, substituted at the 3-position, proved essential for biological activity and in 1948, after synthesizing over 150 compounds, a 4-hydroxycoumarin derivative which was longer acting and more potent than dicoumarol was selected, not for clinical use, but as a rodenticide for development by the Wisconsin Alumni Research Foundation! The compound (**109**) named warfarin (an acronym derived from the name of the institute coupled with "arin" from coumarin), became a household name for rat poison. Concern over the use of oral anticoagulants and the inherent risk of haemorrhage inhibited the development of warfarin as a therapeutic agent. However, in 1951, a US army cadet unsuccessfully attempted to commit suicide by taking massive doses of the compound. The incident prompted further clinical trials which resulted in warfarin being used as the

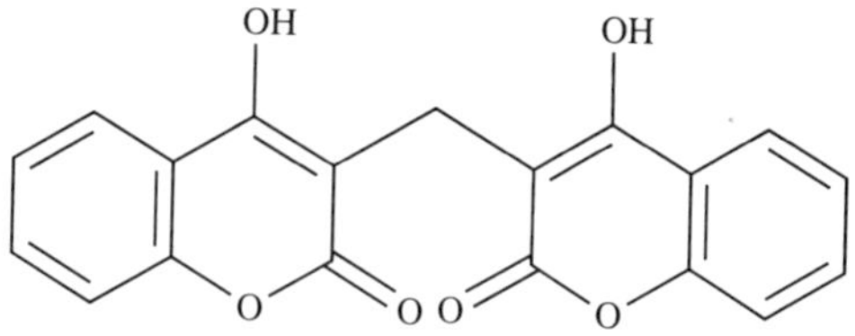

(**107**)

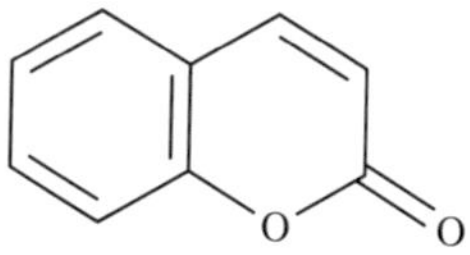

(**108**) coumarin

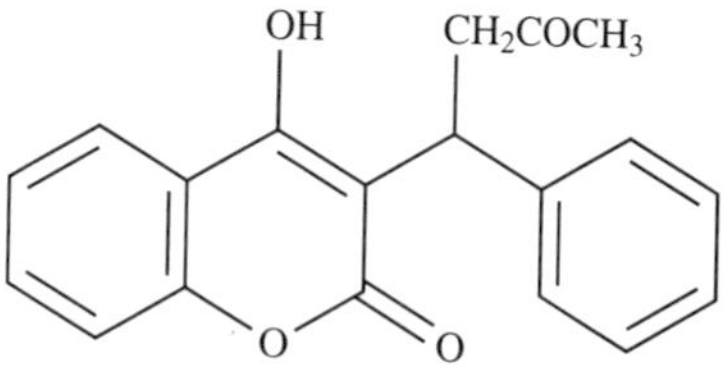

(**109**) warfarin

anticoagulant of choice for prevention of thromboembolic disease (139).

The mode of action of the coumarin anticoagulants involves blocking the regeneration of reduced vitamin K and induces a state of functional vitamin K deficiency, thus interfering with the blood-clotting mechanism (140).

7 ANTIASTHMA DRUGS

7.1 Khellin and Sodium Cromoglycate

The toothpick plant, *Ammi visnaga*, had been used for centuries in Egypt as an antispasmodic agent to treat renal colic and ureteral spasm. In 1879, one of the plant's main constituents was isolated, crystallized and named khellin (**110**) (141). Subsequently, the pure compound was shown to relax smooth muscle and in 1938 the chemical structure was characterized as a chromone derivative (142). In 1945, a medical technician took khellin to treat renal colic and found instead that it acted as a potent coronary vasodilator and relieved his angina (143)! This chance discovery, together with earlier observations, led to khellin being used as a coronary artery vasodilator and for treating bronchial asthma (144). However, its clinical use was severely limited by some unpleasant gastrointestinal side effects.

Five years later, a small British pharmaceutical company called Benger Laboratories, initiated a program to synthesize khellin analogs as potential bronchodilators for treating asthma, and had prepared a series of compounds which relaxed guinea-pig bronchial smooth muscle and protected the animals against allergen-induced bronchospasm (145).

A clinical pharmacologist on Benger's staff, who suffered from chronic asthma, questioned the validity of the animal model and decided instead to test the compounds on himself! He then prepared a "soup" of

guinea-pig fur, inhaled the vapors to induce a reproducible asthma attack and assessed the effects of the synthesised khellin derivatives. Many of the compounds first prepared were insoluble in water and caused nausea and other unpleasant side effects when taken orally. This led to the test compounds being formulated as aerosol sprays and in 1958, an aerosol preparation of a chromone-2-carboxylic acid derivative (111), was found to exert a protectant effect, albeit short lived, against bronchial allergen challenge without showing the bronchodilator activity seen with other compounds. The compound was completely inactive in the guinea-pig asthma model and only afforded its protectant effect in humans when inhaled as an aerosol.

About two new compounds were tested each week and in 1965, after synthesizing some 670 analogs, a bischromone was prepared with gave good protection, even when inhaled up to six hours before bronchial allergen challenge (146). The compound, sodium cromoglycate (112), was obtained by condensing diethyl oxalate with the bis(hydroxy acetophenone) (113) and cyclizing the resultant bis(2,4-diox-

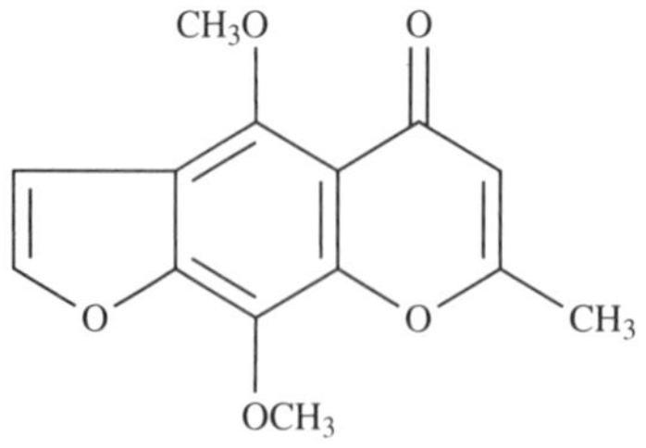

(110) khellin

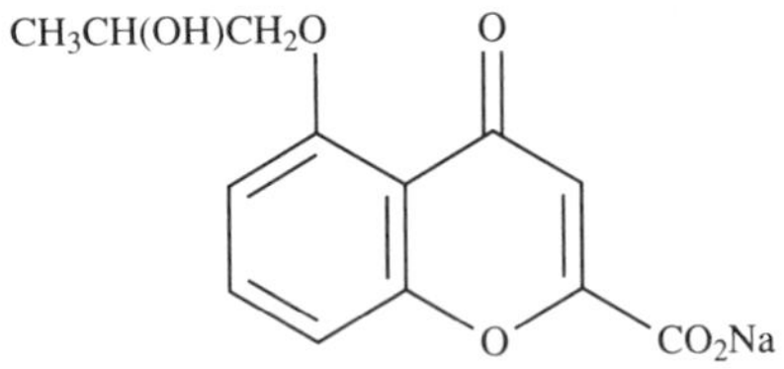

(111)

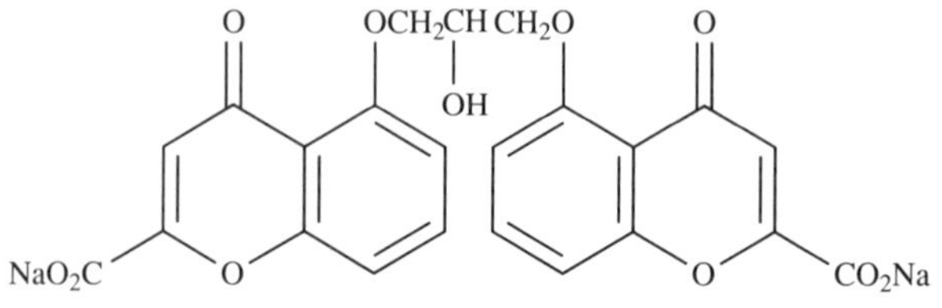

(112) sodium cromoglycate

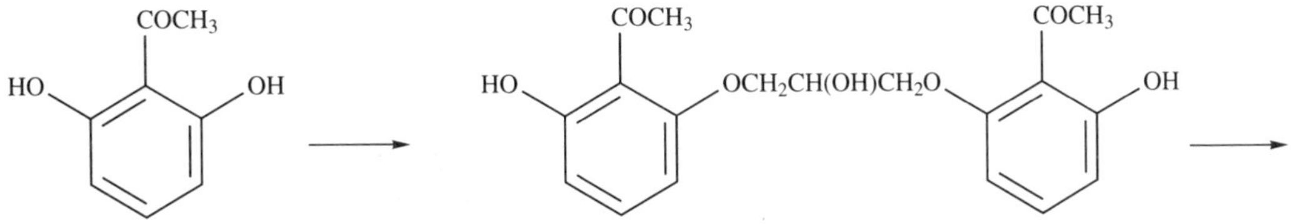

(113)

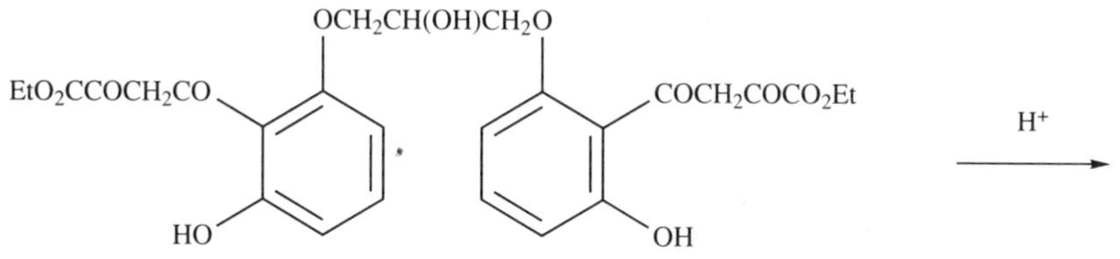

(114)

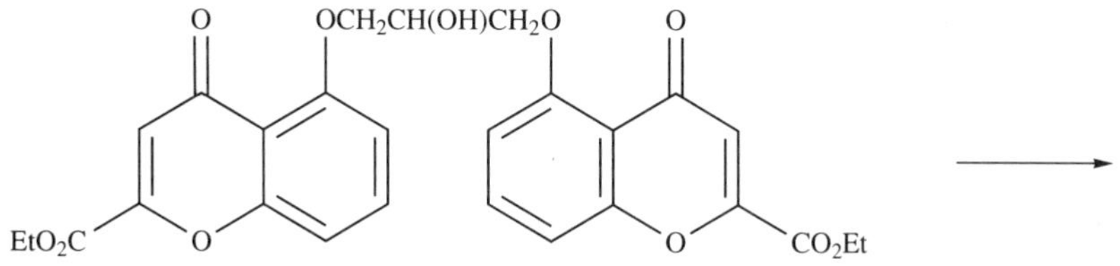

(112)

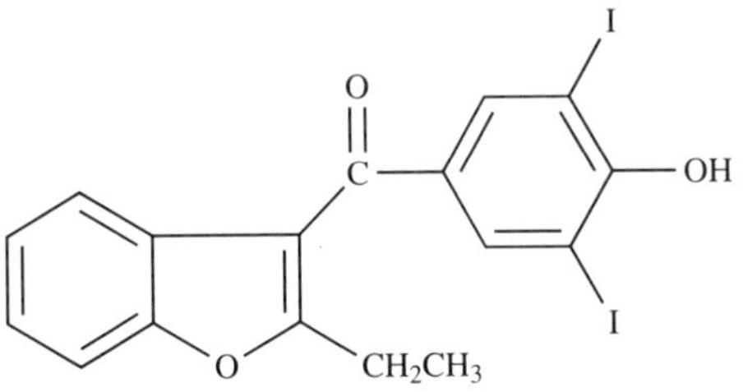

(115) benziodarone

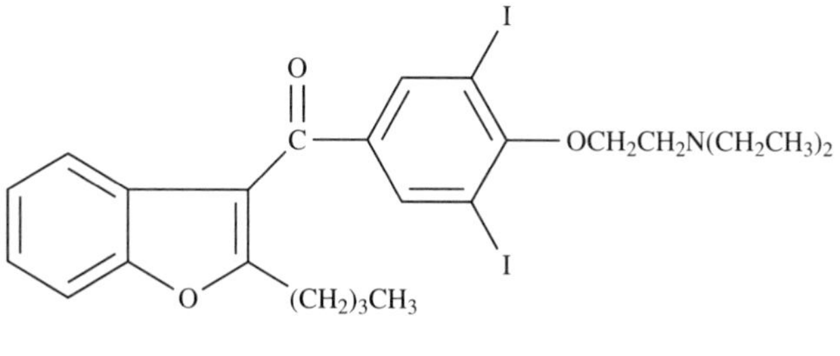

(116) amiodarone

butyric acid) ester (**114**) under acidic conditions (147) (eq. 24.6). The essential chemical features required for activity appeared to be the coplanarity of the chromone nuclei, the flexible dioxyalkyl link and the carboxyl groups in the 2-positions. It is believed to act by stabilizing tissue mast cells against degranulation, thereby preventing release of inflammatory mediators (148).

Sodium cromoglycate entered clinical trials in 1967 and emerged to become a first-line prophylactic treatment for bronchial asthma.

The coronary dilator properties of khellin have not been ignored and at least one successful program was initiated to prepare analogs for testing as potential antiangina drugs (149, 150). Benziodarone (**115**) was the first useful compound to emerge from the Labaz laboratories in Belgium based on the benzofuran ring system. However, the compound caused hepatotoxicity in man and was soon superseded by amiodarone (**116**), a more potent coronary dilator for treating angina. In 1970, the first report of anti-arrhythmic activity in the clinic was published (151) and amiodarone became established for prophylactic control of supraventricular and ventricular arrhythmias during the 1980s (150).

7.2 Ephedrine, Isopenaline and Salbutamol

The Chinese have been using a plant extract known as "ma huang" to treat asthma and hay fever for thousands of years. The extract is prepared from several species of *Ephedra*, a small leafless shrub found in China. Following experiments at the Peking Union Medical College and then at the University of Pennsylvania and the Mayo Clinic in the United States, the active ingredient, ephedrine (**117**), was introduced into western medicine in 1926 as an orally active bronchodilator for the treatment of acute asthma (152, 153).

Ephedrine is related to another natural product which has been used to treat asthma, namely the adrenal hormone adrenaline (**118**) (epinephrine). Adrenaline is a potent agonist of both α- and β-adrenoceptors and thus, produces arterial hypertension as an undesirable side effect. In 1951, a synthetic alternative, isoprenaline (**119**), was introduced and for almost 20 years it was considered the drug of choice for treating bronchospasm associated with acute asthmatic attack (153). Isoprenaline is a specific β-adrenoceptor agonist and although it has no vasoconstrictor activity, the compound does have marked cardiac

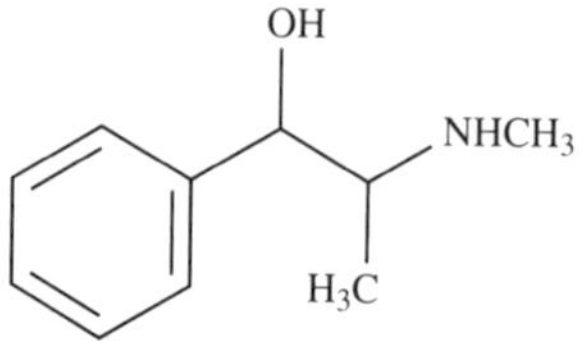

(**117**) ephedrine

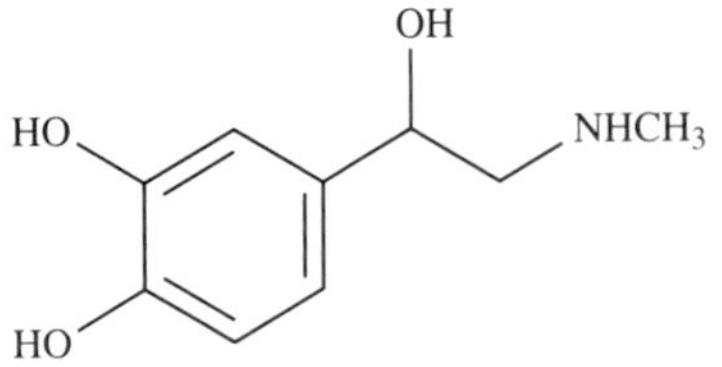

(**118**) adrenaline

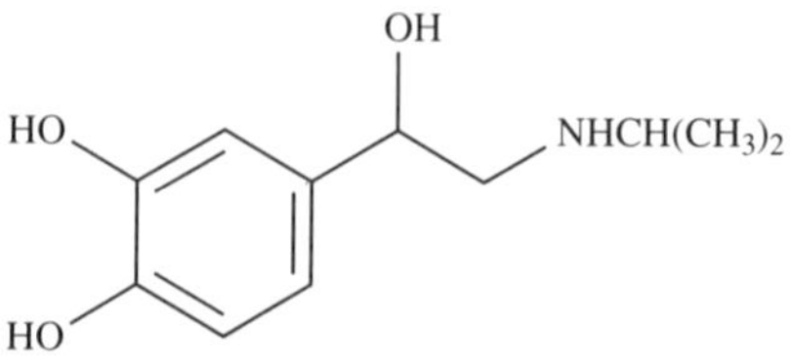

(**119**) isoprenaline

(120) salbutamol

(121) salmeterol

stimulant properties and a short duration of action. Ahlquist's concept (154) of two types of adrenoceptor was developed further by Lands et al. (155) who established the existence of β_1- and β_2-adrenoceptor subtypes. Clear structure activity relationships emerged with the preparation of compounds related to adrenaline and ephedrine; the basic requirement for β-adrenoceptor agonist activity was an aromatic ring substituted by an ethanolamine sidechain, the branched methyl substituent on the sidechain was associated with prolonged duration of action (viz, ephedrine). Whereas aromatic hydroxylation (in isoprenaline) prevented penetration across the blood–brain barrier and thus, prevented stimulation of the CNS (153). However, 1,2-dihydroxy substituents were found to promote enzymic degradation and replacement of the 3-hydroxy group by a hydroxymethyl substituent was required to extend the duration of action. In 1969, salbutamol (120) was launched by Glaxo as a longer-lasting, selective β_2-adrenoceptor agonist for the treatment of the bronchial asthma (156) and recently, a lipophilic ether analog, salmeterol (121), was introduced with

an even longer duration of action which has potential advantage in the prevention of nocturnal asthma.

Despite the many chemical alterations that have been carried out on the phenylethanolamine "template", the key chemical features associated with modern β-agonists can be seen to have originated from the naturally occurring compounds, adrenaline and ephedrine.

8 ANTIPARASITIC DRUGS

8.1 Artemisinin, Artemether, and Arteether

Artemisia annua (sweet wormwood, qing hao) has been used in Chinese medicine for well over one thousand years. The earliest recommendation is for the treatment of hemorrhoids, but there is a written record of use in fevers dated 340AD. Modern development dates from the isolation of a highly active antimalarial, artemisinin (qinghaosu), in 1972, and has been carried out almost entirely in China. Much of the original literature is therefore in Chinese, but there is an excellent review on qinghaosu by Trigg (157) and an account of the uses of *A. annua* (158). This section is largely a summary of these two articles.

Artemisinin (122) is a sesquiterpene lactone with an unusual peroxide bridge. One of the earliest modifications involved catalytic reduction of the peroxide, resulting in loss of one oxygen and total loss of antimalarial activity (157) in the adduct (123). The role of the peroxide bridge in producing antimalarial effects was not fully understood, but it appeared essential for activity, so much of the work on analogs has conserved this structural feature. It may be significant that the peroxide-bridged compound (124), isolated from *Artabotrys uncinatus*, also has antimalarial activity (158). Artemisinin is an excellent antimalarial, approximately equal in potency to chloroquine, with a good thera-peutic index except on the foetus. The preparation of semisynthetic derivatives has been stimulated primarily by a requirement for improved solubility, because ar-temisinin is relatively insoluble in both water and oil.

Reduction of (122) with sodium boro-hydride occurs at the lactone carbonyl, leaving the peroxide intact (157, 158). The resulting cyclic hemiacetal, dihydroar-temisinin (125), which is a more potent antimalarial than the parent compound, shows typical acetal reactivity. In the pres-ence of acid a highly reactive carbocation intermediate allows S_N1 type substitution with a variety of nucleophiles. For exam-ple, boron trifluoride catalyzes reactions with methanol and ethanol to give ar-temether (126) and arteether (127), respec-tively, two of the most important deriva-tives (157). Both are more potent than the parent compound and have improved solu-bility in oil. Artemether has been chosen for development in the West under the name Paluther.

Water solubility can be greatly improved by the standard ploy of esterification with succinic acid and conversion to the sodium salt. Applied to compound (125), this tech-nique gives sodium artesunate (128), a water-soluble prodrug which may be given intravenously (157). It may be assumed that hydrolysis occurs *in vivo* to give back (125) as the active antimalarial, since (126) has been shown to be unstable in aqueous

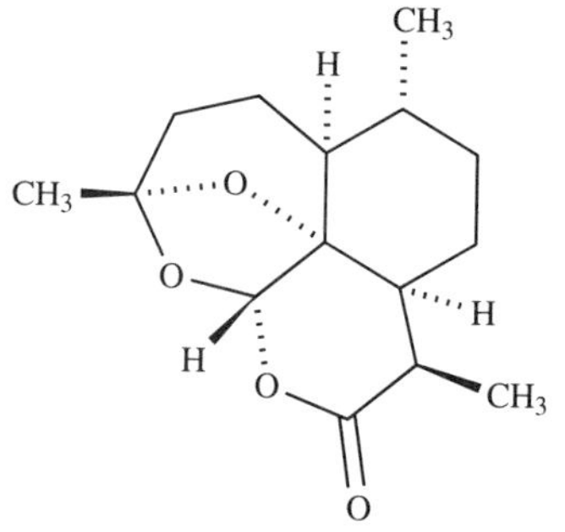

(123)

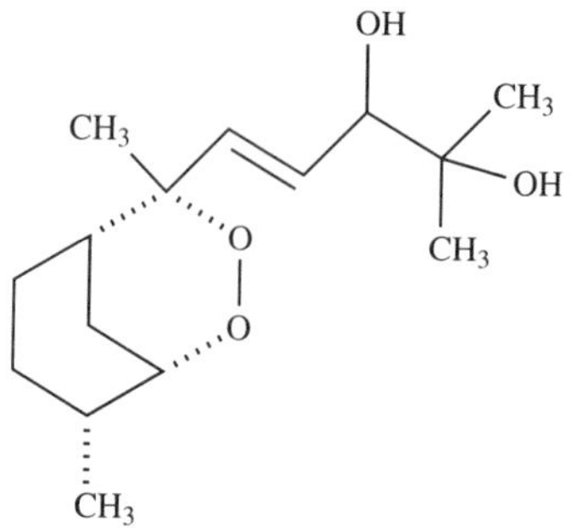

(124)

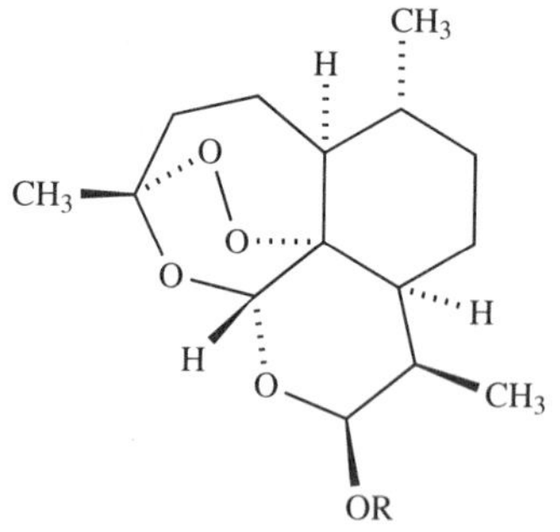

(125) R = H

(126) R = CH₃ artemether

(127) R = CH₂CH₃ arteether

(128) R = COCH₂CH₂COONa

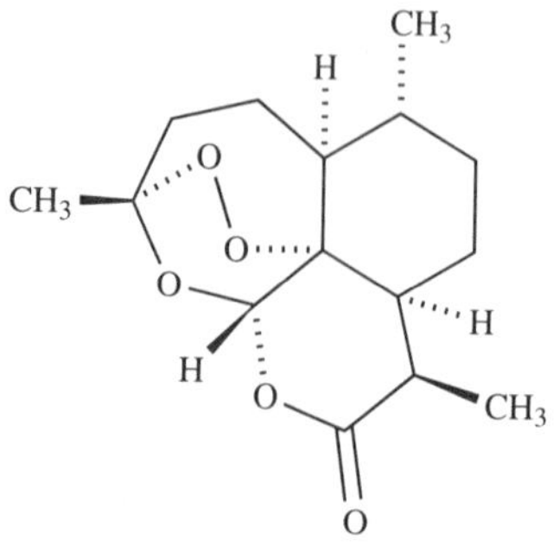

(122) artemisinin

solution and because analogous carboxylic acids with a nonhydrolyzable ether link are relatively inactive.

There are two reasons for the great

interest being shown in artinemisinin and its derivatives. First, there is little cross-resistance with *Plasmodium falciparum* between the members of this series and the quinoline-based antimalarials like chloroquine (159). On the contrary, significant potentiation of effect is observed in combination with chloroquinone analogs such as mefloquine (160). Second, the high lipid solubility of, for example, artemether ensures rapid penetration into the CNS, so these sesquiterpene lactones are first-line drugs for the treatment of cerebral malaria caused by *P. falciparum* (158), which is otherwise fatal.

The mechanism of action of artemisinin has recently been elucidated (161, 162). The drug has a high affinity for hemozoin, a storage form of hemin which is retained by the parasite after digestion of hemoglobin, leading to a highly selective accumulation of the drug by the parasite. Artemisinin then decomposes in the presence of iron, probably from the hemozoin, and releases free radicals which kill the parasite. The peroxide bridge is, therefore, a crucial part of the drug molecule as was suspected from structure-activity studies.

Whole plant extracts often show promising activity which may not be traceable to single components. This is obviously not true of *Artemisia annua* extracts, but it is interesting to note that other constituents, notably methoxylated flavones, have potentiating effects on the antimalarial activity of artemisinin (163).

The reported effect of artemisinin on systemic lupus erythematosus (157) is intriguing, given the history of use of quinine-type antimalarials in this disease.

8.2 Quinine, Chloroquine and Mefloquine

The use of Cinchona bark (e.g., *Cinchona succirubra*) by South American indians to treat fevers and the subsequent importation of the bark into Europe by Jesuit priests in the 17th century is well known (164). At that time malaria was widespread even as far north as eastern Scotland and there was no effective treatment for "the ague". Although quinine (**129**) is not very potent or long-acting, a good sample of Cinchona bark contains about 5% of the alkaloid (165). This high concentration permitted genuinely therapeutic doses of bark to be given and allowed the pure alkaloid to be isolated (166) as early as 1820. During the next hundred years quinine was the only effective treatment for malaria known to Europeans. Without quinine, life in the tropics was impossible for those without natural immunity to malaria. "One thing that was compulsory was the taking of five grains of quinine a day ... And if you didn't take it and got ill your salary was liable to be stopped" (167). Supplies of quinine to Europe were threatened in the First World War, stimulating a major program of research into synthetic analogs.

The chemical techniques available to chemists in the period 1820–1920, while improving rapidly, did not allow a structure to be proposed for quinine with any confidence: the first completely correct proposal (168) came in 1922 and was finally confirmed by total synthesis (169) as late as 1945. However, part structures were known, such as the 6-methoxyquinoline moiety, from long before, and were sufficient to allow the synthesis of mimics. The first clinically successful mimics were the 8-aminoquinolines.

In the early years of the 20th century, synthetic organic chemistry was a young discipline, largely governed by empirical rules. Progress towards synthetic analogs of complex natural structures was governed as much by synthetic feasibility as by a desire for close mimicry. The first quinine analogs were, therefore, a combination of the accessible 6-methoxyquinoline part of the quinine structure, with elements of the first successful antimicrobial agents, such as 9-aminoacridine. Nitration followed by re-

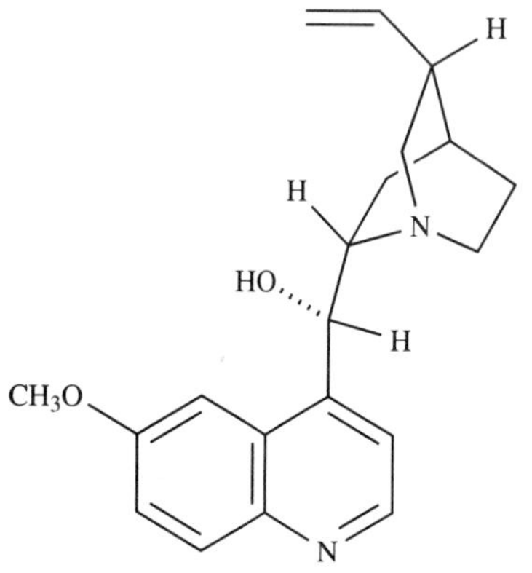

(129) quinine

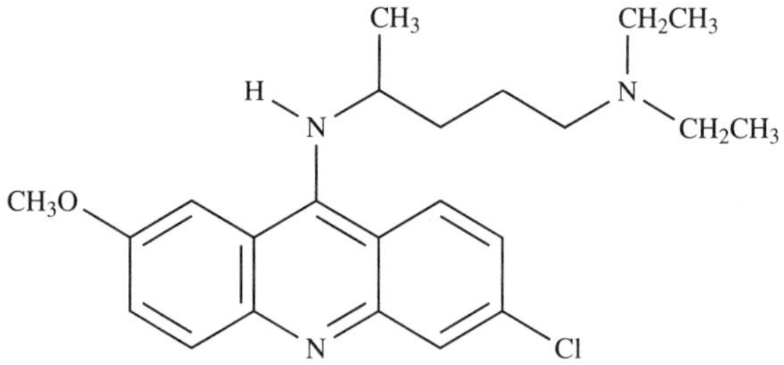

(132) quinacrine

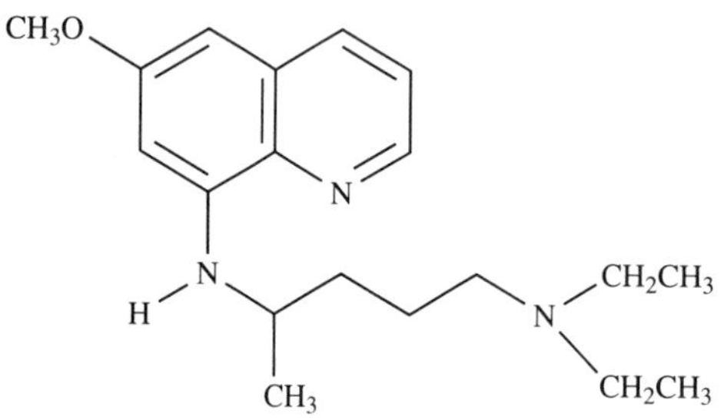

(130) pamaquine

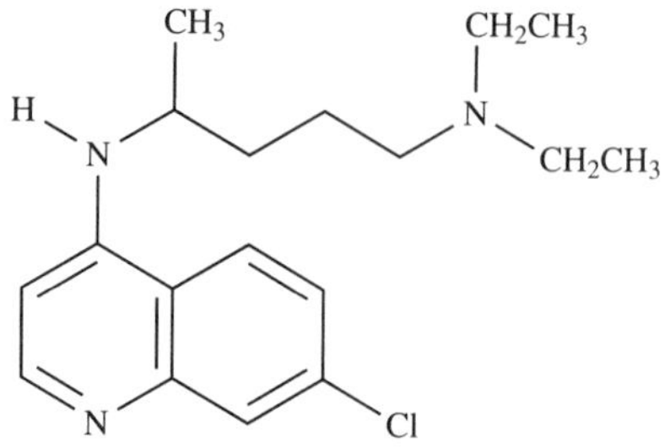

(133) chloroquine

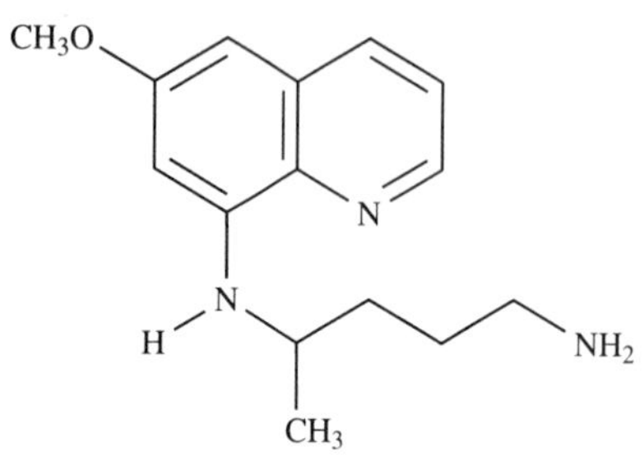

(131) primaquine

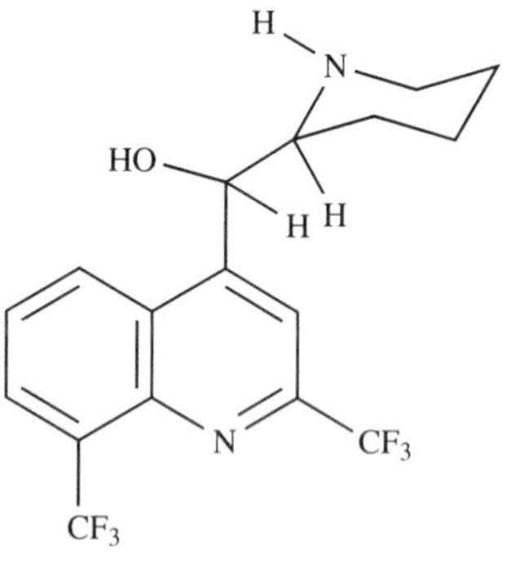

(134) mefloquine

duction could be used to generate a number of new molecules from a variety of
parent heterocycles. It is recorded (170)
that 4-, 6- and 8-aminoquinolines have
antimalarial properties and, quite extraordinarily, two of these chemical classes are

still used today, have quite different uses as
antimalarials, and quite possibly have different modes of action.

The first of the 8-aminoquinolines to be
introduced into medicine was pamaquine
(**130**), not long after the First World War

(171). Despite greater toxicity than quinine, this class of drugs was found to have radical curative ability against the relapsing malarias. Several hundred analogs were tested during World War II and of these, primaquine (131) survives to the present day for short-term use as a radical curative (172).

Quinacrine (132) is an obvious embodiment of the principle outlined above; as a derivative of both quinine and 9-aminoacridine it combined a known antimalarial with a known antimicrobial. The result was a useful, relatively nontoxic antimalarial which, however, stained the skin and eyeballs yellow (173). Despite this side effect and a high incidence of gastro-intestinal disturbance, quinacrine was widely used during World War II by European troops in East Asia. The availability of the results of medicinal chemistry research to both sides in wartime is a curious feature of antimalarial development, highlighted below.

As has been explained, the major stimulus for research into synthetic antimalarials was not so much the therapeutic inadequacy of quinine as the potential lack of availability in times of social upheaval. During World War II, the United States encouraged the planting of Cinchona in Costa Rica, Peru, and Ecuador (173). The total synthesis of quinine was too difficult in the 1940s and in unlikely to become economically viable even in the 1990s. This problem was partly overcome with quinacrine, which was used widely in World War II, but quinacrine has the defects described above. The conceptual derivation of chloroquine (133) from quinacrine is obvious and apparently happened twice, in Germany and the U.S., the latter about ten years after the Germans had discarded the drug as being too toxic! The story of the rediscovery of chloroquine is fascinating, as an account of human muddle and misjudgement, finally leading to an extraordinarily valuable drug (173).

Over decades of sublethal exposure the resistance of all types of malaria has increased to a point where chloroquine no longer offers certain protection. With the partial exception of quinine and dihydroquinine (174), resistance to antimalarials had reached the stage at the time of the Vietnam war where more research was required. The development of mefloquine (134) was a continuation of the World War II effort, with a gap of about 20 years. Resistance to chloroquine had developed widely during that period, but surprisingly less so to quinine, given the obvious similarities in structure. This observation stimulated a re-appraisal of quinolines, known as quinoline methanols, which bear a hydroxy group on the α-carbon of a substituent attached to the 4-position (175). Up to 1944, a total of 177 quinoline methanols had been synthesised and tested, resulting in one compound (135) with activity superior to that of quinine. In human volunteers there was a high incidence of phototoxicity associated with (135), so research on quinoline methanols in 1944 had ceased in favour of the 4-amino series which included chloroquine. Reappraisal of about 100 of the World War II compounds confirmed the high activity and phototoxicity of (135) and also showed the high potency of an analog (136), which had reduced phototoxicity (175). These data, together with results from about 200 newer compounds, fostered the belief that phototoxicity was separate from antimalarial activity. Extensive evaluation of (136) in humans with chloroquine-resistant *Plasmodium falciparum* infections showed promise, but with a significant incidence of toxic reactions: the dose required was also inconveniently large.

Two hypotheses concerning the effect of the 2-phenyl substituent were proposed. One was that metabolic oxidation was blocked at this position, so that duration of action was prolonged: this was considered desirable. Secondly, the UV chromophore was enlarged, which would increase the

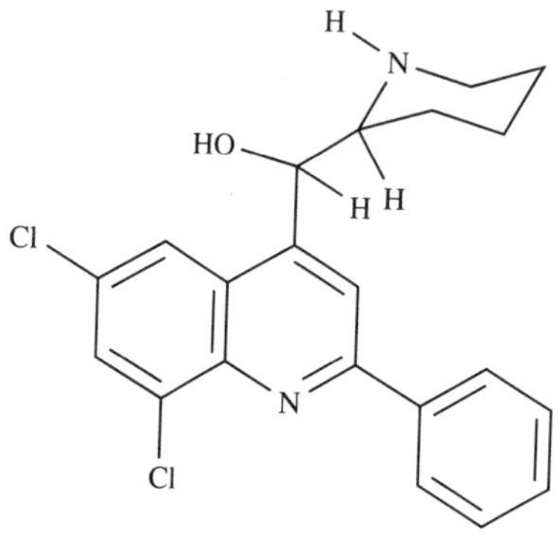

(135)

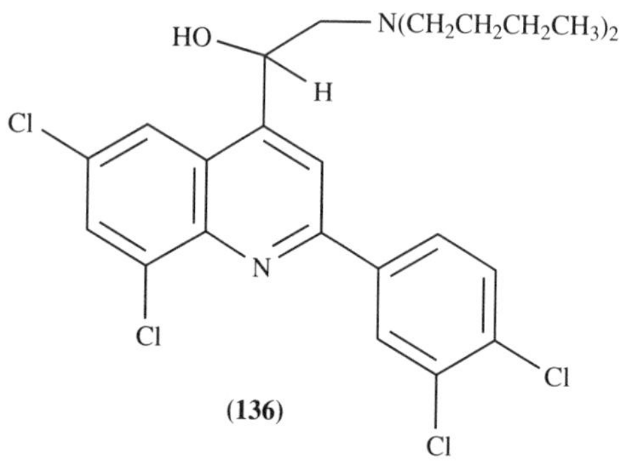

(136)

likelihood of drug-induced photosensitivity. The phenyl substituent was, therefore, replaced by trifluoromethyl in the 2-position (176). Before the first such derivatives were tested, further analogs were prepared with an additional trifluoromethyl group on the benzene ring. This was serendipitous, because the first series of 2-trifluoromethyl analogs had low potency and were also photosensitising. The series with two trifluoromethyl groups, one at position 2 and another in the 6, 7 or 8-position were all potent and free from phototoxicity (177). The most potent was mefloquine (134), a drug which is now regarded as the only effective prophylactic against multidrug resistant *P. falciparum* for visitors to many parts of Asia and southern Africa.

Physicians are pragmatic when choosing therapy for patients whose suffering is not alleviated by accepted methods. A drug which has been shown to be toxicologically safe may be utilized in a new area for the flimsiest of reasons. Thus Page (178) described his use of quinacrine in two cases of lupus erythematosus as being based on "A chance observation...", but he did not describe the observation which led to his decision. He did, however, record that quinine had been tried previously and "prevented extension of the lesions", so this may have been the basis for his rationale. In the event, the beneficial effects of quinacrine were remarkable and appeared to be related to the degree of yellowing of the skin which, as described earlier, is a common side effect of the use of quinacrine in malaria.

Among Page's group of patients with lupus erythematosus were two with rheumatoid arthritis, whose symptoms also responded to treatment with quinacrine. The following year, other physicians (179) conducted a trial of quinacrine on a larger group of patients with rheumatoid arthritis; the results encouraged Haydu (180) to test chloroquine on similar patients, again with positive results. A year later, two more physicians (181) compared quinacrine with chloroquine and found the latter to be better tolerated, the majority of patients gaining some benefit. Both quinacrine and chloroquine caused gastrointestinal disturbances, which led to a trial (182) of hydroxychloroquine (137), an unsuccessful antimalarial but with less effect on the gut,

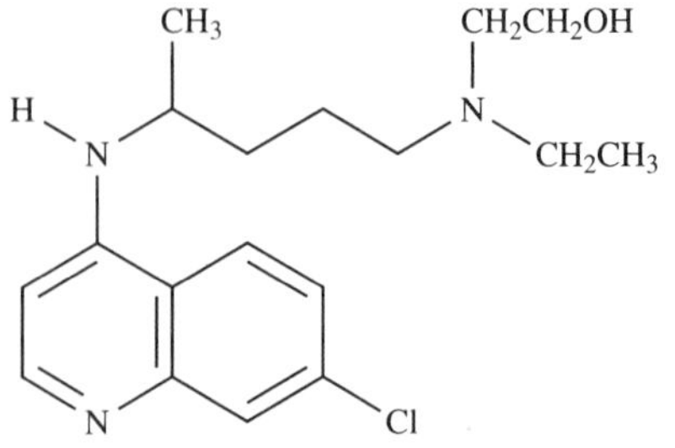

(137) hydroxychloroquine

which allowed larger doses to be given. Hydroxychloroquine has remained part of the standard drug therapy for rheumatoid arthritis ever since.

So far, the choice of quinine-like drugs to treat rheumatoid arthritis has been based on preliminary selection as antimalarials. Since the two types of action are presumably unconnected there might be some value in a screening program aimed directly at rheumatoid disease.

8.3 Avermectins and Milbemycins

There is no major distinction between the avermectins and milbemycins, which are based on the same complex polyketide macrocycle (138): the avermectins are oxygenated at C13 and bear a disaccharide on this oxygen. They have been isolated from cultures of a number of *Streptomyces* species, obtained from all over the world (183).

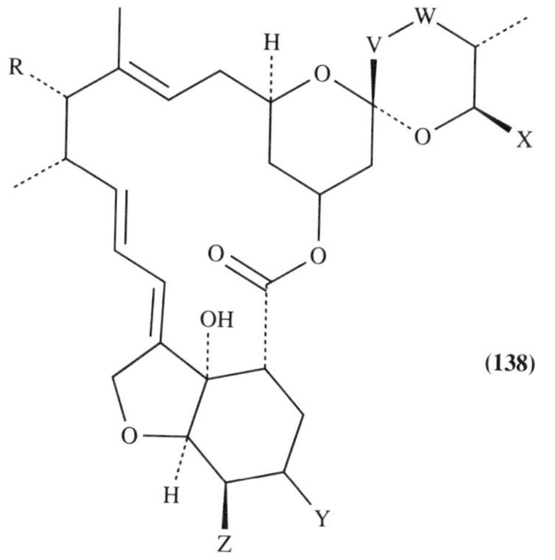

(138)

avermectin R =

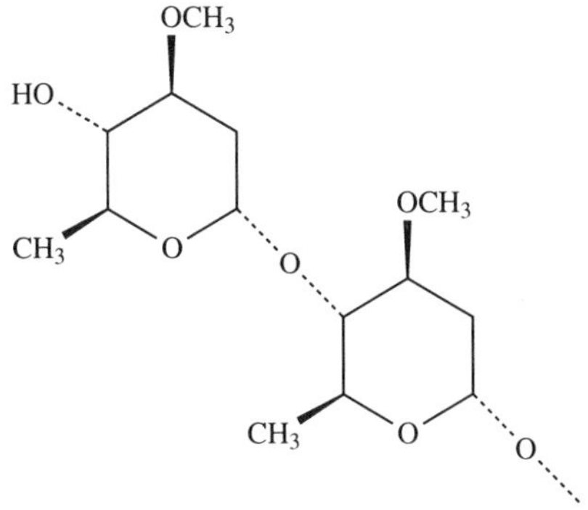

milbemycin R = H

Consult ref. 183 for details of V, W, X, Y, Z in both avermectins and milbemycins.
In the avermectins the series are designated as follows (Y = CH$_3$) :

A, Z = CH$_3$
B, Z = H
a, X = CH(CH$_3$)CH$_2$CH$_3$
b, X = CH(CH$_3$)$_2$
1, V-W = CH=CH
2, V-W = CH$_2$CH(OH)

The avermectins, particularly, have been the subject of intense commercial interest, since they possess potent activity against both nematode and arthropod parasites of livestock (184). A full discussion of structure–activity relationships would be out of place here, not least because the data are voluminous, so we shall concentrate on the development of ivermectin, which has been a major success.

Structural designation of avermectins is quaintly based on three series: A, B, a, b and 1, 2. These are illustrated diagrammatically. Greater activity resides in the B series, with a free OH at position 5. There is little difference in potency between the a and b series. In the more potent B series there are important differences between the 1 series and the 2 series; B_1 is the more active orally while B_2 is the more potent by injection. There are also differences in their spectrum of activity (185). The spectrum of activity was kept as broad as possible by hydrogenation of a mixture of avermectins B_1a and B_1b to give ivermectin (**139**) which contains at least 80% of 22, 23-dihydroavermectin B_1a and not more than 20% of 22,23-dihydroavermectin B_1b.

Ivermectin is used all over the world for treatment and control of parasites in cattle, horses, sheep, pigs, and dogs. It is an oblique commentary on our scale of values that the authors of reference 185 were able to say "...it is not yet known whether ivermectin will be useful in human medicine." There is now a clear indication for the use of ivermectin in onchocerciasis, which causes blindness in tens of thousands of Africans (186–188).

9 CONCLUSION

Natural product samples represent a rich chemical diversity which will continue to be an important source of lead compounds for

(**139**) ivermectin $X = CH(CH_3)CH_2CH_3$ (major) or $CH(CH_3)_2$ (minor)

medicinal chemistry programs and will also provide biochemical tools for mechanistic studies. Advances in molecular biology and automation technology will allow even greater numbers of samples to be tested against more biological targets (189, 190). This fact, coupled with the knowledge that perhaps over 90% of bacteria, fungal, and plant species are still waiting to be investigated (191), means that the medicinal chemist has a unique opportunity to continue utilizing the rich chemical diversity offered by nature.

REFERENCES

1. E. Rodriguez and R. Wrangham, "Zoopharmacognosy: The Use of Medicinal Plants by Animals" in K. R. Downum, J. T. Romeo, and H. A. Stafford, Eds., *Phytochemical Potential of Tropical Plants*, Plenum Press, New York, 1993, pp. 89–105.

2. R. Gerardy and M. H. Zenk, *Phytochemistry*, **32**, 79–86 (1993).

3. M. J. Stone and D. H. Williams, *Molecular Microbiology*, **6** (1), 29–34 (1992).

4. T. Amann and M. H. Zenk, *Tetrahedron Lett.*, **32** (30), 3675–3678 (1991).

5. R. J. Bryant, *Chem. and Ind.*, 146–153 (1988).

6. C. E. Inturrisi, M. Schultz, S. Shin, J. G. Umans, L. Angel, and E. J. Simm, *Life Sci.*, **33** (Suppl. 1), 773 (1983).

7. W. Sneader, *Drug Discovery: The Evolution of Modern Medicine*, John Wiley & Sons, Inc., New York, 1985, pp. 78–80 summarizes the confusion surrounding the early work.

8. A. F. Casy and R. T. Parfitt, *Opioid Analgesics*, Plenum, New York, 1986, p. 407.

9. R. Grewe and A. Mondon, *Chem. Ber.*, **81**, 279 (1948).

10. Ref. 8, p. 153.

11. K. W. Bentley and D. G. Hardy, *Proc. Chem. Soc.*, 220 (1963).

12. G. F. Blane, A. L. A. Boura, A. E. Fitzgerald, and R. E. Lister, *Br. J. Pharmacol.*, **30**, 11 (1967).

13. J. W. Lewis, *Adv. Biochem. Psychopharmacol.*, **8**, 123 (1974).

14. J. Hughes, T. W. Smith, H. W. Kosterlitz, L. A. Fothergill, B. A. Morgan, and H. R. Morris, *Nature*, **258**, 577 (1975).

15. J. A. H. Lord, A. A. Wakerfield, J. Hughes, and H W. Kosterlitz, *Nature*, **267**, 495 (1977).

16. O. Schaumann, *Arch. Exp. Path. Pharm.*, **196**, 109–136 (1940).

17. Ref. 8, pp. 209–301.

18. A. G. Gilman, T. W. Rall, A. S. Nies, and P. Taylor, *Goodman and Gilman's The Pharmacological Basis of Therapeutics*, 8th ed. Pergamon Press, New York, 1990, p. 550.

19. L. Lemberger, *Clin. Pharmacol. Therap.*, **39**, 1 (1986).

20. S. E. Sallan, N. E. Zinberg, and E. Frei, *New England J. Med.*, **293**, 795 (1975).

21. R. K. Razdan, in P. Krogsgaard-Larsen, S. Brogger Christensen, and H. Kofod, Eds., *Natural Products and Drugs Development*, Munksgaard, Copenhagen, 1984, pp. 486–499.

22. L. Lemberger and H. Rowe, *Clin. Pharmacol. Ther.*, **18**, 720 (1976).

23. T. S. Herman, L. E. Einhorn, S. E. Jones, C. Nagy, A. B. Chester, J. C. Dean, B. Furnas, S. D. Williams, S. A. Leigh, R. T. Dorr, and T. E. Moon, *New England J. Med.*, **300**, 1295 (1979).

24. A. Ward and B. Holmes, *Drugs*, **30**, 127–144 (1985).

25. W. A. Devane, L. Hanus, A. Breuer, R. G. Pertwee, L. A. Stevenson, G. Griffin, D. Gibson, A. Mandelbaum, A. Etinger, and R. Mechoulam, *Science*, **258**, 1946 (1992).

26. M. G. Bock, *Drugs of the Future*, **16**, 631–640 (1991) provides a succinct summary.

27. R. S. L. Chang, V. J. Lotti, R. L. Monaghan, J. Birnbaum, E. O. Stapley, M. A. Goetz, G. Albers-Schonberg, A. A. Patchett, J. M. Liesch, O. D. Hensens, and J. P. Springer, *Science*, **230**, 177 (1985).

28. P. R. Dodd, J. A. Edwardson, and G. J. Dockray, *Regul. Pept.*, **1**, 17 (1980).

29. R. B. Innis and S. H. Snyder, *Proc. Natl. Acad. Sci. USA*, **77**, 6917 (1980).

30. D. R. Hill, N. J. Campbell, T. M. Shaw, and G. N. Woodruff, *J. Neurosci.*, **7**, 2967 (1987).

31. R. A. Gregory, *Bioorg. Chem.*, **8**, 497 (1979).

32. P. S. Anderson, R. M. Freidinger, B. E. Evans, M. G. Bock, K. E. Rittle, R. M. Dipardo, W. L. Whitter, D. F. Veber, R. S. L. Chang, and V. J. Lotti, *Int. Cong. Ser. Excerpta, Med.*, **766** (Gastrin Cholecystokinin), 235–242 (1987).

33. D. C. Horwell, A. Beeby, C. R. Clark and J. Hughes, *J. Med. Chem.*, **30**, 729 (1987).

34. M. A. Geotz, M. Lopez, R. L. Monaghan, R. S. L. Chang, V. J. Lotti, and T. B. Chen, *J. Antibiot.*, **38**, 1634 (1985).

35. B. E. Evans, *Z. Gastroenterol. Verh.*, **26**, 269–271 (1991).

36. B. E. Evans et al., *J. Med. Chem.*, **31**, 2235 (1988).

37. I. G. Marshall and R. D. Waigh in A. L. Harvey, ed., *Drugs from Natural Products*, Ellis Horwood, Chichester, 1993, pp. 131–151.

38. H. King, *J. Chem. Soc.*, 1381 (1935).

39. P. Karrer in D. Bovet, F. Bovet-Nitti, and G. B. Marini-Bettolo, Eds., *Curare and Curare-like Agents*, Elsevier, Amsterdam, 1959, pp. 125–136.

40. P. G. Waser, *Helv. Physiol. Pharmacol. Acta*, II, Suppl. VIII (1953).

41. W. C. Bowman, *Pharmacology of Neuromuscular Function*, J. Wright, Bristol, 1990.

42. A. J. Everett, L. A. Lowe, and S. Wilkinson, *J. Chem. Soc., Chem. Commun.*, 1020 (1970).

43. R. B. Barlow and H. R. Ing, *Brit. J. Pharmacol. Chemother.*, **3**, 298 (1948).

44. D. Bovet, F. Bovet-Nitti, S. Guarini, V. Longo, and R. Fusco, *Arch. Internat. Pharmac. Therap.*, **88**, 1–50 (1951).

45. E. P. Taylor and H. O. J. Collier, *Nature*, **167**, 692 (1951).

46. J. B. Stenlake, R. D. Waigh, G. H. Dewar, R. Hughes, D. J. Chapple, and G. G. Coker, *Eur. J. Med. Chem.*, **19**, 441 (1981).

47. R. Hughes in J. Norman, Ed., *Clinics in Anaesthesiology*, Vol. 3, W. B. Saunders, London, 1985, pp. 331–345.

48. J. E. Caldwell, T. Heier, J. B. Kitts, D. P. Lynane, M. R. Fahey, and R. D. Miller, *Brit. J. Anaesth.*, **63**, 393 (1989).

49. R. L. Noble, C. T. Beer, and J. H. Cutts, *Annals of the New York Academy of Science*, 882–894 (1958).

50. I. S. Johnson, H. F. Wright, and G. H. Svoboda, *J. Lab. Clin. Med.*, **54**, 830 (1959).

51. G. H. Svoboda, *Lloydia*, **24**, 173 (1961).

52. A. C. Sartorelli and W. A. Creasey, *Annu. Rev. Pharmacol*, **9**, 51 (1969).

53. K. Gerzon in "Dimeric Cataranthus Alkaloids," in J. M. Cassady and J. D. Douros, Eds., *Medicinal Chemistry*, Academic Press, New York, 1980, pp. 271–317.

54. J. B. Sørensen and H. H. Hansen, *Investigational New Drugs*, **11**, 103–133 (1993).

55. J. Mann, *Murder Magic and Medicine*, Oxford University Press, Oxford, 1992, pp. 213–214.

56. J. Caesar, *The Battle for Gaul*, Book 6, Section 31, A. Wiseman and P. Wiseman translators, Chatto and Windus, London, 1980, p. 126.

57. T. Bryan-Brown, *Quart. J. Pharm. Pharmacol.*, **5**, 205–219 (1932).

58. D. G. I. Kingston, "Taxol and other Anticancer Agents from Plants" in J D. Coombes, Ed., *New

Drugs from Natural Sources*, IBC Technical Services, 1992, pp. 101–108.

59. M. Suffness, "Taxol: From Discovery to Therapeutic Use" in J. A. Bristol, Ed., *Ann. Reports in Med. Chem.*, Vol. 28, Academic Press Inc., 1993, pp. 305–314, provides a good review of the discovery and development of taxol and related derivatives.

60. M. C. Wani, H. L. Taylor, M. E. Wall, P. Coggon, and A. T. McPhail, *J. Am. Chem. Soc.*, **93**, 2325–2327 (1971).

61. P. B. Schiff, J Fant, and S. B. Horwitz, *Nature*, **277**, 665–667 (1979).

62. W. P. McGuire, E. K. Rowinsky, N. B. Rosenhein, F. C. Grunbine, D. S. Ettinger, D. K. Armstrong, and R. C. Donehower, *Ann. Intern. Med.*, **111**, 273–279 (1989).

63. G. M. Cragg, S. A. Schepartz, M. Suffness, and M. R. Grever, *J. Nat. Prods.*, **56** (10), 1657–1668 (1993).

64. D. G. I. Kingston, *Pharmac. Ther.*, **52**, 1–34 (1991).

65. L. Mangatal, M.-T. Adeline, D. Guénard, F. Guéritte-Voegelein, and P. Potier, *Tetrahedron*, **45**, 4177–4190 (1989).

66. J.-N. Denis, A. E. Greene, D. Guénard, F. Guéritte-Voegelein, L. Mangatal and P. Potier, *J. Am. Chem. Soc.*, **110**, 5917–5919 (1988).

67. C. Palomo, A. Arrieta, F. Cossio, J. M. Aizpurua, A. Mielgo, and N. Aurrekoetxea, *Tetrahedron Lett.*, **31**, 6429–6432 (1990).

68. F. Guéritte-Voegelein, D. Guénard, F. Lavelle, M.-T. Le Goff, L. Mangatal, and P. Potier, *J. Med. Chem.*, **34**, 992–998 (1991).

69. K. C. Nicolaou, C. Riemer, M. A. Kerr, D. Rideout, and W. Wrasidlo, *Nature*, **364**, 464–466 (1993).

70. A. Stierle, G. Strobel, and D. Stierle, *Science*, **260**, 214–216 (1993).

71. K. C. Nicolaou, Z. Yang, J. J. Liu, H. Ueno, P. G. Nantermet, R. K. Guy, C. F. Claiborne, J. Renaud, E. A. Couladouros, K. Paulvannan, and E. J. Sorensen, *Nature*, **367**, 630–634 (1994).

72. R. A. Holton et al., *J. Am. Chem. Soc.*, **116**, 1597–1598, 1599–1600 (1994).

73. H. Stähelin and A. von Wartburg in E. Jucker, Ed., *Progress in Drug Research*, Birkhauser-Verlag, Basel, Vol. 33, 1989, pp. 169–266.

74. H. Sähelin and A. von Wartburg, *Cancer Research*, **51**, 5–15 (1991) present a shorter and more readable account.

75. M. G. Kelly and J. L. Hartwell, *J. Natl. Cancer Inst.*, **14**, 967 (1954).

76. I. W. Kaplan, *New Orleans Med. Surg. J.*, **94**, 388 (1942).

77. J. L. Hartwell and A. W. Schrecker in L.

Zechmeister, Ed., *Progress in the Chemistry of Organic Natural Products*, 1958, pp. 83–166 provide a detailed review of the earlier developments and background.

78. V. Podwyssotzki, *Arch. Exp. Pathol. Pharmakol.*, **13**, 29 (1880).

79. J. L. Hartwell and A. W. Schrecker, *J. Amer. Chem. Soc.*, **73**, 2909 (1951).

80. K. S. Pankajamani and T. R. Seshadri, *Proc. Ind. Acad. Sci.*, **36A**, 157 (1952) through *Chem. Abs.* **48**, 2702 (1954). See ref. 77 for a wider discussion.

81. A. Stoll, J. Renz and A. von Wartburg, *J. Amer. Chem. Soc.*, **76**, 3103 (1954).

82. A. Stoll, A. von Wartburg, E. Angliker, and J. Renz, *J. Amer. Chem. Soc.*, **76**, 6413 (1954).

83. A. von Wartburg, E. Angliker, and J. Renz, *Helv. Chim. Acta*, **40**, 1331 (1957).

84. I. Jardine in J. M. Cassady and J. D. Douros, Eds., *Medicinal Chemistry*, Academic Press, New York, Vol. 16, 1980, pp. 319–351 provide a useful review of the middle years.

85. H. Emmenegger, H. Stähelin, J. Rutschmann, J. Renz, and A. von Wartburg, *Drug. Res.*, **11**, 327–333, 459–469 (1961).

86. H. Stähelin, *Planta Med.*, **22**, 336–347 (1972).

87. H. Stähelin, *Med. Exp.*, **7**, 92 (1962).

88. M. Kuhn and A. von Wartburg, *Helv. Chim. Acta.*, **52**, 948 (1969).

89. C. Keller-Juslen, M. Kuhn, A. von Wartburg and H. Stähelin, *J. Med. Chem.*, **14**, 936 (1971).

90. B. H. Long and A. Minocha, *Proc. Am. Assoc. Cancer Res.*, **24**, 321 (1983).

91. A. Fleming, *Br. J. Exp. Med.*, **10**, 226–236 (1929).

92. E. Chain, H W. Florey, A. D. Gardner, N. G. Heatley, M. A. Jennings, J. Orr-Ewing, and A. G. Sanders, *Lancet*, **2**, 226–228 (1940).

93. Ref. 7, pp. 298–315 provides a good review of the discovery and development of penicillin antibiotics.

94. Ref. 18, pp. 1065–1085 summarizes the pharmacological properties of the more important commercial penicillins.

95. J. C. Sheehan, "Molecular Modification in Drug Design," *Advances in Chemistry Series, No. 45*, American Chemical Society, Washington D.C., 1964, pp. 15–24.

96. T. F. Howarth, A. G. Brown, and T. J. King, *J. Chem. Soc., Chem. Commun.*, 266–267 (1976).

97. C. Reading and P. Hepburn, *Biochem. J.*, **179**, 67–76 (1979).

98. A. P. Ball, A. M. Geddes, P. G. Davey, I. D. Farrell, and G. R. Brookes, *Lancet*, **1**, 620–623 (1980).

99. Ref. 7, pp. 321–324 provides an interesting account of this discovery.

100. Ref. 7, pp. 324–300.

101. G. G. F. Newton and E. P. Abraham, *Nature*, **175**, 548 (1955).

102. H. J. Smith, "Design of antimicrobial chemotherapeutic agents" in *Smith and William's Introuction to the Principles of Drug Design*, 2nd ed., Wright, London, 1988, pp. 285–288.

103. E. H. Flynn, Ed., *Cephalosporins and Penicillins Chemistry and Biology*, Academic Press, New York, 1972.

104. G. Albers-Schöhnberg et al., *J. Am. Chem. Soc.*, **100**, 6491–6499 (1978).

105. W. J. Leanza, K. J. Wildonger, T. W. Miller, and B. G. Christensen, *J. Med. Chem.*, **22**, 1435–1436 (1979).

106. A. Imada, K. Kitano, K. Kintaka, M. Muroi, and M. Asai, *Nature*, **289**, 590–591 (1981).

107. R. B. Sykes, C. M. Cimarusti, D. P. Bonner, K. Bush, D. M. Floyd, N. H. Georgopapadakou, W. H. Koster, W. C. Liu, W. L. Parker, P. A. Principe, M. L. Rathnum, W. A. Slusarchyk, W. H. Trejo, and J. S. Wells, *Nature*, **291**, 489–491 (1981).

108. R. B. Sykes, D. P. Bonner, K. Bush, N. H. Georgopapadakou, and J. S. Wells, *J. Antimicrob. Chemother.*, **8**, Suppl. E, 1–16 (1981).

109. R. B. Sykes and D. P. Bonner, "Monobactam Antibiotics: History and Development, in J. D. Williams and P. Woods, Eds., "Aztreonam, The Antibiotic Discovery for Gram-negative Infections," *Royal Soc. Med. Int. Congress and Symposium Ser. No. 89*, Royal Society Medicine, 1985, pp. 3–24.

110. N. Bahal and M. C. Nahata, *Ann. Pharmacother.*, **26**, 46–55 (1992).

111. J. Barber, J. I. Gyi, G. A. Morris, D. A. Pye, and J. K. Sutherland, *J. Chem. Soc. Chem. Commun.*, 1040 (1990).

112. P. Kurath, P. H. Jones, R. S. Egan, and T. J. Perun, *Experientia*, **27**, 362 (1971).

113. S. Omura, K. Tsuzuki, T. Sunazuka, S. Marui, H. Toyoda, N. Inatomi, and Z. Itoh, *J. Med. Chem.*, **30**, 1941 (1987).

114. L. D. Bechtol, V. C. Stephens, C. T. Pugh, M. B. Perkal, and P. A. Coletta, *Curr. Ther. Res.*, **20**, 610 (1976).

115. H. A. Kirst and G. D. Sides, *Antimicrob. Agents and Chemother.*, **33**, 1413–1418 (1989), provide a useful, brief review.

116. P. Luger and R. Maier, *J. Cryst. Mol. Struct.*, **9**, 329 (1979).

117. G. M. Bright et al., *J. Antibiot.*, **41**, 1029 (1988).

118. S. Moromoto, Y. Takahashi, Y. Watanabe and S. Omura, *J. Antibiot.*, **37**, 187 (1984).

119. J. S. Tkacz in J. Sutcliffe and N. H. Georgopapadakou, Eds., *Emerging Targets in Antibacterial and Antifungal Chemotherapy*, Chapman and Hall, New York, 1992, pp. 504–508.

120. J. M. Balkovec et al., *J. Med. Chem.*, **35**, 194 (1992).

121. R. Gordee and M. Debono, *Drugs of the Future*, **14**, 939 (1989).

122. E. E. Slater and J. S. McDonald, *Drugs*, Suppl. 3, 72–82 (1988).

123. A. Endo, M. Kuroda and Y. Tsujita, *J. Antibiot.*, **29**, (12), 1346–1348 (1976).

124. D. J. Gordon and B. M. Rifkind, *Annals of Int. Med.*, **107**, 759–761 (1987).

125. A. G. Brown, T. C. Smale, T. J. King, R. Hasenkamp and R. H. Thompson, *J. Chem. Soc.*, *Perkin Trans. 1*, 1165–1170 (1976).

126. P. R. Vagelos, *Science*, 252, 1080–1084 (1991), gives a brief, chronological account of the discovery of lovastatin.

127. A. W. Alberts et al., *Proc. Natl. Acad. Sci. USA.*, **77**, 3957–3961 (1980).

128. A. Endo, *J. Antibiot.*, **32**, (8), 852–854 (1979).

129. A. W. Alberts, *Am. J. Cardiol.*, **62**, 10J–15J (1988), and references therein.

130. S. M. Grundy, "HMG Co A Reductase Inhibitors: Clinical Applications and Therapeutic Potential" in B. M. Rifkind, Ed., *Drug Treatment of Hyperlipidemia*, Marcel Dekker, New York, 1991, pp. 139–167.

131. W. F. Hoffmann, A. W. Alberts, P. S. Anderson, J. S. Chen, R. L. Smith and A. K. Willard, *J. Med. Chem.*, **29**, 849–852 (1986).

132. S. H. Ferreira, *Brit. J. Pharmacol.*, **24**, 163–169 (1965).

133. S. H. Ferreira, L. J. Greene, V. A. Alabaster, Y. S. Bakhle, and J. R. Vane, *Nature*, **225**, 379–380 (1970).

134. S. H. Ferreira, D. C. Bartelt, and L. J. Greene, *Biochemistry*, **9**, 2583–2593 (1970).

135. M. A. Ondetti, B. Rubin and D. W. Cushman, *Science*, **196**, 441–444 (1977).

136. R. A. Maxwell and S. B. Eckhardt, *Drug Discovery A Casebook and Analysis*, Humana Press, Clifton, New Jersey, 1990, pp. 19–34.

137. D. Potterton, Ed., *Culpeper's Colour Herbal*, Foulsham, London, 1983, p 123.

138. K. P. Link, *Harvey Lectures*, Series 39, 1944, pp. 162–216.

139. K. P. Link, *Circulation*, **19**, 97–107 (1959).

140. Ref. 18, pp. 1317–1322.

141. Mustafa, *C. R. Acad. Sci. Paris*, **89**, 442 (1879).

142. E. Späth and W. Gruber, *Ber. Dtsch. Chem. Ges.*, **71**, 106 (1938).

143. G. V. Anrep and G. Misrahy, *Gaz. Fac. Med. Cairo*, **13**, 33 (1945).

144. G. V. Anrep, G. S. Barsoum, M. R. Kenawy and G. Misrahy, *Lancet*, 557–558 (1947).

145. G. B. Kauffman, *Education in Chemistry*, **21**, 42–45 (1984).

146. Ref. 55, p. 192.

147. H. Cairns, C. Fitzmaurice, D. Hunter, P. B. Johnson, J. King, T. B. Lee, G. H. Lord, R. Minshull, and J. S. G. Cox, *J. Med. Chem.*, **15**, 583–589 (1972).

148. Ref. 18, pp. 630–632.

149. B. N. Singh, *Am. Heart J.*, **106**, 788–797 (1983).

150. B. N. Singh, N. Venkatesh, K. Nademanee, M. A. Josephson, and R. Kannan, *Prog. Cardiovascular Dis.*, **31**, 249–280 (1989).

151. J. van Schepdael and H. Solvay, *Presse Med.*, **78**, 1849–1855 (1970).

152. Ref. 55, pp. 189–191.

153. Ref. 7, pp. 98–105.

154. R. P. Ahlquist, *Am. J. Physiol.*, **153**, 586–600 (1948).

155. A. M. Lands, F. P. Luduena, and H. J. Buzzo, *Life Sci.*, **6**, 2241–2249 (1967).

156. Ref. 136, pp. 333–348.

157. P. I. Trigg, in H. Wagner, H. Hikino, and N. R. Farnsworth, Eds., *Economic and Medicinal Plant Research*, Academic Press, London, Vol. 3, 1989, pp. 19–55.

158. W. Tang and G. Eisenbrand, Eds., *Chinese Drugs of Plant Origin*, Springer-Verlag, Berlin, 1992, pp. 161–175.

159. J. Karbwang, K. N. Bangchang, A. Thanavibul, D. Bunnag, T. Chongsuphajaisiddhi and T. Harinasuta, *Lancet*, **340**, 1245 (1992), report some recent clinical experience to support the data in refs. 157 and 158.

160. A. N. Chawira, D. C. Warhurst, B. L. Robinson, and W. Peters, *Trans. R. Soc. Trop. Med. Hyg.*, **81**, 554 (1987).

161. S. R. Meshnick, A. Thomas, A. Ranz, C.-M. Xu, and H.-Z. Pan, *Mol. Biochem. Parasitol.*, **49**, 181–190 (1991).

162. S. R. Meshnick, Y.-Z. Yang, V. Lima, F. Kuypers, S. Kamchonwongpaisan, and Y. Yuthavong, *Antimicrob. Agents and Chemother.*, **37**, 1108–1114 (1993).

163. B. C. Elford, M. F. Roberts, J. D. Phillipson, and R. J. M. Wilson, *Trans. R. Soc. Trop. Med. Hyg.*, **81**, 434 (1987).

164. A. I. White in C. O. Wilson, O. Gisvold, and R. F. Doerge, Eds., *Textbook of Organic, Medicinal and Pharmaceutical Chemistry*, 7th ed., J. B. Lippincott, Philadelphia, 1977, pp. 247–268.

165. F. A. Flückiger and D. Hanbury, *Pharmacographia, A History of the Principle Drugs of Vegetable Origin, Met With in Great Britain and British India*, Macmillan, London, 1879, pp. 361–362.

166. J. Pelletier and J. Caventou, *Ann. de Chim. et de Phys.*, **XV**, 292 (1820).

167. Annon, quoted by C. Allen, *Tables from the Dark Continent*, Warner, London, 1992, p. 30.

168. P. Rabe, *Berichte*, **55**, 522 (1922).

169. R. B. Woodward and W. E. Doering, *J. Am. Chem. Soc.*, **67**, 860 (1945).

170. F. Schonhofer et al., *Z. Physiol. Chem.*, **274**, 1 (1942).

171. P. Mühlens, *Naturwissenschaften*, **14**, 1162–1166 (1926).

172. Ref. 18, pp. 988–991.

173. G. R. Coatney, *Am. J. Trop. Med. Hyg.*, **12**, 121–128 (1963).

174. Anon, *Bull. World Health Org.*, **61**, 169–178 (1983).

175. L. H. Schmidt, R. Crosby, J. Rasco, and D. Vaughan, *Antimicrob. Agents Chemother.*, **13**, 1011–1030 (1978).

176. R. M. Pinder and A. Burger, *J. Med. Chem.*, **11**, 267 (1968).

177. C. J. Ohnmacht, A. R. Patel, and R. E. Lutz, *J. Med. Chem.*, **14**, 926 (1971).

178. F. Page, *Lancet*, 755 (1951).

179. A. Freedman and F. Bach, *Lancet*, 321 (1952).

180. G. G. Haydu, *Am. J. Med. Sci.*, **225**, 71 (1953).

181. J. Forestier and A. Certonciny, *Rev. Rhum. Mal. Osteoartic.*, **21**, 395 (1954).

182. A. L. Scherbel, S. L. Schuchter and J. W. Harrison, *Cleve. Clin. Q.*, **24**, 98 (1957); see also A. L. Scherbel, *Am. J. Med.*, **75**, 1 (1983).

183. H. G. Daview and R. H. Green, *Chem. Soc. Rev.*, **20**, 211–269 (1991), provide structural details of a large number of analogs.

184. H. G. Davies and R. H. Green, *Nat. Prod. Reports*, 117 (1986).

185. W. C. Campbell, M. H. Fisher, E. O. Stapley, G. Albers-Schonberg, and T. A. Jacob, *Science*, **221**, 823 (1983).

186. K. Awadzi, K. Y. Dadzie, H. Schulz-Key, D. R. W. Haddock, H. M. Gillies, and M. A. Aziz, *Ann. Trop. Med. Parasitol.*, **79**, 63 (1985).

187. B. M. Greene et al., *New Engl. J. Med.*, **313**, 133 (1985).

188. F. A. Drobniewski, *Microbiology Europe*, 24–28 (1993).

189. G. G. Yarbrough, D. P. Taylor, R. T. Rowlands, M S. Crawford, and L. Lasure, *J. Antibiot.*, **46**, 535–544 (1993).

190. W. H. Moos, G. D. Green, and M. R. Pavia, "Recent Advances in the Generation of Molecular Diversity" in J. A. Bristol, Ed., *Ann. Reports in Med. Chem.*, Vol. 28, Academic Press Inc., 1993, pp. 315–324.

191. J. D. Coombes, Ed., *New Drugs from Natural Sources*, IBC Technical Services, London, 1992, pp. 59–62, 93–100.

Index

A antigens, 936
Abbreviated New Drug
    Applications:
    (ANDAs), 255, 272
ABO antigens, 936–937
Abortifacients, 374, 686
Absolute novelty patent
    requirement, 42, 46, 47–48
Absorption:
    carbohydrate-based drugs, 908
    loading doses, 126
    pharmacokinetics of, 115, 117,
    119–120
    prodrugs, 960–964
    and volume of distribution, 120
Academic-industrial collaborations,
    in drug discovery, 32–33
Acarbose, 926–927
Acarviosine, 927
Accelerated Approval Regulations
    of, 1992, 255
ACD, 434, 436–437
ACE, see Angiotensin-converting
    enzyme
2-Acetamido-D-galactosyl-
    transferase, 936
Acetaminophen, 144, 145
    acylated derivatives, 955
    allergy evaluation, 215
    immune response stimulation,
    188
    and thrombocytopenia, 197
Acetate-CoA ligase, 158
Acetazolamide, 970–971
Acetylaminobenzoate, 955
Acetylation, 156–157, 158
Acetylcholine, 790
Acetylcholine receptors, 789
Acetylcholinesterase, 790
Acetylcoenzyme A, role in
    acylation, 157, 158
N-Acetylcysteine, 163
B-(1-6)-N-Acetylglucos-
    aminyltransferase inhibitors,
    929
N-Acetyl-N'-methyl-alanineamide,
    815

N-Acetyl-N'-methyl-glycineamide,
    815
O-Acetyl-propanolol, hydrolysis,
    975
Acetylsalicylic acid, 960
    hydrolysis, 147
N-Acetyl-valine-methylamide, 587
α_1-Acid glycoprotein, 117
Acids, dissociation and ionization
    of, 526–527
Acquired Immune Deficiency
    Syndrome (AIDS), see AIDS
Acrolein, reaction with glutathione,
    164
Actinidin, 535
Active analog approach, 638
Active moiety, prodrugs, 950, 953
Active principle, 953
Active sites, 6, 7, 738
Activity, of ligands, 353
Activity-activity relationships, 540–
    541
Acute toxicity studies, 265
Acyclovir, 735, 906
    and double prodrug concept, 968
    esters, 959
    as prodrug, 961, 965
2-(N-Acyl)amino-2-deoxy-β-D-
    glucopyranosyl, 935
Acylation, 157–158
Acyl-CoA synthetase, 159
Acyl-glucuronides, 153, 155
2-Acylglycerol O-acyltransferase,
    160
N-Acyltransferases, 159
O-Acyltransferases, 160–161
Adamtine, 887
Adaptive least squares, 530
Additivity model, see Free Wilson
    analysis
Additivity of group contributions,
    in QSAR, 503–505
Adenoregulin, 356
Adenosine, as dopamine agonist,
    355
Adenosine deaminase inhibitors,
    755–756

S-Adenosyl-L-methionine, 148
S-Adenosylmethionine
    decarboxylase inhibitors, 770
Adhesion, cellular, 903, 937
Adhesion proteins, cellular, 687–
    690
Adiposins, 927
Adrenaline, 1020
α_2-Adrenergenic clonidine analogs,
    540–541
Adrenergic agents, multiple effects
    of, 6–7
β-Adrenergic receptor, Hansch
    analysis, 536
β_2-Adrenergic receptor, rDNA
    studies, 683–684
β-Adrenergic receptor blockers, for
    glaucoma, 970
β-Adrenergic receptor kinase, 683
β-Adrenoreceptor antagonists, 793
β-Adrenoreceptor partial agonists,
    793
Adrenoreceptors, 370
β-Adrenoreceptors, 374, 375
β_1-Adrenoreceptors, 1021
β_2-Adrenoreceptors, 1021
Adriamycin, 904, 905, 956
Adverse drug reactions, 182. See
    also Allergies
Advocate groups, 287
Aerosol dosage form, 264
Affinity:
    molecular modeling calculation,
    613–617
    oligonucleotide therapeutics,
    865–866
Affinity chromatography, 910
Affinity labels, 762, 766, 767–774
Agarose, 956
Agonists, 353–354
    partial, 357
    QSAR modeling, 502
    structure-aided drug design, 305
Aib, 814, 816
AIDS, 296, 735, 906, 1012. See
    also HIV
    drug discovery criteria, 21

AIDS (*Continued*)
HIV proteinase structure
identification, 321
new drug development for, 257
structure-aided drug design, 321,
332–339
and sulfonamide allergy, 206
AIMB, 547
AKUFVE method, 511
ALADDIN, 448
for molecular modeling, 608,
612, 642
Alanine, in conjugation, 159
Alanine racemase inhibitors, 734,
767
Alanine-scanning mutagenesis,
670–671
Albumin, 117, 185
binding, Hansch analysis, 536
free radical inactivation, 167
Alchemy, 105
Alcohol dehydrogenases, 134–135
Hansch analysis, 536
Alcohols:
conjugation with fatty acids, 158
glucuronidation, 153, 155
oxidation, 137, 144
sulfation, 150–151
Alcohol sulfotransferase, 150
Alcuronium, 992, 993
Aldehyde dehydrogenases, 135,
137
Aldehyde oxidase, 135
Aldehyde reductases, 134–135
Aldehydes, oxidation, 137
Aldoketo reductases, 135
Aldolases, 915
Aldose reductases, 135
Alicyclic amines, sulfation, 151
Alkyl chain homologation, in
analog design, 791–792
Alkylmethyleneamine, 840
Allergies, 182–217. *See also*
Adverse drug reactions
allergy-simulating reactions,
204–207
cross-sensitivity, 212–213
and diseases, 206–207
drug evaluation for, 213–216
"artificial" conjugates, 215
direct immunologic evaluation,
214
hapten-protein conjugates, 215,
216–217
using drug directly, 215–216
in vitro protein reactivity
evaluation, 213

in vivo protein reactivity
evaluation, 213–214
hypersensitivity reactions, 190–
207
classification, 190
immediate *vs.* delayed, 190
types of, 190–198
immunologic assays
cellular immunity, 209
humoral immunity, 207–208
lymphocyte sensitization, 182–
184
macromolecular carriers, 185–
190
bonding nature, 185–186
response to different therapeutic
agent classes, 184–185
Allinger force field, 577
Allopurinol:
and hepatitis, 199
prodrugs, 964–965
and vasculitis, 200
Allosterically regulated receptor
complexes, 353
Allosteric modulators, 356, 359–
361
Allylisopropylacetylcarbamide, and
thrombocytopenia, 197
α receptors, 7
ALS, 530
Alzheimer's Disease, drugs for,
274, 275, 278, 281, 296
AMBER/OPLS, 577, 599, 613
American mandrake, 1001
American Type Cell Culture
Collection, 54
Amide isosteres, 805, 838–847
physical properties, 846 *table*
Amides:
glucuronidation, 153–154, 156
hydrolysis, 147
OPLS charge distribution, 577
oxidation and reduction, 141–143
Amidomethyleneamine, 840
Amidopyrine:
and granulocytopenia, 196
immune response stimulation,
188
Amine *N*-methyltransferase, 148,
149
Amine oxidases, 135
Amine prodrugs, 958–959
Amines:
acetylation, 157, 158
glucuronidation, 154, 156
oxidation and reduction, 141–143
polarization energies, 403

protonation free energies, 407–
408
Amine sulfotransferase, 150
Amino acids:
conjugate formation, 159–160
constrained, in peptidomimetics,
see Peptidomimetics,
constrained amino acids
PCA analysis, 506, 509
D-Amino acids, 833
9-Aminoacridine, 1023
3-Aminobenzaepines, 990
m-Aminobenzoic acid, 809
Aminobiotin, 408–409
γ-Aminobutyric acid, *see* GABA
7-Aminocephalosporanic acid, 1006
cis-4-Aminocrotinic acid, 797
trans-4-Aminocrotinic acid, 797
γ-Aminocycloalkane carboxylic
acids, 826
α-Aminocycloalkane carboxylic
acids, 817–818
β-Aminocycloalkane carboxylic
acids, 825–826
α-Aminocycloheptane carboxylic
acid, 817
α-Aminocyclohexane carboxylic
acid, 817
γ-Aminocyclopentane carboxylic
acid, 826
α-Aminocyclopentane carboxylic
acid, 817
β-Aminocyclopentane carboxylic
acid, 825
α-Aminocyclopropane carboxylic
acid, 817
4-(2-Aminoethyl)-6-dibenzo-
furanpropionic acid, 836
Aminoglycosides, absorption, 908
2-Amino-5-hydroxyindane
carboxylic acid, 831
Aminohydroxy oligonucleotide
backbone, 889
1-Amino-2-(4-hydroxy)-
phenylcyclopropane carboxylic
acid, 831
2-Amino-6-hydroxytetralin-2-
carboxylic acid, 831
2-Aminoindane-2-carboxylic acid,
831
α-Aminoisobutyric acid, 814, 816
p-Aminomethylbenzoic acid, 809
2'-Aminomethylbiphenyl-2-
carboxylic acid, 836
(1*S*,2*S*)-(*E*)-1-Amino-2-
methylcyclopropane carboxylic
acid, 830

6-Aminopenicillanic acid, 1004
Aminopeptidase inhibitors, 845
Aminopeptidase M, 164
1-Amino-2-phenylcyclopropane carboxylic acid, 830
1-Aminoproline, 826
Aminopyrine, and granulocytopenia, 196
8-Aminoquinolines, 1023
Aminosalicylates, and hepatitis, 199
Aminosalicylic acid, and pneumonitis, 203
para-Aminosalicylic acid acetylation, 157
and hemolytic anemia, 196
β-Amino-tetrahydronaphthyl carboxylic acid, 833
2-Amino-tetrahydronaphthyl carboxylic acid, 833
2-Aminotetralin-2-carboxylic acid, 831
Amiodarone, 1019, 1020
Amitriptyline, 59, 787
Amoxycillin, 1004
Amphetamine:
CASE carcinogenicity prediction, 243
methylation, 149
Ampicillin, 955, 1004
esters, 960
and mononucleosis, 206
Amyloid precursor protein, 387
Analgesia, biological basis for, 987
Analgesics, 986–988
Analine mustards, Hansch analysis, 540
Analog design, 783–801
alkyl chain homologation, 791–792
bioisosteric replacement, 785–788
chain branching alteration, 792–793
goals, 784
interatomic distance variation, 799–801
lead compounds in, 783–785
fragment (of lead compound) design, 797–799
rigid analogs, 788–791
conformation "freezing," 788–789
ring position isomers, 792–793
ring size changes, 793–794
stereoisomerism and, 795–797
Analogs, 539–543, 752–757, 783–784, *See also* specific Analogs

Analytical Abstracts, 108
Anandamide, 989
Anaphylatoxins, 204
Anaphylaxis, 182, 183–184, 190–193
Anchor principle, 504
Androgens, C(10)-demethylation, 137
Anesthetics, anaphylactic reactions, 191
Angiotensin:
AiB incorporation, 814
Angiotensin II, 821, 825, 829
Angiotensin II receptor, 375
Angiotensin-converting enzyme, 748, 771
molecular modeling, 622–623
Angiotensin converting enzyme inhibitors, 736, 748, 750, 844, 1016
mechanism-based, 771
prodrugs, 958, 961–962
structure-aided design, 323–324
Angiotensin-converting enzyme inhibitors:
molecular modeling, 624–626, 639–640, 646, 647
natural products, 812
9-Anilinoacridines, 540, 543
Animals, patentability, 49, 50–51
Animal studies:
for direct immunologic evaluation, 214
in drug development, 265–268
in drug discovery, 11, 18, 20
needless studies, 21
oligonucleotide therapeutics, 881–882
for pharmacokinetic characterization, 126
of prodrugs, *vs.* human studies, 952, 974–975
whole animal screens, 701–703, 704
Anomeric effect, 911–912
Antagonists, 354–355
QSAR modeling, 502
structure-aided drug design, 305
types of, 354
Anthracycline antibiotics, 904
Anthramycin, 990
Antiangina drugs, 1020
Antiarrhythmic drugs, 126
Antiasthma drugs, 1017–1021
Antibacterial agents, 956
carbohydrate-based vaccines, 929–931

Antibiotic-producing organisms, by rDNA technology, 666
Antibiotics, 826
carbohydrate-based, 904–906
natural products, 1003–1014
by rDNA technology, 666–667
screening discovery, 12, 1005
Antibodies, 183
antinuclear, 202–203
classes of, 183
formation, 183–190
Anticancer alkylating agents, 164
Anticancer drugs, 736
natural products, 995–1003
nausea from, 988
prodrugs, 966–967
Anticoagulants, 908, 1017
Anticonvulsants:
and aplastic anemia, 206
and granulocytopenia, 196
and hepatitis, 199
lupus-like syndromes, 202
lymphadenopathy from, 205
Antidepressants, 736
Antiepileptics, 736
Antigens, 182–184
Antihistamines, glucuronidation, 156
Anti-immunoglobulin reagents, 196
Antimalarials, 1021–1022
Free Wilson analysis, 541
Hansch analysis, 539
lupus-like syndromes, 202
phototoxicity, 1025–1026
resistance to, 1025
Antimicrobials, 1023
Antinuclear antibodies, 202–203
Antiparasitic drugs, 904
natural products, 1021–1028
Antiproliferative agents, 736
Antipsychotics, 787
Antipyrine, sensitivity to, 205
Antisense oligonucleotides, 691, 891–892 *table*
Antitumor drugs, 736, 956. *See also* Anticancer drugs
Hansch analysis, 539–540
polysaccharides, 934
Antiulcer agents, 967
Antiviral agents, 956
Aplastic anemia, 206
Aprosulate, 924
Arene oxides, 147
Aromatase, 135, 137
Aromatic amine moiety, *O*-substituted, 229 *table*

Aromatic amines:
    acetylation, 157, 158
    glucuronidation, 154, 156
Aromatic azaheterocyclic
    compounds, 141
Aromatic azo compounds, 143
Aromatic hydroxylamides,
    sulfation, 151
Aromatic-hydroxylarylamine
    O-acetyltransferase, 157
Aromatics, oxidation, 140
Aromatic substituents,
    representative parameters, 507–
    508 *table*
Aromatization reactions, 143
Arphamenines, 845
Arsenic, redox reactions of, 144–
    145
Arsenicals, 5, 145–146
Arseno compounds, 146
Arsenoxides, 146
Arteether, 1022
Artemether, 1022
Artemisinin, 1021, 1022–1023
Arthritis, 1026–1027
Arylalkylamine *N*-acetyltransferase,
    157
Arylakylamines, *N*-formylation,
    157
Arylamides, cytotoxicity, 151
Arylamine *N*-acetyltransferase, 156
Arylamine glucosyltransferase, 152
Arylamines:
    cytotoxicity, 151
    N-formylation, 157
((Arylcarbonyl)oxy)propanolamines,
    172
Aryldialkylphosphatases, 137
1-(X-Aryl-3,3-dialkyltriazenes, 539
Arylesterases, 137
Arylformamidase, 157
Arylhydroxamic acid, acetylation,
    157
Arylhydroxylamines, acetylation,
    157, 158
Arylpropionic acids, chiral
    inversion, 161
Arylsufatases, 137
Arylsulfonamidophenethanolamines,
    793
Aryl sulfotransferase, 150
L-Aspartate transcarbamoylase
    inhibitors, 736
Aspartic endopeptidases, 137
Aspartic protease inhibitors, 678–
    679, 680
Aspartic proteinases, 325, 328

Aspercilin, 387, 388, 798–799,
    990–991
Aspirin, 984
    anaphylactic reactions, 191
    immune response stimulation,
        188
    prodrugs, 960
    sensitivity to, 204–205
    trademark loss, 85
Assays:
    immunologic, 207–209
    radioligand binding, *see*
        Radioligand binding assays
    rDNA for reagents, 673–676
    receptor binding, 378–385
    stability-indicating, 262
Asthma, 203–204
Atom-centered point charges, 597–
    598
Atracurium, 993–994
Atrial M$_2$ acetylcholine receptors,
    789
Atrial natiuretic peptides, cyclic
    structures in, 805
α-Atrial natriuretic peptide
    receptor, 684–685
Atropine, 984, 987
Augmentin, 1004
Auranofin, 907
Aurelic acid antibiotics, 904
Australia:
    patentable subject matter, 50
    scientific misconduct handling,
        293
    trade secret protection, 92–93
AUTONOM, 106, 469, 482–483
Autoradiography, receptors, 385–
    386
Avermectins, 904, 905, 918, 1027–
    1028
Avidin-biotin interaction, 408–410
6-Aza pyrimidines, 884–885
4-Azaspiro[2,4]heptane carboxylic
    acid, 820–821
Azetidine-2-carboxylic acid, 819
Azetreonam, 1009
Azithromycin, 1011, 1012
p-Azobenzene arsonates, immune
    response stimulation, 187
Azo compounds, 141, 143
Azothioprine, and pneumonitis, 203
Azoxy compounds, 143
AZT, 167, 296, 906, 963
Azyline, 819

Bacampicillin, 960
Baccatin II, 999

Backbone cyclization (peptides),
    813–814
Backbone modifications,
    oligonucleotide therapeutics,
    867 *table*, 886, 888–890
Bacterial resistance, 537, 672
    enzyme inhibitors and, 737
Bacterial toxins, 920
Bambuterol, 955
B antigens, 936
Barbiturates, glucuronidation, 156
Basal ganglia, 355
Bases, dissociation and ionization
    of, 526–527
Basic research, 13, 21. *See also*
    specific Research methods
Bateman function, 972
BC(DEF) parameters, 512
Beclomethasone, 984
Beilstein's Current Facts in
    Chemistry on CD-ROM, 486
BEL-FREE method, 522
Belladonna alkaloids, 984
Benzamidines, 536
    Free Wilson analysis, 542
Benzene:
    and aplastic anemia, 206
    bone marrow toxicity, 140
Benziodarone, 1019, 1020
Benzo-(a)-pyrene, 209
Benzoate-CoA ligase, 159
1,4-Benzodiazepine, 847
Benzodiazepine CNS depressants, 5
Benzodiazepines, 176, 702–703
Benzodiazepin receptor, Hansch
    analysis, 536
Benzoic acids, amino acid
    conjugation, 159–160
Benzomorphans, 987
    Free Wilson analysis, 542
Benzothiazolines, 356
N-(X-Benzoyl)-glycine methyl
    esters, 535
N-Benzoyl-glycine X-phenyl esters,
    535–536
5-(X-Benzyl)-2,4-diamino-
    pyrimidines, 534–535
Benzylidene, 913
Benzylpenicillin, 1004
Benzyl-penicilloyl-polylysine, 212
α-Benzylproline, 833
Bestatin, 751
BEST Europe, 109
Best mode, in patent specification,
    54–55
BEST North America, 109
Betamethasone, 984

β receptors, 7
β-Sheet structures, 835–836
β-Turn mimics, 833–835
Bicyclic peptides, 813
Bilinear model, 524–525
Binding affinities:
 calculation by molecular
  modeling, 613–615
 carbohydrate-based drugs, 909
Binding assays, receptors, 378–385
Binding-site models, 619–621
Bioavailability, 119–120, 734
 and drug discovery, 18, 19, 24
 prodrugs, 973–974
Bioisosterism:
 and analog design, 785–788
 and *prima facie* obviousness, 59
 and QSAR modeling, 504
Biological materials, patentability,
  49, 50–51
Biophobes, 227
Biophores, 227–232
 contribution of biophore 1 to
  carcinogenicity, 233 *table*
 major biophores with mouse
  carcinogenic potential, 228
  table
Bioprecursors, 173, 174
BIOSIS, 105
Biotech companies, 33
Biotechnology, intellectual property
  issues in, *see* Intellectual
  property
Biotechnology Art Unit (of the
  PTO), 41
Biotin-avidin interaction, 408–410
vic-Bisdehalogenation reactions, 139
α,ω-Bis-trimethylammonium
  polymethylene compounds,
  800–801
Bleomycin, 888
β-Blockers, with ultra-short action,
  172
Blood-brain barrier, 804, 843
 Hansch QSAR analysis, 538
 α-methyldopa carrier system, 967
Blood cells, and clearance, 117
Blood group carbohydrates, 935–
  937
B lymphocytes, 182–184, 186
Board of Patent Appeals and
  Interferences, 62, 63, 64
Bombesin, 839, 843
Bonding, drug-target, *see* Drug-
  receptor binding
Born-Oppenheimer surface, *see*
  Potential surfaces

Boronic acid peptides, 757
Boundary element method, 581
Bovine lens leucine aminopeptidase
  inhibitors, 751
Bovine trypsin, homologous
  modeling, 316
Bradykinin, 821, 825, 828, 832,
  845
 AiB incorporation, 814
Brain natriuretic peptide receptor,
  684–685
Brain penetration (prodrugs), 176
Breast cancer, 922, 999
BRIDGE, 612
Britain, *see* United Kingdom
Bromelain, 535
Bromides, and dermatitis, 198
N^{10}-Bromoacetyl-5,8-dideazafolate,
  776–777
(p-Bromobenzyl)acetic acid, 604
α-Bromo-phenethylamines:
 Free Wilson analysis, 520–521
 Hansch analysis, 517–519, 539
Bromperidol, 338
 molecular modeling, 609
Brookhaven Protein Databank, 607
BRS, 105
Brucellosis, 930
Budapest Treaty, 53, 54
α-Bungarotoxin, 376
Buprenorphine, 987
Busulfan:
 and pneumonitis, 204
 and vasculitis, 200
Butryate-CoA ligase, 158
N-Butyl deoxynojirimycin, 928
O-t-Butylserine, 833
O-t-Butylthreonine, 833
6-O-Butyryl castanospermine, 928
Butyrylcholinesterase, Hansch
  analysis, 536

CA File, 105, 108
Calcineurin, 681
Calcitonin, cyclic structures in, 805
Calcium, as second messenger, 362
Calcium agonists, Hansch analysis,
  537
Calcium channel blockers, 143, 226
Calcium channels, 351
Calicheamicin, 905, 906
Calmodulin, 681, 682
Cambridge Crystallographic
  Database, 108
Cambridge Structural Database
  System, 445, 446
cAMP, 361

Canada, patentable subject matter, 50
Cancellation, of trademarks, 84
Cancer, *see also* Carcinogenicity
 carbohydrate role in metastasis,
  938
 glycosylation pattern, 919–920
Cancer drugs, *see* Anticancer drugs
Candida, 1012–1013
Cannabinoids, 988–989
Cannabis, 988–989
Capping, of RNA, 865, 872–873
Captopril, 150, 167, 736, 1016
 discovery, 662, 663
 immune suppression by, 206
 and nephritis, 201
 structure-aided design, 324
Carba, 841–842
Carbamate prodrugs, 963
Carbamates, Hansch QSAR
  analysis, 538
Carbamazepine, 141
 10,11-epoxide, 141
 glucuronidation, 156
Carbamic acids, glucuronidation, 153
Carbamoyl glucuronides, 155
Carbenicillin, 960
Carbohydrate-based therapeutics,
  902–939
 antibiotics, 904–906
 cardiac glycosides, 906–907, 908
 future directions, 938–939
 glyconconjugates, 903, 919–926
  glycolipids, 919–922
  glycoproteins, 925–926
  proteoglycans, 922–925
 for immunomodulation, 929–935
  antibacterial vaccines, 929–931
  immunostimulants and
   adjuvants, 931–935
 instrumentation, 909–912
 multivalency, 909
 nucleosides, 906
 patent issues, 926
 pharmacology, 907–909
 synthesis, 912–919
 synthetic carbohydrates, 907
Carbohydrate-lectin complexes, 910
Carbohydrates, 902–903
 anomeric effect, 911–912
 branching, 903
 and cellular recognition, 902–903
 as chiral synthons, 917–918
 chromatography, 910
 enzyme inhibitors of, 926–929
  glycosidase inhibitors, 926–928
  glycotransferase inhibitors,
   928–929

2-Carbon chain elongation reactions, 161–163
Carbonic anhydrase, Hansch analysis, 536
Carbonic anhydrase inhibitors, molecular modeling, 615
Carbon monoxide, as second messenger, 362
Carbon oxidation/reduction reactions
sp^3, 137–139
sp and sp^2, 140–141
Carbonyl conjugation reactions, 167–168
Carbonyl reductases, 135, 140
Carboxamides, glucuronidation, 153, 156
Carboxylesterases, 137
Carboxylic acids, glucuronidation, 153
Carboxymethyl-CoA, 755–756
Carboxypeptidase A, 843, 1016
Carcinogenicity:
electrophilic theory of, 226
prediction by mutagenicity, 225
prediction with SAR, 224–246. See also Computer-automated Structure Evaluation
vs. mutagenicity, 224
Carcinogenicity studies:
in drug development, 266–267
in drug discovery, 17
Cardiac glycosides, 906–907, 908
Cardiovascular drugs, natural products, 1014–1017
Career paths, in drug discovery, 31–32
Carfecillin, 960
Carrier-linked prodrugs, 173
Carrier moiety, prodrugs, 950, 953–954
Carvediol, glucuronidation, 155, 156
CASE, see Computer-automated Structure Evaluation (CASE)
CASREACT, 105, 460
CAS Registry File, 107
Castanospermine, 927, 928
Catalase, 137
Catecholamines, 748
Catechol-O-methyltransferase inhibitors, 748
Catechols, 140
Catechol O-transferase, 148
Cathartics, 1001
CAVEAT, for molecular modeling, 608, 612
CAVITY, 604, 605, 607

CCK, see Cholocystokinin
CCK$_5$, 825
CCR, 461, 462
CD4, 669, 670
CD-ROM databases, 484–486
Cefacrol, 1007, 1008
Cefadroxil, 1007, 1008
Cefotiam, 960
Ceftazidime, 1008
Ceftizoxime, 1008
Ceftriaxone, 1008
Cefuroxime, 1007, 1008
Cellular adhesion, 903, 937
Cellular adhesion proteins, 687–690
Cellular hypersensitivity reactions, 190
assays for, 209
Cellular recognition, and carbohydrates, 902–903
Cellular uptake, oligonucleotide therapeutics, 879–881, 887–888
Cellulose, 956
Cephacetrile, 1006
Cephalexin, 1007, 1008
Cephaloglycin, 1007, 1008
Cephaloridine, 1007, 1008
Cephalosporin C, 1006
Cephalosporins, 212, 1006–1009
anaphylactic reactions, 191
Cephalothin, 1006
and hemolytic anemia, 196
and nephritis, 201
Cephalothins, 212
Cephamandole, 1007, 1008
Cephapirin, 1006
Cephradine, 1007, 1008
Ceramide, 919
Cerebral malaria, 1023
Certificate of Correction (patents), 66
cGMP, 361
Chain branching, and analog design, 792–793
Chakrabarty v. Diamond, 49
Chaos theory, 353, 358
Charge-charge interactions, 579
Charge-dipole interactions, 578–579
Charge image method, 581
Charge transfer energy, 402
CHARMM, 322, 613
CHC, 461, 462, 463
CHCD Dictionary of Natural Products on CD-ROM, 484–486
ChemBase, 105–106, 466

Chem3D, 466
ChemDBS-3D, 445, 446–447
ChemDraw, 466
CHEMEST, 469, 477–478
ChemFinder, 466, 467
Chemical Abstracts, 108
Chemical diversity sources, 673 674 table
Chemical information computing software, integrated, 486–489
Chemical information databases, in drug discovery, 14, 105–106
2D Chemical information databases:
commercial, 433–440
in-house, 432–433
vendors, 418–419 table, 434 table
3D Chemical information databases:
commercial systems, 449–452
in-house, 448–449
for molecular modeling, 607–610
vendors, 418–419 table, 450 table
2D Chemical information management software, 417–432
chemical connection file formats, 420–421
chemical structure searches, 421–422
"similarity" searches, 424–425
chemical substructure searches, 422–424
functions and capabilities, 419–427
microcomputer-based, 465–466
specific software systems, 427–432, 428 table
structure registration, 421, 426
vendors, 418–419 table
3D Chemical information management software, 440–448
functions and capabilities, 440–445
"similarity" structure searching, 443–444
specific systems, 445–448
structure registration, 441
structure searching, 441–444
multiple conformations and, 443
vendors, 418–419 table, 445 table
Chemical libraries, 724–730
ligand libraries, 388–390

Chemically-intelligent computing software, 466–484
  SAR spreadsheets, 468–470
  vendors, 469 table
Cheminform, 106, 464
Chemoattractants, 814, 817
ChemOffice, 466
Chemotactic peptide, 843
Chemotherapeutic agents, anaphylactic reactions, 191
ChemReact, 461, 462
ChemSynth, 461, 462
ChemTalk, 105
CHEM-X, 106, 446
  for molecular modeling, 608, 609
Cheng-Prusoff equation, 381
Child-resistant closures, 263
Chirality, and activity, incorrect assumptions about, 795
Chiral synthons, carbohydrates as, 917–918
CHIRAS, 461–463
Chloramphenicol, 644, 955, 1005
  and aplastic anemia, 206
  glucuronidation, 155
  glutathione conjugation, 164
  and granulocytopenia, 196
  as prodrug, 963
  and thrombocytopenia, 197
Chloroform, 510
Chloropromazine, 59
Chloroprothixene, 59
Chloroquine, 537, 1022, 1023, 1024, 1025
Chlorothiazide, and thrombocytopenia, 197
Chlorproamide, anaphylactic reactions, 191
Chlorpromazine, 376
Chlorpropamide, and hepatitis, 199
Chlortetracycline, 1005
Cholecystokinin, 840, 845, 889–890
Cholecystokinin-A receptor antagonists, 798–799, 990–991
Cholecystokinin-B receptor antagonists, 841, 843, 990–991
Cholecystokinin-B receptors, 792–793
Cholesterol-conjugated oligonucleotides, 887
Cholesterol-lowering agents, 690, 736, 966
Cholesteryl ester synthase, 158
Cholinesterase, 137
Chondroitin sulfates, 922
Chromatographic parameters, 511

Chromatography, carbohydrates, 910
Chromium, immune response stimulation, 185, 189
Chromomycin, 904
Chronic toxicity studies, 266
Chymotrypsin inhibitors, 750–751, 778–779
  Hansch analysis, 535–536
  molecular modeling, 613
C.I. vat yellow 4, CASE carcinogenicity prediction, 231–232
Cilazapril, structure-aided design, 324
Cilofungin, 1012, 1013
Cimetidine:
  discovery, 662, 663, 681–682
  and nephritis, 201
Cinchona bark, 1023, 1025
CIPSLINE PC, 105
CIRX, 462, 464
^{13}C isotope labeling, 313–314
Cisplatin, 995
Citrate synthase inhibitors, 755–756
CJACS, 105
CJWILEY, 105
CLAIMS, 108
Claims, in patent specification, 55
Clarithromycin, 1011, 1012
Clavulanic acid, 734–735, 1004
Clearance, 116–119
Clearance approach, prodrug pharmacokinetics, 972–973
Cleavage reagents, oligonucleotide therapeutics, 888
CLF, 462, 464
Clindamycin, anaphylactic reactions, 191
Clinical studies, *see also* Phase I clinical studies; Phase II clinical studies . . . .
  in drug development, 279–300
  in drug discovery, 18–20, 24–25
Clinical Trial Reports, 295
CLOGP, 474
CLOGP-3, 439, 474–476
Clonidine controlled release, 956
Cloning, *see* Recombinant DNA technology
Closure development, 262–264
Clozapine, 368–369
Cluster analysis, 531–532
Clustering methods, 533
Cluster significance analysis, 532
CMC-3D, 450–451
CNS diseases, drug design for, 13–14

CNS drugs, 5
  Hansch QSAR analysis, 538, 540
  natural products, 986–992
COBRA, 547
Codeine, 950, 986
  conjugation with fatty acids, 158
Coenzyme-A, conjugation reactions with, 158–159
Coenzymes, 6
Cofactors:
  in conjugation reactions, 147, 148
  in glucuronidation reactions, 152
  in methylation reactions, 150
  in sulfation reactions, 150
Collaborations, in drug discovery, 32–33
Collagen, 820
Collander equation, 510
Colon-specific drug delivery, 964
Combinatorial approach, to homologous modeling, 319
Combinatorial aspects, of potential surface minimization, 583–585
Combinatorial libraries, 727–728
Committees, in drug discovery, 32
COMPACT, 530
Compactin, 736, 759, 1015
Comparative molecular field analysis, 171, 499, 546–550
  for molecular modeling, 604–605, 630, 646, 648
Compartmental approach, prodrug pharmacokinetics, 971–972
Competitive antagonism, 354
Competitive enzyme inhibitors, 743
Complementarity, 626
Composition of matter, as patentable subject matter, 48, 58–59
Comprehensive Medicinal Chemistry, 106
Compulsory licenses, 77–78
Computational chemistry, 911
Computer-aided drug design, 7
Computer-assisted molecular design (CAMD), 351
Computer-automated Structure Evaluation (CASE), 527. See *also* Biophores
  approach of, 225–227
  database analysis by, 243
  example results, 232–246
  methodology, 227–232
  MULTICASE, 227, 229, 231, 236, 246
  QSAR option, 236–237
  toxicological activities modeled with, 235 table

Computers, 105–106. *See also* Information retrieval
Concanavalin A, Hansch analysis, 536
CONCORD, 448, 450, 547
 for molecular modeling, 608
Condylomata acuminata, 1001
Configurational factors, and structure-metabolism relationship, 170
Conformational analysis, for minimization of potential surfaces, 587–589
Conformational clustering, 586–587
Conformational entropy, 502
Conformational flexibility, 407
Conformational mimicry, 633–635
Congo red, anaphylactic reactions, 191
Conjugation reactions, 132, 147–168
 acetylation, 156–157, 158
 acylation, 157–158
 amino acid conjugate formation, 159–160
 carbonyl conjugation, 167–168
 chiral inversion of arylpropionic acids, 161
 with coenzyme-A, 158–159
 glucosidation, 152, 156
 glucuronidation, 152–156
 glutathione conjugation, 163–167
 and immune response, 185–190
 lipid formation, 160–161
 macromolecular conjugates, 132
 methylation, 148–150
 β-oxidation and 2-carbon chain elongation, 161–163
 phosphorylation, 167
 sterol ester formation, 160–161
 sulfation, 150–152
Constrained amino acids, *see* Peptidomimetics, constrained amino acids
Constrained minimization, 636–637
Contact dermatitis, 185
Container development, 262
Continuation-in-part (CIP) application, 42–43
Contraceptives, 202, 903, 938, 984
Coombs reagents, 196
Cooperative research and development agreements (CRADs), 26–27
Copper ion modulation, by gangliosides, 922
Copyrights, 94
Cord factors, 932–933

CORINA, 547
Corneal absorption, of drugs, 969–971
Correction of patents, 66–67
Corticosteroid esters, 959
Cortisol sulfotransferase, 150
Cosmic force field, 576
Costs, of drug development, 257–258
Coumarin, 1017
COUSIN, 427
Covalently binding enzyme inhibitors, 761–779. *See also* Enzyme inhibitors
CP 96, 345, 388, 726
CQNRYTDLVAIQNKE, 937
Craig diagrams, 532
Creatine kinase inhibitors, 775
Criteria, in drug discovery, 20–25
CRM 197, 931
Cromoglycate, and pneumonitis, 203
CROSSBOW, 427
Crystallization, 308
 "multi-termini" approach, 307
Crystallography, 306, 307–312
 electron density maps, 310
 model building, 310–312
Crystathioninuia, 737
CSD, 450, 451
 for molecular modeling, 607, 608, 609
CSM, 462, 464
CTOP, 825
Curare alkaloids, 992–993
Current Chemical Reactions, 106
Current Facts in Chemistry, 105
Current Facts in Chemistry on CD-ROM (Beilstein's), 486
Current Good Manufacturing Practices (cGMP), 261
N-[*N*-(Cyanoacetyl)-L-phenylalanyl]-L-phenylalanine, 771
Cyclic dermorphins, 807–808, 844
Cyclic enkephalins, 806–807, 807 *table*, 811, 812, 829, 843
Cyclic nucleotides, 361
Cyclic peptide linkages, 811–813
Cyclic somatostatin, 805, 808–809
Cyclization, of peptides, 805–814
Cyclized aromatic amino acids, 831–832
Cyclobis, 377
Cyclophilin, 602–603
 rDNA technology in study of, 680–681
Cyclophosphamide, 968
 and pneumonitis, 204

Cyclosporin, 388, 984
 molecular modeling, 602–603
 rDNA technology for studies of, 679–680
Cyclosporin A:
 cyclic structures in, 805
 NMR, 314
Cyclosporine, 119–120
Cyclotetrazoles, 844
CYP2D6, 967
CYP gene superfamily, 136 *table*
CYP P450 enzymes, 135–136
 in carbon oxidation, 137, 138, 140–141
 in morphine biosynthesis, 984–985
 in nitrogen oxidation, 141
 in oxidative cleavage, 146–147
 in oxygen oxidation, 144
 in sulfur oxidation, 143–144
Cyproheptadine, glucuronidation, 156
γ-Cystathioase inhibitors, 737
Cysteine-*S*-conjugate *N*-acetyltransferase, 164
Cysteine-conjugate β-lyase, 176
Cysteine-*S*-conjugate β-lyase, 164
Cysteine endopeptidases, 137
Cysteinylglycine dipeptidase, 164
Cystic fibrosis, 691
Cytochrome enzymes, 136–136. *See also* CYP P450 enzymes

4-DAMP, rigid analogs, 789
DARC, 429
 substructure searching, 424
DARC-CHCD, 434–435
DARC-PELCO approach, 522
Database management software, 105–106
Databases, 14, 104–106, 416–417, *See also* specific Databases
 CD-ROM, 484–486
 2D chemical information databases, *see* 2D Chemical information databases
 3D chemical information databases, *see* 3D Chemical information databases
 synthetic reaction information databases, *see* Synthetic reaction information management databases
 vendors, 418–419 *table*
Data-Star, 105
Daunomycin, 887
N-Dealkylations, 146
O-Dealkylations, 146

S-Dealkylations, 143, 146
Deaminations, 146
Debrisoquine, metabolism, 170
Decamethonium, 799, 992, 993
Declaration of Interference, 63
Degradation, of RNA, 865
Degranol, 907
Dehalogenation reactions, 139
Dehydrocholate sodium,
    anaphylactic reactions, 191
Dehydrogenases, 134–135, 137
Dehydrohalogenation reactions, 139
Dehydroleucine, 826
Dehydrophenylalanine, 826
Dehydropiperazic acid, 821
3,4-Dehydroproline, 822
6,7-Dehydrotestosterone, 137, 139
Deletion mutagenesis, 364
N-Demethylation, 146, 149
O-Demethylation, 146
Demexiptiline, 787
De novo approach, *see* Free Wilson
    analysis
De novo constants, 516–517
De novo design, of ligands by
    molecular modeling, 610–613
1-Deoxy-*N*-acetyl-D-glucosamine,
    933
Deoxyacyclovir, 961
S-(5'-Deoxy-5'-adenosyl)-1-
    ammonio-4-(methylsulfonio)-2-
    cyclopentane, 770
2'-Deoxycoformycin, 755
2'-Deoxycytidine, 870
5'-Deoxy-5-fluorouridine, 966
2-Deoxy-Gal-β-1,3-GlcNal-β-1,
    x-C$_8$ ester, 928, 929
N-(2-Deoxy-L-leucylamino-β-D-
    glucopyranosyl)-*N*-
    octadecyldodecanamide
    acetate, 935
3-Deoxy-D-*manno*-2-octulosinic
    acid, 929
Deoxynojirimycin, 927
Deoxyoligonucleotides, 887
Department of Agriculture, 253
DEPICT, 431
Deposits, patentable life forms,
    53–54
Depot neuroleptics, 954, 962–963
Dermal delivery (prodrugs), 176
Dermatan sulfate, 922
Dermatitis, 182, 198
Dermorphin, 807, 833
Dermorphin analogs, 816, 831,
    832, 833, 843–844
Derwent World Patents Index, 108
10-Desacetylbaccatin II, 999

Desaminocystein, 809–811
DESBASE, 506
Design patents, 43, 95
13-Desmethyl-13,14-dihydro-*all-
    trans*-retinyl trifluoroacetate,
    747
Development teams, for drug
    discovery, 16
Dexamethasone, 964, 965
Dextran, anaphylactic reactions,
    191
Diacyl-azibicyclo[2,2,2]octane,
    836, 837
Diacylglycerol *O*-acyltransferase,
    160
α,α-Dialkylglycines, 817
Dialog, 105
Diamine *N*-acetyltransferase, 157
2,4-Diaminopyrimidines, 542–543
Diamond v. Chakrabarty, 49
Diazepam:
    discovery, 662
    half-life increase with age, 124
Diazepoxide, discovery, 662
Dibenzylglycine, 817
N-*N*-Di-*n*-butyldopamine, 792
1,3-Dicarbonyl compounds,
    glucuronidation, 154
Dichloroalkane moiety, 230
((3,4-Dichlorobenzyl)oxy)acetic
    acid, 604
Diclofenac:
    glucuronidation, 155
    methylation, 148, 150
Dicoumarol, 1017
3D Dictionary of Drugs, 450, 451
3D Dictionary of Fine Chemicals,
    450, 451
3D Dictionary of Natural Products,
    450, 451
Dictionary of Natural Products on
    CD-ROM (CHCD), 484–486
2',3'-Dideoxycytidine, 906
    phosphorylation, 167
2',3'-Dideoxyinosine, 906
Dielectrics, 579–581
Dienestrol, 796
Diethyldithiocarbamic acid,
    glucuronidation, 156
Diethylglycine, 817
β,β-Diethyl-β-mercaptopropionic
    acid, 810
Diethylstilbestrol, 796
Diflunisal:
    glucuronidation, 155
    sulfation, 151, 152
α-Difluoromethylornithine, 735,
    736

Digitalis glycosides, 984
Digitoxin, 186, 906–907
Digoxin, 120, 906–907, 908
Dihydroartemisinin, 1022
Dihydrodiol dehydrogenases, 135,
    140
Dihydrodiols, 141
trans-Dihydrodiols, 147
Dihydro-β-erythroidine, 376
Dihydrofolate reductase inhibition:
    Free Wilson analysis, 542–543
    Hansch analysis, 534–535
    rDNA technology for studies of,
    677
Dihydrofolate reductase-
    trimethoprim interaction, 410,
    677, 735
Dihydromuscimol, 786
Dihydropyridine carriers, 176
Dihydropyridines, 141, 709
Dihydroxyethylene, 846
3,4-Dihydroxy pipecolic acid, 823
9-(1,3-Dihydroxy-2-propoxy-
    methyl)-guanine, 167
Dilantin, immune suppression by,
    206
2,6-Dimethoxybenzylpenicilloyl-
    polylysine, 212
β,β-Dimethyl amino acids, 829
2-(Dimethylamino)-1-ethyl
    diphosphate, 756–757
N,*N*-Dimethyl-α-bromo-
    phenethylamines:
    Free Wilson analysis, 520–521
    Hansch analysis, 518
N,*N*-Dimethyldopamine:
    as dopaminergic agonist, 792
    semirigid analogs, 789
    sulfonium isostere, 787
Dimethylene desaturation, 137
N,*N*-Dimethyl hydrazino
    oligonucleotide backbone, 888,
    889
β,β-Dimethyl-β-mercaptopropionic
    acid, 810
N,*N*-Dimethylsphingosine, 921
Dimethylsulfoxide, 720
Dimethylthiazolidine-4-carboxylic
    acids, 821, 822
Dimethyltubocurarine, 992
Dinitrogen moieties, reduction, 143
2,4-Dinitrophenyl amino acids,
    immune response stimulation,
    187
2',4'-Dinitrophenyl-2-deoxy-2-
    fluoro-β-D-glucopyranoside,
    777
S-Dioxides, 144

Diphenols, oxidation, 140
Diphenylglycine, 817
Diphenylhydantoin, 194
    CASE carcinogenicity prediction, 234
4,5-Diphenylpyrazolidinones, 990
Diphtheria toxoid CRM 197, 931
Dipole interactions, 403, 501, 578–579
    quantum mechanical treatment, 597–598
N,N-Di-n-propyldopamine, 792
Dipropylglycine, 817
Dipyrone, and hemolytic anemia, 196
DIRECTED DOCK, 322
Directionality, 633
Discipline approach, to drug discovery, 12, 27, 29
DISCO, 642
Discovery of drugs, *see* Drug discovery
Discriminant analysis, 530
2,3-Disialosyl-paragloboside, 921
Disiloxane bridges, 811
Disoogenin, 984
Dispersion interactions, 402, 501, 578
    and enzyme inhibition, 739
Disposition, 131
Dissociation, of acids/bases, 526–527
Distance matrix, 628
Distance range matrix, 628, 629
Distribution:
    carbohydrate-based drugs, 908
    half-life as (poor) indicator of mechanism, 123–124
    pharmacokinetics of, 115–121
Distribution volume, 120–121
1,3-Disubstituted tetrazole rings, 844–845
1,5-Disubstituted tetrazole rings, 634
Disulfide bridge replacement, 812
Disulfiram, 156
Dithiocarboxylic acids, glucuronidation, 154, 156
Dithromycin, 1011
Diversity-based ligand libraries, 389–390
Divisional patent applications, 61–62
DNA:
    drug binding to, 410–411
    immune response stimulation, 186–187

interaction with oligonucleotides, 865–867, 869–871, 875
molecular dynamic modeling, 591
recombinant diversity libraries, 673, 674, 676
triple-stranded structures, 870–871
DNA-DNA hybrids, 865, 867
DNA "fingerprinting," 369
DNA libraries, 676, 877
DNA polymerase, Hansch analysis, 536
DNA-RNA hybrids, 865–866, 873
DOCK, 322, 610, 612
    for molecular modeling, 603, 604
Doctrine of equivalents, 68
L-DOPA, methylation, 148
Dopamine:
    locus map, 633
    uptake inhibition, Hansch analysis, 537
Dopamine agonists, 355
Dopamine β-hydroxylase, 135
Dopamine β-hydroxylase inhibitors, 760
Dopamine receptors, 368, 370, 374, 383
    Hansch analysis, 537
DOPE, 881
D-optimal design methods, 533
Dosage form development, 260–262
Dose adjustment, 122
Dose-response curves, 354, 356
Dosing interval, 122–125
Dosing rate, 121
Dothiepin, 787
DOTMA, 881
Doxepin, 787
DPDPE, 829
Drug absorption, *see* Absorption
Drug allergies, *see* Allergies
Drug candidate proposals, 16
Drug candidates, 15
    failure rate, 20
Drug delivery systems, 173, 174, 956–958, 959–960
Drug design:
    computer-aided, 7
    lead compounds, 5–6
    metabolism modulation by structural variations, 171–172
    prodrugs, *see* Prodrugs
    "rational," *see* Rational drug design and steric interactions, 7

structure-aided, *see* Structure-aided drug design
Drug development, 252–300
    approval and product launch, 299–300
    chemistry, 259–264
    clinical studies, 279–300
        ethics, 292–295
        evaluating adverse events, 291–292
        phase I, 279, 280–282, 295
        phase II, 279, 282–286, 295–296, 297
        phase III, 279, 282–286, 297
        phase IV, 279–280, 286
        regulatory review during, 296–300
        reports, 295
    closure development, 262–264
    container development, 262
    costs, 257–258
    dosage form development, 260–261
    evolution
        commercial environment, 256–257
        regulatory environment, 253–255
        scientific environment, 255–256
    formulation development, 260–262
    investigator selection, 288–290
    overview, 258–259, 259 *table*
    planning, 269–279
        critical components/path, 275–279
        master plan, 272–275
        preclinical-clinical transition, 268–269
        preclinical studies, 264–268
        stopping development, 295–296
        strategy definition, 271–272
Drug discovery:
    chemistry-driven, 662–664
    costs, 20
    criteria, 20–25
    critical path, 22
    defined, 10–12
    external issues, 26–27
    future management strategies, 34–36
    high throughput screening, 709–710
    information retrieval in, *see* Information retrieval
    intellectual property issues, *see* Intellectual property

marketing issues, 19
mass ligand screeing, *see* Mass
  ligand screening
organizational approaches/issues,
  12, 27–34
portfolio management issues, 25–
  26
process development, 23
selectivity screening, 710
stages of, 12–20
  basic research, 13, 21
  clinical development, 18–20,
    24–25
  feasibility studies, 13–15,
    21–22
  nonclinical development,
    16–17, 23–24
  programs, 15–16, 22–23
strategic issues, 20–27
strategies, 706–710
"systems" screening approach,
  698–704, 710
Drug disposition, *see* Disposition
Drug distribution, *see* Distribution
Drug elimination, *see* Elimination
Drug interaction studies, 281
Drug metabolism, *see also*
    Conjugation reactions;
    Functionalization reactions;
    Prodrugs; Xenobiotic
    metabolism
  biological factors affecting, 133–
    134
  carbohydrate-based drugs, 908–
    909
  genetic influences, 216
  Michaelis-Menten kinetics, 118
  modulation by structural
    variations, 171–172
  structure-metabolism relationship,
    168–171
    configurational influences, 170
    electronic factors and
      lipophilicity, 170–171
  studies, in drug discovery, 17–18
Drug Price Competition and Patent
  Term Restoration Act of 1984,
  255, 272
Drug reactions, *see* Adverse drug
  reactions; Allergies
Drug-receptor binding, 400–411,
  713–714
  charge transfer energy, 402
  conformational flexibility, 407
  dispersion attraction, 402
  electrostatic energy, 401–402
  examples, 408–411

exchange repulsion energy, 402
polarization energy, 402
QSAR modeling, 500–503
thermodynamics, 400–401, 404–
  408
Drug receptors, *see* Receptors
Drug recognition sites, 350, 351
Drug resistance:
  enzyme inhibitors and, 737
  Hansch analysis, 537
  rDNA technology for mutant
    library creation, 672, 673
Drugs, *see also* drugs and diseases,
    i.e., AIDS; classes of Drugs,
    such as Antibiotics; and
    specific Drugs
  binding in blood, 117
  brand loyalty, 79–80
  dose-response relationship, 115
  multiple effects of, 6–7
  patent infringement, 69
  peptide esters, as prodrugs, 958–
    959
  pharmacokinetics, *see*
    Pharmacokinetics
  prodrugs, *see* Prodrugs
  reduction to practice
    requirements, 65
3DSEARCH, 608–609
Dummy variables, 516–517
Dummy vectors, 631
DYLOMMS, 605
Dyphylline prodrugs, 952–953

Eadie-Hofstee plots, 742, 746
  competitive inhibition, 743
  noncompetitive inhibition, 745
  uncompetitive inhibition, 744
ECEPP, 613
Echinocandin L-688, 1013
Echinocandins, 1012–1014
E. coli, vaccines, 930
E. coli thymidilate synthetase
  inhibitors, 677
EDTA-oligonucleotide conjugates,
  875
Efficacy, of ligands, 353, 357
Egg-sperm recognition, 902–903,
  937–938
Ehrlich, Paul, 350, 500
Electron density maps, 310
Electronic factors, and structure-
  metabolism relationship, 170–
  171
Electronic parameters, 513–515
Electrophilic theory, of
  carcinogenicity, 226

Electrospray mass spectrometry,
  911
Electrostatic interactions, 401–402,
  501, 502, 578–582
  and enzyme inhibition, 739
  molecular modeling, 605–607,
    628–631, 632–633
  quantum mechanical treatment,
    596–599
Elimination, 115
  first pass effect, 119, 127
  half-life as (poor) indicator of
    mechanism, 123–124
  pharmacokinetics of, 116–119,
    122–125
  prodrugs, 972
Elixir of sulfanilamide tragedy,
  254
Enablement, in patent specification,
  52–54
Enalapril, 736, 961–962, 1016
Enalaprilate, 961–962
Endonucleases, 878
Endorphins, 987
Endothelin, 709–710, 715
Endothiapepsin, 325, 329, 330,
  331
Enforcement:
  of patents, 67–72
  trade secrets, 89–90
England, *see* United Kingdom
English yew, 996–997
Enkephalin mimetics, 620
Enkephalins, 806–807, 829, 843,
  987
  AiB incorporation, 814
Enoxaprin, 923
Ensembles, 589
Enterobacteriae, vaccines, 931
Entropy, 589
Enzymatic synthesis, carbohydrate
  drugs, 915–917
Enzymatic triggers, 959
Enzyme-induced inactivators, 762,
  763–766, 767–774
Enzyme induction, 134
Enzyme inhibition, 134
  Dixon plots, 746
  Eadie-Hofstee plots, *see* Eadie-
    Hofstee plots
  forces involved, 738–740
  Hansch analysis, 534–536
  irreversible binding, 745
  kinetics, 738–739
  Kitz-Wilson plots, 764
  Lineweaver-Burk plots, *see*
    Lineweaver-Burk plots

Enzyme inhibitors, 6, 7
affinity labels, 762, 766, 767–774
classification, 737 *table*
covalently binding, 761–779
mechanism evaluation criteria, 762–767
mechanism-based inhibitors, 762, 763–766, 767–774
medical applications, 734–737
multisubstrate inhibitors, 757–761, 759–761
noncovalently binding, 738–761
forces involved, 738–740
pseudoirreversible inhibitors, 762, 767, 777–779
rapid, reversible inhibitors, 740–748
competitive, 743
design, 740–741
IC_{50}, 745–746
kinetics, 741–742
noncompetitive, 744–745
uncompetitive, 743–744
research applications, 737–738
slow binding inhibitors, 748–751
slow-tight binding inhibitors, 748, 750
structure-aided drug design, 305
tight binding inhibitors, 748
transition-state analogs, 752–757
examples, 755–757
Enzymes:
active sites, 6, 7, 738
basic concepts, 352–353, 738–740
functionalization catalyzing, 134–137
rDNA technology for studies of, 676–681
specificity and selectivity, 132–133
structure elucidation, 6
Ephedrine, 1020
Epidermal growth factor, 921
Epinephrine, 969, 1020
anaphylactic reactions, 193
Epitope mapping, 669–671
Epoxidation reactions, 141
Epoxide hydrolazes, 137, 141, 147
Epoxides, 846
hydration, 147
N-(2,3-Epoxypropyl)-N-amidinoglycine, 775
Equine 2-macroglobulin, 909
Ergodic systems, 590
Erythromycin, 960, 1005, 1009, 1010

Erythromycin estolate, and hepatitis, 199
Erythromycin macrolides, 1009–1012
Erythropoietin, 926
E-Selectins, 937
Esmolol, 172
ESPACE, 105
Esterases, 147
Ester linkages, 811
Esterone, 956
Ester prodrugs, 147, 954–956
Esters, hydrolysis, 147
Estradiol, 966
Estradiol-β-D-xyloside, 925
Estragole, sulfation, 151
Estrogen receptor, Hansch analysis, 537
Ethanol:
conjugation with fatty acids, 158
oxidation, 137
Ethics, in drug development, 292–295
3-Ethoxy-4H-3,1-benzoxazin-4-one, 777
Ethoxyzolamide, 970–971
Ethylene, 841–842
Ethylene oxide, anaphylactic reactions, 192
Ethyl phosphate triesters, 878
ETMC, 641–642
Etoposide, 1002, 1003
Eudragit, 963
European Patent Convention, 73–74
EVAL, 528
Exchange repulsion energy, 402
Excretion, carbohydrate-based drugs, 909
Exonucleases, 878
Expert systems, metabolic scheme prediction, 170
External issues, in drug discovery, 26–27
Extraction ratio, 116, 118
Extrathermodynamic approach, *see* Hansch analysis

Factor analysis, 530
Factorial designs, 533
Fast-ion bombardment, 911
Fatty-acyl-ethyl-ester synthase, 158
FCD, 434, 435
FCD-3D, 450, 451
FDA approval process, 252. *See also* various applications, such as Abbreviated New Drug Applications

Current Good Manufacturing Practices (cGMP), 261
in drug development, 253–255
during clinical trials, 296–300
preclinical-clinical transition, 268–269
and public disclosure of patents, 47–48
stereoisomers policy, 264
and trade secrets, 87
Feasibility studies, in drug discovery, 13–15, 21–22
Feedback modulators, 352
Fenfluramine, 146
amino acid conjugation, 160
Fetindomide, 965
Fibrin, 667–669
Fibrinogen, 667–669
Fibrinolytic enzymes, 958
Fibronectin, 924
Ficin, 535
Field parameter, 513
Filtration assays (radioligand binding), 721
Fine Chemical Directory, 106
First pass effect, 119, 127
FK-506, 388, 679–680, 682
FK binding protein, 680–681, 682
Flavin-containing monooxygenases, 135
Flavodoxin, 811
Flavoproteins, 140–141
Fluorescein, 887
anaphylactic reactions, 191
Fluorinated enzyme inhibitors, 844, 845–846
5-Fluoro-2'-deoxyuridylate, 736
Fluoroketomethylene, 845–846
Fluoroketone, 845–846
trans-Fluoroolefins, 843–844
Flupenthioxol, 963
Fluphenazine, 963
Food and Drug Administration (FDA) approval process, *see* FDA approval process
Food, Drug, and Cosmetic Act of 1938, 254
Foot-and-mouth disease, 935
Force fields, 575–578
quantum mechanical treatment, 598–599
Format (SMD), 420
Formulation:
development, 260–262
and drug discovery, 18
N-Formylation, 157
N-Formyl-L-kynurenine, 157
Forssman antigen, 920

FOUNDATION, 610
Fourier transformation, 309
Fragmin, 923
France:
    patentable subject matter, 50–51
    trade secret protection, 93
Fraxiparine, 923
Freedom of Information Acts, 91–92
Free radical inactivation, by glutathione, 167
Free radicals, toxicity, 177
Free Wilson analysis, 498, 499, 500, 520–522
    applications, 541–543
    relationship to Hansch analysis, 522–523
Freund's complete adjuvant, 931
FRODO, 310–311
Frog oocytes, cloning using, 367
Fuadin, and hemolytic anemia, 196
α-(1-2)-Fucosyltransferase inhibitors, 929
Functional antagonism, 354–355
Functionalization reactions, 132
    enzymes affecting, 134–137
    hydration, 147
    hydrolysis, 147
    oxidation and reduction
        carbon, 137–141
        nitrogen, 141–143
        sulfur and other atoms, 143–146
    oxidative cleavage, 146–147
Functional screening, for CNS diseases, 13–14
Furosemide, 960–961
    and nephritis, 201

G_{D2}, 922
G_{D3}, 922
G_{G3}, 922
G_{M1}, 921
G_{M3}, 921, 922
GABA, 736, 768
    conformational constraint, 814
    congeners, 796
GABA agonists, 796
GABA aminotransferase inhibitors, 736, 767–770
GABA-A receptor agonists, 786
GABA/benzodiazepine, 352
GABA/benzodiazepine receptor, 360, 361, 377
GABA inhibitors, molecular modeling, 643–644
γ-Turn mimics, 835
Gangliosides, 920, 921–922

Gastrin, 840, 843
Gastrointestinal absorption, prodrugs, 960–964
Gear algorithm, 591
GENBANK, 105
Gene therapy, 7
Genins, 908
Genotoxicants, 224
Genotoxic carcinogens, 224
Geographic issues, in drug discovery, 29–30
Germany:
    patentable subject matter, 51
    trade secret protection, 93
GLA-60, 934
Glaucoma, 970–971
D-Glucans, 934
Glucoamylase inhibitors, 926–927
Glucocorticoids, 964
β-D-Glucopyranosyl, 935
Glucose-6-phosphate dehydrogenase deficiency, 198
β-D-Glucose spacers, 847–848
β-Glucosidase, Hansch analysis, 536
β-Glucosidase inhibitors, 777, 778
Glucosidation, 152, 156
β-Glucuronidases, 135
Glucuronidation, 152–156
O-Glucuronidation, 153, 155
N-Glucuronides, 156
S-Glucuronides, 156
β-Glucuronides, 152
Glucuronyltransferase, 152–156
Glutamate, 736
Glutamine, in conjugation, 159
Glutamine N-acyltransferase, 159
Glutamine N-phenylacyltransferase, 159
Glutamyl transpeptidase, 164
Glutathione, 141
    conjugation reactions, 163–167
    free radical inactivation, 167
    in liver-specific drug delivery, 966
    metabolism, 163–167
    redox equilibrium, 163
    selenium's role, 163
Glutathione peroxidase, 163
Glutathione reductase, 135
Glutathione S-transferases, 163
Glycerol trinitrate, hydrolysis, 147
Glycinamide ribonucleotide transformylase inhibitors, 759–760, 776
Glycine, in conjugation, 159
Glycine, N-acyltransferase, 159
Glycine N-benzoyltransferase, 159

Glycolic acid oxidase, Hansch analysis, 536
Glycolipids, 903, 919–922
    as adjuvants, 934–935
N-Glycolylneuraminic acid, 911
Glycomimetics, 917
Glyconconjugates, 903, 919–926
    glycolipids, 903, 919–922
    glycoproteins, 903, 925–926
    proteoglycans, 903, 922–925
Glycopeptide antibiotics, 904
Glycoprotein hormones, 920
Glycoproteins, 903, 925–926
    recombinant, 926
Glycosaminoglycan chains, 922
Glycosidase inhibitors, 926–928
Glycosidation, 914
O-Glycosides, 915
Glycosphingolipids, 919, 921–922
Glycosylation, 914–915
Glycosyl fluorides, 915
Glycosyl 1-phosphates, 916
Glycosylphosphatidylinositols, 919
Glycosyltransferase inhibitors, 928–929
Glycosyltransferases, 916, 928
Glycosyl trichloracetimidates, 914
Glyvenol, 907
GM 1115, 924
Gold:
    and aplastic anemia, 206
    and lupus, 206
    and nephritis, 201
GOLEM, 527–528
GOLPE, 531
Good Clinical Practices (GCP), and drug development, 259, 260 table, 273
Good Laboratory Practices (GLP)
    and drug development, 259, 260 table
    and drug discovery, 18
Good Manufacturing Practices (GMP)
    and drug development, 259, 260 table
    and drug discovery, 18, 24
Goodpasture's syndrome, 204
Goodwill, 79–80
GPAT, 108
GPRLSA, 311
G-protein coupled receptors, 351
    agonist effects at, 358
    allosteric modulation, 356
    model, 364
    QSAR modeling, 501
    rDNA cloning/studies, 364, 369, 372, 373–375, 683–684

Grace period, patents, 42, 56
Granulocytopenia, 182, 196–197
GRID, 499, 545
  for molecular modeling, 604
Grid tyranny, 638
Griseofulvin, lupus-like syndromes, 202
Group contributions, additivity in QSAR, 503
Growth-hormone releasing factor, 840
Guanine deaminase, Hansch analysis, 536
Guanylyl cyclase, 685

H189, 328
H261, 328–329, 330
Half-life, 121, 122–125
  dose lost *vs.* half-lives, 122 *table*
  multiple-dosing, 125
Hallucinogens, Hansch analysis, 540
Haloalkenes, reaction with glutathione, 164–165
Haloethanols, conjugation with fatty acids, 158
5-Halogenated nucleosides, 884
α-Haloketones, 777
Haloperidol, 338, 963
  molecular modeling, 609
Halothan, 139
Halothane:
  and hepatitis, 199
  immune response stimulation, 188
Hammett reaction constant, 498–499, 513
Hansch analysis, 499, 500, 517–520
  applications, 533–541
  activity-activity relationships, 540–541
  relationship to Free Wilson analysis, 522–523
H antigens, 936
Hapten-antibody interactions, Hansch analysis, 536
Hapten-protein conjugates, 215, 216–217
Haptens, 185–188
Hard sphere *exo*-anomeric (HSEA) effect, 911
HASL model, 546
Hecogenin, 984
Hemagglutination, 208
Hemagglutins, 938
Heme-coupled monooxygenases, 135

Hemicholinium, 799
Hemoglobins, 135
  molecular modeling, 604
  oxygen binding curves, 505
Hemolytic anemia, 182, 195–196
Hemozoin, 1023
Heparan sulfate, 922
Heparin, 922–923
  absorption, 908
  anaphylactic reactions, 191
  half-life, 908–909
  low molecular weight, 923–924
  mechanism of action, 923–924
Hepatic clearance, 117–118
Hepatic extraction ratio, 118
Hepatitis, 182, 198
Hepatocytes, 117
Heptachlor, CASE carcinogenicity prediction, 234, 236
Hermetic containers, 262
Heroin, 950–951, 986
  anaphylactic reactions, 191
  sensitivity to, 204
Herpes, 735, 880
Heterocycle modifications, oligonucleotide therapeutics, 878, 884–887
Heteropolysaccharides, 934
Hexestrol, 796
hGH binding, 671
High performance liquid chromatography (HPLC), 511
High-pH anion exchange, 910
High-throughput screening, 390–391, 709–710
Hilar adenopathy, 203–204
HINT, 545
Hippuric acid, 159–160
Histamine:
  anaphylactic reactions, 192
  methylation, 149
Histamine antagonists, molecular modeling, 636–637
Histamine methyltransferase, 148
HIV:
  carbohydrate-based drugs for, 927
  expression, 673
  oligonucleotides for, 871, 891
HIV-1 gp120 receptor, 669
HIV protease inhibitors, 840, 846
  rDNA technology for studies of, 678–679, 680
  structure-aided design, 332–339
HIV proteases, 845
  hydrogen bonding in, 337
  molecular modeling, 600–601, 606, 609, 615–616, 618, 649

rDNA technology for studies of, 678–679, 680
  structure, 321, 333–334
HIV1-RT inhibitors, 747
HIV Tat inhibitors, 673–674
HMG-CoA reductase inhibitors, 736, 758–759, 1014
Hodgkin's disease, 995
Homatropine, 971
Homing receptors, 688
Homologous modeling, 315–320, 617–618
  combinatorial approach, 319
  modeling side chains, 318
  protein folding identification, 318
  satisfaction of spatial restraints method, 318
  simulated annealing, 320
Homologue-scanning mutagenesis, 670
Homopolysaccharides, 934
Homopurine-homopyrimidine sequences, 870
Hoogstein binding, 870
Host cell recognition, 938
H_1-receptor antagonists, Hansch analysis, 536
H_1-receptor antihistaminics, Hansch analysis, 538
HSV-thymidine kinase, Hansch analysis, 536
HTSS/TREE, 466
Human growth hormone, recombinant, 664
Human growth hormone releasing factor, 840
Human growth hormone-somatogenic receptor interaction, 670, 671
Human insulin, recombinant, 664
Human prolactin, recombinant, 671
Humoral hypersensitivity reactions, 190
  assays for, 207–208
Hyaluronan, 922
Hyaluronic acid, 922, 956–957
Hydantoins, 176
  and vasculitis, 200
Hydralazine:
  acetylation, 157
  allergy evaluation, 215
  carbonyl conjugation, 167–168
  immune response stimulation, 188
  lupus-like syndromes, 202, 203
Hydrated polar gate principle, 910
Hydration reactions, 147
Hydrazides, acetylation, 157, 158

Hydrazines:
  acetylation, 157, 158
  carbonyl conjugation, 167–168
  immune suppression by, 206
  oxidation and reduction, 141, 143
Hydrazones, 167
Hydrocodone, 967
Hydrocortisone, 956
Hydrogen bonding, 6, 501, 510
  in carbohydrates, 912
  and enzyme inhibition, 740
  and force fields, 578
  molecular modeling, 604–605
Hydrolazes, 137, 147
Hydrolysis, 147
  of prodrugs, 959–960
Hydromorphone, 967
Hydrophobic effect, 581–582
Hydrophobic fragmental constant, 512
Hydrophobic interactions, 501–502
  in enzyme inhibition, 739–740
  molecular modeling, 605–607
Hydrophobicity, 5. See also Lipophilicity
Hydroquinones, 140
(1S,2R)-cis-21-[[[2-(Hydroxy-amino)-2-oxoethyl]methyl-amino]carbonyl]cyclohexane-carboxylic acid, 748
1-(4-Hydroxybenzyl)imidazole-2-thione, 760
Hydroxychloroquine, 1026–1027
Hydroxyethylene, 846
Hydroxylamides, glucuronidation, 153, 156
Hydroxylamines, 141
  glucuronidation, 153, 155–156
Hydroxylation reactions, 137–138
3′-Hydroxy-4′-methoxy-diclofenac, 148, 150
3-Hydroxy-4-methoxy-5-nitrobenzaldehyde, 748
(R)-(-)-11-Hydroxy-10-methylaporphine, 795
3-Hydroxymorphinian opiod analgesics, 964
β-(4′-Hydroxyphenyl)-proline, 832
Hydroxyprolines, 823
Hydroxypropyl cellulose, 956
α-Hydroxysteroid dehydrogenases, 135
β-Hydroxysteroid dehydrogenases, 135
Hydroxysteroids, sulfation, 151
6β-Hydroxytestosterone, 137, 139

7-Hydroxy-1,2,3,4-tetrahydroisoquinoline carboxylic acid, 831
5-Hydroxytryptamine receptors, 686
Hypersensitivity reactions, see Allergies, hypersensitivity reactions
Hypertension, drug discovery for, 14
Hypolipidemic agents, 159

Ibuprofen, 967
  hybrid liquid formation, 161
IC_{50}, 745–746
ICAM-1, 868, 874, 876, 877
ICAMs, 903
IFN-α (serum)
  half-life, 124–125
  volume of distribution, 121
Ileal M$_3$ acetylcholine receptors, 789
Imidazole, methylation, 149
Imines, 143
Imipenem, 1009
Imipramine, 59, 787
Immobilized enzymes, 917
Immune recognition, glycolipid role, 920
Immune response, 182–190. See also Allergies
  genetic influences, 216
Immunoadhesins, 669, 670
Immunoglobulin E, 183, 184
  anaphylactic reaction mediation, 192
  as evidence of anaphylactic sensitivity, 207–208
  and serum sickness, 194
Immunoglobulin G, 183
  and anaphylactic reactions, 193
  and nephritis, 201
  and serum sickness, 194
  and thrombocytopenia, 197
Immunoglobulin M, 184
Immunoglobulins, 183
Immunologic assays, 207–209
Immunologic memory, 183
Immunomodulation, carbohydrate-based therapeutics, 929–935
Immunostimulants, carbohydrate-based, 931–935
Importance sampling, 593
Inactivation theory, 358–359
$Index$ $Chemicus$, 439–440
Indicator variables, 516–517
Indomethacin:
  and hepatitis, 199
  sensitivity to, 205

Industrial-academic collaborations, in drug discovery, 32–33
Influenza, 938
  vaccines, 930–931
Information Disclosure Statements, 61
Information retrieval, 104–106. See also Computers; Databases; Software
  benefits, 110
  in chemical development, 109
  in compound isolation, characterization, and structure determination, 107–108
  in compound synthesis, 107
  in lead compound optimization, 108–109
  in licensing, 109
  in patent filing, 108
  in product development, 109
  in project initiation, 106–107
Information science, 104–110
Infringent, 67–72
  defenses (of challenger), 69–71
  remedies, 71–72
Inhibitors, see Enzyme inhibitors
Injunctions:
  as infringement remedy, 71–72
  protecting trade secrets, 90
Inosine, 885
INPADOC, 108
In re $Durden$, 59–60
Insecticides, and aplastic anemia, 206
Insulin, 956
  recombinant, 664
Integrated chemical information computing software, 486–489
Integrin receptors, 687–688, 689, 703
Intellectual property, 38–96
  and academic-industrial collaborations, 33
  copyrights, 94
  design patents, 95
  other forms of protection, 94–96
  overview of importance and rewards of, 38–43
  patents, see Patents
  statutory invention registration, 94–95
  trademarks, 78–87
    legislative framework, 79, 81–82, 84, 86–87
    oppositions and cancellations, 83, 84
    registering, 82–84
    selection, 80–82
    worldwide rights, 85–86

Intellectual property (*Continued*)
  trade secrets, 87–94
    and abandoned patent
      applications, 60, 63
    enforcement, 89–90
    and Freedom of Information
      Acts, 91–92
    outside U.S., 92–94
    patent improvements kept as,
      45
    and patents, 90–91
    requirements for, 88–89
Interaction energies, 401–408
Interatomic distance variation, in
  analog design, 799–801
Intercellular adhesion, 903
Intercellular adhesion molecule,
  687
Interference proceedings, patents,
  63–66
Interferons, 183, 920
Interleukin-1α, homologous
  modeling, 316
Interleukin-1β:
  crystal structure, 308
  homologous modeling, 316
  isotope labeling, 313
  NMR, 313, 314
Interleukin-1 (IL-1) cytokine, 14
Interleukin-1RA, 316
Interleukin-2, 7
Interleukins, 183, 894
Intravenous administration:
  and bioavailability, 119
  dose adjustment, 122
Intrinsic activity, 357
Insulin, 956
Inverse agonists, 355
Investigational Exemption to a New
  Drug application (IND), 255
  elements of, 268–269
Investigational New Drug (IND)
  applications, 16
  filing, 18
Investigator's Brochure, 268
In vitro studies, 15, 20, 213
  needless studies, 21
Iodides:
  anaphylactic reactions, 191
  and dermatitis, 198
  and vasculitis, 200
Iodinated dyes, histamine release
  by, 204
Ion-induced dipole interaction, 403
Ionization, of acids/bases, 526–527
Iproniazid:
  and hepatitis, 199
  and vasculitis, 200

Iris, drug distribution in, 971
ISIS, 106, 459, 487–489
ISIS 1082, 871–872, 879, 880, 882
ISIS 1570, 874
ISIS 1753, 872
ISIS 1939, 873, 874
ISIS 2105, 882
ISIS/Base, 105–106, 487, 488–489
ISIS/Draw, 487, 488
ISIS/Host, 489
Isocyanates, reaction with
  glutathione, 165
Isoniazid, 19
  acetylation, 157
  carbonyl conjugation, 167–168
  and hepatitis, 199
  lupus-like syndromes, 202
Isopentyl diphosphate isomerase,
  756, 757
Isoprenaline, 1020
Isopropylidene, 913
Isopropyl phosphate triesters, 878
Isosorbide, glutathione role in drug
  action, 166–167
Isosorbide dinitrate, 907
Isosorbide-5-nitrate, 907
Isothiocyanates, reaction with
  gluthathione, 165
Isotope labeling, 313–314
Isovaline, 814
Italy:
  patentable subject matter, 51
  trade secret protection, 93
Ivermectins, 904, 1028

Japan:
  drug development in, 273
  patentable subject matter, 51
  trade secret protection, 93
JAPIO, 108
JOY, 316

K-13, 812
Kanamycin, 1005
Karaya gum, anaphylactic
  reactions, 191
Kefauver-Harris Amendments,
  254–255
Keratan sulfate, 922
Ketofluoromethylenes, 846
Ketomethylene, 845–846
Ketone reductases, 135
Khellin, 1017–1018
Kidneys, drug clearance by, 118–
  119
Kitz-Wilson plots, 764
Klebsiella, vaccines, 930
Koenigs-Knorr reactions, 914

L-364,286, 990
L-364,718, 990
L-365,260, 991
L-366,509, 388
L-670,207, 357
Labeling, 252–253, 271
Labetalol, 544
α-Lactalbumin, homologous
  modeling, 315
β-Lactam antibiotics, 672
  natural products, 1003–1009
β-Lactamase inhibitors, 734–735
β-Lactamases, mutant library, 672
Laminin, 201
Lanham Act, 79, 81–82, 84, 86–87
Lanthionine bridge, 812
Latent inactivators, 762, 763–766,
  767–774
Latex, anaphylactic reactions, 191–
  192
Laudexium, 993
Lawesson's reagent, 842
Lead compounds, 5–6
  in analog design, 783–785. *See
    also* Analog design
  fragment design, 797–799
  discovery, and receptors, 387–
    391
  in drug discovery, 13, 14, 22
  information science applications,
    108–109
  sources, 388–391
  structure-aided design
    identification, 321
Leap-frog algorithm, 591–592
Lecithin retinol acyl transferase
  inhibitors, 747–748
Leloir pathway, 916
Lentinan, 934
Leucine aminopeptidase, 843
Leudmedins, 703
Leu-enkephalinamide, 841
Leukemia, 995, 1003
Leukocyte adhesion, 703
Lewis X, 919
LHASA, 107
Lh-RH, 840
Licensing, 77–78
  information science applications,
    109
Lidocaine, hydrolysis, 147
Lidocaine analogs, Hansch
  analysis, 539
Life forms, patentability, 49, 50–51
LIG$_{A4}$, 921
LIG$_{A20}$, 921
Ligand binding, NMR studies,
  314–315

Ligand gated ion channels, 351
  allosteric modulation, 356
  cloning, 370, 372, 375–377
  model, 365
  receptor complexes, 360–361
Ligandin, 163
Ligand libraries:
  diversity-based, 389–390
  pharmacophore-based, 388–389
Ligands, *see also* Agonists;
    Antagonists; Radioligand
    binding assays; Receptors
  basic concepts, 352, 353–355
  classes, 353–355
  molecular modeling, *see*
    Molecular modeling
  multiple receptor selectivity, 378,
    621
  occupancy, and receptor
    dynamics, 362
  receptor complexes, 359–361,
    501–503
Ligase chain reaction technique,
    367, 368
Light-resistant containers, 262
Lincosaminide antibiotics, 904
Line organizational structure, and
    drug discovery, 28–29
Lineweaver-Burk plots, 742–746
  competitive inhibition, 743
  noncompetitive inhibition, 745
  uncompetitive inhibition, 744
Lipid A, 933
Lipid formation, 160–161
Lipidic peptide prodrugs, 959
Lipid X, 933
Lipid Y, 933
Lipophilicity, 499
  in molecular modeling, 640
  nonlinear relationships with
    activity, 523–526
  and structure-metabolism
    relationship, 170–171
Lipophilicity parameters, 509–512
  measurement/calculation, 511–
    512
Lipopolysaccharide endotoxins, 933
Lipoprotein(a), 690
Liposomes, 734, 880–881
5-Lipoxygenase inhibitors, 786,
    793
Literal infringement, 68
Liver, drug clearance by, 117–118
Liver alcohol dehydrogenases
    (LADHs), 134
Liver-specific drug delivery, 966
Loading dose, 125–126
Lock and key hypothesis, 350, 500

LOCON, 528
Locus maps, 633
Logiparin, 923
LOGONA, 528
Log P, 499
  estimation, 474
Lomoparin, 923
Long-chain fatty acid-CoA ligase,
    159
Losartan, 662, 663
Lovastatin, 966, 984
  discovery, 662, 663
  mode of action, 1014–1015
Low molecular weight heparins,
    923–924
L-Selectins, 937
LUDI, 610
Lung cancer, 995, 1003
Lupus erythematosus, 202–203,
    1023, 1026
  and gold allergy, 206
Luteinizing hormone-releasing
    factor, 825
Lymphadenopathy, 205
Lymphoblastic leukemia, 995
Lymphocyte function-associated
    molecule, 687
Lymphocyte leukemia, 995
Lymphocyte sensitization, 182–
    184, 186
Lymphocyte tracking, 688–689
Lymphokines, 183
Lymphomas, 995, 1003

MACCS, 106
  for lead compound optimization,
    108
MACCS-3D, 445, 447
  for molecular modeling, 608
MACCS Drug Data Report, 106
MACCS-II, 428, 429–430
  ACD interface, 436–437
  FCD interface, 436
  Index Chemicus interface, 439–
    440
  MDDR interface, 437
  programming languages, 429
  substructure searching, 423
  Therapeutic Patent Fast-Alert
    interface, 439
Machine, as patentable subject
    matter, 48
Macrolide antibiotics, 904
MACROMODEL, 589
Marcomolecular carriers, in
    immune response, 185–190
Macromolecular conjugates, 132
Macromolecular prodrugs, 956–958

MACROSEARCH, 589
Ma huang (Chinese extract), 1020
Mainframe computers, databases
    for, 106
Major histocompatibility complex
    proteins, 183
Management, of drug discovery,
    see Drug discovery
Management career paths, in drug
    discovery, 31–32
Mandalate racemase, 753
Mannich bases, as prodrugs, 956
Mannitol Myleran, 907
α-Mannosides, 938
Manufacture, as patentable subject
    matter, 48
Marketing issues, in drug
    discovery, 19
MarkOut, 469, 470, 471
Markov chains, 594
Marks, *see* Trademarks
Markush structural searches, 107
Mass ligand screening:
  "blind alleys," 706
  future of, 710
  radioligand binding assays, *see*
    Radioligand binding assays
  selectivity of, 699–700
  vs. systems screening, 698
Mass spectrometry, 910–911
Material Safety Data Sheets
    (MSDS), database for, 105,
    108
Matrix organizational structure, and
    drug discovery, 12, 28–29
May apple, 1001
MCD, 528
MCSS, 322
MDDR, 434, 437–438
MDDR-3D, 450, 451
Meat packing, 253–254
Mechanism-based enzyme
    inhibitors, 762, 763–766, 767–
    774
Mecillinam, 960
Medicinal chemistry, 3–7
Medicinal product, 953
Medline, 105
Mefenamic acid:
  and hemolytic anemia, 196
  sensitivity to, 205
Mefloquine, 1023, 1024, 1025,
    1026
Membrane glycosphingolipids, 919
Membrane receptor assays, 381–
    383
Membranes, 510–511
Meningitis, 930

MENTHOR, 448
Meperidine, 798, 987
  rigid analogs, 789–790
Mephenesin, and pneumonitis, 203
Mephenytoin, and hemolytic
  anemia, 196
Meprobamate, and
  thrombocytopenia, 197
2-Mercaptobenzoic acid, 809
6-Mercaptopurine, 150
Mercapturic acids, 164
Mercurials:
  anaphylactic reactions, 191
  and nephritis, 201
MERLIN, 428, 430–432
Mesantoin, immune response
  stimulation, 188
Message-address concept, 847
N-Mesyl-glycine X-phenyl esters,
  535
MetabolExpert, 469, 479–482
Metabolism, see Drug metabolism;
  Xenobiotic metabolism
Metabolites, 131
  functionalized products vs.
    conjugates, 132
  immune response stimulation by,
    187, 188–189
  toxicity, 6
Metalloendopeptidases, 137
METALYSIS, 462, 464
META program, 246
Metazocine, 798
Methadone, 798
Methamphetamine, and vasculitis,
  200
2,3-Methano amino acids,
  β-substituted, 829–831
2,3-Methanomethionine, 831
Methanoprolines, 820
2,3-Methanotyrosine, 831
Methazolamide, 970–971
Methicillin, 1004
  and nephritis, 201
Methimazole, and
  granulocytopenia, 197
Methionine:adenosyl transferase
  inhibition, 643, 760–761
Methotrexate, 537, 677
  and pneumonitis, 204
Methoxyflurane, and hepatitis, 199
Methoxyhydrofuran derivatives,
  793
Methoxyhydropyran derivatives,
  786
N-Methyl-aceteamide, 847
  binding to HIV protease, 606
β-Methyl amino acids, 829

N-Methyl aminohydroxyl
  oligonucleotide backbone, 888,
  889
N-Methyl-D-aspartate receptor,
  360–361
α-Methylated amino acids, 814–
  817
Methylation, 148–150
N-Methylation, 149–150, 823
O-Methylation, 148
S-Methylation, 148, 150
N-Methylation-α-(R&S)-benzyl-o-
  AMPA, 809, 810
Methyldopa, 952
  and hepatitis, 199
  lupus-like syndromes, 202
α-Methyldopa:
  blood-drain barrier transport, 967
  and hemolytic anemia, 196
Methylene-N-acetylamine, 840
Methylenealkylamine, 840
Methyleneamine, 838–840, 846
3,3′-Methylenebis(4-hydroxy-
  coumarin), 1017
Methylene ether, 841–842
Methylene-N-formylamine, 840
Methylene hydroxyamines, 846
Methylene sulfones, 846
Methylenesulfoxide, 840–841
Methylenethioether, 840–841
Methylformamide, 166
N-Methylhydropyridine carriers,
  176, 177
Methyl isocyanate, reaction with
  glutathione, 165
α-Methylleucine, 814
Methylmalonyl-CoA epimerase,
  161
α-Methylnoradrenaline, 967
β,β-(4-Methylpentamethylene)-β-
  mercaptopropionic acid, 810
α-Methylphenylalanine, 814
Methylphosphonates, 871, 874,
  875, 879
  toxicity, 881–882
  in vivo pharmacokinetics, 881–
  882
Methylprednisolone, 964, 965, 974
Methylprolines, 820
2′-O-Methyl pseudoisocytidine,
  870
Methyltransferases, 148–150
α-Methylvaline, 814
2-Methyoxy-6-chloro-9-(5-
  hydroxypenty)amino acridine,
  880–881
Metocurine, 992, 993
Metronidazole, 143, 965

Metronidazole esters, 959
Metropolis algorithm, 589, 594
Mevinolin, 736
Mexico, trade secret protection, 93
Michaelis-Menten kinetics, 118,
  352, 353, 741–742
Milbemycins, 904, 1027–1028
L-Mimosine, 787
MIMUMBA, 547
Minimization of potential surfaces:
  conformational analysis, 587–589
  conformational clustering, 586–
  587
  in molecular modeling, 635–639
  systematic search methods, 583–
  587, 636, 637–638
Minimum effective concentration,
  122
Minimum toxic concentration, 122
Minoxidil, 151–152
Mithramycin, 904, 905
Mitindomide, 965
Mitomycin C, 956
Mivacurium, 994
MK-329, 990
ML-236B, 1014
MM3, 613
Model receptor sites, 644–645
Molar refractivity, 513
Molecular comparison, 631–635
Molecular connectivity indices, 516
Molecular dynamics, 590–592
  hydrophobic effect calculations,
  582
  for potential surface
    minimization, 588
Molecular electrostatic potential,
  598
Molecular mechanics, 575–596
Molecular modeling, 574–575
  approaches:
    molecular mechanics, 575–596
    quantum mechanics, 596–599
  and drug discovery, 11–12
  historical perspective, 574–575
  known receptors, 599–618
    affinity calculation, 613–617
    homology modeling, 617–618
    ligand design, 607–613
    site definition/characterization,
    600–607
  unknown receptors, 618–635
    common pattern determination,
    635–649
  molecular comparisons, 631–635
  pharmacore vs. binding site
    models, 619–627
  similarity searching, 627–631

Molecular modification, 4–5
Molecular Spreadsheet, 469, 473–474
Molecular weight, 515–516
Molecule Spreadsheet, 469, 470–473
MOLFILE, 420
Molkick, 105
MOLPAT, for molecular modeling, 608
Molybdenum hydroxylases, 135
Monoamine oxidase, 135
    amine deamination by, 147
    Hansch analysis, 536
Monoamine oxidase inhibitors, 736
Monoclonal antibodies
    carbohydrates in, 911, 922
    drug coupling to, 173
    to receptors, 377
Mononucleosis, and ampicillin allergy, 206
S-Monooxides, 144
Monooxygenases, 135
    in phosphorus oxidation, 145
    in sulfur oxidation, 143–144
Monooxygenation reactions, 135
Monophosphoryl lipid A, 933–934
Monte Carlo simulations, 592–594
    hydrophobic effect calculations, 582
    for potential surface minimization, 588
Moral issues, in drug discovery, 30
Morphiceptin, 822, 826
    molecular modeling, 637–638, 639
Morphinans, 987
Morphine, 984–985
    analogs, 797–798, 847
    glucuronidation, 155
    prodrugs of, 950–951
    sensitivity to, 204
Morphine alkaloids, 986–988
MOS, 106
MTD, 528, 641
MULTICASE, 227, 229, 231, 236, 246, 527
Multidrug resistance, Hansch analysis, 537
Multiple binding modes, 378, 621
Multiple Copy Simultaneous Search (MCSS) method, 322
Multiple-dose containers, 262
Multiple-dosing half-lives, 125
Multiple Isomorphous Replacement method, 307, 309–310
Multiple salt linkages, 185

Multiple-unit containers, 262
Multisubstrate enzyme inhibitors, 757–761
Multi-termini crystallization, 307
Multivalency, carbohydrate-based therapeutics, 909
Multivariate analysis methods, 530–532
Murabutide, 932
Muramethide, 932
Muramyl dipeptide, 931–932
Muscarinic acetylcholine receptors, 789
    cloning, 366–367, 370, 374, 682
Muscarinic receptor agonists, 790
Muscarinic receptor ligands, Hansch analysis, 536
Muscle relaxants, 992–994
Mutagenic agents, Hansch analysis, 537
Mutagenicity:
    for carcinogenicity prediction, 224
    vs. carcinogenicity, 224
Mutagenicity studies:
    in drug development, 267
    in drug discovery, 17, 23–24
Mutants, 672, 673, 676, 737
MVT-101, 600–601
Myasthenia gravis, 203
Myelobomol, 907
Myeloperoxidase, 137, 140

Nabilone, 989
Nadolal, 970
Nalorphine, 986
Naloxone, 986
Naltrexone, 963
Naphthalene, glutathione conjugation, 164
Naphthylalanine, 833
Naphth-2-yl-amidines, 536
Naproxen, 956
Narcotics, 798
National Library of Medicine, 105
Natriuretic peptide receptor, 684–685
Natural product libraries, 728–730
Natural products, 3–4, 984–1029,
    See also specific Natural product drugs; specific plants
    antiasthma drugs, 1017–1021
    antibiotics, 1003–1014
    anticancer drugs, 995–1003
    antiparasitic drugs, 1021–1028
    cardiovascular drugs, 1014–1017
    CNS drugs, 986–992
    β-lactams, 1003–1009

as lead component sources, 388
    neuromuscular blocking drugs, 992–995
    patentability, 49
    prodrugs, 950
N^α-C^α-cylized amino acids, 818–823
Nebularine, 755
Neomycin, 1005
Nephritis, 182, 200–201
Net atomic charge, 579
Neural networks, 528, 646
Neuroleptics, 368
    depot neuroleptics, 954, 962–963
    glucuronidation, 156
    molecular modeling, 644
Neuromuscular blocking drugs, natural products, 992–995
Neutrophil tracking, 688–689
Newcastle disease virus, 938
New Chemical Entities (NCE), 20
New Drug Applications (NDAs), 254, 296–299
    abbreviated (ANADs), 255, 272
Nickel, contact dermatitis, 185
Nicotinamide, methylation, 150
Nicotinamide N-methyltransferase, 148
Nicotinate glucosyltransferase, 152
Nicotinic acid, 956
Nicotinic cholinergic receptors, 361, 365, 367, 377
Nicotinic receptor agonists, 800
Nifedipine, 709
Nimopidine, 709
NIPALS, 530
^{15}N isotope labeling, 313–314
Nitrates, hydrolysis, 147
Nitrendipine, 709
Nitric oxide, as second messenger, 362
Nitro compounds, 143
Nitrofurantoin:
    anaphylactic reactions, 191
    and hepatitis, 199
    and pneumonitis, 204
Nitrogen:
    isotope labeling, 313–314
    oxidation and reduction reactions, 141–143
Nitroglycerine, 166–167
Nitrosoarenes, 166
Nivaldipine, 143
NMDA receptor, 382
N. meningtidis, vaccines, 930, 931
N^α-Methylated amino acids, 823–825
Nomifesin, and hemolytic anemia, 196

Non-Boltzman sampling, 595–596
Nonclinical development, *see*
    Preclinical development
Noncompetitive antagonism, 354
Noncompetitive enzyme inhibitors,
    744–745
Noncovalently binding enzyme
    inhibitors, 738–761
Nongenotoxic carcinogens, 224
Non-Hodgkin's lymphomas, 995
Nonlinear lipophilicity-activity
    relationships, 523–526
Non-nucleic acid targets, of
    oligonucleotides, 877
Nonobviousness, as patent
    requirement, 55, 57–60
Nonpeptide ligands, for peptinergic
    receptors, 847–848
Nonsteroidal antiinflammatories,
    703
Norapomorphine, 791–792
Norepinephrine:
    rigid analogs, 791
    uptake inhibition, Hansch
        analysis, 537
Norfenfluramine, 146
Normal equations, 528
North American Free Trade
    Agreement (NAFTA), 92, 93
Notice of Opposition (trademarks),
    84
Novel libraries, 727–728
Novelty, as patent requirement, 55,
    56–57
NPC 12724, 706
NSAI drugs, 960
Nuclear magnetic resonance
    (NMR) techniques, 306, 312–
    315
    carbohydrate study, 911, 912
    3-dimensional, 314
    and drug design, 314–315
    isotope labeling, 313–314
    and site modeling, 601–602
Nuclear Overhauser effects, 313,
    912
Nuclease stability, of
    oligonucleotides, 877–878,
    886–887
Nucleic acids:
    immune response stimulation,
        186
    interactions with oligonucleotide
        therapeutics, *see* Oligonu-
        cleotide therapeutics
    as receptors, 6
Nucleosides, carbohydrate-based,
    906

Nucleotide intercalator, 410–411
Nucleotodiyltransferases, 875
Nutrition, and drug metabolism,
    134

Obviousness, as patent
    requirement, 55, 57–60
Occular absorption, of prodrugs,
    969–971
Occupancy-activated
    destabilization, oligonucleotide
    therapeutics, 872–874
Occupancy-only mediated
    mechanisms, oligonucleotide
    therapeutics, 869–872
Occupancy theory, 356–358
n-Octanol/water partition, 509–510
Office Actions (PTO), 62
Office of Research Integrity, 292
Okadaic acid, 918, 919
Oleandomycin, 1005
cis-Olefins, 846
trans-Olefins, 843–844
Oligonucleotides, 864–865
α-Oligonucleotides, 871, 888
Oligonucleotide therapeutics, 864–
    894
    activities, 890–894
        tissue culture, 890–893
        in vivo, 893–894
    backbone modifications, 867
        table, 886, 888–890
    cellular uptake, 879–881, 887–
        888
    cleavage reagents, 888
    heterocycle modifications, 878,
        884–887
    intracellular stability, 878–879
    nonnucleic acid interactions,
        877–878
    nuclease stability, 877–878, 886–
        887
    nucleic acid interactions, 865–
        869
    occupancy-activated
        destabilization, 872–874
    occupancy-only mediated
        mechanisms, 869–872
    RNA receptor sequences and,
        863
    target cleavage, 875–878
    target covalent modification,
        874–875
    target selectivity, 867
    oligonucleotide conjugates, 885–
        886
    pharmacodynamics, 865–877
    pharmacokinetics, 877–883

sugar modifications, 884–887
    toxicology, 882–883
Oligostatins, 927
Olivomycin, 904
Omeprazole, 967
    CASE carcinogenicity prediction,
        237, 238–242
On-line databases, 104–106
On-line vendors, 105
OPC 21268, 388
Ophthalmic drugs, 969–971
Opiate agonists, 226
Opiates:
    anaphylactic reactions, 191
    histamine release by, 204
Opioid peptides, 806, 825, 828,
    829, 838, 839, 840
Opioid receptors, 807, 832
Opium, 984
Oppositions, to trademarks, 83, 84
ORAC, 430, 458–459, 461
ORAC Core Database, 462, 464
Oral administration:
    and bioavailability, 119
    dose adjustment, 122
Oral contraceptives, lupus-like
    syndromes, 202
Orbit, 105
Organ clearance, 117
Organ damage, 194–195
Organizational issues, in drug
    discovery, 12, 27–34
Organosilicon, fluorouracil
    derivatives, 957
Organ-selective prodrugs, 174, 176
ORGSYN, 462, 464
Orientation maps, 622–623, 626,
    637
Ornithine aminotransferase
    inhibitors, 767
Ornithine decarboxylase inhibitors,
    735
Orphan Drug Act of 1983, 255,
    272
Orphan drugs, 255, 272
Orphan receptors, 362, 368
OSAC, 428, 430
Outside funding, and patent
    secrecy, 42
Ovarian cancer, 999
Overproducers, 737
Oxazepam, glucuronidation, 155
Oxidation reactions:
    carbon, 137–141
    nitrogen, 141–143
    sulfur and other atoms, 143–146
β-Oxidation reactions, 161–163
Oxidative cleavage, 146–147

Oxidative dehalogenation, 146
Oxidative desulfurization, 144
Oxidoreductases, 134–137
Oxime oligonucleotide backbone, 889
Oxyphenisatin, and hepatitis, 199
Oxytetacyclin, 1005
Oxytocin, 813, 822, 833, 841
　cyclic structures in, 805
　reduced amide bond incorporation, 840
Oxytocin antagonists, 810, 819, 829

Pacific yew, 997
P. aeruginosa, vaccines, 930
PAF-antagonists, 274
Palytoxin, 918
Pamaquine, 1024–1025
Papain inhibition, Hansch analysis, 535
Papaverine, 984
Papyrus, 105
Parabolic model, 523, 525
Paracetamol, 144, 145, 155
　esters, 959
　and glutathione conjugation, 164
　sulfation, 151
Parenteral administration, prodrugs, 964–966
Paris Convention for the Protection of Industrial Property, 73
Parkinson's disease, 363, 748
Partial agonists, 357
Partial least squares method, 499, 530–532
Partition coefficients, 509–512
　estimation, 474
　measurement/calculation, 511–512
Partition functions, 590
Partition ratio, 765–766
Patent and Trademark Office, 41
　Board of Patent Appeals and Interferences, 62, 63, 64
　examiner requirements, 41
　life form patentability, 49
　Office Actions, 62
　statutory invention registration program, 94–95
Patent Cooperation Treaty, 74–76
Patents, 43–78
　"absolute novelty" requirement, 42, 46, 47–48, 56–57
　compulsory licences, 77–78
　continuation-in-part (CIP) application, 42–43

as cornerstone of intellectual property protection, 40
　correction, 66–67
　design patents, 95
　enforcement, 67–72
　first-to-invent *vs.* first-to-file, 46–47
　grace period, 42, 56
　importance of secrecy before filing, 42
　importance/rewards of, 39
　improvements to previously patented inventions, 45
　improvements to system, 44
　information science applications, 108
　infringement actions, 67–69
　infringement defenses (of challenger), 69–71
　infringement remedies, 71–72
　interference proceedings, 63–66
　invention to priority contests, 41
　life forms, 49
　　deposit requirements, 53–54
　maintenance fees, 67
　outside U.S., 41, 44, 47, 72–78
　　patentable subject matter, 50–51
　　pre-grant opposition, 78
　procedure, 60–63
　　appealing claim rejections, 62–63
　　flow chart of, 60
　　secrecy of, 60
　protection of, 43–44
　protein glycoforms, 926
　public disclosure, 42, 47–48
　reduction to practice, 46
　reexamination, 66–67
　reissue, 66
　requirements, 40–41
　　new and unobvious, 55–60
　　new and unobviousness
　　　35 U.S.C. §102, 56–57
　　　35 U.S.C. §103, 57–60
　　patentable subject matter in U.S., 48–50
　　patentable subject matter outside U.S., 50–51
　　specification, 51–55
　　　best mode, 54–55
　　　claims, 55
　　　enablement, 52–54
　　　written description, 52
　　utility, 49–50
　special applications, 61
　strategy, 44–46
　and trade secrets, 90–91

types, 43
　working requirements, 77–78
PATFULL, 108
Pattern recognition, 499, 527
　in molecular modeling, 635–649
PBr322, 366
PC-Gene, 105
PCMODELS, 469, 474–476
Penicillamine, 829
　and Goodpasture's syndrome, 204
　immune suppression by, 206
　and myasthenia gravis, 203
　and nephritis, 201
Penicillenic acid, 188
Penicillin:
　allergy mechanisms, 209–213
　anaphylactic reactions, 191, 193
　coagulation factor VIII inhibition, 205
　and dermatitis, 198
　development, 1003–1004
　ester prodrugs, 960, 965–966
　and hemolytic anemia, 195–196
　metabolite immune response stimulation, 187, 188
　and nephritis, 201
　and pneumonitis, 203
　and polymyositis, 203
　and serum sickness, 194, 207
　and vasculitis, 200
Penicillin polymers, 211
Penicilloic acid, 188
Penicillopepsin, 325
Penicilloyl, 187, 188
Penicilloylated dextrans, 186
β,β-Pentamethylene-β-mercaptopropionic acid, 809
Pepsin inhibitors, 845
Pepstatine, 325
Peptidases, 147, 804
Peptide antibiotics, cyclic structures in, 805
Peptide cyclization, 805–814
Peptide drug esters, as prodrugs, 958–959
Peptide-like nucleic acids (PNA), 870, 888, 890
Peptide prodrugs, 176
Peptide pseudoreceptors, 644, 645
Peptides, 804
　cyclization, 805–814
　multipole electrostatics model, 579
Peptidomimetics, 619–621
　amide bond isoteres, 838–847
　　1,3-disubstituted tetrazole ring, 844–845

Peptidomimetics (*Continued*)
  ethylene: "carba," 841–842
  fluoroketomethylene, 845–846
  trans-fluorolefins, 843–844
  ketomethylene, 845–846
  methyleneamine, 838–840
  methylene ether, 841–842
  methylenesulfoxide, 840–841
  methylenethioether, 840–841
  miscellaneous isosteres, 846–
    847
  trans-olefins, 843–844
  retro-inverso modifications,
    838
  thioamide, 842–843
  conformational changes, 805
  constrained amino acids, 814–
    833
    α-amino cycloalkane
      carboxylic acids, 817–818
    β-amino cycloalkane
      carboxylic acids, 825–826
    γ-amino cycloalkane
      carboxylic acids, 826
    cyclized aromatic amino acids,
      831–832
    α,α-dialkylglycines, 817
    β,β-dimethyl amino acids, 829
    β-methyl amino acids, 829
    α-methylated amino acids,
      814–817
    miscellaneous mimetics, 832–
      833
    N^a-C^a-cyclized amino acids,
      818–823
    N^a-methylated amino acids,
      823–825
    β-substituted-2,3-methano
      amino acids, 829–831
    substituted proline, 832
    α,β-unsaturated amino acids,
      826–828
  defined, 804–805
  nonpeptide ligands for
    peptinergic receptors, 847–848
  peptide cyclization, 805–814
    backbone cyclization, 813–814
    linkages, 811–813
  secondary structure mimetics,
    833–838
Perinatal/postnatal studies, 267
Periodic boundary conditions, in
  Monte Carlo simulations, 592–
  593
Permeabilizing cell membranes,
  734
Peroxidases, 135, 137
  in oxygen oxidation, 144

Personal computers, databases for,
  105–106
Personal File Systems, 105
Pesticides, and aplastic anemia,
  206
Pethidine, 987
Petition for Cancellation
  (trademarks), 84
PGEM, 366
Pharmaceutical companies, 33–34
Pharmaceuticals, *see* Drugs
Pharmacodynamics, 114, 115
  defined, 114
  key parameters in, 115 *table*
  oligonucleotide therapeutics,
    865–877
  and xenobiotic metabolism, 131,
    133
Pharmacokinetics, 114–128. *See
  also* specific pharmacokinetic
    parameters
  in clinical studies, 126–128
  defined, 114
  environmental science
    applications, 128
  Hansch QSAR analysis, 538–539
  oligonucleotide therapeutics,
    877–883
  parameters important in drug
    distribution, 115 *table*, 115–
    121
  parameters important in
    therapeutic application, 121–
    126
  in preclinical development, 126
Pharmacological antagonism, 354–
  355
Pharmacophore-based ligand
  libraries, 388–389
Pharmacophores, 619–621, 797.
  See also Lead compounds
  and molecular modeling, 619–621
Pharmaprojects, 105
Pharmsearch, 108
Phase I clinical studies:
  in drug development, 279, 280–
    282
    stopping tests, 295
    typical studies, 280 *table*
  in drug discovery, 18–19
  formulation development for, 261
  pharmacokinetic applications,
    126–128
Phase II clinical studies:
  in drug development, 279, 282–
    286
    end of trial conferences, 297
    stopping tests, 295–296

  in drug discovery, 19–20
  formulation development for, 261
  pharmacokinetic applications,
    127
Phase III clinical studies
  in drug development, end of trial
    conferences, 297
  formulation development for, 261
  pharmacokinetic applications,
    127
Phase IIIa clinical studies, 279,
  282–286
Phase IIIb clinical studies, 279,
  286
Phase II reactions, *see* Conjugation
  reactions
Phase I metabolism studies, 261
Phase I reactions, *see*
  Functionalization reactions
Phase IV clinical studies, 279–280,
  286
  pharmacokinetic applications,
    128
Phenacetin:
  cytotoxicity, 151
  and hemolytic anemia, 196
  immune response stimulation,
    188
  and nephritis, 201
Phenanthrenecarbinols, Hansch
  analysis, 539
2,10-Phenanthroline, 875
Phenazone-5,10,di-*N*-oxide, 888
Phenelzine, 736
Phenethylamines, Free Wilson
  analysis, 542
β-Phenethylamines, 787, 791
Phenobarbitol, glucuronidation, 156
Phenol β-glucosyltransferase, 152
Phenolphthalein, and dermatitis,
  198
Phenols:
  glucuronidation, 153
  oxidation, 140, 144
  phosphorylation, 167
  sulfation, 151
Phenothiazine antipsychotics, 787
Phenothiazines:
  and granulocytopenia, 196
  and hepatitis, 199
Phenoxypropionic acids, 544
Phenylacetate-CoA ligase, 159
Phenylalkylenetrimethylammonium
  derivatives, 800
Phenylbutazone:
  and aplastic anemia, 206
  glucuronidation, 156
  and granulocytopenia, 196

and hepatitis, 199
immune response stimulation, 188
and vasculitis, 200
1-(X-Phenyl)-3,3-dialkyltriazenes, 537
Phenylephrine, 969, 971
Phenylethanolamine N-methyl-transferase, 148, 149
Phenylethanolamines, methylation, 149
Phenyl-β-D-glucosides, Hansch analysis, 536
4-Phenylpiperidines, 798, 988
β-Phenylproline, 832
trans-β-Phenylproline, 832
2-Phenylquinolinylmethanols, 541
Phenytoin, 962
glucuronidation, 155, 156
PHIND, 105
Phorbol-12,13-diesters, 525
Phorbol esters, Hansch analysis, 539
Phosgene, reaction with glutathione, 165
Phosphines, 145
3'-Phosphoadenosine 5'-phosphosulfate, 150
Phosphodiester linkages, 811
Phosphodiester oligodeoxy-nucleotides, 878, 879
Phosphodiesters, 875, 880
3-Phosphoglycerate kinase inhibitors, 776
Phospholipids, immune response stimulation, 187
Phosphonaminate, 846
Phosphonate, 846
Phosphonoacetyl-L-aspartate, 736
(Phosphonomethoxy)ethylguanidines, 793
Phosphonotransferases, 875
Phosphoroamidates, 878
Phosphorodiesters, lipophilic substituent conjugation, 887
Phosphorothioate 2'-O methyl oligonucleotides, 887
Phosphorothioates, 874, 875, 876, 878, 879, 881
lipophilic substituent conjugation, 887
toxicity, 881–882
in vivo pharmacokinetics, 881–882
Phosphorus, redox reactions of, 144–145
Phosphorylated compounds, 734
Phosphorylation reactions, 167

Photoallergy, 198
Phototoxicity, 198
Physiological activity, 498
π (lipophilicity parameter), 499, 512
Pilocarpic acid diesters, 970
Pilocarpine, 968, 969, 971
Pipecolic acid, 819
Piperazic acid, 819
Piperidineacetic acid, 826
Pirenzepine, 682
Pivampicillin, 960
Pivmecillinam, 960
PK_{S3}, 921
PKALC, 469, 477
PKFILE, 434, 438
Placenta transfer, Hansch analysis, 538
Plagiarism, 292
Planning, of drug development, 269–279
Plant patents, 43
Plants, patentability, 49, 50–51
Plant Variety Protection Act of 1970, 43
Plasma cells, 183
Plasminogen activator inhibitors, 667–669
Plasminogen activator (t-PA), recombinant, see Tissue-type plasminogen activator
Plastics, for closures, 263
Pneumococcal pneumonia, 930
Pneumocystis carinii inhibition, 735, 1012
Pneumonitis, 182, 203–204
Podophyllin, 1001
Podophyllotoxin, 1001
Podophyllotoxin β-D-gluco-pyranoside, 1001, 1002
Podophyllum, 1000–1003
Poisson-Boltzman equation, 580, 581
Polarizability, 582
Polarizability parameters, 513
Polarization energy, 402
Polyacrylates, 957
Polyadenylation, 865, 873
Polycyclic aromatic amines, N-formylation, 157
Polycyclic hydroxymethylarenes, sulfation, 151
Polyene antibiotics, 904
Polyether antibiotics, 904
Poly-L-(glutamic acid), 956
Poly-D-lysine, 216–217
Poly-L-lysine, 878
3'-Poly-L-lysine oligonucleotides, 880

Polymerase chain reaction (PCR) technique, 367–368, 675–676, 877
Polypurines, 864
Polypyrimidines, 864
Polysaccharide antitumor drugs, 934
Polysaccharide prodrugs, 956
Polysaccharides, immune response stimulation, 186
POMONA92, 434, 438
POMONA92-3D, 450, 451
POMONA MED CHEM database, 438–439
Population pharmacokinetic models, 127
Porcine pancreatic elastase inhibitors, 845
Porphyrin-conjugated oligonucleotides, 875, 887
Portfolio management issues, in drug discovery, 25–26
Postenzymatic reactions, 132, 138
Post-marketing surveillance, 279, 286
Potassium channels, 351
Potency, of ligands, 353
Potential surfaces, 582–583
minimization approaches, 583–589, 635–637
3-PPP, 795
Practolol, lupus-like syndromes, 202, 203
Pravastatin, 1015–1016
Prazosin, 963
Preclinical studies
in drug development, 264–268
in drug discovery, 16–17, 23–24
pharmacokinetic applications, 126
Preformulation, 261
Pregnancy, and drug metabolism, 134
Prima facie obviousness, 58–59
Primaquine, 1024
Principal component analysis, 506, 509, 530
Principal component methods, 533
Prior art, 55–56, 57
duty to disclose, 61
Procainamide, 956
immune response stimulation, 188
lupus-like syndromes, 202, 203
Process, as patentable subject matter, 48, 59–60
Process development, in drug discovery, 23

PROCHECK, 320
Pro-Cite, 105
Prodrugs, 172–178, 735, 950–977
　activation, 173–174
　active moiety, 950, 953
　amines, 958–959
　animal *vs.* human studies, 952,
　　974–975
　bioavailability assessment, 973–
　　974
　carrier moiety, 950, 953–954
　defined, 950
　design considerations, 974–975
　　rationale for design, 974–975
　design objectives, 172–173
　distribution, 966–968
　double prodrugs, 967–968
　drug delivery systems, 956–958,
　　959–960
　esters, 954–956
　examples, 174–177
　future directions, 976–977
　gastrointestinal absorption, 960–
　　964
　　sustained release, 962–964
　　taste, 964
　　tolerance diminishment, 964
　　tolerance improvement, 960–
　　　962
　hydrolysis, 959–960
　lipidic peptides, 959
　macromolecular, 956–958
　Mannich bases, 956
　from natural products, 950
　nomenclature, 953
　occular absorption, 969–971
　　pharmacokinetics of, 971
　parenteral administration, 964–
　　966
　peptide derivative prodrugs, 958
　peptide drug esters, 958–959
　pharmaceutical viewpoint, 952
　pharmacokinetics
　　clearance approach, 972–973
　　compartmental approach, 971–
　　　972
　pharmacokinetic view, 951–952
　principles of, 172–174
　regulatory aspects, 952–953
　reversible/irreversible conversion,
　　967–968
　therapeutic gain, 176
　tissue targeting, 966
　transdermal absorption, 968–969
　urinary elimination, 972
Product development:
　information retrieval in, 109
　issues overview, 114

Product regioselectivity, 133
Product selectivity, 132–133
Product stereoselectivity, 133
Profiling, 710
Progesterone analogs, Free Wilson
　analysis, 543
Programs, in drug discovery,
　15–16, 22–23
Program teams, in drug discovery,
　15, 29
Project teams, in drug discovery,
　35–36
Prolactin (human), recombinant,
　671
Proline, 832
β-Proline, 826
Proline mimetics, 819–822
PRO-LOGP, 469, 476–477
PROLSQ, 311
Promazines, and vasculitis, 200
Propanolol, 970
Propargylglycine, 737
Propranolol, metabolism, 168–169
Proprietary medicinal product, 953
N-n-Propyl-*N-n*-butyldopamine,
　792
Propylene glycol dipelargonate, 510
Propylthiouracil, and
　granulocytopenia, 197
Proresid®, 1003
Prostaglandin-endoperoxide
　synthase, 135, 137
Prostaglandin ketoreductases, 135
Prostaglandins, 969
Protaxols, 999–1000
Protecting Groups, 106
Protein Data Bank, 312, 315, 319
Protein kinase C, 921
　rDNA technology for studies of,
　　676–677
Protein kinase inhibitors, 844
Protein kinases, 361–362
Proteins:
　as macromolecular carriers in
　　immune response, 185–186
　from rDNA technology, 667–673
Proteoglycans, 903, 922–925
Proton-detected heteronuclear
　NMR, 313
Prototype compounds, *see* Lead
　(prototype) compounds
P-Selectins, 937
Pseudoirreversible enzyme
　inhibitors, 762, 767, 777–779
Pseudoknots, in RNA, 867–868
PSIDOM/PsiBase/PsiGen, 466
Psoralen-linked methyl-
　phosphonates, 875

Pure Food and Drugs Act of 1906,
　254
Purine modifications,
　oligonucleotides, 885
Purine-rich oligonucleotides, 870
Pyran, 956–957
Pyridines, 141
Pyridoxal 5′-diphospho-5′-
　adenosine, 776
Pyridoxal phosphate-dependent
　enzymes, 767
Pyrimidine modifications,
　oligonucleotides, 884–885
Pyrimidine-rich oligonucleotides,
　870–871
Pyrrolizidines, 927
Pyruvate cofactor, 770

Qing hao, 1021
Qinghaosu, 1021
QSAR:
　in CASE, 236–237
　dissociation and ionization of
　　acids/bases, 526–527
　drug-receptor interaction
　　modeling, 500–503
　Free Wilson analysis, 498, 499,
　　500, 520–522
　　applications, 541–543
　future directions, 551
　group contribution additivity,
　　503–505
　Hansch analysis, 499, 500, 517–
　　520
　　applications, 533–541
　history, 498–500
　miscellaneous methods, 527–528
　mixed approach, 522–523
　nonlinear relationships, 523–526
　parameters for, 505–509
　　electronic, 513–515
　　indicator variables, 516–517
　　lipophilicity, 509–512
　　miscellaneous parameters,
　　　515–516
　　partition coefficients, 511–512
　　polarizability, 513
　　steric, 515
　statistical methods
　　multivariate analysis methods,
　　　530–532
　　partial least squares analysis,
　　　530–532
　summary, 550–552
　test series design, 532–533
　3D-QSAR, 499, 543–550
　　active site interaction models,
　　　544–546

comparative molecular field analysis, 171, 499, 546–550
for molecular modeling, 630
partial least squares analysis in, 531
stereochemistry and drug action, 543–544
for structure-metabolism studies, 171
Quality of Life measurements, 285
Quantitative drug design, 499
Quantitative structure-activity relationship (QSAR) analysis, see QSAR
Quantitative Structure-Activity Relationships, 500
Quantum chemical parameters, 514
Quantum mechanics, 596–599
Quinacrine, 1024, 1025, 1026
and aplastic anemia, 206
Quinidine:
and hemolytic anemia, 196
and thrombocytopenia, 197
and vasculitis, 200
Quinine, 1023, 1024
and hemolytic anemia, 196
and thrombocytopenia, 197
Quinoline methanols, 1025
Quinone imines, reaction with glutathione, 164
Quinone reductase, 135, 140
Quinones, 140
nonenzymatic reduction, 141
reaction with glutathione, 164

Rabies virus, 938
Radioimmunoassays, 208
Radiolabeled peptides, 383
Radioligand binding, 378, 379–385
Radioligand binding assays, 702, 710–713
assay procedure, 720–721
automation, 724
availability and diversity of, 707
background, 710–713
data analysis, 721–724
equipment for, 715–716
establishing assays, 717–720
examples, 707–708 *table*
ligand selection, 716
problems, 711–712
sample preparation, 720
specificity, 719
theory, 713–714
tissue preparation, 716–717
vs. whole animal screens, 704
Raffinose, 186

Rainforests, as lead compound sources, 388
Ramachandran plots, 312, 320, 586–587
Ramiprilat, 750, 751
Rapamycin, 388
Rapid, reversible enzyme inhibitors, 738–740
Rate theory (receptors), 358
Rational drug design, 11–12, 22, 704–706
future of, 705–706
RD heparin, 923
rDNA technology, see Recombinant DNA technology
REACCS, 106, 107, 109, 429, 454, 455, 458, 459, 461
REACCS-JSM, 462, 464–465
Reaction field theory, 580
Reactions, to drugs, see Adverse drug reactions; Allergies
Reagents, cleavage, 888
Reagents, recombinant:
for new drug screening, 673–676
for structural biology studies, 676
Receptor complexes, 359–361
Receptor mapping, 642–644
Receptors, 6–7. See also Ligands; Radioligand binding assays
allosteric modulation, 356
autoradiography, 385–386
basic concepts, 352–353
binding assays, 378–385
binding to drugs, see Drug-receptor binding
classes, 351–352
desensitization, 353
dynamics, 362–363
identification in drug discovery, 14
interactions and integration, 362
isotope labeling, 315
and lead compound discovery, 387–391
model sites, 644–645
models of, 377
molecular biology of, 363–377
molecular modeling, see Molecular modeling
multiple, 6–7
nomenclature, 377–378
rDNA cloning, 363–377, 386–387, 681–686
cloned receptor expression, 370–373
sequence analysis, 369–370
strategies for, 365–369
structural analysis, 373

second and third messenger systems, 361–362
theories of
inactivation theory, 358–359
occupancy theory, 356–358
rate theory, 358
vs. drug receptors, 352
Recombinant DNA technology, 307, 351–352. *See also* specific recombinant products, such as Human growth hormone, recombinant
alanine-scanning mutagenesis, 670–671
cellular adhesion proteins, 687–690
development of, 664
DNA "fingerprinting," 369
for enzyme studies, 676–681
future directions, 690–691
glycoproteins, 926
homologue-scanning mutagenesis, 670
hybridization techniques, 366
mutant library creation, 672, 673, 676
for new therapeutics, 664–667, 665–666 *table*
polymerase chain reaction (PCR) technique, 367–369, 675–676
protein engineering, 667–673
epitope mapping, 669–671
reagents for new drug screening, 673–676
reagents for structural biology studies, 676
receptor cloning/studies, see Receptors, rDNA cloning
site-directed mutagenesis, 667–673
Red blood cells, carbohydrate role, 935–937
Reduction reactions:
carbon, 137–141
nitrogen, 141–143
sulfur and other atoms, 143–146
Reexamination of patents, 66–67
Reference Manager, 105
Regression analysis, 528–530
Regulatory environment, 253–255. *See also* FDA approval process and prodrugs, 952–953
Reissue of patents, 66
REMOTEDISC, 546
Renal clearance, 118–119
Renin:
homologous modeling, 315
substrate specificity, 325

Renin inhibitors, 811, 812, 840, 841, 844, 845, 846
  glycopeptide conversion, 926
  structure-aided drug design, 323, 325–332
Reproduction studies, in drug development, 267
Reserpine, CASE carcinogenicity prediction, 227–228, 231
Resonance parameter, 513
RESTRAIN, 311
Restriction requirements, patents, 61
(R)-Reticuline, 984–985
Retinoic acid receptors, 369
Retro-inverso modifications, of amide bond isoteres, 838
Retroviruses, 938
Reward issues, in drug discovery, 30
R-factor, 312
RGD peptide antagonists, 810, 829
RGD platelet GPIIb/IIIa receptor agonists, 620
Rheumatoid arthritis, 1026–1027
Rhinovirus inhibition, 687
Rhizopuspepsin, 325
Ribbed melilot, 1016
Ribonucleases, 875
Ribozymes, 875–876
Rifampin, 119–120
Rifamycin, 1005
Rigid analogs, 788–791
Rigid body rotations, and potential surface minimization, 585–586
Rigid geometry approximation, and potential surface minimization, 583
Ring position isomers, 792–793
Ring size changes, in analog design, 793–794
Rings (virtual), in potential surface minimization, 586
Risk issues, in drug discovery, 34
RNA:
  interaction with oligonucleotides, 865–869
    receptor sequences and activity, 876–877
  processing, 865
  structure, 867–869
    disruption, 872
  transcription, 865
RNA intermediary metabolism, 865
RNA libraries, 877
RNA polymerases, 865, 869
RNA-RNA hybrids, 865, 867

RNase H, 873–874
RO 5-3335, 673
RO 24-7429, 673
Romurtide, 932
Rosy periwinkle, 995
Rous sarcoma viruses, 873
Roxithromycin, 1011
Royalties, 78
RP 67580, 388
RTECS, 105
RU 486, 374, 686
RUBICON, 448
Rubisco, x-ray diffraction pattern, 309
Rx-to-OTC switch studies, 286

Safety assessments, 16. *See also* Clinical studies
Safrole, 151
Salbutamol, 1021
Salicin, 984
Salicylate, 956
Salicylic acid:
  amino acid conjugation, 160
  prodrugs, 960
Salicyluric acid, 159–160, 161
Salmetrol, 1021
Salmonella mutagenicity assay, 224, 225, 226, 246
Salutaridine, 984–985
Salutaridine synthase, 984
Sampling algorithms, in Monte Carlo simulations, 593–594
SANDRA, 106, 469, 483–484
Saponins, 935
SAR spreadsheets, 468–470
Satisfaction of spatial restraints method, 318
Saturability, in radioligand binding assays, 719
Scaled particle theory, 580–581
Scale-up, and drug discovery, 18
Scatchard plots, 385, 713
Schild plots, 356, 357
Science Models, 109
Scientific career paths, in drug discovery, 31
Scintillation counting, 390
  for radioligand binding assays, 720
Screening, in drug discovery, 12, 22, 1009
  rDNA for screening reagents, 673–676
SCRIP, 105
SDF, 434, 439
SDF-3D, 450, 451

SDI profile, 107
Secondary meaning, 81
Secondary structure mimetics, 833–838
Second messengers, 361–362
Secretin, 839
Selectins, 688–690, 703
  and cellular adhesion, 937
Selective Dissemination of Information (SDI) profile, 107
Selective organ damage, 194–195
Selectivity, 132–133
  defined, 132
  of ligands, 353
Selectivity screening, 710
Selenenic acids, 146
Seleninic acids, 146
Selenium:
  redox reactions of, 144–145, 146
  role in glutathione metabolism, 163
Selenols, 146
SELEX procedure, 675, 676
Sendai virus, 938
Serine endopeptidases, 137
Serine hydrolazes, 137
Serine protease inhibitors, 845
Serine proteases, homologous modeling, 315
Serious adverse experiences (SAEs), 269, 291–292
Serotonin, 793–794
  uptake inhibition, Hansch analysis, 537
Serotonin antagonists, Hansch analysis, 536
Serotonin 5-HT$_1$ receptors, 718, 794, 795
Serotonin 5-HT$_2$ receptors, 794
Serum albumin, 879
Serum sickness, 182, 193–194
Sex, and drug metabolism, 134
Sex steroids, 362
β-Sheet structures, 835–836
Sialyl Lewis X epitope, 937
SIBIS, 528
Silanes, 145
Silanols, 145
Silicon, redox reactions of, 144–145
Similarity reaction searching, 456
Similarity structure searching:
  2-dimensional, 424–425
  3-dimensional, 443–444
  and molecular modeling, 609
  in molecular modeling, 627–631
Simplex techniques, 532

Simulated annealing, 594
Simvastatin, 966, 1015
Single-dose containers, 262
Site-directed mutageneis, 667–673
  problems with, 705
Site-specific chemical delivery
  systems, 173, 174, 964, 966
Slow binding enzyme inhibitors,
  748–751
Slow-tight binding enzyme
  inhibitors, 748, 750
SMILES, 420–421, 431, 449
Snake toxins, 705, 711
SOCRATES, 427
Sodium artesunate, 1022
Sodium cromoglycate, 1018
Sodium-potassium-ATPase, 907
Soft drugs, 172
Software, 416–417. See also
  numerous specific Software
  programs
  chemically-intelligent computing
    software, 466–484
    vendors, 469 table
  copyright protection, 94
  for database management, 105–
    106
  2D chemical information
    management, see 2D Chemical
    information management
    software
  3D chemical information
    management, see 3D Chemical
    information management
    software
  for structure-aided drug design,
    322
  synthetic reaction information
    management, see Synthetic
    reaction information
    management software
    vendors, 418–419 table
Soil screening, for antibiotics, 1005
Soluble starch, 956
Solvation, 579–581
Somatostatin, 620, 820, 822, 826,
  833, 852
  cyclic structures in, 805, 808–
    809
  glucose spacers in, 847–848
  reduced amide bond
    incorporation, 840
Spare receptors, 353
sp Carbon atoms: oxidation and
  reduction, 140–141
sp² Carbon atoms: oxidation and
  reduction, 140–141

sp³ Carbon atoms: oxidation and
  reduction, 137–139
Special patent applications, 61
Specification, patents, 51–55
Specificity, 132–133, 734
  defined, 132
  oligonucleotide therapeutics,
    866–867
SPECINFO, 105, 108
Sperm-egg recognition, 902–903,
  937–938
Sphingosine, 919, 921
Spindle poisons, 1003
Spiro-DAMP, 789
SPLICE, 610, 611
Splicing, of RNA, 865, 871
S. pneumonia, vaccines, 930
SR 48692, 388, 726
Stability-indicating assays, 262
Standard Drug File, 106
Statine, 325, 329, 331
Statistical mechanics, 589–590
Statutory bars, 56
Statutory invention registration,
  94–95
Stereochemistry:
  and drug action, 543–544
  and structure-metabolism
    relationship, 170
Stereoisomerism
  and activity: incorrect
    assumptions about, 795
  and analog design, 795–797
Stereoisomers, FDA policy toward,
  264
Steric interactions, 7
  molecular modeling, 630–631
Steric parameters, 515
STERIMOL, 506, 515
Sterling-Winthrop antivirals, 616
Steroids, 848
Steroid sulfotransferase, 150
Sterol O-acyltransferase, 158, 160–
  161
Sterol ester formation, 160–161
Steryl glycosides, 919
Stibophen, and hemolytic anemia,
  196
Stimulon, 935
STN, 105
STN Express, 105
Straub tail, 987
Streptavidin, 408–409
Streptococcus pneumonia,
  vaccines, 930
Streptomycin, 904, 1005
  anaphylactic reactions, 191

Structural alerts, 226
Structural biology studies, rDNA
  technology for reagents, 676
Structural diversity sources, 673,
  674 table. See also Chemical
  libraries
Structurally conserved regions, 316
Structurally variable regions, 316
Structure-activity relationship
  (SAR), 223–224, 350–351
  for carcinogenicity prediction,
    224–246. See also Computer-
    automated Structure Evaluation
  database application, 108
  quantitative, see QSAR
Structure-activity relationship
  (SAR) spreadsheets, 468–470
Structure-affinity relationship
  (SAFIR), 351
Structure-aided drug design, 304–
  306
  active site identification, 320–321
  compound optimization, 323
  examples, 323–339
    AIDS drugs, 332–339
    angiotensin converting enzyme
      inhibitors, 323–324
    renin angiotensin system
      inhibitors, 323, 325–332
  homologous modeling for, 315–
    320
  lead compound identification,
    320–321
  lessons learned, 339
  software for, 322
  structural accuracy required, 321
Structure-metabolism relationship,
  168–171
Structure-toxicity relationship, 177
Studies, see specific types of
  Studies: Carcinogenicity
  studies etc.; Animal studies
Subacute toxicity studies, 265–266
Subpart E designation, 297–298
Substance, 953
Substance P, 839, 841, 844, 845
  AiB incorporation, 814
Substance P analogs, cyclic, 813,
  814
Substance P receptor, 378
β-Substituted-2,3-methano amino
  acids, 829–831
Substrate enantioselectivity, 132
Substrate-product selectivity, 133
Substrates, 352. See also Enzymes
  protection, 764, 765
Substrate selectivity, 132

Substructure searches, 422–424
Succinylcholine, 191
Sucralfate, 907
Sucrase inhibitors, 926–927
Sugar modifications,
    oligonucleotide therapeutics,
    884–887
Suicide substrates, 762, 763–766,
    767–774
Sulbactam, 734–735
Sulfadimethoxine, glucuronidation,
    155, 156
Sulfa drugs, Hansch analysis,
    537
Sulfanilamide, Elixir of
    Sulfanilamide tragedy, 254
Sulfates, hydrolysis, 147
Sulfation, 150–152
O-Sulfation, competition with
    O-glucuronidation, 155
Sulfenes, 144
Sulfenic acids, 143–144
Sulfides, metabolism, 143–144
Sulfinamides, 166
Sulfines, 144
Sulfinic acids, 143–144
Sulfinpyrazone, glucuronidation,
    156
Sulfites, anaphylactic reactions,
    191, 192
Sulfobromophthalein, anaphylactic
    reactions, 191
Sulfonamides, 847
    acetylation, 157
    and AIDS, 206
    allergy evaluation, 215
    anaphylactic reactions, 191
    and aplastic anemia, 206
    and dermatitis, 198
    glucuronidation, 154, 156
    and granulocytopenia, 196
    and hepatitis, 199
    and nephritis, 201
    and pneumonitis, 203
    and serum sickness, 194
    and thrombocytopenia, 197
    toxicity, 166
    and vasculitis, 200
Sulfones, 143–144
Sulfonic acids, 143–144
Sulfotransferases, 150–152
Sulfoxides, 143–144
Sulfur, oxidation and reduction
    reactions, 143–146
Sulindac, 967
Super agonists, 357
Suppressor T lymphocytes, 183
Surragate endpoints, 285

Sustained release prodrugs, 962–
    964
Suxamethonium, 992, 993
SV40 T-antigen, 873
Swainsonine, 927
Sweden, patentable subject matter,
    51
Sweet clover, 1016
Sweet wormwood, 1021
SYBYL/3D UNITY, 428–429,
    445, 447, 448, 473, 489
SYNLIB, 453, 458, 459, 461
SYNLIB Master Chemical Reaction
    Library, 463, 465
Synthesis:
    carbohydrate-based therapeutics,
        912–919
    and drug discovery, 18
    information retrieval in, 107
Synthetic carbohydrates, 907
Synthetic libraries, 725–727
Synthetic Methods of Organic
    Chemistry, 106
Synthetic reaction information
    databases, 452–459
    commercial, 460–465
    in-house, 459–460
    vendors, 462–463 *table*
Synthetic reaction information
    management software, 452–
    459
    functions and capabilities, 452–
        457
    reaction registration, 455
    reaction searching, 456
    "similarity" reaction searching,
        452–457
    specific systems, 457–459
    vendors, 458 *table*
Systematic search methods, for
    minimization of potential
    surfaces, 583–589, 636, 637–
    638
Systems screening, 698–704

Tacrin, 275, 295, 296
Talampicillin, 960
Tamoxifen, CASE carcinogenicity
    prediction, 236
Tamper-evident closures, 263
Tartrazine, sensitivity to, 205
Taste, of prodrugs, 964
Taste ligands, 826, 830
Taurine, in conjugation, 159
Taxol, 729
    development of, 997–1000
    prodrugs for, 999–1000
    synthesis, 999–1000

Taxotere, 999, 1000
T cells, *see* T lymphocytes
Team concept, in drug discovery,
    35–36
Technology transfer, 26
TEM-1 β-lactamase, 672, 673
Teniposide, 1002, 1003
Teprotide, 1016
Teratology studies, 267
Terbutaline, 955, 969
Testosterone, 956
    desaturation, 137, 139
    hydroxylation, 137, 139
Tetrachlorodibenzodioxin receptor,
    Hansch analysis, 536–537
Tetracyclines:
    anaphylactic reactions, 191
    lupus-like syndromes, 202
    and vasculitis, 200
Tetrahydrocannabinols, 158, 988–
    989
1,2,3,4-Tetrahydroisoquinoline-3-
    carboxylic acid, 831
Tetrahydroisoquinones,
    methylation, 149
Tetrahymena ribozyme, 875
2,2,5,5-Tetramethylthiazolidine-4-
    carboxylic acid, 821
Tetrazole ring, 1,3-disubstituted,
    844–845
Thalidomide tragedy, 254–255
THC, 158, 988–989
    endogenous receptor for, 989
Thebaine, 987
Theilheimer, 463, 465
T helper cells, 183
Theophylline:
    dosing *vs.* plasma concentration,
        122–123
    methylation, 150
Therafectin, 935
Therapeutic approach, to drug
    discovery, 12, 27–28
Therapeutic Patent Fast-Alert, 434,
    439
Therapeutics, *see* Drugs; specific
    Therapeutics
Thermodynamic cycle integration,
    594–595
    for affinity calculation, 615–617
Thermodynamics, of drug-receptor
    binding, 400–401, 404–408
Thermolysin, 324
Thermolysin inhibitors, 504, 505
    molecular modeling, 615
Thiazides:
    and nephritis, 201
    and vasculitis, 200

Thienamycin, 1008, 1009
Thioacyl halides, 166
Thioamides, 144, 842–843
Thiobiotin, 408–409
Thiocarbonyl compounds, 144
Thioglycosides, 915
Thioketenes, 166
Thiolester hydrolases, 159
Thiol methyltransferase, 148
Thiols:
    glucuronidation, 154, 156
    oxidation, 143
Thiomuscimol, 786
Thiopental, 191
Thiopurine methyltransferase, 148
4-Thiopyrimidines, 884
Thiouracils:
    and granulocytopenia, 196
    lupus-like syndromes, 202
    and thrombocytopenia, 197
    and vasculitis, 200
Thioureas, 144
Third messengers, 361–362
THOR/MERLIN, 428, 430–432
    3-dimensional, 445, 447–448,
        449
    POMONA92 interface, 438
Thrombocytopenia, 182, 188, 197–
    198
Thromboxane A$_2$ receptor
    antagonists, 274
Thromboxane synthetase inhibitors,
    274
Thymidine 5'-[α, β-
    imido]triphosphate, 747
Thymidylate synthase inhibitors,
    736
Thymolysin inhibitors, 754
Thyroid hormone receptors, 369
Thyroliberin, 620, 828
Thyrotropin-releasing hormone, 957
Tight binding enzyme inhibitors,
    748
Tight containers, 262
Timolol, 970
T independent antigens, 186
Tissue targeting, by prodrugs, 966
Tissue-type plasminogen activator
    (t-PA), 926
    recombinant, 667–669
T lymphocytes, 182–184, 186
    immunologic memory, 183
    rDNA technology for studies of,
        681
TNT, 311
Tolbutamide
    and granulocytopenia, 196
    half-life and hepatitis, 124

Toothpick plant, 1017
TOPKAT, 469, 478–479, 480
Topliss operational schemes, 532–
    533
Topoisomerase II inhibitors, 1003
Total Quality Management, 258
Toxication, 133, 177
Toxicity studies, in drug
    development, 265–268
Toxicology studies:
    in drug discovery, 17
    oligonucleotide therapeutics,
        882–883
Toxophoric groups, 177–178
Trademark Counterfeiting Act of
    1984, 79
Trademark Law Revision Act of
    1988, 79, 87
Trademarks, 78–87
    legislative framework, 79,
        81–82, 84, 86–87
    marketing aspects, 79–80
    oppositions and cancellations,
        83, 84
    registering, 82–84
    selection, 80–82
    using properly, 85
    worldwide rights, 85–86
Trademark Trial and Appeal Board,
    84
Trade secrets, 87–94
    and abandoned patent
        applications, 60, 63
    enforcement, 89–90
    and Freedom of Information
        Acts, 91–92
    outside U.S., 92–94
    patent improvements kept as, 45
    and patents, 90–91
    requirements for, 88–89
    risks of, 87–88
Trade Secrets Act, 88, 91
Transcription, 865
Transcriptional arrest, 865, 869–
    871
Transcription initiation complex, 865
Transdermal administration,
    prodrugs, 968–969
Transferases, 147
Transition state analogs, 752–757
Transition state modeling, quantum
    mechanical, 599
Transition state probes, 750
Translation, of RNA, 865
Translational arrest, 865, 871–872
Transport, of RNA, 865
Tranylcypromine, 736
Trehalose 6,6-dimycolate, 932–933

Trestatins, 927
TRH, 823, 825, 828
Tricyclic antidepressants, 787
Tridione, and nephritis, 201
m-Trifluoromethylbenzoic acid,
    146, 159–160
(m-Trifluoromethyl)phenylacetone,
    146
Triglycerides, 962
Trimethoprim, 537, 735
Trimethoprim-dihydrofolate
    reductase interaction, 410,
    677, 735
2,4,6-Trinitrophenyl residues, 186
Triphenylmethane dyes,
    anaphylactic reactions, 191
Triple-stranded DNA, 870–871
Tripos force field, 576
Triterpenoid saponins, 935
Trojan-horse inactivators, 762,
    763–766, 767–774
Tropicamide, 971
Trypsin inhibitors, 536, 757
Tubilin, 995
D-Tubocurarine, 799, 992–993
Tumor-associated carbohydrate
    antigens, 922
Tumor necrosis factor, 7
Tumor necrosis factor alpha, 700–
    701
Tunicamycin, 928
β-Turn mimics, 635, 833–835
γ-Turn mimics, 835
TX synthase, 135
Tyrosinase inhibitors, 787
Tyrosine-ester sulfotransferase, 150
Tyrosine kinases, 361–362

Uncompetitive antagonism, 354
Uncompetitive enzyme inhibitors,
    743–744
Undue experimentation
    requirement, 53
Uniform Trade Secrets Act, 88, 91
Unit-dose containers, 262
United Kingdom:
    patentable subject matter, 51
    scientific misconduct handling,
        293
    trade secret protection, 93–94
United States Patent and Trademark
    Office, see Patent and
    Trademark Office
UNITY, 106
UNITY-3DB, 609
Unobviousness, as patent
    requirement, 55, 57–60

α, β-Unsaturated amino acids, 826–828
Urethane linkages, 811
Uridine 5'-diphosphate chloroacetol, 771–772
Uridine diphosphate galactose 4-epimerase, 771
Uridine-5'-diphospho-α-D-glucuronic acid, 152, 153
Urinary excretion, 118–119
Utility, as requirement for patentability, 49–50
Utility patents, 43

Vaccines, carbohydrate-based, 929–931
Valproic acid:
   glucuronidation, 155
   β-oxidation, 162–163
Vancomycin, 811–812
Vancomycin-peptide complexes, 613–614
van der Waals forces, 402, 577–578
   molecular modeling, 630
Varapamil, 984
Vasculitis, 200
Vasodilatory drugs, 907
Vasopressin antagonists, 810
Vector maps, 633–635
Verlet algorithm, 591
Vesicular stomatitis virus, 871
Vigabatrin, 736
Vinblastine, 995, 996

Vincristine, 995, 996
Vindesine, 995, 996
VINITI, 461
Virginiamycin, 990
Virtual charge method, 581
Virtual rings, in potential surface minimization, 586
Vitamin A, 747
Vitamin B_{12}, anaphylactic reactions, 191
Vitamin D, receptors, 369
Volume mapping, 631–632
Volume of distribution, 120–121
   multiple distribution pools, 121
   steady state, 121
von Willebrand factor, 924
Voronoi binding site models, 545–546

Warfarin, 1017
Water dragging effect, 510
Water/n-octanol partition, 509–510
Well-closed containers, 262
White/Bovill force field, 576
Whole animal screens, 701–703, 704
Willful infringement, 71
WIN 51708, 388
Wiswesser Line Notation (WIN), 420
WIZARD, 547
Working requirements, patents, 77–78
Written description, in patent specification, 52

Xanthine dehydrogenase, 135
Xanthine oxidase, 135
   Hansch analysis, 536
Xenobiotic-macromolecular conjugates, 132
Xenobiotic metabolism, 106, 130, *See also* Conjugation reactions; Drug metabolism; Functionalization reactions
   pharmacodynamic consequences, 133
   reaction types, 131–132
   specificity and selectivity, 132–133
Xenobiotics, 131 *table*
Xenopus 28 S RNA, 872
XPLOR, 311–312, 320
X-ray diffraction, 308–310
   carbohydrates, 910–911
2,4-Xylidene HCl, CASE carcinogenicity prediction, 233, 235–236

Yellow sweet clover, 1016
Yew trees, 996–997

Zero-gravity crystallization, 308
Zidovudine (AZT), 296, 906, 963
   phosphorylation, 167
Zoxazolamine, and hepatitis, 199
Zuclopentixol, 963
Zytostop, 907